FIRST AID FOR THE® EMERGENCY MEDICINE

Oral Boards

Second Edition

EDITORS

DAVID S. HOWES, MD, FACEP, FAAEM
Former Chief, Residency Program Director Emeritus
Section of Emergency Medicine
Professor of Medicine and Pediatrics
The University of Chicago Pritzker School of Medicine
Chicago, Illinois

JOHN R. DAYTON, MD, FACEP, FAAEM
Division of Emergency Medicine
University of Utah Hospital
Assistant Professor of Surgery
University of Utah School of Medicine
Salt Lake City, Utah

JAMES AHN, MD, MHPE
Associate Director, Residency Program
Director, Medical Education Fellowship
Section of Emergency Medicine
Assistant Professor of Medicine
University of Chicago Pritzker School of Medicine
Chicago, Illinois

NAVNEET CHEEMA, MD
Assistant Director, Residency Program
Section of Emergency Medicine
Assistant Professor of Medicine
University of Chicago Pritzker School of Medicine
Chicago, Illinois

JANIS TUPESIS, MD, FACEP, FAAEM
Graduate Medical Education Liaison
University of Wisconsin Global Health Institute
Professor of Medicine
University of Wisconsin School of Medicine and Public Health
Madison, Wisconsin

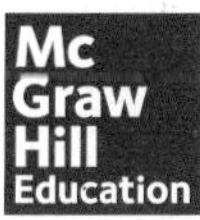

New York Chicago San Francisco Athens London Madrid Mexico City
Milan New Delhi Singapore Sydney Toronto

First Aid for the® Emergency Medicine Oral Boards, Second Edition

1 2 3 4 5 6 7 8 9 DSS 23 22 21 20 19 18

ISBN 978-0-07-183985-3
MHID 0-07-183985-2

NOTICE

Medicine is an ever-changing science. As new research and clinical experience broaden our knowledge, changes in treatment and drug therapy are required. The authors and the publisher of this work have checked with sources believed to be reliable in their efforts to provide information that is complete and generally in accord with the standards accepted at the time of publication. However, in view of the possibility of human error or changes in medical sciences, neither the authors nor the publisher nor any other party who has been involved in the preparation or publication of this work warrants that the information contained herein is in every respect accurate or complete, and they disclaim all responsibility for any errors or omissions or for the results obtained from use of the information contained in this work. Readers are encouraged to confirm the information contained herein with other sources. For example and in particular, readers are advised to check the product information sheet included in the package of each drug they plan to administer to be certain that the information contained in this work is accurate and that changes have not been made in the recommended dose or in the contraindications for administration. This recommendation is of particular importance in connection with new or infrequently used drugs.

This book was set in Times LT Std by Cenveo® Publisher Services.
The editors were Bob Boehringer and Christina M. Thomas
The production supervisor was Rick Ruzycka.
Project management was provided by Surbhi Mittal, Cenveo Publisher Services.

This book is printed on acid-free paper.

Library of Congress Cataloging-in-Publication Data

Names: Howes, David S., editor.
Title: First aid for the emergency medicine oral boards / [edited by] David S. Howes, MD, Professor, Joint Chief and Residency Program Director, Section of Emergency Medicine, The University of Chicago, Chicago, Illinois [and four others].
Description: Second edition. | New York : McGraw-Hill Education Medical, [2018]
Identifiers: LCCN 2018011431| ISBN 9780071839853 (paperback) | ISBN 0071839852 (paperback)
Subjects: LCSH: Emergency medicine—Examinations—Study guides. | First aid in illness and injury—Examinations—Study guides. | BISAC: MEDICAL / Dentistry / General.
Classification: LCC RC86.9 .F574 2018 | DDC 616.02/5076—dc23
LC record available at https://lccn.loc.gov/2018011431

DEDICATION

This book is dedicated to all of the authors who worked so hard to make it happen.

Contents

Contributors

Second Edition Contributors

Michael K. Abraham, MD, MS
Clinical Assistant Professor
Department of Emergency Medicine
University of Maryland School of Medicine
Baltimore, Maryland

Fred Abrahamian, DO, FACEP
Associate Professor of Medicine
David Geffen School of Medicine at University of California, Los Angeles
Los Angeles, California
Director of Education
Department of Emergency Medicine
Olive View-UCLA Medical Center
Sylmar, California

Kip Adrian, MD
Attending Physician
Department of Emergency Medicine
Lutheran General Hospital
Park Ridge, Illinois
Clinical Instructor of Medicine
The University of Chicago
Chicago, Illinois

James Ahn, MD, MHPE
Associate Director, Residency Program
Director, Medical Education Fellowship
Section of Emergency Medicine
Assistant Professor of Medicine
University of Chicago Pritzker School of Medicine
Chicago, Illinois

Eileen M. Allen, MD, FAAP
Attending Physician, Emergency Department
Loyola University Medical Center
Assistant Professor
Section of Emergency Medical Services
Loyola University School of Medicine
Chicago, Illinois

Mark P. Bogner, MD, FACEP
Associate Professor and Residency Program Director
Division of Emergency Medicine
University of Wisconsin School of Medicine and Public Health
Associate Medical Director, UW Health Emergency Services
University of Wisconsin Medical School
Madison, Wisconsin

Philip J. Bossart, MD
Professor of Surgery
University of Utah School of Medicine
Division of Emergency Medicine
Department of Surgery
University of Utah Hospital
Salt Lake City, Utah

Marc Bellazzini, MD
Assistant Professor of Medicine CHS
Director of Medical Informatics
University of Wisconsin
Division of Emergency Medicine
F2/208 Clinical Sciences Center
Madison, Wisconsin

Lindsey Caley, MD
Assistant Professor of Medicine
Virginia Tech Carilion School of Medicine
Roanoke, Virginia
Department of Emergency Medicine/Pediatric Emergency Medicine
Carilion Clinic, Roanoke Memorial Hospital
Roanoke, Virginia

Navneet Cheema, MD
Assistant Director, Residency Program
Section of Emergency Medicine
Assistant Professor of Medicine
University of Chicago Pritzker School of Medicine
Chicago, Illinois

Reb Close, MD
Attending Physician
Division of Emergency Medicine
Community Hospital of the Monterey Peninsula
Clinical Instructor
Department of Emergency Medicine
Olive View-UCLA Medical Center
Sylmar, California

Jamie Collings, MD, FACEP
Program Director
Northwestern University Emergency Medicine Residency
Assistant Professor of Medicine
Northwestern University Medical School
Chicago, Illinois

John R. Dayton, MD, FACEP, FAAEM
Division of Emergency Medicine
University of Utah Hospital
Assistant Professor of Surgery
University of Utah School of Medicine
Salt Lake City, Utah

Gerard S. Doyle, MD, MPH
Assistant Professor, Career Path
Division of Emergency Medicine
University of Utah School of Medicine
Salt Lake City, Utah

H. Megan French, MD, FACEP
Utah Emergency Physicians
Intermountain Medical Center
Salt Lake City, Utah

Fiona Gallahue, MD
Assistant Professor
Division of Emergency Medicine
Attending Physician, Harborview
Medical Center
University of Washington
Seattle, Washington

Christopher A. Gee, MD, MPH
Associate Clinical Professor
Department of Orthopaedics
University of Utah
Salt Lake City, Utah
Associate Program Director
Primary Care Sports Medicine Fellowship
Division of Emergency Medicine
University of Utah Health
Salt Lake City, Utah

Michael Gisondi, MD, FACEP
Associate Residency Director
Assistant Professor of Emergency Medicine
Northwestern University, The Feinberg School of Medicine
Chicago, Illinois

Aleksandr Gorenbeyn, MD, FACEP
Assistant Professor
Department of Emergency Medicine
University of Connecticut School of Medicine
Farmington, Connecticut

Rohit Gupta, MD
Attending Physician
Department of Emergency Medicine
Advocate Christ Hospital
Chicago, Illinois

Gregg Helland, MD, RDMS
Assistant Professor of Medicine
University of Chicago
Chicago, Illinois
Ultrasound Director
Section of Emergency Medicine
University of Chicago
Chicago, Illinois

David S. Howes, MD, FACEP, FAAEM
Former Chief, Residency Program Director Emeritus
Section of Emergency Medicine
Professor of Medicine and Pediatrics
The University of Chicago Pritzker School of Medicine
Chicago, Illinois

Catherine Johnson, MD, FACEP
Department of Surgery
Loyola University
Maywood, Illinois

Alan Kumar, MD, FACEP
Clinical Instructor
University of Chicago Emergency Department
Clinical Instructor
Northwestern Memorial Hospital Emergency Department
Chicago, Illinois
Attending Physician
Lutheran General Hospital Emergency Department
Park Ridge, Illinois

Charles Maddow, MD, FACEP
Assistant Professor and Director of Undergraduate Medical Education
Department of Emergency Medicine
University of Rochester School of Medicine and Dentistry
University of Rochester Medical Center
Rochester, New York

Mária Némethy, MD, FAWM
Attending Physician, Emergency Medicine
PeaceHealth Ketchikan Medical Center
Ketchikan, Alaska

Michael Paddock, DO, MS, FACEP
Senior Staff Physician
Regions Hospital, HealthPartners
St. Paul, Minnesota
Assistant Professor of Emergency Medicine
University of Minnesota
Minneapolis, Minnesota

Joseph Peabody, MD, FACEP
Assistant Professor of Emergency Medicine
University of Illinois at Chicago College of Medicine
Chicago, Illinois
Attending Physician
Department of Emergency Medicine
Advocate Lutheran General Hospital
Park Ridge, Illinois

M. Tyson Pillow, MD, MEd
Emergency Medicine Residency Program Director
Vice Chair of Education
Department of Emergency Medicine
Associate Professor
Baylor College of Medicine
Houston, Texas

Robert Preston, MD, FACEP
Attending Physician, Emergency Medicine
Martin Luther King Jr. Community Hospital
Los Angeles, California

Thomas Regan, MD, FACEP
Associate Professor of Emergency Medicine
University of Connecticut School of Medicine
Farmington, Connecticut

James W. Rhee, MD, FACMT, FACEP, FAAEM
Medical Director
Cedars-Sinai/Marina Del Rey Hospital
Los Angeles, California
Assistant Clinical Professor
UC Riverside School of Medicine
Riverside, California

Anita Rohra, MD, FACEP
Assistant Professor
Director of Simulation
Department of Emergency Medicine
Baylor College of Medicine
Ben Taub General Hospital
Houston, Texas

Philip Shayne, MD
Vice Chair for Education
Associate Professor and Residency Director
Department of Emergency Medicine
Emory University School of Medicine
Atlanta, Georgia

Tara Sheets, MD, FACEP
Assistant Professor of Emergency Medicine
Baylor College of Medicine
Houston, Texas
Assistant Program Director
Emergency Medicine Residency Program
Baylor College of Medicine
Houston, Texas

Richard Sinert, DO
Associate Professor
Research Director
Department of Emergency Medicine
The State University of New York Downstate Medical Center
Brooklyn, New York

Matthew Steimle, DO, FACEP, FAAP
Assistant Professor of Pediatrics
University of Utah School of Medicine
Salt Lake City, Utah
Emergency Ultrasound Director
Division of Pediatric Emergency Medicine
Primary Children's Hospital
Salt Lake City, Utah

Mohammad Subeh, MD, MS
Ultrasound Director, Assistant Medical Director
El Camino Hospital
Mountain View, California
Assistant Clinical Professor
University of California
Irvine, California
Staff Physician
Good Samaritan Hospital
San Jose, California

James I. Syrett, MD, FACEP
Director of Prehospital Care
Department of Emergency Medicine
Unity Hospital
Rochester, New York

Katie Tataris, MD, MPH, FAEMS, FACEP
Assistant Professor of Medicine
Section of Emergency Medicine
University of Chicago Pritzker Medical School
Chicago, Illinois
EMS Medical Director
Chicago South EMS System, Region XI
Chicago, Illinois

N. Seth Trueger, MD, MPH, FACEP
Assistant Professor of Emergency Medicine
Department of Emergency Medicine
Feinberg School of Medicine
Northwestern University
Chicago, Illinois

Janis P. Tupesis MD, FACEP, FAAEM
Graduate Medical Education Liaison
University of Wisconsin Global Health Institute
Madison, Wisconsin
Professor of Medicine
University of Wisconsin School of Medicine and Public Health
Madison, Wisconsin

Flora Waples-Trefil, MD
Clinical Instructor
Section of Emergency Medicine
The University of Chicago
Chicago, Illinois

Michael A. Ward, MD
Department of Emergency Medicine
University of Wisconsin—Madison
Madison, Wisconsin

Daniel Wu, MD
Assistant Medical Director
Grady Memorial Hospital Emergency Care Center
Assistant Professor
Department of Emergency Medicine
Emory University School of Medicine
Atlanta, Georgia

First Edition Contributors

Fred Abrahamian, DO, FACEP
Kip Adrian, MD
Amer Z. Aldeen, MD
Eileen M Allen, MD, FAAP
Marc Bellazzini, MD
Mark P. Bogner, MD, FACEP
Reb Close, MD
Jamie Collings, MD, FACEP
Timothy B. Erickson, MD, FACEP FACEP, FAACT, FACMT
Fiona Gallahue, MD
Michael Gisondi, MD, FACEP
Alexandr Gorenbeyn, MD, FACEP
Rohit Gupta, MD
Mark Hostetler, MD, FACEP
Catherine Johnson, MD, FACEP
Alan Kumar, MD, FACEP
Jason Liebzeit, MD
Charles Maddow, MD, FACEP
Joseph F. Peabody, MD
Thomas J. Regan, MD, FACEP
James W. Rhee, MD
Philip Shayne, MD
Richard Sinert, DO
Janis Tupesis, MD
James I. Syrett, MD, FACEP
Flora Waples-Trefil, MD
Daniel Wu, MD

Preface

First, congratulations are in order! Your decision to purchase this book and prepare for the Oral Board Exam indicates that you have successfully completed the Written Board Exam. This book focuses on preparing you for the next step: Oral Board Exam.

The Oral Board Exam differs significantly from the Written Board Exam. Most physicians have anxiety when they consider the Oral Board Exam process, and this is understandable. Throughout our college, medical school, and residency training, we have taken many written, multiple choice exams and most of us have a high level of comfort with that format. The Oral Board Exam, on the other hand, is totally different. It is verbal, interactive, and you have to be able to think on your feet. To successfully prepare for the exam, you must master not only the material but also this new format. Our goal in writing this book is to help you accomplish both.

The first half of this book is dedicated to covering the material that you can expect on the exam. It includes diagnostic and management algorithms and is organized according to chief complaints and split into adult and pediatric sections.

The second section of this text is composed of 50 practice cases written out as a dialogue between the examiner and candidate. We chose this format in Oral Boards to help you become familiar with the artificial oral testing environment. Reading through the cases should help you become familiar with the testing format. However, there is no substitute for practicing cases out loud. We recommend that after reading clinical chapters in this book, you have a colleague play the examiner and go through several of the cases with you out loud. There is no substitute. The more you practice, the better your performance will be. Good luck!

SECTION 1

TAKING THE BOARDS

CHAPTER 1

Introduction and Technique

David Howes and John Dayton

INTRODUCTION

Congratulations on passing the written board exam!

While the written board exam tests the depth and breadth of your medical knowledge, the oral board exam seeks to validate your patient management skills and your ability to provide rapid, safe, and competent patient care. The oral board exam simulates actual patient encounters to test your ability to gather information, consider likely diagnoses, institute emergent therapy, and execute a diagnostic and therapeutic plan.

The exam focuses on core topics, critical conditions, and infrequent, but life-threatening, conditions. For example, you will need to consider bacterial meningitis when evaluating a patient with headache, fever, and neck stiffness.

Because of the unique format of the test, most physicians have some anxiety when they consider the oral board exam process, and this is understandable. There is no other event in your life that resembles it. You have to learn successful techniques that will help you succeed and be able to think on your feet. The oral exam process is interactive and can provoke anxiety. We recommend that you focus on the following to diminish your anxiety:

1. By passing the written boards, you have already demonstrated that you know the material that will be covered on the oral board exam.
2. The oral exam focuses on a much smaller amount of material than the written board exam. You will have to learn techniques for taking the oral exam, but there is much less material that is covered.
3. The test asks you to simulate and perform tasks that you perform every day. Though there are some test-specific rules, the test attempts to simulate what you do every day—practice emergency medicine.

You are already well prepared for the oral board exam. This book will explain the test, review critical management algorithms, and provide case simulations for you to review. We will teach you language and technique to pass the exam.

TIMING AND LOCATION

The oral board exam is administered every April and October. Upon successful completion of the written board exam, you will be randomly assigned a position in either the April or October administration of the oral board exam. There is some flexibility with the date as you may elect to be on a waitlist to take the exam earlier or delay when you take the oral board exam, but there are fees involved.

Your exam will be administered at the Chicago-O'Hare Marriott during a designated 3 to 5 days period as either a morning or afternoon test. The morning session typically runs from 6:30 AM to 12:30 PM, while the afternoon session runs from 1:30 PM to 7:30 PM. You will be assigned by the American Board of Emergency Medicine (ABEM) to one of these sessions. Along with your test assignment, you will also receive documentation detailing the format and grading of the test and a video demonstrating the testing process. In order to ensure the validity of the test, the board demands absolute secrecy from all participants.

DETAILED DESCRIPTION OF THE EXAM DAY

Your exam will be completed within the 6-hour block to which you are assigned. The 6-hour block includes a half hour orientation, 3 hours of actual testing, and approximately 2 hours of waiting periods.

You must appear at the test site and register before the start of the testing session. Your "Candidate Examination Schedule" is an individualized schedule during your assigned block and will be provided when you register. After registration, the testing session begins with a half hour orientation. The orientation consists of an introduction and welcome, a demonstration of a sample case, a description of ratings and criteria, and an explanation of the logistics of the exam day.

After orientation, you go to the exam location as dictated by your individual schedule. Each patient simulation takes place in a separate hotel room and all of your simulations will take place in a small group of hotel rooms. Each simulation room will be labeled with a letter corresponding to the letters on your schedule. You will be part of a small cohort of 10 to 20 examinees who will take the exam in the same set of rooms. A lounge area will be designated on one of the floors where you can spend your waiting period between simulations. A receptionist will be available on each floor to assist and direct you.

You will go to each simulation room 5 minutes before the simulation is scheduled to begin and wait outside the room. You are not permitted to take anything with you, but paper and pencils will be provided in each room. The examiner will call you into the room when the simulation starts. Each single-patient simulation will take approximately 20 minutes, and the multiple-patient simulations will take approximately 30 minutes. The examiner will begin the simulation, help pace you through it, and end the simulation when either you have completed the simulation or the time is up. After the simulation ends, you must leave any notes you have made in the room and you will either proceed to your next simulation room per your schedule or return to the lounge.

Your testing will consist of six single-patient simulations and two multiple-patient simulations for a total testing time of 3 hours. For each examinee, the order of cases and waiting periods is random. For example, the multiple patient encounters may occur first. You may have a string of cases, then a long waiting period, then a final case to finish up.

THE ORAL BOARD EXAM FORMAT

The oral board exam format consists of five single-patient simulations and two simultaneous-patient simulations. The exam will also include a single-patient test case—this will be used for research and development purposes. You will not know which case is the test casc.

The Patient Simulation

Each patient simulation occurs as a role-playing session between you and the examiner. Though highly artificial, the simulation seeks to mimic what happens in a typical patient encounter. It takes place in a hotel room across a desk. On the desk sits paper and pencil for notes and a light box for viewing x-rays. Your examiner sits behind the desk, behind a placard intended to prevent you from viewing test materials. You play yourself, the examining emergency physician. Your examiner plays all other roles, including the patient, patient's family, emergency medical technicians (EMTs), nurses, and consultant physicians.

After calling you into the room, the examiner will begin by introducing themselves and providing information for the case, including details related to the patient's name, vital signs, and chief complaint. As of 2017, this information will be provided using the eOral case format. This will consist of patient information and results being delivered using an interactive computer screen.

During the introduction of the case, this information can involve audio for emergency medical service (EMS) calls and video of the patient. During the course of the case, this information may include patient records, rhythm strips, updated vital signs, and imaging studies.

To learn more about the new eOral cases format, visit ABEM's Candidate and Video Sample Cases at https://www.abem.org/public/emergency-medicine-(em)-initial-certification/oral-examination/familiarize-yourself-with-the-oral-examination/candidate-video-and-sample-cases.

You will be given paper that shows an outline of the human body on it and has space for taking notes. You can use this note paper to record information related to the case. You will then take a history by asking the examiner questions and issue orders for interventions that you want to take place. As information is ready, the examiner will use the eOral case format or pass you pieces of paper with results of the different lab tests for you to interpret. This may also include electrocardiograms (ECGs) and imaging results to interpret.

At times, the examiner may make the patient's condition change either to simulate evolution of the pathological process, or in response to your interventions. In addition to taking detailed notes on your performance, the examiner will monitor time, keep you moving through the case, and notify you when time has expired.

Throughout the simulation, the examiner will be a pleasant, but neutral, participant. They will try to provide only neutral feedback and avoid changes in voice or facial expressions regarding your performance. In general, the examiner will let you follow any management plan. They will try to make the simulation realistic by having the patient react appropriately to your interventions. You should manage the case expeditiously and efficiently. Case management techniques are discussed later in this chapter. Generally, most patient simulations will reach a conclusion within the time allowed.

Scoring Categories

Each case in the oral board exam is scored individually by assessing eight performance criteria:

1. **Data acquisition:** Assesses your ability to gather an efficient history, perform an appropriate physical examination, and obtain appropriate tests. You can lose points both by missing important data or by gathering too much unnecessary information.
2. **Problem solving:** Assesses your ability to create a differential diagnosis, analyze data accurately to narrow your differential, and draw appropriate conclusions.

3. **Patient management:** Assesses your ability to plan and provide therapy in a timely, efficient, and appropriate manner. Your ability to manage multiple patients is particularly tested during the triple-patient encounters.
4. **Resource utilization:** Assesses your efficiency. Examinees can lose points either for not obtaining required tests or for ordering unnecessary studies. The board does not want examinees to use a "shotgun" approach. You are also being tested on your ability to be resourceful. For example, when dealing with a patient with an unknown ingestion, you should ask to talk to family members at home, EMS personnel, the primary provider, etc to attempt to find out what medications would be available to ingest. Similarly, if you are concerned about pancreatitis, ordering a lipase level only will be scored higher than ordering both amylase (less specific) and lipase (more specific) levels.
5. **Health care provided (outcome):** Assesses the quality of care provided from the patient's perspective and with regard to the national standard of care.
6. **Interpersonal relations and communication skills:** Assesses your ability to communicate with the patients, patients' family, and other health providers. Ideally, communication should be clear and concise.
7. **Comprehension of pathophysiology:** Assesses your understanding of the rationale behind your diagnostic and therapeutic interventions. You will be evaluated on your understanding of the case as you explain the pathology to the patients and their family in layman's terms, and as you consult with your professional colleagues using concise, medical terminology. Your comprehension is assessed during case management and at the end.
8. **Clinical competence (overall):** Assesses your knowledge, competency, and skill, taking into account all aspects of the simulated encounter.

How Tests Are Scored

ABEM has outlined how tests will be scored at https://www.abem.org/public/emergency-medicine-(em)-initial-certification/oral-examination/scoring/rating-scale.

Table 1-1 summarizes how tests are scored.

Critical Actions

For each case, ABEM determines a list of critical actions that must be completed as part of competent management. Each critical action is assigned to a component skill. There are usually four to five critical actions per case. Examples include diagnosing a STEMI by ECG (problem solving), describe how you place a chest tube if a patient has a pneumothorax (patient management), administering pain medications to a patient with a dislocated shoulder (patient management), identifying an allergy to penicillin before administering antibiotics (data acquisition), and explaining to the patient your plan of care in simple, nonmedical language (interpersonal relations).

Additionally, ABEM also determines a list of harmful actions that must be avoided for successful management.

Your performance on each of the component skills is rated on a scale of 0 to 8. Five and six are considered acceptable scores in each area. A flawless performance will earn a score of 8, but is quite rare. It is important to understand that a passing score implies acceptable performance, not perfect performance. The scoring of each component skill depends on completion of critical actions and

Table 1-1. How Oral Board Cases are Scored

Very Acceptable (7,8)
- No missed critical actions and no dangerous actions.
- Correct diagnosis and management.
- Appropriate and efficient history, work-up, and treatment.
- Concern for patient's needs is demonstrated and candidate has appropriate communication with patient, family members, and consultants.

Acceptable (5,6)
- No missed critical actions and no dangerous actions.
- Correct diagnosis obtained, but with mild errors or inefficiencies.
- History, work-up, and treatment are adequate, but not totally complete.
- Adequate concern demonstrated for patient's needs.

Unacceptable (3,4)
- Missed critical actions and no dangerous actions.
- Incomplete history and work-up and correct diagnosis is not obtained.
- Treatment is incomplete and inadequate.
- Lack of concern shown for patient's needs.

Very Unacceptable (1,2)
- Missed critical actions with dangerous actions.
- Inappropriate history and work-up.
- Mismanagement of care as correct diagnosis is not obtained.
- Inappropriate disposition and failure to use appropriate consult.

avoidance of harmful actions. If a critical action is not completed, or if a harmful action is taken, the maximum score that can be assigned is a 4 (a failing score). This can happen for an otherwise flawless performance.

For example, in a case with multiple traumatic injuries, the critical actions could include diagnosis and treatment of a tension pneumothorax (patient management) and diagnosis of a lower extremity fractures (data acquisition). If the examinee makes a rapid assessment of the tension pneumothorax, performs an immediate needle decompression and places a chest tube, but does not identify or treat the leg injuries, they will not score higher than a 4 for data acquisition because they failed to perform a critical action (identify lower extremity fractures).

After assigning scores to each of the component skills, an overall case score is calculated by averaging together the component scores for each case. Scores on each individual case are combined in two ways to determine overall performance. In order to pass the oral board exam, either the average score of all cases must exceed 5.75 or the average of the highest and lowest case scores must exceed 5.0. You will not receive a numerical score; the test is graded as "pass" or "fail." If you do not pass, you will get a report which outlines areas of weakness for further study. ABEM guarantees that you will receive your results by mail within 90 days of the examination.

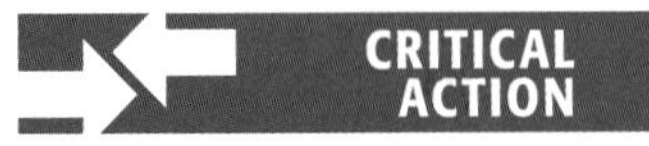

1. Obtain Chest X-ray (DA)
2. Explain Procedure to Patient (IRCS)
3. Treat Chest Pain (PM)
4. Treat Pneumothorax (PM)
5. Evaluate Chest Tube Placement/ Function (PS)

Here is an example of the Critical Actions for ABEM Sample Case 1001 involving a spontaneous pneumothorax at http://www.abem.org/public/docs/default-source/oral-examination-/01_case-summary-and-guidelines.pdf?sfvrsn=2.

Note that these Critical Actions involve several performance criteria including data analysis, interpersonal relations and communication skills, patient management, and problem solving.

While it is important to understand the scoring system to make sure that you address each of the component skills, do not focus too heavily on scoring. If you focus on managing the case properly, the scoring will take care of itself.

CONTENT

The oral board exam tests a significantly narrower range of material than the written board exam. Though ABEM indicates that content can come from anywhere in *The Model of the Clinical Practice of Emergency Medicine* (available at https://www.abem.org/public/publications/em-model/reference), the exam usually focuses on critical and emergent pathology. ABEM states that areas of emphasis include cardiovascular disorders, infection, pulmonary disease, toxicology, trauma, and pediatrics. During an exam, each candidate will manage a total of 12 cases.

With this in mind, you should be familiar with advanced cardiac life support (ACLS), advanced trauma life support (ATLS), and pediatric advanced life support/neonatal resuscitation program (PALS/NRP) protocols. Toxidromes and antidotes are also high yield. It is reasonable to anticipate that two cases will involve cardiovascular disorders, one case will be a toxicology case that will require knowledge of an antidote or other appropriate treatment, and one or two cases will involve trauma. At least one case will require the management of a child.

PASS RATES

The pass rate for the oral board exam is very high. Among residency-trained, first-time test takers, the pass rate is 90% to 93%. With practice and reasonable effort, you will pass.

RECOMMENDED STUDY PLAN

As a practicing emergency physician, finding time to prepare for the oral board exam can be challenging. You are a physician with many responsibilities. You are early in your career and still adjusting to being an attending physician. Having to prepare to jump through another hoop may seem overwhelming.

Relax. You can do it! Having passed the written board exam, you have already demonstrated that you have the knowledge necessary to practice emergency medicine. Preparing for the oral board exam is significantly easier than preparing for the written exam. You have at least three advantages:

1. You are a more seasoned attending with more clinical experience.
2. The material tested on the oral board exam is focused and relevant. The oral board exam tests the critical, emergent problems that you deal with frequently and with which you are familiar.
3. The oral board exam tests your clinical competency and seeks to simulate the same environment in which you practice regularly.

However, despite these significant advantages, the test warrants preparation. To successfully prepare for the exam, you must master the format in which the test is given. Most examinees will immediately focus on the didactic material that is tested, but becoming comfortable with the format of the test is also very important. Remember, you have already reviewed the material on the oral board exam when you prepared for the written exam. It may need to be refreshed, but you know it. The new, unfamiliar activity is taking an oral board exam. The rules of the exam process are new, and oral exams, like all public speaking activities, incite anxiety. Despite the best efforts of the board, the testing atmosphere is artificial. Our recommended study plan addresses both didactics and test taking strategy.

Preparation of Didactic Material

You should be able to review the didactic material for the oral board exam fairly rapidly. A time commitment of 40 hours will allow excellent preparation. We recommend 2 hours a day, 4 to 5 days a week, for 4 weeks. Create a schedule and stick to it.

You have already taken a great first step in preparing by buying this book. Use it as a guide to review the disease processes. Be sure to review ATLS, ACLS, PALS, and NRP algorithms. You will need to know doses of all resuscitation medications.

Preparation for the Exam

In addition to mastering the material, you must also practice the specific format of the oral board exam. This step is vital and you must practice. The second half of this text includes 50 cases for your review. Simply reading the cases should make you familiar with the testing style. Additionally, we recommend live simulation. Find a friend who is taking the test with you and quiz each other. Use cases from this book and elsewhere. If you would like an accurate, live simulation, enroll in an oral board review class (Table 1-2). Better classes have board-certified physicians administering the test in a high fidelity simulation of the actual testing day. We recommend the following practice schedule:

1. Spend 2 weeks reviewing cases to familiarize yourself with the testing process.
2. Get together with a colleague and test each other.
3. Take an oral board review course to fine-tune your skills and to prove to yourself that you are ready.

Table 1-2. Oral Boards Study Resources

Program	Location	Web site	Contact Information
Illinois ACEP Oral Board Review Course	Illinois	https://www.icep.org/cme-conference/oral-board-review/	630-495-6400
Ohio ACEP Oral Board Review Course	Ohio	http://www.ohacep.org/aws/OACEP/pt/sp/cme_oralboard	614-792-6506 info@ohacep.org
AAEM Pearls of Wisdom Oral Board Review Course	Multiple	http://www.aaem.org/education/oral-board-review-course	800-884-AAEM info@aaem.org

Oral Board Instructions

You can think of the oral boards as chess match: it is an artificial environment governed by strict rules with a variety of strategies you can use to win. In this section, I will lay out the rules that govern each section of the exam, as well as strategies that you can use to be successful. In chess, every game is unique, but the same rules and strategies apply to them all. The same is true of the oral boards cases. While every case is a unique interaction between the examiner and examinee, you can apply the technique and methods delineated below to them all.

GENERAL INFORMATION

During the oral boards, most of the cases will be common material that you will most likely be very comfortable and familiar with. However, it is your ability to organize, integrate, and utilize information that is being tested. Communication skills are critical. Remember that a large portion of your score will be based not only on how you handle the medical management of your patient, but also on the way you communicate with your patient, nurses, and consultants. One of the most common mistakes is to focus on medical management and forget to communicate. Here are some key points to remember:

1. Introduce yourself to the patient, family, EMTs, and consultants.
2. Always ask for any missing vital signs. These are usually significant.
3. Do not ignore emotional distress or pain. If your patient appears distressed, the examiner is presenting it that way for a reason. Address it.
4. Explain, and get consent for, all invasive procedures, and also for pelvic or rectal examinations.
5. Always explain test results and disposition to the patient and family.

At the beginning of every case, you will be given a sheet with the patient's name, chief complaint, means of arrival, and vital signs. Remember the patient's name, and use it to address them. Also, make note of the means of arrival. Whoever brought the patient to the hospital (EMS, family members, etc) can give you additional history. If a patient is brought in by EMS, always ask them what they found at the scene and have them stay in the emergency department (ED) so you can speak with them as needed. If the patient has family with them, ask them if they have anything else to add to the history.

Always make your requests for information open-ended as this strategy gives you the best chance of getting key information from the examiner.

Also, make note of the vital signs. There should always be five. One of the first things you should do is request whatever vital signs are missing. Missing vital signs are usually abnormal, and the examiner wants you to request it and address treatment accordingly. If any of the vital signs are abnormal, address that first. Examiners use a similar technique with altered patients who present to the ED by EMS without a glucose level.

APPROACH

The general outline of how to approach the case will be the same for every patient:

1. **Initial assessment:** Assess vital signs (make sure there are five) and get your "first impression" of the patient.

2. **Immediate actions:** Perform a primary survey by checking the airway, breathing, and circulation, disability and exposure, and address any life-threatening concerns or abnormal vital signs. If the patient is unstable, you must stabilize them before moving on to do your complete physical examination and history.
3. **History and physical examination:** Next, perform a secondary survey. If the patient is stable, perform a complete physical examination and history after the initial assessment. Take a history using the AMPLE mnemonic:
   - **A**llergies
   - **M**edications
   - **P**ast medical/surgical history
   - **L**ast meal
   - **E**vents
4. **Diagnostic tests:** After the initial examination and history, order your labs, imaging, and perform any necessary interventions.
5. **Ongoing management and reassessment:** While waiting for your lab results, reassess the patient's vital signs and physical examination.
6. **Disposition:** When your lab results and imaging results return, make any final interventions indicated by the results you receive, call the appropriate specialist, and make your disposition. Speak with the patient and family about your concerns and what you are doing to address them.

Almost all of your patients will be admitted. There are minor presentations managed during the triple cases that may be discharged, but be very cautious about discharging a patient from ABEM General.

We will now address each of these steps in more detail.

1. Initial Assessment

For every case, regardless of the chief complaint and vital signs, your first question should always be, "When I walk into the room, what do I see, hear, and smell?" Making note of all the vital signs and then asking open-ended questions will help you achieve the same kind of first-impression gestalt that you normally get by looking at your patient. The exchange will be similar to the following:

CASE A Lilly Johnson

The examiner gives you the following information:

Patient name: Lilly Johnson

Age: 76

Chief complaint: Shortness of breath

Vitals: BP: 90/40, HR: 118, RR: 35, sat 92% on RA, temp: 38.3°C

Mode of arrival: Brought in by EMS

Candidate: "When I walk into the room, what do I see, hear, and smell?"

Examiner: "You see an elderly, diaphoretic, and pale woman lying in bed with her eyes closed in moderate respiratory distress. She is moaning softly."

This exchange gives you a very clear picture of a patient who is very sick. This impression, coupled with the abnormal vital signs, makes it clear that you are dealing with a woman presenting with sepsis and will require aggressive and immediate interventions.

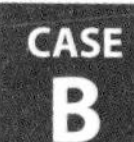

CASE B Bobby Thompson

The examiner gives you the following information:

Patient name: Bobby Thompson

Age: 6

Chief complaint: Abdominal pain

Vitals: BP: 103/48, HR: 118, RR: 45, sat 100% on RA, temp: 36.5°C

Mode of arrival: Brought in by mother

Candidate: "When I walk into the room, what do I see, hear, and smell?"

Examiner: "You see a child who is small and thin for his stated age, lying in bed breathing deeply and rapidly. You smell a fruity odor on his breath."

Again, this first impression, combined with the vital signs, gives you a clear picture of your patient and points you in the direction of diabetic ketoacidosis (DKA) and possibly new-onset diabetes. If you had not asked about the smell, you may not have gotten this impression.

You can already tell, just in these first few seconds, that this child will need fluid resuscitation, lab work, and studies to rule out infection. Getting a good "first impression" of the patients will direct your initial management, as well as your first round of interventions.

2. Immediate Actions

Your immediate actions should be directed toward stabilization of an unstable patient. If the patient appears very stable, your immediate interventions can be as simple as placing the patient on oxygen, cardiac monitors, and placing an intravenous (IV). Almost every patient at ABEM General should get an IV, oxygen by nasal cannula, and be placed on a cardiac monitor.

In a patient who appears ill, your immediate actions will be more complicated. You will start with IV, oxygen, and a monitor, and do a focused primary survey, addressing any needs as they are discovered. We will use Case A above as an example.

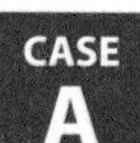

CASE A Lilly Johnson (Continued)

Candidate: "I would like the nurse to place two large-bore IVs, start the patient on 4 L of oxygen by nasal cannula and place the patient on a cardiac monitor. I would like a repeat oxygen sat after the patient is on oxygen, and I would like a rhythm strip when the cardiac monitors are in place. While the nurses are doing this I will evaluate the patient's airway. I ask the patient her name. Is she able to respond to me?"

Examiner: "She does not respond to voice."

Candidate: "Is she responsive to touch?"

Examiner: "When you do a sternal rub, she opens her eyes, pushes at your hand and tells you to go away."

Candidate: "Good. Her airway is intact, and her Glasgow Coma Scale (GCS) is above 8, meaning that she does not need immediate intubation. I would like to listen to her lungs. Do I hear any abnormal sounds like rales, rhonchi, or crackles? Are her breath sounds equal?"

Examiner: "She has decreased breath sounds and rales on her left side. Her right lung is clear."

Candidate: "When I listen to her heart, what do I hear? Is her heartbeat regular? Are the S1 and S2 normal? Murmurs?"

Examiner: "She is tachycardic, but otherwise normal."

Candidate: "I would like to palpate her peripheral pulses and assess her capillary refill."

Examiner: "Her cap refill is prolonged, and her peripheral pulses are thready."

Candidate: "Thank you. What are my repeat vitals and rhythm strip?"

Examiner: "The repeat vitals are BP: 90/40, HR: 120, RR: 30, sat 98% on 4 L nasal cannula, temp: 38.3°C. The rhythm strip shows sinus tachycardia."

Candidate: "Thank you. I would like to give her a 1 L bolus of normal saline and 1 g of Tylenol PR. I would like to change her oxygen to facemask. Can I get another set of vitals after these interventions?"

Examiner: "The repeat vitals are BP: 100/60, HR: 110, RR: 25, satting 100% on facemask, temp: 37.5°C. The patient appears more alert."

Candidate: "Good. I would like to initiate another liter bolus of saline, and while that is running I will do my complete physical examination and history."

There are a few things to take note of in this exchange:

- First, the candidate gets the IV, oxygen, and cardiac monitors placed first. This is always your first intervention.
- Next, the candidate assesses her airway. After her airway is determined to be intact, the candidate moves on to breathing and circulation.
- After the focused examination, the candidate realizes that both the patient's breathing and her circulation are unstable, and they initiate interventions to address both of these problems by starting IV fluids and increasing the patient's oxygen.
- Notice how the candidate frequently reassesses the patient and requests repeated sets of vitals after every intervention. This is very important. You must reassess your patient to be sure that your interventions are having the desired effect.
- After the patient's vital signs begin to normalize, the candidate then states that they will move on to the secondary survey and complete a full history and physical examination.
- Finally, note how the candidate walks the examiner through their thought process. For example, the candidate states aloud, "her GCS is above 8 and her airway is intact, therefore I will not intubate now." This type of verbal outlining is a good habit to get into. The easier it is for the examiner to follow your thought process, the more accurate your score will be.

Let us go through case B now, for another example of initial interventions.

CASE B Bobby Thompson (Continued)

Candidate: "I would like the nurse to place two peripheral IVs, start the patient on 4 L of oxygen by nasal cannula, and place the patient on a cardiac monitor. I would like to start fluids after I get the boy's weight and get a fingerstick glucose. While the nurses are doing this, I will evaluate the patient's airway. I'll ask the patient his name."

Examiner: "My name is Bobby."

Candidate: "Hi Bobby. I am Doctor Emergency and I'm going to make you feel better, okay? I would like to listen to his lungs please. What do I hear—rales, rhonchi, or crackles? Are his breath sounds equal?"

Examiner: "He is tachypneic, taking deep breaths, but the lungs are clear and equal."

Candidate: "When I listen to his heart, what do I hear? Is his heartbeat regular? Are the S1 and S2 normal? Murmurs?"

Examiner: "He is tachycardic, but otherwise normal."

Candidate: "I would like to palpate his peripheral pulses and assess his capillary refill."

Examiner: "His cap refill is slightly prolonged, but his peripheral pulses are normal."

Candidate: "Do I have my weight and fingerstick glucose results yet?"

Examiner: "The boy weighs 20 kg, and his fingerstick glucose is critically high."

Candidate: "Since there is controversy about bolusing children in DKA with insulin, I would like to start fluids with a 20 cc/kg bolus, and also start an insulin drip at 0.1 unit/kg/h. I would like to have q2h glucose measurements. I will complete my history and physical while these orders are being carried out, and then I will order additional lab work. These results will influence whether we need any potassium with the IV fluids. Please draw the blood for labs before initiating the fluids and insulin."

In this example, you can see that the initial management is brief. The candidate orders an IV, oxygen, and monitors, as well as a fingerstick glucose due to the clinical appearance of the patient. Then the candidate evaluates the patient's airway, breathing, and circulation, and initiates IV fluids and insulin. While this patient is very ill, his airway, breathing, and circulation are not critical. It is also important to note that the patient is not tachypneic due to respiratory impairment. The patient is profoundly acidotic and the respiratory changes represent compensation for a metabolic process. The candidate is addressing the tachypnea and tachycardia both by giving fluids and insulin. As in the previous case, the candidate addresses immediate threats to the vital signs, and then moves on to the full history and physical.

It is also useful to note two very effective strategies that the candidate uses in this passage.

- The candidate announces to the examiner what their intentions and logic are behind every decision. Instead of just saying, "Can the patient talk?" the candidate states "I will now evaluate the airway. I'll ask the patient his name." Point out to the examiner how you are structuring your examination according to treatment algorithms. Never pass by an opportunity to show how clever you are!

- The candidate also explains why they are dosing the fluids and insulin as they are. Allow the examiner to see the reasoning behind your actions.

There is room for judgment as to how many lab studies you order before you have completed your full history and physical. We recommend performing studies that are rapid and obviously indicated. For example, check a glucose level in a child with Kussmaul respirations, an upright chest in a patient with a history of ulcers who has peritoneal signs, and an ECG and portable chest x-ray (CXR) in a patient with chest pain. Full laboratory and radiological examinations can wait until you have completed your evaluation. A common strategy is to ask that when the IVs are started that blood be drawn to send for future lab orders.

After your initial primary survey is done, your initial orders given, and your initial management is complete, reassess the patient by asking for vital signs and the patient's appearance. After the patient is stable, you can move on to your secondary survey with a complete physical examination and full history.

3. History and Physical Examination

A simple history will contain all of the following elements:

- **A**llergies
- **M**edications
- **P**ast medical/surgical history and history of **P**resent illness
- **L**ast meal
- **E**vents

In cases that involve surgical and/or trauma patients, it is appropriate for you to obtain a rapid AMPLE history initially and then obtain a full history later if the patient's condition allows it.

Remember that you have several sources for history. Always ask the EMS personnel what they found on the scene, talk to family members to see if they know any more details, request hospital records, and remember that you can call the patient's primary provider. This is especially helpful if the patient is altered, has syncopized, or presenting with psychiatric symptoms.

The physical examination is probably one of the most difficult elements of the exam because no one has ever done a physical examination on a patient that they cannot see. In order to master this skill, you must take a systematic approach and practice it. Begin at the patient's head and work your way down. Don't forget to ask about the scalp, back, skin, and genitals. Similarly, do not forget to do a full neurological examination.

Begin each organ system with an open-ended question such as, "Is there anything remarkable about the HEENT examination?" or, "I would like to examine the lungs now." Leaving open-ended questions allows the examiner to give you as much information as they are able. If the examiner says something such as "Normal," or "The lung examination is unremarkable," that means there are no pertinent findings and you can proceed to the next organ system. Conversely, if the examiner says something such as, "What are you looking for?" then you need to continue to investigate.

You should have a pre-packaged list of questions for each portion of the physical examination that you can modify for individual cases. We've listed our suggestions below. You will not always need to ask all these questions in every case as there will not be time. This list represents the detailed examination that you will do when you are focusing on a certain body part or organ system.

HEENT: Are the pupils reactive and eye movements intact? Is there icterus, injection, or other signs of infection or trauma to the eye? Is the funduscopic examination normal? Are there signs of trauma to the head such as facial instability, rhinorrhea, otorrhea, hemotympanum, or lesions in the mouth? Are the cranial nerves intact? Is the oropharynx normal and are mucous membranes moist? Are there any scalp lesions? If the patient is a neonate you should ask about the fontanelles.

Neck: Is there jugular venous distention (JVD) or tracheal deviation? Is the neck supple; are there any bruises, rashes, or crepitance? Lymphadenopathy or other masses? Is the thyroid normal?

Lungs: Are there normal breath sounds, crackles, rales, or wheezes? Is there any palpable chest-wall deformity, tenderness, or crepitus?

Cardiovascular: Are there any murmurs, rubs, and gallops? Do I hear a normal S1 and S2? Are there friction rubs or distant heart sounds? Are the peripheral pulses symmetric? Is the skin cool or mottled? Are the capillary refill and peripheral pulses normal?

Abdomen: Is the abdomen distended, or tender to palpation? Is it tympanitic? Is there hepato- or splenomegaly? A Murphy sign, McBurney point tenderness, Rovsing sign, or any other surgical findings? Are bowel sounds present on auscultation? Is there rebound, guarding, or signs of peritonitis in any of the four quadrants? On the rectal examination, is there normal tone and a normal prostate (if male)? What color is the stool and is it guaiac negative?

Pelvic (if needed): On bimanual examination is the cervix open or closed? Is the uterus tender or boggy? Are there adnexal masses or tenderness? It there blood? Is there any cervical motion tenderness? Is there any discharge or odor?

Musculoskeletal: Any signs of trauma? Are all peripheral pulses intact and symmetric? Is there any clubbing, cyanosis, or edema? Are there any asymmetries, deformities, or swelling? Does the patient have a Homan sign or calf squeeze tenderness? Any obvious back injury or area of tenderness on palpation?

Neurologic: What is the patient's level of consciousness? Are the cranial nerves intact? Are the muscular strength, sensation, and deep tendon reflexes (DTRs) normal and symmetric in all extremities? Are the Romberg and gait normal? Any pronator drift or dysmetria? Are the Babinskis down-going?

Skin: Any rash, jaundice, or signs of trauma? Any petechiae, purpura, bruising, or joint swelling? Is the turgor normal?

Special considerations in the trauma patient:

- Remember to rock the pelvis (to make sure that it is stable) and check for blood at the urethral meatus.
- Remember to state that you are going to keep the C-spine immobilized and that you will use log-roll precautions while examining the back.

Common mistakes during the history and physical examination portion of the test involve omission. Remember to do a complete neurovascular examination of an injured extremity. **Also, remember to ask about the skin, back, and genitals**. These are often forgotten because we are used to assessing the skin while we are doing the rest of our examinations in the ED. Forgetting to ask about the skin could lead to missing a meningococcal rash, needle tracks, cellulitis, etc.

We will now go through a full history and physical examination for our two examples.

CASE A Lilly Johnson (Continued)

To recap, this is an elderly woman with fever, hypotension, and altered mental status (AMS) who is being resuscitated with 2 L of NS.

Candidate: "As the patient is too confused to give me a history, is there any family at the bedside?"

Examiner: "No."

Candidate: "Did the nursing home send any documentation along with her?"

Examiner: "Yes they did."

Candidate: "Can I review her past medical and surgical history, medications, and allergies?"

Examiner: "She has a history of diabetes, congestive heart failure, hypertension, and dementia. She has no allergies, and she is taking metformin, lasix, aspirin, and captopril. Her only surgery is a hysterectomy."

Candidate: "Can I call the primary provider listed on the nursing home sheet to get the history of present illness?"

Examiner: "Dr. Assisted-Living is on the phone."

Candidate: "Hello, Doctor. This is Dr. Emergency at ABEM General. I have your patient, Lilly Johnson, here in the ED. On arrival, she was febrile, hypotensive with a systolic blood pressure in the 90s, and hypoxic at 92% on room air. We gave a fluid bolus of 1 L and her BP came up to 100, and she is now satting 100% on a facemask. I have not yet ordered diagnostics studies. I was hoping you could tell me more about her and what has been going on with her over the last few days."

Examiner: "Of course. Mrs. Johnson at baseline is a very active and alert woman. When she was so confused this morning I assumed that she may have an infection and sent her into the ED. Sounds like a good thing I did too! Her vitals were normal when she left here!"

Candidate: "Has she had any falls or head trauma, or anything else that could cause her confusion?"

Examiner: "No."

Candidate: "Does she have any history of thyroid or adrenal disease? Is there anything about her history that you think may be helpful to me?"

Examiner: "No."

Candidate: "Thank you very much for your time. When I finish my workup, I will call you with her diagnosis and disposition."

Examiner: "Thank you."

Candidate: "I would like to proceed with my physical examination now. How does the patient look now? Is she in less distress? Can I get another set of vital signs?"

Examiner: "The patient is no longer diaphoretic or in respiratory distress. She appears much more comfortable. Her current vitals, after your second liter bolus, are BP: 120/80, HR: 100, RR: 20, satting 100% on facemask, temp: 37.5°C."

Candidate: "HEENT examination?"

Examiner: "What are you looking for?"

Candidate: "Are the pupils reactive and eye movements intact? Are the sclera icteric? Are there signs of trauma to the head or lesions in the mouth? Is the oropharynx normal and does she have moist mucous membranes? Is there JVD? Is the neck supple and is the thyroid normal?"

Examiner: "The patient has dry mucous membranes, but the rest of her head and neck examination is normal. She has no JVD."

Candidate: "I will listen to her heart and lungs again. Are there any changes to my previous examination?"

Examiner: "The patient still has rales in the left lung. Her heart rate is slower and her pulses are stronger. Her cap refill is normal."

Candidate: "Abdominal examination?"

Examiner: "Normal."

Candidate: "Extremities?"

Examiner: "Normal."

Candidate: "Skin?"

Examiner: "What are you looking for?"

Candidate: "Any rashes, jaundice, or signs of trauma? Any petechiae, purpura, bruising, or joint swelling? Is the turgor normal?"

Examiner: "She has poor skin turgor, but the rest of the derm examination is normal."

Candidate: "Neurological examination?"

Examiner: "What are you looking for?"

Candidate: "First, I would like to assess her GCS."

Examiner: "She currently has a GCS of 15, but she has some mild confusion."

Candidate: "Can she cooperate with a neurological examination?"

Examiner: "She can follow commands."

Candidate: "Are the cranial nerves intact? Are the muscular strength, sensation, and DTRs symmetric in all extremities? I will not assess the gait due to the patient's condition. Is she A&Ox3?"

Examiner: "Her cranial nerves, strength, and sensation are all intact. She is A&Ox2. She thinks that is it 1974."

Candidate: "What are her vital signs now?"

Examiner: "Her current vitals are BP: 120/80, HR: 100, RR: 20, satting 100% on facemask, temp: 37.5°C."

Candidate: "Good. I will order labs tests now."

There are several things to note in this history and physical examination:

- First, as the patient cannot give her own history, the candidate uses the chart, EMS, and the primary provider as sources to obtain a history. Remember that you will always be able to get some kind of history, but in some cases you may have to work more than others.
- Notice how frequently the candidate reassesses the patient. At every break in the case they ask for a set of vital signs and whether the patient appears to be in distress.
- You will also note that in those organ systems in which there are no important physical findings the examiner states that they are "normal." This is a sign for the candidate to move on.
- When the examiner asks, "What are you looking for?" the candidate correctly interprets this as a sign to look for pertinent findings in that organ system and begins to ask several specific questions to obtain more information.
- Use the phrase, "or anything else that seems abnormal" as often as possible, as this leaves the door open to getting more information from the examiner whenever possible.

CASE B Bobby Thompson (Continued)

We will now do a history and physical examination on Bobby Thompson, the 6-year-old with DKA.

Candidate: "May I talk to the mother?"

Examiner: "Go ahead."

Candidate: "Hello Mrs. Thompson. I'm Dr. Emergency. Can you tell me what brings you in today?"

Examiner: "Bobby is just breathing so funny! He also seems really sleepy today and has been complaining for a few days about his belly hurting."

Candidate: "Does Bobby have any medical problems? Does he take any medicines?"

Examiner: "No."

Candidate: "Is Bobby allergic to anything?"

Examiner: "No."

Candidate: "Has he had any fevers?"

Examiner: "No."

Candidate: "Any cough? Nausea? Vomiting or diarrhea?"

Examiner: "No."

Candidate: "Has he been drinking an unusual amount of water or urinating a lot recently?"

Examiner: "You know, now that you mention it, yes. He has been wetting the bed the last few nights and that is not like him."

Candidate: "Thank you Mrs. Thompson. I would like to proceed with my physical examination now. How does the patient look now? Is he in less distress? Can I get another set of vital signs and another fingerstick glucose?"

Examiner: "The patient appears the same. The current vitals are BP: 100/52, HR: 120, RR: 43, satting 100% on RA, temp: 36.5°C. Glucose is still critically high."

Candidate: "HEENT examination?"

Examiner: "What are you looking for?"

Candidate: "Are the pupils reactive and eye movements intact? Are the sclera icteric? Are there signs of trauma to the head or lesions in the mouth? Is the oropharynx normal with moist mucous membranes? Is the neck supple?"

Examiner: "The patient has dry mucous membranes, but the rest of the head and neck examination is normal."

Candidate: "I will listen to his heart and lungs again. Are there any changes to my previous examination? How is the cap refill?"

Examiner: "The patient still has clear lung sounds bilaterally and a regular rate and rhythm. His cap refill is slightly delayed."

Candidate: "Abdominal examination?"

Examiner: "What are you looking for?"

Candidate: "Is the abdomen distended or tender to palpation? Is it tympanitic? Is there any hepato- or splenomegaly? Are bowel sounds present on auscultation? Is there guarding or signs of peritonitis?"

Examiner: "The patient appears uncomfortable and tells you that his 'tummy hurts everywhere,' but his pain does not localize and there is no rebound or guarding. Bowel sounds are present."

Candidate: "Extremities?"

Examiner: "Normal, with the slightly delayed cap refill previously noted."

Candidate: "Skin?"

Examiner: "Normal."

Candidate: "Neurological examination?"

Examiner: "What are you looking for?"

Candidate: "First, I would like to assess his GCS and level of consciousness."

Examiner: "He is tired appearing and irritable, but his GCS is 15."

Candidate: "Are the cranial nerves intact? Are the muscular strength, sensation, and DTRs symmetric in all extremities?"

Examiner: "His cranial nerves, strength, and sensation are intact."

Candidate: "Good. What are his current vital signs?"

Examiner: "The patient appears the same. The current vitals are BP: 100/52, HR: 120, RR: 43, satting 100% on RA, temp: 36.5°C."

Candidate: "I will order labs tests now."

Again, the candidate gets history from a source other than the patient. In this case it is from the mother.

Make sure that you complete the physical examination. If the patient decompensates, becomes unstable, or requires immediate management, address the medical concerns immediately. Once completed, return to the history and physical examination and complete this before you disposition the patient.

Some examinees may get caught up in patient management and forget to finish this critical portion of the exam, especially with the triple cases.

4. Diagnostic Tests

Diagnostic tests can be ordered throughout the exam at any time they seem pertinent. While you can get points taken away for "shotgunning" your patient with excessive labs, do not let that make you afraid to order all the labs you need in order to make your diagnosis and rule out any life-threatening pathology. A good general strategy is to order any rapid and essential diagnostics early during your assessment (fingerstick glucose, ECG, portable CXR, etc) and obtain more invasive and time-intensive diagnostics (CT scans, lab work) after you have completed your evaluation of the patient.

Remember to ask the nurse to draw blood while she is putting in the IV, and hold it for future lab orders.

We will now go through the diagnostics for our two cases.

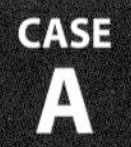

CASE A Lilly Johnson (Continued)

To recap, this is an elderly woman with fever, hypotension, and AMS who is being resuscitated with 2 L of NS.

Candidate: "I would like to order a CBC, basic metabolic panel, CXR (PA and lateral views), blood cultures, urinalysis, ECG, and a set of cardiac enzymes. I would also like to start the patient on 400 mg of Avelox IV for presumed pneumonia. I would also like to start the patient on 100 cc of NS per hour for maintenance. Please have the nurse notify me when the test results come back."

Examiner: "Your lab tests have been sent."

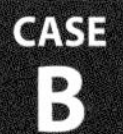

CASE B Bobby Thompson (Continued)

To recap, this is our 6-year-old male with DKA.

Candidate: "I would like to order a CBC, basic metabolic panel with calcium, magnesium, and phosphate. I would also like a CXR (PA and lateral views), blood cultures, and a urinalysis. I would like to repeat the chemistry panel at 4-hour intervals as long as the patient is here in the ED. Have the nurse notify me when the lab tests come back."

Examiner: "Your lab tests have been sent."

There are a few things to note here:

First, always ask the examiner to notify you when the tests come back. This places some responsibility for following up on the examiner.

Another thing to note is that if your patient requires ongoing management, go ahead and order it. Any ongoing order you give relieves you of having to remember to repeat orders in the future.

Finally, remember to involve consultants early. In the real world you may wait to call consultants until you have a definitive diagnosis. However, at ABEM

General, you should call them early in the case. For example, if you have a patient on whom you are doing a computed tomography (CT) to evaluate for appendicitis, call the surgeon to let them know about the patient before you send them for CT. Conversely, do not expect your consultants to add much to your decision making. The surgeon will not give you the answer to the case, they are more likely to say something like, "Well, work the patient up and call me again based on your findings." Regardless, you are expected to call them early to show that you are thinking about definitive care for your patient.

5. Ongoing Management and Reassessment

When your lab results come back, reassess your patient and make any more interventions that need to be made. The examiner may ask you to interpret your test results and you may also be presented with x-ray films, ECGs, etc. You will not be asked to evaluate tests that you would not be expected to be able to read in your normal practice (V/Q scans, magnetic resonance images [MRIs], etc). If you are unable to fully assess a CXR or ultrasound (US), you can ask for a radiology consult, or for a formal read. However, the examiner may take off points if the study is one which you are expected to interpret yourself.

Remember, you will be scored on how well you interpret lab results and whether or not your management is appropriate. Accordingly, if you misinterpret a lab result with critical implications for the patient (a positive troponin, or an ST elevation on the ECG), you will be scored much more harshly than if you miss something which has little relevance, such as slightly elevated potassium in a patient with no suspicious ECG findings. Unlike lab results in the real world, the abnormal levels at ABEM General are not in a bold font or highlighted in any way, but you can ask for reference ranges.

The study results will either be delivered to you via the eOral case format, on a piece of paper, or verbally by the examiner. If you do not have a written report, write the results down on your note paper. You will need those results later when you speak to a consultant or the admitting service.

We will now review this step of the process for our two patients.

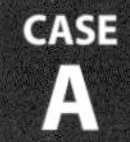

CASE A Lilly Johnson (Continued)

This is an elderly woman with fever, hypotension, and AMS who has presumed pneumonia.

Examiner: "Your lab tests are back.

Na: 152

K: 4.3

Cl: 110

CO_2: 20

BUN: 45

Cr: 1.8

Glucose: 153

WBC: 17

Hg/Hct: 12/36

Platelets: 459

UA: Normal

Cardiac enzymes: <0.03 troponin

Your ECG and your CXR are here. Please interpret them."

(The candidate is given an ECG showing LVH and normal sinus rhythm and a CXR showing large left lobar pneumonia.)

Candidate: "Her lab results are unremarkable, except for mild renal insufficiency which appears to be due to dehydration. Her ECG shows LVH, but no signs of MI, and her CXR shows a left lobar pneumonia. I will continue the patient on Avelox, oxygen, and fluids, and I will admit her to the ICU for further monitoring and treatment."

CASE B Bobby Thompson (Continued)

A 6-year-old male with DKA.

Examiner: "Your lab tests are back.

Na: 152

K: 5.2

Cl: 112

CO_2: 8

BUN: 22

Cr: .8

Glucose: 524

WBC: 25

Hg/Hct: 14/42

Platelets: 459

Ca: 8

Mg: 2.2

P: 1.4

UA: + for leuk esterase, nitrates, bacteria, glucose, and ketones

CXR was normal."

Candidate: "These labs are consistent with severe DKA, probably triggered by a UTI. I will need to replace the magnesium and phosphate. For the UTI, I would like to start ceftriaxone IV. For the low electrolytes, I will have to look up the correct pediatric doses for this. I will speak to the family and then I will admit this child to the PICU."

Again, note how the candidate addresses the issue of pediatric dosing by stating that he will look it up. As long as the medication is not used for resuscitation, you can always call your trusty ABEM General pharmacist if you need dosing, frequency of administration, drug interactions, or contraindications. In the exam, as in real life, it is always better to ask for help when you do not know something than to act without appropriate knowledge and make an error.

6. Disposition

When you are comfortable that your patient has been stabilized, you have to decide on an appropriate disposition. You have three choices: discharge home, admit to the medical floor (with or without specialty consultation), or admit to the intensive care unit (ICU) (with or without specialty consult). Most of your patients will require admission. When working at ABEM General you should be conservative and have a low threshold for admitting patients. If you are concerned that they will need close monitoring, admit them to the ICU. Be very cautious about sending a patient home on exam day. Some of the minor cases during a "triple cases" can be sent home, but it is rare for "single case" patients to be discharged home.

As in the real world, admit the patient by calling the admitting service and giving report. You will then call any specialty consults you require, and finally you should talk to the patient and to the family. If you have time, you may wish to place a call to the primary provider as a courtesy. Do not forget to tell the patient and family their test results and disposition as this will impact your communication score. Use these conversations as a chance to show your understanding of both the case and the patient's pathology.

Be aware that the examiner will often use your consultants as a way of testing your knowledge. If you have a consultant who "pushes back," or does not wish to come in to see the patient in the time frame that you feel is appropriate, state your concern and advocate for your patient. If you think something is indicated, make sure that it happens. If the consultant questions your management, explain your reasoning.

We will now conclude our two cases.

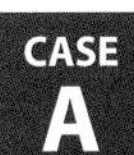

Lilly Johnson (Continued)

This is the elderly woman with sepsis and left-sided pneumonia.

Examiner: "Dr. Intense is on the phone."

Candidate: "Hello Dr. Intense, this is Dr. Emergency. I have a 76-year-old woman here who presented with hypotension at 90/40, and a heart rate of 118. She was satting 92% on room air and had an initial respiratory rate of 35. Her initial temperature was 38.3°C. I put her on a facemask, gave a 2 L bolus with normal saline, and treated her with Avelox and Tylenol. Her vitals now are BP of 120/80, HR of 100, satting 100% on a facemask. Her labs, including a CBC, basic metabolic panel, and cardiac enzymes are normal. She has a white blood cell count of 17, left lower lobe pneumonia on CXR, and blood cultures pending. Her ECG was normal. I would like to admit her to the ICU for monitoring."

Examiner: "Send her up."

Candidate: "May I talk to her primary provider now?"

Examiner: "He is on the phone."

Candidate: "Hello, I wanted to let you know the disposition on Mrs. Johnson. She has left lower lobe pneumonia, and is going to the ICU. Her vitals are currently stable, but I feel that she would benefit from intensive monitoring."

Examiner: "Of course. Thank you for the call. This case is now over."

CASE B Bobby Thompson (Continued)

This is a 6-year-old male with DKA.

Examiner: "Dr. Child is on the phone."

Candidate: "Hello Dr. Child, this is Dr. Emergency. I have a 6-year-old male here with no past medical history who has presented in DKA with a glucose of 524 and an anion gap of 32. His physical examination was remarkable for Kussmaul breathing and his UA was concerning for UTI. I have cultured his urine and initiated treatment with ceftriaxone, IV fluids at twice maintenance, and an insulin drip of 0.1 unit/kg per hour. I am monitoring q2h glucose measurements and q4h metabolic panels. I am also replacing his magnesium and phosphate and will recheck levels. I would like to admit him to the PICU for further care."

Examiner: "Of course. I will see him as soon as he gets up here."

Candidate: "May I talk to the family now?"

Examiner: "Okay."

Candidate: "Mrs. Thompson, the tests that we performed show that your son has diabetes. He will need to come into the hospital in order to get this under control and to get him started on the right medications to control it at home. He also has a urinary tract infection, or UTI, that is being treated with antibiotics. He will be fine, but it will take a few days to make him all the way better. Do you have any questions for me?"

Examiner: "No. Thank you, doctor. This case is over."

This part of the case is often the easiest, as we are all very comfortable presenting patients to our consultants over the phone. Use the conversations to illustrate your thought process related to differential diagnosis and also recognition and treatment of abnormal physical exam findings and study results. Speak as you would if you were really admitting a patient and you should do fine.

7. Managing the Information

As in the real ED, doing well on the oral exam requires being able to organize a large amount of information. In this section we will outline one system for keeping track of the information on exam day. This is not the only system, but can be used as a guideline as you figure out the best system that works for you. Make sure that your system keeps track of the information you will need to do well.

You will be given paper and pencils during the exam. The paper will have a drawing of the human body on the left-hand side, and the rest will be blank. An example of the note paper can be found at the ABEM Web site at http://www.abem.org/public/docs/default-source/oral-examination-/notesheet_candidate_spe.pdf?sfvrsn=2

Use this drawing to mark findings during your physical examination. For example, if you have a trauma victim with multiple injuries, you can mark the location of each one to help you remember to address treatment for each injury. You can also use this drawing to keep track of which parts of the physical examination you have done, and which parts still need to be done.

The right side of the page will be blank. Use this area to organize the case and take notes. One way to do this is to create six boxes with the following headings: history, labs ordered, physical examination, interventions, results, and disposition (Fig. 1-1).

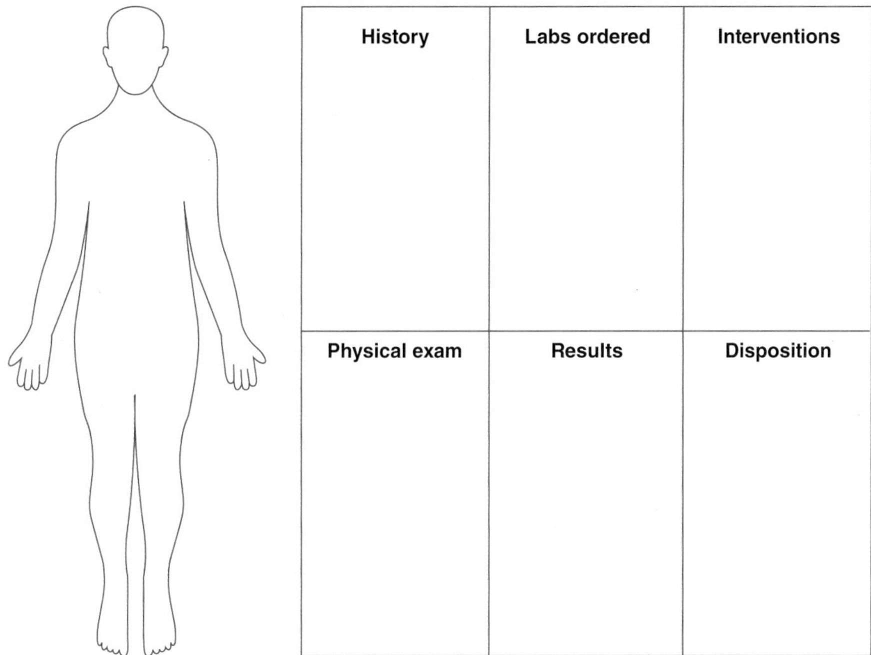

Figure 1-1. Above is an example of one way to organize information during an oral boards case. The paper given to you by the examiner will already have the human figure on it; the boxes and headings you will have to make yourself.

As you advance through the case, you will write down each piece of information that you receive in the appropriate box. For example, in Case A (An elderly woman with LLL pneumonia) the sheet would end up looking like this (Fig. 1-2).

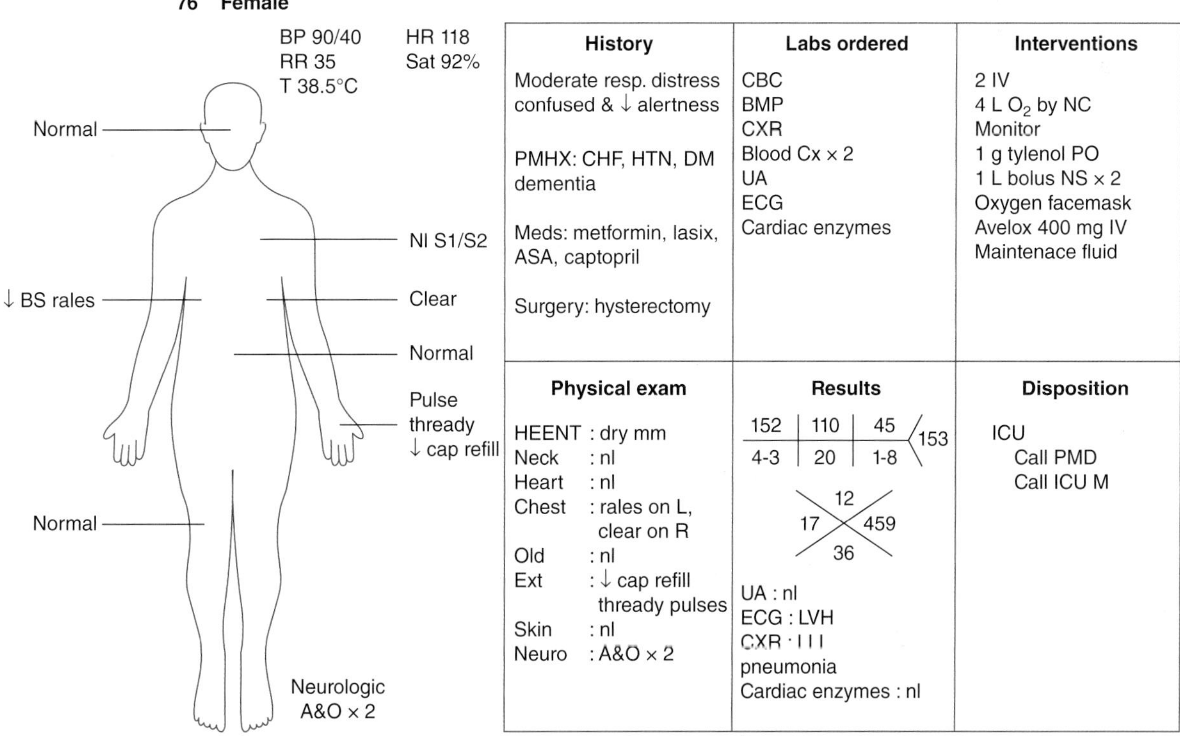

Figure 1-2. Above is an example of the previous sheet with the information from Case A entered. This is how your note paper should look like at the end of the case.

The most important aspect of this system is that it provides you with a framework to help you organize the case, perform all the necessary steps, and follow up on studies that you ordered. For example, you are responsible for the results for every lab test you order. The boxes labeled "labs" and "results" should have the same number of entries before the patient is admitted. Always double-check this. Use this tracking sheet to make sure that you also finish the whole physical examination before you disposition the patient. This is especially important if you were interrupted by something during your evaluation such as a patient crashing or an urgent need from another patient during a "triple case." After you stabilize the patient, remember to come back and finish your exam.

PEARLS

1. Initial Evaluation and General Rules

Remember that patient management is more important than getting every detail right. When a patient has a gunshot wound and hypovolemic shock, stabilize your ABCs first. You should remember to give tetanus shots and antibiotics before disposition, but do not let thinking about those details get in the way of the primary management of the patient.

Remember to set priorities. You should complete the history and physical examination before you send the patient upstairs, but do not delay the management of a critical patient by performing a thorough physical examination before you address a critical concern. If the patient has a potential airway issue, you should manage that before you do anything else. The exam tests your ability to manage patients. If you do not complete your entire history and physical examination before time runs out, but you succeed in stabilizing the patient, then you have addressed the most important aspect of the case.

Remember to perform a primary survey and address any life-threatening concerns as they are discovered. First, make sure they can speak to rule out an airway obstruction. If they cannot, try a jaw thrust, check for foreign body (FB) or secretions, and attempt to clear the airway. If that does not help, use an oral airway and prepare to intubate or perform a cricothyrotomy. Second, listen to breath sounds and assess for any abnormality. Are they symmetric? Are there any rales, wheezing, or areas of decreased breath sounds? Perform needle decompression before obtaining a CXR or moving onto evaluation of circulation. Finally, assess circulation. Palpate peripheral pulses, check cap refill, and look for JVD. Listen to the heart. Is there a regular rate and rhythm? Any murmurs?

In any trauma patient, remember to keep C-spine precautions. Apply a cervical collar (if one is not in place) and use log-roll precautions.

2. Immediate Interventions

No treatment or action will be taken unless you specifically ask the nurses to perform it. This includes things that we take for granted such as getting IV lines established, placing the patient on the monitor, getting vital signs, etc. Remember to ask for everything and assume nothing.

Your orders should be exact. You will need to give the correct dosages, routes, and timing of all drugs. You should know all medications involved in ACLS, PALS, and NRP, but you can state that you will look up the correct dosing and route for all others. When you order an IV, be specific about the gauge and placement location, and remember that small-bore IVs have no place in ABEM General. If the patients are sick enough to need IV access, they need a large-bore IV. When you order your IV line, also order how rapidly you would like fluids delivered.

You can stack orders. For example, in a patient who comes in with profound shock after a car accident which resulted in a partial amputation of their leg, you could give an initial order such as, "I would like two large-bore peripheral IVs and an initial bolus of 2 L of NS. If the patient's blood pressure has not normalized after that initial bolus, I would like to initiate a blood transfusion with two units of packed red blood cells." You do not have to wait and give each order one at a time.

3. History and Physical Examination

Remember that someone will have the information you need to manage your patient. If the patient is unwilling or unable to give you a complete history, you will be able to get that information from another source: the EMTs, family or friends, the patient's primary provider, old records, etc. The examiner will be able to play the role of anyone you wish to speak to. All the information will be available, but you may have to dig for it.

Remember to ask for any recent changes to the patient's medications and be sure that "overdose" is on your differential for every patient with AMS. Request a tox screen, salicylates, acetaminophen, and ethanol (EtOH) levels if there is any question about ingestion.

4. Labs and Reassessment

Remember to reevaluate your patient frequently. Get a set of vitals between each step of the examination: before and after your history, physical examination, lab tests, after any intervention, and before your disposition. If you do not reevaluate frequently enough, your examiner may decide to "crash" your patient due to inappropriate management of ongoing illness.

Patients crash for two reasons: it was planned or you are not managing the case correctly. If the patient crashes at the beginning of the case, it is probably the examiner's way of telling you that you are missing something important. Go back to your ABCs and review your vital signs. Make sure that you have all five. If one is missing, that is likely the one which is causing your patient to crash. If the patient crashes when you have everything done and you are ready to disposition the patient, it is more likely that the crash is a planned part of the case which would happen no matter how good your management was. Do not panic, and do not worry. Restart your primary survey and remember that not all the cases are designed to have the patient survive.

Do not ignore pain. If the patient is in pain, treat it immediately. Likewise, do not ignore emotional distress. There are patients in the exam who may come in for what sounds like a purely medical complaint (right upper quadrant [RUQ] pain) who will have recently attempted suicide (via Tylenol overdose). If you ignore depression, you may miss a very important diagnostic tool, and getting a psychiatry consult in such cases is always a critical action.

Remember to get a pregnancy test in every female of childbearing age.

All trauma patients should get a CXR, pelvis XR, and C-spine imaging.

5. Results and Final Interventions

Give a tetanus shot and consider antibiotics for everyone with a break in their skin.

Assume that you will be asked to interpret at least one x-ray. Usually these will be chest, pelvis, or C-spine films. If you get a film of an extremity fracture, it will usually be a common fracture (Jones, Colles, Lisfranc, etc). A good source for review of emergency imaging is *Emergency Medicine Radiology* by Hawkins and Levy. You will also be expected to be able to interpret basic US images such as FAST scans, RUQ scans, and first-trimester pregnancy imaging.

You should be able to explain and describe the following procedures:

- Indirect and direct laryngoscopy
- Intubation
- Cricothyrotomy
- Needle decompression
- Chest tube placement
- Pericardiocentesis
- Transcutaneous pacing
- Placement of central lines (femoral, subclavian, and internal jugular [IJ])
- DPL and FAST examinations
- Lumbar puncture

6. Disposition

If the consulting service asks the results of tests which you did not order, state that you will order those now and call with the results, and then attempt to explain your reasoning for not ordering the test initially (will results change management, did you check a more specific test, etc). If you are going to discharge someone, make sure that they have appropriate follow-up.

Finally, practice, practice, practice! There is no substitute for practicing cases aloud. We recommend that after you read the clinical chapters in this book that you use the cases section with a colleague to familiarize yourself with exam protocol and strategy. The more you practice, the better your performance will be. Good luck!

SECTION 2

RESUSCITATION AND PROCEDURES

CHAPTER 2

Airway Management

Gregg Helland and James Ahn

INITIAL ASSESSMENT

- Assess airway
  - Is the patient speaking?
  - Is the airway obstructed?
    - Complete obstruction: No gas exchange, no airflow with respiratory effort, no chest wall exertion.
    - Partial obstruction: Stridor, noisy respiration, gagging, debris around mouth.
    - If the airway is completely or partially blocked, consider what is causing the blockage: swelling, blood, foreign body, the tongue, or secretions.
  - Open the airway and reassess
    - Remove any visible foreign material in the anterior oropharynx or reposition the tongue.
    - Head tilt and chin lift maneuver.
    - Jaw thrust maneuver.
    - Place an oropharyngeal or nasopharyngeal airway.
  - The airway must be opened before moving forward as complete obstruction causes death in minutes.
- Assess breathing
  - Check vital signs.
    - RR: Is the patient apneic or agonal? Is the patient tachypneic?
    - Oxygen saturation: Hypoxia?
  - Check for chest wall movement and air movement.
    - Are breaths shallow or deep, regular or irregular?
    - Is air movement present, noisy or quiet, labored?
- Assess mental status
  - Can the patient talk, follow commands, open eyes? Does the patient have a gag reflex?
  - Calculate Glasgow coma score (GCS) (Table 2-1).

Table 2-1. Glasgow Coma Scale

PARAMETER	RESPONSE		SCORE
Eyes	Open	Spontaneously	4
		To verbal command	3
		To pain	2
		No response	1
Best motor response	To verbal command	Obeys	6
	To painful stimulus	Localized pain	5
		Flexion-withdrawal	4
		Decorticate (flex)	3
		Decerebrate (extend)	2
		No response	1
Best verbal response		Oriented, converses	5
		Disoriented, converses	4
		Inappropriate responses	3
		Incomprehensible sounds	2
		No response	1

Reprinted with permission from Gomella LG, Haist SA, eds. Clinician's Pocket Reference. 11th ed. *New York, NY: McGraw-Hill; 2007.*

- The mental status may be altered because of primary respiratory failure and hypoxia or hypercarbia.
- Altered mental status with a GCS <8 may render the patient incapable of protecting the airway and maintaining adequate respiration.

- After assessing the airway, breathing, and mental status, decide whether and what type of ventilatory support the patient requires (this includes noninvasive ventilation such as positive-pressure ventilation).

DON'T FORGET

Tend to the A in ABC, the airway is always assessed and controlled first before moving forward.

BASIC AIRWAY MANAGEMENT

- Nasal cannula
  - Delivers supplemental oxygen.
  - The amount of oxygen cannot be controlled.
  - The amount of oxygen should be titrated to pulse oximeter.
- Non-rebreather (NRB) mask
  - Delivers supplemental oxygen.
  - Although called 100%, NRB masks, the reservoir, and valves actually allow delivery of up to 90% oxygen.
  - Venturi masks allow the amount of oxygen to be carefully titrated.
- Bag valve mask (BVM) ventilation
  - The most important skill in airway management is the ability to ventilate a patient noninvasively with a BVM.
  - In most situations where the airway is not definitively controlled (ie intubation or reversal of underlying process), BVM ventilation can oxygenate and ventilate patients effectively until the airway can be controlled.
  - After a failed intubation, proficient BVM ventilation can provide time to ventilate and oxygenate the patient while preparing an alternative plan for airway control.
  - Technique.
    - Position the head to open the airway: Sniffing position.
    - Place airway adjuncts such as a nasal trumpet or an oropharyngeal airway to keep the airway patient.
    - Ensure a good seal between mask and face: When two people are available, while one person bags, the other person creates a tight seal by placing the heels of both hands on the mask and curling the fingers around the mandible.
    - Assess adequacy of ventilation by observing chest wall excursion, listening for air leaks, feeling resistance with bagging, and monitoring oxygen saturation.

DON'T FORGET

On test day, be aggressive with airway management. Maintain a low threshold to intubate and definitively control the airway.

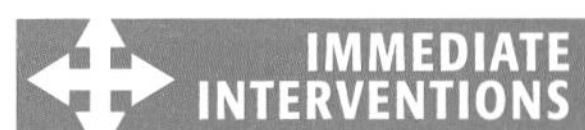

IMMEDIATE INTERVENTIONS

All patients with potential airway compromise get:

- IV
- Cardiac monitor
- Blood drawn for labs

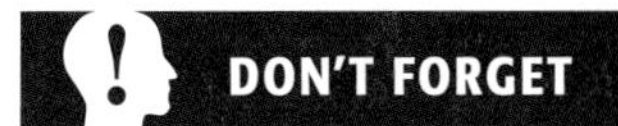

DON'T FORGET

On exam day, all patients with a GCS <8 get intubated.

NONINVASIVE VENTILATORY SUPPORT

- Indications for noninvasive ventilator support (NIVS)
  - Completely patent, nonthreatened airway
  - Awake, interactive patient
    - Must be capable of protecting airway
    - Must be capable of handling secretions
    - Must be cooperative with the equipment
  - Inadequate respiration due to increased work of breathing, decreased respiratory reserve, or compromised gas exchange.
    - Common conditions include asthma, chronic obstructive pulmonary disease (COPD), congestive heart failure (CHF), and pneumonia.
- Methods
  - Continuous positive airway pressure (CPAP)
    - Delivers constant positive-pressure support throughout the respiratory cycle

DON'T FORGET

When ordering supplemental oxygen, indicate how to deliver, how much, and how to titrate.

Mastery of BVM ventilation is a vital skill in real life. When managing difficult airways, BVM keeps the patient alive.

DON'T FORGET

Patients who require ventilatory support but do not meet all of the criteria listed for NIVS need to be intubated.

DON'T FORGET

Always consider prophylactic intubation in patients who are likely to decompensate.

- Bi-level positive airway pressure (BiPAP)
    - Delivers more positive pressure during inspiration and less during expiration.
    - Usual setting is inspiratory positive airway pressure (IPAP) of 10 cm H_2O and expiratory positive airway pressure (EPAP) of 5 cm H_2O.
    - Titrate to patient's ventilatory needs by increasing IPAP in 2 cm H_2O increments.
    - Titrate to patient's oxygenation needs by increasing EPAP in 2 cm H_2O increments.

INDICATIONS FOR INTUBATION

- Respiratory failure or insufficiency
    - Insufficient ventilation
    - Hypoxia
- Inability to protect airway
    - GCS <8
- Threatened airway: If the likely clinical course of the patient's pathology will threaten the airway in the future, then the airway should be controlled early in the case.
    - Predicted loss of ability to protect airway (eg, the mental status of a patient with massive intracranial hemorrhage will likely deteriorate).
    - Impending airway obstruction (eg, a patient with angioedema and increasing swelling, increasing trouble handling secretions, and voice changes will likely develop airway compromise).
    - Impending respiratory failure (eg, the sweaty asthmatic with increasing fatigue and hypercapnia will stop breathing).

INITIAL APPROACH TO INTUBATION

- If the patient is unresponsive, not breathing, or near death, a crash airway is required.
    - Attempt immediate orotracheal intubation with or without medications.
    - If unsuccessful, can the patient be oxygenated and ventilated by BVM?
        - Yes (O_2 sat >90% by BVM): Try difficult airway techniques (as described later in the chapter).
        - No (O_2 sat <90% by BVM): Try failed airway techniques for "cannot intubate, cannot ventilate."
- If the patient is breathing, assess the patient to determine whether a difficult airway is present.
    - Every patient who does not require a crash airway should get a careful airway assessment prior to RSI (rapid sequence intubation).
    - Predictors of difficult airway.
        - Morbid obesity.
        - Limited mouth opening: Inability to open the mouth sufficiently to accommodate three-finger breadths.
        - Hyomental distance: A distance from the hyoid bone to the chin of less than three-finger breadths.
        - Thyrohyoid distance: A distance from the notch in the thyroid cartilage to the hyoid bone of < two-finger breadths.
        - Limited neck mobility.
        - Mallampati score (see Fig. 2-1).
            - The patient opens mouth and sticks out tongue.
            - Visualization of the posterior pharynx is graded from I to IV.
            - Grades I and II predict low intubation failure rates.
            - Grades III and IV predict increasing failure rates.

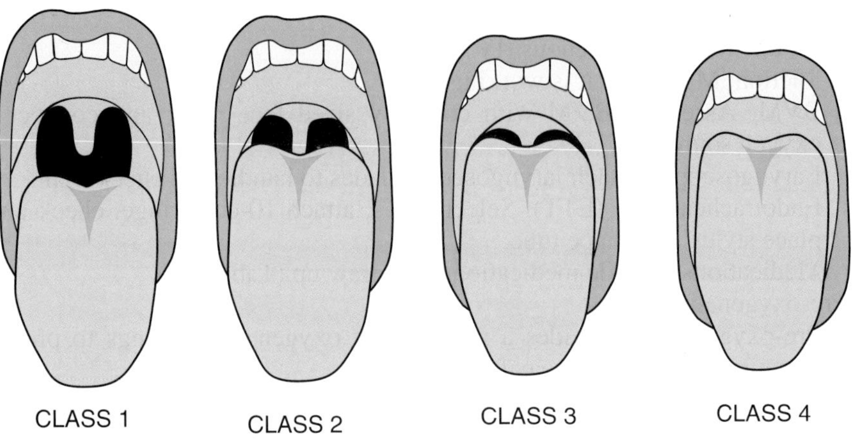

MALLAMPATI CLASSIFICATION

CLASS 1: Soft Palate, Fauces, Uvula, Pillars
CLASS 2: Soft Palate, Fauces, Portion of Uvula
CLASS 3: Soft Palate, Base of Uvula
CLASS 4: Hard Palate Only

A

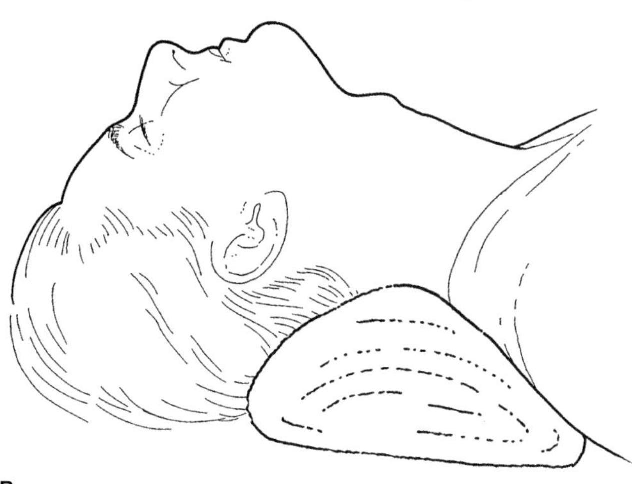

B

Figure 2-1. **(A)** The Mallampati classification. **(B)** The patient is positioned with a rolled towel under the upper shoulders. This position offers excellent exposure, stabilizes the airway structures, and lengthens the cricothyroid membrane. *(A: Reprinted with permission from Brunicardi CF, Anderson DK, Billiar TR, et al.* Schwartz's Principles of Surgery. *8th ed. New York, NY: McGraw-Hill; 2005. B: Reprinted with permission from Reichman RF, Simon RR.* Emergency Medicine Procedures. *New York, NY: McGraw-Hill; 2004.)*

- Upper airway obstructions such as tumor masses.
- If the airway is predicted to be difficult, try the difficult airway techniques (as described later in the chapter).
- Otherwise proceed to RSI.

OROTRACHEAL INTUBATION TECHNIQUE

- Preparation
  - Airway assessment: If predicted to be a difficult airway, should you proceed? Can patient be ventilated by BVM if RSI fails?
  - Patient preparation:
    - Cardiac monitor
    - Blood pressure monitor

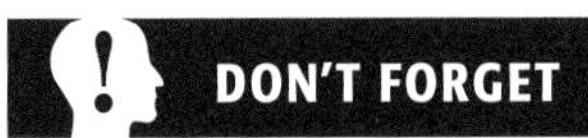

DON'T FORGET

Simplify airway management algorithms for the exam. At ABEM General, all patients should get an initial attempt at orotracheal intubation and if unsuccessful, immediate cricothyroidotomy.

    - Pulse oximeter
    - Functioning intravenous (IV)
  - Suction: Make sure it is working.
  - BVM: Assemble BVM with correctly sized face mask and connect to oxygen source.
  - Laryngoscope: Attach laryngoscope blades to handle and check light.
  - Endotracheal tube (ETT): Select ETTs, attach 10-cc syringe, check cuff, place stylet, and shape tube.
  - Medications: Decide medications and draw up (Table 2-2).
- Pre-oxygenation
  - Pre-oxygenation provides a reservoir of oxygen in the lungs to prevent desaturation during apnea after paralysis.
  - A core principle of RSI is to avoid bagging the patient since bagging forces air into the stomach increasing the risk of aspiration.
  - Provide O_2 by 100% NRB for 3 minutes or if the patient is able to follow commands, have them take 8 breaths with full inhalation and exhalation (vital-capacity breaths).
- Apneic oxygenation
  - During the pre-oxygenation period, place a nasal cannula at the same time and provide 15 L of O_2 per minute and leave the nasal cannula on during the intubation process.
  - Apneic oxygenation can extend the safe apnea time beyond what is provided by traditional pre-oxygenation.
- Premedication
  - Lidocaine and fentanyl to prevent a rise in intracranial pressure (ICP) with intubation.
  - Atropine to prevent bradycardia in children <10 years.
- Paralysis
  - Intubation medications (Table 2-2).
  - Administer a full dose of induction agent to produce loss of consciousness.
  - Follow immediately by a full dose of paralytic.
- Position
  - Move the patient into position to be intubated.
- Placement of ETT
  - Using direct laryngoscopy place the ETT through the vocal cords.
  - Pre-oxygenation combined with apneic oxygenation usually allows 3-8 minutes, or longer, for multiple attempts, if needed, before a patient desaturates below 90%, depending on their acuity and body habitus.
- Proof
  - Look for clouding in ETT.
  - Look for color change on carbon dioxide calorimeter and/or place the patient on an end-tidal carbon dioxide monitor.
  - Listen for breath sounds over both chest walls and the epigastrium.
  - Chest x-ray (CXR).
- Post-tube management
  - Select ventilator settings.
  - Provide sedation to keep the patient comfortable.
  - Consider long-term paralysis if patient needs diagnostic tests and procedures and if frequent neurological examinations are not required.
- Difficult airway techniques
  - Call qualified backup to assist with intubation.
- Awake fiberoptic
  - Rapidly becoming the preferred technique for managing a difficult airway (confirmed or suspected).
  - Advantages: Awake technique allows direct visualization and confirmed tube placement.
  - Disadvantages: Requires experience and expertise, time-consuming.

Table 2-2. Intubation Medications

Agent	Comments	Indications/ Contraindications	Dose/Onset/Duration	Adverse Effects
Premedications				
Lidocaine	Blunts rise in ICP, suppresses cough reflex, and decreases airway irritation.	Neurological protection for suspected ↑ ICP.	1.5 mg/kg IV bolus in adults and pediatrics.	Seizures
Fentanyl	Opioid analgesic decreases reflex sympathetic pain response due to laryngoscopy.	When increase in HR and BP, should be avoided.	1-3 µg/kg IV over 30-60 s in adults and pediatrics.	Hypotension, respiratory depression, chest wall rigidity
Atropine		Pretreatment for all children <10 y	0.02 mg IV 3 min prior to paralysis with succinylcholine; min dose 0.1 mg, max dose 1 mg	
Sedatives				
Etomidate	The preferred agent for induction in the ED; short acting and hemodynamically stable; effective in adults and pediatrics.		**Induction dose:** 0.3 mg/kg IV **Onset:** 20-30 s **Duration:** 10-15 min	Myoclonus, adrenal suppression
Ketamine	An excellent induction agent; the induction agent of choice in asthmatics Advantages: bronchodilator, no respiratory depression, maintenance of airway protection; useful in adults and children.	Contraindicated in patients with elevated ICP because it increases HR and BP by sympathetic stimulation.	**Induction dose** 1-2 mg/kg IV **Onset:** 15-30 s **Duration:** 15-30 min	Increased secretions, emergence reactions, laryngospasm; dose with atropine or glycopyrrolate to reduce secretions
Muscle Relaxants				
Succinylcholine	Advantages include rapid action, short duration, and reliable paralytic effect. Premedicate children with atropine to prevent vagal stimulation and bradycardia.	Contraindications: hyperkalemia, history of malignant hyperthermia, >24 h post burn, >7 d post crush injury, denervation, spinal cord injury. Use with caution in CRF if K^+ is not known.	1.5 mg/kg IV in adults and 1.5-2 mg/kg IV in children. **Onset:** paralysis in 45 s. **Duration:** 8-10 min.	Fasciculations, hyperkalemia, bradycardia, malignant hyperthermia
Rocuronium	Main disadvantage: long duration of action.	Indicated when succinylcholine is contraindicated or preferred by physician.	**Dose (paralysis):** 1 mg/kg IV in adults and pediatrics **Onset:** paralysis in 60 s. **Duration:** 30-60 min	

- Patient selection: Oxygenated patient but does not have to be spontaneously breathing.
- Technique
  - Pre-oxygenate
  - Administer glycopyrrolate 0.1 mg/kg IM/IV to decrease secretions.
  - Anesthetize upper airway oral or nasal depending on route
    - Nebulized lidocaine
    - Topical 4% lidocaine
  - Insert ETT into nare or mouth depending on route.
  - Insert fiberscope through ETT.
  - Advance fiberscope to posterior pharynx, visualize larynx and cords, and advance fiberscope beyond cords on inspiration.
  - Injecting lidocaine through side port will decrease gag reflex and facilitate passage.
  - Advance ETT down past the cords with the fiberscope serving as a guide.

- Awake laryngoscopy
  - Good technique in suspected difficult airway because it employs laryngoscopy, a skill mastered by most emergency department (ED) physicians.
  - Advantages: Awake technique, allows direct visualization, and confirmed tube placement.
  - Disadvantages: Time-consuming, requires careful preparation and anesthesia, higher risk of vomiting and aspiration.
  - Patient selection: Cooperative patient, breathing spontaneously.
  - Technique
    - Pre-oxygenate
    - Anesthetize upper airway.
      - Nebulized lidocaine
      - Topical 4% lidocaine
    - Mild sedation with midazolam.
    - Pain medication with fentanyl.
    - Gently perform laryngoscopy by instructing patient to open mouth.
    - Once cords can be visualized, ETT can be placed, the patient can be paralyzed, or additional sedation can be given.
- Other airway adjuncts for managing difficult airway
  - Bougie
  - Laryngeal mask airway (LMA)
  - Lighted stylet
  - Esophageal/tracheal combitube
- Failed intubation techniques
  - Intubate under controlled circumstances, with help, using difficult airway techniques.
  - "Cannot intubate, cannot ventilate."
    - Cricothyroidotomy (Figs. 2-2 and 2-3).
      - The rescue technique of choice for failed intubation in older children and adults who need immediate airway control.
      - Absolute contraindication: Children <10 years. Relative contraindications: laryngeal or tracheal pathology, coagulopathy, lack of operator experience.
    - Percutaneous transtracheal ventilation (Fig. 2-4).
      - Needle cricothyroidotomy with transtracheal jet ventilation (TTJV) may be used to obtain an airway when cricothyroidotomy is contraindicated or deemed unlikely to succeed.
      - Rescue airway of choice in pediatrics for children <10 years.

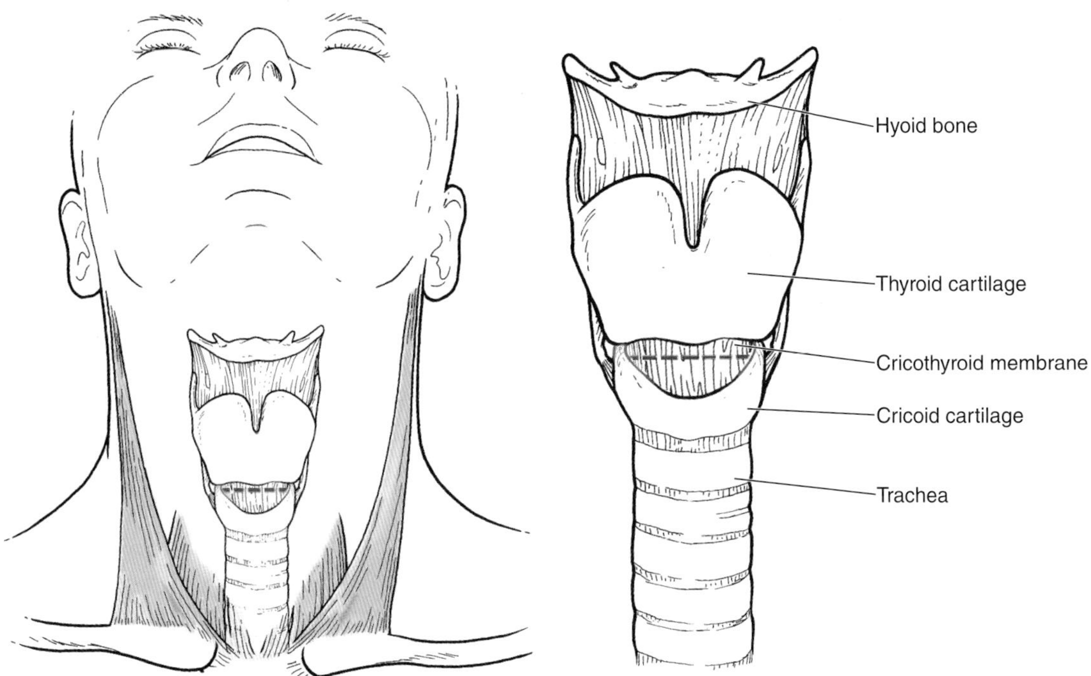

Figure 2-2. The cricothyroidotomy site. The dotted line represents the incision site over the cricothyroid membrane. *(Reprinted with permission from Reichman RF and Simon RR.* Emergency Medicine Procedures. *New York, NY: McGraw-Hill; 2004.)*

    - May be used in adults, but cricothyroidotomy is preferred as it is definitive.
    - Advantages: Fast, simple, less bleeding.
    - Disadvantages: Not a definitive airway, the upper airway must be patent to allow exhalation.
    - Ventilation through needle cricothyroidotomy:
        - BVM: Indicated in all children <5 years.
        - TTJV: Achieves ventilation by utilizing a high-pressure oxygen source to administer tidal volume through rapid, short breaths (inspiration <1 second, expiration 2-3 seconds). Contraindicated in children <5 years. Use with caution as associated with significant complications.
- LMA
    - Not a definitive airway.
    - Advantages: Easy to place and may temporize and enable ventilation.
    - In a "cannot intubate, cannot ventilate" scenarios placing an LMA may temporize and save the patient.
- Pediatric airway management
    - Blade selection: Use only straight blades in children <6 years.
    - Tube size
        - (16 + age [years])/4.
        - Size of pinky predicts the correct internal diameter.
    - Tube type: Uncuffed tubes should be used in children <1 year.
    - Tube depth: Tubes should be advanced to a depth of three times ETT size.
    - Premedication:
        - Atropine 0.01 mg/kg IV (min dose 0.1 mg, max dose 1.0 mg) before succinylcholine in all children <2 years to prevent bradycardia.

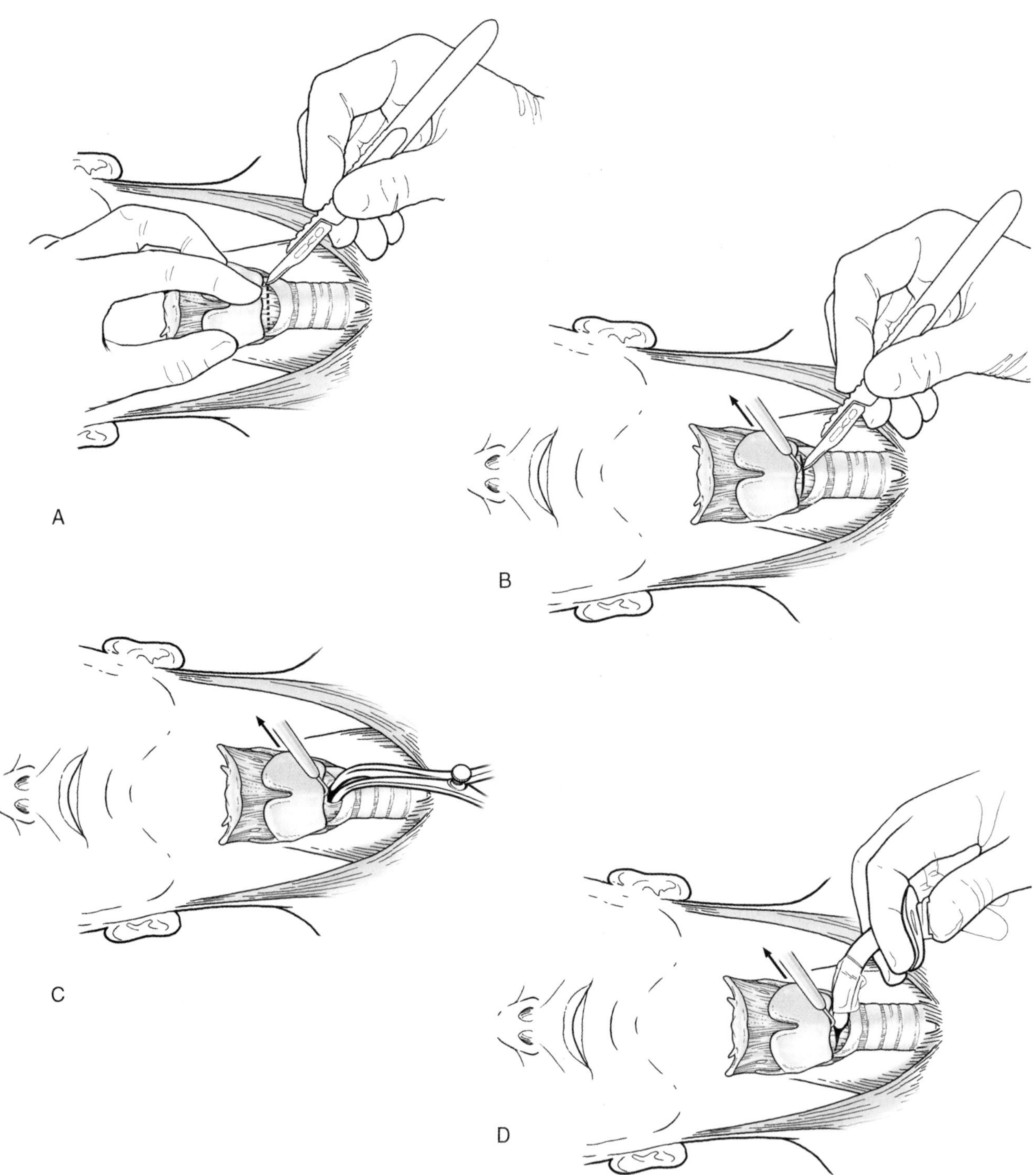

Figure 2-3. **(A)** While immobilizing the larynx, make a 2- to 3-cm vertical incision through the skin and subcutaneous tissue. **(B)** Reidentify the cricothyroid membrane and make a horizontal incision through it. **(C)** Insert a tracheal hook along the scalpel and grasp the inferior border of the thyroid cartilage and dilate the cricothyroid membrane. **(D)** Place the tracheostomy tube, and advance it until it is secure along the skin, insert the inner cannula and connect the patient to a bag-valve mask to ventilate the patient. *(Reprinted with permission from Reichman RF, Simon RR.* Emergency Medicine Procedures. *New York, NY: McGraw-Hill; 2004.)*

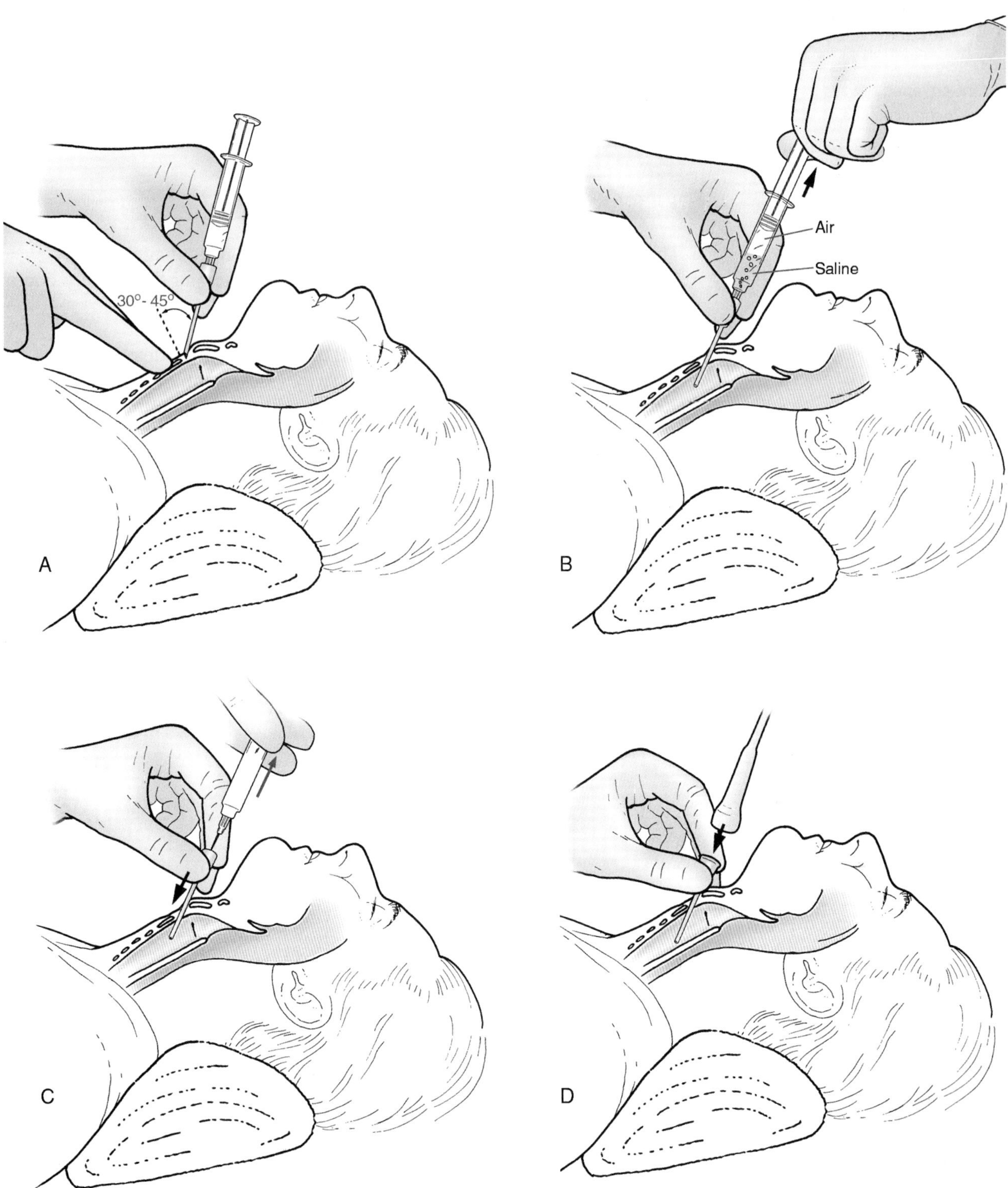

Figure 2-4. **(A)** After placing the patient in a recumbent position and prepping the neck, locate the cricothyroid membrane by palpating the laryngeal prominence, moving inferiorly to identify the cricoid cartilage, and locating the depression between. **(B)** While immobilizing the larynx, insert a 14-gauge syringe attached to a 20-cc syringe. **(C)** As you insert, draw back on the syringe until the plunger pulls back and air is aspirated. **(D)** Advance the 14-gauge catheter into the trachea and connect a 3-mm ETT adapter to the 14-gauge syringe, connect a BVM, and ventilate the patient. After confirming correct placement, if a TTJV system is available, connect it to the 14-gauge angiocath, adjust the pressure to 20 lb/in^2 and adjust it upward as necessary to maintain oxygen saturation. (*Reprinted with permission from Reichman RF, Simon RR.* Emergency Medicine Procedures. *New York, NY: McGraw-Hill; 2004.*)

DON'T FORGET

RSI is the preferred airway management technique.

Memorize an RSI litany: "I will intubate the patient using RSI. I will gather my equipment, pre-oxygenate the patient, premedicate with X (if necessary), wait 3 minutes, sedate and paralyze with etomidate and succinylcholine, place the ETT, confirm tube calorimeter, placement with carbon dioxide auscultation, and CXR, and attach the ventilator.

Always use lidocaine and fentanyl if elevated ICP is a concern.

Use atropine before succinylcholine in all children <2 years.

When a difficult airway is confirmed or suspected, call backup and attempt awake intubation techniques.

After a failed airway, if the patient can be ventilated and oxygenated, then relax. You have time to regroup and plan a new approach with backup.

"Cannot intubate, cannot ventilate" scenarios are feared. In adults perform immediate cricothyroidotomy. In children perform immediate needle cricothyroidotomy.

On the exam state that you will look up doses, tube sizes, and blade selection on the Broselow tape if necessary, but you should know the dosing of RSI medications without having to look them up.

- Percutaneous transtracheal ventilation
  - Cricothyroidotomy is contraindicated in children <10 years given size considerations.
  - Needle cricothyroidotomy is the airway salvage option of last resort in children.
  - Ventilation may be achieved through BVM or TTJV (children >5 years).

WINNING STRATEGIES

- The airway is the A in ABC. Assess it first and manage it aggressively.
- On exam day, maintain a low threshold to intubate and definitively control the airway.
- All patients with a GCS <8 get intubated.
- Consider prophylactic intubation in all patients who may deteriorate.
- Though every patient should get an airway assessment, on test day simplify your airway algorithms. Every patient should get an attempt at orotracheal intubation (RSI or awake) and then surgical or needle cricothyroidotomy.
- RSI is the preferred intubation technique.
- When doing RSI on the test day, use the medications that you normally use and memorize these drugs.
- After a failed airway, if the patient can be ventilated and oxygenated, then relax. You have time to regroup and plan a new approach with backup.
- "Cannot intubate, cannot ventilate." In adults perform immediate cricothyroidotomy. In children perform immediate needle cricothyroidotomy.

CHAPTER 3

Shock

Robert Preston and Phillip Bossart

- There are several classification schemes that attempt to break shock down into tidy categories.
- Traditional: Cardiogenic, neurogenic, hematologic, vasogenic.
- There is also the "etiology" classification: Hypovolemic, cardiogenic, distributive, and obstructive.
- Then there are the old favorites of "warm shock" and "cold shock."
- Extensive overlap occurs between these categories in terms of clinical characteristics, pathophysiologic basis, and descriptive terms.
- For the purpose of emergency medicine (EM) oral boards and the real-world practice of EM, it is best to understand the terminology and then forget the categories. Attempting to classify or categorize shock is not particularly productive in caring for patients, except to the extent that understanding the categories helps in formulating and narrowing your differential diagnosis.

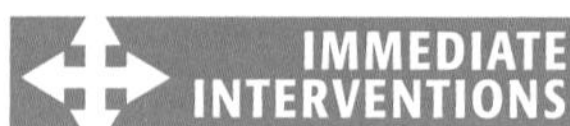

IMMEDIATE INTERVENTIONS

In All Critical Patients

- ABCs = Airway, Breathing, Circulation.
- All patients get two large-bore IVs and 2 L NS bolus.
- All patients get supplemental O_2.
- All patients get placed on a cardiac monitor.
- Obtain ancillary studies early in critical patients: CBC, chemistries including LFTs, cardiac markers, UA, blood cultures, blood gas, lactate, ECG, CXR
- Order tests after history and physical examination in more stable patients.

DEFINITION OF SHOCK

- When oxygen supply is not sufficient to meet oxygen demand in cells, tissues, or organs due to inadequate tissue perfusion, the result is ultimately shock. Cell injury and death occur when this imbalance is extreme and compensatory mechanisms fail. If enough cells die, the organs will fail and the organism will die.
- Our job as emergency physicians is to recognize early shock and prevent failure of compensatory mechanisms while intervening to reverse the underlying cause of imbalance between tissue perfusion and demand.
- The pathophysiology of shock is complex, interesting, and beyond the scope of this text. However, there are certain basic principles and terms that will help (1) identify shock, (2) interpret test results and responses to interventions, and (3) clarify the key concept of goal-directed therapy.

DON'T FORGET

Every 2-3 minutes (at least) ask if the patient's condition has changed (comfort, mental status, vital signs). This way you know if your interventions are working and that you are on (or off) track. If your patient is getting worse, restart primary survey and address problems accordingly.

PATHOPHYSIOLOGY

- Shock is the consequence of an imbalance between oxygen supply and demand leading to inadequate tissue perfusion. The initial response of the organism is to attempt to increase perfusion via compensatory mechanisms. Distressed cells will pull more oxygen off circulating hemoglobin, resulting in a reduced central venous oxygen saturation ($ScvO_2$). As these efforts fail, cells receiving inadequate oxygen convert to anaerobic metabolism and produce lactic acid. At first this lactic acid is "buffered" and pH measurements (eg, via blood gas) may be "normal" in early shock.
- Lactic acidosis is something we can measure and monitor.
- Full blown, clinically obvious shock develops, often quite rapidly, as cellular stress turns into cellular injury and an escalating cycle of cellular injury and death cascades into a systemic inflammatory response syndrome (SIRS) and then multiorgan dysfunction syndrome (MODS) and ultimately death.
- Unless unable to do so (due to drugs or other conditions) the body will initially respond to shock by increasing heart rate (HR) and stroke volume (SV) to increase cardiac output (CO).
- If the patient's system cannot increase HR or SV (β-blockers, heart failure, hypovolemia, or cardiac tamponade), the result will be hypotension. Hypotension may signal shock, or worsening shock; however, this is not always true. Recall that mean arterial pressure (MAP) = CO × systemic vascular resistance (SVR). Thus, if SVR is high (eg, elevated peripheral vascular resistance), even if CO is decreased, hypotension may not immediately occur.
- Shock stimulates a brisk autonomic response. Circulating catecholamines increase and "stress hormones" such as epinephrine, cortisol, norepinephrine,

DON'T FORGET

Shock is the consequence of an imbalance between supply and demand—inadequate tissue perfusion. Shock can be present without hypotension.

Hypotension does not necessarily imply shock if tissue perfusion is adequate.

There is no single lab test or clinical symptom that denotes shock.

SvO_2 is measured via a "Swan-Ganz" catheter.

$ScvO_2$ can be approximated with a central venous catheter.

glucagon, and insulin are released as the system attempts to maintain circulation and substrate supply to vital organs. Antidiuretic hormone (ADH) and the renin-angiotensin axis act to conserve water and sodium.

- The result: Hemoconcentration, acidosis, hyponatremia, hyperglycemia, and prerenal azotemia. Clinically, gut perfusion may be compromised and patients are likely to feel weak, suffer altered level of consciousness, and demonstrate an altered respiratory drive and hyperventilation.
- Manifestations include cold clammy skin, pallor, and weak pulses.
- Since no single lab test or clinical symptom denotes shock, some, all, or none of the expected laboratory abnormalities may occur depending on the duration and severity of shock, the underlying cause of shock, and other factors (illicit drugs, toxins, age and compensatory capacities of the patient, preexisting conditions, etc).
- Similarly, the signs and symptoms of patients in shock vary considerably.

DON'T FORGET

CO = HR × SV

MAP = CO × SVR

SIRS must have two or more of the following:

- Temp >38°C (100.4°F) or <36°C (96.8°F)
- HR >90
- RR >20
- WBCs >12,000 or <4000 or differential with >10% bands

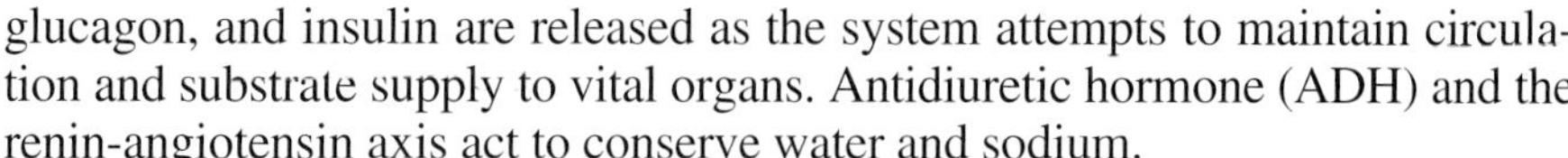

RECOGNIZING SHOCK

- Suspecting shock is the first step toward success. The differential is extensive. Nonetheless, patients presenting in early shock will usually have at least some clinical signs and symptoms, ie, fever or hypothermia, tachycardia, tachypnea, hypotension, pallor, weakness, cool and clammy skin, syncope, etc—and certainly will have some of these findings on examination day.
- We treat early shock by supporting compensatory mechanisms with supplemental O_2, intravascular fluid (IVF) to increase intravascular volume, SV, and CO as well as to replace volume losses.
- Labs and other ancillary studies may not make the diagnosis of shock, but obtaining a broad panel (CBC, chemistries, cardiac markers, UA, blood cultures, lactate, blood gas, ECG, CXR) will provide you with useful hints at the underlying etiology as well as the severity of the shock state.

DON'T FORGET

Expect the patient in shock to have at least some classic signs and symptoms, ie, fever or hypothermia, tachycardia, tachypnea, hypotension, pallor, weakness, cool and clammy skin, syncope, etc. You should recognize shock immediately while rapidly initiating treatment and simultaneously searching for a specific etiology to allow goal-directed management.

You are most likely to encounter cases of cardiogenic, traumatic, and septic shock.

Spend a few minutes on the expanded differential diagnosis of shock given in **Table 3-1**. Many of your oral board cases will come from this list!

IDENTIFY THE CAUSE (TABLE 3-1)

- So, you are faced with a pale, cool, clammy, and tachycardic patient in shock and you have initiated the "immediate interventions" noted in the Pearls section. Now you must attempt to determine the etiology to enable goal-directed, specific interventions.
- Remember to continually return to the patient (reassess) and act immediately if the patient's condition changes, ie, worsening vital signs, mental status changes, complaints of "feeling worse" or "getting weaker" etc.
- **CC:** Suspect shock in patients presenting with trauma, burns, syncope, bee stings, chest pain, shortness of breath, weakness, fever, dehydration, heat illness, hypothermia, severe rash (cellulitis, gangrene, and meningococcemia), bloody or dark stools.
- **HPI:** General description of symptoms/complaints. Onset of illness? Pain? Syncope? Weakness? Sweating? Excessive sweating, urination, appetite changes, headache, neck pain?
- **PMHx:** Pay particular attention to conditions that may aggravate shock, ie, known heart condition, coronary disease, diabetes, steroid dependency, immunocompromised states (steroids, splenectomy, transplant patients, HIV/AIDS, chemotherapy), drug use (endocarditis), pregnancy, thromboembolic risk factors, gastrointestinal (GI) bleeding history, metabolic disorders, renal failure/dialysis, endocrine surgeries/adrenalectomy, pituitary gland disorders, β-blockers, anticoagulation therapy.
- Recent travel (malaria, dengue fever, invasive *Escherichia coli* enteritis, dysentery), tick bites, possible industrial exposures to toxins, gases,

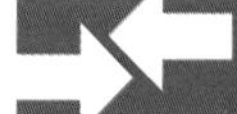

CRITICAL ACTION

Obtain an AMPLE history:

Allergies

Medications

Past medical history

Last meal—in case you have to sedate/intubate

Events leading up to the ER visit

Table 3-1. Differential Diagnosis of Shock

Hypovolemic
- Multiple trauma with hemorrhage: Pelvic and femur fractures, major scalp injury, intra- or retroperitoneal hemorrhage, hemothorax
- Major burns
- GI bleed
- Heat stroke
- Other fluid loss: Excessive exercise/perspiration, diuretic use, the elderly dehydrated patient, nephropathy, diabetes insipidus, ruptured AAA

Cardiogenic
- Tamponade (traumatic or non-traumatic)
- Constrictive pericarditis
- Acute MI with pump failure
- Cardiomyopathy (dilated, restrictive, hypertrophic)
- Valve failure or obstruction
- Aortic injury (dissection, rupture in trauma)
- Arrhythmia

Neurogenic
- Brainstem failure, stroke
- Spinal cord injury and dysfunction
- Autonomic insufficiency

Septic
- Evidence of significant infection, suspected bacteremia, fever, etc plus shock equal to septic shock
- Toxic shock syndrome, bacterial meningitis, dengue fever, endocarditis, staphylococcal infection, "flesh eating bacteria"/necrotizing fasciitis, Fournier gangrene
- Many other specific infections, parasites, malaria, etc.

Others
- Anaphylaxis
- Pulmonary embolus
- Pneumothorax (spontaneous or traumatic)
- Vena cava syndrome
- Myxedema or thyroid storm
- Pheochromocytoma
- Adrenal insufficiency/crisis
- Hypothermia or hyperthermia
- Severe hypo- or hyperglycemia
- Liver failure
- Drugs/toxins (barbiturates, aspirin, heavy metals, cyanide, antihypertensive agents, β-blockers, organophosphates, bioterrorism agents)

cyanide, organophosphates, bioterrorism agents. Students, prisoners, military personnel are at increased risk for meningitis.

- **Physical examination:** General appearance is important. Is the patient ill appearing, toxic, diaphoretic, in pain, confused, obtunded, or weak?
- Complete vital signs including pulse oximetry are of key importance. If the patient is unconscious or unable to give history, beware hypoxia, tachycardia, hypotension, hypothermia, fever, and delayed capillary refill.
- **HEENT:** Trauma? Infection? Bleeding scalp wounds?

- **Neck:** Increased jugular venous pressure (JVP) or flat neck veins, stiffness?
- **Lungs:** Crackles (heart failure, infection)? Wheezing (anaphylaxis, asthma, chronic obstructive pulmonary disease [COPD])? Asymmetric breath sounds (pneumothorax, hemothorax)?
- **Chest wall:** Flail chest? Subcutaneous emphysema?
- **Heart:** Rate, rhythm? Murmurs? Rubs? Gallops?
- **Abdomen:** Ascites? Tenderness (cholecystitis, ascending cholangitis, appendicitis, ruptured spleen, bowel ischemia, bowel obstruction, spontaneous bacterial peritonitis)? Distension? Bowel sounds (absence is most significant suggesting peritonitis)? Palpable abdominal aortic aneurysm (AAA)?
- **Pelvic:** Vaginal bleeding (ectopic or miscarriage)? Pelvic pain (infection, ruptured ectopic, pelvic inflammatory disease [PID])?
- **Rectal:** Bleeding? Mass?
- **Back:** Tenderness on spine, penetrating injury? Flank tenderness (pyelonephritis)?
- **Skin:** Rash (hives, anaphylaxis, insect bites, disseminated meningococcemia, purpura, petechiae)? Warm and dry versus pale, cool, clammy? Capillary refill?
- **Neuro:** Altered mental status? Evidence of stroke—new or old? Weakness? Abnormal reflexes?
- **Psych:** Depression, suicidal, possible overdose, drugs, alcohol use?

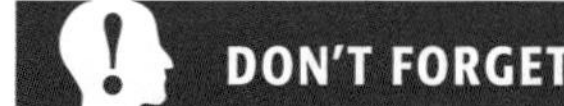

If the patient's condition does not allow for a thorough history, get what you can from the family and EMS personnel and ask for any available "old records."

WINNING STRATEGIES

Key Elements Applying to All Patients

- Supportive care for everyone; see "Immediate Interventions."
- Order tests that will help narrow the differential diagnosis right away in critical patients, after H and P in apparently "stable" patients.
- Obtain history, physical examination, complete vitals—narrow your differential.
- Order more specific tests if need be after completing H and P.
- Continually reassess patient's condition. ABCs.
- If the patient's condition is deteriorating—either you are on the wrong track entirely or you have forgotten a critical intervention.
- Identify and treat the underlying cause of shock.

Specific Treatments/Interventions (Critical Patients)

- Most critically ill patients should be intubated on test day.
- The overall goal in treating shock patients in the emergency room (ER) is restoration of adequate tissue perfusion and oxygenation.
- IVF resuscitation is a critical intervention. Use 2 L initial bolus, then reevaluate. Note that certain patient populations (eg, those with cardiac failure or respiratory compromise) should receive smaller aliquots (250-500 mL) at a time as the fluid may actually cause their condition to deteriorate.
- New recommendation from the most recent Surviving Sepsis Campaign guideline: If patient remains hypotensive after 2 L of crystalloid but is indeed improving, further fluid boluses are permissible before starting pressors.
- A Foley catheter should be placed to monitor urine output—a key parameter to follow to ensure adequate fluid resuscitation >5 mg/kg/h.
- Place an arterial line for accurate blood pressure monitoring.
- Central venous access for monitoring of $ScvO_2$, CO, SVR, and other physiologic parameters is elegant and ultimately the best way to monitor resuscitation via "goal-directed therapy." Specific goals indicating adequate

resuscitation = $ScvO_2$ >70, urine output >0.5 cc/kg/h, central venous pressure (CVP) of 8-12 mm Hg, MAP of 65.

- For all types of shock, treat the underlying condition. This is true for septic, hypovolemic, cardiogenic, anaphylactic and neurogenic shock.
- Neurogenic shock is almost always associated with major trauma—in these cases treat the major trauma issues as you normally would and provide supportive care for "shock" as noted throughout this text.
- Traumatic shock is hypovolemic/hemorrhagic shock until proven otherwise.
- Patients with possible septic shock should receive broad-spectrum antibiotics ASAP after your initial evaluation. Get blood cultures first if possible, but do not delay therapy for more than a few minutes waiting to obtain cultures.
- Patients with suspected septic shock refractory to pressors and those on steroids or with endocrine disorders should receive 100 mg of IV hydrocortisone ASAP. There is good evidence to support at least physiologic dosing of steroids in the initial treatment of septic shock and certainly in potential adrenal insufficiency cases. Steroids may help delay/combat the full blown development of SIRS and later MODS, thereby reducing mortality.
- Transfuse packed red blood cells (PRBCs) as needed to keep hematocrit (Hct) >30.

DON'T FORGET

Remember that measures of supportive care (fluid resuscitation, supplemental oxygen) are cornerstones of treating all critically ill and potentially critically ill patients.

DON'T FORGET

Proper airway management is always a critical action—it is never wrong to intubate a critically ill patient with abnormal/deteriorating vital signs—particularly those with altered mental status or compromised respiratory status, hypoxia, hypotension, significant tachypnea, etc.

Use of Pressors

- Treatment with IV vasopressor therapy should be initiated if all above supportive measures have been implemented—including intravascular volume repletion—and adequate tissue perfusion still cannot be achieved. Ideally "adequate perfusion" is defined by the specific resuscitation goals of $ScvO_2$ >70, urine output >0.5 cc/kg/h, CVP 8-12 mm Hg, MAP 65-90 mm Hg.
- Be aware that treating patients in shock with pressors is a tradeoff: pressors increase both blood pressure and peripheral vasoconstriction. This may actually cause CO to drop.
- The literature supporting use of one pressor over another is generally inconclusive. Based on the most up-to-date expert recommendations, reasonable choices for refractory hypotension and inadequate perfusion include the following:
  - First line:
    - Norepinephrine 1-30 μg/min
  - If first-line agents fail, add:
    - Vasopressin 0.01-0.04 U/min
- Norepinephrine with or without vasopressin may be more useful in septic, neurogenic, other noncardiogenic shock situations as they theoretically are more selective in increasing vasoconstriction with less tachycardia as compared to dopamine or dobutamine.
- Dopamine is no longer recommended as an early pressor choice except in cases where patients may benefit from increased chronotropy.
- Do not start with vasopressin alone as there are no data to support this.

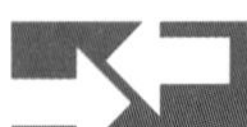

CRITICAL ACTION

Remember your early goal-directed therapy

- Goal-directed treatment should be focused on achieving $ScvO_2$ >70, urine output >0.5 cc/kg/h, CVP 8-12 mm Hg, MAP 65-90 mm Hg. Place a Foley catheter, central line, and arterial line.
- Transfuse PRBCs as needed to keep Hct >30.
- Patients with possible septic shock should receive broad-spectrum antibiotics ASAP.
- Patients with suspected septic shock refractory to pressors and those on steroids or with endocrine disorders should receive 100 mg of IV hydrocortisone ASAP.

Other Considerations (Fig. 3-1)

- Do not forget simple things (eg, rectal Tylenol for fever).
- Do not forget to talk to families, emergency medical technicians (EMTs), and referring physicians.
- Consult the "critical care team" if such exists with all patients in shock—after you have stabilized them and completed all critical interventions.
- If you are at a "smaller hospital with limited resources," most of these patients should be transferred to a major center, ideally by a critical care transport team.

DON'T FORGET

Traumatic shock is hypovolemic/hemorrhagic shock until proven otherwise.

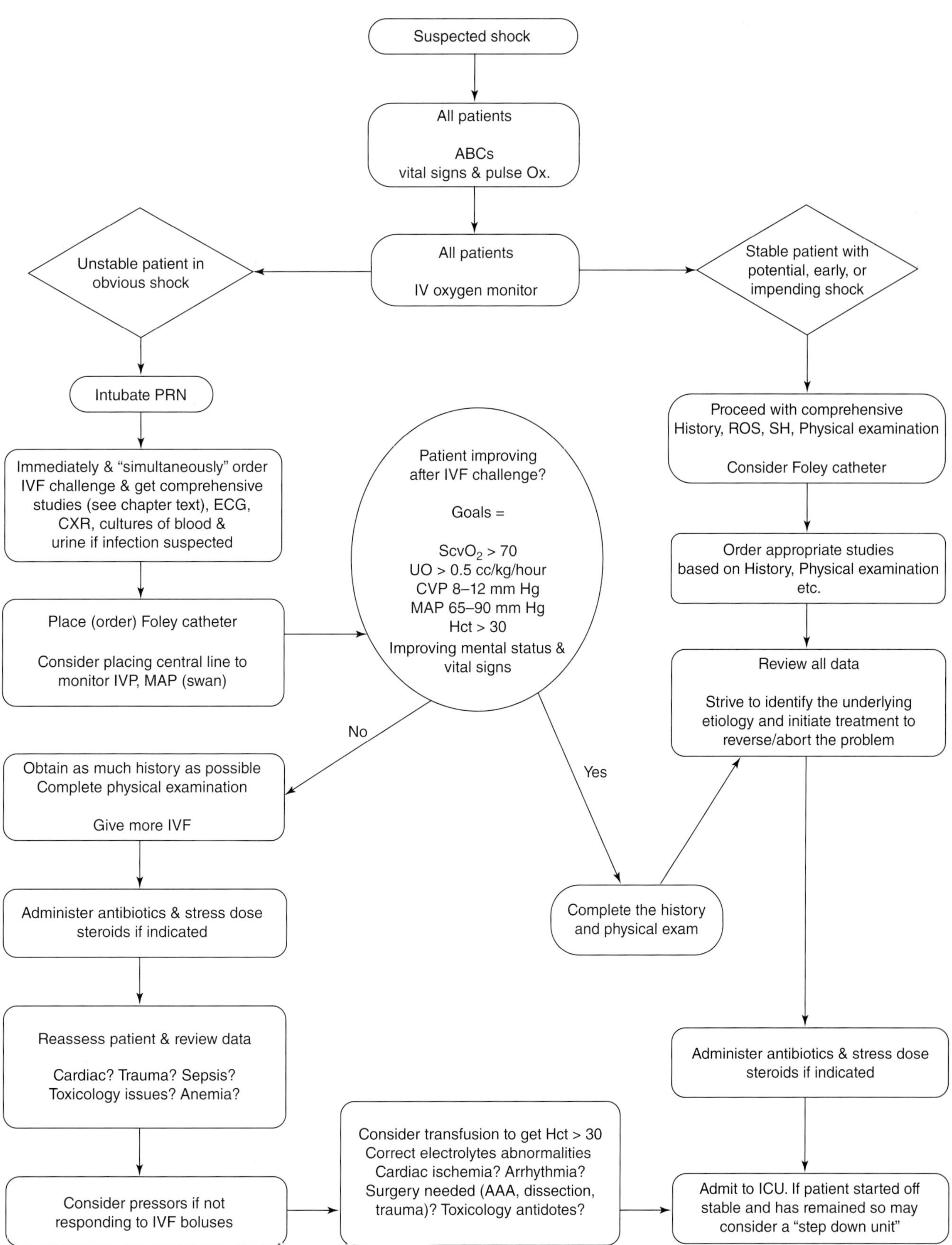

Figure 3-1. Algorithm for diagnosis of shock.

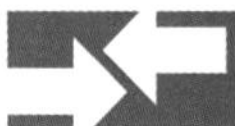

CRITICAL ACTION

- Use vasopressors, inotropes, and vasopressin when all else fails to restore adequate circulation and tissue perfusion:
  - Norepinephrine (vasopressor) is the first choice for septic, hypovolemic and cardiogenic shock.
  - Epinephrine (vasopressor) is the first choice for anaphylactic shock.
  - Dobutamine (inotrope) is also recommended for cardiogenic shock.
  - Vasopressin can be used with norepinephrine.

DON'T FORGET

Hypotension *does not* equal shock, and shock can occur without hypotension.

THE BOTTOM LINE

- Early recognition of shock is a "critical action."
- Understanding the correct definition of shock (inadequate tissue perfusion and oxygenation) and basic pathophysiology facilitates early recognition of shock—serves as a guide for a focused H and P—makes critical interventions for all shock cases intuitive—and allows for a logical, goal-directed approach to resuscitation.
- Hypotension **does not** equal shock, and shock can occur without hypotension.
- The cornerstone of treatment in shock, as with all critical patients, is resuscitation with IVF, oxygen, and supportive measures.
- When in doubt, intubate.
- Place a Foley catheter, central line, and arterial line.
- Goal-directed treatment should be focused on achieving $ScvO_2$ >70, urine output >0.5 cc/kg/h, CVP 8-12 mm Hg, MAP 65-90 mm Hg.
- Make use of history, physical examination, and ancillary studies to determine the underlying etiology of shock (if possible) and direct interventions to correct this underlying problem once identified.
- All septic shock patients get antibiotics—early.
- Initiate pressor treatment if all other measures are failing to restore adequate perfusion. Start with norepinephrine, if this is not enough, add vasopressin.
- All shock patients get admitted to the intensive care unit (ICU).

CHAPTER 4

BLS/ACLS

Katie Tataris and James Ahn

DON'T FORGET

Follow the most recent AHA recommendations when resuscitating a patient as guidelines are updated periodically.

DON'T FORGET

Recently, the American Heart Association (AHA) has placed increased emphasis on early, uninterrupted high-quality chest compressions for cardiac arrest. The 2010 Guidelines recommend initiation of chest compressions before ventilations (CAB instead of ABC) to reflect the importance of chest compressions over airway management.

- During the oral board exam, you may have a critically ill patient requiring resuscitation using the advanced cardiac life support (ACLS) algorithms.
- Be familiar with each of the ACLS algorithms and be able to apply them in clinical scenarios.
- Knowledge of ACLS drugs and doses is expected and you should have these memorized and not need to look them up.

BLS: BASIC LIFE SUPPORT

Assess Responsiveness

- Recognition of cardiac arrest is the important first step.
- You should assess for responsiveness and determine if the patient is alert, responsive to verbal stimuli, responsive to pain, or unresponsive.
- Assess if the patient is breathing normally—agonal or gasping respirations are ineffective.
- If the patient is unresponsive with no breathing or no normal breathing, you should activate the emergency response system and get the automated external defibrillator (AED) or defibrillator.
- If there is no definitive pulse after 10 seconds, begin cardiopulmonary resuscitation (CPR).
- If there is a pulse, start rescue breathing at 1 breath every 5-6 seconds and recheck for a pulse every 2 minutes.

Activate the Emergency Response System

- If you are in a health care setting, activate a "code blue" or cardiac arrest alert. If you are in a public setting, call 911.

C: Circulation

- Begin chest compressions at a ratio of 30 compressions to 2 breaths.
  - Rate of compressions: 100-120 per minute.
  - Depth of compression: At least 2 inches (5 cm) in adults allowing adequate chest recoil.
  - Technique: Place patient on a firm surface. Interlace fingers with one hand on top of the other and place the heel of bottom hand in the center of the patient's chest, over the lower half of the sternum. Keep elbows locked and arms straight and apply force straight down on the sternum.
  - Switch compressors every 2 minutes.
  - Minimize interruptions in chest compressions to maintain cerebral perfusion.

A: Airway

- Open the airway with a head-tilt chin lift.
- If trauma is suspected use a jaw thrust and manual spinal motion restriction (placing one hand on either side of the patient's head to hold it in-line) rather than immobilization devices.
- Use adjuncts such as nasopharyngeal airway (NPA) or oropharyngeal airways (OPA) to maintain patency.

B: Breathing

- Ventilations should be given slowly (over 1 second) to prevent stomach distention.
- Provide sufficient tidal volume to ensure adequate chest rise.
- When an advanced airway is present (endotracheal tube, supraglottic airway), give breaths every 5-6 seconds or 8-10 breaths/min without pausing for ventilations and maintaining continuous chest compressions.
- Avoid hyperventilation as it causes increased intrathoracic pressure.

AED: Automated External Defibrillator

- Early defibrillation using an AED or manual defibrillator is important as ventricular fibrillation (VF) is a common presenting rhythm in adult cardiac arrest.
- When an AED is available, it should be placed by a second provider as the first provider continues chest compressions.
- Defibrillation should take priority in a resuscitation.

ACLS: ADVANCED CARDIAC LIFE SUPPORT

Immediate Goals

- Assess responsiveness.
- Assess ABCs.
- Intravenous (IV), oxygen, monitor.
- Identify arrhythmia.

The ACLS algorithms is built on the BLS initial interventions and provide guidelines for advanced airway placement, drug delivery, and arrhythmia management.

Initial Assessment

Assess responsiveness: Is the patient awake? Can the patient answer questions? Calculate the patient's Glasgow Coma Score (GCS). If the patient is altered, consider whether the change in mental status could be due to a cardiac cause.

Assess breathing: Assess adequacy of breathing. Listen to breath sounds. If the patient is breathing abnormally (labored, too fast), consider whether the source of distress could be due to a cardiac cause.

Assess circulation: Assess the pulse and blood pressure. If the patient has a pulse, is it strong, regular, too fast, or too slow? Does the patient have a normal blood pressure?

Your decision to begin ACLS management protocols will be based on these assessments. Unresponsive or altered patients with abnormal breathing and circulation require ACLS management. ACLS algorithms can be broadly divided into two groups: those that focus on patients with a pulse, and those that focus on patients who are pulseless.

DON'T FORGET

To properly apply ACLS guidelines, answer the following three questions immediately:

1. Is the patient responsive?
2. Is the patient breathing?
3. Does the patient have a pulse?

IMMEDIATE INTERVENTIONS

Pulse Present

- IV, oxygen, cardiac monitor
- Vital signs
- 12-lead electrocardiogram (ECG)
- History
- Physical examination
- Chest x-ray (CXR)

Further management by suspected cause:

1. Chest pain/acute coronary syndrome (see Chap. 8) which may become any of the following:

DON'T FORGET

Always search for reversible causes of cardiac arrest:

- Hypovolemia
- Hypoxia
- Hydrogen ion (acidosis)
- Hypo-/hyperkalemia
- Hypoglycemia
- Toxins
- Tamponade (cardiac)
- Tension pneumothorax
- Thrombosis (coronary or pulmonary)

2. Cardiac Arrest
    i. VF/pulseless ventricular tachycardia (VT)
    ii. Pulseless electrical activity (PEA)/Asystole
3. Bradycardia
    i. First-degree atrioventricular (AV) block
    ii. Second-degree AV block
    iii. Third-degree AV block
4. Tachycardia
    i. Sinus tachycardia
    ii. Supraventricular tachycardia (SVT)
    iii. Atrial fibrillation (AfIb) or atrial flutter
    iv. Monomorphic VT
    v. Polymorphic VT

Pulseless

- Begin CPR.
- Apply cardiac monitor and obtain a rhythm strip.
- Obtain IV or intraosseous (IO) access.
- Use a bag-valve mask with supplement oxygen until endotracheal intubation can be done.
- Identify arrhythmia.
- If the rhythm is VF or pulseless VT, then the patient requires immediate defibrillation.

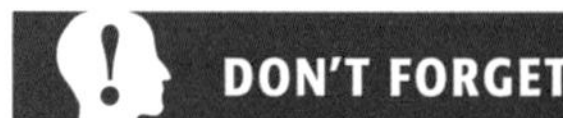

In patients who are breathing with a pulse, you have time to obtain data (history, physical examination, rhythm strip, and ECG), make a diagnosis, and start treatment.

Further management by arrhythmia:

1. VF/pulseless VT
2. PEA/asystole

CARDIAC ARREST ALGORITHMS (FIG. 4-1)

VF/pulseless VT

Principles from BLS remain the same, the emphasis is on early rhythm identification and defibrillation for shockable rhythms.

C: Circulation: High quality, uninterrupted chest compressions for 2 minutes.

A: Airway: Endotracheal intubation is preferred, but a supraglottic airway can be used as a backup option. Attach waveform capnography to confirm and monitor advanced airway placement.

B: Breathing: Once the advanced airway is placed, provide positive pressure ventilation at a rate of one breath every 5-6 seconds, with continuous chest compressions.

D: Defibrillation: Immediate defibrillation on recognition of shockable rhythm. This should take priority in resuscitation above other interventions including medication administration, IV access, and definitive airway management.

- Voltage: Biphasic devices should be shocked initially at 120-200J and then equivalent or higher for subsequent doses. Monophasic devices should be shocked at 360 J.
- After defibrillation, compressions should resume immediately for 2 minutes of high-quality CPR before a rhythm check.

DON'T FORGET

Patients without respiration, a pulse, or a blood pressure need immediate stabilization with defibrillation for shockable rhythms, chest compressions, and airway management.

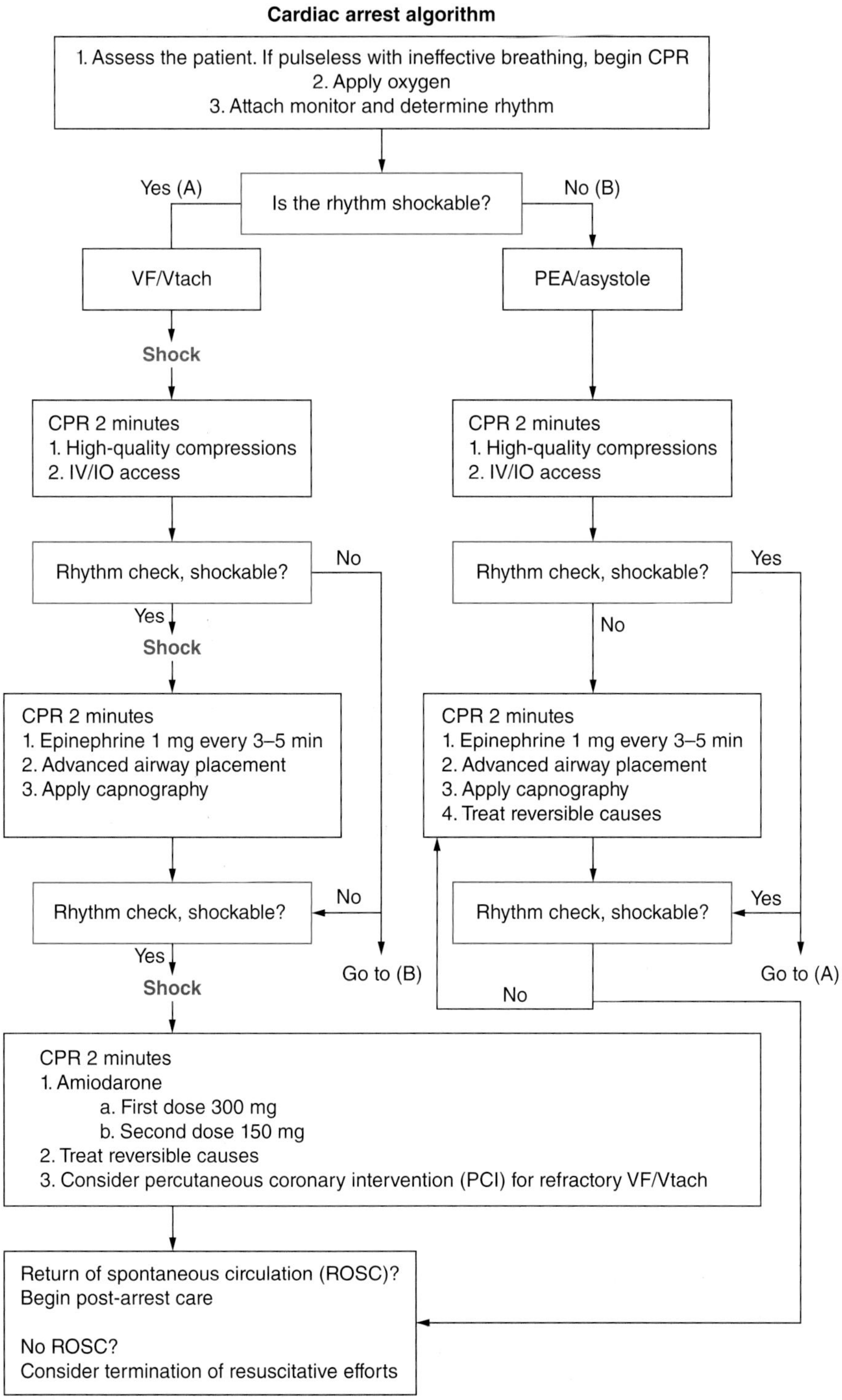

Cardiac arrest algorithm

1. Assess the patient. If pulseless with ineffective breathing, begin CPR
2. Apply oxygen
3. Attach monitor and determine rhythm

Is the rhythm shockable?

Yes (A) → VF/Vtach

No (B) → PEA/asystole

Left side (A): VF/Vtach

Shock

CPR 2 minutes
1. High-quality compressions
2. IV/IO access

Rhythm check, shockable? — No → Go to (B)

Yes → Shock

CPR 2 minutes
1. Epinephrine 1 mg every 3–5 min
2. Advanced airway placement
3. Apply capnography

Rhythm check, shockable? — No → Go to (B)

Yes → Shock

Right side (B): PEA/asystole

CPR 2 minutes
1. High-quality compressions
2. IV/IO access

Rhythm check, shockable? — Yes → Go to (A)

No

CPR 2 minutes
1. Epinephrine 1 mg every 3–5 min
2. Advanced airway placement
3. Apply capnography
4. Treat reversible causes

Rhythm check, shockable? — Yes → Go to (A)

No

Final steps

CPR 2 minutes
1. Amiodarone
   a. First dose 300 mg
   b. Second dose 150 mg
2. Treat reversible causes
3. Consider percutaneous coronary intervention (PCI) for refractory VF/Vtach

Return of spontaneous circulation (ROSC)?
Begin post-arrest care

No ROSC?
Consider termination of resuscitative efforts

Figure 4-1. Adult cardiac arrest.

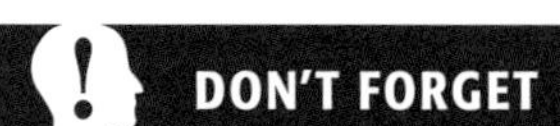

Management of Cardiac Arrest

- Is the rhythm shockable?
- Reassess the rhythm every 2 minutes.
- Drug therapy.
- When advanced airway is placed, the compression-to-breath ratio changes from 30:2 to continuous chest compressions and one breath every 5-6 seconds.

Reassess Rhythm

- Every 2 minutes, the rhythm should be reassessed and defibrillated as indicated.
- If persistent VF/pulseless VT, continue on the left side of the algorithm.
- If PEA/asystole, move to the right side of the algorithm.
- If return of spontaneous circulation (ROSC), begin post-cardiac arrest care by confirming palpable pulse, supporting blood pressure, and managing the airway. Assess for cause of cardiac arrest.

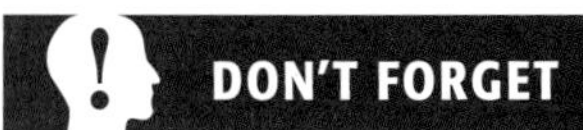

DON'T FORGET

Do not delay defibrillation!

Drug Therapy

- Epinephrine 1 mg IV/IO, may repeat every 3-5 minutes.
- Consider vasopressin 40 U IV push, to replace the first or second dose of epinephrine.
- For persistent VF/pulseless VT unresponsive to defibrillation administer amiodarone 300 mg IV as an initial bolus and 150 mg if needed for a second dose. Lidocaine 1-1.5 mg/kg can also be used.

Return of Spontaneous Circulation (ROSC)

- If a patient has ROSC, post-cardiac arrest care should be initiated.
- Manage hypoxemia and hypotension.
- Consider therapeutic hypothermia for comatose patients.

Pulseless Electrical Activity (PEA)/Asystole

PEA definition: Organized rhythm on monitor but without detectable pulse or blood pressure. This may include electromechanical dissociation (EMD), idioventricular rhythms, bradyasystolic rhythms, post-defibrillation idioventricular rhythms.

Reversible Causes of PEA (5 Hs and Ts)

- Hypovolemia
  - Causes include volume loss or sepsis and require aggressive fluid administration.
  - For hemorrhage, identify source of blood loss and treat.
  - Blood product transfusion may be needed after fluids resuscitation.
- Hypoxia
  - Airway management with proper ventilation
- H^+ ion (acidosis)
  - Identify and treat the cause of acidosis.
  - Sodium bicarbonate 1 mEq/kg IV may be considered.
- Hyperkalemia
  - Calcium carbonate or gluconate IV
  - Insulin 10 U IV push/D50 1 amp
  - Nebulized albuterol
  - Dialysis
- Hypokalemia
  - Usually in the setting of gastrointestinal or renal losses, this alters cardiac tissue excitability and conduction.
  - Replace potassium.
- Hypothermia (accidental)
  - Remove patient from environment and begin rewarming techniques.
- Tamponade, cardiac
  - Pericardiocentesis
- Tension pneumothorax
  - Needle decompression, followed by tube thoracostomy.
- Thrombosis, cardiac (ACS)
  - Percutaneous coronary intervention (PCI) for STEMI patients
- Thrombosis, pulmonary (PE)
  - Empiric fibrinolytic therapy should be considered.
- Toxins
  - Resuscitation of the poisoned patient should follow routine ACLS algorithms. In patients with suspected opiate overdose, naloxone may be useful. For patients with tricyclic antidepressant overdose, sodium bicarbonate may be considered for treatment of wide-complex arrhythmias.

Termination of Resuscitative Efforts

- In patients without ROSC and persistent asystole after resuscitative efforts, consider termination.
- Bedside ultrasound can assist with confirmation of lack of cardiac activity.
- Deliver the death notification to family and provide support for grief.

MANAGEMENT OF BRADYCARDIA

Bradycardia Definition

- Bradycardia typically defined as a heart rate <60 beats/min.
- In most cases of symptomatic bradycardia, the pulse is <50 beats/min. It is important to note if there is "clinically significant bradycardia," or a heart rate that is too slow for the clinical condition.

Bradycardia Algorithm

Initial Actions

- Assess ABCs
  A: Airway: Maintain patent airway
  B: Assist breathing as necessary, apply oxygen if hypoxemic
  C: Apply cardiac monitor and obtain a rhythm strip.
  C: Obtain IV acces
  C: Obtain 12 lead ECG
- Perform history and physical examination
- CXR

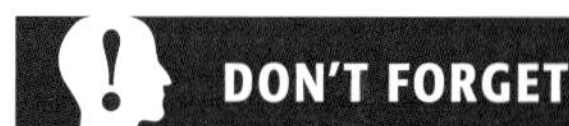

Is the patient stable or unstable?

Is the patient symptomatic or asymptomatic?

Assess for Signs or Symptoms of Poor Perfusion

- Signs: Hypotension, shock, pulmonary congestion, acute heart failure, acute myocardial infarction (MI)
- Symptoms: Ischemic chest discomfort, shortness of breath, acute altered mental status

If signs or symptoms of poor perfusion are present

- The patient should receive immediate treatment and atropine as the first-line drug for symptomatic bradycardia.
- Administer atropine 0.5 mg, repeat every 3-5 minutes to maximum dose of 3 mg.
- Transcutaneous pacing should be initiated in patients who do not respond to atropine.
- Provide adequate analgesia when pacing a patient, as this is a painful procedure.
- Dopamine can also be used, infusion should begin at 2-10 μg/kg/min and titrated to patient response.
- Epinephrine infusion can be started at 2-10 μg/min and titrated to patient response.
- Isoproterenol may also be used.
- Once the patient is stabilized, or proves to be refractory to the above interventions, place a transvenous pacemaker.

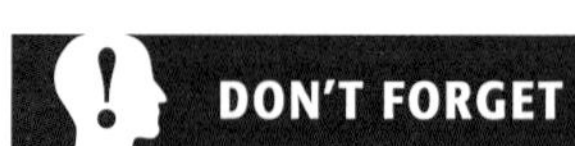

All patients with symptomatic bradycardia get transcutaneous pacing as a bridge to transvenous pacing. On test day, order the transvenous pacer be placed.

If no serious signs or symptoms are present, analyze rhythm

- Type II AV block or third-degree AV block are high-grade conduction abnormalities and may not respond to atropine.

- These patients need transvenous pacer placement, using transcutaneous pacing as a bridge therapy.
- For other bradycardic rhythms, observe the patient and reassess.

MANAGEMENT OF TACHYCARDIA

Tachycardia Definition

- Tachycardia typically defined as a heart rate >100 beats/min.
- In most cases of symptomatic tachycardia, the pulse is >150 beats/min.
- It is important to note if there is "clinically significant tachycardia," or a heart rate that is too fast for the clinical condition.
- Attempt to differentiate if the tachycardia is the primary cause of the patient's symptoms or is a response to an underlying condition (fever or dehydration).

Tachycardia Algorithm

Initial Actions

- Assess ABCs.
- IV, oxygen, cardiac monitor.
- Vital signs.
- 12-lead ECG.
- Targeted history and physical examination.
- CXR.

Assess for Signs or Symptoms of Poor Perfusion due to Tachycardia

- Signs: Hypotension, pulmonary congestion, hypoxia, shock
- Symptoms: Ischemic chest pain, severe shortness of breath, acutely altered mental status

Is the Patient Stable?

- Patient is unstable if any signs or symptoms of poor perfusion or cardiovascular compromise due to tachycardia are present (usually at a rate >150 beats/min).
- Patient is stable if no serious signs or symptoms are present.

Unstable Patients: Immediate Cardioversion

- Discuss procedure with patient, obtain IV access, provide oxygenation.
- Premedicate if possible with sedative ± analgesic.
  - Sedatives: Midazolam, etomidate, ketamine
  - Analgesics: Fentanyl, morphine
- Synchronize shock delivery to QRS complex
  - Energy: 50 J, 100 J, 200 J, 300 J, 360 J
  - Paroxysmal SVTs and atrial flutter often respond to lower energy levels (50-100 J), afib and ventricular tachycardia (VT) frequently require higher settings (200 J). If the initial dose fails to convert, increase the dose in a stepwise fashion.

Stable Patients: Identify Tachycardia

- Is the QRS narrow (<0.12 s) or wide (>0.12 s)?
- Is the rhythm regular or irregular?

Narrow (QRS <0.12 s) Complex Tachycardia

- Regular narrow complex tachycardia
  - Sinus tachycardia

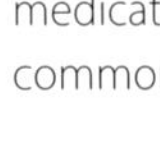

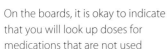

DON'T FORGET

On the boards, it is okay to indicate that you will look up doses for medications that are not used commonly.

DON'T FORGET

When treating tachycardia, assess the patient's stability, determine the rhythm, and then act.

  - SVT
  - Junctional tachycardia, ectopic or multifocal atrial tachycardia
- Irregular narrow complex tachycardia
  - Afib
  - Atrial flutter

Wide (QRS >0.12 s) Complex Tachycardia

- Regular wide complex tachycardia
  - Monomorphic VT
  - SVT with aberrancy
- Irregular wide complex tachycardia
  - Polymorphic VT
  - Afib with aberrancy

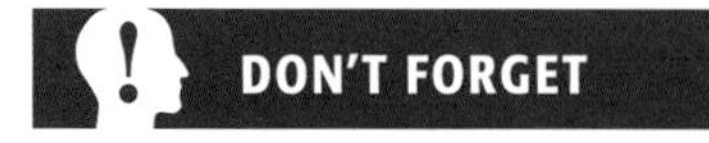

Unstable patients with tachycardia should be cardioverted immediately.

Regular Narrow Complex Tachycardia

- Determine type of narrow complex tachycardia.
  - Sinus tachycardia: Most common cause of regular, narrow complex rhythm. Important to identify and treat the underlying cause with fluids or medication.
  - Paroxysmal supraventricular tachycardia (PSVT): Caused by a reentrant circuit in the cardiac conduction system.
- Vagal maneuvers.
- Adenosine 6 mg IVP through an antecubital vein followed by 20 mL saline flush.
- If no response, double the dose to 12 mg IVP, then 12 mg IVP.
- If vagal maneuvers or adenosine fail to cover PSVT, if there is recurrence, or if these treatments unmask a different form of PSVT (such as afib or atrial flutter), longer AV nodal blocking agents such as calcium-channel blockers (diltiazem or verapamil), beta-blockers can also be used.
- Other rhythms such as junctional tachycardia, ectopic or multifocal atrial tachycardia can be difficult to treat but usually respond to AV nodal blocking agents.
- Wolff-Parkinson-White (WPW) syndrome: Congenital condition of abnormal cardiac conduction tissue between the atria and ventricles, which allows for a reentrant tachycardia circuit.
  - Identification: Shortened PR interval (<120 ms), slurring of QRS upstroke (delta wave), widened QRS complex (>120 ms), ST-T wave changes.
  - This syndrome can cause regular narrow complex tachycardias (AVRT with orthodromic conduction) or both regular and wide complex tachycardias.
  - For known WPW, treatment of PSVT (AVRT with orthodromic conduction) remains the same with vagal maneuvers or adenosine.

Irregular Narrow Complex Tachycardia

Two main rhythms: Afib and atrial flutter, both treated similarly.

- Goal: Rate control
- First-line agents
  - Calcium-channel blockers
    - Diltiazem 0.25 mg/kg IV (usual dose is 15-20 mg) initial dose and may repeat 0.35 mg/kg in 15 minutes (20-25 mg). Maintenance infusion dose is 5-15 mg/h titrated to heart rate.
    - Verapamil: 2.5-5mg IV bolus over 2 minutes, repeat doses of 5-10 mg may be administered to a total dose of 20 mg.
  - Beta-blockers
    - Metoprolol 5 mg IV given every 15 minutes up to three doses.
    - Can also use atenolol, propranolol, esmolol, labetolol.

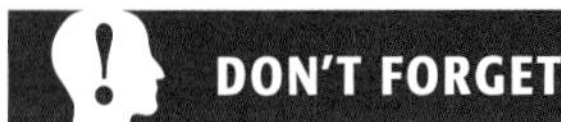

DON'T FORGET

Wide complex tachycardias are difficult to manage and cardiology consultation is important.

- For patients with impaired cardiac function (ejection fraction [EF] <40%)
  - Digoxin load 10-15 μg/kg lean body weight
- Rhythm control: Cardioversion can be considered for new onset afib/atrial flutter with duration <48 hours and proper anticoagulation.

Regular Wide Complex Tachycardia

- Rhythm: Stable monomorphic VT or SVT with aberrancy
- Can administer adenosine for regular, monomorphic, wide complex tachycardia, SVT should convert to normal sinus rhythm (NSR), there should be no effect on VT.
- For presumed VT:
  - Consider immediate synchronized cardioversion.
    - Procainamide 20-50 mg/min IV max dose is 17 mg/kg (Caution! Prolonged QRS and hypotension may result.)
    - Sotalol 100 mg IV over 5 minutes
  - Consider amiodarone 150 mg IV over 10 minutes in patients with poor ventricular function.
  - Lidocaine is second-line therapy.
  - Patients with WPW can present in AVRT with antidromic conduction that causes a wide complex tachycardia that can be mistaken for VT.
  - Stable patients can respond to drug therapy such as amiodarone or procainamide.
  - When in doubt treat as VT.

Irregular Wide Complex Tachycardia

- Rhythm: Afib with aberrancy, pre-excited afib, or polymorphic VT/torsades de pointes
  - Polymorphic VT: Is baseline QT interval normal or prolonged?
  - Normal baseline QT interval.
  - Treat myocardial ischemia.
  - Correct electrolytes and other known precipitants.
  - Medications: Beta-blocker, amiodarone.
- If cardiac function impaired, amiodarone or lidocaine and cardioversion are preferred.
- Long baseline QT interval (torsades de pointes).
- Correct abnormal electrolytes.
- Magnesium IV.
- Other therapies: Overdrive pacing, beta-blockers.
- Caution with patients with WPW!
- Patients with WPW can enter afib or atrial flutter that presents as a wide complex tachycardia ie, >200 beats/min.
- AV nodal blocking agents are absolutely contraindicated and may be harmful (adenosine, beta-blockers, calcium-channel blockers, digoxin) and lead to VT.
- Use procainamide or synchronized cardioversion.

DON'T FORGET

If you do not remember doses off the top of your head, indicate that you will look up dosages for infrequently used medications.

WINNING STRATEGIES

- Memorize and follow the ACLS algorithms.
- Patients without respirations, a pulse, or a blood pressure need immediate resuscitation with CPR, early defibrillation for shockable rhythms, and airway management.
- In patients who have adequate breathing with a pulse, you have time to obtain data (history, physical examination, rhythm strip, and ECG), make a diagnosis, and then implement treatment.

- For VF/VT do not delay defibrillation!
- When treating PEA, look for reversible causes (remember 5 Hs and 5 Ts).
- All patients with symptomatic bradycardia get transcutaneous pacing as a bridge to transvenous pacing. On test day, place a transvenous pacer in your patient!
- When treating tachycardia, assess the patient's stability, determine the rhythm, and then act.
- Unstable patients with tachycardia should be cardioverted immediately.

CHAPTER 5

PALS/NRP

Gerard Doyle and John Dayton

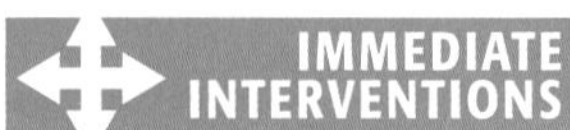

ABCs and IV, O_2, and monitor

IMMEDIATE INTERVENTIONS

- IV access with 18+ gauge needle. Blood should be drawn at this time for laboratory studies.
- Supplemental oxygen via NC or NRB to keep oxygen saturation >95%.
- Early and definitive airway management if needed.
- Cardiac monitor with continuous monitoring.
- Pacer/defibrillation pads.

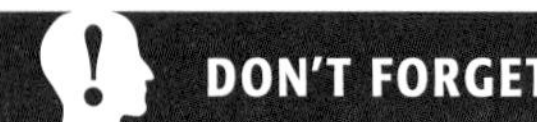

Keep it simple: If patient is breathing adequately, assist as needed. If not, start with positioning:

- Head tilt and chin lift: Perform these only if you do not suspect C-spine trauma

  OR
- Jaw thrust

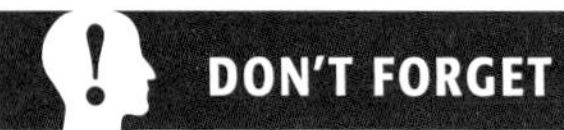

If worsening, assist and intervene.

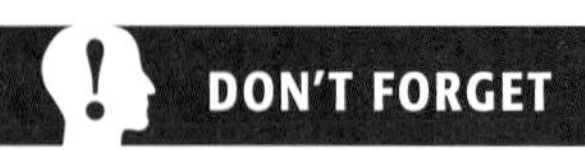

Rescue breathing, especially in prehospital setting, serves as a bridge until definitive airway management is established.

- Mouth-to-mask
- Mouth-to-mouth
- Mouth-to-nose
- Bag-to-mouth

INITIAL ASSESSMENT

- Initial focus on airway, breathing, and circulation (ABC).
- Is the airway patent?
- Is the child breathing spontaneously?
- Does the child have cardiac activity, good perfusion, and strong pulses?

First Priority: Immediate Interventions to Resuscitate Patient

- Standard of care: Basic life support (BLS) including access to emergency medical services (EMS), early cardiopulmonary resuscitation (CPR), early airway intervention, and early defibrillation. This should be followed by advanced cardiovascular life support measures (pediatric advanced life support/neonatal resuscitation program [PALS/NRP]).

BASIC LIFE SUPPORT

Assess Responsiveness

- Most pediatric arrests are due to airway compromise, hypoxia, or circulatory shock.
- Assess for neck injury: Stabilize C-spine and move the patient only if absolutely necessary.

Airway and Breathing

- Standard precautions: Gloves, face shields, etc.
- General maneuvers
  - Remove any foreign material in the anterior oropharynx.
  - Head tilt and chin lift or jaw thrust.
  - Assess breathing: Look for chest rise, listen for air escape during expiration, feel for air flow.
- Oxygen administration
  - Masks: Can deliver between 30% and 50% oxygen to patient with spontaneous ventilation
  - Nasal cannula: Also delivers oxygen to patient with spontaneous ventilation
  - Bag valve masks (BVMs)
    - Can be used for patients who are either spontaneously breathing and for patients who needs assistance with ventilation.
    - Can deliver between 60% and 90% oxygen concentrations.
    - Need to have appropriately sized mask and bag.
    - Be familiar with both one and two-person bagging techniques.
  - Oropharyngeal and nasopharyngeal airways: Use for unconscious patients and after attempts to clear airway is unsuccessful.
  - Laryngeal mask airway (LMA)
    - Supraglottic airway is used to secure airway in an unconscious patient without requiring laryngoscopy.
    - Introduced into pharynx and advanced until resistance is felt.
    - When balloon is inflated, the laryngeal inlet is sealed, improving bag ventilation.
    - Advantages: Ease of use for all ages and prehospital use.
    - Disadvantages: Does not prevent aspiration and is not a "secure" airway—it may become dislodged during transport.
- Endotracheal intubation
  - Indications
    - Glasgow Coma Score (GCS) <8, apnea, inadequate respiratory effort, inability to protect airway, or pending airway failure

- Need for high positive pressures
- Need for paralysis or deep sedation
- Advantages
  - Establishes definitive airway
  - Ability to oxygenate and ventilate
  - Decreased risk of aspiration
  - Inspiratory time, inspiratory pressures, and end-expiratory pressures can be measured and controlled.
- Disadvantage
  - Tube may become dislodged (or obstructed) during transport (common problem on exam day).
- Preparation
  - Pre-oxygenate with nasal cannula or BVM.
  - Choose the correct uncuffed endotracheal tube (ETT) size by using the Broselow tape or this formula: ETT size = (age/4) + 4.
  - Prepare functioning laryngoscope and suction.
  - Prepare post-procedure tools such as end-tidal carbon dioxide (CO_2) detector and device to secure ETT.
  - Position patient to maximize success: "Sniffing position," towel roll under neck and shoulders, with auditory meatus in same plane as sternal manubrium.
  - Stabilize C-spine in trauma patients.
- Rapid sequence intubation (RSI)
  - Pretreatment
    - Atropine at 0.02 mg/kg intravenous (IV) contributes to safety in children <8 by reducing bradycardia when succinylcholine is used.
    - Lidocaine at 1.5 mg/kg IV can be used in cases of suspected head trauma.
  - Sedation
    - Etomidate at 0.3 mg/kg IV protects hemodynamic stability and is neuroprotective.
    - Ketamine at 1-2 mg/kg IV can be used in patients with bronchospasm, asthma, and septic shock.
    - Midazolam at 0.2 mg/kg IV can be used in children with status epilepticus.
  - Paralytic
    - Succinylcholine at 2 mg/kg IV
    - Rocuronium at 1 mg/kg IV instead of succinylcholine in cases of myopathy, hyperkalemia, burn, head/face trauma, or crush injury
- Visualization of passage through cords is the most reliable indicator of successful intubation.
- Depth of insertion should correspond to three times the ETT size used.
- PALS now endorses cuffed ETTs for children <8 years.
- Verification of proper tube placement by CO_2 detector, fogging of tube, bilateral breath sounds, chest rise, and chest x-ray (CXR).

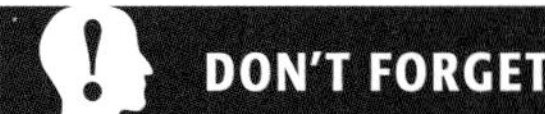

Know which drugs are best for each situation.

Tube size: (Age/4) + 4 or use Broselow tape; cuffed tubes >8

Depth of tube: Three times tube size or (age/2) + 12

Circulation

- Assessing circulation via perfusion and pulses.
- Chest compressions
  - Serial compressions over the lower sternum artificially deliver blood flow by increasing intrathoracic pressure and directly compressing the heart.
  - Initiate in absence of pulse or poor perfusion, or if heart rate (HR) <60 beats/min.
  - Compress to a depth of one-third of the anteroposterior (AP) diameter of the child's chest.

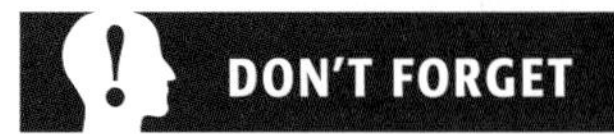

Different chest compression techniques for different ages. Know the difference!

- Infants: Two-thumb technique
- Children: One hand
- Older children: Two hands
- If unsure of rate, use 100+ compressions per minute.

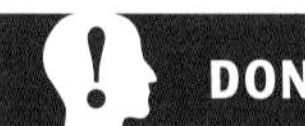

DON'T FORGET

Use normal saline, lactated Ringer solution, or blood products for volume expansion.

- Infants
  - Two-thumb technique: Hands encircle infant's chest with thumbs on the lower sternum
  - 100+ per minute
  - 5:1 ratio for compressions to ventilations
- Children between 1 and 8 years
  - Heel of one hand used to depress sternum 4 cm
  - 100 per minute
  - 30:2 ratio for compressions to ventilations
- Children >8 years
  - Two-handed technique (same as adults) used to depress sternum 5 cm
  - 100 per minute
  - 30:2 ratio for compressions to ventilations
  - Don't ventilate more than 10 breaths/min

DON'T FORGET

Remember which medications can be given via ETT by the LEAN mnemonic:

- Lidocaine
- Epinephrine
- Atropine
- Naloxone

ETT doses are usually higher than those given via IV.

- Establishing vascular access
  - Use the largest, most accessible vein that does not interfere with the rest of the resuscitation.
  - Use large diameter, short-bore catheters as they have the lowest resistance to flow and provide for the most rapid fluid resuscitation.
  - Use an intraosseous (IO) line if you are unable to rapidly place an IV line.
    - Insert into the anterior tibia.
    - Other options include the distal femur, medial malleolus, and anterior superior iliac spine.
    - These can be used to obtain laboratory specimens for chemistries, blood gas analysis, and type and crossmatch.
  - In neonates, consider an umbilical catheter.
- Intravascular fluids
  - Expansion of intravascular volume is critical in patients who have shock from hemorrhagic and distributive shock.
  - Volume expansion is best achieved by isotonic crystalloid solutions such as normal saline and lactated Ringer solution.
  - Fluids containing dextrose should not be used as they do not expand intravascular volume and may cause a hyperglycemia-induced osmotic diuresis.
  - Initial dose of volume resuscitation should be 20 cc/kg.
  - If adequate volume expansion is not achieved with infusion of 60 cc/kg, consider transfusion of blood products and addition of vasopressor medications.
- Defibrillation
  - Use for ventricular fibrillation (VF) or unstable, symptomatic dysrhythmias
  - Paddle size:
    - Infants: 4.5-cm paddles
    - Children: 8-cm paddles

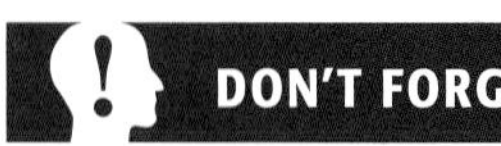

DON'T FORGET

Know: 2 J/kg for defibrillation

  - Positioning of electrodes options:
    - AP
    - Right second intercostal space to the right of the sternum and left mid-clavicular line at level of xiphoid process
  - Defibrillation:
    - Use 2 J/kg for VF.
    - Use 2-4 J/kg on second attempt, and 4 J/kg for all other attempts.

Drugs Used for Cardiac Arrest and Resuscitation

Adenosine

- Use for supraventricular tachycardia (SVT)
  - Temporarily blocks conduction through the atrioventricular (AV) node.
  - Must be given as a rapid IV or IO bolus.

- Need to have rapid post-dose flush to ensure that drug enters central circulation.
- Monitor electrocardiogram (ECG) during administration.
- Dose
  - 0.1 mg/kg IV (6 mg max dose) initially.
  - 0.2 mg/kg IV (12 mg max dose) if initial dose fails.

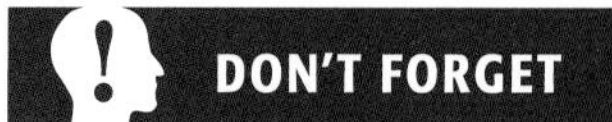

During your Oral Boards exam, you are responsible to know the medications and dosage used for ATLS, ACLS, PALS, and NRP.

If you are unable to remember, ask to use a medical reference or the Broselow tape.

Amiodarone

- Use for ventricular tachycardia (VT) and for SVT if adenosine has failed.
- Produces vasodilation and AV nodal suppression.
- Inhibits outward potassium flow, prolonging QT interval.
- Inhibits sodium channels, prolonging QRS duration.
- Dose
  - Pulseless VT/VF: 5 mg/kg IV bolus
  - Perfusing tachycardias: 5 mg/kg IV over 20-60 minutes
  - Maximum dose: 15 mg/kg/d

Atropine

- Use for bradycardia.
- Accelerates sinus conduction and increases AV conduction.
- Dose
  - 0.02 mg/kg IV and 0.02-0.04 mg/kg ETT
  - Minimum dose of 0.1 mg and maximum dose 0.5 mg in child and 1.0 mg in adolescent
  - Can be given IV, IO, and ETT

Epinephrine

- Use for cardiac arrest, bradycardia.
- Vasoconstriction is most important action.
- Increases aortic diastolic pressure and coronary perfusion pressure.
- Enhances contractility of heart.
- Dose
  - 0.01 mg/kg (0.1 mL/kg of 1:10,000) solution given via IV or IO route
  - 0.1 mg/kg (0.1 mL/kg of 1:1,000) solution given via endotracheal (ET) route
  - 0.1-0.2 μg/kg/min for continuous infusion

Lidocaine

- Sodium channel blocker that decreases automaticity, which suppresses ventricular dysrhythmias
- Dose
  - 1 mg/kg rapid bolus by the IV/IO/ET route
  - 20-50 μg/kg/min continuous infusion

Pediatric Advanced Life Support Algorithms

Pediatric pulseless arrest

1. BLS
   a. Assess and support ABCs.
   b. Intubate if necessary.
   c. Oxygenate.
   d. Attach monitor and defibrillator.

2. Assess and evaluate rhythm.
   a. VF/VT
      i. Defibrillate (2 J/kg once, 4 J/kg for subsequent attempts). Interpose CPR and drug administration between defibrillation attempts: CPR-drug-shock-REPEAT
      ii. Epinephrine, IV/IO/ETT, every 3-5 minutes.
      iii. Reevaluate tracheal tube position, electrode position, and vascular access while doing CPR.
      iv. Antidysrhythmics.
         1. Amiodarone
         2. Lidocaine
         3. Consider magnesium, 25-50 mg/kg IV especially for polymorphic VT, over 10-20 minutes.
      v. Reevaluate rhythm.
      vi. Consider terminating efforts.
   b. Pulseless electrical activity (PEA) or asystole
      i. Epinephrine, IV/IO/ETT, every 3-5 minutes.
      ii. Reevaluate tracheal tube position, electrode position, and vascular access while doing CPR.
      iii. Treat the Hs and Ts.
      iv. Consider terminating efforts.

DON'T FORGET

Always "ABC and electricity"

- Airway
- Breathing
- Circulation
- Shock if needed

DON'T FORGET

For PEA, think of things that you can fix. Think of the "Hs and Ts."

- Hypoxemia
- Hypovolemia
- Hypothermia
  - Hydrogen ion (acidosis)
  - Hypoglycemia
  - Hypo/hyperkalemia

Others:

- Tamponade
- Tension pneumothorax
- Toxins
- Thrombosis: pulmonary (PE) and coronary (MI)

Pediatric bradycardia

1. BLS:
   a. Assess and support ABCs as needed.
   b. Intubate, if needed.
   c. Oxygenate.
   d. Attach to cardiac monitor and defibrillator.
2. Assess cardiovascular stability (poor perfusion, hypotension, altered level of consciousness, and increased respiratory effort).
   a. Stable
      i. Observe.
      ii. Support ABCs.
      iii. Transfer if facility unable to treat critically ill children.
   b. Unstable
      i. Perform chest compressions if HR is <60 after oxygenation.
      ii. During CPR verify ET tube placement, electrode position.
      iii. Epinephrine IV/IO/ETT every 3-5 minutes.
      iv. Atropine 0.02 mg/kg. May be repeated once.
      v. Consider cardiac pacing.
      vi. If patient degenerates into different algorithm, follow that pathway.

DON'T FORGET

Epinephrine, not atropine, is drug of choice in pediatric bradycardia!

Pediatric tachycardia

1. BLS:
   a. Assess and support ABCs as needed.
   b. Intubate, if needed.
   c. Oxygenate.
   d. Attach to cardiac monitor and defibrillator.

2. Assess cardiovascular stability (poor perfusion, hypotension, altered level of consciousness, and increased respiratory effort).
   a. Stable
      i. 12-lead ECG.
      ii. Observe.
      iii. Support ABCs.
      iv. Transfer if facility unable to treat critically ill children.
   b. Unstable
      i. If VT, cardiovert with 0.5-1 J/kg.
      ii. If SVT, give adenosine 0.1 mg/kg IV (may give second dose of 0.2 mg/kg) if stable, or cardiovert with 0.5-1 J/kg.
      iii. Consider antidysrhythmics.
         1. Amiodarone 5 mg/kg IV; may repeat up to 15 mg/kg
         2. Procainamide 15 mg/kg IV; give over 30-60 minutes
         3. Lidocaine 1 mg/kg IV
      iv. If patient degenerates into different algorithm, follow that pathway.

NRP

- Aggressive supportive care and supplemental oxygen will reverse distress, cyanosis, and bradycardia for the majority of patients.
- Make sure to reassess the efficacy of interventions every 30 seconds.
- Initial assessment
  - Warm and dry infant.
  - Clear airway if needed.
  - Assess respirations, pulse, color, cry, and muscle tone.
  - Assess for presence of meconium, and suction any present if newborn has cyanosis or respiratory compromise.
  - If breathing adequately, HR >100, and newborn is warm, give supportive care and allow skin-to-skin contact with mother.
  - If cyanotic, consider blow-by oxygen.
  - If the child is apneic or gasping, HR is <100, or if cyanosis is not relieved by 30 seconds of supplemental oxygen, then suction nose and start positive pressure ventilation (PPV) with BVM at 40-60 breaths/min.
  - If apnea and cyanosis persist for more than 30 seconds after starting PPV, and if HR is <60, then start chest compressions at 90 per minute, in a 3:1 ratio with breaths. A definitive airway and umbilical vein catheter placement should be considered at this time.
  - If the child continues to be in distress, administer 0.1-0.3 mL/kg of 1:10,000 epinephrine.
- Oxygen saturation will initially be low (60%-65%) in full term babies at birth, and saturation will slowly increase to 95% over the next 12-15 minutes. Place the oxygen sensor on the right upper extremity to measure pre-ductal saturation; persistent hypoxia in other limbs suggests congenital cardiovascular defect (Fig. 5-1).

WINNING STRATEGIES

- Know your PALS/NRP algorithms.
- Reassess the patient frequently.
- If the patient does not improve, make sure to take a step back and ensure everything is being done according to the algorithm.
- Epinephrine is the drug of choice in pediatric bradycardia.

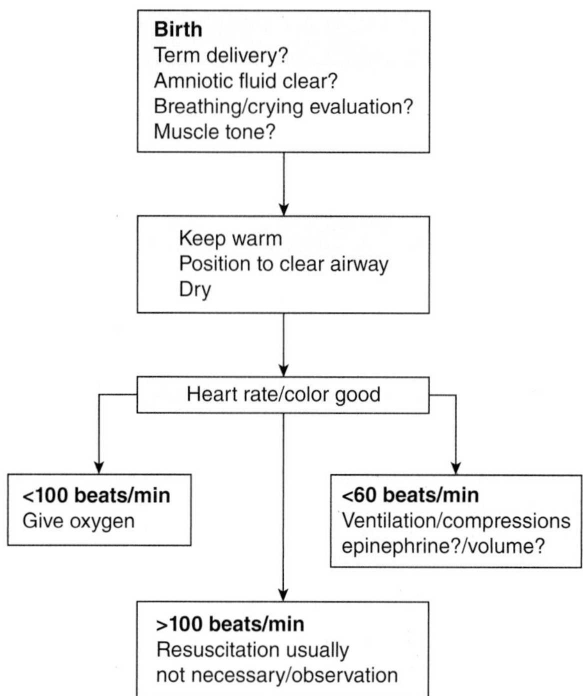

Figure 5-1. Neonatal resuscitation algorithm. (*Data from, Based on recommendations from* Circulation *2005;112:IV-188-IV-195. 2005 American Heart Association. DOI: 10.1161/CIRCULATIONAHA.105.166574.*)

- Remember to defibrillate at 2 J/kg initially in children.
- Use the Broselow tape as reference for weight-based dosing.
- Remember different CPR techniques for different ages.
- For RSI, know which medications are best for each situation.

CHAPTER 6

Common Procedures

Gregg Helland and James Ahn

JOINT INJURIES/REDUCTIONS

Anterior Dislocations of the Glenohumeral Joint

- Usually occurs when arm is in abduction externally rotated.
- Patient presents holding the arm in abduction with slight external rotation.
- Acromion will look prominent and the patient's normal round contour of the shoulder will be lost.
- X-ray: The "Y" view of the shoulder will be diagnostic and will show that the humeral head is displaced inferiorly and medially (Fig. 6-1).
- Axillary nerve should be tested before and after the reduction.

Definitive management

- Pain control
  - Morphine sulfate 2-6 mg intravenous (IV) prn pain q15-30 minutes.
  - Intra-articular injection or conscious sedation as described below.
    - Intra-articular injection: "I will sterilize the affected shoulder area and inject 20 mL of 1% lidocaine into the shoulder joint immediately distally to lateral border of the acromion toward the glenoid cavity."
- Reduction
  - Stimson maneuver: "I will place the patient prone on an elevated stretcher and suspend 5-10 lb of weight from the affected wrist, allowing slow and steady traction to relocate the humeral head. If needed, I will gently externally rotate the patient's arm. After 20 minutes, I will reexamine the patient to see if the dislocation has been reduced."

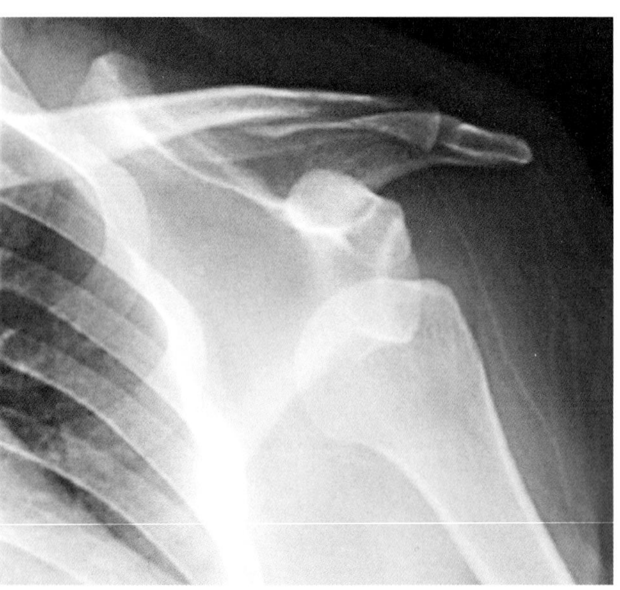

A

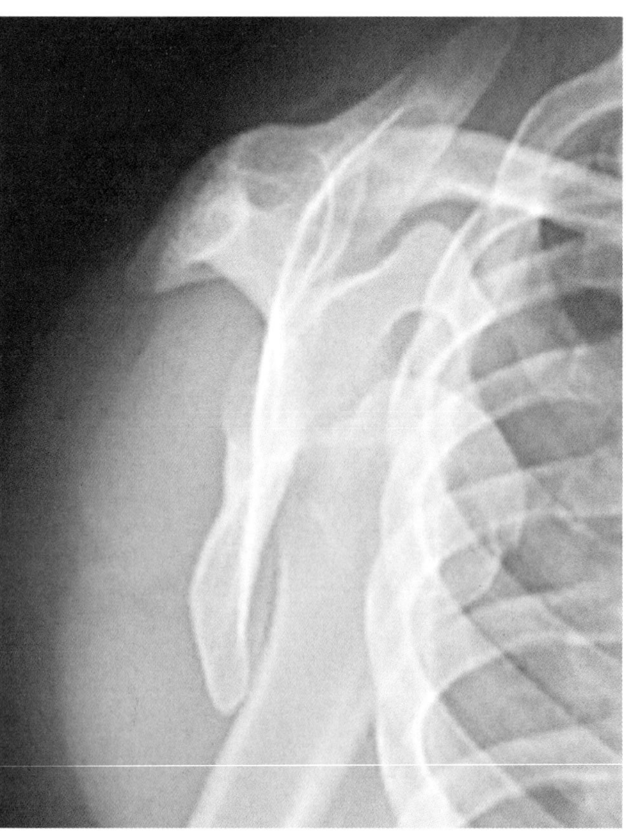

B

Figure 6-1. (**A**) Anterior shoulder dislocation on the AP view. (**B**) Scapular Y view demonstrating an anterior shoulder dislocation. (*Reprinted with permission from Simon RR, Sherman SC, Koenigsknecht SJ.* Emergency Orthopedics: The Extremities. *5th ed. New York, NY: McGraw-Hill; 2007.*)

- Scapular manipulation technique: "I will place the patient in a prone position with the patient's shoulder flexed to 90° and holding 5 lb of weight, then I will push the inferior tip of the scapula medially and dorsally with my thumbs and I will apply traction along the superior aspect of the scapula with my fingers."
- External rotation technique: "I will place the patient supine with the arm adducted and elbow flexed to 90° and gently externally rotate the arm until the forearm is horizontal to the floor. Once the shoulder is fully externally rotated, I will abduct the arm in an overhead position while applying gentle traction to the elbow."
- Traction-counter traction technique: "I will place the patient supine and wrap one sheet around the patient's chest and trunk while having an assistant hold on to that sheet opposite the patient's affected shoulder while I wrap a sheet around the affected arm's flexed forearm and tie it around back. I will apply traction with my body, while my assistant applies counter traction with their body."

DON'T FORGET

Try to explain and obtain consent for all procedures performed at American Board of Emergency Medicine (ABEM) General, but do not delay an emergent procedure to obtain consent.

Disposition

- Place the patient in shoulder immobilizer and get a repeat x-ray to confirm relocation
- Reexamine the patient to look for any new neurovascular deficits post-reduction.
- Consult orthopedics for close follow up.
- Clear discharge instructions.
- Patients should only be discharged if they have fully recovered from any sedation given for reduction.

CRITICAL ACTION

All affected joints should have careful neurovascular examinations—look at joint above and below injury—this will be a critical action.

Posterior Dislocation of the Glenohumeral Joint

- Uncommon injury, <5% of all shoulder dislocation injuries.
- Associated with direct trauma to the anterior shoulder or axial loading of a flexed, adducted, internally rotated arm.
- Consider in all patients after a seizure or electrical shock.
- X-ray: A light bulb appearance of the humeral head may be seen from the obliteration of the greater tuberosity. The acromiohumeral distance is decreased compared to the normal side, and the normal overlap of the humeral head on the glenoid is lost.
- The best radiographic view for diagnosing a posterior dislocation is the axillary view, which allows identification of the glenohumeral relationship. The scapular-Y view can also be helpful.

DON'T FORGET

Order Y views on patients with suspected shoulder dislocations.

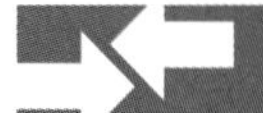

CRITICAL ACTION

Axillary nerve examination: A quick examination testing pinprick sensation and two-point discrimination over the lateral aspect of the deltoid—this will be a critical action.

Definitive management

- Pain control, conscious sedation is usually required.
- Reduction: "After the patient is sedated, I will place traction in an adducted position, in line with the deformity, with the patient in the supine position. I will gently lift the humeral head into the glenoid fossa, avoiding forced external rotation."

Disposition

- Place patient in shoulder immobilizer and get a repeat x-ray to confirm relocation.
- Consult orthopedics for close follow up.
- Reliable discharge instructions.
- Patients should only be discharged if they have fully recovered from any sedation given for reduction.

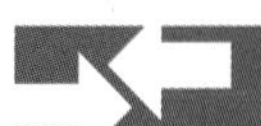

CRITICAL ACTION

Treat the patient's pain. This may be a critical action.

DON'T FORGET

All patients with shoulder dislocations need to be placed in a shoulder immobilizer and followed up with orthopedics.

Fracture/Dislocation of the Distal Radius

- Most common mechanism of injury is a fall on outstretched hand (FOOSH).
- Reduction should only be attempted in the emergency department (ED) if fracture is extra-articular.
- Check patency of radial and ulnar arteries.
- Perform a thorough neurological examination of hand by testing the medial, ulnar, and radial nerve.
- Always check for scaphoid/snuffbox tenderness.

Definitive management

DON'T FORGET

Screen all patients for posterior shoulder dislocation who present after seizure or electrical shock.

- Pain control, local anesthesia, or conscious sedation.
- Reduction: "I will use a hematoma block to perform local anesthesia, or conscious sedation with airway equipment available if needed. I will place the patient's fingers in a finger trap and elevate the wrist with 90° of flexion, and then suspend 10 lb of weight on the elbow for about 5-10 minutes. After this traction, I will apply dorsal pressure over the distal fragments and volar pressure over the proximal fragments. When the proper position has been established, I will remove the weights and immobilize the arm."

Disposition

DON'T FORGET

Get axillary and Y view on patients who you are concerned for posterior shoulder dislocation.

- Place the patient in a wrist splint and get a repeat x-ray to confirm relocation.
- Consult orthopedics for close follow up.
- Clear discharge instructions.
- Patients should only be discharged if they have fully recovered from any sedation given for reduction.

Posterior Hip Dislocation

DON'T FORGET

Intra-articular fracture dislocations are at risk for long-term complications of joint stiffness, post-reduction swelling with secondary compartment syndromes, cosmetic defects, and malunion.

- Significant mechanism of injury with great energy is needed to cause hip dislocations.
- In the hip joint, posterior dislocations are much more common than anterior dislocations.
- Posterior dislocations occur with force applied to a flexed knee, directed posteriorly.
- On examination, the extremity is found to be shortened, internally rotated, and adducted.
- X-rays: Common anteroposterior (AP) and lateral x-rays of hip adequately identify the dislocation, check acetabular and femur views as well (Fig. 6-2).
- In most cases, it is important to obtain emergency orthopedic referral for reduction.

Definitive management

- Conscious sedation
- Reduction: "I will place the patient on a backboard and then I will either lower the patient on the floor on a backboard or straddle the patient's stretcher. I will ask an assistant to keep the patient's pelvis immobilized. I will pull up on the distal calf to apply traction in line with the deformity and gently flex the knee to position of 90°. I will gently pull the hip anteriorly upward with slight external rotation."

DON'T FORGET

Be suspicious for associated acetabular fractures or ipsilateral extremity injuries in the patient who has a hip dislocation.

Disposition

- Based on other injuries identified and always get repeat x-rays after the procedure.
- Orthopedic follow up is essential if patient is discharged.

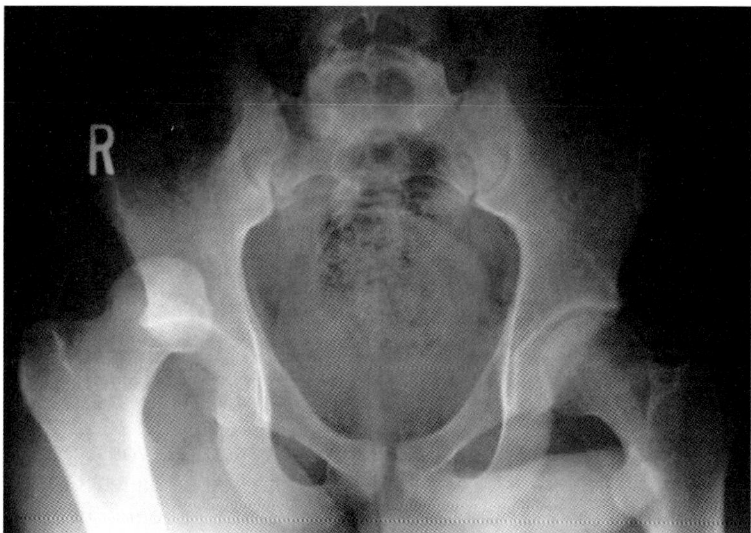

Figure 6-2. AP film of the pelvis showing a posterior dislocation of the hip. (*Reprinted with permission from Simon RR, Sherman SC, Koenigsknecht SJ.* Emergency Orthopedics: The Extremities. *5th ed. New York, NY: McGraw-Hill; 2007.*)

Knee Dislocations

- True orthopedic emergencies: High incidence of popliteal arterial injuries, peroneal nerve injury, and ligamentous/meniscal injury.
- Commonly seen following sporting accidents and falls with posterior dislocation is most common.
- Emergency reduction is indicated, although, frequently patients will have spontaneously reduced prior to evaluation.
- Document neurovascular status pre- and post-reduction.
- Patients with an absent pulse or bruits require immediate vascular surgical consultation for surgical exploration.
- Order a follow-up computed tomography (CT) angiogram and Doppler studies of the affected extremity.

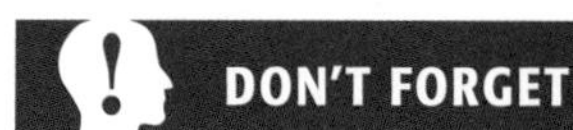

Complications of posterior hip dislocation include sciatic nerve injury and avascular necrosis that increases in direct proportion to the delay in adequate reduction.

Definitive management

- Pain control with morphine sulfate or conscious sedation.
- Reduction: "I will apply traction longitudinally in the line of the deformity while an assistant holds counter traction above the knee. I will then rotate my hand to the undersurface of the tibia and displace it anteriorly into its normal position. I will then order post-reduction films and an arteriogram."

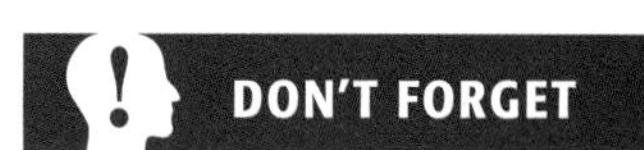

Knee dislocations have a high incidence of popliteal arterial injuries: order post-reduction angiograms.

Disposition

- Patients are admitted for neurovascular examinations.
- Use a knee immobilizer for stabilization and get a repeat x-ray to confirm relocation and evaluate for other injuries.

Ankle Fracture/Dislocation

- Ankle dislocations are usually posterior.
- Commonly associated with fractures of the malleable and distal fibula.
- Do not delay reduction in order to obtain radiograph.

Definitive Management

- Pain control: Use morphine sulfate 2-6 mg IV prn pain q30 minutes.

DON'T FORGET

If three ligaments are unstable, the patient has suffered a knee dislocation and must have further testing to evaluate for vascular injury.

- Reduction: "I will place longitudinal traction on the foot with one hand on the heel and I will put my other hand on the dorsum of the foot. I will ask an assistant to place counter traction on the leg while I place gentle medial pressure until I feel the joint reduce."

Disposition

- Check post-reduction films and neurovascular examination.
- Place posterior mold.
- Consult orthopedic surgery, disposition according to other injuries, stability of joint.

DON'T FORGET

Unstable fracture/dislocations with neurovascular compromise or serious skin tenting (on the verge of breaking skin) should be reduced prior to imaging.

Lumbar Puncture

- Used to evaluate patients for the diagnosis of central nervous system (CNS) infections and for the diagnosis of subarachnoid hemorrhage (SAH).
- Caution/consultation should be considered in patients with possible increased intracranial pressure (elderly, immunocompromised, seizures, altered mental status, and focal neuro deficits), thrombocytopenia or other bleeding diathesis, and spinal epidural abscess.
- A head CT should be done prior to the procedure if a SAH is suspected or if there is an abnormal neurologic or fundoscopic examination.
- Remember not to delay antibiotics if performing a head CT prior to performing the lumbar puncture.
- Procedure: "I will lay the patient on his side perpendicular to the bed/gurney. I will ask the patient to assume the fetal position. Using sterile drape and technique, I will palpate the L4-L5 spinous process, and infiltrate local anesthetic. I will position the spinal needle between the 2 spinous processes and introduce it into the skin with the bevel of the needle facing up. When I see flow, I will measure the opening pressure and collect four tubes of CSF. I will then withdraw the needle and place a dressing over the skin."
- Complications of procedure: Post-spinal tap headache, nerve root trauma, CNS infection, intraspinal hematoma.

DON'T FORGET

If you delay LP by getting a head CT to exclude a mass lesion—the blood cultures should be obtained and antibiotics should be administered empirically before the CT, followed as soon as possible by the LP.

Pericardiocentesis

- ED indications are pericardial tamponade diagnosed by physical examination or ultrasound (US).
- History: Patients with tamponade complain of chest pain, dyspnea, cough, hoarseness of voice, or hiccups. Patients frequently report a history of cancer, lupus, or tuberculosis.
- Physical examination: Tachycardia, tachypnea may develop in acute situations. Jugular vein distention (JVD), narrow pulse pressure can occur in patients with significant pericardial effusion, elevated central venous pressure.
- Nonemergent pericardiocentesis should be performed by cardiologist under fluoroscopy.
- Pericardial tamponade is diagnosed on US by the presence of anechoic pericardial fluid and diastolic collapse of the right ventricle.
- Use caution in patients who are coagulopathic or thrombocytopenic.
- Patients should have a large-bore IV, oxygen, and cardiac monitoring.
- Volume resuscitation of patients is critical.
- Procedure: "I will position the patient at 30°-45° head elevation. I will anesthetize the local site with 3 cc of 1% lidocaine. I will insert a 5-inch spinal needle through the subxiphoid approach on the left side. I will advance the needle and syringe until the needle tip is posterior to the rib cage. While advancing the needle toward the pericardial space under US guidance, I will

DON'T FORGET

Beck triad: Muffled heart tones, hypotension, JVD

aspirate the syringe. I will continue to advance the needle until fluid is aspirated in the syringe."

- Complications: Laceration of a coronary vessel, puncture of the right or left ventricle, bleeding, hypotension, ventricular ectopy, arrhythmia, or acute left ventricular failure with pulmonary edema.

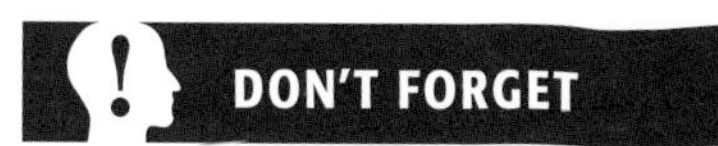

Consult CT/trauma surgeon emergently for trauma patients with cardiac tamponade.

Chest Tube Thoracostomy

- Indicated for patients with spontaneous or iatrogenic simple pneumothorax, tension pneumothorax, penetrating chest trauma, hemothorax, or complicated para-pneumonic effusion.
- Perform bedside lung US for suspected pneumothorax to confirm diagnosis, if available.
- There are no absolute contraindications to tube thoracostomy.
- Chest tube sizes: Spontaneous or iatrogenic pneumothorax: a 16-28 Fr; hemothorax: 32-40 Fr.
- Procedure: "I will place the patient in a supine position with the arm of the involved side placed behind the head. I will prep the area with betadine solution and drape with sterile towels. I will anesthetize the skin superficially and the periosteum deeply one intercostal space below the intercostal space that will be penetrated above the rib in the anterior axillary line of the fifth intercostal space. I will make an incision and then bluntly dissect with a Kelly clamp. I will place the chest tube directing posteriorly and superiorly toward the apex of the lung. I will secure it with sutures and an occlusive dressing and ask the nurse to connect it to a Pleurovac under a water seal of negative 20 cm of water."
- Complications: Unilateral pulmonary edema, lung injury, chest wall bleeding, air leaks, occlusion, subcutaneous emphysema, diaphragmatic/abdominal organ laceration.
- Disposition: Patients should be admitted to a monitored setting with consultation/admission under a trauma and/or cardiothoracic (CT) surgeon.

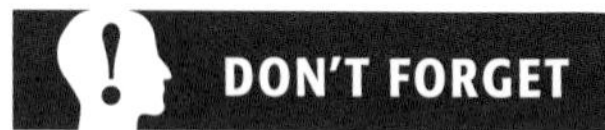

Do not wait for CXR to place chest tube in patients who clinically have a tension pneumothorax.

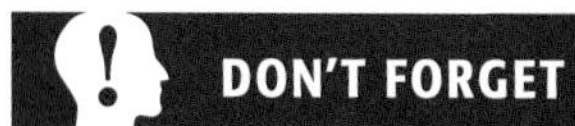

Do not forget to order an x-ray to confirm tube placement.

Cricothyrotomy

- Used when endotracheal intubation is contraindicated, when you anticipate the inability to perform a safe intubation, or when you have a "cannot intubate, cannot ventilate" scenario.
- Absolute contraindications include tracheal transection or when there is significant damage to the larynx or cricoid. Relative contraindications include children <12 years, acute laryngeal diseases, or when there is significant distortion of neck anatomy from swelling, hematoma, or a mass.
- Always make sure to notify your difficult airway consultants (anesthesia, general surgery, otolaryngology [ENT]) as early as possible to have them at the bedside if problems occur.
- Equipment needed: Prepackaged kit or at least a scalpel, appropriately sized tube, tracheal hook, and a suture or tie to secure the tube in place.
- Procedure: "I will hyperextend the neck, if there are no contraindications to do so, and identify the cricothyroid membrane between the thyroid and cricoid cartilage. I will use local anesthetic if time permits and sedate the patient if required. I will make a vertical incision through the skin and then a horizontal incision through the membrane. With the scalpel still in the hole just created, I will insert the tracheal hook and pull the cricoid ring anteriorly and inferiorly. I will then remove the scalpel, insert the tube and secure it. I will then confirm placement as I would with an endotracheal intubation."
- Complications: Failure to intubate, bleeding, infection, and airway obstruction blocking tube placement.

Lateral Canthotomy

- Retrobulbar hemorrhage, usually as the result of trauma, leads to decreased vision, increased intraocular pressure (IOP), and proptosis. A lateral canthotomy can help release the pressure and allow for more time until an emergent ophthalmologic evaluation can be done. This procedure should not be done when a globe rupture is suspected. Make sure you attempt to notify your ophthalmology consultant prior to performing this procedure.
- Equipment: You will need local anesthetic with epinephrine, a straight hemostat, straight scissors, and forceps. This procedure should be done as sterile as the situation allows.
- Procedure: "I will place the patient in a supine position and then infiltrate the lateral canthus with local anesthetic. I will clamp the lateral canthus with the straight hemostat long enough to remove the blood from the tissue and mark the incision line. I will then use the scissors to cut along the crushed tissue straight back to the orbital rim, being careful to avoid the globe. I will then grasp the lower eyelid with the forceps and pull down in order to expose the lateral canthal tendon. I will cut the inferior crus of the tendon and evaluate to see if the pressure has been relieved successfully. If no improvement, I will cut the superior crus as well."
- Complications: Injury to the globe, bleeding, and infection.

Procedural Sedation

- Useful for analgesia and muscle relaxant for brief emergency procedures, joint reductions, hernia reductions, cardioversion, and incision and drainage.
- History
  - PMHx: Screen for comorbidities including chronic obstructive pulmonary disease (COPD), coagulopathies, seizure disorder, obstructive sleep apnea (OSA), alcoholism, congestive heart failure (CHF).
  - Medications: Patients on chronic benzos and narcotics will likely need stronger dose.
  - Allergies
  - Last meal: If the procedure is nonemergent, it is a safe practice to wait >4 hours from last meal before sedating patient.
- Physical examination
  - Vital signs
  - Evaluation of airway (see airway management): Short neck, small mandible, large tongue, trismus, obesity
  - Cardiac/pulmonary examination should identify any potential complications with conscious sedation.
- Preparation: "I would like to prepare for conscious sedation. Please place the patient on a cardiac monitor, pulse oximeter, and oxygen by mask. Please establish an IV. I will need an oral and nasal airway available, bag valve mask, and suction and please keep 2 mg Narcan IV on hand. Draw up 200 μg of fentanyl and 5 mg of versed" (substitute age, weight, and procedure appropriate medications and doses) "I will obtain consent by explaining the risks and benefits."
- Procedure: "After double-checking my suction and airway equipment, I will infuse the medications, administer local anesthesia, and perform the procedure. If oversedation occurs and decreased respirations are noted, I will stimulate the patient, reposition the airway, and assist ventilation with a bag valve mask. Close monitoring will continue until the patient is completely awake and alert."
- Medications: The following medications can be used for procedural sedation. Analgesics and sedative hypnotics are generally used together to provide anxiolysis, amnesia, and pain relief. Each component should be

titrated to the desired target in light of the procedure being performed. Ketamine provides both analgesia and sedation as a single agent.

- Analgesics: Provide pain relief
  - Fentanyl
    - Excellent analgesia with minimal hypotension and sedation at usual doses.
    - Dosage in adults is 50-100 μg, may repeat every 3-5 minutes, and titrate to effect.
    - Dosage in peds is 1-2 μg/kg/dose.
    - Rapid onset 3-5 minutes and 30-60 minutes duration.
    - Complications: Respiratory depression, chest wall rigidity, and apnea.
    - Reversible with naloxone.
  - Morphine
    - Provides analgesia, sedation, and anxiolysis.
    - Dosage in adults is 1-2 mg every 5 minutes, titrate to effect.
    - Dosage in peds is 0.1-0.2 mg/kg/dose.
    - 10-30 minutes are required before its peak effects are seen.
    - Complications: Respiratory depression, hypotension, allergic reactions, itching, nausea, and vomiting.
    - Reversible with naloxone.
- Sedative hypnotics: Provide sedation, amnesia, anxiolysis, and anticonvulsant effects
  - Midazolam
    - One of the most commonly used sedative medications for both adults and peds, as it is safe, effective, and short-acting.
    - Dose in adults is 1-2 mg IV titrated to max of 5 mg; 5 mg/0.07 mg/kg IM.
    - Dose in peds is 0.05-0.1 mg/kg IV titrated to max of 0.6 mg/kg (dosage lower in older kids); intramuscular (IM) 0.1-0.15 mg/kg.
    - Complications: Respiratory depression, hypotension.
    - Reversible with flumazenil.
  - Etomidate
    - Commonly used agent, causes minimal hypotension, frequently used in the ED.
    - Onset of action: 30-60 seconds, peak effect: 1 minute.
    - Duration: 3-5 minutes.
    - Dosage in adults: 0.1-0.2 mg/kg over 30-60 seconds.
    - Not Food and Drug Administration (FDA) approved in children but commonly used.
    - Complications: Nausea, vomiting on emergence, myoclonus, hiccups, adrenal suppression, respiratory depression.
    - Not reversible.
  - Propofol
    - Commonly used sedative in intensive care unit (ICU); becoming more commonly used in ED.
    - Resolves within 5-10 minutes upon discontinuation of the infusion.
    - Not a reliable amnestic, has antiemetic properties.
    - Dosage in adults: 2-2.5 mg/kg given as 40 mg IV q10 seconds until induction onset in young and healthy adults, 1-1.5 mg/kg given as 20 mg IV q10 seconds until induction in the elderly or debilitate.
    - Complications: Cardiovascular depression.
    - Usually analgesic agents are given in addition.
- Dissociative agent
  - Ketamine: Preferred agent for procedural sedation that can be used as a solo agent.
  - "Dissociative" hypnotic that provides sedation and analgesia with minimal respiratory depression.

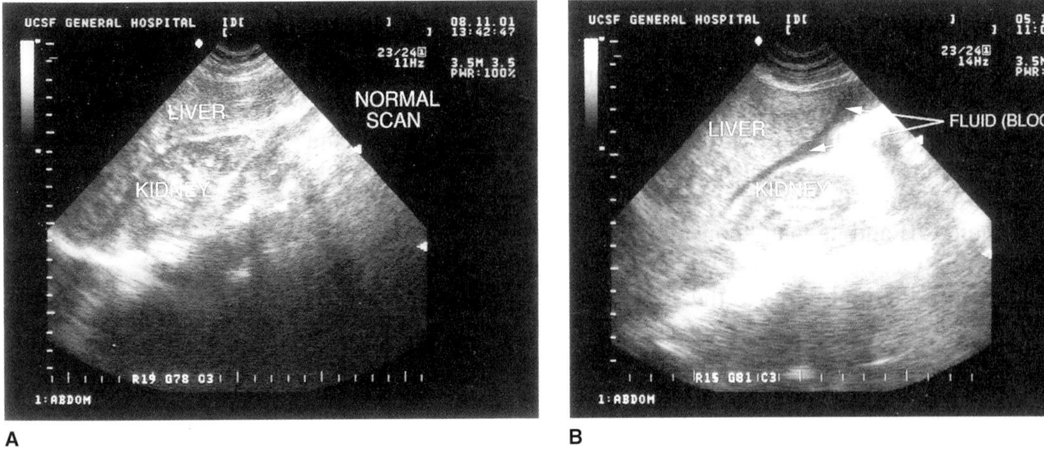

Figure 6-3. **(A)** Normal ultrasound of the right upper quadrant. **(B)** Right upper quadrant ultrasound revealing blood between the liver and the kidney and between the liver and the diaphragm. (*Reprinted with permission from Doherty GM.* Current Surgical Diagnosis and Treatment. *12th ed. New York, NY: McGraw-Hill. 2006.*)

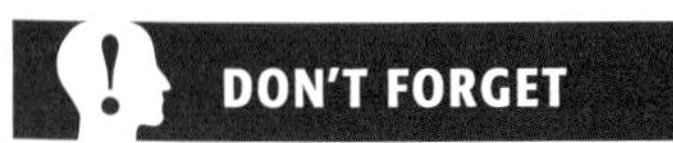

Placing the patient into a Trendelenburg position may increase the amount of blood in the upper abdomen, making it easier to see on FAST scan.

- FAST: Cardiac examination: "I will place the probe at the subxiphoid space and project the probe toward the left nipple, identifying the chambers of the heart looking for any fluid collection that follows the contours of the heart. If this view is indeterminate, or too difficult to obtain, I will obtain a parasternal view by placing the probe in the third or fourth intercostal space just left of the sternum." (Fig. 6-6)

Pelvic-transvaginal US

- Use as an adjunct to the pelvic examination in any women with positive pregnancy test to identify an intrauterine pregnancy (IUP).
- Perform a transabdominal scan before a transvaginal approach, to view the full contents of the pelvis.

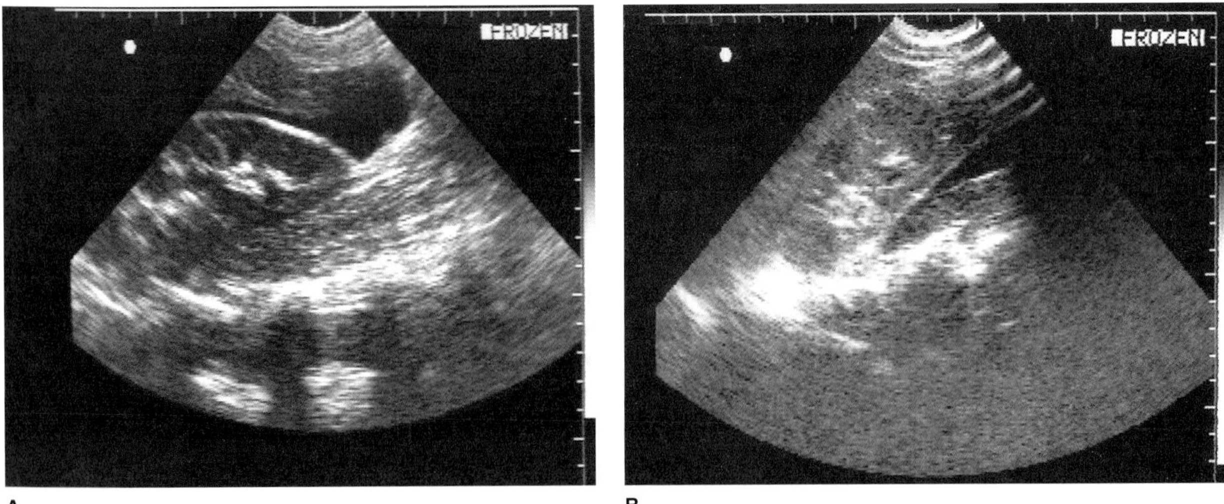

6-4. Free fluid versus retroperitoneal fluid. Right coronal views. **(A)** Free peritoneal fluid in the paracolic gutter (adjacent to the of the right kidney). **(B)** Contained retroperitoneal fluid (pararenal space) overlying the psoas muscle stripe and medial to the *ted with permission from Ma OJ, Mateer JR, Blaivas M.* Emergency Ultrasound. *2nd ed. New York, NY: McGraw-Hill.*

SECTION 3

CARDINAL SYMPTOMS

CHAPTER 7

Fever

Mohammad Subeh and James Ahn

DON'T FORGET

On test day every adult with fever has...

- UTI
- Endocarditis
- Neutropenic fever
- HIV-/AIDS-related illness
- Cellulitis/necrotizing fasciitis
- Thyroid storm
- Intra-abdominal infection
- Pneumonia, or
- Meningitis

...until proven otherwise.

IMMEDIATE INTERVENTIONS

- Oxygen via NC or NRB to keep O_2 >95%.
- Cardiac monitor with rhythm strip.
- 18-gauge IV × 2.
- 0.9% NS 30 cc/kg bolus.
- Draw blood and two sets of blood cultures for lab studies.
- Lactate.
- ECG.
- CXR.
- UA and urine culture.
- Urine pregnancy for any female of childbearing age.
- Initiate empiric antibiotics (don't forget to ask about allergies before starting antibiotics).
- Consider vasopressor initiation via central line in patients with septic shock.
- Bedside ultrasound of the IVC an echocardiogram may be helpful in assessing volume responsiveness.

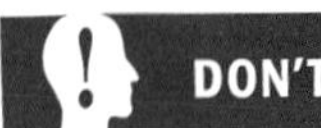

DON'T FORGET

Stabilize any life threats by managing the airway, aggressive fluid resuscitation, and early IV antibiotics ›r bacterial infections. Do NOT move ›rd with the case unless life- ave been stabilized.

INITIAL ASSESSMENT

Focus on age, comorbid conditions—cancer, human immunodeficiency virus (HIV), diabetes, vital signs (VS), including pulse oximetry, general appearance, evidence of rheumatologic disorders, and any potential foci of infection, including skin for cellulitis, perirectal abscess, or infected decubitus ulcers.

INITIAL HISTORY AND PHYSICAL EXAMINATION

History

- History of present illness (HPI)
  - Gradual or sudden onset of fever.
  - Any localizing symptoms—cough, dysuria, headache, urinary symptoms, etc.
  - Joint pains and/or joint swelling.
  - Any new rashes.
  - Recent malaise or other constitutional symptoms.
  - Recent hospitalizations or infections.
  - Recent antibiotics.
  - Recent travel or exposure to ill contacts.
  - Recent sick contacts.
- Past medical history (PMHx)
  - Any comorbid conditions such as cancer, lupus, HIV, diabetes mellitus (DM)?
  - Any risk factors for HIV/AIDS—unprotected sexual exposure? Intravenous drug use (IVDU)? Partner with risk factors for HIV?
  - Any risk factors for endocarditis—Rheumatic heart disease? IVDU? Valve replacement? Mitral valve prolapse (MVP)? Cocaine use?
  - Any recent hospitalizations that could predispose to nosocomial infections?
- Medications
  - If history of cancer, most recent chemotherapy
  - Immunosuppressive agents (eg, steroids, chemotherapy).
- Allergies

Spectrum of sepsis

- Systemic inflammatory response syndrome (SIRS)
  - WBC <4000 cells/mm^3, WBC >12,000 cells/ mm^3, or bandemia >10%.
  - Temp <36°C or >38°F.
  - RR >20 bpm or $PaCO_2$ <32 mm Hg.
  - HR >90 bpm.
- Sepsis
  - Two of four SIRS criteria plus suspected infection.
- Severe sepsis
  - Sepsis plus evidence of end-organ hypo-perfusion (eg, acute kidney injury [AKI], altered mental status (AMS), hypotension, demand cardiac ischemia, lactate elevation).
- Septic shock
  - Severe sepsis plus hypotension despite 30 cc/kg intravenous fluid (IVF) bolus.

Physical Examination

- VS including pulse oximetry.
- Neck: Goiter? Neck stiffness?
- Chest: Lung sounds for rhonchi or diminished breath sounds.

- Cardiovascular (CV): Tachycardia in proportion to fever? New murmur?
- Back: Costovertebral angle (CVA) tenderness?
- Abdomen: Localized tenderness?
- Genitourinary (GU): Fournier gangrene?
- Skin: Evidence of skin breakdown or abscess? Erythema or tenderness of lower extremities? Petechiae? Splinter hemorrhages? Oslers or Janeway lesions? Rashes, especially purpura or petechiae? Vesicular lesions?
- Neuro: AMS? Symmetric motor, sensory, deep tendon relfexes (DTRs)? Kernig or Brudzinski signs?
- Musculo-Skeletal (MSK): Joint swelling, joint tenderness, limited joint range of motion (ROM)

DON'T FORGET

Ask for a detailed history and inspect the patient fully in order to find the source of bacteremia in these patients!

DIFFERENTIAL DIAGNOSIS

The differential for fever in an adult is wide, but the most likely diagnosis in the oral board examination of an adult with fever will be among the following:

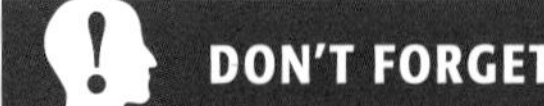

Be certain to ask a detailed social history in these patients (including sexual history and drug abuse history).

UTI

- The term urinary tract infection (UTI) encompasses both upper and lower tract infections from pyelonephritis to simple cystitis. Clinically, this can be determined by duration of symptoms and location of symptoms such as flank pain or dysuria.

Endocarditis

- Damage to the endothelium caused by abnormal hemodynamic states from preexisting valvular or congenital heart defects leads to the development of sterile vegetations composed of platelets and fibrin. Damaged valves can become infected by transient bacteremia, which colonize the vegetations, leading to infective endocarditis (IE).
- The history of any predisposing factor for IE with a fever and a cardiac murmur should lead you to suspect this diagnosis and order a transesophageal echocardiography (TEE). History and physical will help determine if the patient has acute or subacute endocarditis.
- Acute infective endocarditis is characterized by a sudden onset of fever, hematogenous seeding of extracardiac sites, and rapid damage of cardiac structures. This disease will result in mortality within weeks if left untreated.
- Subacute endocarditis has a more indolent course with slow development and progression of cardiac structural damage and rarely spreads to extracardiac sites.

Neutropenic fever

- Most fevers (55%-70%) occurring in cancer patients have an infectious etiology. Patients with neutropenia (fewer polymorphonuclear leukocytes (PMNs) than 500/mm^3) have an increased risk of infection.
- Infection is the number one cause of cancer death and if left untreated in this population has up to 48% mortality. Therefore, any cancer patient with fever and neutropenia should be presumed to have an infection and started on antibiotics as soon as appropriate cultures have been obtained.

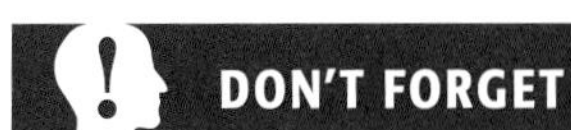

Treat all neutropenic fever patients with broad-spectrum antibiotics as soon as the cultures are sent!

HIV/AIDS

- Fevers associated with HIV infection have a broad differential from acute HIV infection to complications of end-stage AIDS. History and physical along with information from co-historians (family members, private physicians) will be very important in making the diagnosis.
- Do not forget to ask any potential historians (friends or family) you are given to wait in the waiting room so that you can use them as needed!

Cellulitis/necrotizing fasciitis

- Cellulitis is an infection of the skin and subcutaneous tissues characterized by redness, warmth, and swelling. Though usually not life threatening,

cellulitis is a frequently overlooked cause of fever, but can usually be diagnosed easily if the patient is undressed, rolled, and examined completely. Consider performing a bedside soft tissue ultrasound to rule out abscess, which would require an incision and drainage.
- In contrast, deep cutaneous infections and necrotizing infections of the skin constitute a serious threat to life and limb, but may appear benign at initial presentation. The hallmark feature of deep cutaneous cellulitis, Fournier gangrene, and necrotizing fasciitis is crepitus secondary to gas formation.
- Patients with deep cutaneous infections or necrotizing fasciitis are sick and require aggressive resuscitation, early antibiotics, and early surgical consultation and intervention. Mortality may be as high as 75%.

Thyroid storm
- The most severe form of hyperthyroidism, usually following a long history of uncomplicated hyperthyroidism, is a life-threatening disorder if not managed quickly.
- The classic hyperthyroid symptoms have been present for some time-agitation, nervousness, palpitations, and weight loss. Signs to look for include ophthalmopathy, goiter, fever, and tachycardia.
- Be careful to look for evidence of high-output cardiac failure and manage this quickly with beta-blockers and antithyroid treatment!
- Intra-abdominal infection: See Chap. 12
- Meningitis: See Chap. 18
- Pneumonia: See Chap. 10

URINARY TRACT INFECTIONS

Additional History and Physical Examination Findings

- UTIs are the second most common infection encountered by physicians.
- Separate acute uncomplicated cystitis from acute uncomplicated pyelonephritis and complicated UTI cases based on history and physical examination.
- The elderly, pregnant women, immunecompromised, and diabetic patients are more prone to complications such as subclinical pyelonephritis or developing urosepsis.
- The classic symptoms of dysuria, frequency, urgency, flank pain, back pain, hematuria, fever, and suprapubic pain may not be present depending on the patient.
- Ask about urethral or vaginal discharge and do a full GU examination since dysuria may be confused with urethritis.
- Be certain to consider kidney stones as a nidus for infection.

Review Initial Results

- Urine dip: +leukocyte esterase and +nitrites on dipstick suggests UTI.
- Urine analysis
  - Greater than 20 WBC/high-power field on microscopic suggests UTI.
  - RBCs on microscopic suggests a stone as a nidus for infection and will require CT imaging to assess for nephrolithiasis.
- Blood, urea, nitrogen/creatinine (BUN/Cr): Be certain to make sure that the patient has no evidence of renal failure that would place the patient in a high-risk category for urosepsis.
- Urine pregnancy: Pregnant women should receive a different class of antibiotics, longer duration of treatment, and be managed more conservatively than nonpregnant women.

Management Priorities

- Resuscitation for septic patients and intensive care unit (ICU) admission.
- Identify high-risk patients early
  - Pregnant patients.
  - Diabetic patients.
  - Septic patients (two of four SIRS criteria and suspected infection).
- Early IV or PO antibiotics.
- Source control.
- CT abdomen and pelvis to evaluate for urolithiasis.

Definitive Management and Disposition

- Acute uncomplicated cystitis in women
  - 3-day course of PO Trimethoprim/sulfamethoxazole (TMP/SMX) or a fluoroquinolone if not pregnant.
  - 7-day course of antibiotics for diabetic patients, prolonged symptoms (>7 days), recent UTI, age >65 years, or pregnancy.
- Acute uncomplicated pyelonephritis (not pregnant, not septic).
  - 7-10 days of a PO fluoroquinolone.
- Complicated UTI (any patient with underlying neurologic, structural, or medical problems, and male patients).
  - IV antibiotics such as ceftriaxone.
- Aggressive fluid resuscitation.
- Pain control.
- Fever control with ibuprofen or acetaminophen.
- Foley catheter placement if patient has urinary retention.

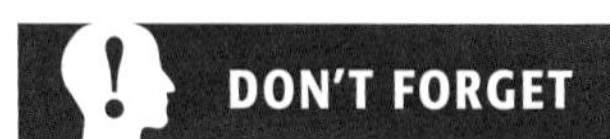

Don't forget to check pregnancy status on all women of childbearing age if you suspect UTI.

Disposition

- Uncomplicated cystitis in pregnant or nonpregnant patients can be discharged home.
- Uncomplicated pyelonephritis in nonpregnant patients who can tolerate oral hydration can be discharged home.
- Complicated pyelonephritis or pyelonephritis in pregnant patients must be admitted for IV antibiotics.
- Patients with infected urolithiasis should be admitted to urology for IV antibiotics and stent placement.
- Patients with severe sepsis or septic shock should be admitted to ICU for aggressive resuscitation, IV antibiotics, and close monitoring.

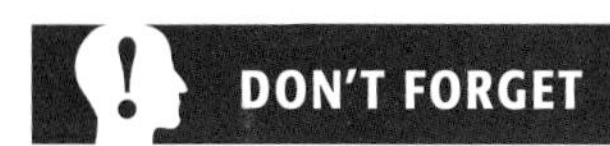

Consider emphysematous pyelonephritis or a perinephric abscess in very ill-appearing diabetic patients with UTI.

ENDOCARDITIS

Additional History and Physical Examination Findings

- Most patients with endocarditis have an underlying cause such as rheumatic or congenital heart disease, calcific degenerative valve disease, prosthetic heart valve, mitral valve prolapse (MVP), a history of IV drug use, or history of endocarditis.
- IV drug use places the patient at high risk for right-sided endocarditis.
- Usually, a subclinical bacteremia precedes the onset of symptoms of bacterial endocarditis by approximately 1 week.
- A number of surgical procedures may result in transient bacteremia including dental, GU, or gastrointestinal (GI) procedures.
- Symptoms of infective endocarditis are nonspecific and diverse with the most common symptoms being malaise (95%) and intermittent fever (85%).
- Early in the presentation, a cardiac murmur is often not present.
- Classic triad associated with endocarditis is fever, anemia, and a heart murmur.

- More than 50% of patients will have some form of vasculitic lesion, including petechiae, splinter hemorrhages, Osler nodes (painful tender nodules on palmar surface of fingertip), or Janeway lesions (painless, erythematous, flat, macular lesions on palm and soles).
- 30% of patients will have splenomegaly.

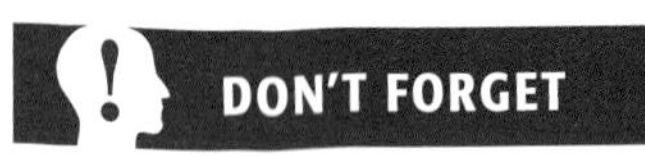

Look for vasculitic lesions if you suspect endocarditis to help make your diagnosis.

Review Initial Results

- Electrocardiogram (ECG): May have conduction abnormalities if an abscess has formed in the myocardium
- Erthrocyte sedimentaiton rate (ESR) or c-reactive protein (CRP): May be elevated, nonspecific.
- Complete blood count (CBC): WBC count may be elevated but this only occurs in 50% of cases.
- Mild anemia is present in most cases.
- Urinalysis (UA): More than 50% of patients with endocarditis have hematuria resulting from embolic lesions of the kidney.
- Bedside ultrasound or transthoracic echocardiography (TTE): Although not the diagnostic test of choice and endocarditis cannot be ruled out with a normal TTE, if a vegetation is seen on a valve, then the diagnosis is made.

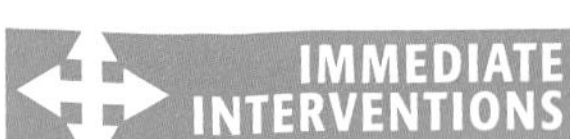

- Three sets of blood cultures.
- TEE to confirm diagnosis.
- Empiric IV antibiotics after cultures are drawn.

Management Priorities

- Obtain three sets of blood cultures prior to antibiotics.
- Empiric IV antibiotics and admission.
- Early consultation with cardiology to set up for definitive diagnostic tests such as TEE that has a negative predictive value of 95%.

Definitive Management

- Empiric antibiotics with vancomycin and gentamicin or ceftriaxone and gentamicin.

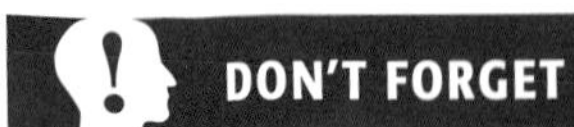

Call cardiology early to set up a TEE once you suspect endocarditis or cardiovascular surgery if you suspect valvular incompetence causing CHF!

Complications

- Severe congestive heart failure (CHF) can occur if there is significant valvular incompetence and requires emergent cardiac surgery.
- Para-valvular leak can occur around a prosthetic valve and requires emergent cardiac surgery.
- Embolic phenomena can occur, causing neurologic deficits or deficits to any organ system.

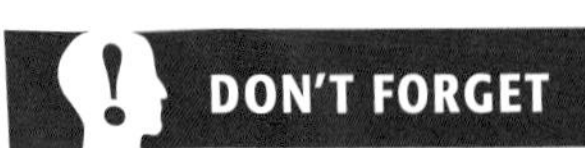

Give antibiotics early to the patients with neutropenic fever or they will go into septic shock on your exam day!

Disposition

- Medical admission to floor for IV antibiotics if patient appears well.
- Cardiac care unit (CCU) admission if patient appears ill and/or requires resuscitation.
- Advocate for the operating room (OR) if severe CHF develops from valvular incompetence or para-valvular leak around a prosthetic valve.

NEUTROPENIC FEVER

Additional History and Physical Examination Findings

- Most fevers occurring in cancer patients have an infectious etiology.
- Neutropenia, defined as fewer PMNs than 500/mm^3, predisposes the patient to an increased risk of infection.
- Fever is the first and sometimes only sign of infection.
- All subtle signs of inflammation or areas of pain should be considered serious as the patient may not be able to mount an aggressive inflammatory response and could be the initial presentation of a necrotizing fasciitis.

- All portals of entry must be inspected carefully including mucous membranes and the perineal region.
- Consider all indwelling catheters as potential sites of infection.
- Pneumonia may be found by auscultation only, if the neutropenia prevents a visible infiltrate from developing.
- Digital rectal examination is relatively contraindicated in neutropenic patients and should be withheld until after the initial antibiotic administration.
- Consider line infections if patient recently had peripherally inserted central catheter (PICC) or port placed or accessed.

Review Initial Results

- CBC-WBC: Multiply the WBC by percentage of PMNs to calculate the absolute neutrophil count (ANC).
- The patient is at very high risk if the ANC is 500/mm^3 or less.
- Chest x-ray (CXR): Look for an infiltrate to suggest pneumonia.
- UA: Review for evidence of UTI specifically WBC, leukocyte esterase, or nitrites.

Management Priorities

- Aggressively resuscitate any unstable patient with IV fluid boluses.
- Blood cultures (×2) and urine culture prior to antibiotics.
- Consider culture of sputum, stool, or wound drainage if productive cough, diarrhea, or wound drainage present, respectively.
- Lumbar puncture (LP) is not part of routine cultures unless patient has signs or symptoms of meningitis or encephalitis.
- Broad-spectrum IV antibiotics.
- Place the patient in an isolation room and request strict hand washing and reverse isolation techniques are practiced.
- Consult infectious disease as part of the workup.
- If the source of fever is identified, be certain to consult the most appropriate specialist to be involved with the case.

Complications

- Neutropenic patients are at high risk for severe sepsis and septic shock; be sure to continuously reevaluate the patients' vital signs.

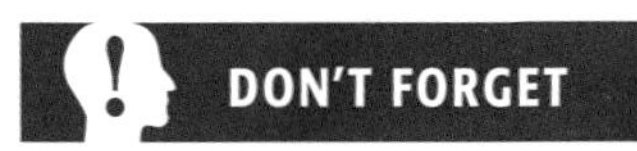

Do not perform a rectal examination on neutropenic patients or you may precipitate bacteremia.

Disposition

- Admit all neutropenic patients with fever to medical floor isolation rooms for IV antibiotics.
- All unstable patients go to the medical intensive care unit (MICU) for close observation and IV antibiotics.

HIV/AIDS

Additional History and Physical Examination Findings

- Fever in HIV has a very large differential, including infectious disease, malignancies, and drug reactions.
- History should include time of diagnosis, any previous AIDS-defining illnesses, recent hospitalizations, any relevant medical history, surgical history, current medications including highly active anti-retroviral therapy (HAART) meds, prophylactic antibiotics, and allergies.
- Also, inquire about the most recent HIV viral load and CD4 counts.
- The patient may not give you a history of HIV but the history may be available through risk factors, historians with the patient, and old records.

- For patients with a fever without a given history of HIV, be certain to ask about common risk factors—any sexual partner with known HIV, unprotected sexual activity, blood transfusions, or hemophilia.
- Ask about any symptoms both from the patient and any historians with the patient, including cough, diarrhea, recent weight loss, and any neurologic changes.
- Hemoptysis suggests pneumococcal pneumonia and/or tuberculosis (TB).
- Nonproductive cough suggests *Pneumocystis jiroveci* pneumonia (formerly *Pneumocystis carinii* pneumonia [PCP]), fungal infection, or neoplasm.
- Examine the oral mucous membranes for evidence of thrush.
- Examine the fundi for evidence of cytomegalovirus (CMV) retinitis.
- Examine the skin for evidence of any skin findings such as Kaposi's sarcoma.

Review Initial Results

- CBC: Look for evidence of neutropenia that would put patient at higher risk for bacterial infections.
- CXR:
  - Focal infiltrates suggesting bacterial pneumonia or diffuse infiltrative process suggesting PCP.
  - Hilar lymphadenopathy with diffuse pulmonary infiltrates suggests *Cryptococcus*, histoplasmosis, mycobacterial pneumonia, or neoplasm.
  - Nodular lesions suggest Kaposi's sarcoma, TB, mycobacterium avium complex (MAC), or toxoplasmosis.
- Pulse oximetry: Oxygen saturation of <95% should prompt further pulmonary workup and suggests PCP or other pulmonary infection.
- Arterial blood gas (ABG): Steroids are required in patients with PCP and a Pa_{O_2} <70 mm Hg or an A-a gradient of >35 mm Hg.
- Lactate dehydrogenase (LDH): Elevated LDH suggests PCP.

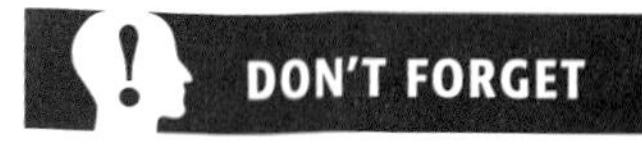

Be sure to ask a detailed social history from the patient and from all historians when treating patients with fever. They may not give you a history of HIV/AIDS until you get more information!

Management Priorities

- First, ensure stability of patient: Airway, breathing, and circulation must be rapidly assessed.
- Any abnormalities with the ABCs should be promptly addressed and rechecked after appropriate intervention.
- Blood should be drawn and sent for CBC, electrolytes, liver function tests (LFTs), lactate, and blood cultures (for aerobic, anaerobic, and fungal).
- UA, urine culture, and CXR should be done.
- Send QuantiFERON Gold test and sputum culture to evaluate for TB.
- Any patient, with no identifiable source of fever with neurologic signs or symptoms, should have an LP after a computed tomography (CT) has been performed. Be sure to obtain an opening pressure!
- Be certain to consult an infectious disease specialist as part of the workup.

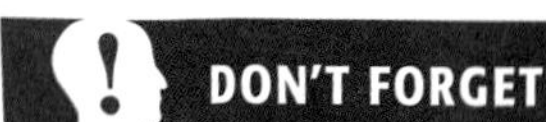

Hypoxia out of proportion to CXR findings in HIV/AIDS = PCP

Complications

- Be certain to continue to recheck these patients for any clinical change after any interventions since they are at high risk for severe sepsis and septic shock.

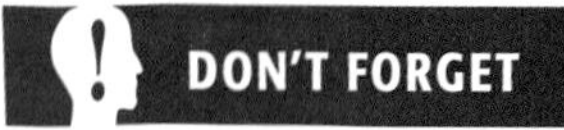

ny HIV patient with
and fever for possible TB
ely etiology is found.

Disposition

- If the patient appears well and has close follow-up ensured by a private physician, discharge can be considered.
- Most of these patients need admission and IV antibiotic therapy tailored to their complaints.
- Have a very low threshold for admitting them , as well as, placing them in respiratory isolation if TB is suspected.

CELLULITIS/NECROTIZING FASCIITIS

Additional History and Physical Examination Findings

- Cellulitis classically presents with redness, warmth, and swelling (Fig. 7-1A).
- The site of infection is painful.
- Lymphangitis or streaking can be observed proximally with lymphadenopathy of the local and regional nodes.
- Crepitant cellulitis usually involves the lower limbs of patients with peripheral arterial disease.
- Fournier gangrene is a necrotizing cellulitis involving the genitalia and perineum occurring in elderly patients with serious comorbidities such as diabetes, CHF, or renal failure.
- Fournier gangrene often develops rapidly; the patient appears systemically ill with high fever.
- The site of infection is severely painful and the skin appears blue-gray.
- Necrotizing fasciitis involves subcutaneous tissue and fascia where the skin appears red and mildly painful and later becomes mottled, discolored, and edematous (Fig. 7-1B).
- Crepitus is a classic sign of necrotizing fasciitis.

Review of Initial Results

- CBC: Elevated WBC count is common.

Risk Stratification

- Cellulitis: High-risk patients are patients with systemic toxicity, diabetes, or involvement of areas such as face, orbit, hand, and perineum.
- Patients with deep cutaneous infections or necrotizing fasciitis are all at high risk.
- The diagnosis of necrotizing fasciitis will be suggested by unstable vital signs, significant comorbidities, and evidence of systemic illness.

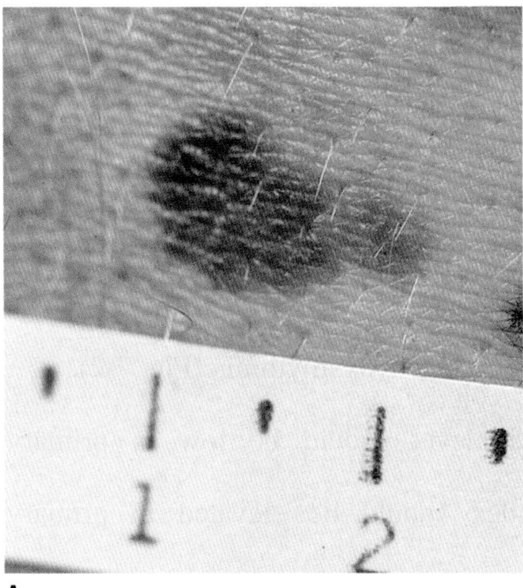

A

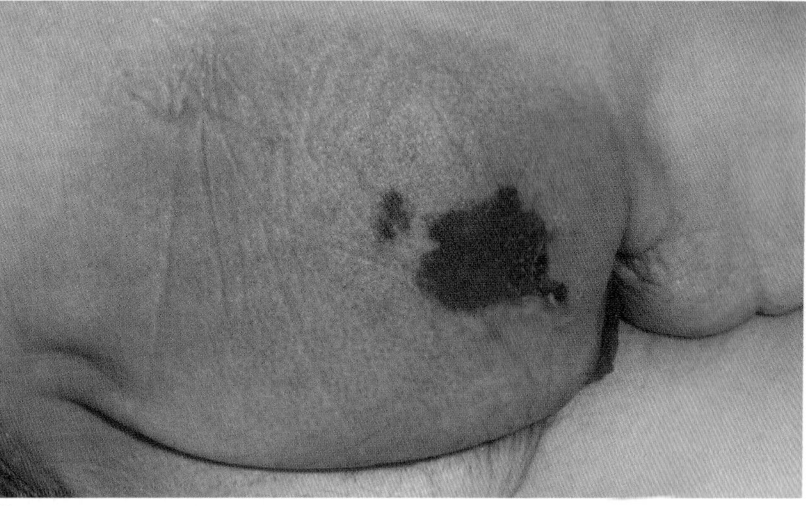

B

Figure 7-1. **(A)** Cellulitis of the left leg characterized by erythema and mild swelling. **(B)** Necrotizing fasciitis of buttock seen as erythema, edema, and progressing area of necrosis. (*Reprinted with permission from Wolff K, Johnson RA.* Fitzpatrick's Color Atlas and Synopsis of Clinical Dermatology. *6th ed. New York, NY: McGraw-Hill; 2009.*)

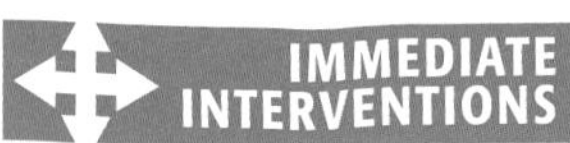

IMMEDIATE INTERVENTIONS

- Soft tissue x-ray of extremity to assess for gas.
- Consider ultrasound to rule out localized infection or abscess.

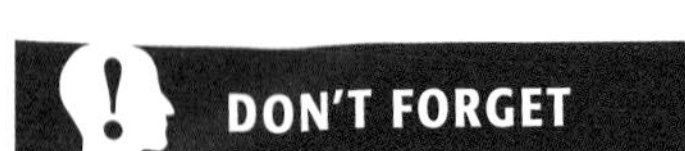

DON'T FORGET

You are unlikely to encounter a patient with simple cellulitis at ABEM General. Suspect necrotizing fasciitis, Fournier gangrene, diabetic foot, or other complicating features.

Definitive Management

- Aggressive fluid resuscitation
- Antibiotics:
  - For simple cellulitis, use nafcillin 2 g IV q6h or cefazolin 1-2 g q6h.
  - For any suspected methicillin-resistant staphylococcus aureus (MRSA) infections, use vancomycin 20 mg/kg IV q12h.
  - For diabetic foot cellulitis, use piperacillin/tazobactam 3.375 g IV q6h and vancomycin 20 mg/kg q12h.
  - For deep cutaneous infections, use piperacillin/tazobactam 3.0 g IV q4-6h and clindamycin 600-900 mg q8h and vancomycin 20 mg/kg q12h.
- Early surgical consultation for operative debridement of necrotizing tissue is mandatory.
- Consider hyperbaric oxygen, in consultation with surgery if immediately available.

Disposition

- All high-risk patients with cellulitis should be admitted to the hospital for IV antibiotics.
- Patients with cellulitis and no high-risk features may be discharged.
- All patients with deep cutaneous infections or necrotizing fasciitis should be admitted to the ICU after a surgical evaluation in the ED.

THYROID STORM

Additional History and Physical Examination Findings

- Classically, the history includes weight loss (20-40 lb), palpitations, agitation, heat intolerance, and nervousness.
- Less common symptoms include chest pain, dyspnea, edema, psychosis, disorientation, diarrhea, and abdominal pain.
- Classic signs include fever, tachycardia, wide pulse pressure, CHF, thyromegaly, tremor, and thyrotoxic stare/lid retraction.
- Less common signs are weakness, shock, somnolence, coma, jaundice, and pretibial myxedema.
- Ask about any precipitating factors of thyroid storm such as infections, recent surgery, emotional stress, or trauma.
- Other precipitating factors may include contrast radiographic studies and drug reactions or complications from diabetes.
- Be certain to palpate the thyroid for thyromegaly since most cases of thyroid storm are secondary to toxic diffuse goiter.
- Be certain to check a fingerstick for elevated blood glucose since hypoglycemia and diabetic ketoacidosis (DKA) can precipitate thyroid storm.

Review Initial Results

- Blood sugar: Hyperglycemia is present in up to 55% of patients.
- ECG may show sinus tachycardia or atrial tachydysrhythmia (Fig. 7-2).
- CXR: To rule out CHF.
- Thyroid-stimulating hormone (TSH) level should be low in primary hyperthyroidism.
- Free T4 level and/or free T4 index should be elevated in primary hyperthyroidism.
- LFTs are often mildly elevated in thyroid storm even without evidence of CHF.

Management Priorities

- Stabilize patients aggressively and address any abnormalities in airway, breathing, or circulation immediately and recheck to ensure adequacy of any interventions made.

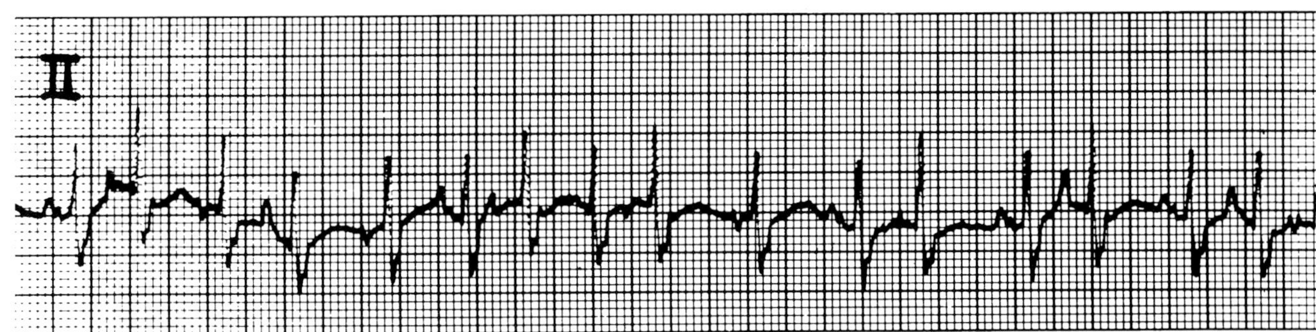

Figure 7-2. Multifocal atrial tachycardia. (*Reproduced with permission from Tintinalli JE, Kelen GD, Stapczynski JS, et al.* Emergency Medicine: A Comprehensive Study Guide. *6th ed. New York, NY: McGraw-Hill; 2004.*)

- Address any CHF early with beta-blockers (beta-blockade not contraindicated in CHF secondary to thyrotoxicosis).
- Investigate and address any precipitating factors for thyroid storm such as infections or DKA.
- Consult endocrinologist as soon as possible.

Definitive Management

- Block peripheral adrenergic stimulation.
  - Beta-blockers are the best drugs to accomplish this blockade.
  - Propranolol is the preferred beta-blocker because of its additional ability to block peripheral conversion of T4 to T3.
  - Propranolol should be given as slow 1-2 mg boluses repeated every 10-15 minutes until the desired effect is achieved.
  - Oral propranolol can then be started at 20-120 mg/dose.
- Prevent peripheral hormone conversion.
  - Propylthiouracil (PTU), propranolol, or dexamethasone all block peripheral conversion of T4 to T3.
  - Dexamethasone is the most effective drug of these and should be given as 4 mg IV every 6 hours.
- Block hormone release.
  - Iodine or lithium can inhibit thyroid hormone release.
  - Iodine is preferred because it is less toxic and easier to titrate.
  - PTU should be given at least 1 hour prior to iodine to prevent organification of the iodine. If iodide is given prior to this 1 hour period, then this can create increased hormone production and worsening of the storm state.
  - Iodine can be given as
    - Lugol solution: 30 drops per day in three to four divided doses PO or by nasogastric tube (NGT)
    - Potassium iodide (SSKI): 5 drops every 6 hours PO or by NGT.
    - Sodium iodide: 1 g slow IV drip every 8-12 hours.
- Inhibit hormone synthesis.
  - PTU and methimazole block thyroid hormone production.
  - PTU is preferred because it also inhibits peripheral conversion of T4 to T3.
  - PTU is given 600-1000 mg PO, followed by 200-250 mg every 4-6 hours.

Complications

- CHF can be caused by thyroid storm and should be treated with oxygen, diuretics, and beta-blocker therapy.

DON'T FORGET

Most patients in thyroid storm have been hyperthyroid for a period of time. Ask all historians about symptoms of hyperthyroidism if patient is unable to provide history.

DON'T FORGET

Most patients in thyroid storm have a precipitating stressor. Remember to check common stressors such as hyperglycemia or infection!

DON'T FORGET

Although beta-blockers are usually not indicated in CHF, thyroid storm causes high-output failure and requires beta-blockade!

DON'T FORGET

Treat thyroid storm in the following order:

1. Decrease adrenergic stimulation—Propranolol (also blocks T4 →T3 conversion)
2. Block new thyroid hormone production—PTU followed by iodine (after 1 hour!)
3. Decrease peripheral T4 → T3 conversion—Dexamethasone

DON'T FORGET

Avoid aspirin in thyroid storm. Salicylates displace thyroid hormone from TBG and make the condition worse!

- Atrial tachydysrhythmias may occur and will likely revert to sinus rhythm after antithyroid therapy is initiated.
- Hyperpyrexia from thyrotoxicosis should not be treated with aspirin because it displaces thyroid hormone from thyroid-binding globulin (TBG).
- Hyperpyrexia should be treated with acetaminophen, ice packs, and hypothermia blankets.
- Dehydration is a common complication caused by fever, diarrhea, and vomiting associated with thyroid storm, and requires fluid replacement.

Disposition

- All patients with thyroid storm should be admitted.
- Any patient with thyroid storm and CV complications (CHF or tachydysrhythmias) should be admitted to the CCU.
- All patients with thyroid storm should have endocrine consultants involved with their care.
- All patients with CV complications of thyroid storm should have cardiology consultation.

WINNING STRATEGIES

- Every patient with fever has a UTI, endocarditis, neutropenic fever, HIV-/AIDS-related illness, thyroid storm, cellulitis, pneumonia, or meningitis until proven otherwise.
- Patients with fever require a complete H + P, including interviewing other historians, to help determine cause of fever.
- Give antibiotics and initiate fluid resuscitation early.
- Evaluate the severity of the septic patient with a lactate level.
- Before treating a female of childbearing age for a UTI, be sure to check a pregnancy test.
- TEE is the test of choice for endocarditis—call the cardiologist early!
- Look for the classic triad in endocarditis of fever, anemia, and heart murmur.
- Assume all neutropenic patients have an infection and impending sepsis until proven otherwise.
- Isolate all patients with HIV/AIDS, fever, and hemoptysis until TB is ruled out.
- Most patients in thyroid storm have had hyperthyroidism for some time; be sure to ask about symptoms of hyperthyroidism.
- Investigate potential stressors for patients in thyroid storm such as infection or hyperglycemia.
- Reassess patients following all interventions.

THE BOTTOM LINE

- The history is often the key to making the diagnosis in these scenarios.
- Call any necessary consultants early.
- Blood cultures, urine and urine culture, ECG, and CXR for every patient with fever.
- Recognize sepsis and initiate early fluids, antibiotics, and source control.
- Treat fever with antipyretics.
- Assume the most life-threatening causes of fever until proven otherwise.

CHAPTER 8

Chest Pain

Seth Trueger and James Ahn

DON'T FORGET

Every CP patient has either

- ACS
- Aortic dissection
- PE
- Pneumothorax

......until proven otherwise.

IMMEDIATE INTERVENTIONS

- Oxygen via NC or NRB to keep O2 >95%.
- Cardiac monitor with rhythm strip.
- 18-gauge IV, 0.9% NS at KVO, draw blood for laboratory studies.
- ECG: Obtain within 10 minutes.
- CXR: Demonstrated to change management in 15%-20% of patients with chest pain.
- Stabilize life threats by managing airway, aggressive resuscitation, and tube thoracostomy.

INITIAL ASSESSMENT

- Focus on age, vital signs (VS), general appearance—cyanosis? Diaphoresis? Lung sounds?
- Identify unstable patients with immediate life threats.
  - Tension pneumothorax
  - Shock

INITIAL HISTORY AND PHYSICAL EXAMINATION

History

- History of present illness (HPI)
  - Onset—Was this exertional?
  - Quality/severity.
  - Location/radiation/migration.
  - Duration.
  - Exacerbating/alleviating factors.
  - Diaphoresis, nausea, vomiting, shortness of breath.
  - Pleuritic component.
  - Lower extremity pain or swelling.
- Past medical history (PMHx)
  - Prior heart disease.
  - Cardiac risk factors: Diabetes mellitus (DM), hypertension (HTN), positive family history (FH), hyperlipidemia (HL), smoking.
- Medications
- Allergies

Physical Examination

- VS (order BP in both arms).
- Neck: Trachea midline, jugular venous distention (JVD), supple, hepatojugular reflux?
- Chest: Breath sounds equal, crackles, wheezes?
- CV: Murmurs, rubs, gallops? Peripheral pulses symmetric?
- Extremities: Cyanosis, edema, tenderness?
- Neuro: Motor, sensory, deep tendon reflex (DTR) symmetric?

DIFFERENTIAL DIAGNOSIS

- Acute coronary syndrome
  - The term acute coronary syndrome (ACS) refers to a spectrum of disease from unstable angina (UA) to acute myocardial infarction (AMI) and applies to patients with active cardiac ischemia, injury, or infarction.
  - Clinically, we divide ACS into ST-segment-elevation myocardial infarction (STEMI), non–ST-segment-elevation myocardial infarction (NSTEMI), and UA in order to maximize the possibility of reperfusion strategies.
  - Immediate electrocardiogram (ECG) is imperative for chest pain (CP).
- Aortic dissection
  - An aortic dissection originates from a tear in the aortic intima and propagates a false lumen distally and often proximally as well. Mortality is 1% per hour for the first 2 days.
  - Dissections of the ascending aorta occur twice as frequently as ones involving only the descending aorta; ascending aortic dissection requires immediate surgical intervention.

- The history, coupled with findings of unequal BP in the arms, and a suggestive chest x-ray (CXR) prompt you to call the cardiothoracic (CT) surgeons! HPI clues include severe exertional onset and ripping/tearing pain, radiation to back.
- Pulmonary embolism
  - An elusive diagnosis that will be more obvious in the examination format than in real life as there will be no apparent myocardial infarction (MI) or dissection and there will be predisposing factors, eg, current or past deep venous thrombosis (DVT) or pulmonary embolism (PE), cancer, prolonged travel or bed rest, a long leg cast, recent trauma or surgery, pregnancy, or obesity. A D-dimer can be ordered, but more definitive testing will be necessary!
- Pneumothorax
  - The PE findings of deviated trachea and unilateral absent breath sounds will give you the ultimate life threat in this category.
  - Immediately decompress a tension pneumothorax based on your PE; if you wait for the CXR, the patient will crash!

DON'T FORGET

DDx Summary

- ECG for ACS.
- CXR for aortic dissection or pneumothorax.
- PE is suggested by nondiagnostic ECG and CXR in a hypoxic patient with atypical chest pain.

ACUTE CORONARY SYNDROME

Additional History and Physical Examination Findings

- The incidence and severity of coronary artery disease (CAD) increases with age. Be extra suspicious of an ACS in elderly patients.
- Classically, the pain is described as being substernal, crushing, or squeezing in quality. Atypical pain is common in ACS and does not preclude the diagnosis.
- Alternate chief complaints that suggest an ACS, especially in the elderly, are syncope, epigastric pain that sounds like reflux or gastritis, shortness of breath, and weakness.
- Radiation of pain to one or both arms increases the likelihood of an ACS, as well as exertional pain, vomiting, and diaphoresis.
- Pleuritic pain, sharp or stabbing pain, or reproducible chest wall pain reduce but do not eliminate the risk of ACS.
- Risk factors increase probability of CAD, but the lack of risk factors does not preclude ACS.
- A prior history of AMI or CAD increases the risk of ACS fivefold.
- Pain that is similar to prior coronary event increases risk an additional threefold.
- The response to a gastrointestinal (GI) cocktail or nitroglycerin cannot be used to rule in or out ACS.
- The physical examination is useful in diagnosing complications of an ACS including congestive heart failure (CHF).

DON'T FORGET

The history in your ACS patient is generally classic on exam day, but they may give you an older patient who presents with a CC of "weak and dizzy" or syncope who also has CP if asked.

Review Initial Results

- ECG: Review the ECG carefully as soon as it is performed even if it interrupts your H/P. Obtain a previous ECG for comparison.
- When reviewing the ECG, ask yourself the following questions:
  - Is the ECG diagnostic of an STEMI?
    - >1 mm (0.1 mV) ST-segment elevation in two or more contiguous ECG leads
    - New left bundle branch block (LBBB)
  - Posterior MI (ST depression V1-V4 with tall R waves) (see Fig. 8-1).
  - Left ventricular hypertrophy (LVH) with strain pattern (be concerned for ACS unless no change) (see Fig. 8-2).

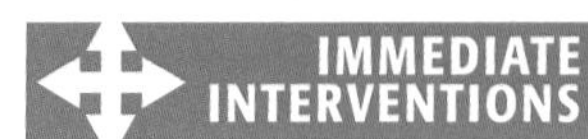

- Chewable ASA 325 mg PO.
- Portable CXR.
- Order CBC, electrolytes, cardiac enzymes, and coags.
- Nitroglycerin 0.4 mg SL q5min (×3 if needed).

- Changes that may confuse the picture (assume the worst).
  - Early repolarization pattern.
  - Pericarditis.
  - Left ventricular (LV) aneurysm.
- Is the ECG diagnostic of ischemia or injury?
  - ST-segment depression.
  - Dynamic ECG changes.
  - T-wave inversion.
  - Peaked T waves.

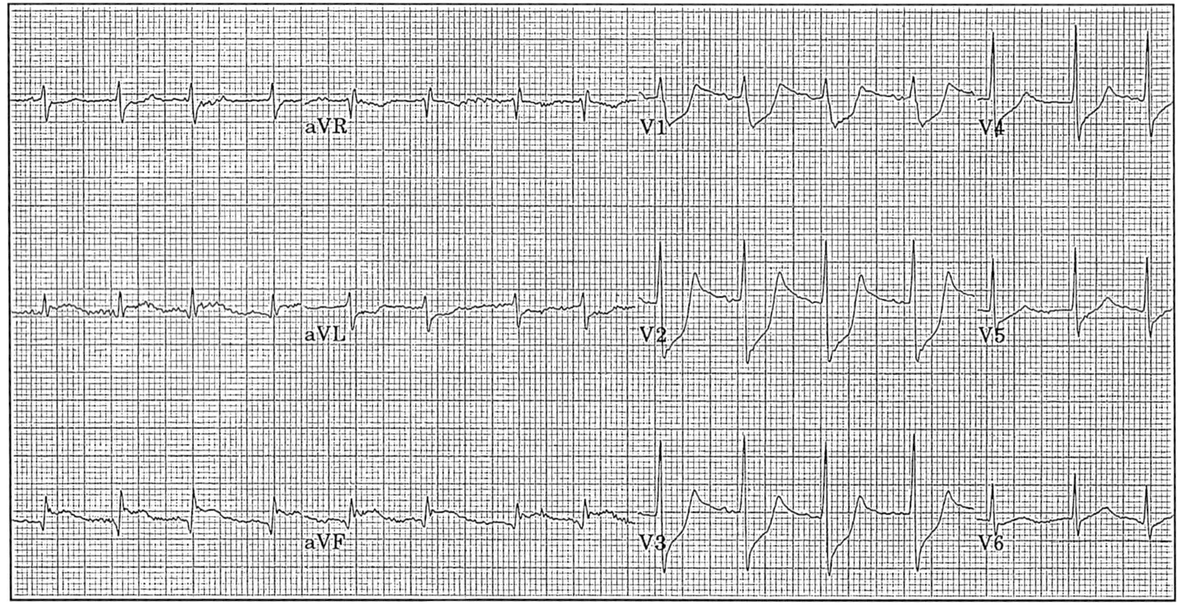

Figure 8-1. ECG with posterior MI pattern. (*Reproduced with permission from Goldschlager NF, Goldman MJ.* Principles of Electrocardiography. *13th ed. New York, NY: McGraw-Hill; 1989.*)

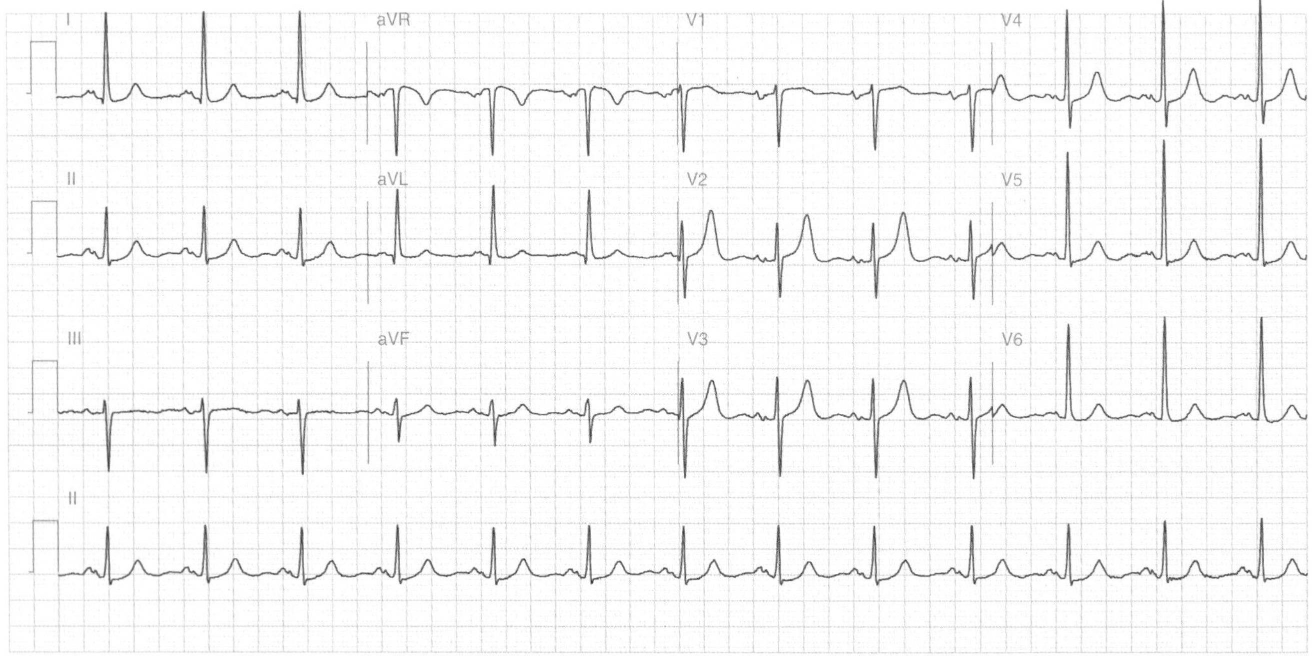

Figure 8-2. ECG with LVH and strain pattern. (*Reprinted with permission from Fauci AS, Braunwald E, Kaspter DL, et al.* Harrison's Principles of Internal Medicine. *17th ed. New York, NY: McGraw-Hill; 2008.*)

- A completely normal ECG (no nonspecific ST changes, no LVH, no old infarcts) has an negative predictive value (NPV) of 99% for excluding MI but cannot be used to exclude UA (if the patient has a concerning story with persistent pain, think dissection or PE but repeat the ECG at least once later).

- CXR:
  - Rule out a widened mediastinum (>8 cm). Aortic dissection into coronaries can cause coronary ischemia and infarction. Instituting anticoagulation and reperfusion therapy for a patient with coronary ischemia or infarction from extension of an aortic dissection is deadly.
  - Look for alternative explanations for pain (pneumonia, rib fracture, pneumothorax, etc).
  - Look for evidence of CHF.
  - Patients with pulmonary edema and an ACS are at high risk.
- Cardiac enzymes:
  - Figure 8-3 shows the pattern of rise and fall of cardiac enzymes in AMI.
  - Cardiac enzymes will not be elevated in patients with UA.
  - The initial set of cardiac enzymes is positive in 70%-80% of patients with STEMI or NSTEMI.

Risk Stratification: Management Priorities

- STEMI
  - High risk of morbidity/mortality.
  - Initiate aspirin and ticagrelor/clopidogrel, anticoagulation, maximize antiplatelet therapy, maximal therapy to reduce oxygen demand, and maximize reperfusion strategy with either thrombolytics or immediate trip to cath lab for percutaneous coronary intervention (PCI).
- NSTEMI/UA
  - Aspirin.
  - Ticagrelor or clopidogrel.
  - Anticoagulation with unfractionated heparin or enoxaparin.
  - Oxygen to keep arterial oxygen saturation (SaO_2) >93%.
  - Nitrates or opiates for CP.

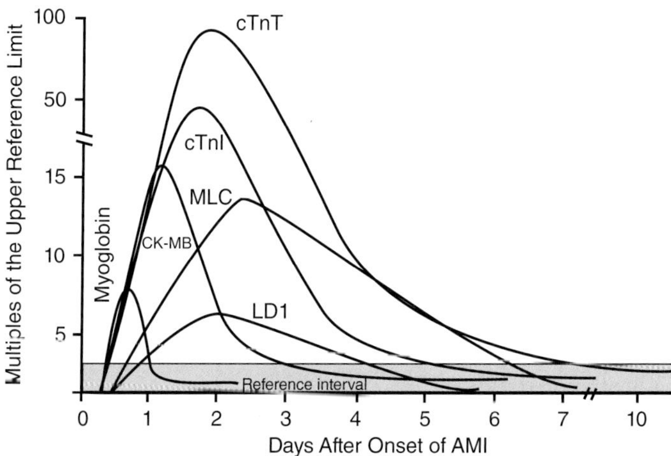

Figure 8-3. Relative timing and levels of cardiac markers in blood after acute myocardial infarction. (*Reprinted with permission from Ma OJ, Cline DM, Tintinalli JE, et al.* Emergency Medicine Manual. *6th ed. New York, NY: McGraw-Hill; 2004.*)

DON'T FORGET

Ask for previous ECGs or old records, including cath reports and/or stress tests.

DON'T FORGET

Make sure to order at least one repeat ECG.

DON'T FORGET

You must check the CXR to assess for widened mediastinum before treating an ACS patient with heparin or thrombolytics.

DON'T FORGET

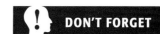

Initiate reperfusion therapy as soon as possible in the STEMI patient—thrombolytics or cath lab for PCI—get cardiology consultant involved. Be prepared to transfer the patient to a PCI-capable facility if necessary.

Definitive Management

Pain control

- Oxygen if hypoxic.
- Nitroglycerin: Sublingual nitrogylcerin (NTG) 0.4 mg, sublingual q5min, (×3 if needed); intravenous (IV) nitroglycerin, start at 20 μg/min and increase by 10 μg/min every 10 minutes until the patient is pain-free or BP drops.
  - Do NOT give in inferior STEMI as these patients are extremely preload-dependent and giving this medication can cause deadly hypotension.
- Fentanyl: 25-50 μg IV q510min until pain is gone.

Antiplatelet therapy

- ASA:
  - Reduces mortality 15%-20%.
  - Chewable 325 mg.
  - Give as early as possible, at home, during emergency medical service (EMS) transport, or upon arrival.
- Ticagrelor or clopidogrel: Indicated in patients who cannot take ASA; give a 180-mg PO or 300-mg PO loading dose, respectively.
- GIIb/IIIa inhibitors:
  - The role is not clearly defined.
  - Clearly indicated for high-risk patients with refractory pain or patients going to cath.
  - Decision to start should be made in conjunction with a cardiologist.

Anticoagulation therapy

- Unfractionated heparin
  - Load with 60 U/kg, then 12 U/kg drip.
  - Check partial thromboplastin time (PTT) in 6 hours and adjust drip.
- Low-molecular-weight heparin (LMWH)
  - Enoxaparin 1 mg/kg subcutaneous (SQ) q12h.
  - In comparison to unfractionated heparin, use of LMWH may decrease recurrent angina, MI, the need for urgent revascularization, and mortality rate.

Reperfusion

- Consult cardiology immediately if reperfusion is indicated.
- Thrombolytics: Not indicated for NSTEMI/UA. PCI preferred, thrombolytics if not available and transfer not possible.
  - Absolute indications (class I):
    - ECG diagnostic of STEMI as indicated above
    - Time to therapy <12 hours
    - Age <75 years
  - Relative indications (class II):
    - Age >75 years
    - Time to therapy 12-24 hours
  - Contraindications.
  - Absolute:
    - Previous hemorrhagic stroke
    - Other stroke or cerebrovascular accident (CVA) within 1 year
    - Active internal bleeding (excluding menses)
    - Known intracranial neoplasm
    - Suspected aortic dissection
  - Relative:
    - Time to therapy >24 hours
    - Uncontrolled HTN (BP >180/110 mm Hg)

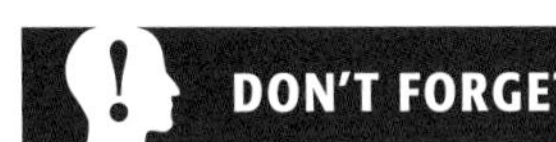

These cases will be classic ACLS—a quick review of ACLS algorithms will serve you well!

    - Pregnancy
    - Recent internal bleeding; peptic ulcer disease (PUD)
    - Recent trauma
  - Dosing: On the oral board exam, ask to look up dosing if needed.
- PCI:
  - Preferred reperfusion strategy if available within 90 minutes
  - Indications
    - Cardiogenic shock in patients <75 years
    - As an alternative to thrombolytics
    - High-risk patients with NSTEMI/unstable angina
    - Refractory CP

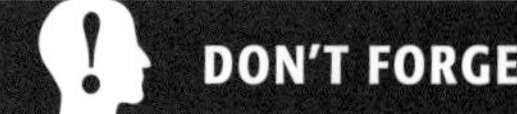

Get a cardiology consultant ASAP in order to initiate reperfusion therapy—give thrombolytics or take patient to the cath lab for PCI.

Frequent Reassessment

- Repeat ECGs every 15–30 minutes and with any change in the pain.
- High-risk features, including persistent or recurrent pain, dynamic ECG changes, or positive enzymes mandate escalation of care.

Complications

Cardiogenic shock

- Institute inotropic and vasopressor therapy.
- Consult cardiologist immediately to arrange PCI and consider intra-aortic balloon pump.
- Transfer the patient if primary PCI is not available within 90 minutes.

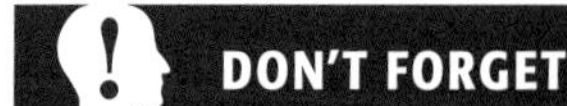

Repeat VS and ECGs are necessary to properly manage these patients.

Conduction disturbances

- Prophylactic lidocaine in uncomplicated AMI is contraindicated.
- Premature ventricular contractions (PVCs)
  - Treat only if PVCs are frequent (>30/min), multifocal, or associated with short runs of V-tach.
  - Optimize anti-ischemic therapy (oxygen, pain control, beta-blockers).
  - Anti-arrhythmic:
    - Amiodarone: Preferred agent if there is LV dysfunction
    - Lidocaine
- Tachyarrhythmia: Manage according to ACLS guidelines.
- Bradycardia: Manage according to ACLS guidelines.
- Indications for transvenous pacing in MI.
  - Mobitz type II second-degree atrioventricular block (AV) block.
  - Bilateral bundle branch block (alternating BBB or RBBB plus alternating LAPF/LPFB).
  - Bifascicular block (RBBB + LAFB or LPFB).
  - Complete heart block.
  - Symptomatic bradycardia.

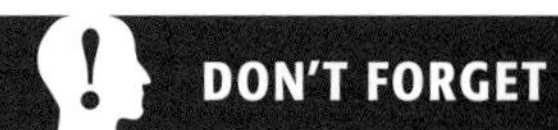

Cardiogenic shock requires inotropic and/or vasopressor therapy, as well as potential aortic balloon pump intervention—coordinate with cardiology.

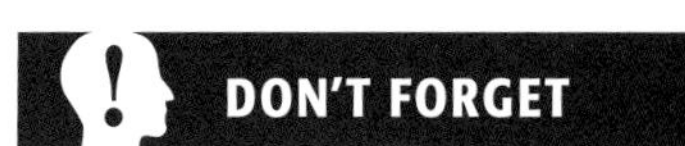

With new AV block place pacer pads and consider floating transvenous pacemaker.

Disposition

- STEMI
  - Admit to critical care unit (CCU).
  - Ensure that the patient is seen in a timely manner.
- High-risk NSTEMI/unstable angina
  - Admit to CCU.
  - Ensure that the patient is seen in a timely manner.
- Moderate-risk NSTEMI/unstable angina
  - Admit to telemetry or CP unit.
  - In-patient rule out with serial enzyme measurements.
  - Risk stratify prior to discharge.

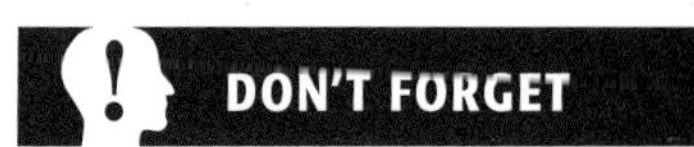

All ACS patients go to the CCU on exam day.

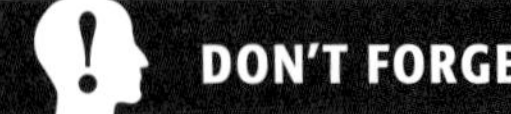

There will be no "low-risk" ACS patients on exam day.

- Low-risk NSTEMI/unstable angina/undifferentiated chest pain
  - No defined management strategy.
  - Management options include
    - Rapid rule out algorithm
    - CP unit
    - Traditional rule out
    - Out-patient cardiac risk stratification

AORTIC DISSECTION

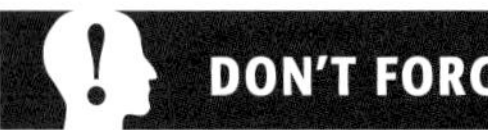

Severe, migratory CP that radiates to or moves from the chest to the back/abdomen is the tip-off to aortic dissection—even more so if there are signs of side branch occlusion, eg, confusion, arm pain, stroke symptoms.

Additional History and Physical Examination Findings

- The CP classically is severe (10/10), of sudden onset with significant exertion, and "sharp, ripping, or tearing" in quality.
- The pain is often migratory and frequently radiates to the back or elsewhere in the chest.
- More than 70% of patients present with CP; other common complaints include syncope, back pain, and abdominal pain. *Side branch occlusions* may result in acute stroke, paraplegia, cardiac ischemia, a cold, pulseless extremity, or cardiac tamponade. Another clue: symptoms above AND below diaphragm, eg, CP with limb ischemia or gut ischemia (GI bleed).
- It has been suggested that 90% of aortic dissections will be appreciated if the following three questions are asked:
  1. Was the onset of the pain sudden and maximal in intensity at the outset?
  2. Does the pain radiate to the back?
  3. Is the pain severe and migratory?
- Common risk factors:
  - Older patients: Increasing age, atherosclerosis, HTN.
  - Young patients: Inflammatory diseases that cause a vasculitis, connective tissue diseases (Marfan syndrome, Ehler-Danlos syndrome), and aortic coarctation.
- Vital signs: BP—usually hypertensive, but ascending aorta involvement may cause hypotension. Check BP in both arms—BP differential >20 mm Hg between the arms or left arm and leg strongly suggestive.
- Is there JVD? Are the lung sounds clear and symmetric? Are there rubs, murmurs, or gallops? Are the peripheral pulses symmetric? Is the motor, sensory examination intact? DTRs equal?

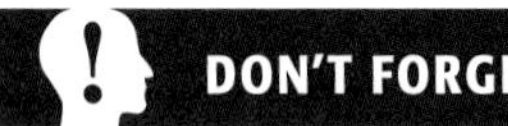

On examination, check pulses in all four extremities and ask for BP in both arms. Ask if there are any murmurs (aortic regurgitation is a classic). If there is a murmur, ask if it is new.

Review Initial Results

- CXR (Fig. 8-4)
  - A completely normal film occurs in only 10% of patients.
  - Abnormal in 80% of patients with type A dissections and 60% of patients with type B dissections.
  - Findings:
    - Widened mediastinum (>8 cm at aortic knob).
    - "Egg shell" sign: Separation of aortic intimal calcifications >5 mm from edge of aortic wall.
    - Indistinct mediastinum/blurred aortic knob (Fig. 8-5).
    - Apical cap.
    - Left pleural effusion.
    - Shift and depression of the left main stem bronchus.
    - Obliteration of aortopulmonary (AP) window.
    - Deviation to left of the trachea or esophagus.
- ECG: Will usually reveal LVH but otherwise nondiagnostic; may have evidence of ACS (in up to 40% of aortic dissections, probably not on exam day)

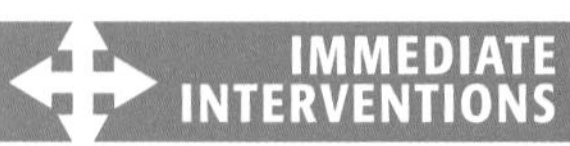

- Second large-bore IV
- Fluid resuscitation if necessary
- Assess stat portable CXR
- CBC, electrolytes, coags, U/A, T & C for 8 U packed RBC
- Pain control with IV narcotics
- HR and BP control

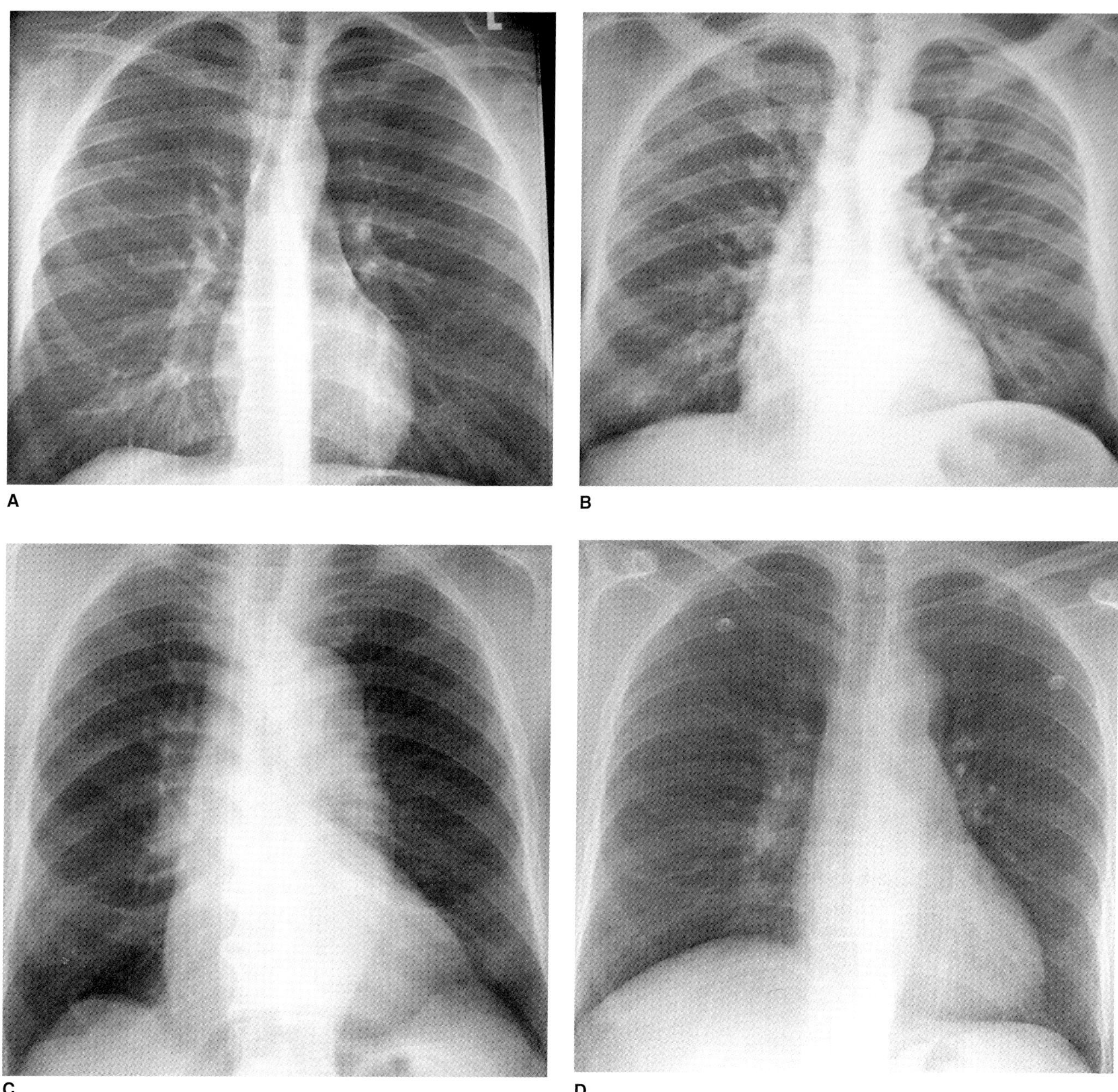

Figure 8-4. Radiographic appearances of the aorta. Aortic enlargement can be graded as mild, moderate, or severe, and is shown in young (age ≤40 years), middle-aged, and older individuals. **Elderly persons** with markedly dilated aortas are at increased risk of dissection (**C** and **F**), although dissection can occur in patients with only mildly or moderately dilated aortas (**D** and **E**), which are "normal" in the elderly (**B**). In a **young person** with chest, back, or abdominal pain, any aortic dilation is abnormal and should prompt consideration of aortic dissection (**G**). A normal narrow aortic contour in a young person substantially reduces the likelihood of dissection (**A**). **(A) Normal aorta** in a 27-year-old man—dissection is unlikely. **(B)** Moderately dilated **tortuous aorta** in a 74-year-old man is "normal for age," although dissection could be present. **(C)** Moderately dilated and elongated, **tortuous aorta** in an 81-year-old man is suspicious for dissection. Chest CT showed no dissection. **(D) Aortic dissection** in a 58-year-old woman. The aorta is only mildly dilated aorta and is "normal for age." **(E) Aortic dissection** in a 61-year-old man. The moderately dilated aorta is indistinguishable from a tortuous aorta that is "normal for age." **(F) Aortic dissection** in a 63-year-old man. The aortic knob is markedly dilated, which is suspicious for dissection. **(G) Aortic dissection** in a 40-year-old man. The moderately dilated aorta is clearly "abnormal for age" and suggests that aortic pathology is present. (*Reprinted with permission from Schwartz DT.* Emergency Radiology: Case Studies. *New York, NY: McGraw-Hill; 2008.*)

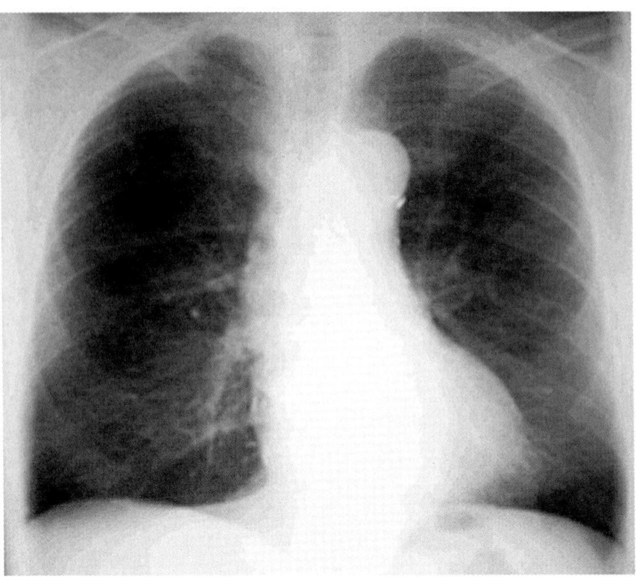

E

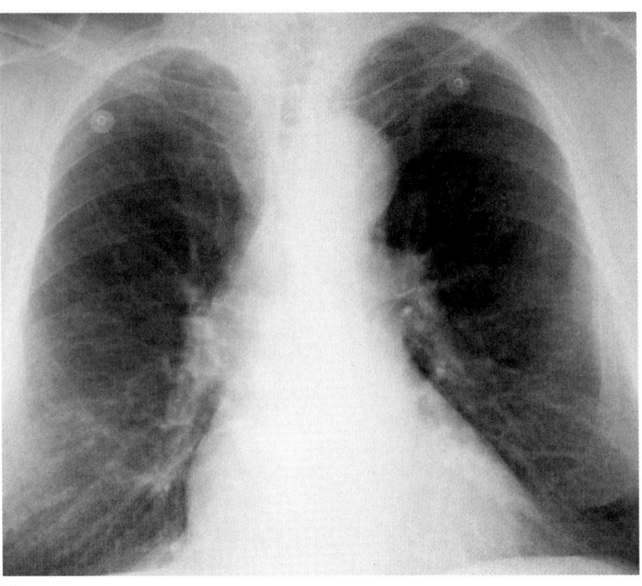

F

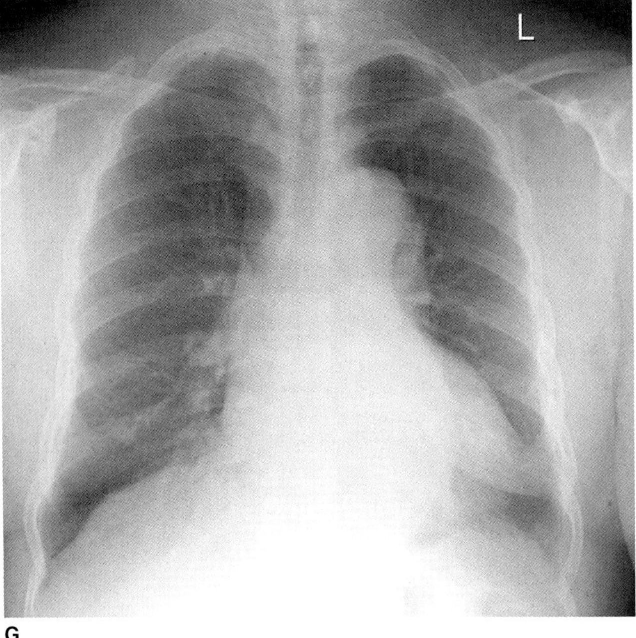

G

Figure 8-4. (*Continued.*)

Risk Stratification: Management Priorities

- Stanford system
  - Type A: Involve the ascending aorta (with or without descending portion) and require surgical repair.
  - Type B: Involve the descending aorta only and are approached with medical management.

Definitive Management

- Resuscitation:
  - Aggressive resuscitation with normal saline (NS) boluses to correct hypotension.
  - Initiate transfusion with packed red blood cells (PRBCs) if patient is in shock.

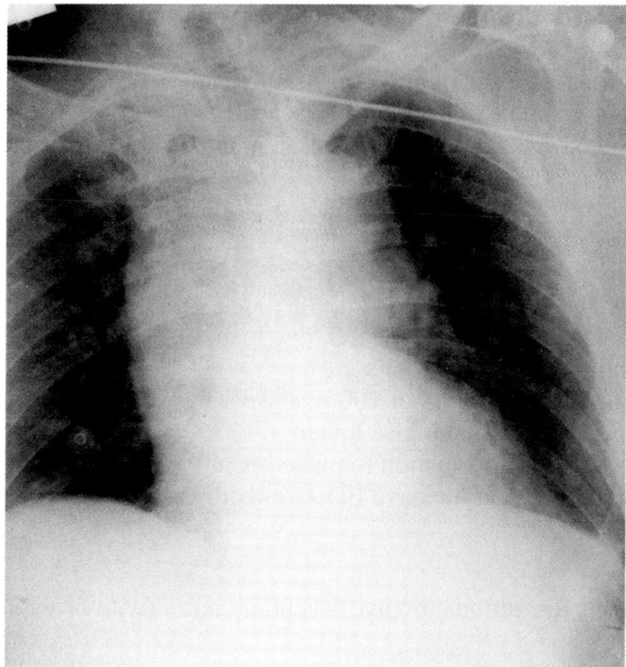

Figure 8-5. AP view of the chest showing a widened mediastinum and an indistinct aortic knob consistent with aortic dissection. (*Reprinted with permission from Hall JB, Schmidt GA, Wood LDH.* Principles of Critical Care. *3rd ed. New York, NY: McGraw-Hill; 2005.*)

- Control HTN and tachycardia.
  - Initiate heart rate (HR) control first or concomitant with HTN control.
- Dual-agent therapies:
  - Metoprolol: 5 mg IV q5min, can use over three doses as long as patient tolerates medication.

  OR
  - Esmolol drip, titrate to HR <60.

  AND
  - Nicardipine drip, titrate to target SBP 100-120.

OR
- Single-agent therapies:
  - Labetalol 20 mg bolus, then a drip at 1-2 mg/min.
  - Target systolic blood pressure (SBP) is 100-120 mm Hg. Target HR is 60 beats/min.
  - If available, place an arterial catheter for BP monitoring.
    - Consult cardiovascular or thoracic surgery and cardiology.
    - Do not allow unstable patients to go to radiology—arrange for definitive diagnostic tests to be performed in the emergency department (ED) under close monitoring.
    - Stable patients may leave the ED for diagnostic radiographic studies if accompanied by physician or nurse.

Further Diagnostic Considerations

- Transesophageal echocardiography (TEE)—an ideal study
  - Very high sensitivity/specificity
  - Safe when done in the ED or operating room (OR) and can be quickly done.
  - No contrast or radiation.

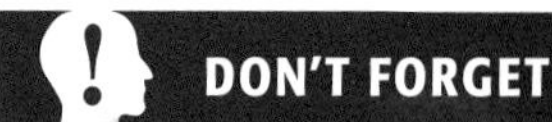

Call for the cardiologist and CV/thoracic surgeon ASAP if you think you have a dissection—call the surgeon again once you demonstrate involvement of the ascending aorta.

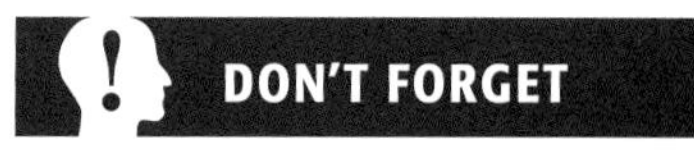

If you have a probable dissection, strive to get the HR to 60 beats/min and the SBP to 120 mm Hg.

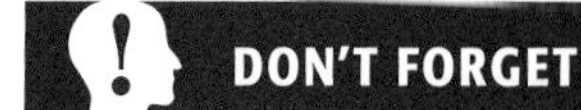

TEE in the ED is the way to go if it is available!

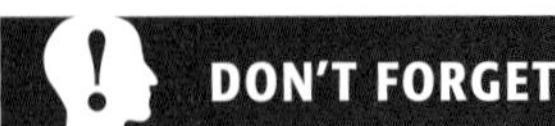

Type A dissections are going to the OR for surgical repair. Type B dissections are going to the ICU for medical management.

  - Provides all of the information surgeon will need.
    - Ascending versus descending alone, ie, need to operate.
    - Assess for presence of aortic insufficiency.
    - Assess for extension to aortic branches.
  - Disadvantages: Operator-dependent; not universally available.
- Rapid sequence CT angiography.
  - Excellent screening test but cannot provide all information necessary to make operative decision.
  - Very sensitive and specific.
  - Universally available.
  - Disadvantages: Need to leave ED, dye load, time-consuming.
- Aortography
  - "Gold standard" though not 100% sensitive as dissection; may be missed if no blood flow through false lumen.
  - Does provide all information to make operative decision.
  - Disadvantages: Need to leave ED, dye load, very time-consuming.

Disposition

- Type A aortic dissections involve ascending aorta (with or without descending portion).
  - Managed operatively.
  - If delay to OR, send patient to intensive care unit (ICU) under the care of a surgeon or critical care physician.
- Type B aortic dissections involve only descending aorta.
  - Managed medically.
  - Admit to ICU.
- When consulting physician for admission, demand that he/she immediately see the patient in the ED.
  - Stabilize and transfer the patient if resources are not locally available.

PULMONARY EMBOLISM

Additional History and Physical Examination Findings

- Dyspnea is the most frequent symptom.
- The classic description of pleuritic pain, dyspnea, and hemoptysis is present in a minority of patients.
- Sudden onset of pain occurs in less than half of patients; the pain typically does not radiate and patients may have pain for days to weeks prior to presentation.
- Major risk factors include
  - Current DVT or prior DVT or PE.
  - Cancer.
  - Immobility caused by travel, prolonged bed rest, or extremity cast.
  - Recent trauma or surgery (especially orthopedic).
  - Pregnancy.
  - Tachycardia.
  - Obesity.
- Physical examination will reveal a patient in respiratory distress who has abnormal VS with tachypnea, tachycardia, and hypoxemia; a low-grade fever may be present. Patient may appear "anxious."
- The chest and cardiovascular examination is usually unremarkable.
- Specifically look for and (will usually find) asymmetric leg swelling (>3 cm differential) or palpable cords.
- A history that screens for melena or a rectal examination to screen for GI bleeding gives bonus points.

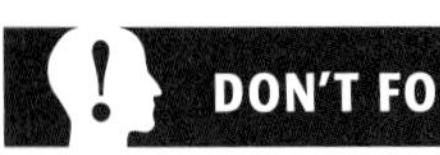

On exam day, the dyspneic patient with atypical CP—a nondiagnostic ECG and CXR, and a risk factor for PE—is a PE!

Review Initial Results

- ECG
  - Many PE patients will have normal ECGs.
  - Common positive findings include:
    - Sinus tachycardia
    - Precordial T-wave inversions
  - S1Q3T3 pattern indicating R ventricle strain is not often present and is nonspecific.
  - Concomminant ST depressions in inferior *and* anterior leads highly suggestive of PE but also nonspecific.
  - Most important to rule out ACS.
- CXR
  - Often normal, though an elevated hemidiaphragm and/or atelectasis are classic findings.
  - Westermark sign: Relative oligemia of the affected lung is rarely present.
  - Hampton hump: A pleural-based wedge-shaped infiltrate (caused by infarction) is rarely present.

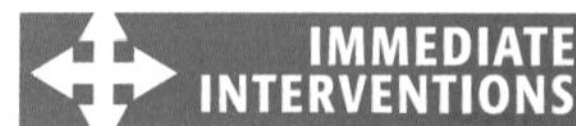

- High-flow mask oxygen.
- Fluid bolus if BP is low.
- Send CBC, BMP, D-dimer (if low risk), coagulation studies.
- Screen ECG and CXR to assess for ACS and aortic dissection.

Risk Stratification: Management Priorities

- The decision to empirically anticoagulate the patient and pursue further diagnostic testing is based on pretest risk stratification.
  - Wells criteria (Table 8-1).

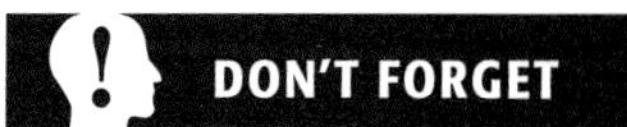

Only stable patients may leave the ED for a confirmatory test for PE.

Risk score

- Wells score > 4.0 points: PE likely
  - Diagnostic imaging is needed.
- Wells score ≤ 4.0 points: PE unlikely
  - If D-dimer is negative, diagnosis excluded.
  - If D-dimer is positive, obtain confirmatory test.

Definitive Management

- Unfractionated heparin 80 U/kg bolus, then 18 U/kg infusion.
- LMWH: Enoxaparin 1 mg/kg SC bid may be an alternative.
- The patient with hypotension who responds to fluids should not leave the ED—anticoagulate and consider alternative diagnostic approach, eg, a bedside echocardiogram to look for signs of right ventricular (RV) strain, troponin (which should have already been ordered to evaluate for ACS) and BNP.

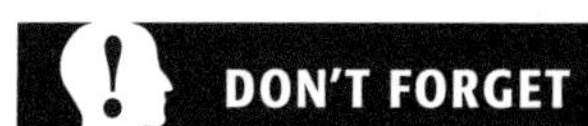

Make sure that you have checked the CXR for signs of dissection (or pneumothorax) prior to anticoagulation.

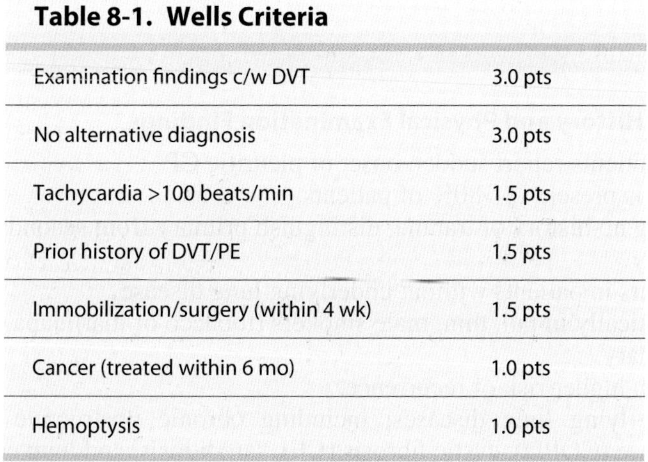

Table 8-1. Wells Criteria

Examination findings c/w DVT	3.0 pts
No alternative diagnosis	3.0 pts
Tachycardia >100 beats/min	1.5 pts
Prior history of DVT/PE	1.5 pts
Immobilization/surgery (within 4 wk)	1.5 pts
Cancer (treated within 6 mo)	1.0 pts
Hemoptysis	1.0 pts

- The unstable patient with signs of cardiovascular collapse should not leave the ED, needs a bedside echocardiogram as noted above and treatment with heparin.
- The patient with a PE and hypotension should be considered a massive PE and be a candidate for thrombolytic therapy —administer tPA, 100 mg over 2 hours (or similar agent) and consult a CV/thoracic surgeon for consideration of thrombectomy, or interventionalist for catheter-directed therapy.

DON'T FORGET

Persistently unstable patients need a bedside echo to confirm RV strain, heparin, and thrombolytics and call a CVT surgeon.

Further Diagnostic Considerations

- D-Dimer.
  - Only useful for low-risk patients (Wells ≤4.0)—if normal, can exclude PE-DVT.
- Computed tomography pulmonary angiography (CTPA).
  - Test of choice as it is widely available, fast, safe, and has an excellent specificity for PE and other pathology.
  - Sensitivity for small, peripheral clots lower, but addition of complementary CT extremity runoff study—now routine in many centers—helps improve testing yield.
  - Disadvantages: Dye/radiation exposure; patient leaves ED.
- V/Q scan
  - Helpful if normal—safely excludes the diagnosis, thus a good screening test in many patients.
  - Unfortunately up to 75% of patients receive nondiagnostic interpretations (intermediate, indeterminate, or low probability) and need further testing.
  - High probability scan has a 90% PPV and rules in the diagnosis in most patients.
  - Advantages: No exposure to contrast dye.
  - Disadvantages: Frequently not diagnostic, patient leaves ED.
- Lower extremity Doppler ultrasound
  - Sensitive and specific for thigh DVTs.
  - May be helpful when initial study is nondiagnostic. A positive study for acute DVT strongly supports the diagnosis of PE in the patient with hypoxemia.

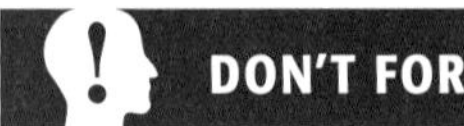

DON'T FORGET

Most stable patients with high risk of PE should initially receive heparin and confirm the diagnosis with CT.

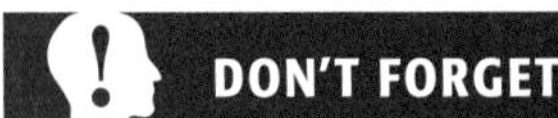

DON'T FORGET

Err on the side of an ICU admission for most PE patients.

Disposition

- On exam day, all patients with confirmed PE should be admitted for anticoagulation and monitoring.
- Patients with diagnostic signs of submassive PE such as elevated troponin, BNP, or lactate, or right heart strain on echo, ECG, or CTPA and patients with persistent hypoxemia, tachycardia, or tachypnea should be admitted to the ICU under the care of an intensivist.
- Stable patients may be admitted to a telemetry bed.

PNEUMOTHORAX

Additional History and Physical Examination Findings

- 95% of patients report sudden onset of pleuritic CP.
- Dyspnea is present in >80% of patients.
- Assuming no history of trauma, distinguish primary from secondary causes:
  - Primary
    - Occurs in patients without underlying lung disease
    - Classically in tall, thin, male smokers (tobacco or marijuana)
  - Secondary
    - Much higher risk of recurrence.
    - Underlying lung diseases, including chronic obstructive pulmonary disease (COPD), cystic fibrosis (CF), sarcoidosis, and lung cancer.
- Patients with a prior history of pneumothorax often have a recurrence.

DON'T FORGET

Is a pneumothorax the reason why your asthma or COPD patient is not responding to treatment?

- The patient with simple pneumothorax often has tachypnea and hypoxemia. Other abnormal vital signs, especially hypotension, suggest tension pneumothorax—immediately assess for tracheal deviation and JVD—when present, confirm with chest examination and treat accordingly.
- Chest examination will reveal decreased breath sounds on the affected side with hyperresonance to percussion.
- Consider bedside ultrasound to demonstrate absence of lung sliding in equivocal patients (unlikely on test day).

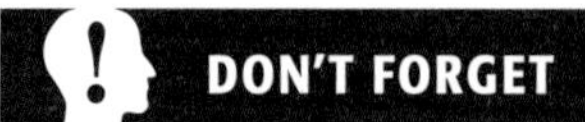

The patient with sudden, unilateral, pleuritic CP and dyspnea must be immediately assessed for tracheal deviation and JVD; if present, confirm absent breath sounds and treat for tension pneumothorax with immediate needle decompression.

Review Initial Results

- CXR
  - Ask for upright CXR if possible.
    - 75%-85% sensitive and nearly 100% specific.
    - A pneumothorax appears as a continuous pleural line that is collapsed away from the ribs with the absence of lung markings beyond the line.
    - Small pneumothorax is <10% of total lung volume.
    - On exam day, all pneumothoraces will be medium, large, or under tension.
    - A tension pneumothorax should never be diagnosed by CXR—the only CXR obtained in a patient with tension pneumothorax should demonstrate a reinflated lung post chest tube placement which was performed after needle decompression.
- ECG: To exclude other causes of CP (Fig. 8-6).

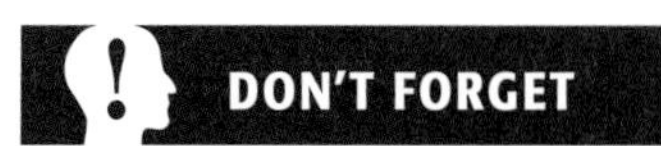

- Unless tension PTX, patient should have ECG before CXR.

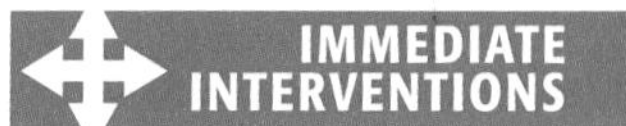

- Oxygen: 100% facemask (improves reabsorption of pleural air).
- Send blood for CBC, BMP, coags.

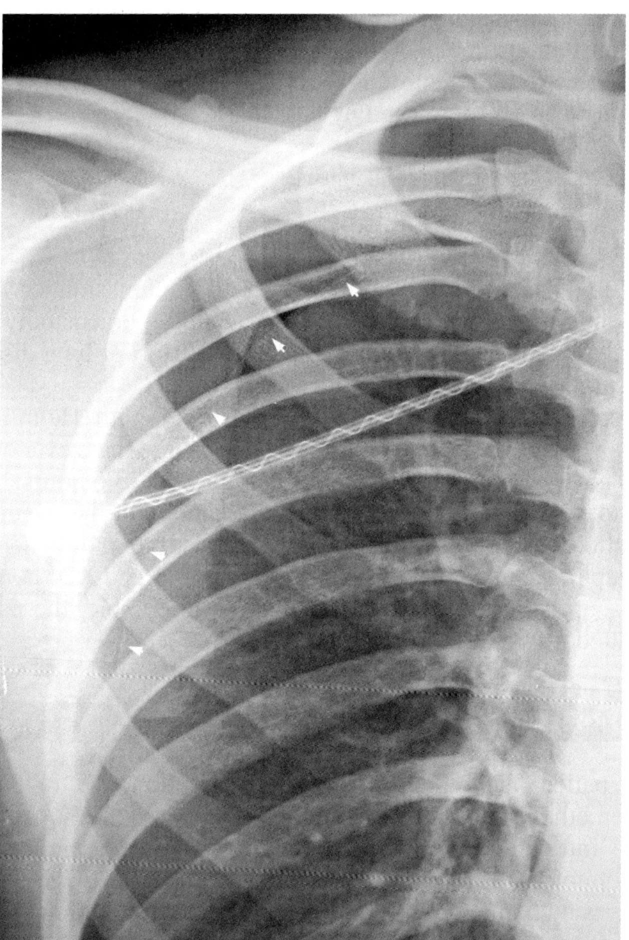

Figure 8-6. In this patient, a pneumothorax can be seen along the right pleural margin, the side of the patient's chest pain (*arrowheads*). (*Reprinted with permission from Schwartz DT.* Emergency Radiology: Case Studies. *New York, NY: McGraw-Hill; 2008.*)

Risk Stratification: Management Priorities

- Tension pneumothorax: Tracheal deviation, JVD, and diminished breath sounds get your attention—focused H&P, then needle, then tube.
- Symptomatic pneumothorax—This is the only other pneumothorax you will see on exam day; it may be primary or secondary, moderate to large, and a first-time or recurrent episode—these get a chest tube and admission.
- A small (<10%), primary, first-time pneumothorax (<25% patients in real life)—unlikely to appear on the oral board exam, though in real life this distinct group of patients can be managed conservatively.

Definitive Management

- Tension pneumothorax
  - Immediate needle decompression: 14-gauge needle, midclavicular line, second intercostal space.
  - Chest tube thoracostomy with pleurovac to wall suction.
  - CXR to confirm tube placement and re-expansion of lung.
- Symptomatic pneumothorax
  - Chest tube thoracostomy:
    - Traditional thoracostomy with pleurovac to wall suction.
    - Pigtail catheter thoracostomy with Heimlich valve (a one-way valve that allows air to vent but not reenter the pleural space).
  - Repeat CXR immediately to confirm tube placement and re-expansion of lung. If no re-expansion, reposition or remove and replace with chest tube.
- Small, primary, first-time pneumothorax
  - Observation: No intervention is required.
  - Keep patient on 100% oxygen by face mask.
  - Repeat CXR in 6 hours.
  - If increased in size, manage as above.

DON'T FORGET

One more time: Unilateral CP—assess for tracheal deviation and JVD; confirm diminished breath sounds—needle, then chest tube, CXR follows.

Disposition

- Patients with tension pneumothorax require ICU admission.
- Admit stable patients with traditional chest tube thoracostomy to the floor setting (order telemetry if they have underlying heart or lung disease).
- Thoracic surgery consultation for everyone.
- Management with pigtail catheter thoracostomy with Heimlich valve or observation without intervention may enable discharge (but never on exam day).
  - Patients must be monitored in ED for a minimum of 6 hours.
  - CXR prior to discharge cannot show enlargement of the pneumothorax.
  - Close follow-up must be arranged with a CT surgeon or general surgeon.
  - Follow-up physician must order a repeat CXR after 12-24 hours.
  - If follow-up is doubtful or if the patient is unreliable, the patient should be admitted for a 24-hour observation.

DON'T FORGET

On exam day, everyone gets a chest tube. And no one goes home!

WINNING STRATEGIES

- Every CP patient has either ACS, aortic dissection, PE, or pneumothorax until proven otherwise.
- Immediate interventions in all CP patients: IV-O_2-monitor-ECG oxygen, cardiac monitor with rhythm strip, IV, and immediate ECG. Obtain a CXR right away as it changes management in 15%-20% of patients with CP.
- Stabilize life threats by managing airway, aggressive resuscitation, and tube thoracostomy.
- The history in your ACS patient is generally classic on exam day, but they may give you an older patient who presents with a CC of "weak and dizzy" or syncope who also has CP if asked.

- Get the cardiologist involved in reperfusion strategies, and expect that the patient with an AMI will require you to go through at least one "complication" algorithm.
- You must check the CXR to r/o widened mediastinum before treating an ACS or any other patient with heparin or thrombolytics.
- You cannot repeat VS or ECG too often.
- Repeat ECGs are vital to properly managing ACS patients.
- Cardiogenic shock requires pressor therapy and potentially aortic balloon pump intervention—coordinate with cardiology and ICU.
- With new AV block, place pacer pads and consider floating transvenous pacemaker.
- All ACS patients go to the CCU on exam day.
- Severe, migratory CP that radiates to or moves from the chest to the back/abdomen is the tip-off to aortic dissection—even more so if there are signs of side branch occlusion, eg, confusion, arm pain, CVA symptoms—check pulses in all extremities and get a BP in both arms.
- TEE for all unstable patients in the ED is the way to go if it is available!
- T & C for 8 U packed RBC in the dissection patient.
- Call for the cardiologist and CV/thoracic surgeon ASAP if you think you have a dissection—call the surgeon again once you demonstrate involvement of the ascending aorta and don't take no for an answer.
- The dyspneic patient with atypical CP—a nondiagnostic ECG and CXR and a risk factor for PE—is a PE!
- Only stable patients may leave the ED for a confirmatory test for PE.
- Persistently unstable patients need a bedside echo to confirm RV strain, heparin, and thrombolytics and call a CVT surgeon.
- The patient with sudden, unilateral, pleuritic CP and dyspnea must be immediately assessed for tracheal deviation and JVD; if present, confirm absent breath sounds and treat for tension pneumothorax with immediate needle decompression, then a chest tube, and then a CXR.
- On exam day, all patients with pneumothorax get a chest tube and no one goes home!

CHAPTER 9

Syncope and Palpitations

Michael Paddock and James Ahn

DON'T FORGET

Every patient with syncope has a life-threatening etiology until proven otherwise.

On test day, the patient with syncope will have

- Neurologic emergency (seizure, ICH, CVA)
- Cardiac emergency (aortic stenosis, aortic dissection, arrhythmia)
- Orthostatic hypotension (GI bleeding, severe anemia)

Syncope is a transient loss of consciousness with a temporary loss of postural tone. Its etiology spans benign conditions to life-threatening cardiac conduction abnormalities and arrhythmias. Syncope is a symptom of an underlying disorder rather than representing a disease itself. It is therefore important to quickly assess the patient and identify potentially life-threatening conditions that require immediate management. You will need to rapidly ascertain the underlying etiology and keep a broad differential diagnosis throughout the patient's course.

INITIAL ASSESSMENT

- Focus on patient's age, general appearance, and vital signs.
- Immediately assess an electrocardiogram (ECG) for rate, rhythm, intervals (PR, QRS, QTc), and pathognomonic waveforms (Brugada, Wolff-Parkinson-White [WPW], epsilon wave, ventricular hypertrophy).
- Repeat ECGs throughout the patient's course and place the patient on continuous cardiac telemetry.

INITIAL HISTORY AND PHYSICAL EXAMINATION

History of Present Illness

- The history and physical examination can identify the potential cause of syncope in 45% of patients in whom a primary disorder can be identified.
- Obtaining the history of events immediately prior to, during, and after a syncopal episode is crucial to forming a diagnosis and risk stratification.
- Determine if the event occurred during exertion or at rest and if the patient was supine, seated, or standing.
- What was the patient doing when the event occurred?
- Did the patient experience chest discomfort, shortness of breath, or severe headache prior to the event?
- Was there a feeling of nausea, warmth, or tunnel vision?
- How rapid was the onset?
- Was there generalized seizure activity noted by bystanders?
- How quickly did the patient fully recover?
- Has the patient had similar episodes in the past?
- Questions aimed specifically at the time preceding, during, and immediately after the event are important in further defining the etiology of syncope.
- Additionally, a detailed history will aid in differentiating a true syncopal event from a seizure or hypoglycemic episode.
- Remember to ask bystanders or paramedics what happened during the event if it was witnessed.

Past Medical History

- One of the most important questions to ask the patient is if they have a history of heart disease.
- Left ventricular dysfunction, arrhythmia, valvular disease, or congenital heart disease?
- Does the patient have a pacemaker?
- Does the patient have a history of seizure disorder that may mimic a syncopal episode?

Family History

- If the patient is young, a family history may assist in identifying more serious causes of syncope.

- Is there is family history of sudden cardiac death that may be related to prolonged or shortened QT interval?
- Is there a history of connective tissue disease such as Marfan syndrome?
- Is there any congenital heart disease or known family history of WPW syndrome?

Medications

- Medications should be reviewed with emphasis on drugs that may cause QT prolongation, bradycardia, conduction blocks, and orthostatic hypotension.
- Nonprescription medications, herbal remedies, nutritional supplements, and illicit drug use should also be reviewed.

Allergies

- Pertinent allergies should be noted.

Physical Examination

- Vital signs: Obtain a complete set of vital signs (including temperature).
- General: Is the patient awake and alert or do they appear to be confused or slow to respond after the event (postictal period)?
- Head and neck: Note signs of head trauma, tongue biting, bruits, jugular venous distention (JVD). Note pupil examination for signs of intracranial hemorrhage (ICH) or toxidromes.
- Pulmonary: Note crackles or tachypnea.
- Cardiovascular: Note rhythm, rate, regularity, murmurs, and symmetry of pulses.
- Extremities: Is there edema or unilateral leg swelling or pain present?
- Neuro: Look for new focal neurologic deficits including cranial nerves and focal weakness or sensory changes.

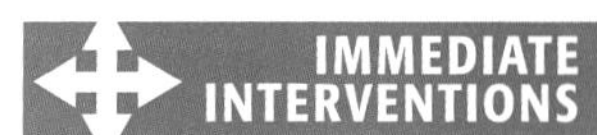

- Oxygen (if hypoxic)
- Continuous cardiac telemetry monitoring
- IV access
- ECG

DIFFERENTIAL DIAGNOSIS

- Reflex-mediated syncope
  - Reflex or neurally mediated syncope is thought to arise from excessive afferent discharge from mechanoreceptors found in the left ventricle, viscera, or arterial circulation. This stimulus results in a reflex-mediated increase in parasympathetic tone which results in vasodilation, relative or absolute bradycardia, and hypotension. This is the most frequent cause of syncope in patients without structural heart disease.
  - Vasovagal syncope, situational syncope, and carotid sinus hypersensitivity are examples of reflex-mediated syncope. Neurally mediated syncope is thought to be a relatively benign disorder except in patients who are predisposed to injury from trauma such as the elderly or those taking anticoagulants.
- Orthostatic hypotension syncope
  - Syncope caused by orthostatic hypotension has a mean prevalence of 8%. This may be caused by intravascular volume depletion such that occurs with diuretic use, hemorrhage, decreased oral fluid intake, and vomiting or diarrhea.
  - Medications that cause a reduction in preload or afterload such as nitroglycerine and alpha-antagonists, respectively, may result in orthostatic hypotension.
  - Primary or secondary autonomic dysfunction from conditions, such as Parkinson disease, Addison disease, diabetic neuropathy, alcoholic neuropathy, and physical inactivity may result in orthostasis.
  - Obtaining positional (orthostatic) blood pressures is no longer necessary nor specific for the diagnosis of orthostatic hypotension. However,

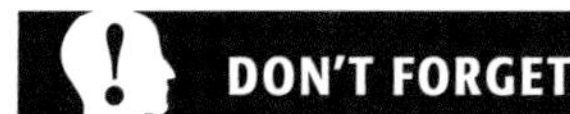

A very thorough history will direct your evaluation and management to rule out life-threatening causes. Make sure to ask bystanders, family members, and paramedics the details of the event.

syncope should not be attributed to orthostatic hypotension if symptoms are not reproduced with a trial of position changes, and an alternate etiology of syncope should be sought. Obtain blood pressure in both arms to evaluate for thoracic aortic dissection.

- Neurologic syncope
  - Neurologic syncope has a mean prevalence of 10% and may include disorders such as transient ischemic attacks (TIAs), migraine, subclavian steal, or certain types of seizures such as atonic or temporal lobe epilepsy.
  - It is important to remember that true seizure does not fit the accepted diagnosis of syncope.
  - Migraine or TIA may result in syncope by loss of adequate perfusion to the vertebrobasilar circulation and reticular activating system.
- Cardiovascular syncope
  - Cardiovascular syncope may be subcategorized into organic heart disease and arrhythmia.
  - Aortic stenosis, pulmonary embolism, pulmonary hypertension, hypertrophic cardiomyopathy, atrial myxoma, aortic dissection, myocardial infarction, and cardiac tamponade are all considered organic heart disease.
  - Arrhythmias that should be considered in cardiovascular syncope include bradycardia, sick sinus syndrome, second- or third-degree heart block, pacemaker malfunction, ventricular tachycardia, WPW syndrome, Brugada syndrome, hypertrophic cardiomyopathy, prolonged QTc (precursor to torsade de pointes), and supraventricular tachycardia.
  - Cardiovascular syncope is the most serious and potentially the most life-threatening form of syncope. Thus, a high index of suspicion should be maintained by the emergency physician.
- Unknown syncope
  - The cause of syncope is unknown in 13%-41% of cases after initial evaluation. The disposition of these patients should be based on risk of other underlying medical conditions and risk assessment for further morbidity and mortality.
  - Patients at high risk are with the following characteristics: age >60 years; a history or physical examination findings of congestive heart failure (CHF) or ventricular arrhythmia and chest discomfort or signs and symptoms compatible acute coronary syndrome; physical examination findings suggestive of valvular heart disease; and abnormal ECG findings such as ischemia, arrhythmia, QT prolongation, or bundle branch block. These patients should be admitted to the hospital.

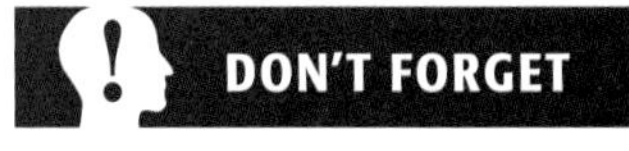

DDx Summary

- Reflex-mediated syncope
- Orthostatic hypotension syncope
- Psychiatric syncope
- Neurologic syncope
- Cardiovascular syncope
- Unknown syncope

REFLEX-MEDIATED SYNCOPE

Additional History and Physical Examination Findings

Reflex-mediated syncope may be caused by vasovagal syncope, situational syncope such as cough, micturition, defecation, as well as by carotid sinus hypersensitivity or intense pain. Vasovagal syncope is usually preceded by diaphoresis, nausea, dizziness, and a sensation of feeling flushed or warm. This type of syncope may occur as a result of a strong emotional response or intense pain as may be perceived with venipuncture. Situational syncope may immediately follow urination, defecation, or cough.

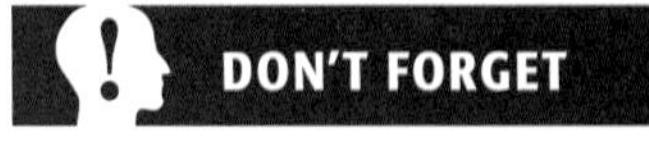

If atypical signs or symptoms are present in a patient you suspect of reflex-mediated syncope, continue your evaluation looking for other possible life-threatening causes.

Carotid sinus sensitivity can be triggered by pressure applied to the neck such as with shaving, a tight collar, or neck tie. An exaggerated response defined by asystolic arrest for greater than or equal to 3 seconds may be elicited by carotid sinus massage. This maneuver may be performed safely in patients without carotid bruits, recent myocardial infarction, and history of ventricular tachycardia, or recent stroke.

Review Initial Results

ECG: A 12-lead ECG should be reviewed if there is suggestion of an alternate cause of syncope or the patient is determined to be at high risk for cardiovascular complications.

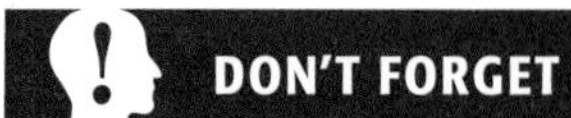

Always evaluate the patient for traumatic injuries after a syncopal event. Have a low threshold for imaging (which may include a CT of the head) in the elderly patient. While CT is not necessary to evaluate all causes of syncope, you should carefully consider traumatic ICH associated with the event.

Risk Stratification: Management Priorities

- Low risk: Patients with clearly defined reflex-mediated syncope.
- High risk: Elderly patients or patients taking anticoagulation.

Definitive Management

Definitive management is sometimes difficult for reflex-mediated syncope. It is best to advise the patient to attempt to avoid precipitating factors such as wearing tight clothing around the neck in carotid sinus hypersensitivity. Patients should be advised to lay supine when undergoing venipuncture or other painful procedures. Male patients may also be advised to urinate while seated on the toilet rather than standing.

Complications

Complications from trauma should be sought in and evaluated for all patients who have experienced a syncopal episode.

Disposition

Patients who do not have significant trauma and who have a clearly low-risk etiology for their syncopal episode may be discharged and instructed to follow-up with their primary care physician.

ORTHOSTATIC HYPOTENSION SYNCOPE

Additional History and Physical Examination Findings

Syncope caused by orthostatic hypotension should be suspected when the patient has loss of postural tone shortly after arising from a seated or supine position. BP should be checked in the supine position after lying flat for 5 minutes and again after standing for a period of 2-3 minutes. Syncope should only be attributed to orthostatic hypotension if the patient's symptoms are reproduced with positional change testing.

The history should focus on factors that would contribute to intravascular volume depletion such as vomiting, diarrhea, bleeding, decreased intake of fluids, or diuretic use. Medications should be reviewed for agents that would lead to orthostatic hypotension such as alpha-blocking agents. A history of diabetes, Parkinson disease, adrenal insufficiency, or alcoholism should be elicited as a possible etiology for autonomic dysfunction and orthostatic hypotension.

Review Initial Results

Vital signs should be reviewed and, if symptoms are not reproduced, an alternate etiology for syncope should be sought. If gastrointestinal (GI) bleeding is suspected, a complete blood count (CBC) and a fecal sample for blood should be obtained.

Risk Stratification: Management Priorities

Risk stratification and management depends on the severity of orthostatic hypotension symptoms and etiology. Patients at high risk are those with acute hemorrhage or moderate to severe volume depletion. Those with GI hemorrhage should have immediate large-bore intravenous (IV) access established and be type- and cross-matched for blood. Those with moderate to severe intravascular volume depletion should have IV crystalloid fluids administered.

Definitive Management

Patients with significant intravascular volume depletion should receive IV fluid resuscitation. Those with hemorrhage should receive IV fluid and packed red blood cells (PRBCs).

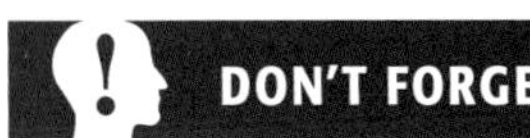

DON'T FORGET

Do not attribute syncope to orthostatic hypotension if the examination does not reproduce the symptoms.

Patients with mild intravascular volume depletion caused by diuretic use should be instructed to increase oral intake by mouth and reduce the dose of medication. Patients with orthostasis caused by alpha-blocking agents may either reduce the dose or take the medications before bed to reduce symptoms.

Patients with orthostasis due to autonomic dysfunction should be advised to increase oral fluid intake and arise from a seated or supine position slowly and with caution. Addition of a mineralocorticoid may help in refractory cases or those where adrenal insufficiency is a concern.

Frequent reassessment: Patients with significant volume depletion or hemorrhage should have frequent reassessment of vital signs.

Complications: Complications from trauma should be sought in all patients who have experienced a syncopal episode.

DON'T FORGET

Look for hemorrhage in a patient with orthostatic hypotension.

Disposition: Patients who are orthostatic and have evidence of hemorrhage or significant dehydration should be admitted to the hospital. If patients are unstable or refractory to attempts at initial stabilization, they should be admitted to the intensive care unit (ICU). Patients who are stable after intervention in the emergency department (ED) and do not have significant comorbidity may be discharged with outpatient follow-up after appropriate instructions have been given.

DON'T FORGET

- Suspect ICH in a patient with headache and syncope.
- A new focal neurologic deficit after a syncopal event should prompt CNS imaging.
- Nonspecific "twitching" during syncope should not lead you to diagnose seizure.
- Patients with syncope and signs and symptoms of "vertigo" should undergo evaluation for vertebrobasilar insufficiency and possible vertebrobasilar dissection.

NEUROLOGIC SYNCOPE

Additional History and Physical Examination Findings

True syncope should be distinguished from conditions that mimic a syncopal event such as an unwitnessed generalized seizure or drop attack. Bystanders, if available, should be questioned regarding witnessed seizure activity or signs suggestive of a postictal state. Muscular contractions (myoclonic jerking), not representing true seizure, can sometimes be seen after cerebral hypoperfusion following syncope. The patient should be evaluated for trauma to the tongue that may suggest occurrence of a seizure. Sudden onset of severe headache prior to the syncopal event may suggest subarachnoid hemorrhage (SAH).

A thorough neurologic examination should be performed and focal neurologic deficits documented. Patients should be asked if they experienced any difficulty speaking, diplopia, or difficulty with balance suggestive of vertebrobasilar hypoperfusion prior to the event.

Review Initial Results

Computed tomography (CT) should be obtained if the history is suggestive of ICH. Lumbar puncture (LP) should be performed in patients suspected of SAH with negative head CT. Magnetic resonance structural and vascular imaging of the brain should be obtained if the history or physical examination suggests vertebrobasilar hypoperfusion.

Risk Stratification: Management Priorities

Those patients with focal neurologic findings and history suggestive of ICH or vertebrobasilar insufficiency should receive priority imaging and subspecialty consultation.

Definitive Management

Patients with SAH should have immediate neurosurgical consultation and aggressive control of hypertension. Patients with vertebrobasilar insufficiency should be treated in consultation with neurology depending on etiology, ie, dissection, thromboembolism, or migraine.

Frequent Reassessment

Patients with ICH should be monitored closely for any signs of airway compromise.

Disposition

Those with vertebrobasilar insufficiency, ICH, and poorly controlled seizures should be admitted to the hospital.

CARDIOVASCULAR SYNCOPE

Additional History and Physical Examination Findings

- Syncope that occurs after exertion should raise concerns for hypertrophic cardiomyopathy with outflow obstruction, aortic stenosis, unstable angina, or myocardial infarction.
- The murmur associated with hypertrophic cardiomyopathy is typically heard best along the left sternal boarder during systole and is increased by maneuvers that decrease preload such as Valsalva and standing. The murmur is decreased by squatting and isometric handgrip. This diagnosis should be suspected in the young athlete with exertional syncope. Sudden cardiac death is typically related to malignant arrhythmia precipitated after exertion.
- Aortic stenosis may have many etiologies, including bicuspid aortic valve, rheumatic disease, or valvular calcification. The murmur of aortic stenosis is systolic, crescendo-decrescendo, and heard best at the right sternal boarder and typically radiates to the carotid arteries.
- Long QT syndrome may be congenital or acquired and should be suspected in patients with exertional syncope, or in those patients taking drugs that may prolong the QT interval such as many antiarrhythmic agents, older second-generation antihistamines, erythromycin, certain quinolones, and cisapride. Prolonged QT interval may lead to syncope or sudden cardiac death by precipitating torsade de pointes.
- Short QT syndrome has also been described as a predisposing factor to syncope and sudden cardiac death by inducing tachyarrhythmias or ventricular fibrillation.
- The Brugada syndrome (incomplete right bundle branch block [RBBB] associated with ST segment elevation with a "saddle" appearance in the precordia leads) is associated with syncope and sudden cardiac death in those with structurally normal hearts.
- Cardiac tamponade should be suspected in patients with elevated jugular venous pressure, muffled heart sounds, and narrow pulse pressure.
- Syncope has been reported in 13% of patients with aortic dissection. Cardiac tamponade, stroke, and proximal dissection are independently associated with syncope in aortic dissection. Factors that should raise suspicion for aortic dissection include chest pain that radiates to the back, unequal

DON'T FORGET

- Exertional syncope should alert you to possible hypertrophic cardiomyopathy with outflow tract obstruction, aortic stenosis, or acute coronary syndrome.
- Review the ECG for conduction blocks, bradyarrhythmia, QT-interval abnormalities, ischemia, infarct, or signs of organic heart disease.

DON'T FORGET

- Patients with chest discomfort and syncope should be evaluated for aortic dissection, acute coronary syndrome, or pulmonary embolism.
- Do not discharge patients with syncope and a cardiovascular etiology.

DON'T FORGET

High-risk patients:

- History or examination consistent with heart disease
- Chest pain consistent with cardiovascular etiology
- ECG suggestive of ischemia, alteration in QT interval, or conduction block
- Age >60 years
- Family history of unexplained sudden death
- Exertional syncope

BPs in the upper extremities, diastolic murmur of aortic regurgitation, and physical characteristics such as a tall thin person with a family history of connective tissue disease such as Marfan syndrome or sudden death.

- Pulmonary embolism should be suspected in patients with a history of previous thromboembolic disease, unexplained asymmetrical leg swelling, family history of thromboembolic disease, contraceptive use, adenocarcinoma, or immobility. Patient presenting with tachypnea, hypoxia, hypotension, or pleuritic chest pain before or after syncope should be suspected of pulmonary embolism.
- The physical examination should also be directed at noting the rate and regularity of the pulse. This may uncover a tachyarrhythmia or bradyarrhythmia or suggest conduction block.

Review Initial Results

- Telemetry: Review a rhythm strip to identify arrhythmia or conduction disturbance.
- ECG: Left ventricular hypertrophy may be a clue to structural heart disease including hypertrophic cardiomyopathy and aortic stenosis.
  - Long QT syndrome is characterized by QTc prolongation of >0.45 seconds in men and 0.46 seconds in children and women (Fig. 9-1A).
  - Short QT syndrome is characterized by a QT interval of ≤280 ms or QTc of ≤300 ms.
  - Brugada syndrome should be suspected in patients with downsloping ST-segment elevation in V1 and V2 and QRS pattern resembling a RBBB (Fig. 9-1B).
  - Electrical alternans or a low-voltage pattern may suggest pericardial effusion and possible tamponade (Fig. 9-1C).
  - Look for signs of ischemia characterized by ST-segment depression or T-wave inversion. Look for signs of infarct suggested by peaked T waves, ST-segment elevation, or new Q waves.
  - Look for signs of WPW syndrome suggested by the upsloping delta wave of the QRS complex or short PR interval (Fig. 9-1D).
  - Evaluate the ECG for significant conduction blocks as in type II second-degree heart block and complete heart block (Fig. 9-1E).
  - New onset tachycardia, RBBB, or right axis deviation may be associated with pulmonary hypertension and pulmonary embolism.
- Chest x-ray (CXR): Cardiac enlargement on an x-ray obtained may suggest structural heart disease and can be a clue to hypertrophic cardiomyopathy, left ventricular failure, aortic stenosis, or pericardial effusion.
  - A wide mediastinum or abnormal aortic contour may suggest aortic dissection.
  - The CXR in pulmonary embolism may exhibit atelectasis, elevated hemidiaphragm, and small pleural effusion or may appear normal. Although focal oligemia or pleural-based opacity pointing away from the pleura may be more specific for pulmonary embolism, these findings are rare.
  - Cardiac ultrasound: A point-of-care cardiac ultrasound performed by the trained emergency physician may help in identifying a pericardial effusion and tamponade.
  - Other: CT or ventilation perfusion scanning should be done in patients suspected of pulmonary embolism.

Risk Stratification: Management Priorities

- Patients with syncope and a clear cardiovascular etiology are at relatively high risk for increased morbidity and mortality and should be admitted to the hospital. As always, management priorities are airway, breathing, and circulation. Identify life-threatening arrhythmia by immediate telemetry monitoring and treat it, based on advanced cardiac life support (ACLS) protocols.

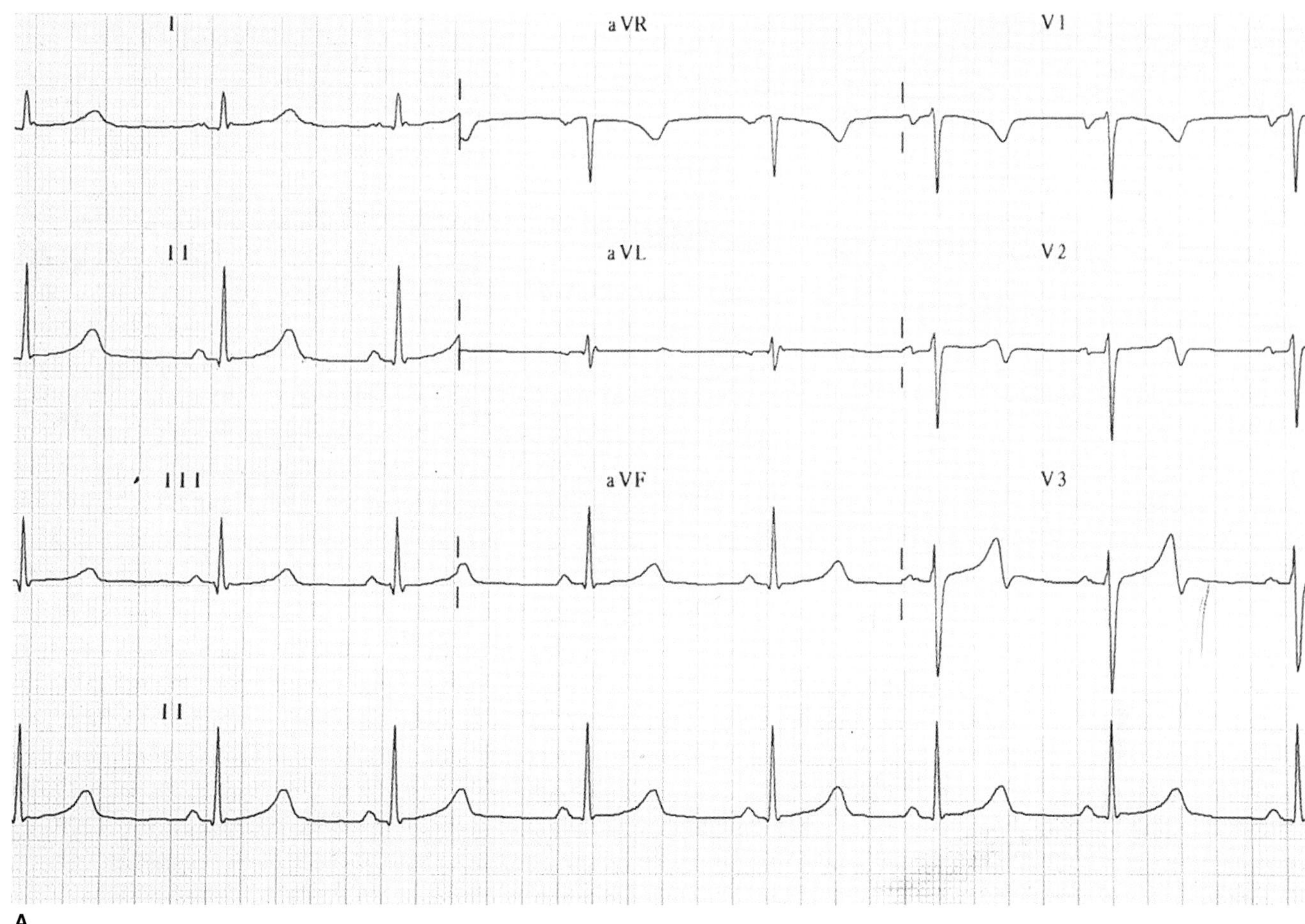

Figure 9-1. **(A)** A QT interval of 0.48 seconds is seen in a 10-year-old patient presenting with syncope following exercise. His family history was positive for heart disease (his father died an unexplained death at age 35); his family history was negative for deafness. **(B)** Twelve-lead ECG typical of Brugada syndrome shows characteristic downsloping ST-segment elevation in leads V1 and V2 and QRS morphology, resembling a right bundle branch block. **(C)** ECG showing low voltage in the limb leads (<5 mm). There is slight beat-to-beat variation in the QRS amplitude of leads V1, V4, and V5 (electrical alternans). **(D)** Atrial fibrillation in Wolff-Parkinson-White syndrome. **(E)** Type II second-degree atrioventricular block. Surface ECG; leads I, aVF, and V1 and intracardiac electrograms from the right atrial (RA), proximal, and distal His bundle electrogram (HBE) catheters are shown. Surface ECGs show that the PR intervals are constant at 0.2 second with a left bundle branch block morphology of the QRS complex, and the fourth P wave is not followed by a QRS complex. The HBEs reveal that the site of block of the fourth P wave is below the HBE. ([A] *Reproduced with permission from Shah BR, Lucchesi M*. Atlas of Pediatric Emergency Medicine. *New York, NY: McGraw-Hill; 2006. [B, D] Reproduced with permission from Tintinalli JE, Kelen GD, Stapczynski JS, et al*. Emergency Medicine: A Comprehensive Study Guide. *6th ed. New York, NY: McGraw-Hill; 2004. [C] Reproduced with permission from Schwartz DT*. Emergency Radiology: Case Studies. *New York, NY: McGraw-Hill; 2008. [E] Reproduced with permission from Fuster V, O'Rourke RA, Walsh R, Poole-Wilson P*. Hurst's The Heart. *12th ed. New York, NY: McGraw-Hill; 2008.*)

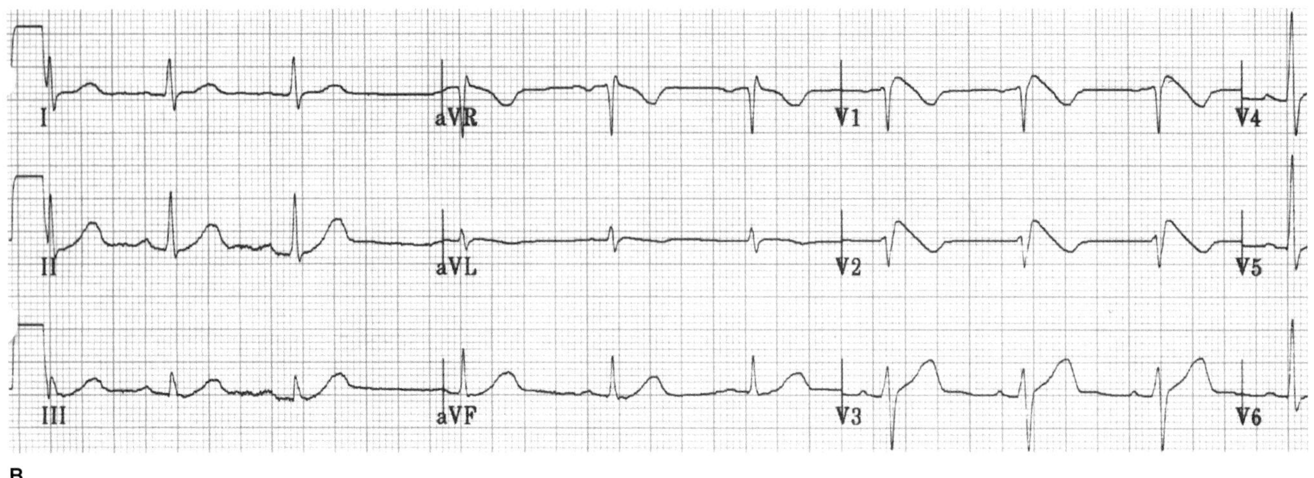

B

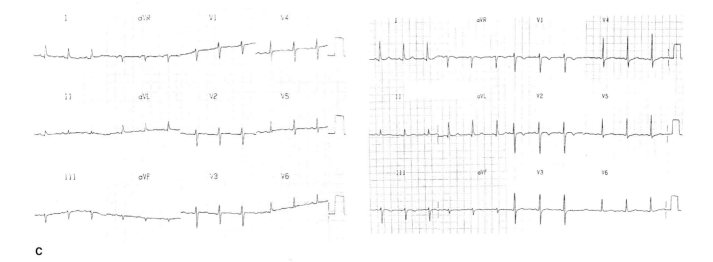

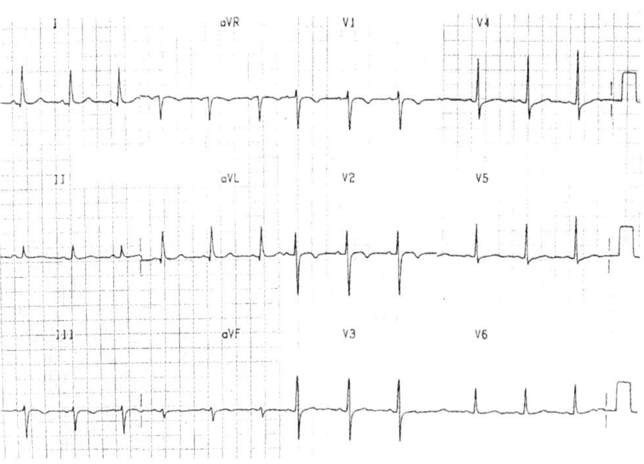

C

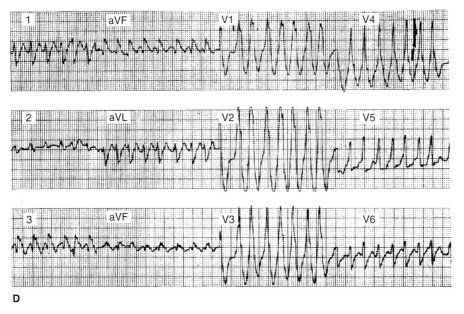

D

Figure 9-1. (*Continued.*)

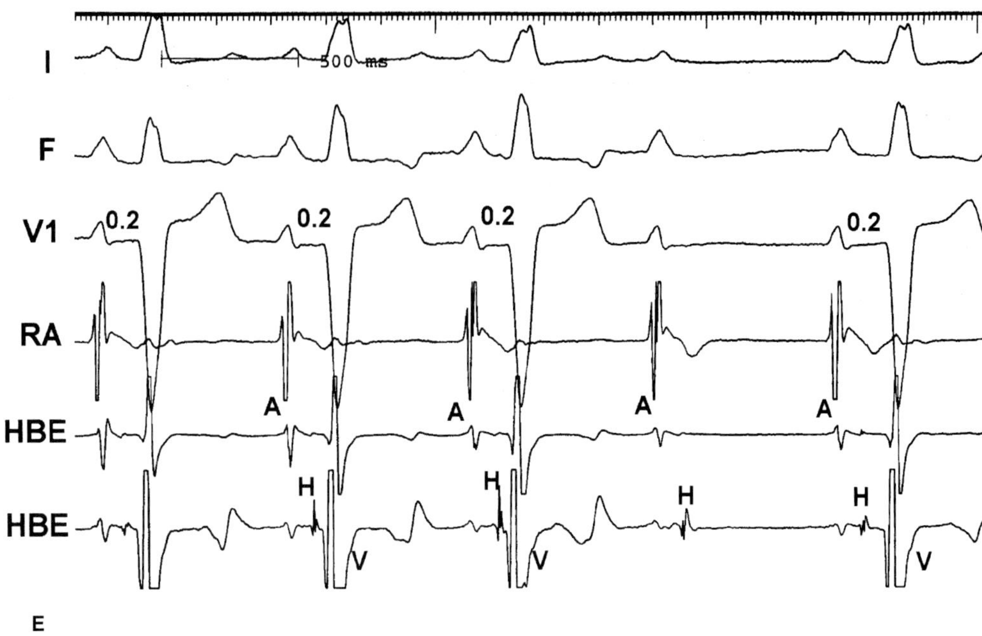

Figure 9-1. (*Continued.*)

Definitive Management

- Patients with suspected hypertrophic cardiomyopathy should undergo echocardiography. Medical management includes initiation of beta-blockers and referral for possible internal defibrillator placement. Patients should be given strict instructions not to engage in strenuous physical activity.
- Patients with aortic stenosis and syncope should be admitted for evaluation of valve replacement.
- Patients with acute coronary syndrome or unstable angina should be stabilized in the ED and immediately referred to for coronary intervention.
- Patients with disorders of the QT interval should undergo evaluation of serum potassium, calcium, and magnesium. Medications that are thought to alter the QT interval should be discontinued after consultation with the patient's primary care physician. If the disorder of the QT interval is thought to be congenital, other family members should be tested and the patient be referred to for possible internal defibrillator placement.
- Patients with Brugada syndrome should be referred to for possible internal defibrillator placement.
- If patients are diagnosed with cardiac tamponade, an immediate crystalloid fluid challenge should be given and preparations be made for pericardiocentesis. Cardiology and cardiothoracic surgery should be consulted.
- Patients with proximal or type A aortic dissection need immediate surgical intervention and rapid control of heart rate and BP. Shearing forces should be controlled with IV esmolol first, then reduce BP with IV nicardepine.
- Patients with pulmonary embolism and syncope should be treated with heparin and admitted to the ICU. Evaluation for right ventricular strain by ECG, bedside echocardiography, or troponin/ brain-type natriuretic peptide (BNP) elevations may warrant cardiology or interventional radiology consultation for thrombolysis systemically or targeted (mechanically). ECG may show right ventricular strain pattern (ST depression or T wave inversion inferiorly). Bedside echocardiography may reveal right ventricle dilation. Systemic thrombolysis should be considered in consultation with a critical care physician if targeted therapies are not available.
- Transcutaneous pacing should be started in patients with bradyarrhythmias who are unstable and refractory to medical management. Patients should be prepared for transvenous pacing via the right internal jugular route.

Frequent Reassessment

- Patients should be continuously monitored by telemetry and vital signs be frequently checked.

Disposition

- Patients with a clear cardiovascular etiology or other life threatening etiologies for syncope should be admitted to the hospital.

WINNING STRATEGIES

- Every patient with syncope has a life-threatening etiology until proven otherwise.
- Immediate intervention in all patients with syncope should include IV access, telemetry monitoring, oxygen, and stat ECG on exam day.
- Obtain a BP in both arms and a CXR in patients with syncope and chest pain.
- Do not attribute syncope to a psychiatric etiology in a young healthy female with "hyperventilation." Consider pulmonary embolism!
- Review the patient's medications. Some medications may cause conduction disturbances and QT-interval prolongation, or, may lead to orthostasis.
- Do not attribute syncope to orthostasis if the patient does not have reproducible symptoms.
- Always look for trauma (head injury or otherwise) in the patient who has experienced a syncopal episode, especially in the elderly.
- Your history and cardiovascular examination (including ECG) will be one of the most important factors in narrowing your differential diagnosis.
- Patients with a clear cardiovascular etiology and a syncopal event should not go home.
- Do not automatically attribute syncope to a seizure if minor "twitching" is noted during the event.
- Headache and syncope mean ICH until proven otherwise.
- Do a thorough neurologic examination.
- If a patient has clear reflex-mediated syncope associated with additional complaints such as chest pain, work it up! Do not be satisfied with a neurocardiogenic etiology.
- Evaluate the patient for hemorrhage when orthostatic syncope is diagnosed.
- Place pacer pads on the patient with bradycardia and clinically significant heart block. Prepare for placement of a transvenous pacer.
- Patients with a history or physical examination suggestive of CHF, valvular disease or ventricular arrhythmia, and syncope should be admitted to the hospital.
- Patients with chest pain suspicious for cardiac etiology or ECG findings of ischemia, significant conduction block, abnormal QTc interval, or arrhythmia should be admitted to the hospital.
- Patients with syncope who are >60 years, have a history of coronary artery disease or congenital heart disease, exertional syncope or a family history of sudden death should be admitted to the hospital on exam day.
- Patients should be instructed not to drive if they are thought to be at risk for recurrent syncope.

THE BOTTOM LINE

- Every patient with syncope has a life-threatening etiology until proven otherwise.
- Immediate intervention in all patients with syncope should include IV access, telemetry monitoring, oxygen, and immediate ECG on exam day.
- Elderly patients, patients with heart disease, and exertional symptoms or concerning abnormalities on ECG associated with syncope should be admitted to the hospital.

CHAPTER 10

Shortness of Breath

Navneet Cheema

INITIAL ASSESSMENT

- Get a full set of vital signs (VS). Is the patient hypoxic? Febrile?
- Immediate supplemental oxygen and ventilatory support if needed.
- Identification of immediate life threats is important. Pericardial tamponade? Tension pneumothorax? These require immediate intervention!
- A wide and complex variety of potential etiologies here, many of which are immediately life-threatening. Focus on age, VS, past medical history (PMHx), and examination to narrow down causes and focus treatment efforts.

DON'T FORGET

On test day, the patient will have

- Volume overload/CHF
- Asthma/COPD exacerbation
- PE
- MI
- Pneumonia
- Pneumothorax
- Pericardial effusion
- Metabolic derangement

INITIAL HISTORY AND PHYSICAL EXAMINATION

History

- History of present illness (HPI)
  - Onset (gradual vs acute/sudden)
  - Associations (travel, trauma, exposures, sick contacts)
  - Aggravating/alleviating factors (exertion, position, oxygen)
  - Duration
  - Noncompliance with medications or dietary restrictions
  - Smoking and illicit drug use
- PMHx
  - Prior lung disease such as asthma or chronic obstructive pulmonary disease (COPD)?
  - History of coronary artery disease (CAD), congestive heart failure (CHF), or recent myocardial infarction (MI)?
  - Cardiac risk factors: diabetes mellitus (DM), hypertension (HTN), family history, high cholesterol, smoking
  - History of malignancy? Immunosuppressed state? Renal failure?
  - Previous hospitalizations or intubations?
- Medications
  - Specifically, diuretics, inhalers, home oxygen?
- Allergies

IMMEDIATE INTERVENTIONS

- Oxygen via NC or NRB to keep O_2 >95%
- Cardiac monitor
- 18-gauge IV, 0.9% NS at KVO, draw blood for laboratory studies
- Immediate ventilatory support if needed!

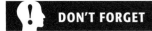

Physical Examination

- VS (obtain on a complete set including respiratory rate [RR], O2 sat, and temperature)
- BP increased? Decreased?
- Skin: Diaphoresis, cyanosis, pallor?
- Neck: Trachea midline, jugular venous distention (JVD), stridor, hepatojugular reflux?
- Chest: Breath sounds equal, crackles, wheezes, rubs?
- CV: Murmurs, rubs, gallops? Peripheral pulses symmetric?
- Abdomen: Distended (limiting ventilation), firm? Bowel sounds? Kussmaul respirations? (Could indicate potential acidosis.)
- Extremities: Cyanosis, edema, asymmetric swelling/ tenderness?
- Neuro: Motor, sensory, deep tendon reflexes (DTRs) symmetric, mental status?

DON'T FORGET

Remember to use BiPAP to stabilize the acutely ill patient, but be prepared to intubate if the patient deteriorates.

DIFFERENTIAL DIAGNOSIS

- Asthma
  - Patients typically will present with shortness of breath, cough, and wheezing, and have a history of asthma. Possible exacerbants include infection, allergen exposure, medication noncompliance, and illicit drug use.
  - These patients require prompt treatment with bronchodilators, steroids, magnesium, and possible epinephrine.

DON'T FORGET

Be careful to differentiate dyspnea from hyperpnea (increased ventilation secondary to acidosis or metabolic requirements).

- COPD exacerbation
  - A chronic lung disease grouping that includes components of bronchospasm, airway inflammation, and airway collapse (emphysema). Precipitants include infection, allergen exposure, and medication noncompliance.
  - As these patients are typically older adults, beware of comorbid conditions such as MI and pulmonary embolism (PE). Consider pneumothorax with acute sudden exacerbations.
- CHF/pulmonary edema
  - These patients will typically present with shortness of breath which is usually increased with exertion or lying down. Most will have a previous history of CHF and be on diuretics. They are typically hypertensive with crackles in their lungs and elevated jugular venous pressure (JVP). Exacerbants include medication adjustments or noncompliance, ischemia, or valvular disease.
- Pericardial tamponade
  - Results from increased fluid in the pericardial sac which interferes with cardiac output and diastolic filling.
  - Patients will typically present with dyspnea and decreased exercise tolerance.
  - Suspect highly in any patient with thoracic trauma or with history of renal failure, lupus, or malignancy.
- Pneumonia
  - Usually presents with fever, cough, and possibly hypoxia. May require ventilatory support.
  - A vast array of causes exist: use PMHx, travel history, exposure history, social history, and comorbidities to narrow down the causes and select appropriate antibiotic treatment and disposition.
- Pulmonary embolism
  - Consider in the patient with shortness of breath or chest pain and no evidence of CHF, pneumonia, or MI. Suspect also with predisposing factors, eg, current or past DVT or PE, cancer, prolonged travel or bed rest, recent trauma or surgery, and pregnancy or obesity.
- Pneumothorax
  - Suspect tension pneumothorax in patients with dyspnea, decreased unilateral breath sounds, and deviated trachea.
  - Immediate intervention is the key here...don't wait for the chest x-ray (CXR)! (Refer to Chap. 8.)
- Noncardiogenic pulmonary edema
  - A complex phenomenon of increased pulmonary capillary membrane permeability usually secondary to causes such as overwhelming sepsis, drug overdose, altitude illness, and inhalation injuries (Fig. 10-1).
  - Can be very difficult to distinguish clinically from cardiogenic edema.

DON'T FORGET

Always consider other diagnoses such as MI and PE in short-of-breath patients with history of asthma.

DON'T FORGET

In the COPD patient with sudden deterioration, think spontaneous pneumothorax.

DON'T FORGET

Immediately isolate any patient with suspected TB.

Immediate needle decompression of the chest in any patient with suspected tension pneumothorax!

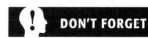

ASTHMA

Additional History and Physical Examination Findings

- Patients usually present with dyspnea, cough, wheezing, and chest tightness, and have a history of asthma.
- Typical findings include increased RR, wheezing, and prolonged expiration.
- Exacerbation is often preceded by upper respiratory tract infection (URTI), new allergen exposure, medication change or noncompliance, or illicit drug use.
- Higher-risk patients have had previous intensive care unit (ICU) admissions, previous intubations, illicit drug use, and recent emergency department (ED) visits.
- Hypoxia, accessory muscle use, diaphoresis, inability to lie down or speak in more than single words, peak flows <50% predicted/personal best are indicative of more severe exacerbation.
- Paradoxical respirations and altered mental status are indicative of imminent arrest.

DON'T FORGET

Beware of the "silent chest" in asthma—a sign of impending respiratory failure!

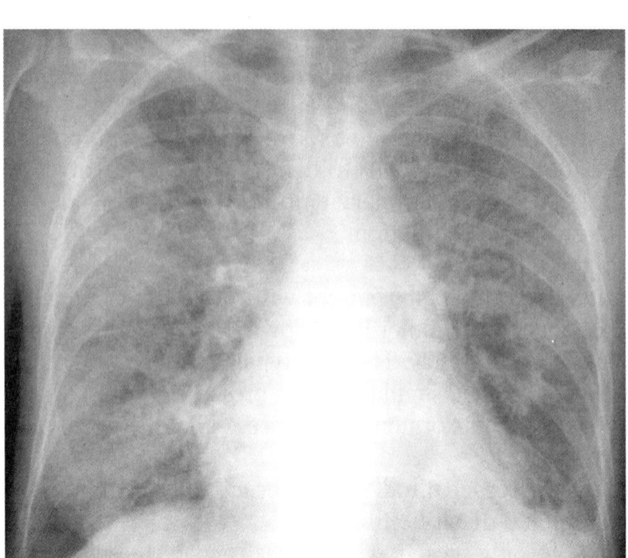

Figure 10-1. Noncardiogenic pulmonary edema. Diffuse airspace edema without a central distribution in a patient following an overdose of heroin. (*Reprinted with permission from Schwartz DT.* Emergency Radiology: Case Studies. *New York, NY: McGraw-Hill; 2008.*)

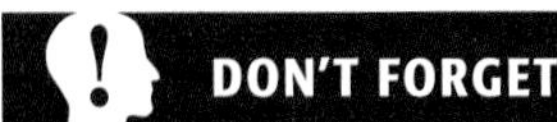

DON'T FORGET

Reserve testing in the asthmatic for the patient with a severe exacerbation, unclear diagnosis, or significant comorbidities.

Review Initial Results

- Peak flow measurements: Use initially and periodically to monitor for improvement.
- CXR: Usually not necessary in a simple exacerbation unless there is suspicion for a complication such as pneumothorax or pneumonia.
- Typically will reveal hyperexpanded lungs.
- Electrocardiogram (ECG): Again, not necessary unless unclear diagnosis or elderly patient or patient with comorbidities. Can reveal right ventricular strain pattern which typically resolves with clinical improvement.

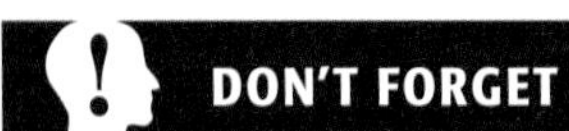

DON'T FORGET

Immediate intubation and mechanical ventilation if imminent respiratory arrest

Risk Stratification: Management Priorities

- Historical risk factors include prior sudden severe attacks, previous ICU admissions and intubations, recent ED visits or hospitalizations, or illicit drug use.
- Objective features of severe exacerbation include heart rate (HR) >120 beats/min, RR >40 breaths/min, accessory muscle use, upright position, agitation, hypoxia, and inability to speak more than single words.
- Immediate treatment and frequent reevaluation are vital!

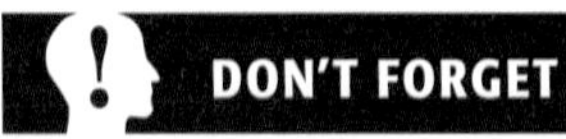

DON'T FORGET

Employ a ventilatory strategy of permissive hypercapnia to avoid complications.

Definitive Management

- Oxygen: High-flow via non-rebreather mask (NRB) mask if hypoxic.
- Inhaled beta-agonists: Typically by nebulizer. Albuterol 2.5 mg every 30-60 minutes × 3 or continually for severe exacerbations.
- Anticholinergics: Ipratropium bromide 0.5 mg every 4-6 hours for moderate to severe exacerbations.

- Corticosteroids: Indicated for all but the mildest of exacerbations. Prednisone 50-60 mg PO for most, methylprednisolone 80-125 mg intravenous (IV) for severe exacerbations or patients unable to tolerate PO.
- Epinephrine: Helpful in severe exacerbations, especially if unable to inhale beta-agonists. Dose at 0.2-0.5 mL 1:1000 intramuscular (IM) or subcutaneous (SQ), every 5-10 minutes up to three doses.
- Magnesium sulfate: 1-2 g IVPB over 30 minutes may be helpful in severe exacerbations.
- Heliox: An 80:20 or 70:30 mixture of helium and oxygen, resulting in a less dense gas allowing improved airflow and gas exchange. May reduce work of breathing and buy time to avoid intubation.
- Continuous positive airway pressure/bilevel positive airway pressure (CPAP/BiPAP): Face mask–administered ventilation with CPAP or BiPAP—may be beneficial and reduce work of breathing.
- Intubation/mechanical ventilation: The last resort for asthmatic patients in impending respiratory failure.
  - Ketamine is the preferred agent for induction because of its bronchodilatory effects.
  - Succinylcholine or rocuronium recommended for initial paralysis.
  - Ventilatory strategy of permissive hypercapnia important to minimize barotrauma and breath stacking.
    - Use high fraction of inspired oxygen (FIO_2).
    - Low tidal volumes 6-8 mL/kg to prevent barotrauma.
    - Low ventilatory rate to allow for proper exhalation (<10/minutes).
    - Low or no positive end-expiratory pressure (PEEP) needed.
    - In-line bronchodilator treatments.

Frequent Reassessment

- Monitor peak flow measurements, HR, RR, O2 sat, respiratory effort, and degree of wheezing to assess improvement.
- If ventilated, frequent reassessments of VS, peak airway pressures, and arterial blood gases (ABGs) are key.

Complications

- Respiratory arrest: Treat with mechanical ventilation.
- Pneumothorax: Stat CXR if suspected, immediate decompression if suspected tension pneumothorax, definitive treatment with chest tube.
- Hypotension/cardiac arrest: Often can be caused by increased intrathoracic pressure from breath stacking, especially if mechanically ventilated.
- Treat hypotension with bolus of IV 0.9 NS.
- If no improvement or cardiac arrest, consider temporary removal from ventilator to allow for complete exhalation during the resuscitation.
- If no response, consider pneumothorax and empiric bilateral chest tubes.

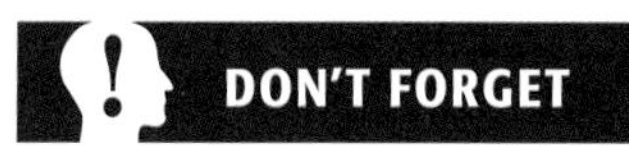

Breath-stacking and elevated intrathoracic pressure can lead to cardiac arrest in ventilated asthmatics. Disconnect ventilator to allow exhalation during resuscitation.

Disposition

- If good response to treatment (stable VS, peak flow >70% pred., lower risk), may discharge home with 4-6 additional days of steroid treatment. Ensure proper metered-dose inhaler (MDI) technique and adequate medication supply.
- If incomplete response (peak flow 50%-75% pred., some wheezing), consider admission to medical or observation unit.
- If poor response/no response, definite hospital admission, ICU admission if continued signs of respiratory distress or requiring very frequent or continuous bronchodilator treatments.

COPD EXACERBATION

Additional History and Physical Examination Findings

- Assess RR, temp, BP, HR, O_2 sat.
- Lung auscultation for unequal breath sounds, crackles, wheezes, diminished heart tones, murmurs, leg edema.
- If patient presenting with acute sudden dyspnea and deterioration, consider diagnosis of pneumothorax.
- If subacute deterioration, over hours to days, consider worsening bronchospasm, superimposed respiratory infection, cardiovascular events, PE, small pneumothorax.

Review Initial Results

- CXR
  - Definitely recommended as radiographic abnormalities are common (pneumothorax, pneumonia, atelectasis).
- ECG
  - Also important to reveal signs of arrhythmia or possible cardiac ischemia.
  - Will likely reveal evidence of right ventricular hypertrophy (RVH) or cor pulmonale.
- B-type natriuretic peptide (BNP)
  - May help differentiate between a CHF or COPD exacerbation.
- ABG
  - Is helpful in assessing respiratory status, particularly if moderate to severe respiratory distress?
  - Look for acute or chronic respiratory acidosis.
- Additional labs
  - Complete blood count (CBC) and basic metabolic panel (BMP).
  - Creatinine kinase (CPK), troponin to rule out MI.
  - Sputum cultures and rapid influenza studies.

Risk Stratification: Management Priorities

- All patients in moderate to severe respiratory distress need cardiac monitoring and pulse oximetry. Consider CPAP or BiPAP.
- Immediate intubation and mechanical ventilation if respiratory arrest imminent.

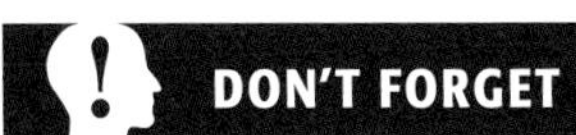

Provide high-flow oxygen initially to all hypoxic patients; wean FiO_2 down as condition allows.

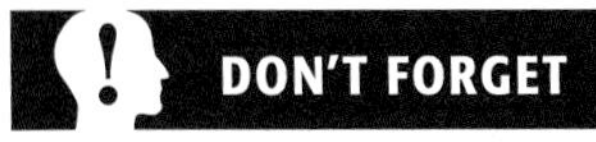

Give corticosteroids and antibiotics to all COPD patients on test day.

Definitive Management

- Oxygen
  - Important initial therapy for all hypoxic patients
  - Wean oxygen to maintain a saturation >90%
- Bronchodilators
  - Most effective if bronchospastic component to the COPD
  - Albuterol 2.5 mg via nebulizer every 30 minutes or continuously
- Anticholinergics
  - Ipratropium bromide provides additional bronchodilation: use 0.5 mg via neb every 4 hours
- Corticosteroids
  - Typically beneficial as there is usually some inflammatory component.
  - Prednisone 60 mg PO for stable patients
  - Methylprednisolone 80-125 mg IV for hospitalized patients
- Antibiotics
  - Typically indicated as empiric therapy for all COPD exacerbations.
  - Consider beta-lactam and macrolide or extended spectrum fluoroquinolone.

- Face mask ventilation with CPAP or BiPAP.
  - Consider in a patient with severe respiratory distress as it can prevent intubation and allow time for definitive treatments to become effective.
- Intubation and mechanical ventilation
  - Treatment of last resort.
  - As with asthma, permissive hypercapnia is the rule with tidal volumes 6-8 mL/kg, rate 8-10 breaths/min, high-flow oxygen, little or no PEEP.

Complications

- Especially from mechanical ventilation, include pneumothorax, breath stacking, and cardiac arrest.

Disposition

- Consider admission for all patients with significant deterioration from baseline or if failure to improve in the ED.
- ICU admission if requiring ventilatory assistance.

CONGESTIVE HEART FAILURE/PULMONARY EDEMA

Additional History and Physical Examination Findings

- Can be sudden or gradual in onset.
- Patients will often present with dyspnea, typically with exertion or lying flat.
- Inquire about previous history of CHF, medication changes or noncompliance, coronary artery disease, or dietary indiscretions.
- Typically present with tachypnea, hypertension, elevated JVP, crackles and wheezes in lung fields, and S_3 or S_4 heart sound, and possible lower extremity edema.
- Hypotension is an ominous sign and signifies a critical exacerbation. Also consider tamponade.
- Can result from many disease processes such as HTN, ischemia or MI, other cardiomyopathies, valvular dysfunction, renal failure, or occasionally "high-output" failure such as with profound anemia.
- On test day, will typically see patient with left heart failure manifesting as pulmonary edema. Can also present with right heart failure with hepatic congestion and leg edema.

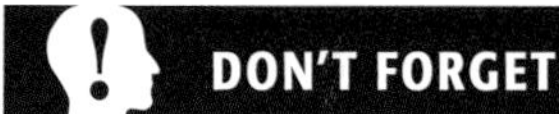

As with asthma, employ a ventilator strategy of permissive hypercapnia to minimize adverse events.

Review Initial Results

- ECG
  - Important study here—assess for evidence of acute MI/ischemia or conduction disturbances.
  - Often will see evidence of left ventricular hypertrophy (LVH), atrial hypertrophy, or atrial fibrillation.
- CXR
  - Findings will progress as pulmonary vascular pressures increase.
  - Begins as vascular redistribution to the upper lobes progressing to interstitial edema and finally alveolar pulmonary edema (Fig. 10-2).
  - Can also see cardiomegaly.
- Laboratory testing
  - Check blood urea nitrogen (BUN)/creatinine to exclude renal failure.
  - Cardiac enzymes/troponin to exclude MI.
  - May see lactic acidosis caused by decreased tissue perfusion.

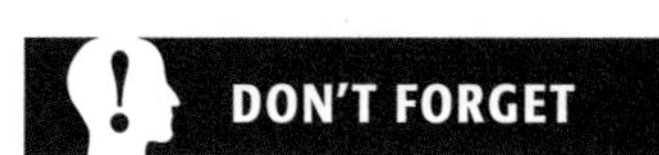

Hypotension is an ominous sign and signifies a critical exacerbation. Also consider tamponade.

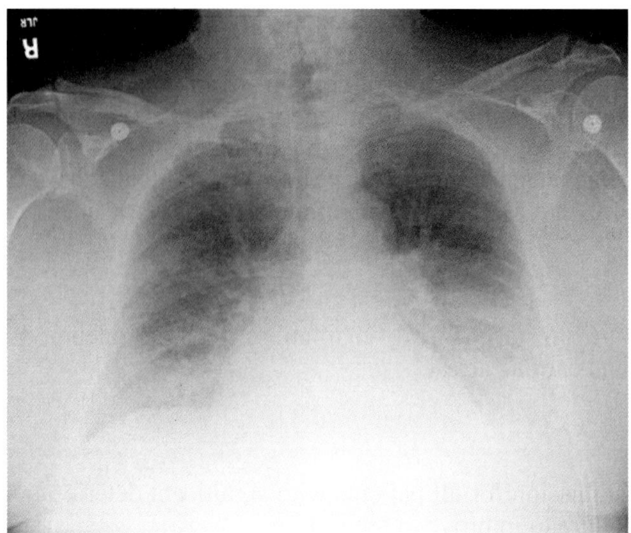

Figure 10-2. Pulmonary edema. Note indistinct vasculature, perihilar opacities, and peripheral interstitial reticular opacities. While this is an anteroposterior film making cardiac size more difficult to assess, the cardiac silhouette still appears enlarged. *(Reprinted with permission from Fauci AS, Braunwald E, Kaspter DL, et al.* Harrison's Principles of Internal Medicine. *17th ed. New York, NY: McGraw-Hill; 2008.)*

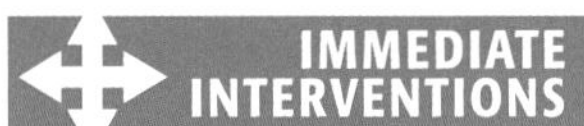

IMMEDIATE INTERVENTIONS

- High-flow mask oxygen
- Immediate ventilatory assistance if needed
- IV access
- Diuretics, nitrates, and morphine as BP allows
- Send CBC, BMP, cardiac enzymes, BNP
- Stat bedside ECG and CXR

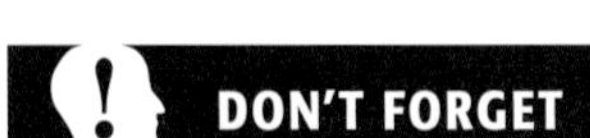

DON'T FORGET

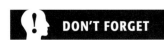

Most patients respond fairly rapidly to treatment, so consider CPAP/BiPAP first in the patient with respiratory distress unless obtunded or arrest is imminent.

- BNP
  - A fairly sensitive and specific study which can add to the diagnostic assessment. Typically elevated above 100 in pulmonary edema/LV dysfunction (can see levels in the thousands with severe exacerbations).

Risk Stratification: Management Priorities

- Assess these patients immediately and provide oxygen, pharmacologic therapy, and ventilatory assistance if needed.
- Higher-risk patients are those with hypotension, severe respiratory distress, and acute MI.
- Mainstays of treatment include
  - Decreasing cardiac workload through decreasing preload and afterload
  - Diuresis
  - Improving cardiac output
  - Assisting oxygenation and ventilation

Definitive Management

- IV access, high-flow oxygen, cardiac monitor, and pulse oximetry.
- Immediate ventilatory assistance with CPAP/BiPAP or intubation and mechanical ventilation if signs of respiratory distress (most respond rapidly to treatment).
- Loop diuretics (furosemide/bumetanide).
  - Allow significant reduction of volume and pulmonary congestion and provide preload reduction.
  - Furosemide 40-80 mg IV or bumetanide 2-4 mg IV.

- Nitrates
  - Potent vasodilators which decrease preload and afterload and reduce cardiac work.
  - Can administer in several forms, including sublingual (SL), topically, or intravenously via infusion.
  - Infuse at 10-20 μg/min and increase as needed.
  - Avoid if hypotensive.
- Afterload reduction
  - Recent data suggest that angiotensin-converting enzyme (ACE) inhibitors or hydralazine in combination with nitrates may have additive benefit in acute pulmonary edema.
  - Consider giving captopril 12.5-25 mg SL, enalapril 1.25 mg IV, or hydralazine 10 mg IV to the severely hypertensive patient in pulmonary edema.
- Morphine sulfate
  - Provides analgesia, reduction in catecholamine response, and preload reduction.
  - Dose at 2-5 mg IVP repeatedly as needed.
  - Careful if hypotensive.
- Dopamine
  - Produces increased inotropy and chronotropy.
  - Has dose-dependent effects with maximal beta-adrenergic effects at 5-15 μg/kg/min. Higher doses cause increased vasoconstriction.
- Dobutamine
  - Primarily a beta-1-receptor agonist with some beta-2 activity.
  - Acts to increase cardiac output with also some vasodilatation (careful with low blood pressure, can make it lower).
- Intra-aortic balloon pump or left ventricular-assist devices.
  - The last resort for cardiogenic shock.

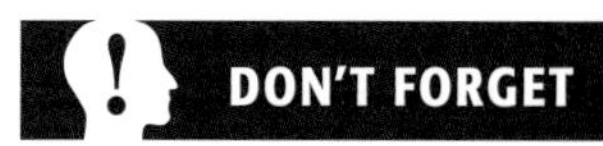

Avoid topical nitrates if very diaphoretic or evidence of decreased tissue perfusion as absorption can be erratic.

Frequent Reassessment

- Follow VS and clinical status as well as urine output for signs of improvement.
- Be ready to modify treatment as status can improve quickly.

Complications

- Respiratory failure: Manage with intubation and mechanical ventilation.
- Cardiogenic shock: Manage with vasopressors or Intra-aortic balloon pump/ Left ventricular assist device (IABP/ LVAD).
- Cardiac arrest or arrhythmias: Manage as per ACLS guidelines.

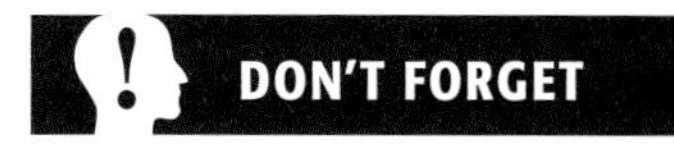

Hypotensive patients with CHF will most likely require IV vasopressor therapy with dopamine and/or dobutamine. If severe CHF, consult cardiology from the ER.

Disposition

- Severe exacerbations such as those requiring vasopressors or persistent ventilatory assistance, or acute MI with CHF should be admitted to the ICU.
- Patients with stable VS that improve can be admitted to cardiac or medical floor.

CARDIAC TAMPONADE

Additional History and Physical Examination Findings

- Patients present typically with weakness and shortness of breath.
- Take a good history of any recent trauma or cardiovascular procedure or bleeding disorder which could produce hemopericardium.
- If no trauma/procedure, need a good history of conditions which can cause pericardial effusions such as malignancy, renal failure, and systemic lupus erythematosus (SLE).

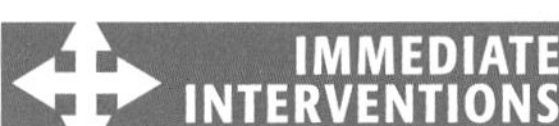

- Two 18-gauge IV lines, high-flow O_2, monitor, fluid bolus.
- ECG, CXR, and labs sent.
- Stat bedside echo or ultrasound (see Fig. 10-3).
- Obtain immediate cardiothoracic surgery consult if suspected.
- Bedside pericardiocentesis if arrest imminent.
- Beck's triad of elevated JVP, hypotension, and diminished heart tones is present in only about one-third of patients and usually is a very late sign just before cardiac arrest.

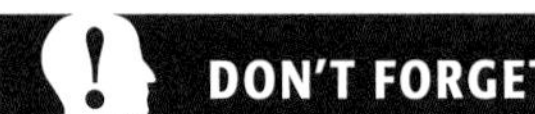

Remember with trauma and acute hemopericardium only a small amount of pericardial fluid is needed to cause tamponade.

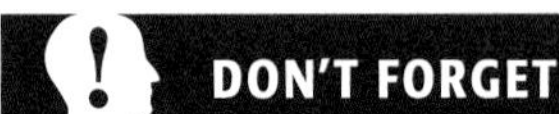

The definitive treatment here is surgical; mobilize the surgeon/surgical team immediately.

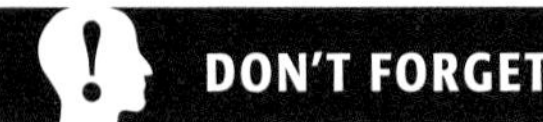

Consider pneumonia in the weak elderly patient, even without cough or shortness of breath.

- A high index of suspicion is needed as the disease can mimic many other presentations such as tension pneumothorax, CHF, hypovolemia, or PE.
- Physical examination can reveal tachycardia, pulmonary edema, hepatocongestion, elevated JVP, narrow pulse pressure, pulsus paradoxus >25 mm Hg, muffled heart tones, and hypotension as a late finding.
- Suspect in any PEA arrest, especially if traumatic.
- Have a high index of suspicion in a patient with any thoracic trauma, especially stab wounds.

Review Initial Results

- ECG: Can see low voltage, ST elevation, or electrical alternans (beat-to-beat alteration in R-wave amplitudes).
- CXR: May reveal enlarged cardiac silhouette or "epicardial fat pad" sign (lucency representing water density between heart and pericardium).
- Echocardiogram/bedside cardiac ultrasound: Evaluate for pericardial fluid (especially posterior) or diastolic collapse.

Risk Stratification: Management Priorities

- All tamponade patients are high risk and require immediate evaluation and surgical intervention.

Definitive Management

- IV access, high-flow oxygen, monitor.
- 0.9-NS fluid bolus to augment cardiac output.
- Arrange for immediate cardiothoracic surgery consult for pericardial window and drain.
- Bedside pericardiocentesis.
  - Consider if unstable or imminent cardiac arrest.
  - Perform with 18-gauge spinal needle and if possible ultrasound guidance or with V lead of ECG attached.
  - Insert needle just below xiphoid process at 30°-45° angle to the skin, aiming at the left shoulder blade.
  - If cardiac arrest, consider thoracotomy (especially if penetrating trauma).

Disposition

All patients are high risk and will need to go to the operating room (OR) for definitive treatment. No one goes home.

PNEUMONIA

Additional History and Physical Examination Findings

- Patients present typically with cough, fever, and dyspnea.
- Elderly patients can present with nonspecific symptoms such as altered mental status, weakness, or simply not feeling well.
- Key historical elements include age, travel/exposures, residence in a nursing home or recent hospitalization, aspiration risks, underlying lung disease, human immunodeficiency virus (HIV), or immunosuppression.
- Physical examination should focus on overall status, signs of respiratory distress/failure, and other diagnostic clues such as rash, sore throat, lymphadenopathy/splenomegaly, thrush, wasting, etc.

Review Initial Results

- CXR: The key diagnostic test here (Fig. 10-3).

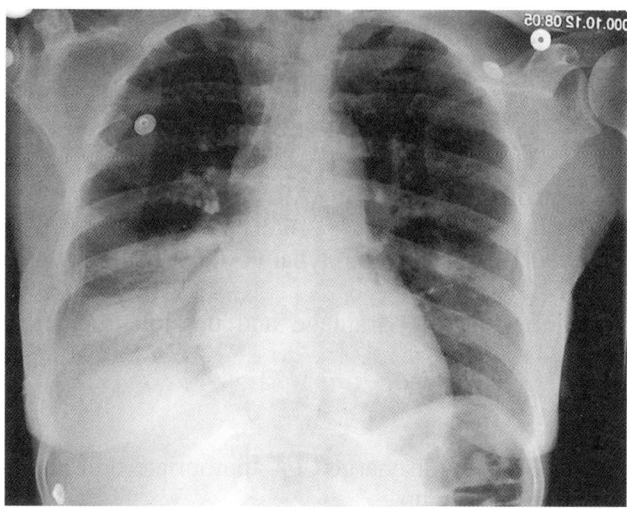

Figure 10-3. Right lower lobe pneumonia. (*Reprinted with permission from Stone CK, Humphries RL.* Current Diagnosis and Treatment in Emergency Medicine. *6th ed. New York, NY: McGraw-Hill; 2008.*)

- Infiltrate distribution can be suggestive (not diagnostic) of certain pathogens.
  - Segmental or lobar infiltrate with air bronchograms suggests bacterial pneumonia.
  - Interstitial infiltrates often seen with atypical pneumonias such as *Pneumocystis jiroveci* pneumonia (formerly *Pneumocysiis carinii* pneumonia; PCP), mycoplasma, or viral.
  - Diffuse patchy infiltrates with atypical and viral pneumonias.
  - Cavitary masses with tuberculosis (TB), fungi, staph, anaerobes.
- CXR can be nondiagnostic or normal appearing especially in the immunosupressed or dehydrated.
- CBC: Can see leukocytosis, leukopenia, neutropenia, or lymphopenia (as in acquired immunodeficiency syndrome [AIDS]).
- Sputum Gram stain and cultures:
  - May be helpful in diagnosis.
  - Rapid influenza and respiratory syncytial virus (RSV) testing of sputum helpful in winter months.
  - Immunosuppressed or AIDS patients may require bronchoscopy.
- Serologic tests for Legionella, cytomegalovirus (CMV) also helpful, but usually not immediately available.

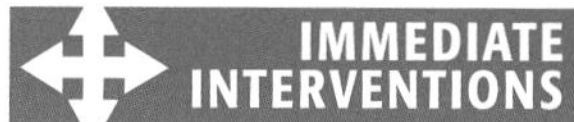

IMMEDIATE INTERVENTIONS

- IV, oxygen as needed, cardiac monitor
- Blood for labs and cultures
- Immediate ventilatory assistance if needed
- Immediate respiratory isolation if TB suspected
- CXR PA and lateral or bedside if critically ill
- Appropriate and timely antibiotic selection

Risk Stratification: Management Priorities

- Provide immediate oxygen and ventilatory support as needed.
- High-risk patients include the elderly, immunocompromised, underlying lung disease, or those with respiratory distress.
- Prudent broad-spectrum antibiotic selection guided by history and examination and ancillary data.
- Immediate respiratory isolation if suspect TB.

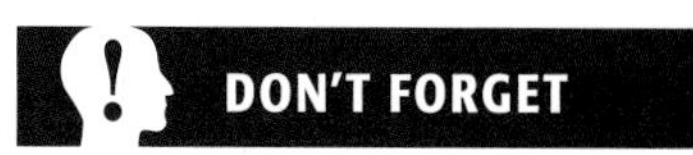

DON'T FORGET

Use history, examination, CXR, and lab data to guide initial, broad-spectrum antibiotic therapy. Infectious disease consult if critically ill or immunocompromised patient.

Definitive Management

- IV, oxygen, monitor.
- Immediate ventilatory assistance if needed.

- Appropriate antibiotic therapy (see Table 10-1 for common major causes).
- If critically ill patient or immunocompromised, AIDS, or transplant patient, consider ED infectious disease consult.

Complications

- Respiratory distress/failure: Treat with CPAP/BiPAP or intubation and mechanical ventilation as needed.
- Sepsis: May need advanced hemodynamic monitoring, fluid resuscitation, and vasopressors.
- Empyema: Requires pleural drainage and possible thoracic surgery and decortication.

Disposition

- Low-risk patients can be discharged on appropriate oral antibiotic therapy and with outpatient follow-up.
- Consider admission for those at moderate to high risk of complications.
  - RR >30 breaths/min, systolic blood pressure (SBP) <90 mm Hg, HR >120 beats/min, partial pressure of oxygen (Pao_2) <60 mm Hg
  - Evidence of sepsis or dehydration
  - Elderly, immunocompromised, underlying lung disease or malignancy, cardiovascular disease
- ICU admission for those with impending respiratory failure or septic shock.

Table 10-1. Initial Antibiotic Decision Making

Patient type	Usual Pathogens	Initial Antibiotic
Normal host/community acquired	Typical and atypical bacterial pathogens	Second- or third-gen. cephalosporin + macrolide or Extended-spectrum fluoroquinolone
	If aspiration suspected	Clindamycin or Amp/sulbactam
Recently hospitalized or nursing home patient or if neutropenic	Usual pathogens plus nosocomial	Cefepime or Imipenem (+ possible addition of aminoglycoside)
	If aspiration suspected	Piperacillin/Tazorac or Clindamycin + ciprofl oxacin or aminoglycoside
AIDS patient	*Pneumocystis carinii*	Trimethoprim sulfa (also add corticosteroids if hypoxic—Pao_2 <70 mm Hg)
Influenza A		Oseltamivir (potential benefit in the first 48 h)
Cystic fibrosis	Pseudomonas	Tobramycin and piperacillin

WINNING STRATEGIES

- In patients presenting with shortness of breath, there are multiple possible causes, most of them serious and potentially life-threatening.
- Always provide immediate supplemental oxygen and ventilatory assistance to any patient in respiratory distress or imminent respiratory failure. Don't wait for the ABG or CXR!
- Use history and physical examination to narrow down causes of dyspnea and initiate definitive treatments.
- Be careful to distinguish dyspnea from hyperpnea (increased ventilation) which could indicate an underlying acidosis such as diabetes ketoacidosis (DKA) or toxic alcohol ingestion.
- In patients with dyspnea and a history of asthma or COPD, always consider other diagnoses such as MI, PE, or pneumothorax.
- In the COPD patient presenting with sudden acute deterioration, think spontaneous pneumothorax.
- Beware of the "silent chest" in asthma…a sign of impending respiratory failure!
- You can't fake diaphoresis!
- Employ a strategy of permissive hypercapnia with intubated and mechanically ventilated asthmatics and COPD patients to avoid complications and cardiac arrest.
- Provide high-flow oxygen to all hypoxic patients initially (even in COPD), then wean down as able.
- Give corticosteroids and antibiotics to all COPD exacerbation patients on test day.
- For the hypertensive CHF/pulmonary edema patient, begin immediate treatment with oxygen, diuretic, nitrate, afterload reduction, and morphine.
- Most CHF patients respond to treatment fairly rapidly, so consider CPAP/BiPAP first in the patient with respiratory distress (unless obtunded or arrest imminent).
- Avoid topical nitrates in CHF if very diaphoretic or evidence of decreased tissue perfusion as absorption can be erratic.
- Hypotensive patients in CHF are critically ill and will require urgent vasopressor therapy and a cardiology consult. Also, beware of cardiac tamponade in these patients!
- Beck's traid of elevated JVP, hypotension, and diminished/muffled heart tones is rarely present in cardiac tamponade, and hypotension is a late sign of imminent cardiac arrest in these patients.
- Involve surgeon immediately in tamponade, bedside pericardiocentesis if arrest is imminent.
- With acute hemopericardium, only a small amount of additional pericardial fluid can cause tamponade.
- Consider pneumonia in the weak/"not feeling well" elderly patient, even without a cough.
- In pneumonia, use history, examination, and CXR findings to guide initial broad-spectrum antibiotic therapy. Consider infectious disease consult if critically ill or AIDS or immunocompromised patient.

THE BOTTOM LINE

Many possible causes of dyspnea, nearly all are immediately life-threatening and require immediate evaluation and intervention.

- Provide immediate supplemental oxygen and ventilatory assistance to patients in respiratory distress.
- Use history, examination, and stat bedside testing to narrow down causes and begin initial treatment.

CHAPTER 11

Sore Throat/Dysphagia

Navneet Cheema

DON'T FORGET

Every sore throat/dysphagia patient has

- Epiglottitis
- Ludwig angina
- Angioedema
- Peritonsillar abscess
- Retropharyngeal abscess
- Foreign body (especially in child) . . . until proven otherwise.

INITIAL ASSESSMENT

- Focus on airway, breathing, and circulation (ABCs). Keep immediate life threats in mind first.
- Ask for a full set of vitals with every patient, including pulse, BP, respirations, temperature, oxygen (O_2) saturation, and glucose.
- Large-bore intravenous (IV) × 2, O_2, monitor in every patient.
- Draw labs and hold for orders.

Case-Specific Recommendations

- Identify unstable patients with airway compromise (eg, muffled voice, dysphonia, air hunger, stridor, drooling, hypoxia).

INITIAL HISTORY AND PHYSICAL EXAMINATION

History

- History of present illness (HPI)
  - Fever
  - Progressive sore throat
  - Neck pain
  - Swelling
  - Dysphagia/odynophagia: Can the patient handle secretions, sputum, liquids, or solids?
  - Respiratory distress
  - Absence or presence of cough
- Past medical history (PMHx)
  - Odontogenic infection
  - Poor dental hygiene
  - Recent dental extraction
  - Tongue piercing
- Medications
  - Is the patient taking an angiotensin-converting enzyme (ACE) inhibitor?
  - Any new medications?
- Allergies

Physical Examination

- General appearance
  - Ill appearing
  - Sitting position (bolt upright, tripod)
  - Obvious respiratory distress
- Vital signs (including pulse oximetry)
  - Fever
  - Tachycardia
  - Tachypnea
- Head, eye, ear, nose, throat (HEENT) examination
  - Tongue (swelling, elevation, protrusion)
  - Lip swelling
  - Poor dental hygiene
  - Trismus
  - Submandibular or sublingual swelling with brawny induration
  - Oropharynx: Normal appearing, red, purulent exudate, unilateral or bilateral swelling, uvular deviation
  - Moist mouth with excessive drooling
- Neck
  - Swelling
  - Hoarse voice, change in voice

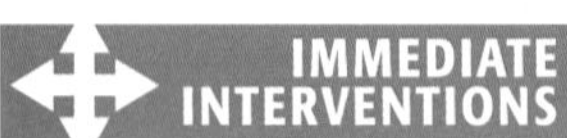

- Intubation equipment must be available at the bedside.
- Be prepared to perform cricothyroidotomy.
- Oxygen to keep O_2 saturations ≥95%.
- Immediate ENT consultation.

- Stridor
- Lymphadenopathy

- Lungs/heart
  - Tachypnea
  - Tachycardia

DIFFERENTIAL DIAGNOSIS

- Ludwig angina
  - Progressive infection of the floor of the mouth leading to tongue elevation and airway obstruction. Typically, a complication of a dental infection, procedure, trauma to the floor of the mouth, piercing, lacerations, or fractures.
  - The infection starts in the submandibular space and extends to the soft tissues of the mouth and neck (Fig. 11-1).
  - Airway compromise can be rapid and make oral tracheal intubation impossible. Must have surgical airway equipment immediately available at the bedside.
- Epiglottitis
  - The incidence has decreased in children due to *Haemophilus influenzae* type b vaccination, and is currently seen more often in adults. Potential microorganisms causing the infection include *Streptococcus pyogenes, Streptococcus pneumoniae,* and *Staphylococcus aureus.*

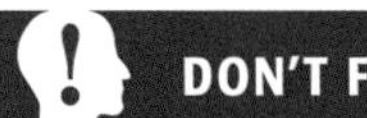

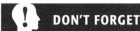

DON'T FORGET

DDx Summary

- Swelling of the floor of the mouth with tongue elevation or protrusion suggests Ludwig angina.
- A febrile, toxic appearing patient (especially a child) with drooling and stridor and a normal appearing oropharynx has epiglottitis.
- Painless swelling of the lips, tongue, or oropharynx, especially in a patient on an ACE inhibitor, suggests angioedema.
- Unilateral swelling with redness, purulent discharge, and deviation of the uvula suggests PTA.

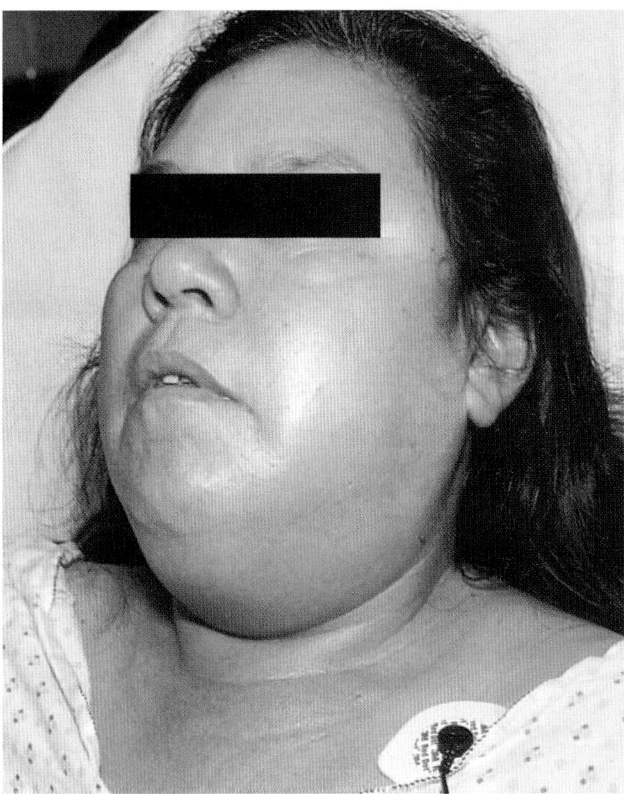

Figure 11-1. Ludwig angina. Note the diffuse submandibular swelling and fullness. Direct palpation of this area would reveal a characteristic brawny induration. Potential airway compromise is a key concern in all patients with Ludwig angina. (*Reproduced with permission from Knoop KJ, Stack LB, Storrow AB.* Atlas of Emergency Medicine. *2nd ed. New York, NY: McGraw-Hill; 2002.*)

- Patients may develop rapid airway compromise, especially children because of a narrower airway, and as a result any irritating procedures (IV, blood draw, throat examination) should be delayed until the airway is secure.
- Diagnosis is made by direct visualization, utilizing fiber-optic bronchoscopy in the operating room (OR). Soft tissue lateral neck radiographs can be performed in selected patients with the physician at the bedside (Fig. 11-2).

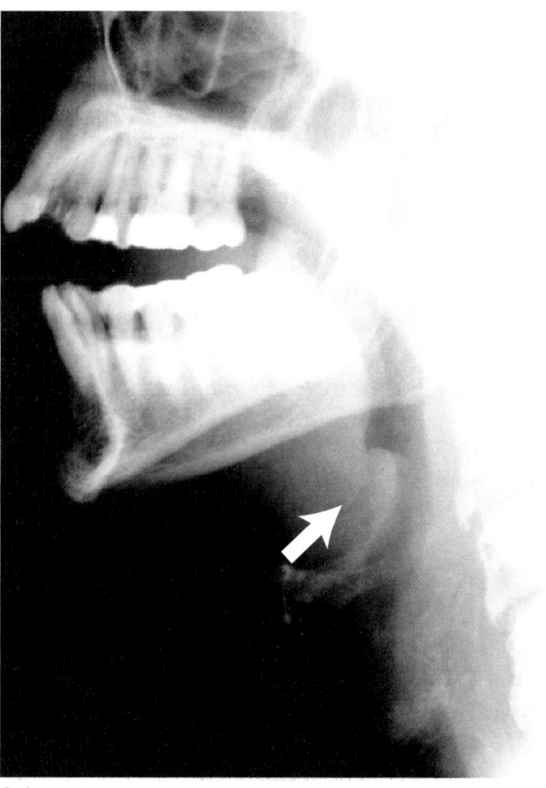

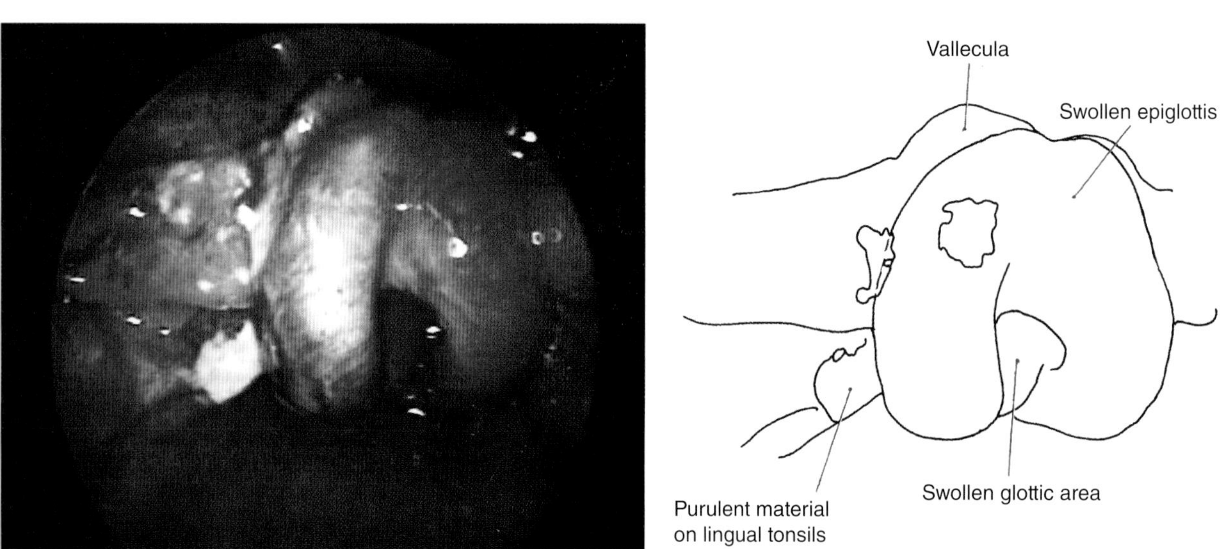

Figure 11-2. **(A)** Lateral radiograph demonstrating thumbprinting of the epiglottis consistent with epiglottitis. **(B)** Fiber-optic laryngoscopy showing a red, edematous epiglottis and glottic area with marked airway compromise in an adult with epiglottitis. (*[A] Reproduced with permission from Tintinalli JE, Kelen GD, Stapczynski JS, et al.* Emergency Medicine: A Comprehensive Study Guide. *6th ed. New York, NY: McGraw-Hill; 2004. [B] Reproduced with permission from Knoop KJ, Stack LB, Storrow AB.* Atlas of Emergency Medicine. *2nd ed. New York, NY: McGraw-Hill; 2002.*)

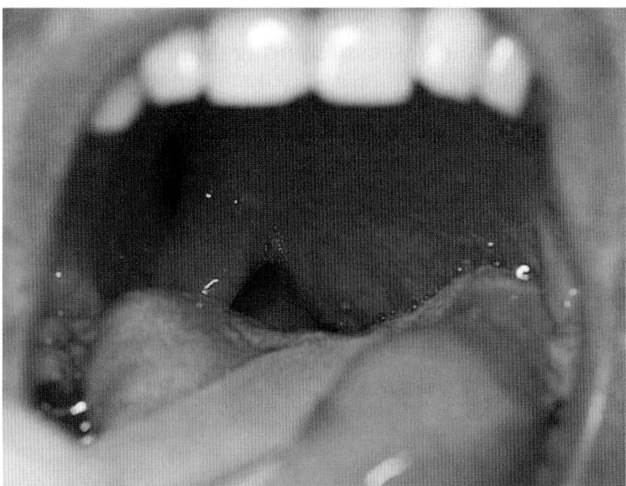

Figure 11-3. Acute peritonsillar abscess showing medial displacement of the uvula, palatine tonsil, and anterior pillar. Some trismus is present, as demonstrated by patient's inability to open the mouth maximally. (*Reproduced with permission from Knoop KJ, Stack LB, Storrow AB.* Atlas of Emergency Medicine. *2nd ed. New York, NY: McGraw-Hill; 2002.*)

- Angioedema: See Chap. 23 for a discussion of urticaria/anaphylaxis/angioedema.
- Peritonsillar abscess (PTA)
  - A PTA occurs as a complication of acute pharyngitis from group A streptococci (GAS) or infectious mononucleosis. The PTA can occur at any age, but is more common in teenagers and young adults.
  - The abscess collects between the tonsillar capsule and the superior constrictor muscle of the pharynx. Polymicrobial in origin, PTAs must be incised and treated with antibiotics (Fig. 11-3).

LUDWIG ANGINA

Additional History and Physical Examination Findings

- History of toothache or recent dental procedure on the lower molars.
- Patients who inject IV drugs into neck veins are also at risk.
- Common complaints are neck pain and swelling.
- Dysphagia with difficulty controlling oral secretions secondary to pain as well as swelling of the tongue.
- Dysphonia.
- Dyspnea and stridor are ominous signs.
- Infection may rapidly progress, resulting in septic shock (be prepared for this and manage aggressively).
- Brawny edema and swelling are seen on examination and are the keys to diagnosis.

Review Initial Results

- History and physical examination should lead to the diagnosis.
- Plain soft tissue lateral neck radiographs may show submandibular soft tissue swelling and gas.

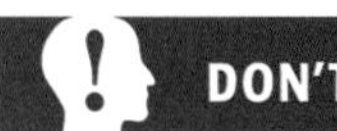

DON'T FORGET

Submandibular swelling with tongue elevation or protrusion should make you suspect Ludwig angina.

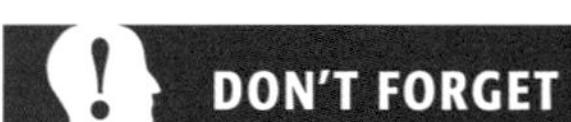

IMMEDIATE INTERVENTIONS

- Soft tissue series of the neck if the patient is stable. X-rays should be done in the ED.
- Consider CT scan of the neck in stable patients.
- Obtain IV access, begin NS, and draw blood for the laboratory.
- Order CBC with differential, blood cultures, and electrolytes.

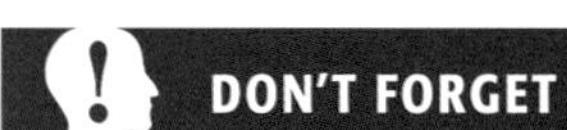

DON'T FORGET

Airway control is paramount. Have cricothyroidotomy tray at the bedside. Infection is polymicrobial in origin with a predominance of oral flora. Obtain emergent ENT consultation. Admit to ICU.

DON'T FORGET

For the purpose of oral boards, if you cannot remember the proper antibiotic(s) or dosage(s), it is acceptable to say, "I will look it up in a reference."

- A stable patient may have a computed tomography (CT) scan with IV contrast to delineate cellulitis from abscess requiring drainage.
- Panorex or mandible radiographs may be used to identify tooth abscess (rarely performed).

Risk Stratification: Management Priorities

- Airway control is paramount; you should immediately call for a cricothyroidotomy tray to be at the bedside.
- Administer IV antibiotics.
- Ear, nose, throat (ENT) specialist needs to evaluate the patient immediately.

Definitive Management

- Resuscitation
  - Airway control
    - Predicted difficult airway.
    - Do not use rapid sequence intubation (RSI).
    - Consider awake laryngoscopy or fiber-optic intubation.
  - Supplemental oxygen
  - Hemodynamic stabilization
  - Aggressive IV fluid resuscitation
- Treatment
  - Infection is polymicrobial in origin with a predominance of oral flora (primarily anaerobes and gram-positive organisms such as *Streptococcus* and *Staphylococcus* species).
    - Clindamycin (600-900 mg IV q8h), or
    - Ampicillin/sulbactam (3 g IV q6h), or
    - Cefotetan (2 g IV q12h)
  - Emergent ENT consultation.
  - Unstable patients should never leave the emergency department (ED) for studies.
  - Stable patients may leave the ED if accompanied by a registered nurse (RN) or medical doctor (MD).

Complications

- Asphyxia from sudden airway obstruction
- Septic shock
- Carotid invasion
- Jugular vein thrombosis
- Mediastinitis
- Empyema

Disposition

- Intensive care unit (ICU) admission for all.
- May need surgical drainage of abscess.

EPIGLOTTITIS

Additional History and Physical Examination Findings

- Abrupt onset of fever and sore throat.
- Patient appears toxic.
- Stridor, voice change, drooling.
- Can have tenderness over the anterior neck.
- Oropharyngeal examination is often normal with a patient complaining of severe throat pain.

- Patient tends to sit erect and/or refuse to lie flat.
- Preceding upper respiratory tract infection symptoms (eg, cough) are uncommon.

Review Initial Results

- Ask for complete vital signs including pulse oximetry.
- Do not send an unstable patient to x-ray.

Risk Stratification: Diagnosis and Management

- For unstable patients, the diagnosis is made in the OR.
- Airway control is paramount. You should immediately call for a cricothyroidotomy or tracheostomy tray.
- Unstable patients require definitive airway control prior to any further interventions. Employing a double setup in the OR or ER, both ENT and anesthesia should be present, so the airway can be controlled through direct or fiber-optic laryngoscopy or emergent tracheostomy.
- Stable patients can be risk-stratified, using soft tissue x-rays of the neck and direct or fiber-optic laryngoscopy (see Fig. 11-2A).
- In epiglottitis, soft tissue lateral neck radiographs may show a swollen epiglottis that appears flat and squat (like a thumbprint sign at the base of hypopharynx).
- In epiglottitis, indirect or direct laryngoscopy may show a cherry red and swollen epiglottis (must have airway management equipment at the bedside).
- After securing the airway, IV antibiotics should be administered rapidly.

Definitive Management

- Resuscitation
  - Definitive airway control is indicated for all children and unstable adults. Stable adults may be managed with close observation and frequent reevaluation in the ICU. For the oral board exam, obtain definitive airway control for all patients.
  - Supplemental oxygen.
- Treatment
  - IV antibiotics:
    - Ceftriaxone 50 mg/kg qd IV or
    - Cefotaxime 50 mg/kg/d IV, divided q6h
  - Nebulized racemic epinephrine may be helpful.
  - Be prepared to perform cricothyroidotomy.
  - Emergent ENT and anesthesia consult.
  - All patients with immediate airway threats should go to the OR for diagnosis and treatment.
  - Unstable patients should never leave the ED for studies.
  - Stable patients my leave the ED if accompanied by an RN or MD.

Complications

- Meningitis
- Retropharyngeal abscess

Disposition

- All patients are admitted to the ICU.

PERITONSILLAR ABSCESS

Additional History and Physical Examination Findings

- Fever and sore throat for 2 days or more.
- Odynophagia and dysphagia.

DON'T FORGET

Suspect epiglottitis in a patient with sore throat who is febrile, toxic appearing, and drooling, and stays in a tripod position and has a normal appearing oropharynx.

DON'T FORGET

Patients may develop rapid airway compromise. Any irritating procedures (IV, blood draw, throat examination) should be delayed until the airway is secure in unstable adults and children.

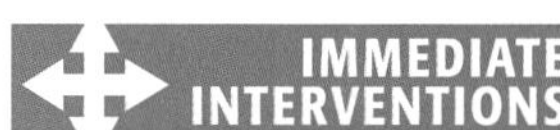

IMMEDIATE INTERVENTIONS

In adults, it is usually safe to begin therapy with

- 18-gauge IV, start NS.
- Collect blood and order CBC with differential, complete metabolic profile, and blood cultures.
- Soft tissue x-ray (AP and lateral) of the neck.
- Direct or indirect laryngoscopy, preferably in the OR.

DON'T FORGET

Have various size intubation tubes available at the bedside.

DON'T FORGET

Unstable patients should never leave the ED for studies.

DON'T FORGET

On the oral board exam, all patients with epiglottitis should be managed with definitive airway control.

- Unilateral pain that radiates to the ipsilateral ear.
- Drooling and trismus may occur, but voice change and stridor are uncommon and suggest other etiologies.
- Can have tenderness over the anterior neck.
- Oropharyngeal examination is abnormal.
- The ipsilateral soft palate is red and swollen; the tonsil is displaced medially; the uvula is displaced laterally; and the breath may be foul-smelling (see Fig. 11-3).
- Preceding upper respiratory tract infection symptoms (eg, cough) are uncommon.

Review Initial Results

- Ask for complete vital signs including pulse oximetry.
- Do not send an unstable patient to x-ray.

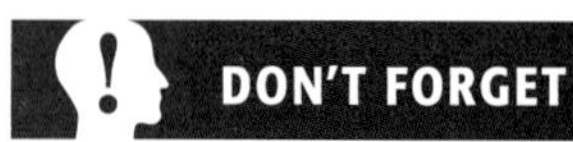

You may have a patient with a PTA as one case in a triple encounter.

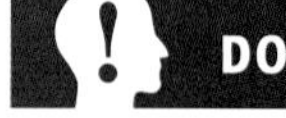

DON'T FORGET

If you do not I&D PTAs in your practice setting, it is reasonable to refer the patient to ENT for further management.

Definitive Management

- Airway compromise is usually not an issue.
- Treatment.
  - IV antibiotics for polymicrobial infection:
    - Clindamycin (600-900 mg IV q8h)
    - Ampicillin/sulbactam (3 g IV q6h)
  - Incision and drainage
    - Keep airway equipment on hand.
    - Provide oxygen and suction to patient.
    - Anesthesia with local, nebulized lidocaine, and direct application of viscous 4% lidocaine.
    - Localize abscess with needle aspiration.
    - Stab incision with number 11 blade to open abscess.

Complications

- Deep space infection of neck and face

Disposition

- Most patients can be managed as outpatients.
- Home with oral antibiotics.
- Close outpatient follow-up in 1-2 days with ENT.

WINNING STRATEGIES

- Every patient presenting with sore throat/dysphagia must have an assessment for airway patency.
- Unstable patients should never leave the ED for studies.
- Supplemental oxygen to keep O_2 saturations ≥95%.
- Submandibular swelling, tongue elevation, and protrusion should prompt you to suspect Ludwig angina.
- With Ludwig angina, peritonsillar abscess, or epiglottitis, initiate IV antibiotics early.
- Consider epiglottitis in a child who is febrile, toxic, and drooling, and stays in a tripod position.

THE BOTTOM LINE

- Do not compromise airway management for any diagnostic test in an unstable patient.
- Have surgical airway equipment at the bedside.
- Obtain immediate ENT consultation.

CHAPTER 12

Abdominal Pain

Thomas J. Regan and Aleksandr Gorenbeyn

INITIAL ASSESSMENT

- Focus on age, vital signs (VS), general appearance: Icterus/jaundice? Moving in pain versus lying still? Rigid versus soft abdomen?
- Identify unstable patients with immediate life threats:
  - Shock
  - Acute (surgical) abdominal findings

DON'T FORGET

On examination day, every patient with abdominal pain has

- Perforated viscus
- Intestinal obstruction
- Peritonitis or any other *-itis* except for gastroenteritis
- Mesenteric ischemia
- Ovarian torsion in a female of childbearing age
- Testicular torsion in a young adult male until proven otherwise

INITIAL HISTORY AND PHYSICAL EXAMINATION

History

- History of the present illness (HPI)
  - Onset
  - Quality/severity
  - Location/radiation/migration
  - Duration
  - Associated symptoms: nausea/vomiting/fever/chills/appetite/dysuria
  - Exacerbation/relief
- Past medical history (PMHx)
  - Prior abdominal/pelvis surgeries
  - Prior cardiovascular disease
  - Hx of gastric/duodenal ulcers/dyspepsia
  - Indwelling intra-abdominal devices
  - Hx of sexually transmitted diseases (STDs)/sexual activity as appropriate
  - Drug/alcohol use
- Medications
- Allergies

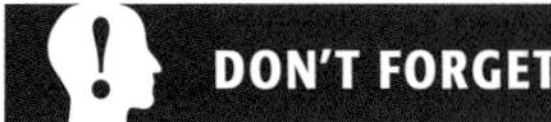

DON'T FORGET

Remember that abdominal pain can be cardiac.

Physical Examination

- VS
- Head, eyes, ears, nose, and throat (HEENT): Scleral icterus? Dry mucosa?
- Chest: Breath sounds equal?
- Cardiovascular (CV): Murmurs, rubs, gallops? Peripheral pulses present?
- Abdomen: Distended? Increased/decreased bowel sounds? Rigid or soft? Tenderness to palpation/rebound tenderness? Guarding? Hernias?
- Rectal: Trace/gross blood? Stool in vault? Melena?
- Pelvic: Cervical motion tenderness (CMT)? Adnexal tenderness? Masses?
- Scrotal examination: Swelling? Tenderness? Penile discharge? Hernias?
- Extremities: Cyanosis/edema?
- Neuro: Mental status? Gross motor/sensory?
- Skin: Jaundice?

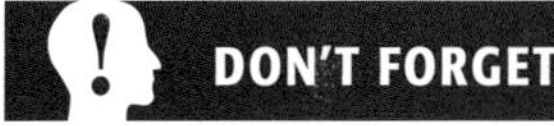

DON'T FORGET

Abdominal pain and shock are

- Mesenteric ischemia
- AAA rupture
- GI hemorrhage
- Severe pancreatitis
- Cholangitis
- Perforated viscus
- MI
- Pulmonary embolism

Think broad and early about life-threats!

Differential Diagnosis

- Peritonitis/Spontaneous bacterial peritonitis (SBP)/Peritoneal dialysis (PD) related
  - Peritonitis refers to the infection in the peritoneum that is usually caused by gastrointestinal (GI) tract flora. Most commonly, peritonitis develops from a ruptured viscus such as bowel or appendix with spillage of intestinal contents in the peritoneal cavity and resulting inflammation and infection.
  - SBP refers to bacterial infection of ascites, usually in a setting of liver cirrhosis and portal hypertension.
  - Patients on PD are prone to peritonitis because of the possibility of skin flora, entering the peritoneal cavity through the catheter.

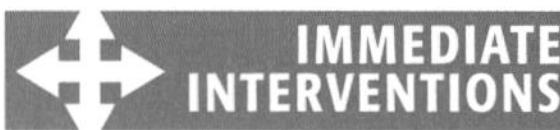

- Oxygen via NC to keep sat >95%
- Cardiac monitor
- 18 gauge IV, IV crystalloid bolus
- Draw blood for labs.
- ECG: For any male aged > 45 or female > 55 or anyone with CV history/risks
- Upright abdominal x-ray: Probably the best first test in suspected bowel obstruction/perforation.
- Stabilize life-threats by managing airway, providing aggressive fluid resuscitation.
- Provide pain relief with potent short-acting analgesics.

  - While peritonitis from a ruptured viscus and as a complication of PD usually presents as a rapid and progressive worsening of abdominal pain with rigidity and rebound tenderness, SBP can be subacute. Peritoneal tap is necessary and is diagnostic in equivocal cases. Upright chest x-ray (CXR) or lateral decubitus x-ray will be necessary if patient with peritoneal signs is believed to have a ruptured bowel.
- Perforated viscus
  - Perforated viscus can be in a number of areas. Classically, peptic ulcer disease (PUD) is a predisposing factor (50% of cases). Occasionally, perforation of large bowel occurs because of diverticular disease or a neoplastic process.
  - Sudden onset of abdominal pain with rapidly ensuing rigidity and other peritoneal signs are a textbook description. This history coupled with free air seen on the upright CXR is diagnostic irrespective of where perforation occurred.
- Mesenteric ischemia
  - Mesenteric ischemia is an intra-abdominal catastrophe that is almost as lethal today as it was 50 years ago (mortality 59%-93%). The superior mesenteric artery (SMA) is most commonly affected. It can be caused by arterial embolism, arterial thrombus, venous thrombosis, or a nonocclusive mesenteric ischemia (NOMI).
  - Classic presentation: Acute abdominal pain occurring in the presence of heart disease, while examination reveals (at least initially) a soft and minimally tender or nontender abdomen. Remember "pain out of proportion" on examination.
- Intestinal obstruction
  - Abdominal pain with distention, tenderness, and vomiting is the classic presentation.
  - Intestinal obstruction most frequently occurs secondary to adhesions, incarcerated hernias, and neoplasms.
  - Small bowel obstructions are much more frequent than large bowel obstructions. The latter are more likely to be secondary to cancer. Sigmoid and cecal volvulus are less frequent, but more likely to require surgery.
  - In most cases, flat and upright abdominal x-rays provide diagnosis, but computed tomography (CT) scanning might be needed to further define an etiology.
- Appendicitis
  - Appendicitis is inflammation/infection of appendix that can happen at any age, though the elderly have higher mortality (2.3% vs 0.2%). Perforations are also more common in the elderly.
  - Classic presentation is anorexia, fever, right lower quadrant (RLQ) pain, and elevated white blood cell (WBC) count.
  - A variety of atypical presentations are possible, requiring high index of suspicion.
  - Diagnosis is often clinical, but observation or advanced radiologic imaging may be required.
- Pancreatitis
  - Pancreatitis is a potentially fatal disease with mortality of 5%-10%. Alcohol and gallstones are the most common etiologies, but neoplastic processes are frequent in elderly and should be considered.
  - Severe epigastric pain with radiation to the back, nausea and vomiting, as well as jaundice can be a typical presentation.
  - Disease is diagnosed clinically and laboratory studies help to support the diagnosis. In chronic cases CT scan or ultrasound (US) may help. Ranson criteria help with prognosis.

- Cholecystitis/cholangitis
    - Both cholecystitis and cholangitis result from acute obstruction of a portion of the biliary system.
    - Cholecystitis describes focal gallbladder inflammation, resulting from complete obstruction of the gallbladder outlet.
    - Cholangitis describes acute retrograde inflammation and infection of the bile and intrahepatic ducts secondary to complete biliary obstruction in the presence of bacteria and can commonly be complicated by sepsis.
- Diverticulitis/abscess
    - Diverticulitis is the most common complication of diverticular disease and results from microperforations of the diverticulum. The subsequent inflammatory event results in a localized colonic wall reaction, but can progress to microperforation, which is then walled off, forming a diverticular abscess. Free perforation with generalized peritonitis is relatively uncommon.
- Pelvic pain/pelvic inflammatory disease (PID)/tubo-ovarian abscess (TOA)
    - PID is an important cause of ectopic pregnancy, infertility, and chronic pelvic pain. It results from ascending polymicrobial infection (*Neisseria gonorrhoeae* and/or *Chlamydia trachomatis*, and anaerobes) via the vagina and cervix.
    - Although rarely life-threatening, if left untreated the infectious process may spread causing peritonitis or abscess formation (ie, TOA). The seriousness of the acute and chronic problems associated with PID makes early diagnosis and treatment imperative.
- Ovarian torsion
    - Ovarian torsion is an uncommon event usually occurring because of ovarian enlargement from some secondary cause (ie, large simple cyst or large ovarian tumor), enabling the now pedunculated structure to twist on its pedicle and compromise the ovarian blood supply.
    - Ovarian torsion often involves torsion of the fallopian tube as well. If left untreated, this situation can progress to anoxic ovarian degeneration and eventual gangrenous necrosis.

DON'T FORGET

Someone with liver cirrhosis, fever, and abdominal pain may be a classic SBP patient, but beware of a patient who has history of alcoholism and presents with dyspnea and worsening mentation.

DDx Summary

- ECG for ACS/arrhythmia because it can be present in the abdominal pain patient.
- Paracentesis to diagnose SBP.
- Upright CXR or lateral decubitus abdominal x-ray to diagnose obstruction or perforation.
- Angiogram for suspected mesenteric ischemia.
- Appendicitis is suspected on clinical grounds of fever, vomiting, and pain eventually localizing to RLQ.
- Know Ranson criteria for pancreatitis patients.

PERITONITIS/SBP/PD RELATED

Additional History and Physical Examination Findings

- Patients with ascites secondary to liver cirrhosis have a 29% yearly risk of SBP. Be suspicious of it in a patient with history of cirrhosis or of prior SBP. Incidence of peritonitis related to PD is one episode every 15 patient-months.
- Classically, the patient will have fever, abdominal pain, and diffuse abdominal tenderness. However, peritoneal signs may be absent in a patient with ascites and perforated viscus because parietal and visceral layers of peritoneum are separated by ascitic fluid. A PD patient with abdominal pain and cloudy effluent has PD-related peritonitis until proven otherwise.
- Alternative chief complaints suggesting SBP include subacute functional decline or worsening of baseline encephalopathy.
- Risk factors increasing the probability of SBP include prior SBP, recent known increase in ascites, any infection such as urinary tract infection (UTI), concomitant upper GI hemorrhage, recent paracentesis (SBP can be iatrogenic), serum bilirubin >3.2 mg/dL, or platelet count <98,000/cc.
- The response to paracentesis cannot be used to exclude SBP—microscopy/cell counts of the fluid obtained are needed.
- The physical exam is useful in diagnosing complications such as chronic heart failure (CHF), pleural effusions, or tamponade.

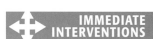

IMMEDIATE INTERVENTIONS

- Bolus of crystalloid IV.
- Send CBC, lytes, LFTs, coags, ammonia level, UA, and possible β-hCG.
- Order CXR to rule out pneumonia/pleural effusions.
- Paracentesis for peritoneal fluid and send it for cell counts, Gram stain, cultures, albumin, bilirubin, LDH levels.
- Send PD effluent for cell counts, Gram stain, and cultures.
- Order antibiotics.

DON'T FORGET

You must continue with paracentesis even if febrile person with cirrhosis and ascites is diagnosed with UTI or pneumonia.

DON'T FORGET

Although some literature suggests paracentesis is safe even with underlying coagulopathy, correct severe coagulopathy prior to paracentesis on test day.

DON'T FORGET

- SBP is mainly a monomicrobial infection:
  - *Escherichia coli* 37%
  - *Klebsiella* 17%
  - *Pneumococcus* 12%
- Surgical peritonitis is usually polymicrobial.
- PD-related peritonitis:
  - *Staphylococcus epidermidis* 40%
  - *Staphylococcus aureus* 10%
  - *Streptococcus* species 15%-20%
  - Gram-negative bacteria 15%-20%

Review Initial Results

- Review electrocardiogram (ECG) and abdominal and chest films.
  - Any evidence of cardiac ischemia/acute coronary syndrome (ACS) (they can fool you on the examination day). (See Chap. 8 for management.)
  - Any evidence of obstruction/perforated viscus or pneumonia/pleural effusions.
- Review labs: Complete blood count (CBC) often not helpful, but WBC could be elevated, especially in surgical peritonitis. Review electrolytes, blood urea nitrogen (BUN), and creatinine for abnormalities that may need attention. Elevated ammonia and coagulopathy may signal worsening liver failure or development of hepatorenal syndrome.
- Review paracentesis or PD fluid results (see Risk Stratification: Management Priorities next). When performing paracentesis, you can use US for guidance if available. You must use US to diagnose ascites first if they have not been previously diagnosed, history is suspicious, and if no perforated viscus is identified.

Risk Stratification: Management Priorities

- Surgical peritonitis: From perforated viscus of any magnitude, abscess, appendicitis, etc (see subsequent sections)
  - High mortality even with appropriate early antibiotics.
  - Immediate surgical consult and admission to operation room (OR).
- SBP: Paracentesis shows >500 WBCs or 250 polymorphonuclear leukocytes (PMNs)/cc
  - Gram stain is rarely helpful in identifying specific bacteria.
  - High-risk patients: Worsening renal function (Cr >3) is the best predictor of death and worsening of encephalopathy.
    - Intravenous (IV) antibiotics, admission, and reassessment of antibiotic response in 48 hours
  - Low-risk patients: Normal renal function, minimal encephalopathy, no shock, hemorrhage, or ileus
    - Outpatient management of certain low-risk SBP patients with PO antibiotics can be considered (eg, quinolones), but unlikely to be seen on test day.
- PD-related peritonitis: Effluent cell counts reveal >100 leukocytes/cc or >50 PMNs/cc
  - All PD patients get rapid PD fluid exchanges with antibiotics added to the dialysate, but no IV antibiotics.
  - PD patients appearing well with no signs of shock/sepsis can be considered for discharge; all others are admitted.

Further Diagnostic Considerations

- If clinical peritonitis is not 100% evident (patient is tender but not rigid), no free air is identified, patient is not deteriorating, and patient's blood work has normal WBC count, a contrast abdominal pelvis CT can be obtained in conjunction with surgical consultant.
- If ascites diagnosis is uncertain or when a quick US cannot be obtained, a CT scan of abdomen and pelvis may be obtained.

Definitive Management

- Pain control: Control patient's pain during workup and prior to definitive diagnosis or prior to consultant involvement
  - Short-acting potent opioid analgesics are preferred to allow for frequent reassessments (eg, fentanyl).
- Fluid resuscitation: Assume patients with peritonitis are dehydrated on presentation and infuse crystalloid. Monitor vital signs. With any evidence of shock, order second IV and more fluids, followed by antibiotics, vasopressors, or blood products as needed.

- Antibiotics:
  - Surgical peritonitis (most likely polymicrobial):
    - Third-generation cephalosporin (eg, ceftriaxone) or quinolone to cover gram negatives and metronidazole to cover anaerobes
  - SBP:
    - Third-generation cephalosporin or quinolone if patient is getting admitted. To be narrowed once cultures return. Total duration is 5 days.
    - Oral quinolone if outpatient management is considered.
  - PD-related peritonitis:
    - First-generation cephalosporin or vancomycin is added to the dialysis fluid.
    - Treatment continues for 7 days after first negative culture of the effluent is obtained (average 10 days).

DON'T FORGET

Appropriate pain management is easy to overlook, but it can also earn you valuable and easy points toward your overall score.

Frequent Reassessment

- Monitor vital signs and pain levels often to avoid missing subtle signs of deterioration and decompensation.

Complications

- Septic shock:
  - Evidenced by hypotension and tachycardia that are poorly or not responsive to fluids alone.
  - Frequently reassess the airway and breathing while instituting more fluids, antibiotics (if not done yet), and vasopressors.
  - Push immediately for intensive care unit (ICU) admission or immediate transfer to OR if appropriate.

Disposition

- Surgical peritonitis:
  - Must go to OR.
  - In the unlikely scenario of "no surgeon is available for next 3 hours," patient needs to be stabilized and transferred to an appropriate facility.
  - If clinical peritonitis is not 100% evident, an observation admission can be considered.
- SBP:
  - Admit all high-risk patients to medicine.
  - Any hemodynamic instability/shock to the ICU.
  - Low-risk patients can be discharged if adequate close follow-up is available, patients or their families seem reliable, and the patient is willing.
  - If paracentesis is negative (PMNs <250/cc), then treat other infections and admit using risk criteria; if no infections but febrile or encephalopathic, patient needs admission; if entire workup is negative, patient looks and feels better; discharge with close follow-up.
- PD-related peritonitis:
  - Unstable, ill appearing patients and those who cannot be ensured a close follow-up need admission to medicine.
  - All others can be discharged with close follow-up.

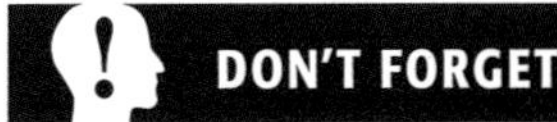

Err on the side of admitting all patients with peritonitis.

INTESTINAL OBSTRUCTION

Additional History and Physical Examination Findings

- Of all intestinal obstructions, 50% are associated with postoperative adhesions and 15% are associated with hernias and neoplasms.
- Classically, pain is episodic and crampy, poorly localized, and crescendo-decrescendo in nature, with accompanied hyperactive bowel sounds, abdominal distention, and bilious vomiting.

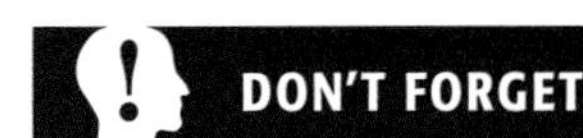

Absence of hyperactive bowel sounds does not rule out obstruction.

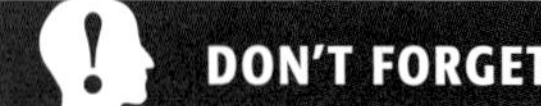

Physical exam alone cannot completely rule out bowel strangulation. Be suspicious if there is a tender mass at the inguinal femoral triangle or in the abdominal midline. Associated erythema is ominous for strangulated bowel.

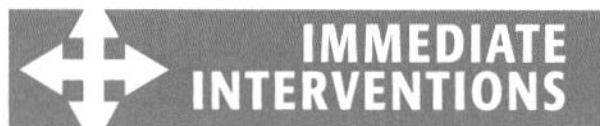

- Bolus of crystalloid IV.
- Send CBC, lytes, LFTs, coags, UA, and possible β-hCG.
- NGT to suction if obstruction confirmed on x-rays.
- Early surgical consultation.
- Consider antibiotics if prolonged symptoms, fever, and obvious small bowel obstruction or volvulus present.
- Control pain and nausea/vomiting.

- A more distal obstruction has slower time of onset, more constant pain, and delayed onset of vomiting that can be feculent. Inability to pass flatus may accompany symptoms.
- Risk factors for intestinal obstruction include prior abdominal surgery (especially GI tract or gynecologic), hernias, and known or suspected neoplasms. Age >50, history of constipation, vomiting, and abdominal distention also increase the probability of obstruction.
- Improvement of pain with passage of gas or stool or after vomiting cannot be used to exclude an obstruction since decompression is the key initial treatment and will provide temporary improvement.
- The physical exam will not only help in detecting bowel sounds, distention, masses, and hernias, but is also useful to diagnose hypovolemia, peritonitis, or sepsis.

Review Initial Results

- ECG: Needs to be obtained in an older patient with upper abdominal pain. Review first for any suggestion of ischemia or infarction.
- Review abdominal x-ray series: Diagnostic in 50%-60% of cases and suggestive in another 20%-30%.
  - Can see distended loops of bowel proximal to site of obstruction, followed by normal or collapsed bowel distal to the obstruction plus multiple air-fluid levels (Fig. 12-1).
  - The more dilated loops that are present, the more distal the site of obstruction.
  - Can also detect sigmoid or cecal volvulus and some abdominal masses.
  - Other findings could be that of generalized ileus or a sentinel bowel loop, usually indicating another local inflammatory process (eg, pancreatitis).
  - Presence of free air indicates perforated viscus and the need for emergent surgery.

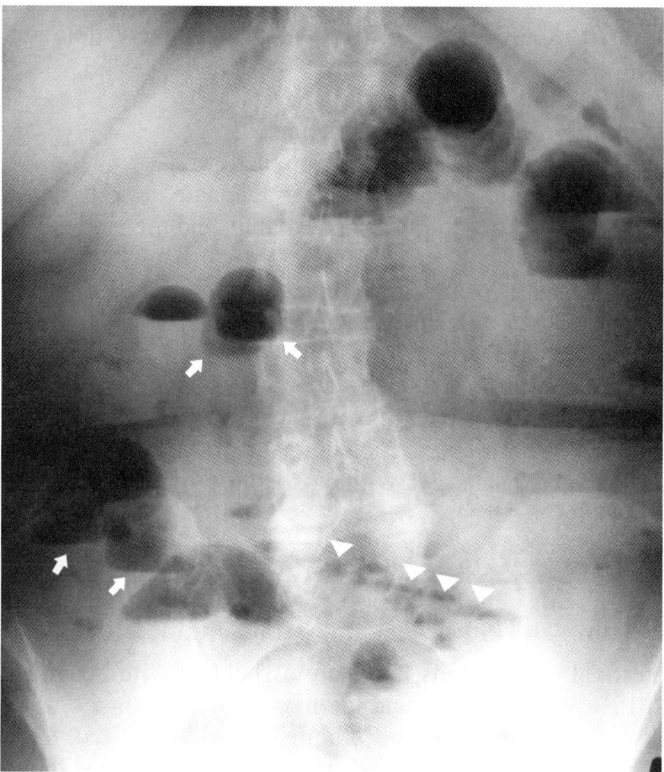

Figure 12-1. X-ray of the abdomen with air-fluid levels.

Risk Stratification: Management Priorities

- Small bowel obstruction: Adhesions and hernias are most common culprits.
  - Prolonged symptoms carry risk of bowel ischemia or infarction. Suspect it when initially intermittent and colicky pain becomes constant and severe.
  - Patients without prior abdominal surgeries may have an incarcerated mesenteric hernia that can become strangulated. Elderly are especially at risk.
  - Obtain early surgical consultation, especially if patient is febrile and has signs of shock or peritonitis—such patients need to go to OR.
  - Admission for everyone.
- Large bowel obstruction: More common in elderly because of diverticular disease and neoplasms.
  - More likely to be slow symptom onset and more constant pain from the beginning, but continuing worsening of pain suggests bowel ischemia.
  - Sudden onset of severe and unremitting pain suggests volvulus.
  - Obtain early surgical consult in all cases, especially if patient is febrile and has signs of shock or peritonitis—such patients need to go to OR.
  - Admit everyone, as most patients will require surgical management.
- Adynamic ileus: Can be secondary to
  - Abdominal trauma, extraperitoneal infection or inflammation (eg, pancreatitis), hypokalemia, renal colic, and opioids may cause abdominal pain and vomiting, imitating an obstructive picture.
  - Abdominal x-rays may not show a clear obstruction, but labs may be helpful to determine the cause.
  - If hydrated and still cannot tolerate PO, admission is warranted, usually to medical service.

Further Diagnostic Considerations

- If obstruction is suspected and x-rays are inconclusive, order an abdominal-pelvis CT with contrast (helpful to define obstructions as well as to diagnose hernias).

Definitive Management

- Pain and vomiting control: Control patient's pain during workup and prior to definitive diagnosis or consultant involvement
  - Short-acting potent opioid analgesics are preferred to allow for frequent reassessments (eg, fentanyl).
  - Prochlorperazine or ondansetron are preferred to control nausea.
  - Coordinate with a consultant—if they can see patient quickly, pain medications may mask examination findings. Patients with obvious peritonitis will be hard to get pain-free, so medicate to comfort.
- Fluid resuscitation: If patient has been vomiting, assume dehydration.
  - Infuse crystalloid.
  - If patient is in shock, at least 2 L need to be given before vitals are reassessed.
  - If no or poor response to fluids, order antibiotics and possibly vasopressors and get emergent surgical evaluation.
- Antibiotics: Administer if peritonitis or bowel ischemia is suspected, patient is becoming unstable, or surgery is planned.
  - Third-generation cephalosporin or quinolones to cover gram negatives and metronidazole or clindamycin to cover anaerobes.
- Nasogastric tube (NGT) insertion: Decompression, bowel rest, and fluid hydration can be curative in up to 75% of cases.
- Surgical intervention: Immediate with peritonitis or any evidence of bowel strangulation (eg, acidosis, septic patient, etc) or if initial 48 hours of NGT decompression fail.
- Adynamic ileus: Treat an underlying disease process.

DON'T FORGET

When obstructed intestine has more fluid than gas, look for the "string of pearls" sign—small pockets of gas that are trapped between valvulae conniventes of the small bowel and appear as an oblique series of round radiolucencies on upright film.

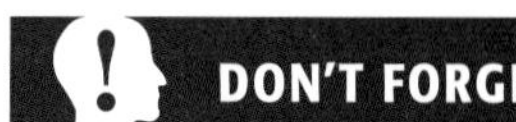

On the examination day, you are likely to make a diagnosis of obstruction by plain abdominal x-rays. If the patient starts to deteriorate, bowel strangulation is probably the cause, and the next step is surgical consult and OR, not CT (even if consultant insists).

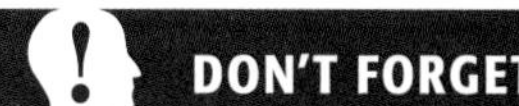

Do not rely on WBC count to call a consultant or to make a diagnosis. However, WBC >20,000/cc should make you suspect bowel infarction, intra-abdominal abscess, or peritonitis.

DON'T FORGET

Oliguria and lactic or other metabolic acidosis are predictors of secondary complications from bowel obstruction.

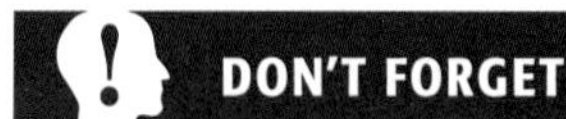

All unstable or debilitated patients and those going to OR require Foley placement.

DON'T FORGET

Pseudo-obstruction (Ogilvie syndrome) may also mimic bowel obstruction. It affects lower colon most commonly and is diagnosed by seeing large amount of gas without air-fluid levels in the large intestine. Anticholinergics or tricyclics are often the culprits. Colonoscopy is preferred for an early intervention.

DON'T FORGET

Metoclopramide is a promotility agent and may make obstruction worse, though this has never been proven.

DON'T FORGET

Patients in shock most likely have a combination hypovolemic and septic shock. Consider antibiotics early.

DON'T FORGET

Classic: Pain out of proportion to the examination findings lasting >2 hours in anyone >50 years of age should raise your suspicion for mesenteric ischemia.

DON'T FORGET

Development of abdominal distention and diffuse abdominal tenderness, followed by involuntary guarding and rebound tenderness means bowel is becoming necrotic. Frequent reexamination is a must!

Frequent Reassessment

- Monitor vital signs and pain levels often to avoid missing subtle decompensation or transition from a simple bowel obstruction to a strangulated bowel.

Complications

- Bowel necrosis: When developing peritoneal signs are missed, there is a great chance of bowel necrosis. Surgical intervention is needed.
- Septic shock: Even in absence of bowel necrosis, bacteria can translocate from the gut to the blood stream, but bowel necrosis almost guarantees sepsis if not aggressively treated. ABCs, fluids, and antibiotics followed by surgical management.

Disposition

- All are admitted to surgery, but if it is adynamic ileus and underlying cause is not surgical, admit the patient to appropriate service.
- Unstable patients need go to the OR directly or initially to the ICU and then OR.
- Transfer all unstable patients if definitive management is delayed for any reason.

MESENTERIC ISCHEMIA

Additional History and Physical Examination Findings

- Approximately 50% caused by arterial embolism, 15% each caused by arterial and venous thrombosis, 20% caused by NOMI
- Median age of patients is 70 years and mortality is 59%-95%.
- Classically, the presentation involves acute onset of severe, poorly localized abdominal pain, GI tract emptying, and underwhelming findings on the abdominal examination—flat, soft, and often nontender.
- Alternatively, less severe and vague abdominal pain or unexplained abdominal distention or GI bleeding in lieu of pain may be the only indications of acute mesenteric ischemia (AMI).
- Risk factors
  - Arterial embolism: Coronary artery disease (CAD) (postmyocardial infarction [MI] thrombi, CHF), valvular heart disease (rheumatic mitral valve disease, nonbacterial endocarditis), chronic atrial fibrillation, aortic aneurysms or dissection, s/p coronary angiography.
  - Arterial thrombosis: Elderly, diffuse atherosclerosis, and hypertension.
  - Venous thrombosis: Hypercoagulable states (sickle cell disease, malignancy, protein C or S deficiency, etc), inflammatory conditions (pancreatitis, cholangitis), blunt abdominal trauma, CHF, decompression sickness.
  - NOMI: Low-flow states (CHF, cardiogenic shock, postcardiopulmonary bypass, dysrhythmias), proceeding hypotensive episode (shock), drug-induced splanchnic vasoconstriction (digoxin, vasopressors, cocaine abuse).
  - The physical exam will help in excluding other diagnoses and may help in identifying a precipitating cause, but examination of the abdomen will generally be normal early in the course of disease. Occult heme-positive stool can be present early. Gross bleeding signifies bowel necrosis.

Review Initial Results

- ECG:
  - ACS and cardiogenic shock can cause NOMI, but also could be an alternative diagnosis.
  - Presence of atrial fibrillation is a risk factor for mesenteric embolism.

- X-rays: Plain abdominal films are often obtained first, especially if pain and vomiting are present to rule out free air and obstruction, but most likely they will be normal early on.
  - Subtle signs: Adynamic ileus, distended air-filled loops of bowel, bowel wall thickening
  - Late signs: Pneumatosis intestinalis or presence of gas within portal venous system
- Labs: Most patients will have lab abnormalities, such as elevated WBC count, elevated lactic acid levels, or elevated amylase. Normal values do not exclude a diagnosis of mesenteric ischemia. Abnormal values are usually present when bowel infarction has already occurred.

Risk Stratification: Management Priorities

- Arterial embolism: Most commonly involves SMA because of the anatomy. Diagnosis is most reliably made by angiogram.
- Arterial thrombosis: SMA is most often implicated as well, and angiography is needed to diagnose.
- Venous thrombosis: It could be diagnosed by CT or by angiography.
- NOMI: It is diagnosed by angiogram. It is often present in admitted patients.

Further Diagnostic Considerations

- Proceed to an abdominal-pelvis CT scan if labs and x-rays don't help you, but suspicion is still high.
- CT will be most helpful to exclude other diagnoses or to diagnose venous thrombosis. It will pick up on bowel abnormalities only once bowel has infarcted (ie, too late).

Definitive Management

- Pain and vomiting control: Control patient's pain during workup and prior to definitive diagnosis or consultant involvement.
  - Short-acting potent opioid analgesics are preferred to allow for frequent reassessments (eg, fentanyl).
  - Prochlorperazine or odansetron are preferred to control nausea.
  - Coordinate with a consultant. Patients with obvious peritonitis will be hard to get pain-free anyway, so medicate to comfort.
- Fluid resuscitation:
  - Infuse crystalloid: If patient is in shock, at least 2 L need to be given before vitals are reassessed.
  - Order blood products if hemorrhage is present.
  - Order antibiotics as patient may be septic.
  - Vasopressors are the last resort and alfa-agents should be avoided, while ionotropes are preferred.
- Correct dysrhythmias, CHF, and other metabolic abnormalities as much as possible.
- Antibiotics: If peritonitis or bowel ischemia is suspected, patient is or becoming unstable, or surgery is planned.
  - Third-generation cephalosporin to cover gram negatives and metronidazole or clindamycin to cover anaerobes
- NGT insertion: Nonfunctioning intestine will be overloaded with secretions and inflammatory/dead cells. May help with vomiting.
- Arterial embolism: Start papaverine infusion, observe for peritoneal signs that would require OR (if major embolus, to OR for embolectomy or resection).
- Arterial thrombosis: If no peritoneal signs and good collaterals seen on angiography, observe. If peritoneal signs or collaterals are absent, patient needs to go to OR for resection and/or reconstruction.

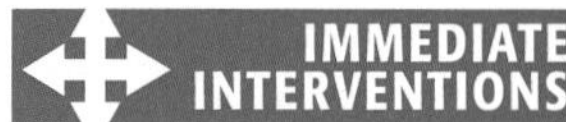

- Fluid resuscitation with crystalloid
- Send CBC, lytes, LFTs, coags, amylase, lipase, lactate level, type and screen, UA, possible β-hCG.
- NGT to suction can be helpful to decompress bowel.
- Emergent surgical consult
- Control pain and nausea.
- Antibiotics are used commonly if mesenteric ischemia is suspected, but no good scientific data exist to support the practice.
- Order angiogram if your index of suspicion is high (order on examination day!).

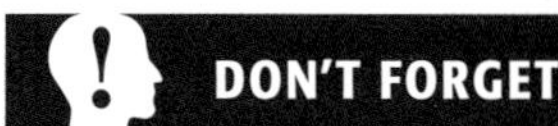

Most abdominal x-ray abnormalities show up only when transmural bowel damage has already occurred.

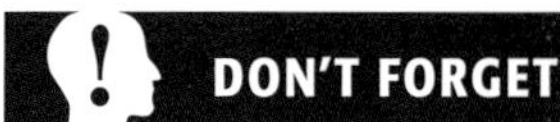

Major embolus: Proximal to take off of ileocolic artery from the SMA. Minor embolus—distal to the ileocolic artery origin.

DON'T FORGET

Postprandial abdominal pain can be equivalent of intestinal angina and precede arterial mesenteric thrombosis by several months.

- Venous thrombosis: Without peritoneal signs—anticoagulation with or without thrombolytics. With peritoneal signs—patient needs to go to OR for resection. Further management depends on extent of ischemic bowel found and resected, but eventual anticoagulation will be needed.
- NOMI: Papaverine infusion for everyone, but if peritoneal signs develop, patient needs to go to OR.

Frequent Reassessment

- Monitor vital signs frequently.
- You may need invasive hemodynamic monitoring if you are to start papaverine infusion.
- Reexamine patient often when patient decompensates, while you are resuscitating or ordering tests, or when examiner seemingly stalls you.

DON'T FORGET

Though NOMI is usually caused by splanchnic vasoconstriction consequent to a preceding cardiovascular event, it may appear hours to days after the event because vasoconstriction persists after the precipitating event has been corrected.

Complications

- Missed bowel necrosis or delay in surgical treatment may lead patient to develop septic shock, preceded by severe metabolic acidosis.
  - Pay attention when a patient becomes more tachypneic, develops altered mentation, drops blood pressure, becomes very tachycardic, or spikes a fever. Control ABCs, give antibiotics, and send to OR.
- All patients are at risk of secondary complications such as renal failure and respiratory failure, or exacerbation of their underlying illnesses (eg, new MI). Severe acidosis may lead to a cardiac arrest.

DON'T FORGET

Papaverine is a vasodilator that could give systemic hypotension if not targeted to occluded mesenteric circulation.

Disposition

- All are admitted to surgery, and if unstable, go to ICU.
- All on papaverine infusion need to go to ICU, but all with peritoneal signs go to OR.
- If no surgeon is available or there is a delay, transfer your patient (remember that after 12 hours of ischemia bowel necrosis is almost universal, while timely treatment within 12 hours leads to almost 100% recovery of bowel function, though other complications can still cause significant mortality).

PERFORATED VISCUS

DON'T FORGET

More likely than not, your surgical consultant will not be available or will give you hard time until you make a diagnosis, no matter of your level of suspicion. Thus, do not delay and go for angiography!

Additional History and Physical Examination Findings

- Fifty percent of cases happen in people who have PUD.
- Classically, patients complain of sudden onset of diffuse abdominal pain, with rapid development of peritoneal signs such as tenderness, guarding, and rigidity, as well as fever.
- Alternatively, patients with chronic diseases such as inflammatory bowel disease (IBD) or diverticulosis can have more indolent onset of abdominal pain with acute abdomen being a late presentation preceded by fever, vague discomfort, and anorexia. Vomiting may or may not be present.
- Iatrogenic bowel perforation from endoscopies and colonoscopies are more common today because of widespread use of these diagnostic modalities.
- Risk factors: PUD, foreign body ingestion, IBD (Crohn's disease or ulcerative colitis), chronic steroid use, bowel malignancy, diverticular disease, recent endoscopy, sigmoidoscopy, or colonoscopy.
- The physical exam will be useful in detecting acute abdomen/peritonitis, but will also help to diagnose patients in shock and in need of airway control.

Review Initial Results

- Review ECG as most people will be older—rule out ACS. Especially in a patient with shock as cardiogenic shock is always on the differential.

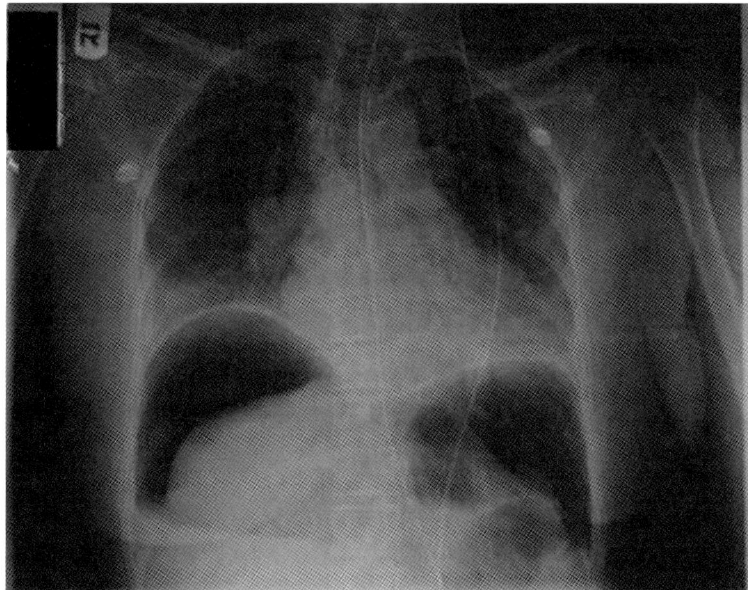

Figure 12-2. Upright chest x-ray showing free air under the diaphragm. *(Reprinted with permission from McPhee SJ, Papadakis MA.* Current Medical Diagnosis and Treatment 2009. *48th ed. New York, NY: McGraw-Hill; 2009.)*

- Review chest and abdominal films after ABCs are stabilized.
  - Upright CXR/abdominal x-ray: Look for a free air under the diaphragm signifying perforation (Fig. 12-2).
  - Lateral decubitus film (debilitated or intubated patients for whom true upright film is impossible): Look for free air collecting above the liver.
  - Look for other abnormalities: Air-fluid levels, severely dilated loops of small/large bowel, toxic megacolon in IBD patient, and pneumatosis intestinalis.
- Review labs: Often unhelpful. Early on WBC count can be normal and does not rule out the diagnosis.

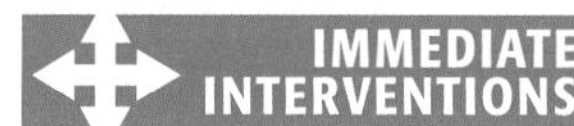

IMMEDIATE INTERVENTIONS

- Bolus of crystalloid IV.
- Send CBC, lytes, LFTs, lipase, amylase, coags, type and screen, UA, possible β-hCG.
- Emergent surgical consult once free air is seen or patient exhibits signs of peritonitis/sepsis.
- Control pain.
- Order antibiotics.

Risk Stratification: Management Priorities

- Stomach and duodenum perforations:
  - PUD is the main culprit and management is surgical.
  - Low pH of stomach and part of duodenum contents leads to extreme pain on perforation and almost immediate peritonitis.
- Rest of small bowel:
  - pH is higher, so presentation could be less acute.
  - Foreign bodies, IBD, and tumors are the most common causes, but perforations overall are infrequent.
  - Surgical management required.
- Large bowel:
  - High bacterial load. With microperforations slower progression of illness is possible.
  - May only get free fluid (ascites) without free air.
  - More often requires CT scan for diagnosis.
  - Diverticular disease, tumors, and IBD are the culprits.
  - Surgical management is required.
- Foreign bodies: More often happen in children, but can happen in patients with mental illnesses as self-mutilating or suicidal gestures.

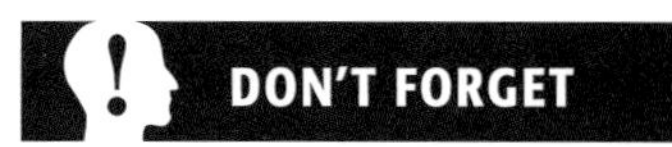

DON'T FORGET

Duodenum is a retroperitoneal organ. If perforation occurs at its posterior wall, pain could be in the back and peritonitis may be absent.

 **DON'T FORGET**

Transverse colon is the most frequent site of toxic megacolon. Dilatation of over 6 cm is abnormal, but most often see dilatation in excess of 8 cm.

 **DON'T FORGET**

Twenty-five percent of those with toxic megacolon perforate.

 **DON'T FORGET**

CT will define subtle free air if present as well as masses, ascites, obstruction, diverticultis, or even a site of perforation.

  - More likely to perforate at the narrow points of the GI tract. These include upper esophageal sphincter, level of aortic arch, gastroesophageal junction, pylorus, duodenal sweep, ileocecal valve, or rectum. The first two are likely to present with chest pain.
  - Surgical intervention once perforation has occurred regardless of the site.

Further Diagnostic Considerations

- If films appear normal or nonspecific and the patient seems to have peritoneal signs but otherwise is stable, order abdominal-pelvis CT with IV contrast while calling a surgeon.

Definitive Management

- Pain and vomiting control: Control patient's pain during workup and prior to definitive diagnosis or consultant involvement.
  - Short-acting potent opioid analgesics are preferred to allow for frequent reassessments (eg, fentanyl).
  - Prochlorperazine or odansetron are preferred to control nausea.
  - Coordinate with a consultant—if they can see the patient quickly, pain medications may mask examination findings. Patient with obvious peritonitis will be hard to get pain-free, so medicate to comfort.
- Fluid resuscitation:
  - Infuse crystalloid: At least 2 L in hemodynamically unstable patients before vital signs are reassessed.
  - Order blood products (if any suspicion of bleeding) or vasopressors as needed.
- Antibiotics: If peritonitis or bowel ischemia is suspected or patient is becoming unstable.
  - Third-generation cephalosporin or quinolone to cover gram negatives and metronidazole or clindamycin to cover anaerobes.
- All cases of perforation will require surgical management once diagnosed.
- Postprocedural perforation: If no peritonitis is present, but free air is identified, an observation admission is warranted with frequent repeat examinations.

Frequent Reassessment

- Monitor vital signs frequently.
- Reexamine patient often when patient decompensates, while you are resuscitating or ordering tests, or when examiner seemingly stalls you.

Complications

- Perforation leads to peritonitis, which in turn can lead to sepsis and septic shock.
- Be aggressive in maintaining ABCs, involve surgery early, and treat with antibiotics immediately.

Disposition

- All are admitted to surgery.
- All need to go to OR immediately or very soon.
- Unstable patients may need to go to ICU first, but if there is a delay in surgeon's availability, transfer patient out if sepsis is impending.

APPENDICITIS

Additional History and Physical Examination Findings

- Seven percent will develop appendicitis during lifetime. It can present at any age.

- Classically, patient presents with anorexia, nausea and vomiting, fever, RLQ abdominal pain, and elevated WBC.
- Atypical presentations are common especially in elderly, including low-grade or no fever, diffuse abdominal pain, and no leukocytosis. Appendicitis can masquerade as a UTI.
- In pregnant females, the pain of appendicitis is commonly above the RLQ location.
- Improvement of pain, especially if followed by vital signs worsening, is suggestive of the appendix rupture and cannot be ignored.
- The physical exam is useful in making a clinical diagnosis, detecting diffuse peritonitis (eg, after rupture of appendix) and excluding gynecologic etiologies in females (eg, ectopic, TOA, ovarian torsion).

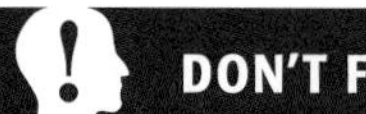
DON'T FORGET

In females of reproductive age, ovarian torsion on the right side can mimic appendicitis and must be excluded.

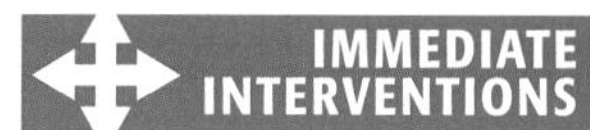
IMMEDIATE INTERVENTIONS

- Bolus of NS IV.
- Send CBC, lytes, possibly LFTs, lipase, coags, type and screen (equivocal examination), UA, possible β-hCG.
- Emergent surgical consult if peritonitis detected.
- Control pain/vomiting.
- Antibiotics if peritonitis is evident.

Review Initial Results

- Review ECG in an older patient, especially if pain is diffuse as ACS must be ruled out.
- Abdominal x-rays are indicated if any suspicion of perforation (eg, diffuse peritonitis) or obstruction (history of abdominal surgeries with intact appendix).
- Labs may help in ruling out other diagnoses (eg, pancreatitis); however, a normal WBC can be present, especially in elderly, making the diagnosis more clinical.

Risk Stratification: Management Priorities

- Young, RLQ pain, anorexic, elevated WBC—surgical consult
- Young, non-specific findings/symptoms—RLQ ultrasound in children or observation especially if tolerating PO. Use CT judiciously in this age group.
- Older, with tender abdomen, especially if diffuse—surgical consult
- Older, non-specific findings/symptoms—CT abdomen-pelvis
- Anyone with diffuse peritoneal signs, especially if prolonged course, abnormal vitals, or history of transient pain improvement—immediate surgical consult.

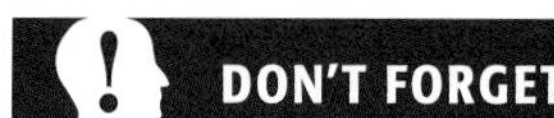
DON'T FORGET

Clinical picture will most often drive the index of suspicion. Obtain a surgical consult early, as a ruptured appendix is a disastrous complication.

Definitive Management

- Pain and vomiting control: Control patient's pain during workup and prior to definitive diagnosis or consultant involvement.
  - Short-acting potent opioid analgesics are preferred to allow for frequent reassessments (eg, fentanyl).
  - Prochlorperazine or odansetron are preferred to control nausea.
  - Coordinate with a consultant: If they can see patient quickly, pain medications may mask examination findings. Patient with obvious peritonitis will be hard to get pain-free, so medicate to comfort.
- Fluid resuscitation: If patient has been vomiting, he/she is dehydrated.
  - Infuse crystalloid: At least 2 L in hemodynamically unstable patients before vital signs are reassessed.
  - If no or poor response to fluids, order antibiotics and possibly vasopressors and get emergent surgical evaluation.
- Antibiotics: If peritonitis or bowel ischemia is suspected, patient is becoming unstable, or surgery is planned.
  - Third-generation cephalosporin or quinolone to cover gram negatives and metronidazole or clindamycin to cover anaerobes
- Appendicitis requires appendectomy in OR as soon as diagnosis is made.

Frequent Reassessment

- While a patient with suspected appendicitis is being worked up, several repeat examinations are necessary as the disease course has relatively rapid progress (eg, pain may now localize to RLQ, patient may spike a fever or start vomiting).

DON'T FORGET

Sudden and brief improvement of pain may suggest ruptured appendix. Peritonitis will follow.

- If patient decompensates or an examiner seemingly stalls you, go back and reexamine the patient.

Complications

- Ruptured appendix leads to peritonitis, which leads to sepsis and septic shock.
- Be aggressive in maintaining ABCs, involve surgery early, and treat with antibiotics immediately if any suspicion of peritonitis.

Disposition

- All are admitted to surgery and need to go to OR.
- Unavailability of surgeon requires patient transfer.
- It is not unreasonable to discharge a younger (not elderly) patient who has mild pain, nonfocal examination, normal labs, and is tolerating PO with the condition of their return for repeat evaluation within 8-12 hours (unlikely to be an option on the examination day).

DON'T FORGET

Severity of pain does not correlate with severity of disease in pancreatitis.

PANCREATITIS

Additional History and Physical Examination Findings

- Ninety percent of cases are caused by cholelithiasis or alcohol abuse.
- Other causes are multiple and include drugs, trauma, toxins, infections, neoplasms, cystic fibrosis, pregnancy, and collagen vascular diseases.
- Classic presentation includes severe steady epigastric or left upper quadrant (LUQ) abdominal pain, radiating to the back, nausea and vomiting, as well as fever and/or jaundice.
- Acute presentation may include hypovolemic shock and multisystem organ failure because of vomiting, fluid third spacing, and vasodilatation.
- The physical exam will reveal epigastric tenderness, but rarely peritoneal signs. Abdominal distention and hypoactive bowel sounds can be present from associated ileus. Abnormal vitals are frequently seen.

DON'T FORGET

- Grey Turner sign (bluish discoloration of the flanks) and Cullen sign (bluish discoloration around umbilicus) are rare signs of hemorrhagic pancreatitis.

Review Initial Results

- Review ECG in an older patient, especially if pain is diffuse as ACS must be ruled out.
- Abdominal x-rays are indicated if any suspicion of perforation (eg, diffuse peritonitis) or obstruction (history of abdominal surgeries with abdominal distention and vomiting).
- Labs: Elevated lipase is the most specific test. Elevated liver enzymes or bilirubin may indicate gallstone or other common bile duct obstruction etiology for the pancreatitis.

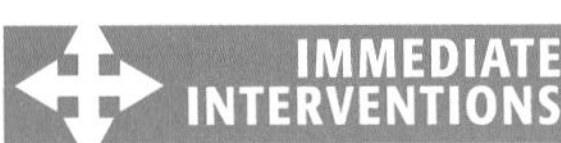

IMMEDIATE INTERVENTIONS

- Bolus of NS IV in a vomiting/dehydrated patient.
- Send CBC, lytes, LFTs, LDH, lipase, coags, type and screen, UA, possible β-hCG
- Emergent surgical consult if peritonitis is detected.
- Control pain/vomiting.

Risk Stratification: Management Priorities

- Ranson criteria for predicting mortality risk from acute pancreatitis (acute presentation):
  - Age >55, blood glucose >200 mg/dL, WBC >16,000/mm3, aspartate transaminase (AST) >250 U/L, lactate dehydrogenase (LDH) >700 U/L.
  - Additional criteria (at 48 hours) include Hct fall of >10%, rise in BUN by >5 mg/dL, total calcium <8 mg/dL, arterial Po2 <60 mm Hg, fluid sequestration >6 L, base deficit >4 mEq/L.
- Three or fewer criteria predict <1% mortality, four criteria predict 16 % mortality, five criteria predict 40% mortality, and more than 6 predict 100% mortality.

DON'T FORGET

Calcification of the pancreas on plain x-rays is suggestive of chronic disease.

Further Diagnostic Considerations

- Abdominal US may help define biliary obstruction as well as show pancreatic changes, though it cannot be used to diagnose acute pancreatitis.
- Abdominal-pelvis CT may be needed to grade the degree of pancreatic inflammation (especially in chronic cases), further help with defining pancreatitis etiology, and to screen for other diagnoses in equivocal presentations.

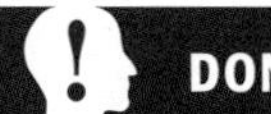

DON'T FORGET

Pancreatic inflammation may cause small bowel ileus demonstrated as a sentinel loop on plain x-rays.

Definitive Management

- Ninety percent recover spontaneously and require only supportive measures unless gallstone obstruction or neoplasm present.
- Pain and vomiting control: Control patient's pain during workup and prior to definitive diagnosis or to consultant involvement.
  - Short-acting potent opioid analgesics are preferred to allow for frequent reassessments (eg, fentanyl).
  - Prochlorperazine or odansetron are preferred to control nausea.
- Fluid resuscitation: If patient has been vomiting or appears dehydrated.
  - Resuscitate with crystalloid: At least 2 L in hemodynamically unstable patients before vital signs are reassessed.
  - If patient is in shock, fluid resuscitation may need to be augmented with vasopressor therapy.
- Biliary pancreatitis: If there is persistent biliary obstruction as could be evidenced by US, endoscopic retrograde cholangiopancreatography (ERCP) and decompression are needed urgently—contact gastroenterology immediately.
- Antibiotics: Not routinely indicated in mild to moderate cases, but can be given if secondary infection is suspected.
  - Third-generation cephalosporin or quinolones to cover gram negatives and metronidazole or clindamycin to cover anaerobes or
  - Ampicillin/sulbactam or other combination penicillin or
  - Fluoroquinolone if penicillin/cephalosporin allergic (eg, levofloxacin)
  - Imipenem or Zosyn (piperacillin and tazobactam) preferred for necrotizing pancreatitis

DON'T FORGET

In chronic pancreatitis, all labs may be normal despite pain and similar examination findings as in acute pancreatitis.

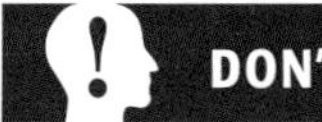

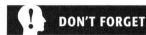

DON'T FORGET

Chronic pancreatitis has similar goals in management except that focus is to rule out other disease processes, especially pseudocysts or abscesses requiring surgical intervention.

Frequent Reassessment

- Patient may continue sequestering fluid and requires fluid resuscitation—reassess patient during workup.
- Complications as delineated below may develop and may need intervention prior to definitive disposition is made.

Complications

- Pulmonary: Pleural effusions, hypoxemia, acute respiratory distress syndrome (ARDS) (high mortality)
- Cardiovascular: Myocardial depression
- Metabolic: Hypocalcemia, hyperglycemia, coagulopathy and disseminated intravascular coagulation (DIC), acidosis from hypovolemia, and poor perfusion
- Other: Hemorrhage, renal failure, pseudocyst, abscess

DON'T FORGET

Pancreas may sequester many liters of fluid and, therefore, resuscitation may involve massive infusion of fluids.

Disposition

- Mild to moderate cases with patients, who are well appearing, able to tolerate PO fluids, have no evidence of biliary involvement, have good pain control, and meet three or fewer Ranson criteria, can be treated as outpatients (will not happen on the examination day).
- Patients not meeting guidelines above will be admitted, usually to medicine.

DON'T FORGET

No one with pancreatitis goes home on examination day at ABEM General Hospital.

DON'T FORGET

Cholangitis and acute cholecystits can present in a similar fashion, although fever and signs of sepsis are more likely to be seen in cholangitis.

DON'T FORGET

Charcot triad is noted in only 25% of cholangitis patients.

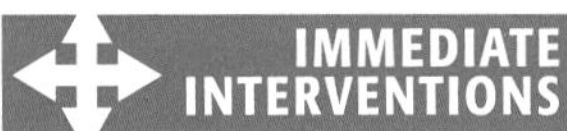

IMMEDIATE INTERVENTIONS

- Second large-bore IV if shock is suspected
- Fluid resuscitation if necessary
- CBC, electrolytes, LFT, lipase, coags
- RUQ ultrasound

DON'T FORGET

Accurate diagnosis of most biliary disorders almost always requires the aid of US.

DON'T FORGET

RUQ ultrasound demonstrates 95% of stones when present and can see stones as small as 2 mm. Absence of stones and normal gallbladder make this diagnosis unlikely.

- Patients in shock or developing secondary complications of the disease will require ICU admission.
- Any evidence of peritonitis requires surgical consult/intervention.

CHOLECYSTITIS/CHOLANGITIS

Additional History and Physical Examination Findings

- The risk of gallstone formation increases with female gender, parity, obesity, family history of gallstones, certain medications (ie, clofibrate and exogenous estrogen), prolonged fasting, rapid weight loss, and non–African Americans.
- Certain diseases also increase the risk of gallstone formation, including cystic fibrosis, intestinal malabsorbtion syndromes, and hemolytic anemias including sickle cell disease.
- Most prominent complaint will be acute or gradual onset of epigastric or right upper quadrant (RUQ) pain, commonly associated with nausea and vomiting. Pain may radiate to the base of the scapula. Fever and chills may also be present.
- Physical exam findings may reveal tachycardia without fever for cholecystitis, although fever usually present with cholangitis. RUQ pain is the most prominent finding as well as Murphy sign. Jaundice is only occasionally seen on initial presentation.
- Findings of RUQ pain, fever, and jaundice (Charcot triad) compatible with cholangitis can also be seen with acute cholecystitis.

Review Initial Results

- CBC, electrolytes, and liver function tests (LFTs) with lipase should be ordered. Of note: Normal WBC count and LFTs are often found in acute cholecystitis, but not in cholangitis. Lactate can be considered if sepsis/acidosis is suspected.
- ECG should be done in elderly patients with epigastric pain to exclude MI or ischemia.
- Plain abdominal x-rays are not recommended since helpful findings of calcified gallstones, gas in the gallbladder, or RUQ sentinel loop are uncommon.
- RUQ ultrasound is the most useful test (Fig. 12-3). No evidence of stones in the gallbladder is highly accurate for ruling out cholecystitis, while findings of gallstones, thickened gallbladder wall, and pericholecystic fluid are highly diagnostic of cholecystitis. Cholangitis will show intrahepatic duct dilatation as well as a common bile duct or gallstone.

Risk Stratification: Management Priorities

- Acute cholecystits:
  - Fluid depletion is usually seen secondary to nausea and vomiting.
  - Although microbial infection is usually not initially present, antibiotics are recommended.
- Cholangitis:
  - Fluid resuscitation with crystalloid is usually needed for hemodynamic stabilization. Vasopressors may be required if severe shock is present.
  - Early broad-spectrum antibiotic should be initiated since sepsis is a significant complication.
  - Early surgical consult should be initiated.

Definitive Management

- Antiemetics: If vomiting is present, antiemetics can help reduce further fluid depletion.

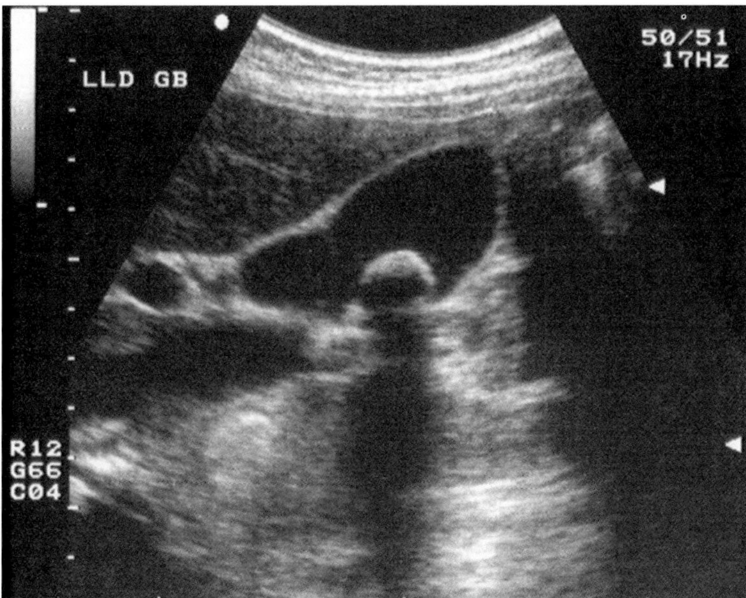

Figure 12-3. Gallstones. Longitudinal sonogram through the right upper quadrant. The gallbladder contains both sludge and stones (arrows). The gallstones are characteristically seen as highly reflective structures that cast an acoustical shadow. *(Reprinted with permission from McPhee SJ, Papadakis MA.* Current Medical Diagnosis and Treatment 2009. *48th ed. New York, NY: McGraw-Hill; 2009.)*

- Pain control: If the diagnosis is certain, it provides comfort to the patient preoperatively.
- Hemodynamic stabilization: Accomplished by crystalloid infusion. May need to add vasopressors if significant shock is present.
- Antibiotics: Administration is recommended for both disease processes. Single broad coverage can be used for acute cholesystitis (eg, second- or third-generation cephalosporin, quinolone, etc) with or without metronidazole, but cholangitis requires broad-spectrum coverage with double or triple antibiotics specifically targeting gram-negative organisms and anaerobes (eg, third generation cephalosporin and metronidazole, or piperacillin/tazobactam, or imipenem/cilastatin).
- Surgical consultation in the emergency department (ED); early surgical consultation if shock is present.

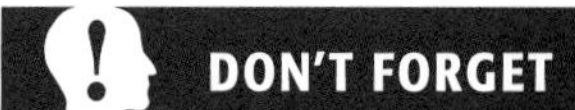
DON'T FORGET

Cholangitis has a high mortality rate if left untreated or inadequately treated.

Frequent Reassessment

- Repeat vital signs to assess hemodynamic status and response to treatment. Be ready for early development of sepsis.

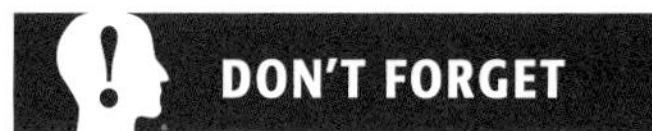
DON'T FORGET

The most frequently encountered organisms in both diseases include *E. coli, Enterococcus, Klebsiella*, and Bacteroides.

Further Diagnostic Considerations

- Hepatobiliary iminodiacetic acid (HIDA) scan is considered the "gold standard" for diagnosing acute cholecystitis. Findings would include filling of the hepatic and common bile duct visualized with no filling of the gallbladder after 1 hour of IV of technetium infusion.

Disposition

- Acute cholecystitis: Usually admitted to the surgical floor until symptoms have improved with probable cholecystectomy during the hospital stay.

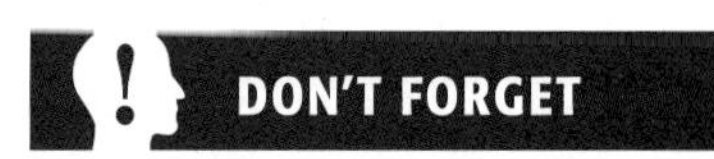
DON'T FORGET

On examination day, all patients with cholecystitis and persistent pain or cholangitis are admitted.

DON'T FORGET

Fifty percent of the US population by age 65 has diverticulosis, but only 10%-20% ever becomes symptomatic.

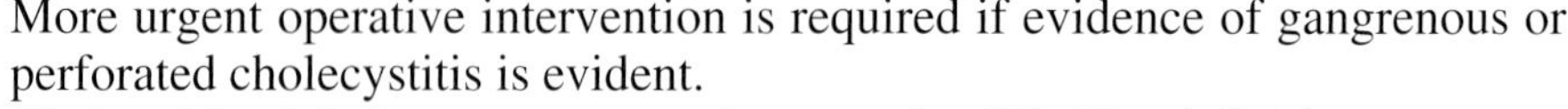

More urgent operative intervention is required if evidence of gangrenous or perforated cholecystitis is evident.

- Cholangitis: Admit to surgery service or to the OR. The definitive treatment of cholangitis is early biliary decompression, and can be accomplished by endoscopic retrograde cholangiopancreatiography (ERCP), percutaneous transhepatic cholangiography (PTHC), or surgery. Ensure that the patient is seen in a timely manner.

DIVERTICULITIS/ABSCESS

Additional History and Physical Examination Findings

- The risk of diverticulitis is directly related to the presence of diverticulosis. Risk factors for diverticulosis include age >40 years, and consumption of diet low in fiber. The patient may also relate a history of having a colonoscopy or barium enema in the past that showed diverticulosis. The patient may also relate a history of prior diverticulitis.
- The most common presenting complaint is abdominal pain, initially vague and generalized, but quickly localizing to the left lower quadrant. Pain is described as constant, dull, and crampy.
- Other presenting symptoms include change in bowel habits (either constipation or diarrhea) and tenesmus. If diverticular inflammation occurs in the area of the bladder or ureter, urinary frequency and dysuria may result. If it occurs adjacent to small bowel, nausea and vomiting, abdominal distension, and inability to pass gas can occur indicating the presence of an ileus or partial small bowel obstruction.
- Physical exam of diverticulitis frequently demonstrates a low fever.
- Abdominal examination reveals localized tenderness in the left lower quadrant and commonly accompanied by voluntary guarding and localized rebound.
- Rectal examination often displays either general tenderness or tenderness on the left side of the rectum. Stool guaiac will be positive for occult blood in more than 50% of patients.
- Severe localized pain, fever, and signs of localized rebound and guarding may indicate the presence of an actual diverticular abscess. Rupture of an abscess can lead to signs of generalized peritonitis with diffuse abdominal pain, high fever, guarding, and rebound tenderness, with the patient wanting to maintain immobility lying on one side with the hips flexed.

DON'T FORGET

Majority of diverticula occur in the sigmoid colon, but can occasionally involve more proximal parts of the colon.

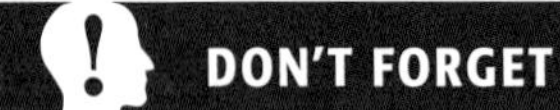

DON'T FORGET

Patients with a prior diverticulitis episode have a 10%-25% risk of recurrence.

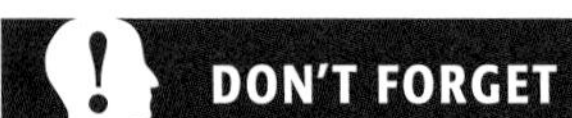

DON'T FORGET

In patients aged >50 years with RLQ pain, diverticulitis should always be a diagnostic consideration because of the possibility of redundant sigmoid colon.

Review Initial Results

- CBC should be ordered, but is only elevated in 36% of patients with active diverticulitis.
- CT scan of the abdomen: Although abdominal-pelvic US may be useful, the most common imaging study is a CT of the abdomen-pelvis (without rectal contrast). Both studies may reveal colonic wall thickening, localized mesenteric inflammation, or an abdominal fluid collection indicating abscess formation.

DON'T FORGET

High-grade fever may indicate abscess formation or onset of generalized peritonitis.

Risk Stratification: Management Priorities

- In very mild episodes of diverticulitis with no signs of systemic infection (ie, low-grade fever, tolerating fluids, mild pain, no evidence of abscess, etc), patients can be sent home on oral antibiotics, analgesics, liquid diets, and close follow-up. In more moderate to severe cases, or if there is evidence of abscess formation, admission is required with IV fluid, analgesics, IV antibiotics, and frequent reexamination.

- Although most episodes of diverticulitis are localized, there is the unlikely risk of the diverticulum to fully perforate and spill the abscess contents into the free peritoneal space causing generalized peritonitis. This will result in severe abdominal pain, high fever, generalized abdominal guarding and rebound, and the possibility of sepsis.

Definitive Management

- IV fluid: Crystalloids may be required if nausea and vomiting is present for fluid replacement. If peritonitis is present, treatment of shock may be required with crystalloids and possibly vasopressors.
- Analgesics: If patient has a mild episode of diverticulitis, oral analgesics may be sufficient. Otherwise, parental pain medication is required.
- Antibiotic therapy: Broad-spectrum antibiotics coverage should be instituted in the ED and specifically targeting colonic flora (ie, third generation cephalosporin or quinolone plus flagyl).
- Surgical consultation should be obtained if moderate or severe diverticulitis is evident or if abscess is present. Prompt consultation is needed if peritonitis is apparent.

Further Diagnostic Studies

- Sigmoidoscopy or colonic barium contrast studies are generally not recommended until the acute inflammatory episode has subsided.

Disposition

- If patient has only mild diverticulitis with no evidence of abscess, patient can be discharged on liquid diet, oral antibiotics, and close follow-up.
- If diverticulitis is moderate to severe, the patient should be admitted to surgery for IV fluid, parental antibiotics, and pain control with frequent reexamination. If evidence of abscess formation, percutaneous drain can be placed or surgical drainage can be performed.
- If evidence of diffuse peritonitis, patient requires IV antibiotics, hemodynamic stabilization, and immediate surgical intervention.

PELVIC PAIN/PID/TOA

Additional History and Physical Examination Findings

- Common risk factors: Adolescence, multiple sexual partners, lower socioeconomic status, non-Caucasians, presence of intrauterine device (IUD), recent dilation and curettage (D&C)/abortion/birth, recent menses, history of STD, and prior history of PID.
- Lower abdominal pain is the most frequent symptom, with onset usually developing shortly after menses. Pain is gradual in onset, but increases over hours or days. Pain is generally bilateral, steady, dull, or sharp, and can be aggravated by motion or sexual intercourse.
- Associated symptoms can include vaginal discharge, dysuria/urgency/frequency (secondary to urethral irritation), and vaginal spotting. Fever, chills, anorexia, and nausea and vomiting may also be present.
- Physical exam findings reveal vaginal discharge, exquisite CMT, and bilateral or unilateral adnexal fullness and tenderness. Localized guarding and rebound tenderness may also be present.
- TOA results from an infected tube that involves an ovary with pus accumulation, resulting in a tender, nonmobile, poorly defined pelvic mass. It presents with severe, constant, and diffuse abdominal pain, but later will localize to the abscess site. GI or genitourinary (GU) symptoms may occur from extrinsic pressure from the abscess impinging on surrounding structures.

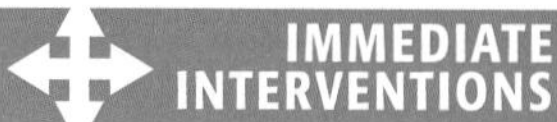

IMMEDIATE INTERVENTIONS

- Second large-bore IV if generalized peritonitis or sepsis is suspected
- Fluid resuscitation if necessary
- CBC, electrolytes, coags, UA, possible β-hCG
- CT scan of the abdomen with IV and PO contrast

DON'T FORGET

Most episodes of diverticulitis are not severe and will respond to medical management alone. On examination day, however, all patients require a surgical consult while in the ED.

DON'T FORGET

Patients who are immunodeficient, taking steroids or other immunosuppressive drugs, or the elderly may not develop the classic inflammatory findings of peritonitis and are therefore at high risk. These patients are never sent home.

DON'T FORGET

No patient with diverticulitis will be discharged from ABEM General Hospital on examination day.

DON'T FORGET

PID is rare in pregnancy after the 12th week.

DON'T FORGET

TOA formation complicates 15% of PID cases.

DON'T FORGET

Findings of fever, abdominal pain, and a unilateral adnexal mass strongly suggest TOA requiring imaging.

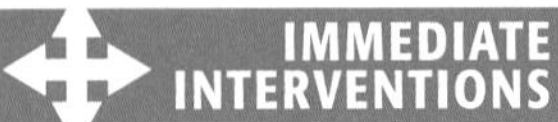

IMMEDIATE INTERVENTIONS

- Second large-bore IV if sepsis is suspected
- Fluid resuscitation if necessary
- CBC, electrolytes, UA, urine pregnancy testing
- LFTs if LUQ pain accompanies presentation

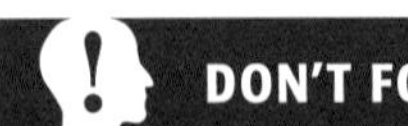

DON'T FORGET

PID is the most common condition confused with ectopic pregnancy.

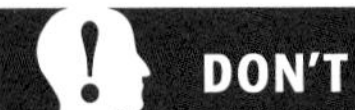

DON'T FORGET

False diagnosis of acute appendicitis may be mistakenly made when torsion of the right ovary results in RLQ pain and is accompanied by nausea and vomiting.

DON'T FORGET

TOA is treated with antibiotics alone without surgical drainage in 75% of cases.

- Peritoneal involvement can spread to include perihepatitis (Fitz-Hugh-Curtis syndrome). This syndrome occurs secondary to discharged pus from the fallopian tubes tracking up the right pelvic gutter to the liver. These patients present complaining of days of acute PID-type pain with the sudden onset of additional severe pleuritic, sharp, RUQ pain. Physical exam reveals profound tenderness over the liver, some lower abdominal tenderness, CMT, and vaginal discharge.

Review Initial Results

- WBC is often elevated with a left shift.
- Urinalysis (UA) with urine β-human chorionic gonadotropin (β-hCG) should be performed.
- Although required, cervical culture for *N. gonorrhoeae* and *Chlamydia* will not be useful in the acute setting. Gram stain may detect the presence of *N. gonorrhoeae*, but lack of findings does not rule out gonorrheal infection.

Risk Stratification: Management Priorities

- PID infection can lead to chronic pain, infertility, or ectopic pregnancy in 25% of cases. Antibiotic treatment should be initiated ASAP.
- TOA should be strongly considered if the patient presents with symptoms of PID but also has evidence of a unilateral pelvic mass. TOA should also be considered in patients previously diagnosed with PID, but demonstrating a lack of response to standard antibiotic therapy after 36-48 hours. Rupture of a TOA should be suspected if the patient presenting with PID symptoms complains of sudden, severe, diffuse, abdominal pain that is associated with shock.

Definitive Management

- PID is treated with antibiotics, antiemetics, and pain relief. Most can be managed as an outpatient after initial ED visit. PID may at times warrant hospitalization and parental antibiotics. Consider admission if
  - Temperature >38°C (or >100.4°F)
  - WBC >12,000/mm^3
  - Immunocompromised (ie, HIV, diabetes, etc)
  - Presence of an IUD
  - Nausea/vomiting precluding oral antibiotics
  - Suspected or confirmed TOA
  - Diffuse peritonitis
  - Evidence of shock
  - Upper peritoneal symptoms indicating perihepatitis
  - Failure to respond to oral antibiotics within 36-48 hours
  - Unclear/uncertain diagnosis
- Antibiotics: Instituted as early as possible and should provide empiric broad-spectrum coverage of the likely pathogens plus vaginal flora:
  - Outpatient: IM/IV ceftriaxone (one dose) plus oral doxycycline for 14 days
  - Inpatient: IV cefotetan or cefoxitin plus doxycycline, or aminoglycoside plus clindamycin
- Antiemetics/pain control: For patient comfort.
- Ob/gyn consultation in the ED if admission is considered or 2-day follow-up is required after initiation of treatment and discharge.

Further Diagnostic Considerations

- Pelvic/vaginal US or abdominal-pelvic CT is required if there is a concern for TOA.

Disposition

- Admission to ob/gyn if clinically warranted for PID treatment. If TOA present, antibiotic therapy with possible surgical or CT/US-guided percutaneous drainage.
- For mild cases of PID that do not fit admission criteria, discharge with oral antibiotics and gyn follow-up with 36-48 hours.

OVARIAN TORSION

Additional History and Physical Examination Findings

- Ovarian torsion can occur at any age, but most cases occur in women in their mid-twenties. A significant number (20%) of ovarian torsion cases occur during pregnancy, commonly at 8-16 weeks, and especially in patients who received ovarian stimulation. A previous history of ovarian torsion also increases a patient's risk.
- Patients present with acute, severe, unilateral, lower abdominal, and pelvic pain which can be either sharp and intermittent or dull with sporadic sharp exacerbations. The right ovary has a greater tendency to twist than does the left ovary. Often the patients relate an onset of pain with an abrupt change of position. Patients may also relate a history of similar intermittent episodes preceding the most acute episode representing previous spontaneous detorsion.
- Commonly, nausea/vomiting is present (up to two-thirds of cases). Fever is uncommon, but may occur if adnexal/ovarian necrosis has occurred.
- Physical exam reveals unilateral, extremely tender adnexal pain, with a palpable mass noted in more than 90% of patients. Pain may radiate to the flank, back, or groin. Most patients have CMT and adnexal tenderness. If gangrenous necrosis has occurred, findings of frank peritonitis may be present.

Review Initial Results

- CBC: Patient may or may not have a leukocytosis on presentation.
- UA: Obtained to assess for other causes of pain (urinary infection or renal calculi).
- β-HCG: Assesses pregnancy status.
- Vaginal US should reveal the pathologic condition predisposing to torsion such as ovarian enlargement >10 cm, and/or the presence of an adnexal mass. The ovary/adnexa may appear as a twisted mass, either solid or cystic in nature. Visualization of the twisted vascular pedicle is highly predictive.
- Doppler flow study: It may show an absence or severe decrease of arterial or venous flow within the twisted adnexa. This is highly predictive or torsion. However, normal flow studies do not exclude torsion, since 50%-60% of surgically confirmed cases had a normal Doppler flow.

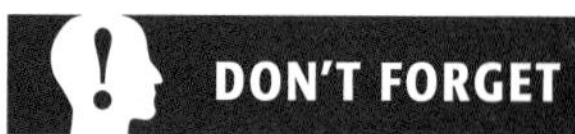

Normal Doppler flow does not exclude torsion, since half of all cases have a normal study.

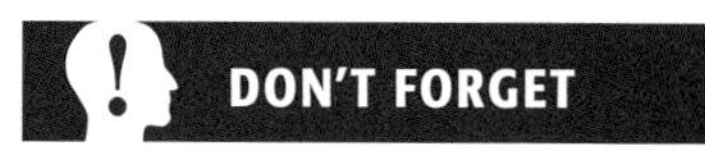

The diagnosis of ovarian torsion is often missed, and ovarian salvage is rare.

Risk Stratification: Management Priorities

- Early ob/gyn consultation should be initiated if the diagnosis of ovarian torsion is strongly considered. Ovarian torsion is a gyn emergency since delay in diagnosis can have significant consequences. Missed diagnosis is common with the correct preoperative diagnosis made in only 18%-64% of cases. Consequences of a missed or late diagnosis include reduced fertility, increased risk of ectopic pregnancy, and infection/necrosis of the ovary with resulting peritonitis and shock.
- Early surgical consultation is needed if evidence of diffuse peritonitis is seen on initial examination.

Definitive Management

- Antiemetics: If vomiting present.
- Pain control: It provides comfort to the patient preoperatively.

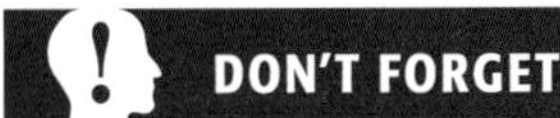

The definitive management of torsion is surgery ASAP in order to retain future fertility.

- Hemodynamic stabilization: Accomplished by crystalloid infusion. If diffuse peritonitis with shock is present, vasopressors may also need to be considered.
- Antibiotics: Most symptoms of ovarian torsion result from ischemia, but if fever and peritoneal signs are evident, broad-spectrum antibiotics should be instituted to cover abdominal flora.
- Early ob/gyn consultation in the ED since prompt management is vital to avoid ischemic necrosis and loss of affected ovary.

Disposition

- Admit to ob/gyn service for either diagnostic laparoscopy if the diagnosis is uncertain, or for laparoscopic or surgical detorsion of the ovary, or oophorectomy if the ovary is not viable.

WINNING STRATEGIES

- Every patient with abdominal pain has a perforated viscus, intestinal obstruction, peritonitis, mesenteric ischemia, pancreatitis, and ovarian or testicular torsion until proven otherwise.
- Reassess your patients frequently!
- Beware of ACS presenting with upper abdominal pain/GI complaints.
- Patients older than 45 for men and 55 for women who present with epigastric pain need an ECG included in their immediate interventions as well as IV, cardiac monitor, and crystalloid infusion.
- Obtain upright CXR and abdominal x-ray series in patients with abdominal pain, vomiting, and suspicion for intestinal obstruction or perforation.
- Expect most abdominal pain patients to develop peritonitis, rapid hemodynamic, or cardiac decline somewhere in the process of workup.
- Involve surgery early in all instances, but expect consultants to ask you for complete workup before agreeing to see/admit a patient.
- Administer antibiotics in all cases where the diagnosis of peritonitis is suspected, either as a primary problem or as a secondary complication.
- SBP can be classic with fever and abdominal pain in a cirrhotic patient or can present with a subacute decline in function and mentation without fever or severe pain.
- Paracentesis is the key to diagnosis of SBP, even if alternative diagnoses such as UTI or pneumonia have already been made.
- PD patients will need a cell count of their effluent if it is not obviously cloudy to diagnose peritonitis.
- Surgical peritonitis of whatever cause usually reveals exquisite tenderness, guarding and/or abdominal rigidity in addition to rapidly ensuing sepsis. Involve surgery immediately.
- All SBP- and PD-related peritonitis patients get admitted on the examination day.
- Perforated viscus can be diagnosed with upright chest/lateral decubitus abdominal films in 50% of cases—don't forget it.
- Beware of more indolent presentations that can be present with large bowel perforations.
- Pain that is out of proportion to the examination findings in a person older than 50, especially with any history of CAD or PVD is suspicious for mesenteric ischemia.
- Screen patients with suspected mesenteric ischemia for risk factors: Digoxin use, atrial fibrillation, hypovolemic state, CHF, etc.
- The best way to diagnosis mesenteric ischemia is an angiogram. If this test is "unavailable," abdominal x-rays or CT abdomen should be ordered.

- Involve surgery immediately after initial resuscitation is done and initial studies are performed if mesenteric ischemia is suspected.
- Reassess mesenteric ischemia patients frequently as they will develop peritonitis once bowel becomes necrotic. If this is suspected to have happened, administer antibiotics and call surgery (if not already consulted).
- Mesenteric ischemia patients will ultimately require surgery in almost all cases. They will likely need admission to the ICU.
- Adhesions and hernias are the most common culprits in intestinal obstruction. Constipated elderly patients with extreme pain and distention have a volvulus until proven otherwise.
- NGT is indicated in most cases of obstruction, especially if vomiting is present.
- Surgical consult needs to be obtained early in cases of suspected obstruction.
- Strangulated hernia causing obstruction can become ischemic and eventually lead to peritonitis—reassess frequently.
- All patients are admitted to surgery, though not all will require OR for the bowel obstruction.
- Expect atypical appendicitis presentations instead of classic presenting symptoms of anorexia, vomiting, fever, and abdominal pain in RLQ.
- Females of childbearing age with abdominal pain need a pregnancy test. These patients are considered pregnant until proven otherwise.
- Beware of pregnant females with RUQ pain that may be appendicitis.
- Sudden pain relief of a brief duration is suggestive of appendix perforation, especially if followed by peritonitis and vital sign deterioration.
- US, not CT, is initial imaging of choice in children for appendicitis diagnosis.
- If any doubt of appendicitis diagnosis, CT scan should be ordered and surgery contacted.
- In pancreatitis, pain can be severe, but abdominal examination will be relatively benign.
- Pancreatitis sequesters fluid, so patients can easily go into shock—resuscitate aggressively.
- US can help with identifying pancreatitis etiology.
- Neither US nor CT can exclude diagnosis of pancreatitis, especially early on, but for chronic cases CT can be helpful to grade the degree of inflammation/damage.
- Most patients without acute biliary obstruction or mass effect will be admitted to medicine. On the examination day expect them to be sick enough to require ICU care.
- Accurate diagnosis of biliary disorders will require some imaging study, with US being the most useful test.
- On examination day, all patients with cholecystitis and persistent pain or cholangitis are admitted. Both cases will require antibiotics and fluid resuscitation.
- In older patients presenting with RLQ pain, both appendicitis and diverticulitis should be considered.
- On examination day, all patients with diverticulitis will require surgical consultation while in the ED.
- Patients presenting with PID and a pelvic mass or patients still with PID symptoms after 2 days of appropriate treatment have a TOA until proven otherwise and need an imaging study.
- Women presenting with RLQ pain, nausea, and vomiting should all have ovarian torsion as part of their differential.
- A normal Doppler flow study does not rule out ovarian torsion. Gyn consult should still be obtained.

CHAPTER 13

GI Bleed

Aleksandr Gorenbeyn and Thomas J. Regan

DON'T FORGET

All patients with GI bleeds get two large-bore IVs or a central line.

INITIAL ASSESSMENT

- Focus on airway, breathing, circulation (ABCs). Keep immediate life-threats in mind first.
- Ask for a full set of vitals with every patient, including pulse, blood pressure (BP), respirations, temp, O_2 sat, glucose, and finger stick hemoglobin.
- Large-bore IV × 2, O_2, monitor for every patient.
- Draw labs and hold for orders.

IMMEDIATE INTERVENTIONS

- Intubation if airway is compromised
- Two large-bore IVs (18-gauge or larger in antecubital veins)
- NS bolus
- Supplemental oxygen
- Cardiac monitor
- Type and cross
- Blood for CBC, lytes, PTT/INR, LFTs

INITIAL HISTORY AND PHYSICAL EXAMINATION

History

- History of the present illness (HPI)
  - Onset of symptoms
  - Hematemesis
  - Hematochezia
  - Melena
  - Estimated amount of blood loss
  - Abdominal pain
- PMHx (patient medical history)
  - History and type of previous gastrointestinal (GI) bleed?
  - History of alcohol abuse?
  - History of bleeding disorders?
  - Blood type?
  - Prior transfusions?
  - Hepatitis?
  - Liver failure?
  - Renal failure?
- Medications
  - Anticoagulation therapy
  - Aspirin
- Allergies

DON'T FORGET

DDx Summary

- It may be difficult to determine exact source of bleeding.
- On the test, a GI bleed is most likely to be from
  - Ulcer
  - Varices
  - Diverticulosis
  - Angiodysplasia

Physical Examination

- Vital signs with focus on blood pressure and heart rate
- Head, ears, eyes, nose, and throat (HEENT): Jaundice? Dehydration? Pale conjunctivae?
- Chest: Tachycardia? Murmurs?
- Abd: Pain, hepatosplenomegaly? Rebound or guarding?
- Extremity: Capillary refill, cyanosis, cool or well perfused?
- Rectal: Melena? Gross or occult blood?
- Neuro: Alteration in mental status?

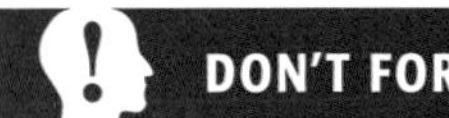

DON'T FORGET

Determining the source of bleeding should always be secondary to stabilization of the patient.

DIFFERENTIAL DIAGNOSIS

- Upper GI bleed
  - Bleeding that occurs proximal to the ligament of Treitz is classified as upper GI (UGI) bleeding. Possible etiologies include peptic ulcer disease, gastritis, esophageal varices, and a Mallory-Weiss tear. Ulcers, including gastric, duodenal, and stomal, comprise about 60% of cases and are the most common cause.
  - Risk factors for ulcer include nonsteroidal anti-inflammatory drug (NSAID) use, *Helicobacter pylori* infection, and heavy alcohol consumption. Gastroesophageal varices result from portal hypertension, most often from cirrhosis.

- As a group, variceal bleeds carry the highest morbidity and mortality.
- Mallory-Weiss syndrome is UGI bleeding caused by a mucosal tear in the cardio-esophageal region. They classically occur after repeated retching and are usually self- limited.

- Lower GI bleed
  - The most common cause of lower GI bleeding is a UGI bleed. Proximal bleeding should be considered even if the blood is red. Bleeding sources distal to the ligament of Treitz include diverticular disease, angiodysplasia, colon cancer, inflammatory bowel disease, gastroenteritis, hemorrhoids, and anal fissures. While hemorrhoids are the most common cause of all lower GI bleeds, a hemorrhoidal bleed is unlikely to be encountered on the oral board examination.
  - Angiodysplasia is the most common cause when the etiology is not obvious, especially in the elderly. Thought to be the result of a diverticulum eroding into an artery, diverticulosis causes painless bleeding that can be massive. The other causes of lower GI bleed are unlikely to result in massive hemorrhage.

DON'T FORGET

Melena indicates the blood has been in the GI tract for at least 14 hours and is probably from a source distant to rectum.

DON'T FORGET

Initial focus should be on assessment of hemodynamic status and volume resuscitation.

UPPER GI BLEED

Additional History and Physical Examination Findings

- Clinical assessment is often poor at determining source but history and symptoms can suggest location.
- Hematemesis (bright red blood) suggests a brisk UGI bleed and coffee ground emesis suggests a slow bleeding source.
- Melena on rectal examination suggests a UGI source because the black color is from the effect of acid on hemoglobin.
- History of aspirin, NSAID, or anticoagulation therapy
- History of previous bleeding episode, peptic ulcer disease, chronic alcohol use, or cirrhosis
- History of cancer, renal disease, or bleeding disorders
- Signs of liver failure, including jaundice, ascites, spider angiomas, and palmar erythema
- Frequent nosebleeds or retching prior to presentation?

DON'T FORGET

Check an ECG on all elderly patients for related cardiac ischemia/infarction.

DON'T FORGET

Hgb/Hct level may not reflect the true level of anemia in patients with brisk bleeds.

Review Initial Results

- Hemoglobin level to assess degree of anemia
- Prothrombin time (PT)/ partial thromboplastin time (PTT) and international normalized ratio (INR) to assess liver function
- Electrolytes: Elevated blood urea nitrogen (BUN) suggests GI bleed.
- Electrocardiogram (ECG)

DON'T FORGET

Factors associated with high morbidity include hemodynamic instability, repeated hematemesis, bright red blood per rectum, age >60, and coexistent systemic disease.

Risk Stratification: Management Priorities

- Overall mortality rate is around 10%.
- Most deaths occur in the elderly and in patients with liver disease.
- Elderly and cardiac patients are susceptible to cardiac complications caused by loss of oxygen-carrying capacity.
- Patients with cardiac symptoms and bleeding should be transfused immediately.
- Mortality is higher in elderly patients.

DON'T FORGET

All patients with GI bleeding get an NG tube on test day.

Definitive Management

- ABCs
- Intravenous fluid (IVF) resuscitation

DON'T FORGET

During the examination, stating that you will look up the dose of an uncommon medication is acceptable.

DON'T FORGET

If an EGD is indicated and your GI consultant tries to delay the procedure, advocate strongly on behalf of your patient.

DON'T FORGET

Patients can deteriorate very quickly. Early intervention to stabilize the patient and frequent reassessment Is mandatory.

DON'T FORGET

With adequate supportive care, the majority of patients with UGI bleed not related to portal hypertension causes will stop bleeding within 48 hours.

- Transfuse if severely anemic (<7 g/dL) or if the vital signs are unstable.
- Transfuse cardiac patients if hemoglobin is <10 g/dL.
- NG tube to determine if upper or lower GI bleed
- Supplemental oxygen
- Transfuse bleeding patients with FFP if INR is abnormal.
- Administer omeprazole 80 mg intravenous (IV) bolus followed by 8 mg/h IV for UGI bleeding.
- Administer octreotide 50 μg IV bolus followed by 50 μg/h IV for 24 hours to patients with suspected portal hypertension bleeding.
- Consider vasopressin 0.2-0.6 U/h in case of variceal hemorrhage with exsanguination.
- Consult GI specialist to arrange UGI endoscopy.
- Indications for emergent endoscopy:
  - Persistent hypotension or tachycardia despite fluids and blood transfusion
  - Persistent bleeding (continued hematemesis, bright red blood on NG aspirate, bright red blood per rectum)
  - High suspicion of variceal bleed

Frequent Reassessment

- Continuous monitoring of vital signs is imperative.
- Repeat hemoglobin to assess stability of patient with brisk bleeding.
- Reassess mental status, especially in the elderly.
- After stabilizing the patient, identification of the bleeding source should be undertaken.

Complications

- Cardiovascular collapse caused by volume loss
- Respiratory failure secondary to aspiration of blood
- Hepatic encephalopathy in liver failure patients

Disposition

- All patients with UGI bleeding should be admitted.
- All patients with ongoing bleeding, hemodynamic instability, clotting disorders (either primary or secondary to anticoagulant use), altered mental status, or unstable comorbid disease (heart disease, renal disease, liver disease) should be admitted to the intensive care unit (ICU).
- All patients with melena should be admitted to an ICU.
- If a patient has completed full evaluation with endoscopy in the emergency department (ED), admission to the floor may be considered.

LOWER GI BLEED

Additional History and Physical Examination Findings

- As in UGI, clinical assessment is often poor at determining source, but history and symptoms can suggest location.
- Hematochezia suggests lower GI source, but 5%-10% of patients will have an UGI source.
- History of aspirin or NSAIDs suggests a UGI source.
- Concomitant anticoagulation therapy greatly increases risk and must be discovered.
- History of previous bleeding episodes including need for transfusion and interventions.
- History of constipation, change in bowel habits or hemorrhoids.

- History of colon cancer, diverticular disease, renal disease, or bleeding disorders
- Anorectal examination/anoscopy to look for hemorrhoids and anal fissures

Review Initial Results

- Hemoglobin level to assess degree of anemia
- PT/PTT and INR to assess liver function and use of anticoagulants
- Electrolytes: Elevated BUN suggests GI bleed
- ECG

Risk Stratification: Management Priorities

- Lower GI bleeds account for up to a third of all GI bleeds.
- Bleeds from lower GI sources generally have a lower mortality than UGI bleeding.

Definitive Management

- ABCs
- Initial management must focus on the stabilization of the patient.
- IVF resuscitation
- Transfuse if severely anemic (<7 g/dL) or unstable vital signs
- Transfuse cardiac patients if hemoglobin <10 g/dL
- NG tube to determine if upper or lower GI bleeds
- Supplemental oxygen
- Transfuse bleeding patients with FFP if INR is abnormal, correct with vitamin K.

Frequent Reassessment

- Continuous monitoring of vital signs is imperative.
- Repeat hemoglobin to assess stability of patient with brisk bleeding.
- Reassess mental status, especially in the elderly.
- After stabilizing the patient, identification of the bleeding source should be undertaken.

Additional Interventions

- Colonoscopy is the procedure of choice for diagnosis and therapy after the lower GI bleed has stopped.
    - Identifies bleeding site in 75%-95% of cases.
    - Therapy with cautery or local epinephrine injection may help if bleeding is from diverticular source.
    - May not be possible if bleeding is massive and the use of colonoscopy in active bleeding is controversial.
- Angiography is used for therapy and diagnosis.
    - Indicated for continuous, severe, or massive lower GI bleeding that prevents colonoscopy.
    - Therapeutic interventions include vasopressin infusion and arterial embolization.
    - Can detect bleeding rates as low as 0.5 mL/min.
    - May provide diagnosis when other modalities do not reveal a source.
- Radionuclide scanning with technetium 99m-labeled red blood cells is useful for diagnosis and is often used as a screening test before angiography.
    - Roughly localizes site of bleeding and can detect slow bleeds with rates as low as 0.1 mL/min and intermittent bleeds.
    - May be used as a screening test prior to angiography because of its increased sensitivity for slow bleeding.

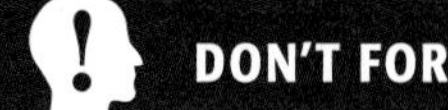

Melena suggests a large, upper GI bleed. These patients should be assumed to be unstable and are always admitted to an ICU.

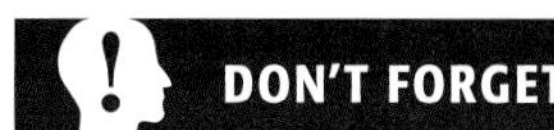

Always ask about Coumadin (warfarin), Xeralto (rivaroxaban), and other anticoagulants and correct INR early in management.

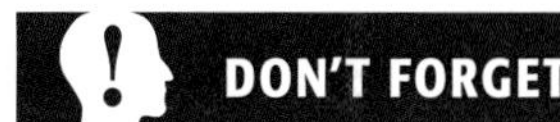

In severe anemia, supplemental oxygen via NRB at 100% is equivalent to transfusing 1-1.5 U of blood.

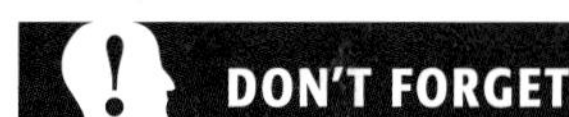

Frequent reassessment is needed because patient's condition can deteriorate rapidly.

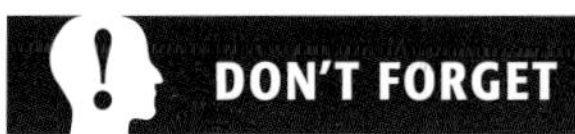

The majority of lower GI bleeds stop spontaneously, but a workup should still be undertaken to identify the source.

Complications

- Cardiovascular collapse caused by volume loss
- Cardiac complications caused by massive blood loss and strained oxygen-carrying capacity

Disposition

- All patients with active lower GI bleeding should be admitted especially on test day.
- All patients with ongoing bleeding, hemodynamic instability, clotting disorders (either primary or secondary to anticoagulant use), altered mental status, or unstable comorbid disease (heart, renal, or liver disease) should be admitted to an intensive care setting.

WINNING STRATEGIES

- Always focus on the ABCs and volume resuscitation before identifying source of bleed.
- Two large-bore IVs on all patients with active GI bleeds.
- Elderly patients or patients with a cardiac history should have an ECG to look for ischemia/infarction secondary to anemia.
- Be aggressive in transfusing elderly patients with comorbidities, cardiac patients, and patients with unstable vital signs.
- NG tube and rectal examination on all patients on examination day.

CHAPTER 14

Back Pain

Aleksandr Gorenbeyn and Thomas J. Regan

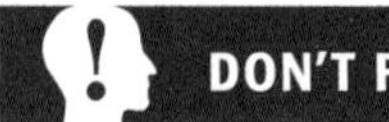

DON'T FORGET

Until proven otherwise, every patient with back pain has

- Abdominal aortic aneurysm (AAA)
- Epidural abscess
- Cauda equina syndrome

INITIAL ASSESSMENT

- Focus on ABCs. Keep immediate life-threats in mind first.
- Ask for a full set of vitals with every patient, including pulse, blood pressure (BP), respirations, temp, O_2 sat, glucose, finger stick hemoglobin (Hgb).
- Large-bore IV × 2, O_2, monitor in every patient.
- Draw labs and hold for orders.

Case-Specific Recommendations

- Focus on age, vital signs (VS), general appearance (level of discomfort).
- Identify unstable patients with immediate life threats including shock or neurologic deficits.

INITIAL HISTORY AND PHYSICAL EXAMINATION

History

- History of the present illness (HPI)
  - Onset
  - Quality/severity
  - Location/radiation/migration
  - Aggravating or relieving factors
- Review of systems (ROS)
  - Associated neurologic complaints—eg, weakness, numbness, loss of bladder/bowel control
  - Associated fever/chills
  - Weight loss, night sweats
- Past medical history (PMHx)
  - Hypertension (HTN)
  - Arteriosclerosis
  - Immunosuppression
  - Connective tissue (ie, Marfan syndrome)
- Psychosocial history (PSHx)
  - Recent spinal neurosurgery
  - Recent epidural catheter
  - Recent lumbar puncture (LP)
- Family history: AAA? Cancer?
- Medications
- Allergies
- Social history: Intravenous (IV) drug abuse

IMMEDIATE INTERVENTIONS

- Oxygen via NC
- Cardiac monitor
- 18-gauge IV with NS KVO
- Draw blood for labs
- Stabilize life-threats by managing airway, providing aggressive fluid resuscitation.

PHYSICAL EXAMINATION

- General appearance
- VS
- Neck: Stiffness, localized pain
- Cardiovascular (CV): Pulses in all four extremities, femoral bruits
- Abd: Pain, guarding, rebound, pulsatile mass, abdominal bruit, ecchymosis
- Back: Focal thoracic or lumbar pain, flank ecchymosis
- Extremities: Mottled, cool, decreased lower extremity pulses, femoral bruits
- Rectal: Decreased tone
- Genitourinary (GU): Scrotal ecchymosis
- Neuro: Extremity strength, sensation, gait, reflexes

DIFFERENTIAL DIAGNOSIS

- Abdominal aortic aneurysm (AAA)
  - Aortic aneurysm occurs as a result of destruction of the aortic wall media layer causing a gradual localized dilation of the aortic wall, most occurring below the level of the renal arteries.
  - Pain can result from impingement of the aneurysm on surrounding structures, or from the sudden onset of leaking or rupture. Rapid identification of the latter is imperative to institute rapid surgical repair.
- Epidural abscess
  - This is a potentially devastating infection of the epidural space along the posterior aspect of the spinal canal, most commonly occurring in the thoracic and lumbar areas. It is caused by either direct extension of a contiguous infected focus, or by hematogenous seeding from a distant source.
  - Examples of contiguous sources are osteomyelitis, psoas abscesses, decubitus ulcers, and recent neurosurgical sites. The most common hematogenous source would be a cutaneous site, but abdominal, pulmonary, and urinary sources are also recognized.
  - Depending on the virulence of the causative organism, clinical signs may develop either slowly or rapidly.
- Cauda equina syndrome
  - Referring to a serious complication of lumbar disc disease, cauda equina syndrome is a neurologic emergency. It results from compression of several nerve roots in the cauda, disc herniation, mass lesion, fracture with hematoma, or from infection.
  - Presenting with back pain, leg pain, loss of sensation in the saddle distribution, and bowel and bladder retention (or incontinence), cauda equina syndrome must be diagnosed immediately and surgically decompressed to prevent permanent disability. Refer to Chap. 20 for full discussion.
- Pyelonephritis
  - A frequent cause of flank pain especially in women, pyelonephritis is an infection of the kidney.
  - Uncomplicated pyelonephritis is unlikely to appear on the oral board exam. If part of the oral boards, pyelonephritis will usually be complicated by sepsis, an obstructing ureteral stone, or immunocompromised status. For further discussion, refer to Chap. 7.
- Ureterolithiasis
  - The classic kidney stone is a common cause of severe back and flank pain.
  - Often presenting in dramatic manner with severe, colicky back and flank pain that radiates to the groin, nausea and vomiting, and diaphoresis, ureterolithiasis is treated with fluids and pain medication. It is unlikely to be the cause of back pain on the oral boards.
- Gastrointestinal (GI) etiology
  - Various GI problems including pancreatitis, penetrating ulcers, and cholecystitis can present with back pain. For further discussion, refer to Chap. 12.

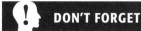

DON'T FORGET

DDx Summary

- Sudden back pain or abdominal pain in an elderly patient with risk factors should evoke strong suspicion of AAA.
- Back pain, unrelieved by position, and accompanied by fever and/or neurologic signs is an epidural abscess until proven otherwise.
- Back pain that seems like musculoskeletal back pain except with objective neurologic compromise and urinary/bowel symptoms is spinal cord compression until proven otherwise.

DON'T FORGET

A postvoid residual of >150-200 mL is the most sensitive finding for spinal cord involvement.

ABDOMINAL AORTIC ANEURYSM

Additional History and Physical Examination Findings

- The risk factors for AAA include family history of AAA, connective tissue disorders (ie, Marfan and Ehlers-Danlos syndromes), and atherosclerotic risk factors (ie, age, HTN, diabetes, smoking, hypercholesterolemia).
- The most common presenting symptom of symptomatic AAA is back or abdominal pain. Common associated symptoms are dizziness or syncope.

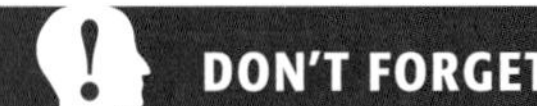

DON'T FORGET

Syncope followed by severe abdominal or back pain should immediately evoke a suspicion of ruptured AAA.

DON'T FORGET

Hypotension and back pain in an elderly patient is a ruptured AAA and should mandate placement of large-bore IVs, type and cross for 10 U of blood, and immediate consultation with a vascular surgeon.

DON'T FORGET

Urgent consultation with the vascular surgeon should take precedence over obtaining any radiographic study when the diagnosis of ruptured AAA is suspected. Do not send a suspected AAA who is unstable to the CT scanner to die!

- Pain is usually sudden and severe, and may be described as ripping or tearing.
- Pulsatile abdominal mass can be felt in 77% of ruptured aneurysms.
- Asymmetrical or absent femoral pulses are highly suggestive, but are not commonly found on examination.
- Retroperitoneal bleeding from a ruptured AAA may be seen as periumbilical, flank, perineal, or scrotal ecchymosis on examination.

Review Initial Results

- Radiographic evaluation may unnecessarily delay operative repair, and therefore the decision to obtain them must be made carefully.
- AAA may be detected on anteroposterior (AP)/lateral plain films in 55%-85% of cases, and is most commonly identified as a calcified, bulging aorta. However, do NOT send your patient for an x-ray out of the department during the oral board exam when suspecting an AAA.
- Bedside ultrasound (US) can detect AAA in almost 100% of cases, but cannot reliably detect rupture (Fig. 14-1).

Risk Stratification: Management Priorities

- Symptomatic but stable patients with suspected AAA may undergo a definitive diagnostic study after consultation with vascular surgery.
- Symptomatic unstable patients with suspected AAA should undergo immediate operative repair. Resuscitative measures should be initiated, but should not delay transfer to the operating room.

Definitive Management

- Resuscitation with normal saline (NS) boluses and early blood transfusion if the patient remains hypotensive.
- Rapid surgical management is the most important treatment option in the setting of significant hypotension.

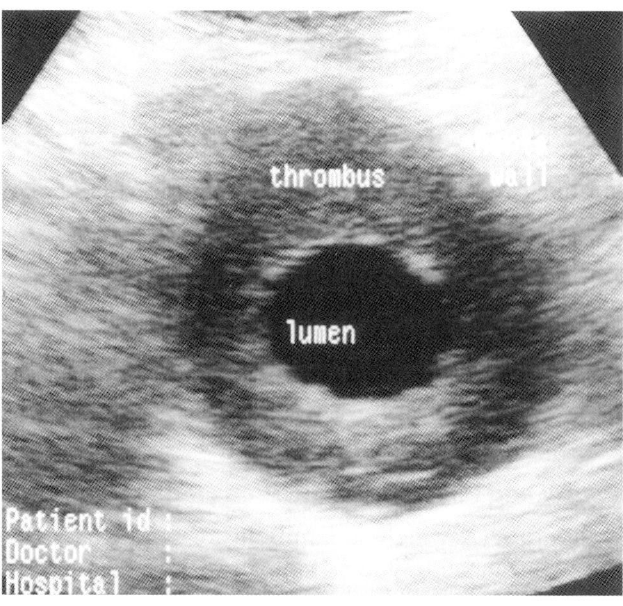

Figure 14-1. Abdominal aortic aneurysm with intraluminal thrombus. (*Reprinted with permission from Tintinalli JE, Kelen GD, Stapczynski JS, et al.* Emergency Medicine: A Comprehensive Study Guide. *6th ed. New York, NY: McGraw-Hill; 2004.*)

Frequent Reassessment

- Vital signs should be checked every 15 minutes in anticipation of possible hypotension.

Further Diagnostic Considerations

- Computed tomography (CT) scan with contrast is just as sensitive as US in detecting presence of AAA, and can better demonstrate the anatomic detail of the aneurysm as well as any associated intra-abdominal rupture or intra-abdominal or retroperitoneal bleed.

Disposition

- When consulting vascular surgery, demand that the patient be seen in the emergency department (ED).
- Symptomatic patients are managed operatively, and should be held in the emergency room (ER) only until the operating room is ready.

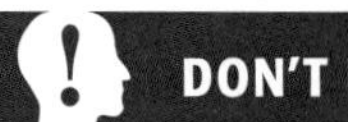

DON'T FORGET

Obtain a bedside US early to evaluate for AAA.

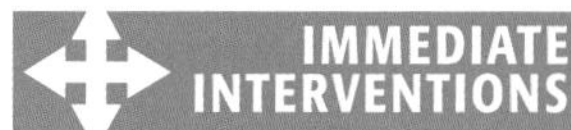

IMMEDIATE INTERVENTIONS

For AAA

- Second large-bore IV.
- Fluid resuscitation if necessary.
- CBC, electrolytes, coags, UA, T&C for 10 U PRBC.
- Immediate consultation with vascular surgeon.

EPIDURAL ABSCESS

Additional History and Physical Examination Findings

- Risk factors include concurrent skin infection, IV drug use, recent back surgery, recent epidural catheter or LP, or recent minor back injury.
- The most prominent symptom is back pain which can range from dull to severe and is initially well localized over the site of the infection. A classic point of history is that the pain is not relieved by rest. Pain can be present for a couple of days to a couple of weeks. As local nerve roots are compressed with the progressing infection, the pain may become radicular in nature.
- Because the dura mater is not adherent to the posterior vertebral column, there are minimal anatomic barriers to prevent the abscess (and thereby the pain) to gradually extend over a number of vertebral spaces.
- Patient may give a history of having intermittent fever/chills. Fever, although common, may be absent on examination.
- Weakness, sensory loss, and areflexia can also occur below the site of the lesion, and can eventually lead to paralysis within hours to days. Bowel and bladder dysfunction may also be present.

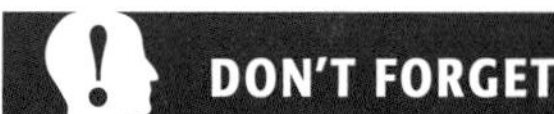

DON'T FORGET

Although common, fever does not need to be present on initial presentation.

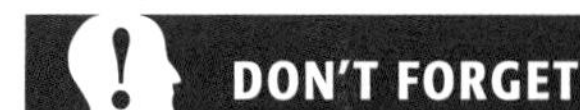

DON'T FORGET

A thorough neurologic examination (including motor, sensory, and reflexes) should be obtained on all patients with localized back pain and fever.

Review Initial Results

- Elevated white blood cells (WBC) usually present.
- Thoracic/spinal radiographic findings may not be helpful; findings of compression fracture, paravertebral mass, or of osteomyelitis may be seen, but these findings may take from 10 days to 2 weeks to appear.
- Erythrocyte sedimentation rate (ESR) will be elevated, even in light of a normal WBC, but the result may take too long to come back, especially in the setting of progressive neurologic findings.
- Blood cultures should be sent; they are positive in 60%-90% of cases, and can help direct and appropriate antibiotic regime during hospitalization.

Risk Stratification: Management Priorities

- Diagnosis is made by clinical impression and by ordering the appropriate imaging test.
- Neurosurgical consult should be made early in the course of evaluation, especially if neurologic deficits are evident.
- Initiation of antibiotic treatment should not be delayed while awaiting an imaging study in a patient with a high suspicion of an epidural abscess.

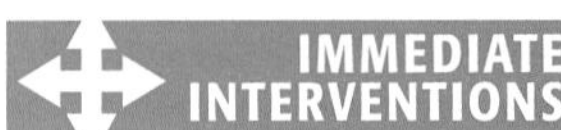

IMMEDIATE INTERVENTIONS

For epidural abscess

- Complete blood count (CBC), electrolytes, blood cultures, and sedimentation rate.
- Early dose of antibiotics if epidural abscess is strongly considered, especially if neuro deficits are present.
- Second large-bore IV and fluid resuscitation if shock evident.

DON'T FORGET

Get a neurosurgery consult ASAP when the clinical impression indicates the diagnosis of epidural abscess is likely.

Epidural abscess is fatal in absence of antibiotic therapy.

Staphylococcus aureus accounts for most cases, and should be remembered when choosing an appropriate antibiotic regime.

Plain CT scan does not exclude the diagnosis of epidural abscess.

Definitive Management

- Antibiotics: Empirical antibiotic therapy should include coverage of gram-positive cocci, particularly staphylococci (including methicillin-resistant Staphylococcus aureus [MRSA]), and gram-negative bacilli.
  - Vancomycin: 1 g IV q12h
  - Cefepime 1g IV q12h or similar
- Steroid therapy: Not found to be useful in epidural abscess.
- IV fluid: Treatment for sepsis/shock may be required with infusion of crystalloids and possibly vasopressors.
- Pain control: For patient comfort.

Frequent Reassessment

- Repeat neurologic examinations should be performed to assess for any new sensory/motor loss or the evolution of symptoms.
- Repeat VS frequently to pick up any indication of sepsis/shock.

Further Diagnostic Considerations

- LP is not recommended.
- Magnetic resonance imaging (MRI) with gadolinium is the study of choice. If not available, CT myelogram would be the next alternative.

Complications

- The chance of partial or complete recovery is inversely related to the amount of neurologic sequelae at the time of diagnosis and treatment.
- Most complications result from cord compression and can include sensory loss, motor weakness or paralysis, and bowel or bladder dysfunction.

Disposition

- Admit to neurosurgery for IV antibiotics and possible decompression and laminectomy.

WINNING STRATEGIES

- Every back pain is an AAA, epidural abscess, or cauda equina syndrome until proven otherwise.
- Immediate intervention in all back pain patients includes oxygen, cardiac monitor, and IV access.
- Stabilize life threats by managing airway and aggressive resuscitation if shock is evident.
- The history in your AAA patient may be classic on examination day (older patient with a history of arteriosclerotic disease complaining of sudden onset of abdominal or back pain), but you may get a younger patient with a history of a connective tissue disease.
- Always be suspicious of normal or low BP in an elderly patient with history of HTN complaining of back pain—it's an AAA with rupture until proven otherwise.
- Syncope followed by back or abdominal pain should raise your suspicions of the presence of ruptured AAA.
- You cannot repeat the VS too often in order to pick up developing signs of shock (hemorrhagic in AAA; septic in epidural abscess).
- Development of shock will require crystalloid and blood in AAA versus crystalloid and pressors in epidural abscess.
- Type and cross for 10 U of packed red blood cells (PRBC) in suspected cases of ruptured AAA.

- Do not let the patient with suspected ruptured AAA leave the ED for CT unless vascular surgeon has already been consulted and the patient is being accompanied by yourself or the vascular surgeon. In fact, the imaging test to perform is an emergency bedside US.
- In suspected ruptured AAA, immediate consultation with the vascular surgeon is important before ordering any imaging studies.
- In suspected epidural abscess, initial dose of antibiotics and immediate consultation with neurosurgery is important before any imaging studies.
- Repeat the neurologic examination in patients with suspected epidural abscess to detect evolving spinal cord impingement on examination day. Inform neurosurgery immediately if this occurs.
- Prioritize and address all life threats first, but don't forget to treat the patient's pain when appropriate.

CHAPTER 15

Painful Extremity

Megan French and David Howes

INITIAL ASSESSMENT

- Focus on age, level of distress, abnormal vital signs (VS).

INITIAL HISTORY AND PHYSICAL EXAMINATION

History

- History of present illness (HPI): "How do they look?"
  - Onset (acute vs subacute vs chronic)
  - Quality/severity/paresthesias/paralysis
  - Location (joint-based vs distal extremity)
  - Range of motion (active/passive)
  - Fevers?
  - Recent trauma, fracture, or procedures?
  - Any systemic symptoms? (Lung or abdominal involvement)
- Past medical history (PMHx)
  - Immune compromised state?
  - Diabetes?
  - Atrial fibrillation?
  - Risk factors for deep venous thrombosis (DVT)
  - Arthritis or other inflammatory disorders
  - Medications
  - Allergies

DON'T FORGET

For the painful extremity, to ensure a proper diagnosis/treatment plan definitive interventions will follow a thorough H&P.

Physical Examination

- VS
- Cardiac: Atrial fibrillation? Valvular murmurs?
- Neuro: Paresthesias, paralysis
- Extremities:
  - Pulses
  - Skin color or breakdown
  - Capillary refill
  - Pain
  - Tense compartments?
  - Anticoagulated?
  - Joint effusion/redness/warmth/range of motion
  - Tenderness along tendon sheaths
  - Signs of chronic arterial or venous disease (diminished hair on legs, shiny hyperpigmented skin, ulcerations, and edema)
  - Calf tenderness

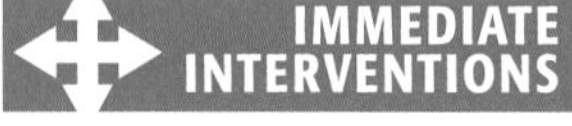

- IV, O_2, monitors
- Labs for CPK, coags, CBC, BMP
- Palpate or Doppler pulses in affected extremity

DIFFERENTIAL DIAGNOSIS

DON'T FORGET

DDx Summary

On the oral board examination, patients with a painful extremity will have

- Arterial embolism
- DVT
- Septic joint

- Arterial embolism: Vascular emergency that requires coordinated care between the emergency physician, radiologist, and vascular surgeon. Mortality is high even with prompt diagnosis and limb salvage time is often <6 hours from onset of symptoms. The finding of a pulseless or greatly diminished pulse in an extremity requires a quick response to avoid amputation.
- DVT: Virchow triad of stasis: Injuries to the vessel wall and hypercoagulable states still apply. Clinical symptoms vary and examination findings have limited predictive value. When the diagnosis is in question, a duplex ultrasound of the involved extremity is a must.
- Septic joint: The differential of traumatic/inflammatory/septic joint is almost never made clinically in the world of oral boards. A detailed history

will provide clues as to the likely etiology and aspiration with fluid analysis will be confirmatory.
- Acute compartment syndrome (ACS): History of recent trauma or fracture coupled with pain out of proportion to examination and tense compartments/pain with passive stretch and/or paresthesias constitutes a surgical emergency and warrants immediate orthopedic consultation and/or measurement of compartment pressures followed by admission.

ARTERIAL EMBOLUS

Additional History and Physical Examination Findings

- Most patients have a history of atrial fibrillation.
- Most are not anticoagulated.
- Prosthetic valves are also risk factors.
- The history will be one of sudden severe pain.
- Risk factors include past heart disease, strokes, smoking, high cholesterol, diabetes, and hypertension.
- The classic six Ps: Pain, pallor, polar (poikilothermia), pulselessness, paresthesias, and paralysis are almost never all present.
- A history of prior trauma or instrumentation makes the possibility of fistulas and aneurysms more likely.

Review Initial Results

- Handheld Doppler: If you are unable to palpate a pulse, a handheld Doppler should be used to confirm the absence of one.
- Blood work:
  - Renal function is helpful prior to angiography to assess for risks of contrast administration.
  - A complete blood count (CBC) will give information about platelets and blood count.
  - Coagulation studies will assess prior anticoagulation efficacy or give baselines prior to instituting heparin therapy.

Risk Stratification: Management Priorities

- Acute arterial embolus
  - High morbidity and mortality.
  - True vascular emergency.
  - Initiate antiplatelet therapy and consider heparin/low-molecular-weight heparin (LMWH) in consultation with vascular surgeon.
  - Confirm embolus with angiogram after consulting vascular surgeon.
- Arterial insufficiency
  - Total occlusion of a previously severely diseased artery with well-developed collateral circulation is often a subclinical event.
  - Patients presenting with decreased but intact pulses and early signs of arterial insufficiency require an urgent evaluation as well.
  - Practical considerations make the oral board test evaluation of arterial insufficiency without acute occlusion an unlikely event.

Definitive Management

- Fluid resuscitation to improve limb perfusion
- Pain control:
  - Morphine sulfate: Use 4-8 mg intravenous (IV) q10min until pain is gone.
- Antiplatelet therapy (aspirin [ASA])

DON'T FORGET

Having a second limb to compare examination findings makes for an easy diagnosis.

DON'T FORGET

The classic six Ps are pain, pallor, polar (cold), pulselessness, paresthesias, and paralysis.

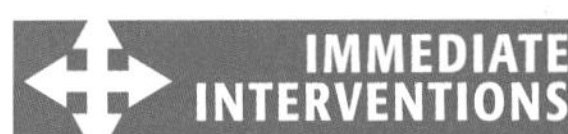
IMMEDIATE INTERVENTIONS

- Handheld Doppler
- 18-gauge IV and heplock
- Send blood for CBC, electrolytes, PT/ PTT/ INR
- ECG

- Anticoagulation therapy:
  - Unfractionated heparin (only in consultation with vascular surgeon associated with possible angiogram). Load with 60 U/kg, then 12 U/kg drip.
  - LMWH: Enoxaparin 1 mg/kg subcutaneous (SQ) q12h if renal function is not impaired.
- Reperfusion
  - Consult vascular surgeon immediately.
  - Possible angiogram for surgical planning.

Disposition

- Admit to intensive care unit (ICU) for postoperative care.

DEEP VENOUS THROMBOSIS

Additional History and Physical Examination Findings

- Risk factors include hereditary hypercoaguable states, pregnancy, immobilization (casts, illness, and long travel), malignancy, trauma, indwelling vascular catheter, or recent surgical/intravascular procedure.
- Physical examination findings include pain, warmth, redness, swelling, and tenderness but are rarely all present.
- Rule out systemic symptoms of chest pain or shortness of breath which would make pulmonary embolus a possibility.

Review Initial Results

- Vital signs
  - Confirm normal O_2 saturation and heart rate as to help rule out possibility of pulmonary embolus.

Risk Stratification: Management Priorities

- If the diagnosis is in question and an immediate duplex ultrasound cannot be obtained, treatment for the possibility of cellulitis can be considered as well as prophylactic anticoagulation if there are no contraindications.

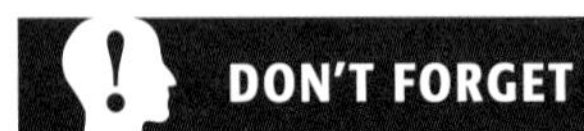

Absence of physical examination findings with a history of appropriate symptoms does not rule out DVT.

Definitive Management

- Duplex ultrasound is the diagnostic test of choice to rule in or out the presence of DVT (Figs. 15-1 and 15-2).
- Venography, long considered the gold standard, has fallen out of favor because of its invasive nature and comparable results on duplex ultrasound.
- Anticoagulation therapy:
  - Unfractionated heparin (only in consultation with vascular surgeon associated with possible angiogram).
    - Load with 60 U/kg, then 12 U/kg drip.
  - LMWH.
    - Enoxaparin 1 mg/kg SQ q12h, only if the patient has no preexisting renal impairment.

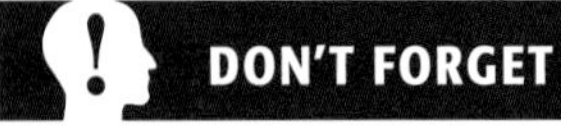

Risk Factors for DVT:

- Tenderness
- Paralysis/bed-ridden
- Recent surgery
- Cancer
- Leg swelling
- Recent travel
- Priory history of PE/DVT

Disposition

- Although outpatient management in stable patients is becoming more routine, admission is still an acceptable plan (especially at ABEM General).

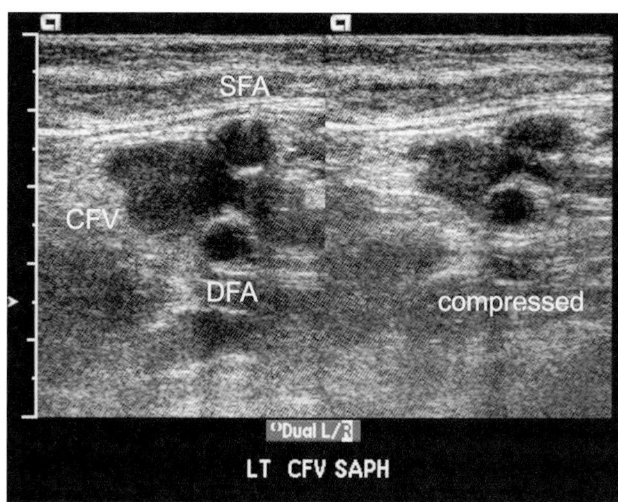

Figure 15-1. Split screen image of the left common femoral vein (CFV) near saphenous junction. The superficial and deep branches of the femoral artery are labeled (DFA, SFA). The CFV contains echoes that represent clot, and does not fully collapse with compression, as seen on the right side of the image. (*Reproduced with permission from Ma OJ, Mateer JR, Blaivas M.* Emergency Ultrasound. *2nd ed. New York, NY: McGraw-Hill; 2008.*)

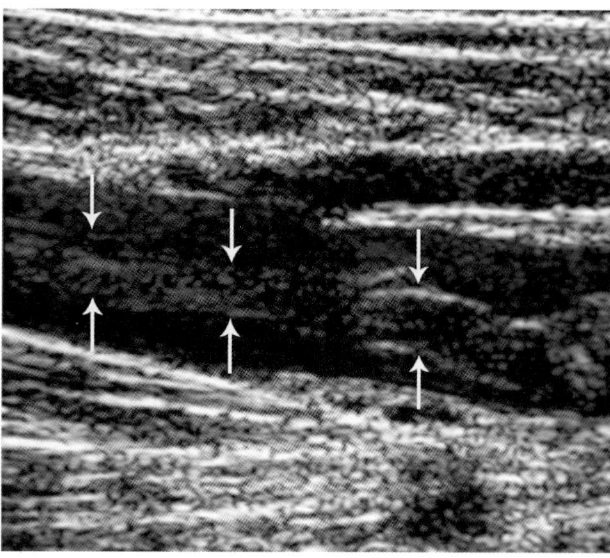

Figure 15-2. Arrows show a freely floating thrombus in the femoral vein. In this portion of the image, the clot does not come in contact with the anterior or posterior wall of the vein. (*Reproduced with permission from Ma OJ, Mateer JR, Blaivas M.* Emergency Ultrasound. *2nd ed. New York, NY: McGraw-Hill; 2008.*)

SEPTIC JOINT

Additional History and Physical Examination Findings

- Patient's complaint will be that of joint pain as opposed to extremity pain.
- History of sexual activity is important in teenagers and young adults.
- The pain is classically severe, exacerbated by any movement of the involved joint.
- The joint is usually warm, red, and tender, has limited range of motion, and has evidence of a joint effusion.

Risk Stratification: Management Priorities

- The most useful tool in diagnosis of a joint disorder is synovial fluid analysis.
- Normal synovial fluid
  - Clarity: Transparent
  - Color: Clear
  - White blood cells (WBC): <200/mm^3
  - Polymorphonuclear leukocytes (PMNs): <25%
  - Culture: Negative
  - Crystals: Negative
- Noninflammatory synovial fluid
  - Clarity: Transparent
  - Color: Yellow
  - WBC: <200-2000/mm^3
  - PMNs: <25%
  - Culture: Negative
  - Crystals: Negative
  - Differential diagnosis (DDx): Osteoarthritis (OA), trauma

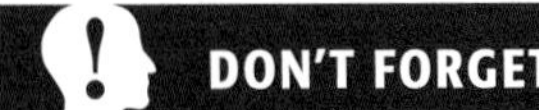

DON'T FORGET

The absence of constitutional symptoms (fevers, etc) should not preclude the diagnosis of septic joint.

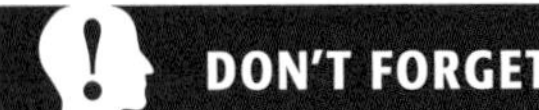

DON'T FORGET

In reality, there is considerable overlap in synovial fluid findings between the various types of arthritis and clinical consideration is warranted.

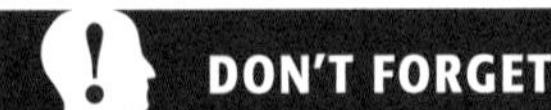

DON'T FORGET

Kanavel signs: Finger held in passive flexion, sausage digit, tenderness along flexor sheath, pain with passive extension. Flexor tenosynovitis is a surgical emergency.

- Inflammatory synovial fluid
  - Clarity: Cloudy
  - Color: Yellow
  - WBC: <200-50,000/mm^3
  - PMNs: >50%
  - Culture: Negative
  - Crystals: Possible
  - DDx: Gout, pseudogout, rheumatoid arthritis (RA), Lyme, lupus
- Septic synovial fluid
  - Clarity: Cloudy
  - Color: Yellow
  - WBC: >50,000/mm^3
  - PMNs: >50%
  - Culture: >50% positive
  - Crystals: None
  - DDx: Septic or gonococcal arthritis
- In small joints where arthrocentesis is difficult, other useful tests include erythrocyte sedimentation rate (ESR), C-reactive protein (CRP), and CBC with differential, or use an ultrasound for guided aspiration.
- If the involved extremity is the finger, look for the possibility of flexor tenosynovitis.
  - Clinical diagnosis based on the four Kanavel signs
    - Finger held in passive flexion
    - Sausage-like swelling of the digit
    - Tenderness along the flexor sheath
    - Pain with passive extension of affected finger

Definitive Management

- Arthrocentesis is the procedure of choice to aid in diagnosis.
- If septic arthritis, parenteral antibiotics and OR washout are the treatments of choice.
- Consult with an orthopedic surgeon for the possibility of arthroscopy or open surgical drainage.
- If flexor tenosynovitis is considered,
  - Consult hand surgeon.
  - Immobilize and elevate extremity.
  - Parenteral antibiotics.

Disposition

- After joint aspiration, if septic arthritis cannot be excluded, admission, antibiotics, and orthopedic surgery evaluation should be the course of action.
- If diagnosis or septic joint or flexor tenosynovitis is made, admit.

ACUTE COMPARTMENT SYNDROME

ACS is a condition that develops when increased pressure within a myofascial compartment exceeds perfusion pressure of the tissues within that compartment resulting in ischemia and compromised function of structures within that compartment.

History and Physical Examination Findings

- Patients may have a history of recent trauma or long bone fracture.
- Postsurgical anticoagulation may contribute to this process.
- Chronic exertional compartment syndrome may present as severe pain and taut compartments following exercise. However, it is difficult to diagnose in the emergency department (ED) setting and is unlikely to be on the exam.

- Common presentations include pain in the forearm or lower leg, though it has been described in the thigh, hand, abdomen, thorax, and eye.
- In children, supracondylar fractures are the most common cause.
  - One quarter of ACS results from soft tissue and/or vascular injuries alone, without fracture.
  - The gold standard for diagnosis is measuring the compartment pressure, which is elevated at 30 mm Hg below the diastolic pressure.
  - Pain may develop as pressure approaches 25-30 mm Hg within the compartment (capillary flow is compromised resulting in ischemia).
  - The classic presentation: Pain out of proportion to exam (early finding). Pain with passive stretch (early finding). Paresthesias (late in the course). Pulselessness (very late in the course). Tense compartments to palpation. Diminished sensation. Muscle weakness.
  - Left untreated, ACS can result in paralysis, sensory deficits, mal or nonunion of fractures, or possibly limb amputation.

DON'T FORGET

Having a second limb to compare examination findings makes for an easy diagnosis. ACS can occur in the presence of an open fracture. Open fascia does not entirely decompress the compartment.

DON'T FORGET

The classic six Ps are pain, pallor, polar (cold), pulselessness, paresthesias, and paralysis. Pain out of proportion to exam and pain with passive stretch are the earliest findings in ACS. Maintain a high degree of suspicion.

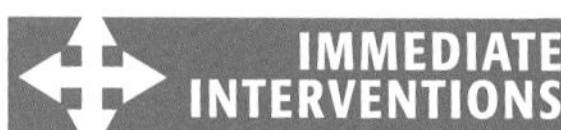

IMMEDIATE INTERVENTIONS

- Handheld Doppler, physical examination, maintain a high degree of suspicion
- 18-gauge IV and heplock.
  IV placement and labs: electrolytes, CPK, CBC, electrolytes, PT/PTT/INR.
  Elevate the affected extremity to the level of the heart
- Contact orthopedic surgery for continued assessment or measure compartment pressures

Review Initial Results

- ACS is diagnosed based on clinical suspicion and physical examination findings. Diagnosis is confirmed by measuring the compartment pressure with a handheld manometer (Stryker device).
- Compartment pressures should ideally be measured prior to fasciotomy. A normal measure may allow for observation instead of immediate compartment decompression.
- Elevating the affected extremity to the level of the heart may help improve symptoms and reduce compartment pressures while optimizing arterial perfusion.
- Most clinicians will not act to decompress the compartment until the pressure reaches 30 mm Hg within the diastolic pressure.
- Lab findings: Creatine phosphokinase (CPK) will likely be elevated. Obtain a basic metabolic panel (BMP) to evaluate for hyperkalemia that can occur with myocyte necrosis. Blood may be present on urine dip (as myoglobinuria).
- If no Stryker device is available, an arterial line set up may be used to measure compartment pressures.

Management Priorities

- Identify early ACS with physical examination findings of pain out of proportion to exam.
- Palpate or Doppler pulses, ask to feel the compartments on examination.
- High morbidity and constitutes a true orthopedic emergency.
- Elevate presenting part to the level of the heart.
- Place IV and draw labs: CPK, electrolytes, consider urinalysis (UA) for blood (myoglobin), coags
- Control pain with morphine 4-8 mg IV q10min until pain is improved.
- Initiate orthopedic consult or consider readying monometer device.

Definitive Management

- Pain control:
  - Morphine sulfate: Use 4-8 mg IV q10min until pain is gone.
- Elevate presenting part to the level of the heart.
- Consult orthopedic surgery or ready handheld manometer.
  - Check all compartments (extremity involved will likely be lower leg), don't forget the deep posterior compartment, which is the one most often missed.
  - Pressure is elevated if >20-30 mm Hg—pain occurs when capillary perfusion pressure is exceeded—Fasciotomy is indicated if the pressure is within 20-30 mm Hg of the diastolic pressure.

Disposition

- Admit to Ortho for serial examinations.
- Fasciotomy followed by admission is the definitive management.

WINNING STRATEGIES

- For the painful extremity, immediate interventions (airway, fluid bolus, ACLS protocols, etc) are rarely needed initially, so take a good history and physical examination (H&P) to ensure a proper diagnosis/treatment.
- The finding of a pulseless or greatly diminished pulse in an extremity requires a quick response to avoid amputation.
- The classic six Ps are pain, pallor, polar, pulselessness, paresthesias, and paralysis.
- Absence of physical examination findings, despite a history of appropriate symptoms, does not rule out DVT.
- Pain out of proportion and pain with passive stretch are the earliest and most sensitive findings in ACS.
- Duplex ultrasound is the diagnostic test of choice to rule in or out the presence of DVT.
- The absence of constitutional symptoms (fevers, etc) should not preclude the diagnosis of septic joint.
- There is considerable overlap in synovial fluid findings between the various types of arthritis, and clinical consideration and conservative management is warranted.
- Kanavel signs of flexor tenosynovitis: Finger held in passive flexion, sausage-like swelling of the digit, tenderness along flexor sheath, pain with passive extension.

THE BOTTOM LINE

- A thorough H&P is paramount to diagnoses and treatment of the painful extremity.
- On exam day, tap all hot joints.
- Admit anyone with suspected compartment syndrome for serial monitoring.

CHAPTER 16

Altered Mental Status: Toxicology Emergencies

Navneet Cheema and James Rhee

INITIAL ASSESSMENT/INTERVENTION

- Vital signs (VS): Make sure to obtain a complete set of vitals including temperature and oxygen saturation.
- Mental status: Agitated, depressed, comatose.
- Signs of trauma: If any question, immobilize cervical spine.
- Coma cocktail: DON'T.
  - **D**exi: Check finger stick glucose or administer parenteral glucose.
  - **O**xygen: Check for hypoxemia or administer oxygen.
  - **N**aloxone: Administer naloxone especially for respiratory depression.
  - **T**hiamine: Administer thiamine 100 mg intravenous (IV) to prevent or treat Wernicke encephalopathy if patient appears malnourished.

INITIAL HISTORY AND PHYSICAL EXAMINATION

- History
  - History of the present illness (HPI): Often times unavailable through the patient; need to establish through other means—family, friends, witnesses, paramedics, nursing home, primary care physician, and medical records.
  - Patient medical history (PMHx): Especially to give hints of possible ingestions or conditions (eg, schizophrenia → lithium overdose, neuroleptic malignant syndrome (NMS); chronic pain syndrome → opioid overdose, tricyclic antidepressant [TCA] overdose, etc).
  - Medications/herbs/supplements/drugs: One of the most important components of the history as this may help make the diagnosis—sometimes takes a little bit of sleuthing—examine medical records, send paramedics back to the scene for clues, and call friends, family, and pharmacy—don't forget about other medications that may be in the house (eg, grandma's calcium channel blocker, dog's TCA, etc).
  - Social history: Work history is especially important as this may lead to source of exposure.
  - Allergies: Medication and food allergies.
- Physical examination
  - VS: Make sure to obtain a complete set of vitals including temperature and oxygen saturation.
  - General: What does the patient look like? Are there any distinct odors detected (eg, ethanol (EtOH), fruity, garlic, bitter almonds)?
  - Head: Any signs of trauma such as hematomas, lacerations, or abrasions?
  - Eyes: Assess pupils for size, symmetry, and reactivity; look for nystagmus; evaluate for papilledema.
  - Cardiovascular: Tachycardic or bradycardic?
  - Respiratory: Any tachypnea or crackles?
  - Abdomen: Bowel sounds? Hemaemesis, melena, or hematochezia? Distended bladder?
  - Extremities: Any rigidity?
  - Neuro: Assess for mental status, seizure activity, muscle tone, and tremor.
  - Skin: Any cyanosis? Hot or cold? Dry or wet? Flushed? Puncture marks or needle tracks?

Additional History and Physical Examination Findings

- In the setting of an ingestion or potential ingestion, the history is frequently unreliable; however, it can be useful if obtained carefully.
- Find out all drugs taken: prescription, over-the-counter (OTC), vitamins, herbs, illicit drugs, and supplements.
- May need to solicit information from family, friends, or paramedics.

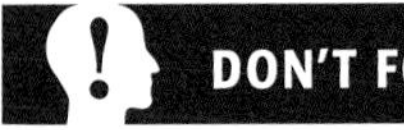

DON'T FORGET

Poisoning and drug overdose (general approach): ABCDEF

- Airway
- Breathing
- Circulation
- Decontamination: Skin, eye, and/or gastric
- Enhanced elimination: Urinary alkalinization, multiple-dose activated charcoal, hemodialysis/perfusion
- Focused therapy: Therapies for specific toxins, antidotes

- Ask about environment patient was found in—presence of pill bottles, drug paraphernalia, or odors.
- Look up medical records, call patient's primary physician and their pharmacy.
- If found in work environment, then contact people at the work site for relevant information.
- Physical examination findings may yield important diagnostic clues.
- Vitals signs
  - Bradycardia (PACED)
    - **P**ropranolol (or other beta-blockers), poppies (opiates)
    - **A**nticholinesterase drugs
    - **C**lonidine, calcium channel blockers
    - **E**thanol (or other alcohols)
    - **D**igoxin
  - Tachycardia (FAST)
    - **F**ree base or other forms of cocaine
    - **A**nticholinergics, antihistamines
    - **S**ympathomimetics (cocaine, amphetamines), solvent abuse
    - **T**heophylline
  - Hypothermia (COOLS)
    - **C**arbon monoxide (CO)
    - **O**piates
    - **O**ral hypoglycemics, insulin
    - **L**iquor
    - **S**edative-hypnotics
  - Hyperthermia (NASA)
    - NMS, nicotine
    - **A**ntihistamines
    - **S**alicylates, sympathomimetics
    - **A**nticholinergics, antidepressants
  - Hypotension (CRASH)
    - **C**lonidine, calcium channel blockers
    - **R**eserpine or other antihypertensive agents
    - **A**ntidepressants, aminophylline
    - **S**edative-hypnotics
    - **H**eroin or other opiates
  - Hypertension (CT SCAN)
    - **C**ocaine
    - **T**hyroid supplements
    - **S**ympathomimetics
    - **C**affeine
    - **A**nticholinergics
    - **N**icotine
  - Rapid respiration (PANT)
    - **P**hencylidine, paraquat, pneumonitis (chemical)
    - **A**spirin and other salicylates
    - **N**oncardiogenic pulmonary edema
    - **T**oxin-induced metabolic acidosis
  - Slow respiration (SLOW)
    - **S**edative-hypnotics
    - **L**iquor
    - **O**piates
    - **W**eed (marijuana)
- Pupils
  - Miosis (COPS)
    - **C**holinergics, clonidine
    - **O**piates, organophosphates

    - **P**henothiazines, pilocarpine
    - **S**edative-hypnotics
  - Mydriasis (SAW)
    - **S**ympathomimetics
    - **A**nticholinergics, antihistamines, antidepressants
    - **W**ithdrawal (alcohol, opiate, sedative-hypnotic)
- Skin
  - Diaphoretic (SOAP)
    - **S**ympathomimetics
    - **O**rganophosphates
    - **A**spirin and other salicylates
    - **P**hencyclidine
  - Dry skin
    - Antihistamines
    - Anticholinergics
  - Bullae
    - Barbituates and other sedative-hypnotics
    - CO
  - Acneiform rash
    - Bromides
    - Chlorinated aromatic hydrocarbons
  - Flushed or red appearance
    - Anticholinergics
    - Boric acid
    - CO
    - Cyanide
  - Cyanosis
    - Ergotamine
    - Nitrates
    - Nitrites
    - Aniline dyes
    - Phenazopyridine
    - Dapsone
    - Any agent causing hypoxemia, hypotension, or methemoglobinemia
- Neurologic
  - Seizures (OTIS CAMPBELL)
    - **O**rganophosphates
    - **T**CAs
    - **I**soniazid, insulin
    - **S**ympathomimetics
    - **C**amphor
    - **A**nticholinergics
    - **M**ethylxanthines (theophylline, caffeine)
    - **P**hencyclidine
    - **B**enzodiazepine withdrawal, botanicals (water hemlock)
    - **E**tOH-related
    - **L**ithium, lidocaine
    - **L**ead, lindane
- Odors: Ask the examiner about any unusual scents.
  - Bitter almonds → cyanide
  - Wild carrots → cicutoxin (water hemlock)
  - Fruity → isopropanol, diabetic ketoacidosis (DKA)
  - Garlic → organophosphates, arsenic, selenium
  - Gasoline → petroleum distillates
  - Mothballs → camphor, naphthalene
  - Pears → chloral hydrate
  - Oil of wintergreen → methyl salicylate

Table 16-1. Physical Signs and Symptoms of the Most Common Toxidromes

Toxidrome	BP	HR	RR	Temperature	Mental Status	Pupil Size	Peristalsis	Diaphoresis	Other
Sympathomimetic	↑	↑	↑	↑	Altered	↑	↑	↑	Flushed skin
Anticholinergic	↕	↑	↕	↑	Altered	↑	↓	↓	Dry skin, urinary retention
Cholinergic	↕	↓	↕	nl	Altered	↓	↑	↑	DUMBELS
Opioid	↓	↓	↓	nl	Altered	↓	↓	↓	
Opioid withdrawal	↑	↑	nl	nl	Normal	↑	↑	↑	N/V, rhinorrhea, piloerection
Sedative-hypnotic	↓	↓	↓	↓	Altered	↕	↓	↓	
Alcohol withdrawal	↑	↑	↑	↑	Altered	↑	nl	↑	

- Rotten eggs → sulfur dioxide, hydrogen sulfide
- Peanut butter → vacor (rodenticide)

- Toxidromes: A collection of symptoms associated with certain classes of poisons. Table 16-1 summarizes the classic toxidromes.
- Cholinergic
  - Symptoms are caused by excessive stimulation of muscarinic and nicotinic acetylcholine receptors.
    - Muscarinic effects (easily remembered by the mnemonic DUMBELS): Defecation, urination, miosis, bronchorrhea, bronchospasm, bradycardia, emesis, lacrimation, and salivation
    - Nicotinic effects: Fasciculations, seizures, altered mental status
  - Commonly seen by agents which cause cholinesterase inhibition and subsequent accumulation of acetylcholine
    - Pesticides including organophosphates insecticides and carbamates
    - Therapeutic cholinesterase inhibitors such as physostigmine, pyridostigmine, neostigmine, and edrophonium
    - Nerve agents such as sarin, VX, soman, and tabun
- Anticholinergic
  - Symptoms are caused by agents that block acetylcholine at muscarinic receptors.
  - Physical findings include elevated temperature, delirium, mumbling speech, tachycardia, dry and flushed skin, dry mucous membranes, urinary retention, decreased or absent bowel sounds, mydriasis (Fig. 16-1), and blurred vision. Seizures and coma may also occur.
  - A simple mnemonic, "hot as a hare, blind as a bat, dry as a bone, red as a beet, mad as a hatter" describes many of the features of the anticholinergic toxidrome.
  - Examples of agents which block acetylcholine at muscarinic receptors:
    - Atropine
    - Antihistamines
    - Antiparkinson medications such as benztropine and trihexyphenidyl
    - Topical mydriatics
    - Antispasmodics such as Donnatal (belladonna alkaloids/phenobarbital and dicyclomine).
    - Muscle relaxants such as cyclobenzaprine
    - Belladonna alkaloids such as scopolamine and hyoscyamine
    - Cyclic antidepressants also cause anticholinergic symptoms.
    - Plants that contain belladonna alkaloids include jimson weed, deadly nightshade, and henbane.

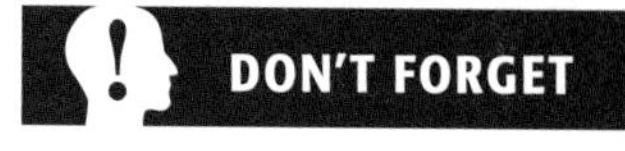

Cholinergic toxidrome = DUMBELS

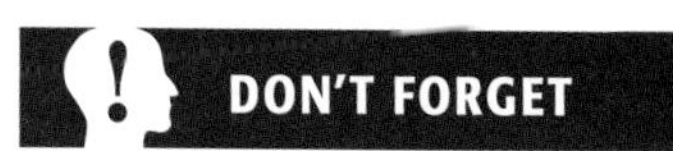

Anticholinergic toxidrome = Hot as a hare, blind as a bat, dry as a bone, red as a beet, mad as a hatter

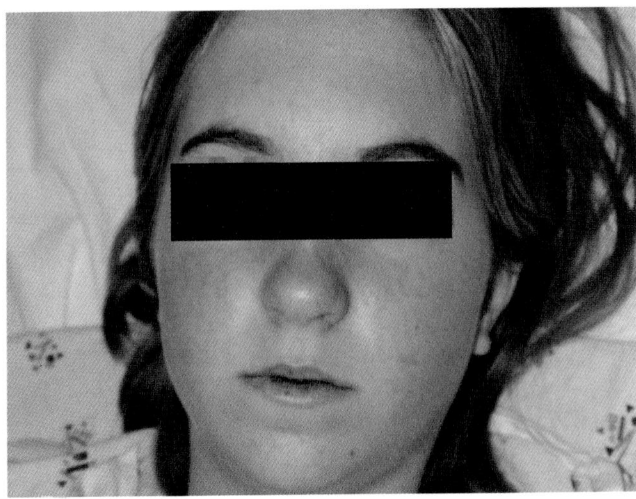

Figure 16-1. Anticholinergic mydriasis; mydriasis and flushing are some of the characteristic findings of anticholinergic toxidrome. (*Reproduced with permission from Knoop KJ, Stack LB, Storrow AB.* Atlas of Emergency Medicine. *2nd ed. New York, NY: McGraw-Hill; 2002.*)

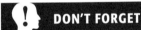

- Sympathomimetic
  - Physical examination findings include hypertension, diaphoresis, tachycardia, tachypnea, hyperthermia, and mydriasis. Restlessness, agitation, excessive speech, tremors, and insomnia also occur. Severe cases are associated with dysrhythmias and seizures.
  - This symptom complex may be difficult to distinguish from the anticholinergic toxidrome. Whereas sweating and normal to hyperactive bowel sounds are associated with sympathomimetic overdose, the anticholinergic toxidrome is manifested by dry skin and diminished bowel sounds.
  - Drugs or toxins that can give you a sympathomimetic picture include
    - Sympathetic agonists such as cocaine and amphetamine.
    - Decongestants such as phenylpropanolamine, ephedrine, and pseudoephedrine.
    - Methylxanthines such as theophylline and caffeine may cause many of these findings by enhancing catecholamine release.
    - Beta-2 adrenergic receptor agonists.
    - Methylphenidate.
    - *Ephedra* species such as ma huang.

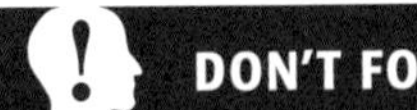

DON'T FORGET

Keys to differentiating a sympathomimetic from and anticholinergic toxidrome

- Sympathomimetic: Wet skin, hyperactive bowel sounds
- Anticholinergic: Dry skin, diminished bowel sounds, urinary retention

- Opioid
  - The classic triad of opioid intoxication is
    - Mental status depression
    - Respiratory depression
    - Pinpoint pupils
  - Other physical examination findings may include bradycardia, hypotension (rare), hypothermia, hyporeflexia, and needle marks.
  - Opioids commonly associated with this toxidrome include
    - Morphine.
    - Heroin.
    - Fentanyl and its analogues.
    - Oxycodone.

        - Hydromorphone.
        - Propoxyphene.
    - Meperidine, pentazocine, and dextromethorphan may cause central nervous system (CNS) and respiratory depression but are often associated with dilated pupils.
    - Central alpha-2 receptor agonists such as clonidine and imidazoline derivatives that act on the locus ceruleus of the CNS cause many of these same symptoms in the overdose setting.
- Sedative-hypnotic
    - Sedative-hypnotic overdoses are associated with hypotension, bradypnea, hypothermia, mental status depression, slurred speech, ataxia, and hyporeflexia.
    - Bullous skin lesions have been reported in some patients with sedative-hypnotic overdoses.
    - Paradoxical excitement is seen with some of the sedative-hypnotics, especially in very young and elderly patients.
    - The sedative-hypnotics include
        - Barbiturates.
        - Benzodiazepines.
        - Chloral hydrate.
        - Ethchlorvynol.
        - Zolpidem.
    - Of course, EtOH intoxication may also present with many of these symptoms.
    - Ingestion of neuroleptics, cyclic antidepressants, and skeletal muscle relaxants may also cause significant sedation.

Review Initial Results

- Basic metabolic panel (BMP): Check for anion gap.
    - Calculate
        - $Na - (Cl + HCO_3) = $ Anion gap
    - Normal anion gap = 8-12 mEq/L.
    - Causes of high anion gap acidosis (ACAT MUDPILE).
        - **A**lcoholic ketoacidosis
        - **C**yanide, CO
        - **A**spirin and other salicylates
        - **T**oluene
        - **M**ethanol, metformin
        - **U**remia
        - **D**KA
        - **P**araldehyde, phenformin
        - **I**ron, isoniazid
        - **L**actic acidosis
        - **E**thylene glycol
    - Serum osmolality: Compare against the calculated one for presence of an osmolal gap.
    - Calculate serum osmolarity.
        - 2(Na) + BUN/2.8 + Glu/18 + EtOH/4.6
    - Osmolal gap
        - Serum osmolality minus calculated serum osmolarity
        - Normal is a value <10 mOsm/L.
        - Note that an increased osmolal gap may be helpful, but does not absolutely exclude the presence of an osmotically active substance.
    - Causes of high osmolal gap (MAD PIE)
        - **M**ethanol
        - **A**cetone

        - **D**iuretics (mannitol)
        - **P**ropylene glycol
        - **I**sopropanol
        - **E**thylene glycol
- Chest x-ray (CXR).
    - Noncardiogenic pulmonary edema (MOPS)
        - **M**eprobamate, methadone
        - **O**piates, organophosphates
        - **P**henobarbital, propoxyphene, phenothiazines
        - **S**alicylates, smoke inhalation, solvents
    - Cardiogenic pulmonary edema
        - Beta-blockers
        - Calcium channel blockers
        - Type 1a antiarrythmics
- Kidney, ureter, and bladder (KUB).
    - Certain agents may be visible on abdominal films (CHIPES).
        - **C**hloral hydrate
        - **H**eavy metals
        - **I**ron
        - **P**ackers
        - **E**nteric-coated or sustained-release
        - **S**alicylates
- Tox screen
    - Usually only tests for common drugs of abuse
    - Rarely, if ever, affects acute management of patient

Risk Stratification: Management Priorities

- Risk is generally based on the specific toxin, the quantity of toxin, and the route of toxin exposure.
    - For example, drinking 10 mL of oil of wintergreen (98% methyl salicylate) carries toxicity >10 mL of children's ibuprofen (100 mg/5 mL).
- It is important to note that some overdoses may present in delayed fashion and may require a prolonged period of monitoring, prophylactic treatment, and/or confirmatory testing.
    - Sustained-release preparations
    - Acetaminophen
    - Toxic alcohols
    - Brodifacoum (anticoagulant found in rat poison)
    - Certain mushrooms
    - Iron
    - Paraquat

Definitive Management

- Management of any unknown poisoning should begin with the basic supportive measures.
- Decontamination
    - Skin and eye decontamination
        - In patients with dermal exposures, all clothing should be removed and skin thoroughly irrigated.
        - Emergency care providers should wear gloves and protect themselves from dermal absorption.
        - Ocular exposures to acids and alkali should be irrigated with copious amounts of normal saline solution until a neutral pH is achieved.

- Gastric decontamination
  - Activated charcoal
    - It has become the first-line agent for patients who have ingested a potentially toxic amount of drug.
    - It binds to a wide variety of toxins and decreases subsequent absorption by the gastrointestinal (GI) tract.
    - Efficacy decreases with time—best if administered within 1 hour of ingestion.
  - Dose
    - Administer by mouth or nasogastric (NG) tube.
    - Conventional dose is 1 g/kg. In an adult, usually 75-100 g.
    - Ideally, charcoal to toxin ratio should be at least 10:1.
  - Contraindications
    - Unprotected airway
    - Hydrocarbon ingestion (as greatest toxicity from this ingestion is aspiration)
    - Caustic ingestion
    - Nonintact (anatomically) GI tract
  - Activated charcoal doesn't bind well to certain substances (PHAILS).
    - **P**esticides
    - **H**eavy metals
    - **A**cids/alkalis/alcohols
    - **I**ron
    - **L**ithium
    - **S**olvents
- Syrup of Ipecac
  - Used to be used to induce emesis, and was once the preferred technique for gastric emptying.
  - Should NOT be used on examination day.
- Cathartics
  - Most common types are osmotic cathartics (Sorbitol) and saline (magnesium citrate, magnesium sulfate, and sodium sulfate).
  - Intended to decrease absorption by accelerating expulsion through the GI tract.
  - However, no research data to support cathartic use.
  - On examination day, would consider administering with the first dose of activated charcoal only.
  - Do NOT administer multiple doses of cathartic.
  - Contraindications
    - Absent bowel sounds, recent abdominal trauma, recent bowel surgery, obstruction or perforation.
    - Corrosive ingestion.
    - Volume depletion, hypotension, or electrolyte imbalance.
    - Magnesium-containing cathartics should not be used in renal failure, renal insufficiency, or heart block.
    - Very young (<1 year) or very old.
- Gastric lavage
  - Not as commonly employed anymore because of lack of evidence of efficacy and the availability of activated charcoal.
  - Indications
    - Ingestion of a potentially life-threatening amount of poison taken within the last 60 minutes.
- Contraindications
  - Depressed level of consciousness
  - Corrosive ingestions

- Hydrocarbon ingestions
- Patients at risk of GI hemorrhage or perforation (eg, recent surgery, history of varices, etc)
- Factors that strengthen the role for gastric lavage
  - Life-threatening overdose
  - Doesn't bind to activated charcoal—remember "PHAILS"
  - No effective antidote
  - Ingestion within 1 hour
  - Example: A 40-year male with no medical problems presents 30 minutes after ingesting 65 mg of colchicine (this lethal ingestion has no effective antidote).
- Procedure
  - Airway protected: Patient is either intubated or awake, alert, and cooperative.
  - Position: Left lateral decubitus and in Trendelenburg.
  - For adults, insert 36-40 French orogastric or nasogastric tube and lavage with 200 mL aliquots of saline until clear.
- Whole bowel irrigation (WBI)
  - Potential to reduce drug absorption by rapidly cleansing the entire GI tract.
  - Indications
    - Sustained-release or enteric coated drugs (eg, sustained-release calcium channel blockers, illicit drug packets)
    - Drugs not well absorbed by charcoal (eg, arsenic, iron, lithium)
  - Contraindications
    - Bowel perforation
    - Bowel obstruction
    - GI hemorrhage
    - Ileus
    - Unprotected airway
    - Hemodynamic instability
    - Intractable vomiting
  - Procedure
    - NG tube placement
    - Instillation of a polyethylene glycol solution (eg, GoLYTELY at 1.5-2 L/h in adolescents/adults, 1 L/h in 6-12 years olds, 500 mL/h in 9 months-6 years olds.
- Enhanced elimination
  - Urinary alkalinization
    - Alteration of urine pH enhances elimination of certain drugs by altering drug ionization and "ion-trapping" the toxin in the urine by preventing reabsorption into the plasma compartment.
    - Helpful for enhancing elimination of weak acids such as salicylates, phenobarbital, and chlorpropamide.
    - Procedure
      - Mix three 50-mL amps containing 50-mEq sodium bicarbonate into 1 L D5W (*not 0.9% NaCl*). Run at 150-250 mL/h (2-3 mL/kg/h).
      - Start a KCl-rider with 40-mEq potassium chloride when using a bicarbonate drip as soon as it is known that the patient is not hyperkalemic. If the patient is hypokalemic, alkalinization of urine is not possible.
    - Contraindications
      - Patients with renal dysfunction.
      - When the necessary fluid volumes may compromise fluid and respiratory functions.
- Multiple-dose charcoal
  - Thought to enhance elimination by interrupting enteroenteric, enterohepatic, or enterogastric circulation of select drugs (ABCDQ).

DON'T FORGET

Don't forget! Do not use repeated doses of cathartics with repeated doses of activated charcoal—especially the young and old who may develop electrolyte derangements and *die*.

- **A**minophylline or theophylline
- **B**arbiturates (specifically phenobarbital)
- **C**arbamazepine
- **D**apsone
- **Q**uinine

- Contraindications
  - Unprotected airway
  - Vomiting
  - Decreased bowel sounds or signs of bowel obstruction
  - Combative patient
  - Corrosive ingestion
  - Hydrocarbon ingestion
  - WBI
- Procedure
  - Adult
    - Initial dose: 1 g/kg aqueous charcoal (may consider use of a cathartic such as magnesium citrate or 1 g/kg of Sorbitol with the first dose of charcoal).
    - Repeat doses: 25-50 g of aqueous charcoal q2-4h (do not use a cathartic, such as Sorbitol, with repeat doses).
  - Child
    - Initial dose: 1 g/kg aqueous charcoal (may consider use of a cathartic, such as magnesium citrate or 1 g/kg of Sorbitol, with the first dose of charcoal).
    - Repeat doses: 0.5 g/kg of aqueous charcoal q2-4h (do not use a cathartic, such as Sorbitol, with repeat doses).
    - The total dose of activated charcoal is determined by consideration of agents ingested, serum concentration, and clinical status of the patient.
- Hemodialysis
  - Extracorporeal measure to enhance elimination of toxic substance.
  - Toxins that are more amenable to removal by hemodialysis have certain characteristics:
    - Low protein binding
    - Small volume of distribution
    - Water solubility
    - Low molecular weight
  - Common toxins that are accessible to hemodialysis (I STUMBLE).
    - **I**sopropanol
    - **S**alicylates
    - **T**heophylline
    - **U**remia
    - **M**ethanol
    - **B**arbituates
    - **L**ithium
    - **E**thylene glycol
  - In general, consult a nephrologist immediately if patient is significantly symptomatic and is suspected to have taken a toxin readily accessible by hemodialysis.
- Hemoperfusion
  - An extracoporeal measure that may be slightly more effective at removing toxins that readily bind to charcoal.
    - Theophylline
    - Barbiturates
    - Carbamazepine
  - However, lack of availability should not keep a patient from undergoing hemodialysis.

Table 16-2. Poisonous Agents and Their Antidotes

Antidote	Toxin
N-acetylcysteine	Acetaminophen and possibly carbon tetrachloride
Ethanol/fomepizole	Methanol/ethylene glycol
Flumazenil	Benzodiazepines
Oxygen/HBO	Carbon monoxide
Naloxone/nalmefene	Opioids
Physostigmine	Anticholinergics
Atropine/pralidoxime	Organophosphates
Methylene blue	Methemoglobinemia
Nitrites and thiosulfate	Cyanide
Deferoxamine	Iron
BAL (chelating agent)	Arsenic/lead
Succimer (chelating agent)	Lead/mercury/arsenic
Digitalis-specific Fab fragments	Digoxin
Crotolid-specific Fab fragments	Crotalid envenomations
Glucagon	Beta-blockers
Sodium bicarbonate	TCAs and other sodium channel blockers
Calcium/insulin/dextrose	Calcium-channel antagoni

- Antidotes: see Table 16-2.
- Geared toward specific toxins.
- Need to identify the toxin, either by history and examination or by laboratory evaluation.

Complications

- Seizures
  - Benzodiazepines should be the first-line treatment for the management of toxin-related seizures.
  - Barbiturates should be used next.
  - Phenytoin and fosphenytoin are generally not indicated as these may in fact decrease the seizure threshold for some toxins (eg, theophylline).
  - Consider administration of pyridoxine if seizures are intractable and patient may have ingested isoniazid.
- Hypotension
  - Fluid resuscitation with isotonic crystalloid
  - Pressors as needed
    - Note that dopamine may be ineffective in some patients with depleted neuronal stores of catecholamine (eg, disulfiram, TCA overdose, etc).
    - Norepinephrine may be more effective.

- Consider specific antidotes.
  - Sodium bicarbonate for tricyclic or other sodium channel blocking drug overdose if QRS is wide
  - Glucagon for beta-blocker overdose
  - Calcium and euglycemic hyperinsulinemia for calcium antagonist overdose
  - Digitalis-specific Fab fragments (antigen-binding fragments) for digoxin or other cardiac glycoside overdose
- Electrocardiogram (ECG) abnormailities
  - QRS widening
    - May be indicative of sodium channel blockade from TCAs or another agent.
    - Treat with sodium bicarbonate to overcome the blockade.

Disposition

- Any patient with a change in mental status from poisoning or overdose should be admitted to the intensive care unit (ICU).
- Any patient who intentionally overdosed on a substance mandates psychiatric consultation or inpatient psychiatric admission (provided that the patient has been medically cleared).

ACETAMINOPHEN

Additional History and Physical Examination Findings

- May be part of a mixed ingestion—especially since many OTC cold preparations have acetaminophen (APAP) as a component.
- Important to establish time of ingestion for acute overdose as this will guide treatment.
- Toxic dose is 140 mg/kg (7-10 g) for adults and 200 mg/kg for children.
- Classically, in acute overdoses, the patient will go through four phases of acetaminophen toxicity.
  - Phase 1: First 24 hours
    - May be asymptomatic
    - Usually GI complaints—nausea, vomiting, mild abdominal pain, loss of appetite, generalized malaise
  - Phase 2: 24-48 hours
    - Asymptomatic or with abdominal pain
    - Transaminases, coagulation tests, bilirubin start to rise
  - Phase 3: 72-124 hours
    - Hepatic necrosis
    - Jaundice
    - Encephalopathy
    - Renal failure
    - Death
  - Phase 4: 5-14 days
    - Recovery (if patient did not die or get liver transplant)

Review Initial Results

- Acetaminophen level
  - Cannot use levels before 4 hours to determine toxicity.
  - Toxic level at 4 hours is 150 mg/mL or greater.
  - Use Rumack-Matthew nomogram (Fig. 16-2) to identify need for treatment if the level obtained is past 4 hours.
    - Note that the nomogram cannot be used after 24 hours and is not valid for chronic toxicity.

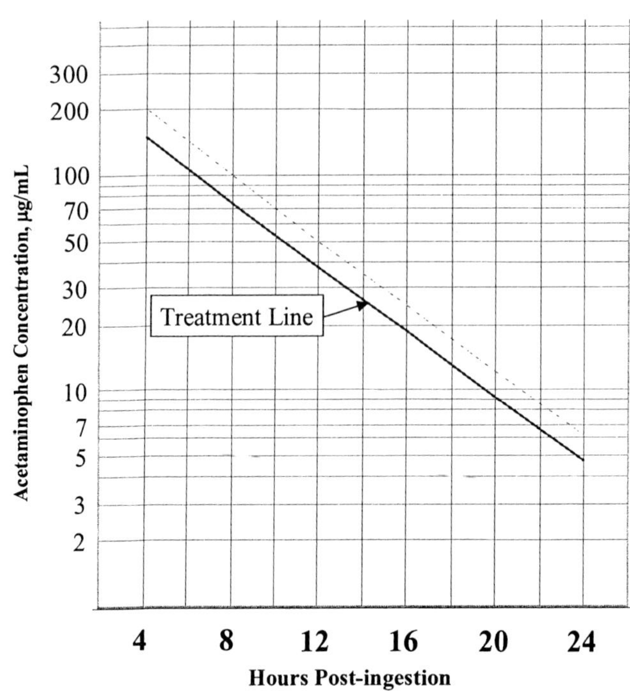

Figure 16-2. Rumack Matthew nomogram for acetaminophen poisoning. (*Reproduced with permission from Tintinalli JE, Kelen GD, Stapczynski JS, et al.* Emergency Medicine: A Comprehensive Study Guide. *6th ed. New York, NY: McGraw-Hill; 2004.*)

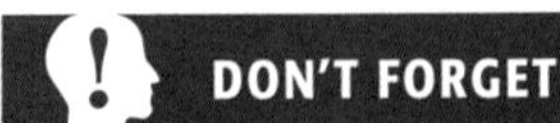

- AST and ALT in the thousands should make you think of a toxic cause—namely APAP.
- Survival approaches 100% if NAC is given within 8 hours for an acute APAP ingestion.
- Every APAP overdose gets NAC on examination day.

- Coagulation studies
  - Coagulopathy may be apparent in late presenters or from repeated supratherapeutic ingestion.
- Liver function tests
  - Expect to start seeing elevation of transaminases and bilirubins 24 hours after exposure.
- Metabolic panel and arterial blood gas (ABG)
  - Acetaminophen toxicity can cause renal failure as well.
  - Serum pH
  - Acidemia portends poor prognosis.

Risk Stratification: Management Priorities

- King's College Criteria predicts the need for potential liver transplant.
  - Acidosis (pH<7.30 after adequate fluid resuscitation)
  - Coagulopathy INR>6.5
  - Creatinine >3.4 mg/dL
  - Grade III/IV hepatic encephalopathy

Definitive Management

- Activated charcoal if patient presents early after ingestion
- N-acetylcysteine (NAC)
  - Replenishes glutathione stores.
  - Optimal efficacy if given within 8 hours.
  - If patient presents 8 hours after ingestion, administer NAC right away without waiting for a level.

  - 140 mg/kg PO for the first dose.
  - May need to administer antiemetics.
  - Consider NG tube if patient is still unable to tolerate drinking the NAC.
  - 70 mg/kg PO q4h × 17 doses after the initial loading dose.
- Liver transplant: Definitive treatment for those who have acetaminophen-induced fulminant liver failure.

Complications

- Coagulopathy
  - Replenish coagulation factors with fresh frozen plasma (FFP).
  - Resuscitate with PRBCs and isotonic crystalloid for hemorrhage.
- Renal failure
  - Correct electrolyte derangement.
  - May need hemodialysis.

Disposition

- Patients with toxic acetaminophen levels need to be admitted for the whole course of NAC.
- Patients who are symptomatic from delayed acetaminophen ingestion or from coingestions need to be monitored in an ICU setting.
- If patient meets King's College Criteria, then the patient needs to be monitored in an ICU setting—ideally at a transplant center.

SALICYLATES

Additional History and Physical Examination Findings

- Exposure to salicylate-containing products
  - Remember that many cold preparations may contain aspirin.
  - BenGay (methyl salicylate), Pepto-Bismol (bismuth subsalicylate), and others also contain salicylate compounds.
- Signs and symptoms
  - Tinnitus: Hear any ringing?
  - Tachypnea/hyperpnea
  - Diaphoresis
  - Fever
  - Altered mental status
  - Seizures

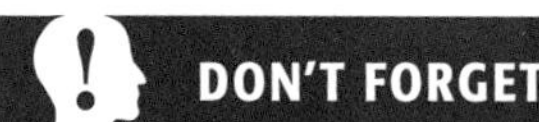

- Anyone with tinnitus: Think salicylates.
- Classic acid-base disturbance: Primary respiratory alkalosis with a high-anion-gap metabolic acidosis

Review Initial Results

- ABG
  - Respiratory alkalosis from direct stimulation of medulla.
  - Metabolic acidosis caused by uncoupling of oxidative phosphorylation and subsequent lactic acidosis.
  - Metabolic alkalosis from vomiting, tachypnea, and diaphoresis leading to volume contraction.
- BMP
  - Will reveal an anion gap.
- Aspirin (ASA) level
- CXR
  - Evaluate for noncardiogenic pulmonary edema.

Risk Stratification: Management Priorities

- ASA level
  - In acute ingestions levels, ASA level of 90-100 mg/dL is indicative of very serious salicylate toxicity.

- Noncardiogenic pulmonary edema
  - Indicates serious salicylate toxicity.
- Altered mental status or seizures
  - Also correlates with severe salicylate toxicity.

Definitive Management

- Activated charcoal
  - May need to give multiple doses to achieve maximal binding capacity.
    - Remember ideal ratio of charcoal to toxin is 10:1.
- Urinary alkalinization
  - Salicylates are weak acids, so are prime candidates for this method of enhanced elimination.
- Hemodialysis
  - Indications
    - Altered mental status
    - Seizure
    - Noncardiogenic pulmonary edema
    - Aspirin level >100 mg/dL in acute ingestions
    - Aspirin level >60 mg/dL in chronic ingestions

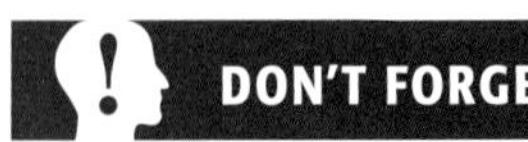

Don't overload the patient with sodium when alkalinizing the urine, ie, don't mix sodium bicarbonate in normal saline.

Further Reassessment

- Urine or serum pH should be checked every 2 hours while undergoing urinary alkalinization to monitor adequacy of the treatment—pH should be ~7.5.
- Potassium should be checked every 2 hours and replenished as needed.
- ASA level should be checked every 2 hours.
  - Aspirin absorption can be somewhat erratic as bezoars may form.
  - Need to follow serial ASA levels to monitor absorption.

Complications

- Mechanical ventilation
  - If patient needs subsequent mechanical ventilation, it is imperative that they get hyperventilated otherwise life-threatening salicylate toxicity may ensue.
  - Ideally, match the ventilator settings to the patient's level of respiration prior to mechanical ventilation (eg, if patient was breathing at a rate of 30 and taking large tidal volumes prior to intubation, set the ventilator to the same rate with a relatively large tidal volume).

Disposition

- Significant ASA ingestions should be admitted to the ICU.
- Asymptomatic patients with low salicylate levels may be discharged after a period of observation—usually 6 hours should suffice provided that they didn't take an enteric-coated or sustained-release preparation.

BETA-BLOCKER/CALCIUM CHANNEL BLOCKER

Additional History and Physical Examination Findings

- Past medical history of cardiac disease or hypertension.
- Or a child playing at grandma's house who has cardiac disease or hypertension.
- History of ingestion.
- May present with hypotension and bradycardia.

Review Initial Results

- ECG: May demonstrate bradycardia with ventricular escape.
- Digoxin level: This is the main differential in the diagnosis if this is an unknown ingestion and the patient presents with hypotension and bradycardia—need to rule out cardiac glycoside toxicity, so this level should be normal or not detected.
- Glucose
  - Elevated: May be a marker for calcium channel blocker toxicity.
  - Low: May be a marker for beta-blocker toxicity.

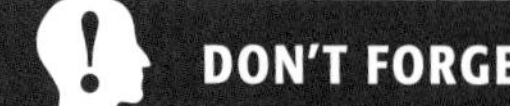

- Patients with hypotension and bradycardia → think beta-blocker, calcium channel blocker, digoxin, or clonidine.
- Glucose low with beta-blockers, glucose high with calcium channel blockers.

Risk Stratification: Management Priorities

- Consider any patient who presents following an acute overdose of these agents as someone who will likely die without intervention—not just for oral boards.
- If presenting early, it is imperative that gastric decontamination be immediately performed as this may prevent the toxicity that will surely ensue.

Definitive Management

- Early after ingestion (within 1 hour)—immediate gastric decontamination after initial stabilization
  - Activated charcoal
  - Consider WBI for sustained-release preparations.
- Hypotension and/or bradycardia
  - Isotonic crystalloid boluses.
  - Atropine 0.5 to 1 mg IV.
  - Glucagon 5-10 mg IV: If positive response, then can infuse continuously at 1-5 mg/h—titrate to effect. Most effective for beta-blocker overdoses.
  - Calcium chloride (10 mL of a 10% solution) or calcium gluconate (10 mL of a 10% solution) IV administration every 5 minutes as needed. Most effective for calcium channel blockers.
  - Hyperinsulinemia is a promising new therapy for the treatment of severe calcium channel blockers overdoses; may require the coadministration of glucose to maintain a euglycemic state; administration consists of an IV infusion of regular insulin at a rate of 0.5 to 1 IU/kg/h (note that this can be up to >10 times the infusion rate used to manage DKA).
  - Consider external or internal pacemaker for symptomatic bradycardia.
  - Consider intra-aortic balloon pump, if medical treatment of cardiovascular instability fails.

Further Reassessment

- Continuous monitoring to assess efficacy of therapies instituted.
- Check serum glucose and potassium frequently if patient is getting hyperinsulinemia treatment.

Complications

- Hypercalcemia: However, unclear if this has untoward effects in the setting of a calcium channel blocker overdose—it, in fact, may be therapeutic.

Disposition

- Patients with a symptomatic overdose of a beta-blocker or calcium channel blocker require ICU admission.
- Asymptomatic patients who have ingested a sustained-release preparation need to be observed in a monitored setting for at least 24 hours with calcium, atropine, and glucagon by bedside.

CARDIAC GLYCOSIDE (DIGOXIN)

Additional History and Physical Examination Findings

- Digoxin ingestion.
- Ingestion of certain plants: Foxglove, oleander, lily of the valley, etc.
- Licking toads.
- May have fatigue, nausea, vomiting, abdominal pain, confusion, and mental status changes.
- Yellow vision change.

Review Initial Results

- Digoxin level: For this to reflect a true distribution level, this level needs to be drawn 6 hours following an acute ingestion.
- Potassium: Check for hyperkalemia.
- ECG: Evaluate for dysrhythmia suggestive of cardiac glycoside toxicity (Fig. 16-3).
    - Bidirectional ventricular tachycardia is pathognomonic for cardiac glycoside toxicity.
    - Other rhythms suggestive of toxicity include atrial tachycardia with block, nonparoxysmal junctional tachycardia, atrial fibrillation with a slow, and regular ventricular rate (atrioventricular [AV] dissociation).

Risk Stratification: Management Priorities

- Hyperkalemia portends a grave prognosis in the setting of digoxin toxicity and is an indication for administration of digoxin-specific antibodies.
- Dysrhythmias and heart block also portend a poor prognosis.
- Chronic toxicity usually does worse.

Definitive Management

- Gastric decontamination if presenting early from an acute ingestion.
    - Activated charcoal

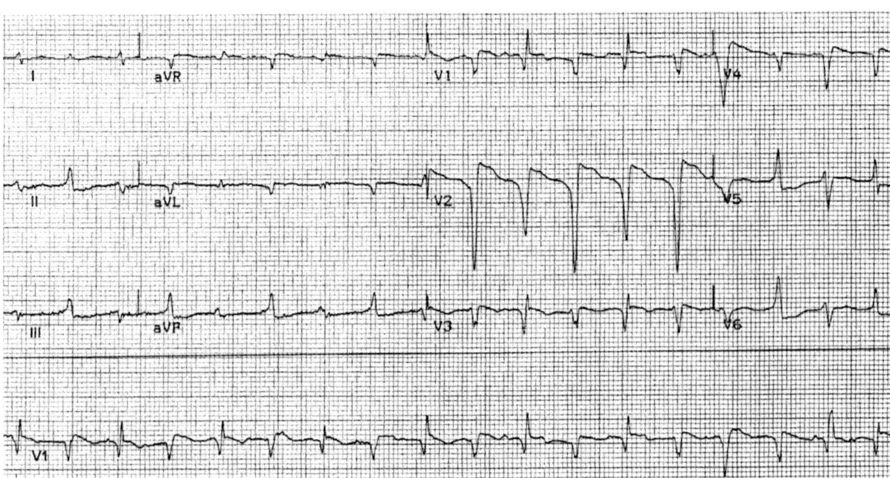

Figure 16-3. Bidirectional ventricular tachycardia; an example of bidirectional ventricular tachycardia that occurred in a patient with digoxin toxicity. (*Reproduced with permission from Knoop KJ, Stack LB, Storrow AB.* Atlas of Emergency Medicine. *2nd ed. New York, NY: McGraw-Hill; 2002.*)

- Digoxin-specific antibodies
  - Indications
    - Life-threatening cardiovascular instability.
    - Life-threatening dysrhythmias.
    - Potassium >5.0 mEq/L in an acute overdose.
    - Serum digoxin concentration ≥10 ng/mL at 6 hours.
    - Ingestion of 10 mg in a digoxin naive adult.
    - Ingestion of 4 mg in a digoxin naive child.
  - Dose
    - Quick estimation of number of vials needed.
      - [Serum digoxin concentration × Wt(kg)]/100.
    - Empiric dose
      - Acute overdose in an adult or child who has cardiovascular instability and no digoxin level is available: 10-20 vials.
    - For acute ingestion of the known amount
      - 1 vial binds to 0.5 mg of digoxin.

Further Reassessment

- Note that serum digoxin levels will not be useful in management of therapy after digoxin-specific antibody Fab fragments are administered.

Complications

- Hyperkalemia
  - Do *NOT* treat with calcium as this may lead to a "stone" heart.
  - Treat with digoxin-specific antibodies.

Disposition

- Symptomatic adult patients with an elevated 6-hour serum digoxin concentration, who receive antidotal or supportive therapy for cardiovascular instability, will require admission to the ICU.
- Asymptomatic adults with an elevated 6-hour serum digoxin concentration, who are hemodynamically stable, may be monitored in a telemetry unit with digoxin-specific antibodies at the bedside.
- Children with an elevated 6-hour serum digoxin concentration will require the PICU.
- Asymptomatic patients of an acute ingestion with a 6-hour serum digoxin concentration that is within the therapeutic range may be medically cleared.

DON'T FORGET

Do *NOT* give calcium to treat hyperkalemia in patients who are digoxic—the patient may die.

THEOPHYLLINE

Additional History and Physical Examination Findings

- Main pharmacologic effects
  - Endogenous catecholamines resulting in stimulation of adrenergic receptors digoxin toxic.
  - Antagonizes adenosine receptors which reverse histamine release and bronchoconstriction.
  - Inhibits phosphodiesterase which leads to increased levels of cyclic adenosine monophosphate (cAMP), leading to more adrenergic stimulation.
- Signs/symptoms include
  - Respiratory: Tachypnea, respiratory failure from fatigue, shortness of breath (SOB).
  - Cardiovasular: Tachydysrhythmia, hypotension, palpitations.
  - CNS: Agitation, anxiety, seizures, mental status change.
  - Dermal: Diaphoresis.

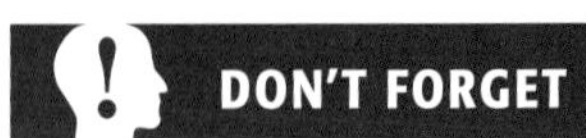

Patient with theophylline toxicity will have a sympathomimetic toxidrome.

- GI: Nausea, vomiting, abdominal cramping.
- Metabolic: Hypokalemia, hyperglycemia, metabolic acidosis, respiratory alkalosis, hyperthermia, and leukocytosis.

Review Initial Results

- Theophylline level, complete blood count (CBC), electrolytes, blood urea nitrogen (BUN)/Cr, glucose, magnesium, calcium, phosphorus, and ECG.

Risk Stratification: Management Priorities

- Chronic toxicity, in general, carries greater risk for major toxicity than from an acute exposure.
    - Within this group, it seems that the risk of major toxicity is correlated with age.
- With acutc toxicity, the peak theophylline level seems to predict risk of major toxicity.

Definitive Management

- Decontamination
    - Activated charcoal
    - Consider WBI if the patient presents <1 hour from ingestion without symptoms of toxicity and has ingested sustained release theophylline.
- Enhanced elimination
    - Multiple-dose activated charcoal
        - 25-50 g (without Sorbitol) every 2 hours
        - If WBI has been started for decontamination, it must be discontinued if activated charcoal is to be used.
    - Hemodialysis is indicated if
    - Theophylline level ≥90 μg/mL in acute ingestions
    - Cardiovascular instability
    - Seizures
    - Failure of conservative measures
    - Theophylline level ≥40 μg/mL if chronic toxicity

Further Reassessment

- Assess theophylline level every 2 hours until two decreasing levels in a row are obtained.
- Repeat electrolytes every 4-6 hours.
- Cardiac monitoring at all times.
- Discontinue activated charcoal or hemodialysis when the patient has no signs or symptoms of toxicity and the theophylline level is <20 μg/mL.

Complications

- Hypertension and supraventricular tachycardia (SVT) can be treated with a short-acting beta-adrenergic antagonist (eg, esmolol).
- Seizures can be treated with benzodiazepines and/or phenobarbital. Phenytoin is less effective at treating toxin-induced seizures.
- Electrolytes such as potassium should be aggressively replaced if a ventricular dysrhythmia is present, but in most circumstances, treatment with a beta-antagonist may be all that is needed. Replace other electrolytes as needed.
- Hypotension: IV fluids.
    - Adults, 1-2 L IV NS bolus if hypotensive
    - Children, 20 cc/kg IV NS bolus if hypotensive
- Acidosis and hyperglycemia resolve when the toxic effects of theophylline are treated.

Disposition

- Theophylline-poisoned patients who are symptomatic or have elevated or rising theophylline levels should be admitted to an ICU setting.
- All sustained-release ingestions should be admitted to a monitored setting or the ICU.
- An asymptomatic patient who ingested immediate release theophylline, and has two serum levels drawn 6 hours apart in the therapeutic range and trending downward, is not considered theophylline toxic.

VALPROIC AID (DEPACON, DEPAKENE, DEPAKOTE)

Additional History and Physical Examination Findings

- Valproic acid (VPA) is used to treat seizure disorders and bipolar affective disorders. Other uses include migraine headache prophylaxis and minor urinary incontinence. VPA increases the availability of gamma-aminobutyric acid (GABA) and may mimic GABA at postsynaptic receptor sites.
- Signs and symptoms include:
  - CNS: Drowsiness, confusion, obtundation, and profound coma and encephalopathy.
  - Respiratory: Respiratory depression/failure.
  - Cardiovascular: Tachycardia and hypotension.
  - GI: Nausea and vomiting, pancreatitis, and hepatotoxicity.

Review Initial Results

- Serum VPA level: Therapeutic range is 50-100 mg/L.
- Electrolytes may have hypernatremia and hypocalcemia.
- BUN, creatinine, glucose.
- Anion gap: May be high in severe overdoses.
- ABG in severe overdoses.
- Liver function tests.
- Serum ammonia: Hyperammonemia (>60 μmol/L) occurs in 35%-45% of patients on chronic VPA.
- Lipase: Can develop pancreatitis.
- Consider a CXR and CT of brain head.

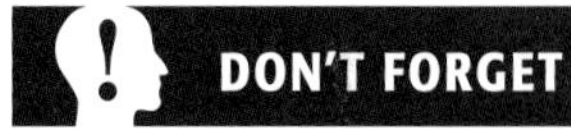

DON'T FORGET

Check the ammonia level: It might be high in VPA overdose.

Risk Stratification: Management Priorities

- VPA level
  - Concentrations >450 mg/L will most likely result in significant clinical effects.
  - Levels >850 mg/L are more likely associated with coma, respiratory depression, aspiration, or metabolic acidosis.

Definitive Management

- Supportive care
- Decontamination
  - Activated charcoal (1 g/kg). Consider repeat doses 25-50 g to maximize binding capacity.
  - WBI may be considered in large ingestions of sustained-released products.
  - Gastric lavage is considered in a life-threatening ingestion presenting within 1 hour. Caution: The potential for airway loss and possible seizure activity during gastric lavage exists in these patients.

- Enhanced elimination
  - Hemodialysis and hemoperfusion
    - Consider in patients with massive overdose, profound acidosis, or metabolic disturbances.
    - Usually reserved for patients with rapid deterioration, evidence of hepatic dysfunction, continued absorption of the drug, and serum levels in excess of 1000 mg/L.
- Focused therapy
  - L-carnitine (controversial)
    - Possibly beneficial to patients with VPA-induced hepatic dysfunction or hyperammonemia.
    - Doses of 100 mg/kg over 30 minutes (maximum 6 g) followed by 15 mg/kg IV over 10-30 minutes every 4 hours until clinical improvement.

Further Reassessment

- VPA level: Must be repeated every 2 hours until two levels are noted to be declining.
- Aggressive airway management and ventilatory care if indicated.
- Hypotension: Idiopathic ventricular fibrillation, pressors as indicated.
- Monitor oxygen saturation, blood pressure (BP), and cardiac rhythm.
- Replace electrolytes as needed.

Complications

- Bone marrow suppression may occur roughly in 3-5 days following acute massive overdose.
  - Characterized by leukopenia, thrombocytopenia, and anemia.
  - Usually resolves spontaneously within days.
- Seizures
  - Treat seizures with benzodiazepines or barbiturates.
  - Phenytoin/fosphenytoin is considered less effective at treating toxin-induced seizures.

Disposition

- Admit symptomatic patients and those with intentional ingestions.
- Progressive CNS or respiratory depression warrants intensive care monitoring.
- Discharge patients only after an accidental ingestion and multiple levels have been drawn to reveal a peak level trending downward, and the patient is asymptomatic.

TRICYCLIC ANTIDEPRESSANTS

Additional History and Physical Examination Findings

- TCAs are one of the most common classes of medications responsible for fatal overdoses.
- Main pharmacologic effects:
  - Sodium channel blockade causes toxicity similar to class 1a antidysrhythmics.
  - Reuptake inhibition of norepinephrine and dopamine leads to depletion of neurotransmitters.
  - Alpha-blockade contributes to hypotension.
  - Anticholinergic effects contribute to confusion, delirium, and seizures.

- Signs/symptoms:
  - Airway: The airway may be compromised because of seizures and CNS depression.
  - Pulmonary: Respiratory depression in severe cases
  - Cardiovascular: Major site of toxicity; may see tachycardia (early), wide QRS complexes (later), bradycardia (very late), and hypotension that may be refractory to fluid boluses.
  - CNS: Agitation may be an early finding; the patient may develop seizures and/or coma in severe poisoning.
  - GI: Decreased bowel sounds, may see delayed gastric emptying.

Review Initial Results

- ECG: Tachycardia, QRS prolongation (concerning when >120 milliseconds); QTc prolongation, terminal portion of R wave in aVR may be prolonged (concerning if >40 milliseconds); may also see incomplete right bundle branch block, right axis deviation (Fig. 16-4).
- TCA levels: Correlate poorly with symptoms and are not useful for the routine management of the TCA overdose.

Risk Stratification: Management Priorities

- ECG is prognostic.
  - QRS duration of >100 milliseconds has increased risk of seizures.
  - QRS duration of >160 milliseconds has increased risk of ventricular dysrhythmias.
  - Large R wave (>3 mm) in aVR is associated with seizures and ventricular dysrhythmias.

Definitive Management

- Gastric decontamination
  - Activated charcoal

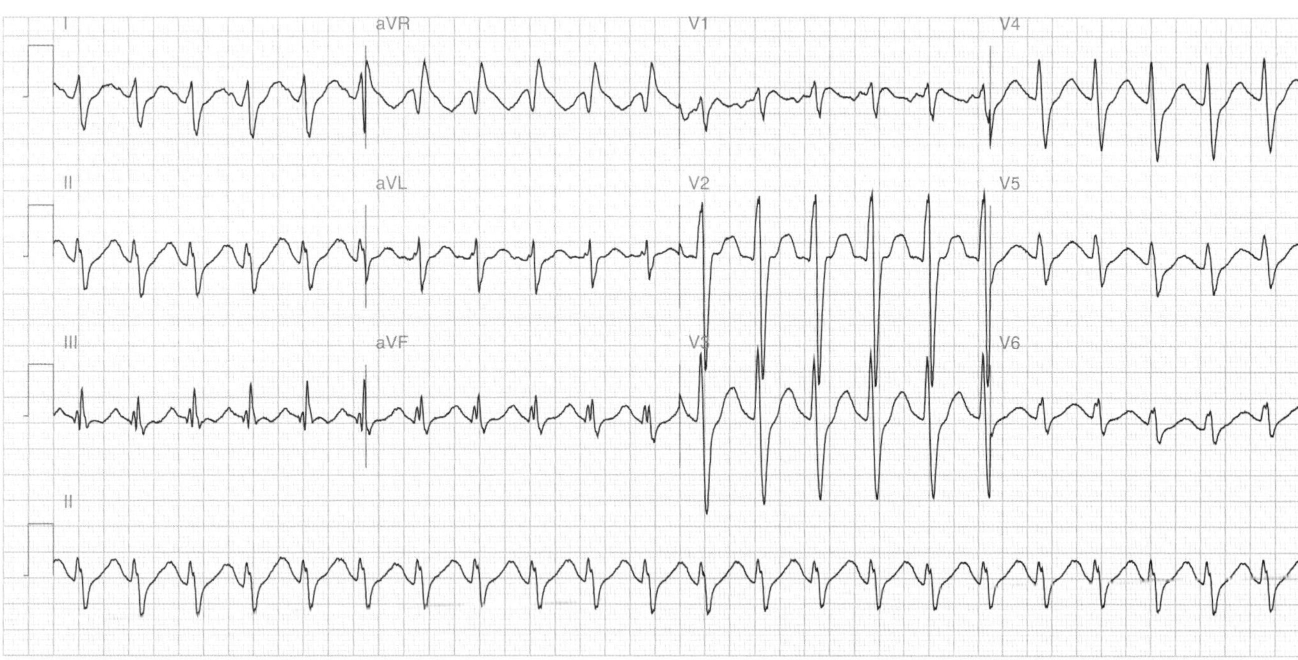

Figure 16-4. Sinus tachycardia; intraventricular conduction delay with a rightward QRS axis. QT interval is prolonged for the rate. The triad of sinus tachycardia, a wide QRS complex, and a long QT suggest TCA overdose. Terminal S wave (rS) in I, and terminal R wave (qR) in aVR are also seen in this condition. (*Reproduced with permission from Fauci AS, Braunwald E, Kaspter DL, et al.* Harrison's Principles of Internal Medicine. *17th ed. New York, NY: McGraw-Hill; 2008.*)

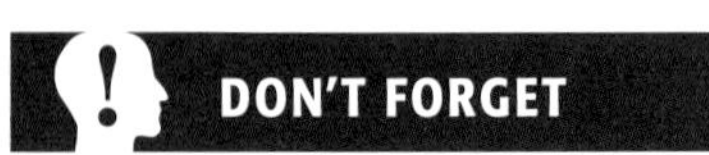

- Get the ECG—the most important diagnostic and prognostic test.
- Do *NOT* give physostigmine to treat the anticholinergic effects from a TCA overdose—this may lead to asystole and death.

DON'T FORGET

Do NOT give flumazenil to TCA overdose → seizures.

- Serum alkalinization and/or sodium loading are used to overcome the cardiac effects of sodium blockade.
  - Sodium bicarbonate 1-2 mEq/kg IV push (bolus); may repeat until QRS normalizes and VS improve; hold if pH >7.55.
- Consider hyperventilation (if the patient is intubated) to a pH of 7.45-7.55.
- Do *NOT* give physostigmine to treat patient's anticholinergic symptoms as this may precipitate asystole.

Further Reassessment

- Monitor with serial ECGs for improvement of QRS widening.
- Monitor serial serum pH to prevent severe alkalemia during therapy.

Complications

- Cardiac dysrhythmias
  - May consider lidocaine or magnesium for refractory ventricular dysrhythmias.
  - Avoid class 1a antidysrhythmics such as quinidine, disopyramide, and procainamide for TCA-induced dysrhythmias, as these medications may potentiate the sodium channel blockade and QT prolongation.
- Hypotension
  - Administer fluid boluses and sodium bicarbonate as initial therapy.
  - If refractory hypotension, consider vasopressors.
    - Theoretically, norepinephrine is more effective than dopamine for catecholamine-depleted patients.
    - For patients who remain severely symptomatic despite aggressive management, consider cardiopulmonary bypass support—shouldn't get this far on examination day though.
- Seizures
  - Treat seizures with benzodiazepines or barbiturates.
  - Phenytoin/fosphenytoin is considered less effective at treating toxin-induced seizures.

Disposition

- Admit patients with signs of toxicity, including persistent tachycardia.
- If any ECG or mental status changes are present, admit to the ICU.
- May discharge patients who are asymptomatic without any signs of toxicity after 6 hours.

ANTIPSYCHOTICS

Additional History and Physical Examination Findings

- Multiple classes within this group including
  - Phenothiazines: Chlorpromazine (Thorazine), prochlorperazine (Compazine), promethazine (Phenergan)
  - Butyrophenone: Droperidol (Inapsine), haloperidol (Haldol)
  - Dibenzodiazepine: Quetiapine (Seroquel), olanzapine (Zyprexa)
  - Other atypical: Risperidone (Risperdal), ziprasidone (Geodon)
- In general, effects described with the use of antipsychotic medications include
  - Antiadrenergic
    - Hypotension
  - Anticholinergic
    - Anticholinergic toxidrome

- Antidopaminergic
  - Extrapyramidal reactions
    - Dystonic reactions
    - Neuroleptic malignant syndrome
- Sodium channel blockade
  - QRS prolongation

Review Initial Results

- ECG: Evidence of QT prolongation, torsade de pointes, QRS prolongation

Risk Stratification: Management Priorities

- NMS is associated with significant mortality.

Definitive Management

- Gastric decontamination with activated charcoal if presents early after ingestion.
- Consider multiple doses of charcoal for sustained-release preparations.
- Treat dystonic reactions with diphenhydramine or benztropine.
- Sodium bicarbonate may be used if patient has evidence of QRS prolongation.
- IV fluids to maintain blood pressure, if hypotensive.

Complications

- Neuroleptic malignant syndrome—refer to separate section.

Disposition

- Patients with NMS require an ICU admission.
- Admit patients with profound CNS depression, cardiovascular toxicity, and those requiring airway stabilization.
- After an appropriate observation period and mental status stability are ensured, patients may be medically cleared.
- Psychiatric consultation for suicidal patients is appropriate.

LITHIUM

Additional History and Physical Examination Findings

- Always consider lithium toxicity if patient has a history of psychiatric illness (and you don't know their medications) and presents with altered mental status.
- Acute ingestion of lithium may cause nausea and vomiting early on with delayed systemic findings of tremor, weakness, ataxia, slurred speech, weakness, and other primarily neurologic symptoms.
- Severe symptoms include altered mental status, coma, seizures, agitation, delirium, and hyperthermia.
- Recent gastroenteritis symptoms or volume depletion can precipitate lithium toxicity in patients who are on lithium chronically.

Review Initial Results

- Lithium level
- Electrolytes: Hypernatremia and dehydration may occur because of lithium-induced nephrogenic diabetes insipidus.
- ECG: May reveal prolonged QT or inverted T waves.

Risk Stratification: Management Priorities

- Any patient with altered mental status, seizures, or coma is very ill, and prompt treatment needs to be initiated to prevent permanent neurologic morbidity.
- Acute on chronic toxicity fare the worst.

Definitive Management

- Initial IV fluid resuscitation with isotonic crystalloid—if patient is dehydrated, lithium will be reabsorbed by the kidneys.
- Gastric decontamination
  - Consider gastric lavage for recent large ingestion as activated charcoal does not bind to lithium very well.
  - WBI may be considered if patient presents early after acute ingestion.
- Hemodialysis
  - Indications
    - Altered mental status
    - Seizures
    - Coma
    - Renal impairment
    - Cardiovascular toxicity
    - Lithium level >4.0 mEq/L in acute ingestion
    - Lithium level >2.5 mEq/L with chronic toxicity

Further Reassessment

- Measure lithium levels every 2 hours.
- Following hemodialysis, lithium level should be checked 6 hours after dialysis has been completed, as redistribution of lithium within the body occurs.

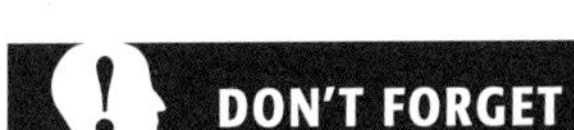

- Gastric lavage if patient presents early and has no contraindications—lithium does not bind to charcoal, can be lethal, and has no antidote.
- Think about dialysis!

Complications

- Neuroleptic malignant syndrome
- Nephrogenic diabetes insipidus

Disposition

- Admit all symptomatic lithium overdoses.
- Admit all with a significant ingestion of lithium (>40 mg/kg).
- Admit all patients who ingested a sustained-release preparation for observation.
- Patients who are asymptomatic with normal lithium levels 6 hours after ingestion of an immediate release preparation may be discharged—either to psychiatrist if this was a suicide attempt, or home if accidental.

IRON

Additional History and Physical Examination Findings

- Iron formulation
  - Ferrous sulfate contains 20% iron.
  - Ferrous fumarate contains 33% iron.
  - Ferrous gluconate contains 12% iron.
- There are five clinical stages of iron poisoning.
  - Stage 1: The corrosive effects of iron cause vomiting and diarrhea, which may be bloody. These symptoms will begin within 2-6 hours of ingestion.
  - Stage 2: There may be apparent improvement of symptoms over 12 hours.
  - Stage 3: Abrupt onset of coma, shock, seizures, metabolic acidosis, coagulopathy, hepatic failure, and death.

- Stage 4: Hepatic failure may occur 2-3 days post-ingestion.
- Stage 5: If the patient survives, scarring form the corrosive injury may result in stricture or obstruction.

Review Initial Results

- Iron level
  - Total serum iron level will peak 2-6 hours post-ingestion.
  - Total iron-binding capacity (TIBC) is unreliable in acute iron overdose.
- ABG: Persistence of metabolic acidosis is the most important marker of ongoing toxicity.
- KUB: Iron pills may be seen.
- CBC: Leukocytosis >15,000 mm^3 may be marker for toxicity.
- Glucose: Serum glucose >150 mg/dL may be marker for toxicity.
- Other useful studies include
  - Electrolytes, glucose, BUN, creatinine, liver function tests, ABG, and coagulation studies

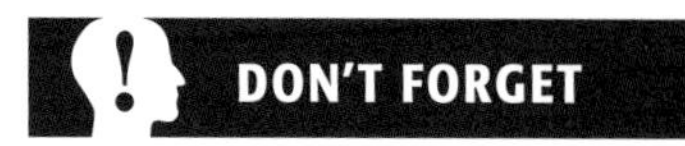

Don't be reassured by improvement in symptoms—may just be stage 2.

Risk Stratification: Management Priorities

- Ingestion
  - <20 mg/kg: Minimal to no toxicity
  - 20-30 mg/kg: Mild to moderate toxicity
  - 40-60 mg/kg: Potentially serious
  - >60 mg/kg: Potentially lethal
- Shock/coma carries a 10% mortality even with antidotal therapy and supportive care.

Definitive Management

- Decontamination
  - Orogastric lavage may be helpful in life-threatening ingestions presenting within 1 hour.
  - Activated charcoal does not bind well to iron and is not recommended.
- Enhanced elimination
  - WBI if radiopaque iron pills are present in the GI tract on radiography.
- Supportive measures
  - IV crystalloid, pressors for hypotension.
  - Benzodiazepines if seizures occur.
- Antidotal therapy
  - Deferoxamine, up to 15 mg/kg/h IV infusion is indicated for patients with severe intoxication (shock, severe acidosis, and/or serum iron >500 µg/dL).
    - Caution should be used when administering deferoxamine, because rapid boluses may cause hypotension.
  - Continue the infusion until acidosis and other clinical signs of toxicity are resolved.

Further Reassessment

- Iron levels should be repeated every 4-6 hours until the level peaks and starts to decrease.
- Continue to monitor patient's acid-base status.
- Check urine color—it should turn "vin rose"—this represents the iron-deferoxamine complex (ferrioxamine).

Complications

- GI strictures from the corrosive effect of iron
- Prolonged (>24 hours) administration of deferoxamine therapy has been associated with acute respiratory distress syndrome (ARDS) and *Yersinia*

enterocolitica sepsis. If therapy is needed for >24 hours, may consider an 8- to 12-hour hiatus before continuing deferoxamine therapy.

Disposition

- Asymptomatic patients with peak iron levels <350 µg/mL without evidence of systemic toxicity (eg, acidosis) may be discharged.
- Any patient with signs of systemic iron toxicity should be admitted to the hospital.
- Patients with shock, coma, or metabolic acidosis should be admitted to an ICU.
- Admitted patients should be reevaluated in 2 weeks for assessment of the GI tract.

LEAD

Additional History and Physical Examination Findings

- History of pica, eating paint chips
- Increased risk in children who live in old homes
- Characteristic exposure in adults is through inhalation (eg, sanding paint in old home without proper respiratory precautions).
- Major systems affected are the hematopoetic system, the nervous system, the kidneys, and the reproductive system—symptoms include:
  - Neurologic: Encephalopathy, coma, seizures, ataxia, foot and wrist drop can be seen with severe lead poisoning. Headache, impaired cognition, and lethargy are seen with mild poisoning.
  - GI: Abdominal pain, constipation, and anorexia.
  - Heme: Pallor, anemia.
  - Renal: Nephropathy may occur with chronic lead exposure.
  - Reproductive: Diminished sperm production, increased rates of miscarriage, and preterm delivery.

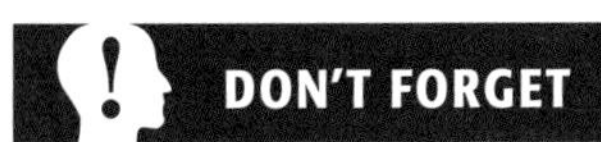

Consider in patients with microcytic anemia and abdominal pain.

Review Initial Results

- Venous blood lead level.
- CBC: May see basophilic stippling.
- Ferritin may reveal concomitant iron deficiency.
- KUB may reveal radiopaque densities.
- Knee x-rays in children may reveal lead lines (Fig. 16-5).
- Although not immediately available, elevated levels of free erythrocyte protoporphyrin (FEP) or zinc protoporphyrin (ZPP) may occur because of lead's inhibition of heme synthesis and are a marker for chronic toxicity.

Risk Stratification: Management Priorities

- Seizures or encephalopathy caused by lead toxicity are medical emergencies.

Definitive Management

- Most important measure—remove patient from source of exposure.
  - This measure may require inpatient admission and social services.
- Treatment is different based on whether patient is a child or an adult.
- Pediatric treatment
  - Lead level 10-19 µg/dL
    - Reduce child's lead exposure; close follow-up; repeat lead level in 1-3 months
  - Lead level 20-44 µg/dL
    - Complete pediatric evaluation within 10 days with attention to identifying the source of exposure; repeat lead level in 1-4 weeks.

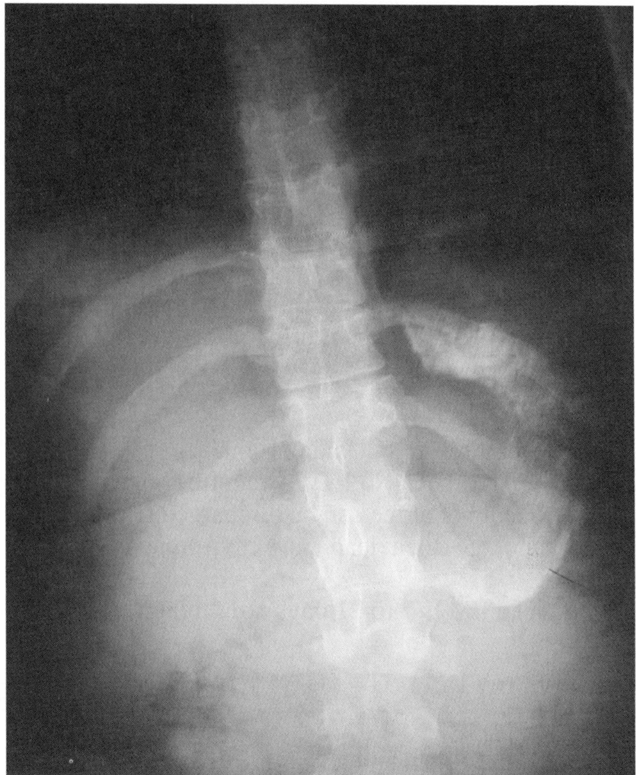

Figure 16-5. Lead lines seen in a pediatric patient with chronic lead poisoning. The increased radiographic densities on the metaphyseal growth plates demonstrate radiologic growth retardation. (*Reproduced with permission from Knoop KJ, Stack LB, Storrow AB.* Atlas of Emergency Medicine. *2nd ed. New York, NY: McGraw-Hill; 2002.*)

- Lead level 45-69 μg/dL—treatment with succimer.
  - Succimer 10 mg/kg/dose or 350 mg/m^2/dose orally tid for 5 days, then reduce to 10 mg/kg/dose or 350 mg/m^2/dose bid for 14 days.
  - Hospitalization may be needed for children with blood lead levels of 45 μg/dL or greater, so that the child can receive chelation in a lead-safe environment.
- Lead level >70 μg/dL—acute medical emergency—child should be hospitalized for treatment with BAL and $CaNa_2EDTA$.
  - BAL 300 mg/m^2/d IM divided q4h
  - $CaNa_2EDTA$ 1000 mg/m^2/d IV (start 4 hours after BAL)
- Acute encephalopathy—acute medical emergency—child should be hospitalized for treatment with BAL and $CaNa_2EDTA$.
  - BAL 450 mg/m^2/d IM divided q4h
  - $CaNa_2EDTA$ 1500 mg/m^2/d IV (start 4 hours after BAL)

- Adult treatment
  - Lead level <70 μg/dL
    - Remove from source of lead exposure.
  - Lead level 70-100 μg/dL or mild symptoms
    - Succimer 10 mg/kg/dose or 250-350 mg/m^2/dose orally tid for 5 days, then bid for 14 days.
  - Lead level >100 μg/dL or with symptoms of lead poisoning or encephalopathy—the patient needs both BAL and $CaNa_2EDTA$.
    - BAL 300-450 mg/m^2/d IM divided q4h
    - $CaNa_2EDTA$ 1000-1500 mg/m^2/d IV (start 4 hours after BAL)

Further Reassessment

- Recheck blood lead levels 7-21 days after treatment is completed. The chelation therapy only gets rid of the lead in the blood. Total body burden may be much greater. Subsequently after completion of therapy, lead levels may go back up again requiring reinitiating treatment, so on examination day, don't forget that these patients need follow-up if you are discharging them.

Complications

- Long-term sequelae occur more in children as high lead levels affect neurologic development—lead exposure has been associated with lower IQs.

Disposition

- Encephalopathy requires an ICU admission.
- Treatment with BAL and $CaNa_2EDTA$ requires hospitalization.
- Treatment with succimer alone can be discharged to a lead-safe environment.
  - If patient cannot go to a lead-safe environment, they will need to be hospitalized.
- Recheck blood lead levels 7 to 21 days after treatment is completed.

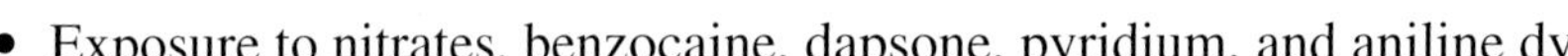

METHEMOGLOBINEMIA

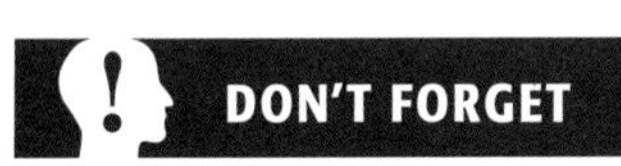

DON'T FORGET

A patient who becomes cyanotic after a procedure using topical anesthetic → think methemoglobinemia.

Additional History and Physical Examination Findings

- Exposure to nitrates, benzocaine, dapsone, pyridium, and aniline dye
- Patient appears cyanotic.
  - No response to oxygen administration
  - Chocolate brown blood on blood draw. (Ask the examiner, what color does the blood look like as it is being drawn?)

Review Initial Results

- Pulse oximetry
  - Will trend toward 85%
- CBC
  - Anemia will exacerbate methemoglobinemia.
- ABG
  - Po_2—likely normal
- Methemoglobin level
  - 1%-2% → normal
  - 15%-20% → cyanosis, chocolate brown blood
  - 20%-50% → dyspnea, exercise intolerance, syncope
  - 50%-70% → dysrhythmias, seizures, coma
  - >70% → death

Risk Stratification: Management Priorities

- Based on level and symptoms and underlying medical problems

Definitive Management

- Oxygen
- Methylene blue
  - Indications
    - Methemoglobin levels are >20%, symptomatic (headache, SOB, chest pain, dizziness, nausea, confusion, seizures, coma), and/or with concurrent medical illness (heart disease, lung disease, anemia).
    - Methemogobin level >30%

  - Contraindicated in patients with glucose-6-phosphate dehydrogenase (G6PD) deficiency as may induce hemolysis.
  - Administer 1-2 mg/kg IV over several minutes.
- Exchange transfusion and hyperbaric oxygen (HBO) should be considered for refractory cases.

Further Reassessment

- Goals of treatment
  - Resolution of symptoms
  - Methemoglobin level <20%

Complications

- Worsening methemoglobinemia—may be indication for exchange transfusion.
- Hemolysis may occur from methylene blue administration if a large dose is given or patient is G6PD deficient.

Disposition

- Admission to the ICU is appropriate for symptomatic cases, especially if exchange transfusion is being considered.

CARBON MONOXIDE

Additional History and Physical Examination Findings

- Exposure.
  - Combustion: Fire, heater, car exhaust.
  - Methylene chloride (paint stripper) is metabolized to CO following ingestion.
- Signs and symptoms range from headache, nausea, vomiting, and dizziness to chest pain, syncope, seizures, coma, and death.

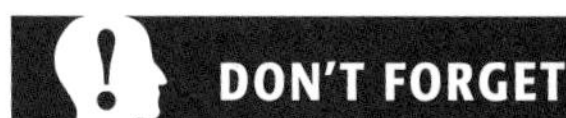

Family comes in for headaches and nausea during the late fall/early winter time → think CO.

Review Initial Results

- Carboxyhemoglobin (COHb) level—either a venous or arterial specimen
- Pregnancy test in females of childbearing age
- ECG: Evaluate for evidence of myocardial ischemia
- ABG
- BMP
- Creatine phosphokinase (CPK): Evidence of rhabdomyolysis
- CT head: May have cerebral edema or basal ganglia defects

Risk Stratification: Management Priorities

- Mild
  - Symptoms: Headache, nausea, dizziness.
  - Signs: Vomiting.
- Moderate
  - Symptoms: Confusion, slow thinking, SOB, weakness, blurred vision.
  - Signs: Tachycardia, tachypnea, weakness, myonecrosis, ataxia, cognitive defects.
- Severe
  - Symptoms: Chest pain, palpitations, severe disorientation, hypotension, syncope.
  - Signs: Dysrhythmias, ECG changes, drowsiness, seizures, acidosis, obtundation, pulmonary edema, coma, brain changes on CT head.
  - If the patient doesn't die, they may have persistent neurologic sequelae.
    - HBO treatment may decrease these sequelae.

Definitive Management

- All patients need oxygen!
- 100% oxygen by face mask until asymptomatic if patient is not pregnant.
- If the patient is pregnant, they should be on 100% NRB for 5 times the length of time needed for the CO level to be <5%.
- Indications for possible HBO treatment:
    - Pregnancy with fetal distress
    - Any history of loss of consciousness
    - Level >25%
    - Neurologic symptoms other than simple headache
    - Abnormal neurocognitive testing
    - Ischemic ECG changes or other cardiac complications
    - Any patient graded as severe poisoning

DON'T FORGET

Half-life of CO is 4-5 hours on room air, 80-90 minutes on 100% oxygen, and 20-30 minutes with HBO.

Further Reassessment

- Repeat COHb level every 2-4 hours until level is <10% or <5% for pregnant patients.

Complications

- Delayed neurologic sequelae: Patient may have persistent cognitive impairment following CO poisoning.

Disposition

- Admit all patients with severe symptoms.
    - May need the ICU for patients with seizures, acute coronary syndrome (ACS), coma.
- Discharge nonpregnant patients who are asymptomatic with a COHb level <10%.

CYANIDE

Additional History and Physical Examination Findings

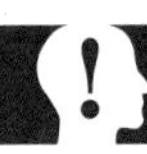

DON'T FORGET

- Think about cyanide (in addition to CO) when a patient presents from a fire and has profound metabolic acidosis.
- If getting bright red blood from a venous stick, think cyanide.

- Exposure
    - Inhalation: Combustion of wool, plastics, and other natural and synthetic products can lead to the production of hydrogen cyanide.
    - Ingestion: Chemicals used in photography, jewelry making, and electroplating may contain cyanide.
    - Metabolism: Nitroprusside, acetonitrile, acrylonitrile, cyanogenic glycosides (eg, peach pits, apricot pits, apple seeds), and laetrile
- Signs and symptoms
    - CNS: Headache, seizures, coma.
    - Cardiovascular: Bradycardia, hypotension.
    - Respiratory: Pulmonary edema.
    - GI: Hemorrhagic gastritis.

Review Initial Results

- ABG: Profound acidemia.
- Mixed venous gas: "Arterialization" of venous blood—the oxygen content of the venous blood is almost the same as the arterial blood as the body is not utilizing oxygen on the cellular level because of cyanide, inhibiting oxidative phosphorylation.
- Lactate: Significantly elevated.

Risk Stratification: Management Priorities

- Cyanide is very potent, and patients with significant toxicity usually die very quickly.
- Ingestion of as little as 200 mg of sodium or potassium cyanide may be fatal.
- Not as common to see cyanide toxicity from nitroprusside or ingestion of amygdalin.

Definitive Management

- Decontamination
  - Inhalation
    - Remove the patient from exposure.
  - Dermal
    - Remove all clothing.
    - Decontaminate skin.
  - Gastric
    - Activated charcoal
- Cyanide antidote kit
  - Indication
    - Signs and symptoms of toxicity from the known or suspected cyanide exposure.
  - Amyl nitrite
    - Indicated when IV access delayed or not possible.
    - Crush 1-2 capsules into gauze.
    - Have patient inhale amyl nitrite through gauze, or place gauze within facemask, over intake valve of bag-valve-mask device or port access to endotracheal (ET) tube during assisted ventilation.
    - Alternate every 30 seconds with 100% oxygen.
    - Discontinue use when IV access obtained and sodium nitrite given. If no IV access within 3 minutes, give the second capsule.
  - Sodium nitrite
    - Induces methemoglobinemia, which combines with cyanide to form cyanmethemoglobin, thus drawing the cyanide groups from their site of primary toxicity, cytochrome oxidase.
    - Adult: 300 mg over 5 minutes or more (10 mL of a 3% solution)
    - Pediatrics: 0.33 mL/kg of a 3% solution
    - Table included with this kit to dose based on hemoglobin if hemoglobin is known.
  - Sodium thiosulfate
    - Thiosulfate transfers sulfur group to cyanmethemoglobin to form thiocyanate which is less toxic and excreted in the urine.
    - Adult: 12.5 g over 10 minutes (50 mL of a 25% solution).
    - Pediatrics: 1.65 mL/kg of a 25% solution.
  - Vitamin B_{12} (cyanocobalamin)
    - Adults: 5 g IV over >15 min
    - Peds: 70 mg/kg over > 15 min

Further Reassessment

- Monitor BP and slow infusion rate of sodium nitrite if hypotension develops.

Complications

- Methemoglobinemia
  - If levels are >30%, do not use methylene blue, consider exchange transfusion.
- Hypotension
  - Fluid boluses and slow rate of sodium nitrite if this occurs.

Disposition

- Admit all symptomatic patients.

HYDROCARBON AND PETROLEUM DISTILLATES

Additional History and Physical Examination Findings

- Typical history is ingestion of lamp oil, kerosene, gasoline, or mineral seal oil.
- Low viscosity agents with low surface tension place the patient at the greatest risk for aspiration.
- Signs and symptoms:
  - Respiratory: Coughing, gagging, choking tachypnea, dyspnea, cyanosis, rales, hemoptysis, pulmonary edema, pneumatoceles, lipoid pneumonia, or respiratory arrest may develop if aspiration occurs.
  - GI: Nausea, vomiting abdominal pain.
  - CNS: Confusion, ataxia, headache, lethargy.
- Important to ascertain the exact ingestion—certain hydrocarbons have unique toxicities associated with them (CHAMP).
  - **C**amphor: Can cause seizures.
  - **H**alogenated hydrocarbons: Such as carbon tetrachloride which can cause hepatotoxicity, or methylene chloride that can cause CO poisoning.
  - **A**romatic hydrocarbons: Such as benzene which is extremely carcinogenic.
  - **M**etal-containing hydrocarbons: Such as leaded gasoline.
  - **P**esticide-containing hydrocarbons.

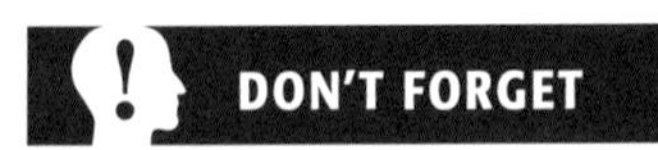

Think aspiration in all cases and don't cause any more aspiration!

Review Initial Results

- ABG: Evaluate for hypoxemia and ventilation status.
- CXR: Typical findings of pneumonitis.

Risk Stratification: Management Priorities

- Patients with any respiratory symptoms at any time may be indicative of aspiration which may develop into severe pneumonitis.

Definitive Management

- Gastric decontamination in any form is controversial and should not be used in most cases as the most significant complication from most hydrocarbon ingestions is severe aspiration pneumonitis.
  - Activated charcoal does not bind to hydrocarbons very well, but administration may be entertained if there exists a toxic coingestion.
  - If patient presents immediately following a large ingestion of a hydrocarbon with inherent systemic toxicity, they may try to aspirate the contents of the stomach with a small NG tube.

Further Reassessment

- Monitor respiratory status.
- Keep the patient on continuous pulse oximetry.
- Repeat CXR: May have delayed findings up to 6 hours post ingestion.

Complications

- Inhalation of hydrocarbons may be associated with myocardial sensitization to catecholamines.
  - Don't scare the patient—this may lead to cardiac dysrhythmias and sudden death.

  - Don't give the patient exogenous catecholamines—epinephrine, norepinephrine.
  - Dysrhythmias may be treated with beta-blockers.

Disposition

- ICU admission for all patients with significant symptoms as their symptoms require mechanical ventilation if they are not already.
- Following an accidental ingestion of a simple hydrocarbon without systemic toxicity, patients with no respiratory symptoms, normal CXR, and normal oxygenation can be discharged home after a 6-hour observation period.

ORGANOPHOSPHATES/NERVE AGENTS

Additional History and Physical Examination Findings

- Exposure to organophosphate pesticide, carbamate pesticide, or nerve agent.
- May have garlic odor.
- Cholinergic toxidrome.

Review Initial Results

- Diagnosis should be made based on toxidrome recognition alone.
- Other helpful tests
  - BMP: The patient may have electrolyte derangements caused by excessive fluid losses.
  - CXR: The patient may have pulmonary edema.
  - ECG
- May send plasma pseudocholinesterase and red blood cell acetylcholinesterase activity levels for confirmatory testing.
  - These levels need to be drawn prior to pralidoxime administration to be accurate. However, this should not delay treatment.

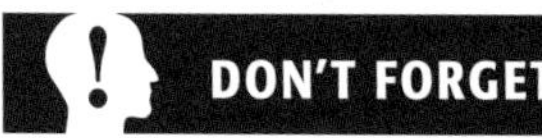

Patients need to be decontaminated otherwise you will wind up having multiple patients to manage, including yourself!

Risk Stratification: Management Priorities

- Unless a clear history is obtained, be prepared for a possible mass casualty.

Definitive Management

- Atropine
  - Administer 0.5-2 mg initially and repeat frequently.
  - May need to give large amounts (up to 100 mg or more).
  - Titrate to secretions/bronchospasm/bronchorrhea.
- Pralidoxime (2-PAM)
  - Regenerates enzyme activity.
  - Most effective when given early.
  - Administer 2 g (20-40 mg/kg in children) IV bolus, followed by continuous infusion 250-500 mg/h (5-10 mg/kg/h in children).

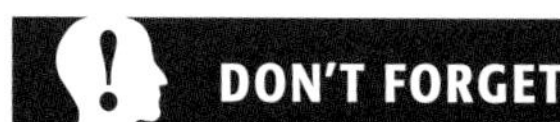

- Don't use succinylcholine for RSI → prolonged paralysis.
- Large amounts of atropine may be needed—up to 100 mg or more!

Further Reassessment

- Monitor patient's toxidrome.
- Watch for seizures and respiratory arrest.
- Rehydrate and replenish electrolytes as needed.

Complications

- Paralytic agents
  - If patient needs to undergo intubation with rapid sequence intubation, use a nondepolarizing agent as the patient will not be able to break down succinylcholine.

Disposition

- Symptomatic patients need an ICU.
- Asymptomatic patients need to be observed for at least 12 hours to monitor for delayed-onset symptoms.

ETHYLENE GLYCOL

Additional History and Physical Examination Findings

- Ethylene glycol is a toxic alcohol commonly found in antifreeze, de-icing solutions, brake (hydraulic) fluids, solvents, fire extinguishers, inks, and air conditioner systems.
- Ethylene glycol is metabolized via alcohol dehydrogenase to glycoaldehyde which subsequently goes on to form toxic metabolites.
- Symptoms/signs:
  - Airway: Airway protection may be compromised secondary to CNS depression.
  - Pulmonary: Tachypnea, hyperventilation, and respiratory depression.
  - CNS: Depression, ataxia, coma, and irritability.
  - Cardiovascular: Tachycardia, labile BP, dysrhythmias.
  - GI: Nausea and vomiting.
  - Renal: Renal failure, crystalluria (possibly).

Review Initial Results

- BMP: Evaluate for a high anion gap.
- Serum calcium may be low.
- UA: May have evidence of calcium oxalate crystals.
- ABG: Acidemia develops as a natural progression of ethylene glycol ingestion.
- Measure serum osmolality (freezing point depression method).
  - Calculate osmolarity: (2 [Na] + [BUN]/2.8 + [glucose]/18 + [ethanol]/4.6).
  - Calculate osmolal gap (measured-calculated).
    - Ethylene glycol is osmotically active and may result in a significant osmolal gap.
    - Normal osmolal gap may, in fact, be toxic because of individual variability in serum osmolality.
    - Acid metabolites are not osmotically active, yet will result in an elevated anion gap.
    - Early presentation may result in an elevated osmol gap while late presenters may only have an elevated anion gap.
    - Some patients may present with both an osmolal gap and an anion gap metabolic acidosis.
  - Consider estimating serum ethylene glycol (mg/dL) by multiplying 6.2 × osmolal gap.
- Stat ethylene glycol level: A level of >20 mg/dL is associated with serious toxicity.

Risk Stratification: Management Priorities

- The extent of toxicity is proportional to the degree of metabolism of ethylene glycol.
  - Do not let continued metabolism of ethylene glycol proceed as this makes the patient more toxic.

Definitive Management

- Decontamination
  - Activated charcoal doesn't bind significantly to ethylene glycol.

- Antidotal therapy: Goal is to block ethylene glycol from being metabolized.
  - Alcohol dehydrogenase inhibition with either fomepizole or EtOH.
    - Fomepizole: Loading dose 15 mg/kg IV followed by 10 mg/kg q12h for 4 doses, then 15 mg/kg q12h until ethylene glycol <20 mg/dL. Increase dosing to q4h during hemodialysis.
    - EtOH: Load and maintenance drip to reach goal of 150 mg/dL.
- Adjunctive therapy: Glyoxylic acid (toxic metabolite formed from ethylene glycol metabolism) is also metabolized to nontoxic metabolites through the aid of thiamine, magnesium, and pyridoxine.
  - Pyridoxine may enhance metabolic conversion of glyoxylic acid to glycine.
    - 50 mg IV/IM q6h until intoxication is resolved.
  - Thiamine acts as a cofactor in the metabolism of glyoxylic acid.
    - 100 mg slow IV (over 5 minutes) or IM; repeat q6h.
  - Folic acid, if methanol ingestion is a possibility.
    - 50 mg IV q4h for 6 doses may be considered.
- Enhanced elimination
  - Hemodialysis: Removes both ethylene glycol and toxic metabolites. Considerations include suspected ethylene glycol poisoning with significant acidosis, an elevated osmolal gap, a serum ethylene glycol level >20 mg/dL. Ideally, hemodialysis should be continued until all ethylene glycol is removed, in addition to stability of any acid-base disorder.

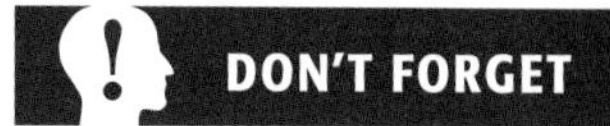

Inhibiting alcohol dehydrogenase with EtOH or fomepizole will be a critical action on examination day.

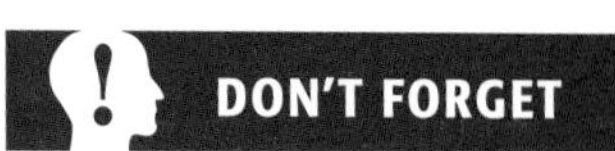

If patient is significantly acidemic → dialysis.

Further Reassessment

- Airway stabilization and ventilatory management as indicated.
- Fluids to correct hypotension.
- Pressors for severe hypotension unresponsive to fluids.
- Sodium bicarbonate for profound acidosis.
- Follow and correct any electrolyte or glucose abnormality.

Complications

- Renal failure

Disposition

- Admit any patient requiring antidotal therapy.
- Patients who are being treated with an EtOH infusion, hemodialysis, or have hemodynamic instability warrant admission to an ICU.
- Patients clinically stable and treated with fomepizole do not need intensive care.
- Discharge only after documentation of an undetectable ethylene glycol level and serial laboratory analysis reveals stability—psychiatric consultation may be considered for suicidal patients.

METHANOL

Additional History and Physical Examination Findings

- Methanol (wood alcohol) is a common ingredient in many solvents, windshield-washing solutions, antifreeze, anti-icing agents, and varnish/paint removers.
- Methanol is metabolized via alcohol dehydrogenase to formaldehyde which subsequently goes on to form the toxic formic acid.
- Symptoms/signs:
  - Airway: Airway protection may be compromised secondary to CNS depression.
  - Pulmonary: Tachypnea, hyperventilation, and respiratory depression
  - CNS: Depression, ataxia, coma, and irritability

- Cardiovascular: Tachycardia, labile BP, dysrhythmias
- GI: Nausea and vomiting
- Ophthalmic: Blindness, blurred or "snow field" vision, hyperemic optic discs, mydriasis, and papilledema

Review Initial Results

- BMP: Evaluate for a high anion gap.
- ABG: Acidemia develops as formic acid forms.
- Measure serum osmolality (freezing point depression method).
  - Calculate osmolarity (2 [Na] + [BUN]/2.8 + [glucose]/18 + [ethanol]/4.6).
  - Calculate osmolal gap (measured-calculated).
    - Methanol is osmotically active and may result in a significant osmolal gap.
    - Normal osmolal gap may, in fact, be toxic because of individual variability in serum osmolality.
    - Formic acid is not osmotically active, yet will result in an elevated anion gap.
    - Early presentation may result in an elevated osmolal gap while late presenters may only have an elevated anion gap.
    - Some patients may present with both an osmolal gap and an anion gap metabolic acidosis.
  - Consider estimating serum methanol level (mg/dL) by multiplying 3.2 × osmolal gap.
- Stat methanol level: A level >20 mg/dL is associated with serious toxicity.

Risk Stratification: Management Priorities

- The extent of toxicity is proportional to the degree of metabolism of methanol.
  - Do not let continued metabolism of methanol proceed as this makes the patient more toxic.

Definitive Management

- Decontamination
  - NG aspiration of methanol after recent ingestion may be considered.
  - Activated charcoal doesn't bind significantly to methanol.
- Antidotal therapy: Goal is to block methanol from being metabolized to formic acid.
  - Alcohol dehydrogenase inhibition with either fomepizole or EtOH
    - Fomepizole: Loading dose 15 mg/kg IV followed by 10 mg/kg q12h for 4 doses, then 15 mg/kg q12h until ethylene glycol <20 mg/dL. Increase dosing to q4h during hemodialysis.
    - EtOH: Load and maintenance drip to reach goal of 150 mg/dL.
  - Folic acid enhances the metabolism of formic acid to water and carbon dioxide.
    - 50 mg IV q4h for 6 doses may be considered.
- Enhanced elimination
  - Hemodialysis: Rapidly removes both methanol and formic acid. Considerations include suspected methanol poisoning with significant metabolic acidosis, an elevated osmolal gap, a serum methanol level >20 mg/dL. Ideally, hemodialysis should be continued until all methanol is removed.

DON'T FORGET

Inhibiting alcohol dehydrogenase with EtOH or fomepizole will be a critical action on examination day.

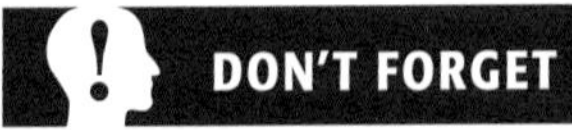

If patient is significantly acidemic → dialysis.

Further Reassessment

- Airway stabilization and ventilatory management as indicated.
- Fluids to correct hypotension.
- Pressors for severe hypotension unresponsive to fluids.
- Sodium bicarbonate for profound acidosis.
- Follow and correct any electrolyte or glucose abnormality.

Complications

- Blindness

Disposition

- Admit any patient requiring antidotal therapy.
- Patients who are being treated with an EtOH infusion, hemodialysis, or have hemodynamic instability warrant admission to an ICU.
- Patients clinically stable and treated with fomepizole do not need intensive care.
- Discharge only after documentation of an undetectable methanol level and serial laboratory analysis reveals stability—psychiatric consultation may be considered for suicidal patients.

OPIOIDS

Additional History and Physical Examination Findings

- Exposure to an opioid.
- Demonstrates opioid toxidrome.
- Meperidine, in addition to opioid toxidrome, is associated with seizures and may also precipitate serotonin syndrome.
- Propoxyphene is an opioid analgesic with unique toxicity in addition to opioid toxidrome.
  - CNS: Seizures may occur.
  - Cardiovascular: Mild hypotension is common; myocardial depression may develop with severe poisoning.

DON'T FORGET

- Propoxyphene can cause cardiac toxicity and seizures.
- Meperidine can cause seizures and serotonin syndrome.
- Give naloxone right away to avoid having to intubate a patient.
- Give up to 10 mg of naloxone, especially for methadone and fentanyl.

Review Initial Results

- Urine toxicology screen may be positive for opioids, but doesn't rule out exposure if negative.
  - Methadone, fentanyl, and propoxyphene don't show up on urine toxicology screen.
  - Diagnosis is based on toxidrome recognition.
- CXR: Opioids may cause noncardiogenic pulmonary edema.
- ECG: Propoxyphene can cause a sodium channel blockade with subsequent increase in QRS duration—also may cause various dysrhythmias, including tachycardia, bradycardia, ventricular dysrhythmias, and atrioventricular blocks.

Risk Stratification: Management Priorities

- Meticulous attention to airway and ventilation as apnea followed by hypoxemia is the most significant complication of opioid toxicity.

Definitive Management

- Naloxone: If rapidly available and given immediately, may obviate need for intubation/mechanical ventilation.
  - Initial naloxone dose:
    - 0.1 mg/kg up to 2 mg in children
    - 0.4 mg to 2 mg in non–opiate-habituated adults
    - 0.4 mg in opiate-habituated adults
  - If inadequate response, consider escalating doses until a single (noncumulative) dose of 10 mg is administered.
  - For long-acting ingestions, consider a titrated naloxone infusion starting at 2/3 of full response dose per hour.
- Sodium bicarbonate may be administered for QRS interval prolongation or hypotension associated with propoxyphene.
  - Sodium bicarbonate 1-2 mEq/kg IV push (bolus); may repeat until QRS normalizes and VS improve

Further Reassessment

- Assess for efficacy of treatment.
  - Reversal of CNS depression
  - Reversal of respiratory depression
  - Normalization of VS

Complications

- Withdrawal may be precipitated in opiate-habituated patients.
- Short duration of naloxone activity (<30 minutes) may require additional doses of antidote if clinical signs of intoxication recur.
- Check for noncardiogenic pulmonary edema as this may develop after naloxone administration.

Disposition

- Patients with noncardiogenic pulmonary edema, hypotension, dysrhythmias, and respiratory depression should be admitted.
- Patients who are not suicidal and asymptomatic may be discharged after an appropriate period of observation following naloxone treatment.

DON'T FORGET

Usually get this toxidrome from diphenhydramine.

ANTICHOLINERGIC

Additional History and Physical Examination Findings

- Multiple agents can bring about anticholinergic symptoms.
  - Usually results from diphenhydramine or TCA overdose
- Will exhibit anticholinergic toxidrome.

Review Initial Results

- ECG: Primarily to evaluate for possible TCA overdose (refer to Sec. Tricyclic Antidepressants).

Risk Stratification: Management Priorities

- Need to determine the cause of toxidrome because if caused by TCA, much greater toxicity.

Definitive Management

- Decontamination
  - Gastric lavage: May be considered with significant ingestions if patient presents within an hour of ingestion. Delayed lavage may be considered outside of the 60-minute window as the anticholinergic effects may delay gastric emptying.
  - Activated charcoal
- Supportive care:
  - Support airway, breathing, and circulation.
  - Treat seizures with benzodiazepines or barbiturates.
    - Phenytoin/fosphenytoin is considered less effective at treating toxin-induced seizures.
  - Consider treatment of prolonged QRS or wide-complex dysrythmias with sodium bicarbonate (1 to 2 mEq/kg).
    - Endpoint of therapy would include cessation of arrhythmia and narrowing of QRS complex.
  - CNS excitation: Consider benzodiazepines for sedation of patient.
  - Movement disorders (eg, dystonia, choreoathetoid movements):
    - Benzodiazepines may be used for treatment of anticholinergic-induced movement disorders.

- Hyperthermia:
  - Cool mist and fans are the most effective means of external cooling.
  - Benzodiazepines may be of use to decrease muscular rigidity and agitation that may contribute to the hyperthermic condition of the patient.
  - Severe poisoning and hyperthermia may require intubation with neuromuscular blockade; a continuous EEG will be needed to monitor for occult seizure activity while the patient is paralyzed.
- Antidotal therapy
  - Physostigmine (Antilirium) may be considered for severe poisoning.
    - Physostigmine may be used as a diagnostic agent to distinguish anticholinergic delirium from other causes of altered mental status.
    - Reversal of anticholinergic signs and symptoms for an extended period of time is not possible because the duration of action of physostigmine is only 20-60 minutes.
    - Coma may be reversed dramatically with this antidote, but physostigmine generally is not recommended just to keep a patient awake.
    - Physostigmine may be used to treat seizures and severe agitation unresponsive to supportive measures; however, safety and efficacy for these indications have not been firmly established.
    - Physostigmine generally is not recommended in patients with suspected TCA overdose or in a patient with an ECG suggestive of TCA overdose.

Further Reassessment

- Keep agitation under control.
- Keep patient normothermic.
- Control seizures.

Complications

- Heart block may be brought about by physostigmine administration.

Disposition

- Admit all symptomatic patients.
- Patient who need active cooling, benzodiazepines for agitation, or seizure control should be admitted to the ICU.
- Discharge patient who are asymptomatic after a 6- to 8-hour observation period.

COCAINE AND AMPHETAMINES (METHYLPHENIDATE, METAMPHETAMINE)

Additional History and Physical Examination Findings

- Sympathomimetic toxidrome
- Other signs/symptoms
  - Chest pain caused by aortic dissection or myocardial ischemia or infarction.
  - Dyspnea caused by pneumothorax or pneumomediastinum.
  - Agitation or seizures.
  - Abdominal pain caused by bowel necrosis or ischemia.

Review Initial Results

- ECG: The patient is probably tachycardic; evaluate for signs of other dysrhythmias or any evidence of ischemia.
- BMP: Assess patient's electrolyte status and renal function.
- CXR: Evaluate for pneumothorax or pneumomediastinum, especially if patient was smoking and now complains of chest pain and dyspnea.

- KUB: Look for packets if suspected (the young tachycardic, diaphoretic patient with seizures who was transported by ambulance from the airport).
- CPK: Especially in patients with agitation and hyperthermia to assess for rhabdomyolysis.
- Head CT: Especially if altered mental status, seizure, agitation, or neurologic deficit.

DON'T FORGET

Ask for the temperature in any suspected case of cocaine overdose.

Risk Stratification: Management Priorities

- Hyperthermia on presentation correlates with higher mortality—don't forget to assess temperature on examination day.
- Other severe effects include altered mental status, seizures, cardiac dysrhythmias, myocardial ischemia or infarction, acute renal failure, and rhabdomyolysis.

Definitive Management

- Gastric decontamination
  - Activated charcoal if significant ingestion and presenting in a timely manner.
  - WBI should be considered for body packers (patients who smuggle massive amounts of cocaine inside rubber packets that are contained within their GI tract).
- Agitation
  - Treat with benzodiazepines.
  - Avoid haloperidol as it may aggravate hyperthermia.
- Hypertension
  - Initially treat with judicious amounts of benzodiazepines.
  - If hypertensive emergency, consider nitroprusside.
  - Do not give a beta-blocker as this may lead to a paradoxical elevation of BP due to unopposed alpha-adrenergic stimulation.
- Myocardial ischemia/infarction
  - Treat as for ACS.
  - One caveat: Consider avoiding beta-blockers.
- Hyperthermia
  - Cool mist and fans are the most effective means of external cooling.
  - Benzodiazepines may be of use to decrease muscular rigidity and agitation that may contribute to the hyperthermic condition of the patient.
  - Severe poisoning and hyperthermia may need intubation with neuromuscular blockade; a continuous EEG will be needed to monitor for occult seizure activity while the patient is paralyzed.

Further Reassessment

- Continuous cardiac monitoring.
- Frequent assessment of core body temperature if initially hyperthermic.
- Follow CPK levels in patients with hyperthermia.
- If patient had rhabdomyolysis, need to maintain adequate hydration status which may require monitoring urine output.

Complications

- Rhabdomyolysis
- Acute renal failure
- Cardiac dysfunction
- Cerebral injury

Disposition

- Any patient with evidence of complications needs admission.
- Significant hyperthermia, seizures, and myocardial infarction should go to an ICU.

- Patients may be discharged following an appropriate observation period (longer period for sustained-release preparations) if asymptomatic with normal VS and normal mental status.

SEROTONIN SYNDROME

Additional History and Physical Examination Findings

- Serotonin syndrome most commonly occurs following the use of combinations of serotonergic agents, but is also reported in patients following a single dose, therapeutic dosing, or overdose of serotonergic agents.
- Drugs implicated in causing serotonin syndrome include monoamine oxidase inhibitors, SSRI, and amphetamines (eg, ecstasy).
- When other etiologies are excluded and a serotonergic agent has been used, the following clinical findings suggest the diagnosis of serotonin syndrome:
  - Musculoskeletal: Muscular rigidity.
  - Autonomic: Hyperthermia, autonomic instability, and diaphoresis may be seen.
  - Neurologic: Altered mental status, agitation, hyperreflexia, tremor, incoordination, and myoclonus.
  - GI: Diarrhea.

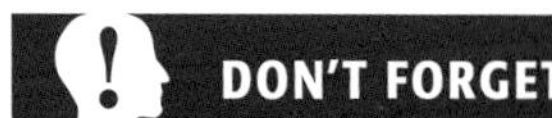

DON'T FORGET

Consider serotonin syndrome in patients with altered mental status, autonomic instability, rigidity and history of using multiple serotonergic agents (eg, selective serotonin reuptake inhibitor [SSRI] + Ecstacy).

Review Initial Results

- No specific laboratory tests are used to diagnose serotonin syndrome.
- Following CPK, urinalysis, renal, hepatic function, and disseminated intravascular coagulation (DIC) profile may be useful as the patient with serotonin syndrome may develop lactic acidosis, rhabdomyolysis, renal and hepatic dysfunction, and DIC.

Risk Stratification: Management Priorities

- Time will resolve the syndrome, but meticulous supportive care is required to prevent complications.

Definitive Management

- Withdraw offending agent(s)
- Supportive care is the mainstay of treatment.
  - Rapid external cooling with fans and mist if hyperthermia exists.
  - Benzodiazepines for muscular rigidity, agitation.
  - Neuromuscular blockade along with intubation may be needed for severe cases.
- Drug therapy
  - Cyproheptadine may be effective.

Further Reassessment

- Serial CPKs to monitor for rhabdomyolysis.
- Continuous core temperature monitoring.

Complications

- Rhabdomyolysis
- DIC
- Hepatic dysfunction
- Renal dysfunction
- Lactic acidosis

Disposition

- Serotonin syndrome resolves in most patients within 24-48 hours after the removal of the offending agent. Any patient with serotonin syndrome should be admitted to the hospital.

NEUROLEPTIC MALIGNANT SYNDROME

DON'T FORGET

NMS looks like serotonin syndrome with altered mental status, autonomic instability, rigidity (lead-pipe)—key difference is patient is on a neuroleptic agent.

Additional History and Physical Examination Findings

- NMS presents with a spectrum of findings.
  - Neurologic: The patient may see agitation, confusion, or coma. Movement disorders such as chorea, lead-pipe rigidity, dystonia, dysphagia, tremors, and opisthotonus.
  - Hyperthermia
  - Cardiovascular: Autonomic instability with labile BP and heart rate.
  - Renal: Acute renal failure from acute tubular necrosis caused by hypoperfusion or rhabdomyolysis.
  - Musculoskeletal: Rigidity and tremors may be seen.

Risk Stratification: Management Priorities

- Patients with NMS carry a 20% mortality.

Review Initial Results

- ECG: May show tachycardia, but no specific ECG changes are associated with this disorder.
- BMP: May show a metabolic acidosis or renal failure.
- Specific antipsychotic levels are not helpful.
- Total CPK and urinalysis (for blood, casts, or other signs of renal injury).

Definitive Management

- Discontinue the medication suspected of causing NMS.
- Active cooling for hyperthermia.
  - Cool mist and fans are the most effective and easiest means.
  - As a significant amount of hyperthermia may be generated by increased muscle activity, paralysis using a nondepolarizing agent such as vecuronium may also be necessary.
  - Benzodiazepines to treat rigidity and assist in sedation and relaxation.
- IV hydration to maintain adequate urine output and renal function.
- Consider alkalinizing urine if rhabdomyolysis is present.
- Antidotal therapy:
  - Currently, there is no universally effective antidote. However, there are some agents that are utilized on the basis of treating the relative dopamine depletion that is the pathophysiologic cause of NMS.
    - Bromocriptine: 2.5-5 mg PO tid

Further Reassessment

- Core body temperature: Continue to monitor, cool patient until normothermic.
- CPK: Serial measurements may be needed as rhabdomyolysis may be a delayed finding.

Complications

- Rhabdomyolysis: Treat with IV fluids and possible urinary alkalinization to help protect the kidneys.

Disposition

- Patients with NMS require intensive supportive care, so they need to be admitted to an ICU.

WINNING STRATEGIES

- All APAP overdoses get NAC.
- Acute ASA overdose has a classic acid-base disturbance and characteristic symptoms—start treatment right away prior to ASA level if the patient is symptomatic.
- Recognize hypotension and bradycardia may indicate beta-blocker or calcium channel blocker overdose; should consider digoxin as well.
- Digoxin-specific Fab fragments to any hyperkalemic patient with digoxin toxicity.
- Theophylline: If seizure, cardiovascular instability → dialysis.
- Valproic acid: Check the ammonia level.
- TCAs: Sodium bicarbonate for QRS widening until QRS narrows.
- Antipsychotics: Usually self-limited, but beware NMS.
- Lithium: Dialyze any patient with altered mental status and elevated lithium level.
- Iron: Toxicity correlates to acidemia—don't be fooled by the quiescent phase.
- Lead: Usually chronic—patients with encephalopathy need ICU admission and chelation therapy with BAL and $CaNa_2EDTA$.
- Methemoglobin: Patient with an oxygen saturation of 85% and not responding to oxygen → think methemoglobinemia.
- Carbon monoxide: Starting to get cold outside and people who live together who present with headaches, nausea → think CO.
- Cyanide: Beware the chemist who comes by ambulance comatose and severely acidemic—may be cyanide.
- Hydrocarbons: Kid who gets into lamp oil and starts coughing is bad news—may have aspiration or chemical pneumonitis, requiring ventilatory support.
- Organophosphates/nerve agent (eg, atropine)—don't forget about 2-PAM as well.
- Ethylene glycol/methanol: Recognize in the patient with altered mental status and high anion gap acidosis—start treating right away while waiting for confirmatory testing.
- Opioids: If the picture fits → Naloxone (up to 10 mg)—until patient is awake and doesn't need to be intubated.
- Anticholinergic: Dry, crazy, hyperthermic, and flushed—keep them comfortable with benzodiazepines; physostigmine doesn't add much value.
- Cocaine: Watch for rhabdomyolysis.
- Serotonin syndrome: Need to consider it in patient who has altered mental status and is on multiple serotonergic drugs.
- Neuroleptic malignant syndrome: Consider in the rigid, hyperthermic patient with altered mental status and taking antipsychotic agents, that is, after ruling out meningitis!

CHAPTER 17

Altered Mental Status: Environment and Endocrine

Navneet Cheema and James Rhee

INITIAL ASSESSMENT/INTERVENTION

- Age:
  - Pediatric: Consider accidental ingestions.
  - Adult: Consider intentional overdose, recreational misadventure.
  - Geriatric: Consider iatrogenic, sepsis, intracerebral hemorrhage.
- Vital signs (VS): Make sure to obtain a complete set of vitals including temperature and oxygen saturation.
- Mental status: Agitated? Depressed? Comatose?
- Signs of trauma: If any question, immobilize C-spine.
- Coma cocktail: DON'T.
  - **D**exi: Check fingerstick glucose or administer parenteral glucose.
  - **O**xygen: Check for hypoxemia or administer oxygen.
  - **N**aloxone: Administer naloxone especially for respiratory depression.
  - **T**hiamine: Administer thiamine 100 mg intravenously (IV) to prevent or treat Wernicke encephalopathy if patient appears malnourished.

DON'T FORGET

On test day, the patient will have AEIOU: TIPS

A: *Alcohol, abuse*
E: *Epilepsy, electrolyte disorders, encephalopathy, endocrine*
I: *Insulin*
O: *Oxygen*
U: *Uremia*
T: *Trauma, temperature, tumors*
I: *Infections*
P: *Psychiatry, poisoning*
S: *Shock, stroke, subarachnoid hemorrhage*

INITIAL HISTORY AND PHYSICAL EXAMINATION

History

- History of present illness (HPI): Often times unavailable through the patient—need to establish through other means—family, friends, witnesses, paramedics, nursing home, primary care physician, medical records.
- Past medical history (PMHx): Especially to give hints of possible ingestions or conditions (eg, diabetes → hypoglycemia, diabetic ketoacidosis [DKA]; schizophrenia → lithium overdose, neuroleptic malignant syndrome; chronic pain syndrome → opioid overdose, tricyclic antidepressant [TCA] overdose; etc).
- Medications/herbs/supplements/drugs: One of the most important components of the history as this may help make the diagnosis—sometimes takes a little bit of sleuthing—call friends, pharmacy, and physicians; send paramedics back to the scene, medical records—don't forget about other medications that may be in the house (eg, grandma's calcium channel blocker, dog's TCA, etc).
- Social history: Work history is especially important as this may lead to source of exposure.
- Allergies: Medication and food allergies.

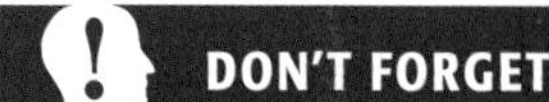
DON'T FORGET

Any patient with altered mental status needs prompt airway evaluation.

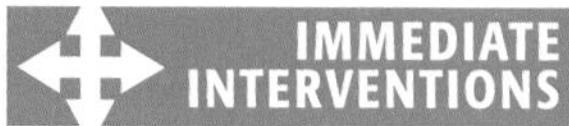
IMMEDIATE INTERVENTIONS

- IV, oxygen, cardiac monitor
- C-spine immobilization

Physical Examination

- VS: Make sure to obtain a complete set of vitals including temperature and oxygen saturation.
- General: What does the patient look like? Are there any distinct odors detected (eg, ethyl alcohol [EtOH], fruity, garlic, bitter almonds)?
- Head: Any signs of trauma such as hematomas, lacerations, or abrasions?
- Eyes: Assess pupils for size, symmetry, and reactivity; look for nystagmus; evaluate for papilledema.
- Ears: Any hemotympanum or blood in the ear canal?
- Nose: Any residue of powder or soot around nares?
- Mouth: Any tongue lacerations? Mucous membranes dry or moist? Any irritation or corrosions?
- Cardiovascular: Tachycardic or bradycardic?
- Respiratory: Any tachypnea or crackles?
- Abdomen: Note bowel sound activity; any hematemesis, melena, or hematochezia? Distended bladder?
- Extremities: Any rigidity?

- Neuro: Assess for mental status, seizure activity, muscle tone, and tremor.
- Skin: Any cyanosis? Hot or cold? Dry or wet? Flushed? Puncture marks or needle tracks?

DIFFERENTIAL DIAGNOSIS

The differential diagnosis for altered mental status is broad.

- **A:** Alcohol, abuse
  - Obviously, alcohol in excess can cause altered mental status. Conversely, patients who are dependent on alcohol can present with delirium tremens. In children, alcohol suppresses the liver's ability to make glucose; therefore, alcohol intoxication increases susceptibility to hypoglycemia and altered mental status.
  - Child abuse may be associated with altered mental status caused by head trauma or diffuse brain injury.
- **E:** Epilepsy, electrolyte disorders, encephalopathy, endocrine
  - Nonconvulsive seizures or postictal states can cause altered mental status.
  - Electrolyte disorders involving sodium, calcium, potassium, or magnesium can cause altered mental status secondary to dehydration, shock, and altered neuron function.
  - Encephalopathy affects the cerebral hemispheres, often resulting in confusion and behavioral changes. In children, encephalopathy may be caused by Reye syndrome, which can arise when parents give a child aspirin during an episode of varicella or flu-like illness. There are many other causes of encephalopathy, including herpes, cytomegalovirus, and human immunodeficiency virus (HIV).
  - Endocrine primarily refers to diabetic problems, including hypoglycemia and hyperglycemia. Other endocrine problems, including thyroid disorders and adrenal insufficiency may also result in altered mental status.
- **I:** Insulin
  - Insulin deficiency leading to DKA may result in altered mental status especially in children. Conversely, insulin excess, which may occur either because of insulin overdose or because of inadequate food intake, can cause hypoglycemia with signs suggestive of shock.
- **O:** Oxygen
  - Lack of oxygen to the brain will cause altered mental status. There are many possibilities for poor oxygen delivery to the brain including poor perfusion (shock states), displacement of oxygen from hemoglobin (carbon monoxide), inability of hemoglobin to bind to oxygen (methemoglobinemia), low levels of surrounding oxygen (high-altitude), ventilation-perfusion (V/Q) mismatch, pulmonary embolism (PE), etc.
- **U:** Uremia (and other metabolic causes)
  - In renal failure, uremia arises when abnormal levels of urea nitrogen, a waste product of nitrogen metabolism, accumulate in the blood.
  - Other metabolic causes of altered mental status include hepatic problems, adrenal insufficiency, and congenital enzyme defects.
- **T:** Trauma, temperature, tumors
  - Head trauma that results in brain injury may cause increased intracranial pressure, hemorrhage, or a concussion. Any traumatic injury that causes hypoxemia or shock, including that arising from child abuse, will generally have altered mental status as a presenting sign.
  - Abnormal body temperature (hypothermia or hyperthermia) is frequently associated with altered mental status.
  - Tumors or other mass lesions of the brain or brain stem may cause altered mental status as well.

- **I:** Infection
  - Meningitis, encephalitis, sepsis, and post-infectious encephalopathy can cause altered mental status.
- **P:** Psychiatric, poisonings
  - Psychiatric causes of altered mental status exist, but factitious altered mental status is rare in younger children; this should be a diagnosis of exclusion.
  - Many different poisonings may result in altered mental status—keep in mind that these toxic events may be either from accidental or intentional ingestion.
- **S:** Shock, stroke, subarachnoid hemorrhage
  - Shock is frequently associated with altered mental status.
  - Stroke is a possible etiology of altered mental status—especially if it affects the reticular activating system.
  - Subarachnoid hemorrhage can also cause altered mental status.

For discussion of the management of the poisoned, overdosed, or intoxicated patient, please refer to the Chap. 16. The remainder of this chapter will be devoted to nontoxicologic causes of altered mental status.

HYPERTHERMIA

Additional History and Physical Examination Findings

- Heat exhaustion
  - Elevated temperature
  - Dizziness and headache
  - Nausea and vomiting
  - Diaphoresis (lack of sweating is one of the classic signs of heat stroke)
  - Other heat-related symptoms: Heat syncope, heat cramps, heat tetany
  - Normal mental status
- Classic heat stroke
  - Typically affects elderly, chronically ill during heat waves.
  - Patients on diuretics and anticholinergics are also prone to this condition.
  - Symptoms are similar to heat exhaustion with the following:
  - Temperature usually >106°F (41°C)
  - Anhydrosis
  - Tachypnea
  - Altered mental status
- Exertional heat stroke
  - Affects younger patients who are overcome by heat production—typically athletes, military recruits.
  - Symptoms are similar to heat exhaustion and classic heat stroke.
    - Temperature usually >106°F (41°C)

Review Initial Results

- Basic metabolic panel (BMP), calcium, magnesium, phosphorus: Many possible electrolyte derangements caused by sweating, and the possibility of rhabdomyolysis and renal failure.
- Liver function tests (LFTs): They are consistently elevated with heat stroke.
- Urinalysis (UA): It may be heme positive with no red blood cells (RBCs) in the setting of rhabdomyolysis.
- Creatine phosphokinase (CPK): Evaluate for rhabdomyolysis.
- Urine myoglobin.

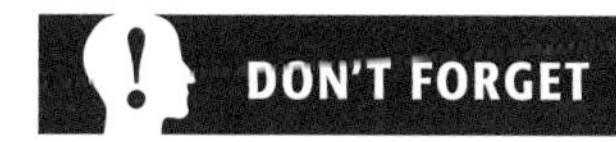

Don't forget to evaluate for rhabdomyolysis.

Risk Stratification: Management Priorities

- Heat stroke is a true medical emergency.
- Heat exhaustion.
  - Risk of death is related to peak temperature and exposure.
    - If treated early, mortality = 10%-15%
    - If treated late, mortality = 80%

Definitive Management

DON'T FORGET

Get the patient cool as fast as possible. Lowering body temperature is the definitive treatment of heat shock—all other treatments are supportive.

- Cooled IV hydration to maintain adequate urine output and renal function.
- Remove from offending environment.
- Active cooling measures for heat stroke.
  - Cool mist and fans—probably the most effective and easy to do.
  - Ice bath immersion is also very effective but difficult to do.
- After adequate fluid resuscitation, consider alkalinizing urine if rhabdomyolysis is present.
- Antipyretics are ineffective.

Further Reassessment

- Continuous core body temperature monitoring.

Complications

- Rebound hypothermia
- Rhabdomyolysis

Disposition

- Patients with true heat stroke should be admitted to the intensive care unit (ICU).

HYPOTHERMIA

Additional History and Physical Examination Findings

- Evaluate for precipitant and predisposing risk factors as these factors may need to be addressed during the patient's treatment.
  - Hypoglycemia
  - Sepsis
  - Alcohol
  - Overdose
  - Endocrinopathy
- Signs and symptoms correlate with degree of hypothermia.
  - Mild: 90-95°F (32-35°C)
    - Shivering
    - Dysarthria
    - Ataxia
    - Lethargy and altered mental status
    - Tachypnea
    - Tachycardia
  - Moderate: 86-90°F (30-32°C)
    - Shivering ceases
    - Stupor
    - Bradycardia
    - Mydriasis
    - Dysrhythmias

- Severe: <86°F (<32°C)
    - No shivering
    - Coma
    - Hypotension
    - Fixed and dilated pupils
    - Cold skin
    - Ventricular tachycardia (VT) or asystole

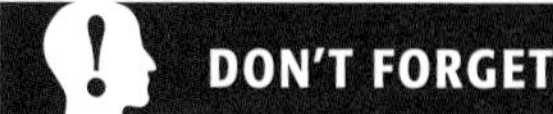

DON'T FORGET

Don't forget to evaluate for rhabdomyolysis.

Review Initial Results

- Temperature: Need core body temperature.
- Glucose: Check right away for hypoglycemia.
- Arterial blood gas (ABG): Because the pulse oximetry probably won't be helpful given the amount of peripheral vasoconstriction that the patient has when significantly hypothermic.
- Electrocardiogram (ECG): This may reveal Osborne waves (J point deflection in same direction as QRS complex); atrial fibrillation and sinus bradycardia are also common findings.
- Coagulation studies: Patient may still be coagulopathic in the setting of normal prothrombin time/partial thromboplastin time (PT/PTT).
- Computed tomography (CT) head: Especially if patient has evidence of traumas.

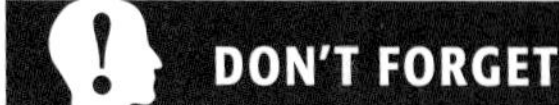

DON'T FORGET

If patient is cold and not shivering (ask if the patient is shivering on exam day), you need to use active measures to rewarm the patient.

Risk Stratification: Management Priorities

- Mild: Passive external rewarming measures only.
- Moderate: Passive external rewarming in addition to active external rewarming.
- Severe: Passive external rewarming, active external rewarming, and active internal rewarming—call cardiac or thoracic surgeon right away if considering.
- Potassium: Levels >10 mEq/L have been associated with poor prognosis.

Definitive Management

- Passive external rewarming
    - Remove wet clothing
    - Warm blankets
- Active external rewarming
    - Only to truncal areas to avoid core temperature "afterdrop" which occurs when peripheral vasodilation from rewarming extremities will cause the return of cooler, peripheral blood to core
    - Mechanical warming blanket
    - Heat lamps
    - Hot water bottles (45-65°C) to axilla and groin
- Active internal rewarming
    - Warm IV fluids (45°C)
        - As this measure is fairly noninvasive, use this modality for the less severe forms of hypothermia as well.
    - Warm humidified oxygen (45°C)
        - Doesn't rewarm as much as it prevents heat loss—again a fairly noninvasive measure that should be used judiciously in the less severe forms of hypothermia
    - Warmed gastric lavage via nasogastric (NG) tube.
    - Warmed bladder irrigation via three-way Foley.
    - Warmed peritoneal irrigation via diagnostic peritoneal lavage (DPL) catheter.
    - Warmed thoracic cavity irrigation via chest tubes.
    - Warmed hemodialysis.
        - Would also remove certain toxins, help correct acid–base status and electrolyte derangements.

DON'T FORGET

Don't forget to check the blood glucose as hypoglycemia is one of the most common causes of hypothermia.

- Cardiopulmonary bypass
  - Most effective means to rewarm core temperature.
  - Consider this immediately especially if patient is in cardiac arrest.
  - Call cardiac or thoracic surgeon immediately if considering.

Further Reassessment

- Continuous monitoring of core body temperature: If patient not warming up adequately, need to consider more aggressive modalities—also may want to empirically administer hydrocortisone and/or levothyroxine to treat a possible underlying endocrinopathy.
- Assess if mental status has improved. If it is not improving, consider the precipitating factors that led to the patient's condition.

Complications

- Dysrhythmias: Treat as per ACLS guidelines.
  - Best (and only definitive) treatment is rewarming the patient.
  - Defibrillate ventricular fibrillation (VT) a maximum of three times if patient's core temperature is <30°C.
  - Bretylium has traditionally been the drug of choice for ventricular dysrhythmias in the setting of hypothermia.

Disposition

- Patients who require active rewarming measures need to be admitted—the most appropriate level of care for moderate to severe hypothermia is an ICU.
- Patients who presented for mild hypothermia who have been warmed back to normal temperature, are asymptomatic, have a clear cause for the hypothermia that has been corrected may be considered for discharge.

HIGH-ALTITUDE ILLNESS

Additional History and Physical Examination Findings

- Recent altitude gain: >2500 m (8200 ft)
- Acute mountain sickness (AMS):
  - Symptoms typically occur and develop 6-10 hours after ascent.
  - Usually resolves within 4 days.
  - Symptoms:
    - Dizziness, fatigue, lassitude
    - Shortness of breath (SOB), exertional dyspnea
    - Headache: Occipital or bitemporal throbbing headache—worse in morning, when supine, and after exercise
    - Nausea, vomiting
    - Decreased urine output, edema
    - Insomnia
- High-altitude pulmonary edema (HAPE)
  - Mild symptoms
    - Dry cough
    - Exertional dyspnea
    - Fatigue
    - Localized rales
  - Moderate symptoms
    - Periodic (Cheyne-Stokes) breathing during sleep
    - Tachycardia and tachypnea
    - Dyspnea at rest

- Severe symptoms
  - Orthopnea
  - Generalized rales
  - White, watery, frothy fluid
  - Impaired cerebral function, mental status changes
  - Cyanosis: Unable to raise oxygen saturation to >90% even after treatment with high-flow oxygen.
- High-altitude cerebral edema (HACE)
  - Altered mental status
  - Ataxia
  - Muscle weakness
  - Bladder dysfunction
  - Papilledema and retinal hemorrhage (5%-40%)
  - Seizures (rare)

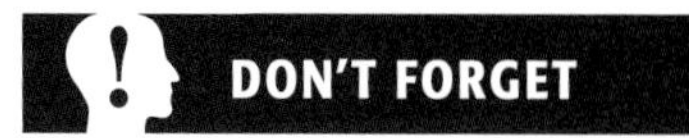

Definitive treatment is descent for all high-altitude illnesses.

Review Initial Results

- Pulse oximetry: Marked hypoxemia is a common finding in HAPE.
- ABG: May see hypoxemia and respiratory alkalosis with HAPE.
- ECG: May see tachycardia.
- Chest x-ray (CXR): In HAPE may demonstrate homogenous or patchy opacities in one or both lungs.
- Head CT especially for altered mental status despite descent and treatment.

Risk Stratification: Management Priorities

- AMS: Generally self-limited.
- HAPE: Immediate descent if moderate to severe symptoms.
- HACE: Medical emergency, needs immediate descent.

Definitive Management

- AMS
  - Stop ascent.
  - Mild cases are usually benign and self-limited.
    - Symptomatic care.
    - Acetazolamide 125-250 mg PO q12h will accelerate acclimatization.
  - If symptoms are severe or persistent, then descend.
- HAPE
  - Descend as soon as possible with minimal exertion.
  - Supplemental oxygen.
  - Positive pressure ventilation and beta-agonist inhalers may be helpful.
  - If descent is not possible or oxygen is unavailable,
  - Portable hyperbaric chamber
  - Nifedipine 10 mg PO, then 30 mg sustained release PO q12h
  - Add dexamethasone if neurologic deterioration occurs.
- HACE
  - Immediate descent.
  - Supplemental oxygen.
  - Dexamethasone 8 mg IV and then 4 mg q6h.
  - Portable hyperbaric chamber if descent delayed.
  - Acetazolamide 125-250 mg PO q12h if descent delayed.
  - Furosemide 40-80 mg IV may help reduce brain edema.

Further Reassessment

- Cases of HAPE or HACE need a reassessment 24 hours after discharge if not admitted.

Disposition

- Mild cases of AMS with no further symptoms for 6-12 hours after descent may go home.
- Patients with good saturation and resolving symptoms may be discharged.
  - Patients should be reevaluated in 24 hours.
  - Educate patient to return if any further SOB.
- Admit patients with significant desaturation, persistent mental status changes or neurologic deficits.

ENDOCRINE: MYXEDEMA COMA

Additional History and Physical Examination Findings

- Typical signs and symptoms include
  - Altered mental status or coma
  - Hypothermia
  - Bradycardia
  - Hypotension
  - Generalized non-pitting edema
  - Dry, coarse hair
  - Cool, dry, puffy skin
  - Deep tendon reflexes (DTRs) with a prolonged lag phase
  - May see a thyroidectomy scar—need to ask specifically when examining the neck.

Review Initial Results

- Thyroid function tests will unlikely be readily available for initial review, but should still be sent as the act of sending the confirmatory test will be a critical action.
  - High thyroid-stimulating hormone (TSH)
  - Low free T4
- ECG may reveal profound bradycardia.
- BMP: This may show hyponatremia as well from syndrome of inappropriate secretion of antidiuretic hormone (SIADH).

Risk Stratification: Management Priorities

- Myxedema coma is a life-threatening condition that needs immediate treatment.
- Hyponatremia is indicative of a poor prognosis.

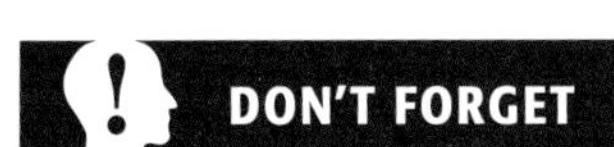

Don't forget to treat for possible adrenal insufficiency as well.

Definitive Management

- Thyroid hormone replacement
  - Thyroxine 4 μg/kg IV bolus, then 100 μg IV 24 hours later, and then 50 μg every 24 hours until tolerating oral agents.
- Stress dose steroids for likely concomitant adrenal insufficiency.
  - Hydrocortisone 100 mg IV

Further Reassessment

- Identify precipitating cause (usually infection) and treat appropriately.

Complications

- Hypotension
  - Treat with IV fluid boluses.
  - Pressors only if needed as this may precipitate a dysrhythmia.
    - Response to pressors may be poor unless thyroid hormone is replaced.

- Hypothermia
  - Initiate passive warming measures, eg, warm blankets.
- Hypoglycemia
  - Correct accordingly with parenteral glucose.

Disposition

- Patients with myxedema coma need to be admitted to the ICU.

HYPOGLYCEMIA

Additional History and Physical Examination Findings

- Common signs and symptoms include
  - Tachycardia (progresses to bradycardia as symptoms get more severe)
  - Diaphoresis
  - Anxiety and tremor
  - Hunger
  - Altered mental status or coma (that's why "D" is in the "DON'T coma cocktail")
  - Hypothermia
- Etiology
  - Excess parenteral insulin
  - EtOH
  - Oral hypoglycemics
  - Insulinoma
  - Adrenal insufficiency
  - Hypothyroidism
  - Liver disease
  - Chronic renal failure
  - Hypothermia

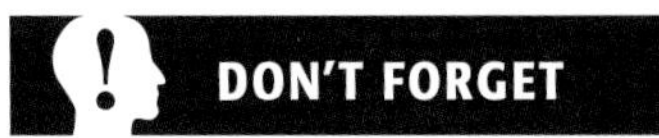

Identify the cause of hypoglycemia; this will be a critical action.

Review Initial Results

- Blood glucose <50 mg/dL.
- Temperature: Treat hypothermia.
- Thyroid function tests may be sent if hypothyroidism is being considered.

Risk Stratification: Management Priorities

- Need to determine underlying reason for patient's condition.

Definitive Management

- Dextrose administration:
  - PO administration of simple sugars if the patient is awake and alert.
  - If unresponsive or mental status depression, IV administration.
    - Adults: 1-2 mL/kg D50W IV
    - Children: 2-4 mL/kg D25W IV
    - Neonates: 5 mL/kg D10W IV
- Glucagon if unable to establish IV—1 mg intramuscularly (IM)—do not need to use if IV is established—hopefully on exam day, the nurses will be able to start a line.
- Hypoglycemia caused by sulfonylureas—in addition to above measures, may try using the following agents:
  - Octreotide
    - Octreotide may be given if an IV dextrose infusion fails to correct hypoglycemia (especially if sulfonylurea overdose is suspected).
    - Adults: 50-100 μg subcutaneously (SC) or IV q6-12h.
    - Children: 1-10 μg SC or IV q6-12h.

Further Reassessment

- Frequent repeat blood glucose measurements to assess adequacy of treatment.

Disposition

- If patient is asymptomatic after correction and etiology is clear, then can discharge patient home.
- A patient who ingests sulfonylureas should be admitted to the hospital if it is a deliberate overdose, complicated by hypoglycemia, or the patient is a young child.
  - Ingestion of just one tablet of a chlorpropamide, glipizide, or glyburide can produce profound hypoglycemia in a child, and delayed (up to 16 hours) onset of hypoglycemia with these agents has been reported. Therefore, observation for a period of at least 12-24 hours postingestion is recommended.
- Patients who have an unclear etiology of hypoglycemia, ongoing neurologic deficits, or a suspected intentional overdose warrant admission.

ACUTE ADRENAL INSUFFICIENCY

Additional History and Physical Examination Findings

- Try to determine precipitant.
  - Infection
  - Cessation of steroid therapy
  - Drugs/medications (remember that etomidate can cause adrenal insufficiency)
  - Trauma
  - Burns
  - Pregnancy
- Characteristic signs and symptoms include
  - Abdominal pain, nausea, vomiting, anorexia
  - Orthostatic hypotension, syncope
  - Mental status changes, delirium, seizures
  - Weakness, fatigue, lethargy
  - Hyperpigmentation of skin (may be a clue on exam day)
  - Hypoglycemia

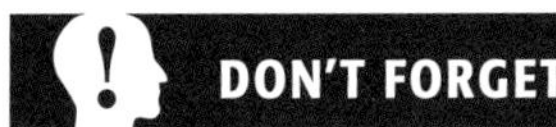

Consider meningococcemia if otherwise previously healthy, and now with acute adrenal insufficiency and sepsis—need to administer antibiotics right away.

Review Initial Results

- While not available for initial review, make sure that you draw and send a serum cortisol and a serum adrenocorticotropin (ACTH).
- Electrolytes: Characteristic picture is that of hyponatremia with hyperkalemia.
- Calcium: May have hypercalcemia.
- Hypoglycemia is characteristic, and may be severe.
- Elevated blood urea nitrogen/creatinine (BUN/Cr), azotemia from dehydration.

Risk Stratification: Management Priorities

- Patients with an adrenal crisis are critically ill and need initiation of glucocorticoid replacement right away—even without a definitive diagnosis. On exam day you may need to recognize this syndrome and start treating it right away.

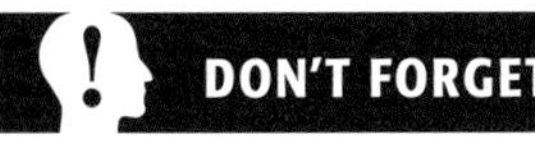

Treat adrenal shock immediately, do not delay while waiting for complicated labs to come back. Your electrolytes and examination should be enough justification.

Definitive Management

- Glucocorticoid replacement: Hydrocortisone (standard) or dexamethasone (will not interfere with cosyntropin stimulation test).
  - Hydrocortisone: 100 mg IV q6h for 24 hours, then gradually taper dose as patient improves, and change to oral maintenance dose (usually prednisone 7.5 mg/d).
  - Dexamethasone: 4 mg IV q12h

- IV fluids—normal saline (NS) for volume expansion—bolus 2 L on exam day especially if patient is hypotensive.
- Dextrose as needed for hypoglycemia.
- Treat the underlying condition/precipitant.

Further Reassessment

- Continuous cardiac monitoring.
- Frequent checks of electrolytes and glucose
- If not performed as part of initial evaluation because of the emergent patient encounter, may want to instruct the nurse to send a cosyntropin stimulation test.

Complications

- Refractory shock: Treat with more fluids, pressors, and glucocorticoids.
- Hyperkalemia-induced dysrhythmias: Treat hyperkalemia with calcium, insulin/glucose, and sodium bicarbonate.

Disposition

- Admit all patients with adrenal insufficiency. Unstable or potentially unstable patients need to go to the ICU.

DIABETIC KETOACIDOSIS

Additional History and Physical Examination Findings

- History of type 1 diabetes mellitus (DM)—however, sometimes patients will present with no history of DM (usually pediatric patients), or you may not know if patient's mental status is impaired—thus the importance of checking blood glucose right away as this may help lead to the diagnosis.
- Signs and symptoms:
  - Polyuria, polydypsia, polyphagia
  - Abdominal pain
  - Dehydration
  - Tachycardia
  - Kussmaul respiration
  - Altered mental status
  - Fruity odor
- Evaluate for precipitating cause as well:
  - Infection
  - Insulin deficiency
  - Myocardial ischemia or infarction
  - Intra-abdominal process: Pregnancy, pancreatitis, ischemic bowel

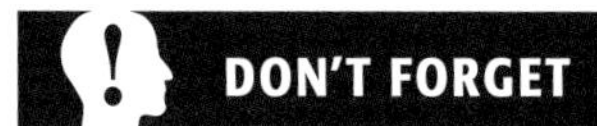

If glucose not >250 mg/dL, then consider another cause of anion gap acidosis, eg, alcoholic ketoacidosis.

Review Initial Results

- DKA diagnosis criteria:
  - Glucose >250 mg/dL
  - pH <7.3
  - Serum HCO_3 <15 mEq/L
  - Moderate ketonuria and ketonemia
- Anion gap.
- Sodium: Pseudohyponatremia may occur if glucose significantly high.
  - Corrected sodium = Na + [0.016 × (Glu – 100)]
- Potassium: Hyperkalemia may be present intitially because of extracellular shifts from acidemia.
  - This should correct on its own with IV fluids and insulin.
  - Patient most likely has a total body deficit of potassium.

- UA: Ketonuria, glycosuria—evaluate also for possible urinary tract infection (UTI) as precipitant.
- Urine ketones: Realize that may not represent true ketoacidosis as this only measures for acetone and acetoacetate—beta-hydroxybutyrate is not measured.
- Calcium, magnesium, and phosphorus may be low.

Risk Stratification: Management Priorities

- Poor prognostic factors
  - pH <7
  - High insulin requirements
  - Persistently high serum glucose
  - Persistently depressed mental status
  - Fever

Definitive Management

- Intravascular expansion and rehydration.
  - Replace intravascular deficit with 2 L of 0.9% NS solution over 1-2 hours.
  - Switch to 0.45% NS after initial bolus—titrate to fluid status or urine output.
  - Switch to D5 0.45% NS when serum glucose falls to 250 mg/dL.
- Insulin replenishment.
  - Regular insulin 0.1 U/kg IVP, followed by regular insulin drip at 0.1 U/kg/h.
- Potassium (K).
  - K >5.5 mEq/L
    - Hold K.
    - Check K every 2 hours.
  - K 3.3-5.5 mEq/L
    - Give 20-30 mEq to keep serum K at about 4-5 mEq/L.
  - K <3.3 mEq/L
    - Hold insulin.
    - Give K (40 mEq in adults) per hour until K >3.3 mEq/L.
- If arterial pH <6.9, consider administering sodium bicarbonate.
- Search for and treat precipitating factor(s).

Further Reassessment

- Monitor vitals, blood glucose, urine output, and potassium every hour until resolution of acidosis, closure of anion gap, and discontinuation of the continuous infusion of insulin.

Complications

- Cerebral edema: Possible association with sodium bicarbonate administration and overly aggressive hydration.

Disposition

- Admit all DKA.
- Patients with significant acidosis, altered mental status, and extremes of age need to go to ICU.
- Discharge patients who have been treated in the emergency department (ED) with resolution of acidemia, no evidence of anion gap acidosis, clear mentation, tolerating PO, and a clearly identified precipitant that has been corrected. This likely will not occur during the oral board exam.

HYPEROSMOLAR HYPERGLYCEMIC STATE

Additional History and Physical Examination Findings

- Occurs in type 2 diabetics: Typically older debilitated patients
- Typical signs and symptoms:
  - Polydipsia, polyuria, polyphagia
  - Coma or altered mental status
  - Profound dehydration, tachycardia, hypotension
  - Focal neurologic signs

DON'T FORGET

Classic scenario is patient with type 2 DM and renal insufficiency at nursing home with mental status changes that has been getting progressively worse over days to weeks.

Review Initial Results

- Diagnostic criteria:
  - Glucose >600 mg/dL (usually >1000 mg/dL).
  - Absence of ketoacidosis.
  - Serum osmolality >350 mOsm/kg or >320 mOsm/kg with at least mild derangement in mental status.
- UA: Glycosuria, check for signs of UTI.
- BUN/Cr: Evidence of prerenal azotemia.
- Sodium: Pseudohyponatremia may occur if glucose significantly high.
- pH normal.
- CXR evaluation for pneumonia as a precipitant.
- ECG evaluation for acute coronary syndrome (ACS) as a precipitant.

Definitive Management

- IV fluids: This is the main therapeutic intervention.
  - Use 0.9 NS rapidly 1-2 L over 1-2 hours to stabilize BP and to maintain an adequate urine output—more if needed.
  - Use 0.45% NS if patient's serum osmolality is >320 mOsm/L, if patient is hypertensive or if patient's serum sodium is >155 mEq/L.
  - Replace half of estimated volume deficit during the first 12 hours, the rest during the next 24 hours (too rapid correction may cause cerebral edema).
    - Average deficit is 8-12 L.
  - Add dextrose to solution when glucose is 250 mg/dL.
- Regular insulin drip at 0.05 IU/kg/h.
  - Insulin requirements less than those in DKA—some patients may not even require insulin.
  - Want to avoid overaggressive correction of serum glucose as this can lead to hypotension and shock.

Further Reassessment

- Frequent reassessment of volume status and mental status.
- Monitor glucose: Lower, no faster than 100-200 mg/dL/h.
- Discontinue insulin when <350 mg/dL.

Complications

- Cerebral edema: It may occur if not frequently checking electrolytes.
- Hypernatremia: It may occur from using isotonic crystalloid even after volume resuscitation.
- Arterial thrombosis: It occurs because of hyperosmolar state—look for signs of myocardial infarction, mesenteric ischemia, or pulmonary embolism.

Disposition

- Patients with hyperosmolar hyperglycemic state require ICU admission.

HYPERNATREMIA

Additional History and Physical Examination Findings

- Most commonly associated with dehydration.
- Identify hypovolemia, euvolemia, or hypervolemia.
  - Hypovolemia: Dry mucous membranes, tachycardia, poor urine output
  - Euvolemia
    - Central diabetes insipidus (DI)
      - Head trauma
      - Tumor
      - Infection
      - Cerebrovascular accident (CVA)
      - Aneurysm
    - Nephrogenic DI
      - Medications: Lithium, amphotericin
      - Metabolic: Hypercalcemia, severe hypokalemia
      - Other: Polycystic kidney disease, sickle cell disease
  - Hypervolemia: Peripheral edema, pulmonary edema
- Signs and symptoms of hypernatremia are primarily neurologic.
  - Tremor, weakness, ataxia, altered mental status, seizures

Review Initial Results

- Serum sodium
- Electrolytes
- BUN/Cr
- Glucose
- UA
- CT head

DON'T FORGET

Don't correct free water deficit too quickly → cerebral edema/seizures.

Risk Stratification: Management Priorities

- Most common cause is dehydration, so first priority is to rehydrate.

Definitive Management

- Hypovolemic hypernatremia
  - Replace volume deficit first with NS boluses.
  - Once volume repleted, start correcting free water deficit with D5W or 0.45% NS.
    - Calculate water deficit.
      - Water deficit = 0.6 (weight in kilogram) × (actual Na – desired Na)/(actual Na)
    - Replace half the deficit in the first 24 hours, then the remainder over the next 48 hours.
  - Avoid rapid correction which is associated with cerebral edema.
- Isovolemic hypernatremia
  - Central DI:
    - Restrict Na.
    - May require vasopressin (DDAVP).
  - Nephrogenic DI:
    - Restrict Na.
    - Discontinue any medications that may be responsible—may require dialysis.
- Hypervolemic hypernatremia
  - Dialysis or diuretics to remove excess volume
  - Following volume removal administer D5W.

Further Reassessment

- Assess serum sodium and volume status frequently.
  - Sodium reduction should be <0.5 mEq/L/h—cerebral edema results from correcting sodium too rapidly.

Disposition

- Admit all Na >150 mEq/L.
- Admit all Na >160 mEq/L or symptomatic patients to the ICU.
- Discharge Na <150 mEq/L if asymptomatic.

HYPERCALCEMIA

Additional History and Physical Examination Findings

- Predisposing conditions:
  - Malignancy (most common)
  - Hyperparathyroidism
  - Dysproteinemias
  - Vitamin D intoxication
  - Milk-alkali syndrome
  - Sarcoidosis
- Signs and symptoms are nonspecific.
  - Mental status changes: Apathy, depression, malaise, obtundation, psychosis, seizure, coma
  - Muscle weakness
  - Anorexia, nausea, abdominal pain, constipation
  - Polyuria, natriuresis, dehydration
  - Nephrolithiasis

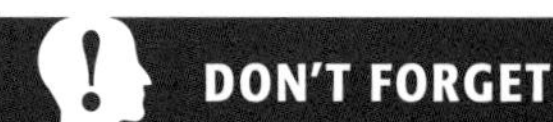

Consider hypercalcemia in any patient presenting with nonspecific symptoms and history of malignancy.

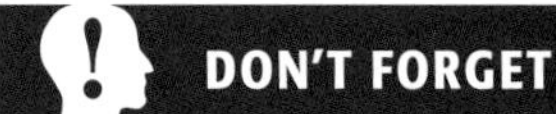

Remember the mnemonic stones (nephrolithiasis), moans (lethargy, altered mental status), groans (abdominal pain, pancreatitis), and psychiatric overtones (delirium, psychosis).

Review Initial Results

- Labs
  - Total calcium: Usually >12 mg/dL if symptomatic
    - Corrected Ca = Measured Ca × (4 − albumin concentration)
  - Ionized Ca
  - BMP
  - Alkaline phosphatase
  - Consider parathyroid hormone (PTH), T4, thyroid-stimulating hormone (TSH)
- ECG
  - Shortened QT interval
  - QRS widening
  - Heart block

Definitive Management

- IV fluids: 1-2 L over the first 2-3 hours to restore volume, then adjust to a urine output of 100-150 mL/h.
  - Furosemide: 40 mg IVP q2h if patient has renal insufficiency or heart failure to prevent fluid overload.
  - Calitonin 6 units/kg SC if calcium is >14 mg/dL or symptomatic.
  - Hydrocortisone: 100 mg IV q6h.
    - Helpful in hypercalcemia associated with malignancies.
- Dialysis for renal failure.

Further Reassessment

- Careful monitoring of volume status and calcium—check frequently.

Complications

- Nephrolithiasis
- Pancreatitis
- Cardiac conduction system blocks

Disposition

- Admit patients who are symptomatic or have corrected calcium >13 mg/dL.
- Admit patients to ICU if corrected calcium >14 mg/dL or if patient is severely symptomatic.
- Discharge asymptomatic patients whose calcium is <13 mg/dL and who have a clearly identified underlying cause which is being treated.

WINNING STRATEGIES

- Everyone with altered mental status gets a coma cocktail.
  - Dextrose (unless rapid blood glucose checked and normal)
  - Oxygen
  - Naloxone
  - Thiamine (if malnourished)
- Hyperthermia: Get the patient cool and check for rhabdomyolysis.
- Hypothermia: If in cardiac arrest, get bypass ready.
- High-altitude illness: Descent is definitive therapy.
- Myxedema coma: Don't forget to treat adrenal insufficiency.
- Hypoglycemia: Why is the patient hypoglycemic?
- Adrenal insufficiency: Treat right away—dexamethasone, if no time to do stimulation test.
- DKA: Fluids, insulin; treat underlying precipitant.
- Fluids, fluids, fluids, maybe insulin; treat underlying precipitant.
- Hypernatremia: Correct the volume deficit and you are half way there.
- Hypercalcemia: Need to consider this diagnosis in your patients with malignancy and nonspecific complaints.

CHAPTER 18

Headache

Michale Abraham and Tyson Pillow

INITIAL ASSESSMENT

- History is usually the key to evaluating and diagnosing headache syndromes. Most patients will have normal neurologic examinations and/or only very subtle findings. Make sure to take a little extra time to ask about risk factors, and be sure to consider all of the life-threatening causes of headache, even when the diagnosis seems clear.
- Patients will usually be stable, but may decompensate if prompt diagnosis and treatment is not initiated.
- Remember to manage pain appropriately.

DON'T FORGET

It is almost never "just a headache" during your oral board exam.

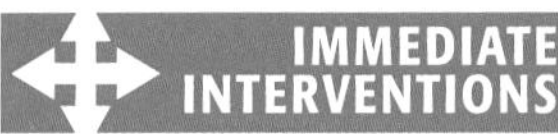

IMMEDIATE INTERVENTIONS

- IV, O_2, and monitor if the patient is unstable.
- **Do a thorough neurologic examination!** Be alert for any signs of blunt head trauma.
- Most of the people you see on exam day will need a STAT head CT and an LP (± depending on the CT read).

INITIAL HISTORY AND PHYSICAL EXAMINATION

History

- History of present illness (HPI)
  - Type of headache, difference from previous headaches.
  - Location
  - Severity
  - Onset (gradual vs sudden/thunderclap)
  - Duration
  - Aggravating/relieving factors
  - Events leading up to headache
  - Sensitivity to light
  - Neck pain
  - Fever
  - Nausea/vomiting
  - Recent illness/sick contacts
- Past medical history (PMHx)
  - Migraines
  - Malignancy
  - Immuno-compromise
- Social history
  - Recent travel
  - Environmental exposure
  - Drug use

Physical Examination

- General appearance
  - Febrile?
  - Level of discomfort?
  - Altered mental status (AMS)?
  - Glasgow Coma Score (GCS)?
- Head, eye, ear, nose, and throat (HEENT) examination
  - Signs of trauma?
  - Sinus or temporal pain/pressure?
  - Nystagmus?
  - Vision changes, papilledema?
- Neck
  - Signs of meningismus?
- Cardiovascular (CV)
  - Tachycardia?
  - Hypertension (HTN)?
- Skin
  - Rashes?

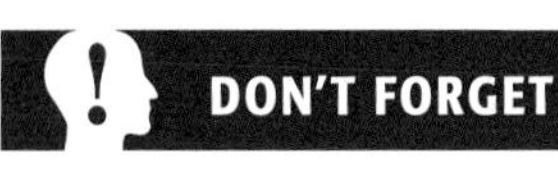

DON'T FORGET

History and physical are the key to diagnosis!

- Neurologic
  - Orientation
  - Cranial nerves, including visual field testing.
  - Cerebellar examination—including gait!
  - Motor examination
  - Sensation
  - Reflexes

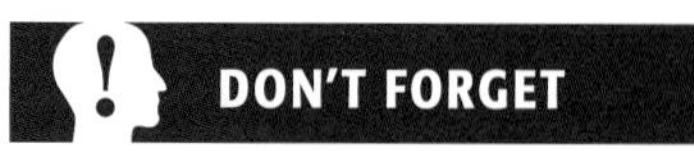

On exam day the patient will have

- SAH
- Meningitis
- Temporal arteritis
- Subdural hematoma
- Hypertensive encephalopathy
- Idiopathic intracranial HTN

PAIN MANAGEMENT

In general, antiemetics such as prochlorperazine and metoclopramide are very effective at improving the patient's pain, as well as controlling symptoms of nausea and vomiting, but should not be used as a "therapeutic trial." If necessary, narcotic analgesics can be added to the regimen for severe, refractory pain. Medications such as ergotamines, nonsteroidal anti-inflammatory drugs (NSAIDs), etc can be used after serious, life-threatening illnesses have been otherwise ruled out.

- Prochlorperazine 10 mg IV/PO q6-8h
- Metoclopramide 10 mg IV/IM/PO q6-8h
- Ondansetron 4 mg IV/PO q 4-6h
- Morphine 0.1 mg/kg IV/IM q30min-1 h PRN pain
- Dilaudid 1-2 mg IV/IM q30min-1 h PRN pain
- Decadron 4-6mg IV × 1

DIFFERENTIAL DIAGNOSIS

- Subarachnoid hemorrhage (SAH)
  - Classically, this presents as a sudden, "thunderclap" headache. It is estimated that approximately 1% of all nontraumatic headaches that present to the emergency department (ED) will be SAHs, with 85% of these due to aneurysms.
  - SAH can present with normal vitals, normal examination, and improve with pain meds, so do not rule out the diagnosis on examination alone (Fig. 18-1).

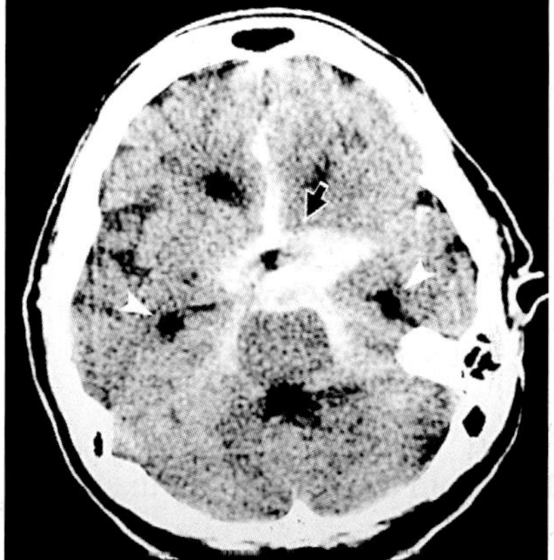

A SAH in suprasellar cistern

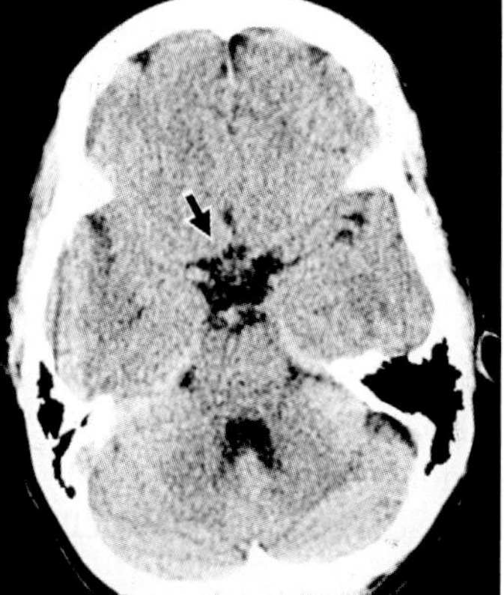

B Normal suprasellar cistern

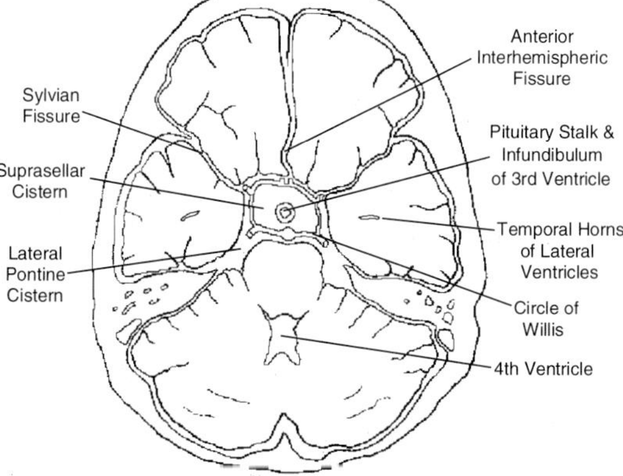

C Suprasellar cistern anatomy

Figure 18-1. Massive SAH fills the suprasellar cistern (pentagonal cistern [black arrow]). Blood extends anteriorly to the anterior interhemispheric fissure, laterally to the left Sylvian fissure, and posteriorly to the lateral pontine cisterns. The temporal horns of the lateral ventricles are dilated (arrowheads) indicative of hydrocephalus. (*Reprinted with permission from Schwartz DT.* Emergency Radiology: Case Studies. *New York, NY: McGraw-Hill: 2008.*)

- Meningitis
  - Infection of the meninges generally occurs as a complication of bacteremia, but can primarily extend from infection of the sinuses or the inner ear; much less common since widespread administration of pneumococcal and meningococcal vaccines.
  - Varied presentations, including headache, seizures, lethargy, neck stiffness, as well as other symptoms.
- Temporal arteritis
  - A vasculitis of the arteries that is also known as giant cell arteritis. Seen almost exclusively in patients >50 years. Women are affected much more commonly than men.
  - It presents with throbbing headache and unilateral temporal pain. No affect on mortality but can cause loss of vision because of optic neuritis in up to 50% of patients.
- Subdural hematoma
  - Intracranial bleed caused by rupture of the bridging veins. This diagnosis should be considered in any patient with new or persistent headache with acute or remote history of head injury.
  - Those at highest risk include elderly, alcoholics, and those on anticoagulants.
- Hypertensive encephalopathy
  - As diastolic pressure and mean arterial pressure (MAP) increase, the pressure on the cerebral vasculature increases and can overwhelm normal autoregulation.
  - This may initially cause headaches, dizziness, mild nausea, and photosensitivity. If this process progresses, then end-organ damage may eventually occur leading to hypertensive encephalopathy (altered mental status, stroke, etc).
- Idiopathic intracranial HTN
  - Classically seen in obese females. Characterized by elevated opening pressure on lumbar puncture (LP) with normal neuroimaging.
  - Headaches are gradual onset, associated with progressive vision loss, can require neurosurgical interventions.

SUBARACHNOID HEMORRHAGE

Additional History and Physical Examination

- Thunderclap, abrupt, or onset in <1 hour, headache.
- Family history of cerebral or coronary aneurysms.
- Recent history of similar, severe headaches.
- HPI can prioritize the diagnosis of SAH, but no combination of history and physical examination findings should rule out SAH without appropriate testing.

Review Initial Results

- Noncontrast computed tomography (CT) of brain: 93%-99% sensitive within the first 24 hours of headache onset, but sensitivity drops to 80% by day 2 and 50% by day 7.
- LP: Gold standard to rule out SAH.
  - Persistently elevated red blood cells (RBCs) from tubes 1 to 4 are diagnostic of SAH.
  - A traumatic tap may give falsely elevated RBCs in the cerebrospinal fluid (CSF) analysis, but this should decrease by at least 25% in tube 4.
  - Xanthochromia can be seen 12 hours after onset.

Definitive Management

- Blood pressure (BP) management:
  - Goal systolic of 140 mm Hg and/or MAP of 110 mm Hg.

  - Reduces mortality.
  - IV nicardipine is the drug of choice for BP management as it is titratable, and may contribute to the prevention of vasospasm.
- Neurosurgical consult.
  - Oral nimodipine is preferred treatment for prevention of vasospasm.
- CT angiography or magnetic resonance imaging/angiography (MRI/MRA): Visualize arterial system and identify any lesions to be clipped or coiled.

Complications

- Rebleeding and vasospasm are the main complications.
- Up to 25% of SAH rebleed within 2 weeks.
- Complications can also occur from the LP itself, but serious complications are rare.

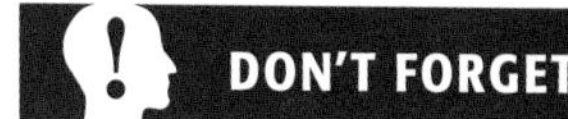

SAH can present with a normal examination and normal vitals. Do not rule out subarachnoid by the patient's appearance, or response to treatment, alone.

Disposition

- Admit to a neurosurgical intensive care unit (ICU).

TEMPORAL ARTERITIS

Additional History and Physical Examination

- History of polymyalgia rheumatica.
- Temporal pain.
- Jaw claudication may be present.
- Pain with brushing/combing hair.
- Vision problems.
- Perform a thorough examination, including visual acuity.

Review Initial Results

- Erythrocyte sedimentation rate (ESR): Usually elevated >50 mm/h.
- C-reactive protein (CRP) elevation.
- Temporal biopsy is necessary to definitely establish the diagnosis, but do not delay treatment.

Definitive Management

- High-dose corticosteroids.
- Pain management.
- Consultations to ophthalmology and rheumatology.

Complications

- Vision loss.

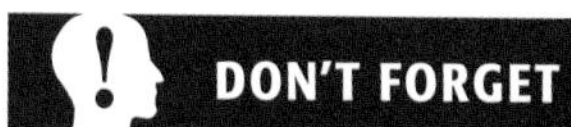

Start steroids for the treatment of temporal arteritis even before the diagnosis is confirmed—this can be a vision-saving intervention.

Disposition

- In well-appearing patients with no vision changes, patients can be discharged home on high-dose steroids with the next day follow-up.
- If there are any systemic symptoms, vision changes, or compliance/social issues, admit to facilitate further treatment.

SUBDURAL HEMATOMA

Additional History and Physical Examination

- History of trauma, even mild trauma can precipitate a subdural hematoma.
- Persistent or worsening nausea, dizziness, or severe headache.
- Anticoagulant use.

Review Initial Results

- CT head: Even if trauma was sustained and initial CT was negative, consider second CT to r/o delayed bleeding (Fig. 18-2) especially in patients on novel oral anticoagulants.
- Prothrombin time/partial thromboplastin time/international normalized ratio (PT/PTT/INR) for any patient on anticoagulants.
- Type and screen.

Definitive Management

- Reverse anticoagulation with fresh frozen plasma (FFP): In patients on anti-coagulation with obvious neurologic deficits, FFP should be started before CT scan if possible.
- Management to prevent increased intracranial pressure (ICP):
  - BP control.
  - Consider mannitol or hypertonic saline with signs of herniation.
  - If intubated, consider mild hypocapnia (Pco_2 32-35 mm Hg) with signs of herniation.

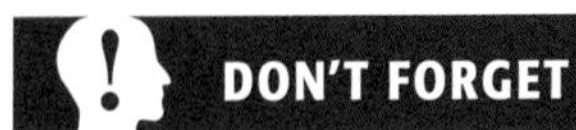

DON'T FORGET

Chronic subdural bleeding can occur over weeks. Always consider a CT scan with a history of trauma, especially in the elderly, diabetics, or those on anticoagulants.

Complications

- Include midline shift, obtundation, herniation, coma.

Disposition

- Neurosurgical consult and admission to ICU.
- Possible evacuation of hematoma.

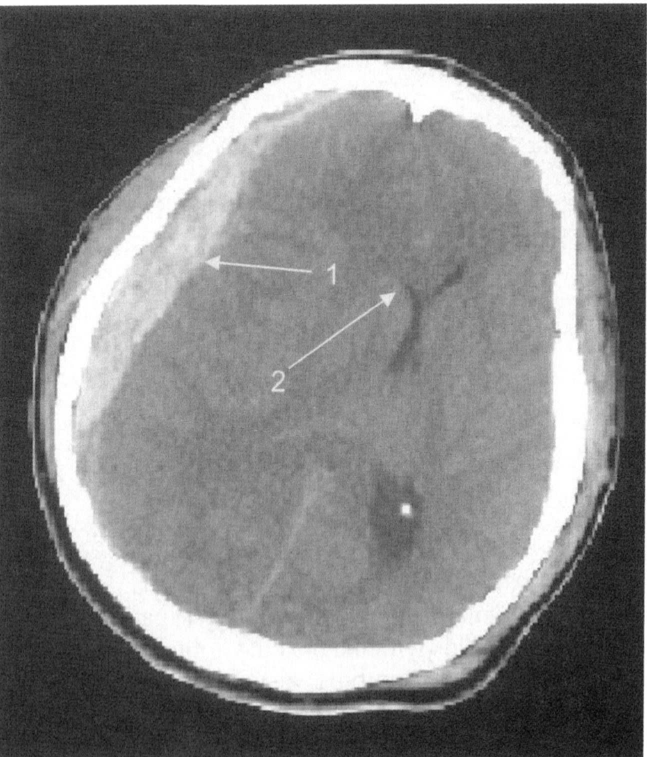

Figure 18-2. Computed tomography scan of a subdural hematoma (arrow 1). Note that the hematoma crosses the suture lines. Arrow 2 demonstrates midline shift. (*Reprinted with permission from Tintinalli JE, Kelen GD, Stapczynski JS, et al.* Emergency Medicine: A Comprehensive Study Guide. *6th ed. New York, NY: McGraw-Hill; 2004.*)

HYPERTENSIVE ENCEPHALOPATHY

Additional History and Physical Examination

- History of HTN
- Vision problems
- Change in mental status
- Noncompliance with medications
- Papilledema
- S_3/S_4, rales

Review Initial Results

- Make sure to evaluate for signs of end-organ damage in other body systems besides the brain.
- CT Head to rule out other causes of encephalopathy.
- Electrocardiogram (ECG).
- Cardiac enzymes (based on symptoms).
- Brain natriuretic peptide (BNP) (based on symptoms).
- Basic metabolic panel (BMP).
- Urinalysis (UA).
- Chest x-ray (CXR) (based on symptoms).

Definitive Management

- No treatment is necessary for simple asymptomatic HTN.
- In general, encephalopathy does not occur until the diastolic BP is >115-130 mm Hg.
- The goal of treatment is to control BP >24-48 hours.
- If symptomatic, decrease the MAP by 10%-25% acutely and reevaluate.
- Optimize perfusion, and supplement with O_2 as necessary.
- Invasive BP monitoring is warranted.
- Pharmacologic agents:
  - Nicardipine: Calcium channel blocker; 5-15 mg/h IV.
  - Labetalol: Alpha- and beta-blocker; start at 20 mg IV and then use 20-80 mg IV until desired BP or max 300 mg. Can start 2 mg/min IV.
  - Hydralazine: Centrally acting agent, somewhat labile, so use with caution; 5-10 mg IM/IV q2-4h.
  - Nitroglycerin: Drug of choice when angina or pulmonary edema is also present. 0.4 mg SL q5min or initial dose of 10-100 μg/min IV.
  - Sodium nitroprusside: Dose of 0.5-10 μg/kg/min.

Complications

- Decreasing MAP >25% can lead to cerebral ischemia.
- Nitroglycerin and nitroprusside may cause cerebral shunting and vasogenic edema which may worsen ICP. Use with caution.
- Nitroprusside can cause cyanide toxicity after prolonged use of (usually) >48 hours.

Disposition

- Admit to the ICU for tight BP management and neurologic assessments.

IDIOPATHIC INTRACRANIAL HYPERTENSION AKA PSEUDOTUMOR CEREBRI

Additional History and Physical Examination

- History of "chronic" headaches
- Vision problems

- Obesity
- Multiple ED visits with no definitive diagnosis
- Papilledema

Review Initial Results

- CT head if no previous imaging studies
- LP with opening and closing pressure

Definitive Management

- Acetazolamide may temporize symptoms.
- In general LP is diagnostic and therapeutic.
- If visual changes, emergent ophthalmologic and neurosurgical consultation for optic sheath fenestration or ventriculoperitoneal (VP) shunt placement.

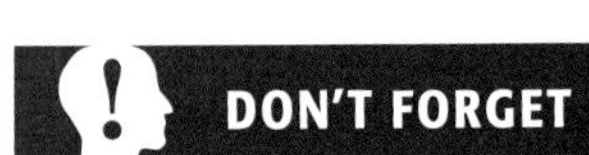

This is a diagnosis of exclusion as all other causes of headache should be evaluated and ruled out.

Disposition

- Admit to the hospital for pain management and neurologic assessments.

MENINGITIS AND ENCEPHALITIS

Additional History and Physical Examination

- Headache is most likely accompanied by fever and meningismus on boards.
- Travel, age, immunocompromised status and exposure to sick contacts are all key elements of the history.
- Physical examination should assess for Kernig and Brudzinski signs.
- Patients may or may not present with a rash—as it may be a late finding.

Review Initial Results

- LP: Gold standard to evaluate .
- Noncontrast (CT) of brain: Required before LP if the patient has any focal neurologic findings or a complete neurologic examination is not possible.
- Elevated white blood cells (WBCs) with neutrophil predominance, high protein, and low glucose are indicative of bacterial meningitis.
  - Encephalitis will usually have moderately elevated WBCs with mononuclear with mild to moderate elevation in protein and normal glucose. Presence of RBCs is consistent with herpes simplex virus (HSV) encephalitis.

Definitive Management

- Antibiotics are the mainstay of treatment for bacterial meningitis.
- Empiric steroids can be given in conjunction with antibiotics if pneumococcal meningitis is suspected.
- Antibiotics should not be held for a formal diagnosis ie, start before CT/LP if you have a high suspicion.
  - Neonates—ampicillin + gentamycin ± vancomycin
  - Adults—ceftriaxone ± vancomycin
  - Immunocompromised or elderly—ceftriaxone ± vancomycin + ampicillin
- Dexamethasone for adult patients
    - Give 10 mg IV 15 minutes prior to first dose of antibiotics.
- Encephalitis is difficult to diagnose in ED. Will need high suspicion based on travel or environmental exposure.
  - HSV encephalitis is an emergency and will require prompt treatment with IV acyclovir.

Complications

- Significant morbidity and mortality if untreated or delays in treatment.
- Hearing loss, developmental delays, death.

Disposition

- Admit to a hospital neonatal intensive care unit (NICU) if neonatal, otherwise admit to appropriate level of care based on acuity.

DON'T FORGET

Start the antibiotics as soon as the diagnosis is suspected.

WINNING STRATEGIES

- History is the key!
- SAH can present with a normal examination and normal vitals. Do not rule out subarachnoid by the patient's appearance alone.
- Start steroids for the treatment of temporal arteritis even before the diagnosis is confirmed.
- Chronic subdural bleeding can occur over weeks. Always consider a CT scan with a history of trauma, especially in the elderly, diabetics, or those on anticoagulants.
- Hypertensive emergency is a diagnosis of exclusion as all other causes of headache should be evaluated and ruled out.
- Do not lower BP >10%-25% in the first day or it may cause cerebral ischemia.
- Give antibiotics before imaging or the LP when suspecting meningitis.
- Remember to control pain.

CHAPTER 19

Weakness

Anita Rohra and Tyson Pillow

DON'T FORGET

On examination day, every patient with a chief complaint of "weakness" without fever will have one or more of the following:

- Acute renal failure
- Rhabdomyolysis
- Cardiac ischemia
- Severe anemia
- Electrolyte abnormalities
  - Hyperkalemia
  - Hypokalemia

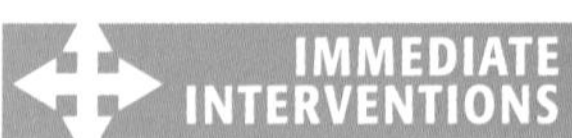

- Oxygen via NC or NRB to keep O_2 >95%.
- Cardiac monitor with rhythm strip.
- Finger stick blood glucose.
- 18-gauge IV.
- Draw blood for laboratory studies.
- Urinalysis and urine dipstick.
- ECG.

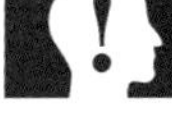

DON'T FORGET

Any patient with hypokalemia/hyperkalemia/acute renal failure or rhabdomyolysis will likely have some "red flags" in their history to cause you to suspect the diagnosis since many of the symptoms and physical examination signs are nonspecific.

Generalized weakness is a common, nonspecific complaint, especially in the elderly. It can have a wide differential diagnosis, spanning from the benign to acutely life-threatening diagnoses. When approaching a patient with weakness, it is important to work in an organized manner, take a detailed history, perform a thorough physical examination, and order all appropriate, indicated tests.

INITIAL ASSESSMENT

- Focus on age, comorbid factors, vital signs (VS), lung sounds, peripheral edema, evidence of anemia.
- Identify any unstable patients with immediate life-threats.
  - Threats to airway.
  - Cardiac dysrhythmias.
  - Fluid overload.

INITIAL HISTORY AND PHYSICAL EXAMINATION

History

- History of the present illness (HPI)
  - Any extreme exercise or exertion recently?
  - Any history of fluid losses (ie, vomiting/diarrhea)?
  - Any recent gastrointestinal (GI) abnormalities?
  - Any genitourinary (GU) abnormalities: Dysuria or difficulty urinating?
  - Any history of dark-colored urine?
  - Any change in medications or doses of medications?
- Past medical history (PMHx)
  - Any history of abdominal mass?
  - Any recent exposure to radiographic contrast agents or exogenous toxins?
  - Any history of chronic urinary tract infection (UTI)?
  - History of recent MI? Burn? Trauma?
  - Potential obstructive problems? (Enlarged prostate, neurogenic bladder, or renal calculi?)
- Medications
  - Any new medications including angiotensin-converting enzyme (ACE) inhibitors?
  - Chronic overuse of nonsteroidal anti-inflammatory drugs (NSAIDs)?
- Allergies

Physical Examination

- VS
- Neck: Jugular venous distention (JVD)?
- Chest: Rales?
- Back: Costo-vertebral angle (CVA) tenderness?
- Abdomen: Any masses palpable?
- Rectal examination: Any prostate enlargement?
- Extremities: Pedal edema?
- Neuro: Motor, sensory, deep tendon reflex (DTR) symmetric? Any slowed mental ability from baseline? Asterixis?

DIFFERENTIAL DIAGNOSIS

- Acute renal failure
  - The term acute renal failure (ARF) refers to any precipitous decline in kidney function. There are myriad causes for ARF, but they all lead to azotemia, the accumulation of nitrogenous end-products of metabolism.

- In evaluating a patient with ARF, it is important to try to determine if there is a pre-renal, intrinsic renal or post-renal/obstructive etiology that can be addressed.
- Rhabdomyolysis
  - A diagnosis that should be suspected in any patient with trauma to skeletal muscle. The damage to the muscle causes release of intracellular contents into the extracellular fluid and circulation.
  - ARF may occur as a result of rhabdomyolysis. Risk factors for rhabdomyolysis are the use of statin drugs, prolonged compression injuries, compartment syndromes, extreme exertion, electrical burns, hyperthermia, myopathies, seizures, infections, electrolyte abnormalities, hypoxia, and certain drugs or toxins.
- Cardiac ischemia: See Chap. 18.
- Electrolyte abnormalities
  - Hyperkalemia
    - True hyperkalemia is usually caused by enhanced potassium absorption, impaired potassium excretion, shifts of potassium out of the cells into the serum, or, rarely, increased potassium intake.
    - Most commonly, renal insufficiency is a cause for hyperkalemia since potassium cannot be excreted effectively without functioning kidneys.
  - Hypokalemia
    - The most common causes of hypokalemia are increased potassium excretion via GI or renal losses or transcellular potassium shifts. Hypokalemia is rarely caused by decreased dietary intake.
    - Suspect this diagnosis if the patient has recently been prescribed diuretics or has had significant GI losses.
- Anemia: See Chap. 12.

ACUTE RENAL FAILURE

Additional History and Physical Examination Findings

- The incidence of renal insufficiency increases with age. Be suspicious of ARF in elderly patients.
- NSAIDs have become a common toxic etiology for ARF, so be suspicious of renal failure in patients using NSAIDs daily.
- Try to determine if the patient has pre-renal, post-renal, or intrinsic renal failure based on history.
- Common pre-renal causes of ARF are volume loss, cardiac insufficiency, sepsis, or liver failure.
- Common post-renal causes of ARF are prostatic hypertrophy or functional bladder neck obstruction. Consider placing a Foley catheter in every male patient to rule out urinary retention. Placing the Foley catheter can often relieve the obstruction in these cases.
- Common intrarenal causes are classified by the portion of the nephron that is involved and include acute interstitial nephritis, glomerulonephritis, and acute tubular necrosis (ATN).

Review Initial Results

- Electrocardiogram (ECG)
  - Review immediately.
  - Assess for evidence of hyperkalemia (Fig. 19-1).
- Chest x-ray (CXR)
  - Look for evidence of a cardiac etiology, such as evidence of congestive heart failure (CHF).
  - Look for signs of volume overload.
    - Pleural effusions.

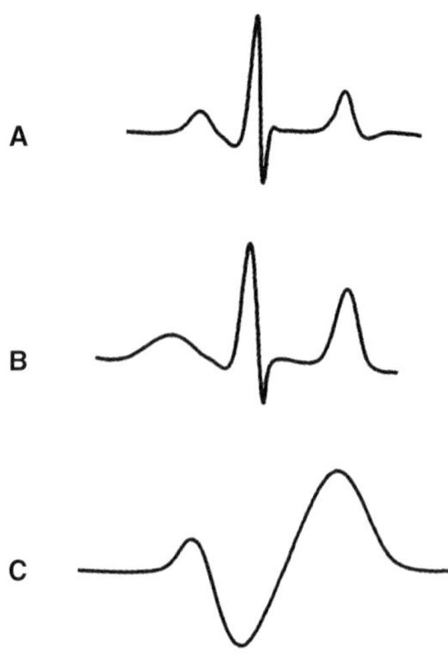

Figure 19-1. ECG changes in **hyperkalemia**. **(A)** Normal ECG. **(B)** ECG with peaked T waves, prolonged PR interval, and widened QRS, seen in moderate hyperkalemia (potassium >7.0 mEq/L). **(C)** "Sine wave" ECG seen at potassium levels >8 mEq/L. (*Reproduced with permission from Strange GR, Ahrens WR, Lelyveld S, Schafermeyer RW.* Pediatric Emergency Medicine: A Comprehensive Study Guide. *2nd ed. New York, NY: McGraw-Hill; 2002.*)

    - Bilateral interstitial infiltrates.
    - Enlarged cardiac silhouette.
  - Look for evidence of pericardial effusion, such as an enlarged cardiac silhouette or a water bottle heart.
- Bedside ultrasound
  - Look for pleural effusions, pericardial effusion, decreased ejection fraction.
- Urinalysis (UA) with microscopic examination
  - Prerenal: High specific gravity, otherwise normal.
  - Intrinsic renal disease: May see white blood cells (WBC) casts from acute interstitial nephritis, red blood cells (RBC) casts from glomerulonephritis, or muddy brown casts from ATN.
  - Suspect myoglobinuria if the UA is positive for blood, but no RBCs are seen on microscopic examination.
- Blood urea nitrogen (BUN)/Creatinine (Cr): A high BUN/Cr ratio is consistent with prerenal failure.
- Potassium: Hyperkalemia can develop rapidly after onset of ARF and may be asymptomatic.
- Calcium: Hypocalcemia may complicate ARF.
- Magnesium: Hypermagnesemia may complicate ARF as a result of decreased renal elimination.
- Phosphate: Hyperphosphatemia may complicate ARF as a result of decreased renal elimination.

Management Priorities

- Stabilize the patient if there is any derangement of airway, breathing, or circulation.
- Correct hyperkalemia as rapidly as possible.
- Identify and address the etiology of the renal failure, if possible.
- Pre-renal causes such as hypovolemia or blood loss should be addressed.

- Post-renal causes should be addressed with relief of the obstruction by Foley catheter if possible. Place the Foley catheter and check a post-void residual. Follow urine output.
- Identify and treat any metabolic derangements caused by the renal failure such as hyperkalemia.
- Consult a nephrologist early to arrange possible dialysis if needed.

Frequent Reassessment

- Repeat ECG and repeat potassium level if hyperkalemia requires medications.
- Check urine output after Foley placement.
- Check lungs if patient is receiving fluid boluses prior to reordering more boluses.

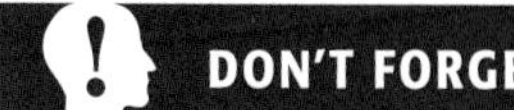

- ECG evidence of hyperkalemia must be treated immediately with calcium gluconate to avoid cardiac arrest.
- Any patient with ARF and history consistent with an obstructive etiology should have a Foley catheter to attempt to relieve the obstruction.
- Assume all patients with ARF have hyperkalemia until proven otherwise.

Complications

- Cardiovascular collapse secondary to untreated hyperkalemia.
- Fluid overload if patient is unable to excrete fluids and is not dialyzed.

Disposition

- All ARF patients need medical admission for workup.
- Indications for emergent dialysis and intensive care unit (ICU) admission:
  - Fluid overload, causing hypoxia and requiring airway support.
  - Severe acidosis.
  - Hyperkalemia.
  - Uremia with evidence of pericarditis, pericardial effusion, or encephalopathy.

RHABDOMYOLYSIS

Additional History and Physical Examination Findings

- Presenting symptoms of rhabdomyolysis are often complaints of myalgias, generalized weakness, malaise, stiffness, and dark urine.
- History is very important, especially any history of alcohol or drug abuse, recent trauma, infection, compression injuries, hyperthermia, electrical shock, or excessive exertion.
- Patients may complain of nausea, vomiting, or abdominal pain.
- Altered mental status may be present secondary to severe renal failure and uremia.
- Creatine kinase (CK) is the best marker of disease. CK levels start to rise between 2 and 12 hours of muscle injury, and peak levels occur within 24-36 hours.
- Disseminated intravascular coagulation (DIC) can occur in patients with acute rhabdomyolysis.

Review Initial Results

- ECG: Review for signs of hyperkalemia (see Fig. 19-1).
- CK level: Greater than 5 times normal is considered diagnostic.
- Serum myoglobin: Should be sent but may be a false negative.
- Urinalysis: Brown urine with a large amount of blood on dipstick, but few or no RBCs on microscopic examination is a classic finding.
- BUN/Cr: May be normal or may be elevated.
- Potassium: Hyperkalemia is a common complication of rhabdomyolysis.
- Calcium: Hypocalcemia is the most common metabolic abnormality in rhabdomyolysis.
- Liver function tests (LFTs): May be elevated from muscle injury alone.

Management Priorities

- Stabilize any patient with derangements in the airway, breathing, or circulation.
- Observe and recheck input and outputs on these patients since they need large amounts of fluids.
- Renal failure is a common complication of rhabdomyolysis; consult nephrology for possible dialysis.
- Hyperkalemia is a common complication of rhabdomyolysis, keep patient on a cardiac monitor and do not allow them to leave the emergency department (ED) without a physician.

DON'T FORGET

Most patients with rhabdomyolysis have a history that suggests this diagnosis. The history may reveal a prolonged episode of lying on the ground, severe exertion, or trauma from lightening or prolonged compression injury.

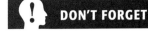

Definitive Management

- Intravenous (IV) fluids.
  - Aggressive IV fluids are the cornerstone of therapy. Patients with rhabdomyolysis need up to 20 L of fluid in the first 24 hours.
  - IV fluids should be administered in frequent 1000-cc boluses until the patient is fluid-repleted and dehydration is corrected. Then IV fluids should be infused at a rate of 250 mL/h.
  - The goal of IV fluid therapy is to maintain a urine output of 200-300 mL/h.
  - Careful track must be kept of I's and O's to ensure that the patient does not become fluid-overloaded.
  - Normal saline is the favored initial fluid. Avoid potassium or lactate containing fluids.
- Consider alkalinizing the urine with sodium bicarbonate infusion.
  - To administer add either 1 amp (44 mEq) to 1 L of 0.5 NS or 2-3 amp to 1 L of D5W (dextrose 5% in water) and infuse at a rate of 100 mL/h.
  - Titrate the infusion to maintain a urine pH >6.5.
- Use a Foley catheter to accurately track urine output.
- Address electrolyte abnormalities.
  - Manage hyperkalemia as discussed under Sec. Hyperkalemia.
  - Hypocalcemia: Only give calcium to symptomatic hypocalcemic patients (eg, signs of tetany). Calcium administration may raise intracellular Ca levels and promote further muscle injury.
- Emergently consult nephrology.
- Consider dialysis.
  - Indicated for patients with ARF.
  - Oliguric patients require dialysis.

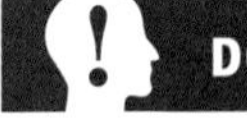

DON'T FORGET

Renal failure can occur from rhabdomyolysis, so consult nephrology early in case the patient needs dialysis!

Frequent Reassessment

- Be certain to pay attention to input and outputs and watch urine output.
- Reassess lung sounds for evidence of fluid overload.

Complications

- Hyperkalemia.
- Hypocalcemia.
- Renal failure requiring emergency dialysis.

Disposition

- Admit all patients with rhabdomyolysis to the hospital.
- Toxic-appearing patients or patients with uncorrected hyperkalemia or ARF may require the ICU.

HYPERKALEMIA

Additional History and Physical Examination Findings

- Classically cardiovascular and neurologic dysfunction are the primary manifestation of hyperkalemia.
- Neurologic symptoms include cramps, weakness, paralysis, paresthesias, and tetany.
- Cardiovascular dysfunction includes a variety of dysrhythmias, including second- and third-degree heart block, wide-complex tachycardia, ventricular fibrillation, or asystole.
- Hyperkalemia may be a result of renal failure, or any situation that causes large amounts of potassium to be released from damaged cells, such as rhabdomyolysis, severe burns, or hemolysis.

Review Initial Results

- ECG: Look for classic changes of hyperkalemia (see Fig. 19-1).
  - Peaked T waves.
  - Disappearance of P waves.
  - Widening or slurring of QRS.
- BUN/Cr.
- Urinalysis: Review carefully to be certain that rhabdomyolysis is not a cause for renal failure.

Management Priorities

- Cardiac dysrhythmias and cardiac arrest can occur with hyperkalemia, so be sure the patient is on a cardiac monitor and treated with calcium for any ECG disturbances.
- Most emergent therapies for hyperkalemia only temporize by shifting potassium and antagonizing its effects at the cardiac membrane. Dialysis is the only rapid, definitive therapy that removes potassium and decreases the whole body potassium burden. Exchange resins remove potassium, but work slowly. Do not delay arranging dialysis for severe hyperkalemia.

Definitive Management

- Immediately infuse 10 mL of a 10% solution of either calcium chloride or calcium gluconate over 2 minutes.
  - By antagonizing the effect of potassium on the cardiac membrane, calcium is immediately cardio-protective.
  - Calcium is the fastest acting antagonist, but its effects are short lived (20-40 minutes).
  - Do not use calcium if the patient is on digitalis because hypercalcemia can potentiate the toxic cardiac effects of digitalis.
  - Calcium chloride has more calcium per milliliter, but is more toxic to tissue if it extravasates.
- Dextrose and insulin: Administer 1 amp of D50 (50 g of glucose), then 5 U of IV regular insulin.
  - Promotes a shift of potassium into cells.
  - Dextrose should be administered to all patients with blood glucose <250 mg/dL to avoid hypoglycemia.
  - Duration of action 4 to 6 hours.
- Beta-2 agonists promote shift of potassium into cells.
  - Duration of action approximately 2 hours.
  - Nebulized albuterol treatments can be given continuously if severe hyperkalemia.

DON'T FORGET

- Any patient with suspected hyperkalemia by history and ECG findings should be treated rapidly and aggressively!
- Assume all patients with hyperkalemia will need dialysis and call the nephrologist early. On examination day, all patients with hyperkalemia will need dialysis.
- Do not give calcium to patients on digoxin without checking the drug levels as it may potentiate a lethal dysrhythmia!

- Exchange resins: Administer 20 g of sodium polystyrene sulfonate (Kayexalate) PO or PR.
  - Exchanged resins remove potassium from the body.
  - One gram of Kayexalate can remove approximately 1 mEq of potassium.
  - For oral or rectal administration, onset of action does not occur for at least 1 to 2 hours.
- Dialysis: For patients with severe hyperkalemia especially if caused by renal failure, hemodialysis is the only definitive management.

Frequent Reassessment

- Repeated ECGs or rhythm strips should be obtained to be certain that any cardiac abnormalities are resolving.
- Recheck a neurologic examination on the patient if there were any neurologic deficits caused by hyperkalemia.
- Patients with poor cardiovascular reserve should be rechecked for evidence of fluid overload during treatment of their hyperkalemia.
- Should repeat treatment with calcium, beta-agonists, insulin, and glucose if symptoms recur.

Disposition

- Patients with hyperkalemia should be admitted to a monitored bed, likely to the ICU if they are severe.

HYPOKALEMIA

Additional History and Physical Examination Findings

- Hypokalemia is usually relatively asymptomatic until potassium serum concentrations are at 2.5 mEq/L.
- Rarely is hypokalemia caused by decreased dietary intake unless this is coupled with other factors, causing loss of potassium (GI losses) or intracellular shifts of potassium (increased insulin doses or beta-agonists).
- Classic signs of hypokalemia are CNS changes, muscular abnormalities in the extremities, cardiac manifestations, and muscular paralysis if potassium <2 mEq/L.
- CNS symptoms include lethargy, depression, irritability, and confusion.
- Muscular symptoms include paresthesias, fasciculations, depressed DTR, myalgias, and generalized weakness.
- Cardiovascular manifestations can include any abnormal rhythm or ectopy.
- ECG findings include T-wave flattening, ST-segment depression, and U waves.
- Intestinal smooth muscle may also be affected, causing nausea, vomiting, abdominal distension, or paralytic ileus.

DON'T FORGET

ECG findings of

- Flattened T waves
- ST-segment depression
- U waves

.....are hypokalemia until proven otherwise.

Review Initial Results

- ECG: Look for classic findings of hypokalemia (Fig. 19-2).
  - Flattened T waves.
  - ST-segment depression.
  - U waves.
  - May also show any dysrhythmia or ectopy.
- Electrolytes: Potassium level <3.5 mEq/L is diagnostic.
- Metabolic alkalosis may be seen as intracellular potassium is exchanged for hydrogen ions.
- Abdominal x-ray: May show a paralytic ileus.

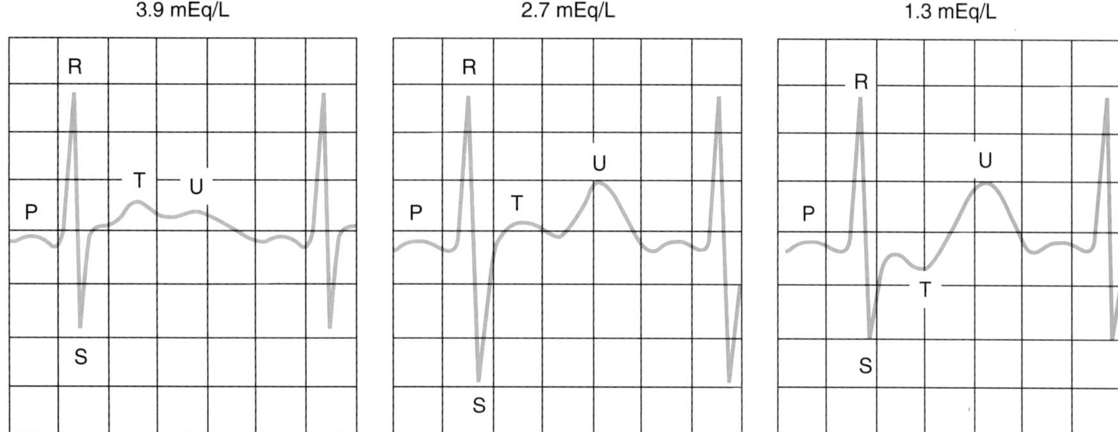

Figure 19-2. ECG effects of hypokalemia. Note progressive flattening of the T wave, an increasingly prominent U wave, increased amplitude of the P wave, prolongation of the PR interval, and ST-segment depression. (*Reproduced with permission from Morgan GE, Mikhail MS, Murray MJ.* Clinical Anesthesiology. *4th ed. New York, NY: McGraw-Hill; 2006.*)

Management Priorities

- Identify instability in airway, breathing, and circulation and address these issues.
- Identify cardiac dysrhythmias, stabilize, keep patient on a cardiac monitor, and continue close observation!
- Replete potassium.
- Identify the cause of the hypokalemia.

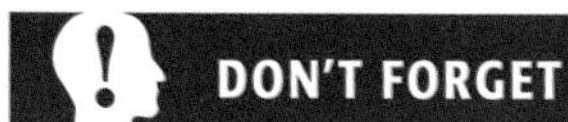

Patients receiving high-dose IV potassium therapy need large-bore IVs or central lines and need to be observed on cardiac monitors.

Definitive Management

- Potassium supplementation
  - Oral supplementation is the preferred route. Administer 20 mEq of potassium every 60 minutes until desired result.
  - Some patients will not be able to receive oral potassium and will require IV supplementation.
  - IV supplementation should occur no faster than 20 mEq/h unless the patient is severely impaired.
  - IV supplementation at >20 mEq/h needs to be given through a large-bore IV or central line because of venous irritation associated with potassium.
  - Patients receiving large doses of IV potassium need to be kept on a cardiac monitor.
- Address the reason the patient became hypokalemic.

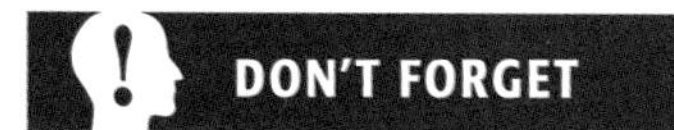

Remember to check the ECG for long QT as well as check for concomitant hypomagnesemia.

Complications

- Cardiac dysrhythmias including ventricular fibrillation and asystole.
- Rhabdomyolysis can occur with severe hypokalemia.

Disposition

- If mild hypokalemia (K 3.0-3.5 mEq/L) and asymptomatic, discharge the patient with potassium supplementation and close follow-up.
- If the patient is symptomatic or has severe hypokalemia (K <2.5 mEq/L) with no cardiac abnormalities, admit to floor for IV potassium supplementation.
- If the patient is severely ill or with cardiac abnormalities, admit to the ICU for cardiac monitoring, intensive IV potassium supplementation and observation.

WINNING STRATEGIES

- On examination day, every patient complaining of weakness without fever will have ARF, rhabdomyolysis, or electrolyte abnormalities such as hyper- or hypokalemia until proven otherwise.
- Immediate interventions for patients with weakness include oxygen, cardiac monitor, fingerstick for blood glucose level, IV, UA and urine dip, and an ECG.
- Any patient with hypokalemia/hyperkalemia/ARF or rhabdomyolysis will likely have some "red flags" in their history to cause you to suspect the diagnosis since many of the symptoms and physical examination signs are nonspecific.
- Once you have established the patient has ARF, rhabdomyolysis, or hyperkalemia, call the nephrologist immediately so that if dialysis is indicated, they are already involved with the patient.
- Look at the ECG for evidence of hyperkalemia which includes peaked T waves, disappearance of P waves, and widened QRS complexes. Also look for evidence of hypokalemia which includes flattened T waves, ST-segment depression, and U waves.
- Any patient with suspected hyperkalemia by history and ECG findings should be treated rapidly and aggressively with calcium, insulin, glucose, nebulized albuterol, and Kayexalate.
- Any patient with ARF and history consistent with an obstructive etiology should have a Foley catheter to attempt to relieve the obstruction.
- Assume all patients with renal failure have hyperkalemia and vice versa until proven otherwise.
- Do not give calcium to patients on digitalis since hypercalcemia can potentate the toxic cardiac effects of digitalis.
- Most of the patients with rhabdomyolysis will have histories that suggest it. Generally, prolonged episode of lying on the ground, severe exertion, trauma from lightening or prolonged compression injury.
- Urine dip positive for blood and a UA with few or no RBCs is always going to be myoglobinuria suggesting rhabdomyolysis.
- Assume all patients with rhabdomyolysis will have renal failure and consult the nephrologist early.
- A patient receiving high-dose IV potassium therapy needs a large-bore IV or a central line and needs to be observed on a cardiac monitor.

THE BOTTOM LINE

- Always get an ECG.
- Consult nephrologist early for ARF, hyperkalemia, and rhabdomyolysis!

CHAPTER 20

Paralysis

Anita Rohra and Tyson Pillow

INITIAL ASSESSMENT

- Start with the ABCs and be prepared to secure the airway if necessary.
- Most causes of paralysis will be sub-acute in nature, but be prepared for deterioration in the patient's mental status.
- Once the patient has undergone initial stabilization, focus on the details of the history to guide diagnosis and treatment.

DON'T FORGET

Always assess the airway first and be prepared for a decline in mental status.

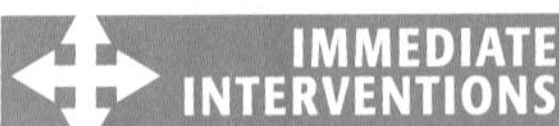

- IV, O_2, and monitor if the patient is unstable.
- Do a thorough neurologic examination. Be alert for any signs of blunt head trauma.
- Most of the people you see on examination day will need a stat head CT +/−an emergent MRI.
- Obtain a point of care glucose level.

INITIAL HISTORY AND PHYSICAL EXAMINATION

History

- History of the present illness (HPI)
  - Level of consciousness
  - Onset
  - Severity
  - Location
  - Progression
  - Duration
  - Aggravating/relieving factors
  - Weakness
  - Sensory changes
  - Recent illness/sick contacts
- Past medical history (PMHx)
  - History of cerebrovascular accident (CVA)
  - History of cancer
  - Hypertension (HTN)
  - Diabetes mellitus (DM)
- Social history
  - Recent trauma
  - Smoking
  - Drug use

Physical examination

- General appearance
- Head, eyes, ears, nose, and throat (HEENT)
  - Signs of trauma
  - Gag reflex
  - Facial droop
  - Ptosis
- Cardiovascular (CV)
  - Tachycardia
  - HTN
- Neurologic
  - Level of consciousness
  - Orientation
  - Cranial nerves
  - Cerebellar examination
  - Motor weakness
  - Sensation
  - Reflexes

DON'T FORGET

Focus on the details of the history including exact time of onset and progression to help narrow the differential and treatment plan.

On Examination day the patient will have

- Stroke
- Spinal cord compression
- Guillian-Barré syndrome
- Myasthenia gravis

DIFFERENTIAL DIAGNOSIS

- CVA
  - Ischemic stroke

- Transient ischemic attack (TIA)
- Basilar artery occlusion
- Hemorrhagic stroke
- Spinal cord compression
- Guillain-Barré Syndrome (GBS)
- Myasthenia gravis (MG)

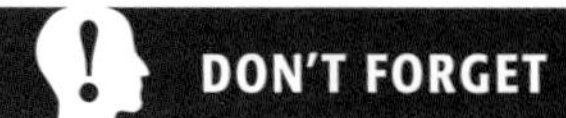

Clearly delineate the precise onset time if available to properly identify thrombolytic candidates.

Cerebrovascular Accident

- Despite advances in modern medicine, stroke remains one of the leading causes of morbidity and mortality. Although there is a large spectrum of disease severity, there are primarily two types of stroke syndromes: hemorrhagic and ischemic.
- Ischemic stroke accounts for approximately 80% of strokes. Arterial obstruction leads to hypoperfusion and ischemia in the vessel's distribution. This can result from thrombosis associated with underlying atherosclerosis and plaque rupture or embolism, most commonly from atrial fibrillation. Other causes include collagen vascular diseases, autoimmune diseases, and hypercoagulable states, but these are much more rare.
- Hemorrhagic stroke accounts for the other 20% of strokes, with intracerebral hemorrhage (ICH) occurring more often than subarachnoid hemorrhage (SAH). The emergency department (ED) management of ICH is identical to SAH except that intravascular interventions (clipping/coiling aneurysms) are not necessary for ICH. Management of SAH is outlined in detail in Chap. 18.

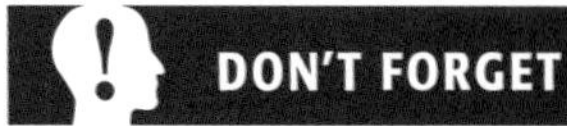

If the patient is a tPA candidate, aggressively manage the BP to <185/110 mm Hg. If the patient is not a tPA candidate, then the BP can be as high as 220/120 mm Hg without treatment.

ISCHEMIC STROKE

Additional History and Physical Examination

- Smoking history.
- Peripheral vascular disease.
- Previous strokes.
- Palpitations or irregular heart beat.
- Onset of symptoms (exact timing if available).
- No historical item can reliably distinguish ischemic versus hemorrhagic stroke, so obtaining the computed tomography (CT) scan of the brain as soon as possible will guide management.
- Dilated pupils.
- Thorough neurologic examination.

Review Initial Results

- CT noncontrast of brain: Obtain as soon as possible after the ABCs have been stabilized. The goals of management depend on the type of stroke present (Fig. 20-1).
- MRI: Limited usefulness in the acute setting caused by lack of availability, increased time involved, and increased time for interpretation.
- Baseline labs: Including coagulation studies, complete blood count (CBC), urinalysis (UA). Infection, hypoglycemia, and metabolic derangements can reproduce symptoms of previous stroke.
- Electocardiogram (ECG): Evaluate for atrial fibrillation and possible embolism as a cause of stroke.

Definitive Management

- ABCs: Ensure that the patient is able to protect their own airway and manage appropriately. Also make sure to assess the patient frequently as their status may deteriorate.

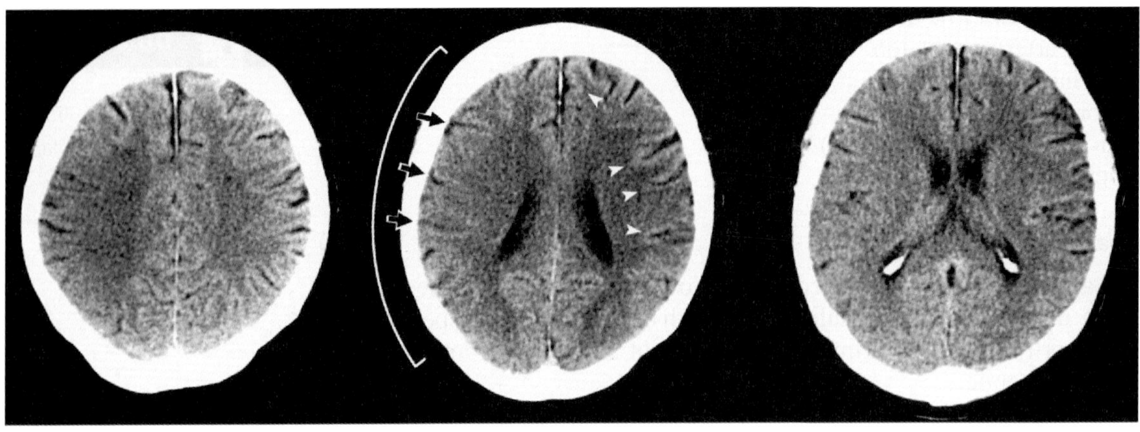

A

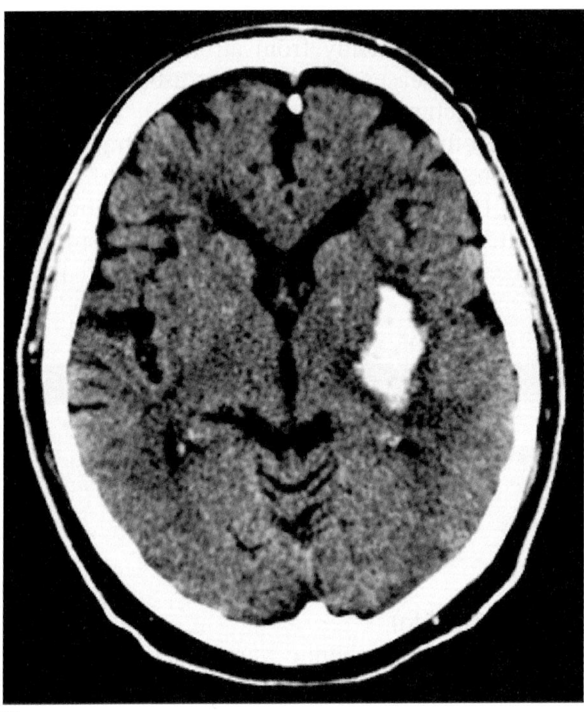

B

Figure 20-1. **(A)** Extensive early ischemic change in right MCA area; on the left cerebral hemisphere, the cortical gray-white differentiation is normal (white arrowheads), whereas on the right, there is a loss of that differentiation (curved white line). Slight mass effect causing effacement of the cortical sulci (black arrows) is also seen. **(B)** Acute hemorrhagic stroke; a large basal ganglion bleed on CT taken less than 3 hours after the onset of hemiparesis. (*Reprinted with permission from Schwartz DT.* Emergency Radiology: Case Studies. *New York, NY: McGraw-Hill; 2008.*)

- Determine whether the patient is a candidate for thrombolytics.
  - Ischemic stroke (no hemorrhage on CT scan) of <6 hours onset
    - Perform the National Institutes of Health Stroke Scale (NIHSS) assessment.
    - Make sure the patient meets both the inclusion and exclusion criteria. Important factors in these criteria include BP control to ≤185/110 mm Hg, rapidly improving symptoms, or only minor symptoms.
    - Make sure to have a thorough conversation of risks and benefits with the patient and/or family.

        - Administer alteplase: 0.9 mg/kg IV to max of 90 mg. Give 10% as bolus then the remainder over 60 minutes.
- You may also confer with your consulting neurologist and/or neuro-interventionalist to discuss endovascular options.
    - If the patient is not a candidate for thrombolytics, then supportive care is the mainstay of therapy.
    - BP management should not be started unless >220/120 mm Hg. The elevated BP may be a protective mechanism to help maintain cerebral perfusion pressure.
    - Aspirin: Started within 24 hours of presentation to the hospital.
    - Blood glucose control
- Transient ischemic attack: By definition, stroke symptoms that resolve within 24 hours are termed TIA. Patients that have a TIA are at a very high risk of having a subsequent stroke within the next 2 days (approx 4%-10%).
    - Admit all TIA patients for an expedited workup.
    - BP control.
    - Antiplatelet medications.
    - Statin drugs.
    - ECG: Rule out other atrial fibrillation/flutter or other arrhythmias.
    - Echocardiogram.
    - Carotid Doppler (Fig. 20-2).
- Basilar artery occlusion: 20% of ischemic strokes involve the posterior circulation. Symptoms include facial numbness or weakness, ataxia, and vertigo. The optimal time frame for treatment of basilar stroke is not known. Because of the high morbidity and mortality of cerebellar strokes, consider intra-arterial thrombolytics and endovascular treatments up to 24 hours after onset of symptoms.
- Pharmacologic agents for BP control:
    - Nicardipine: Calcium channel blocker. 5-15 mg/h IV.
    - Labetalol: Alpha- and beta-blocker. Start at 20 mg IV and then use 20-80 mg IV until desired BP or max 300 mg. Can start 2 mg/min IV.

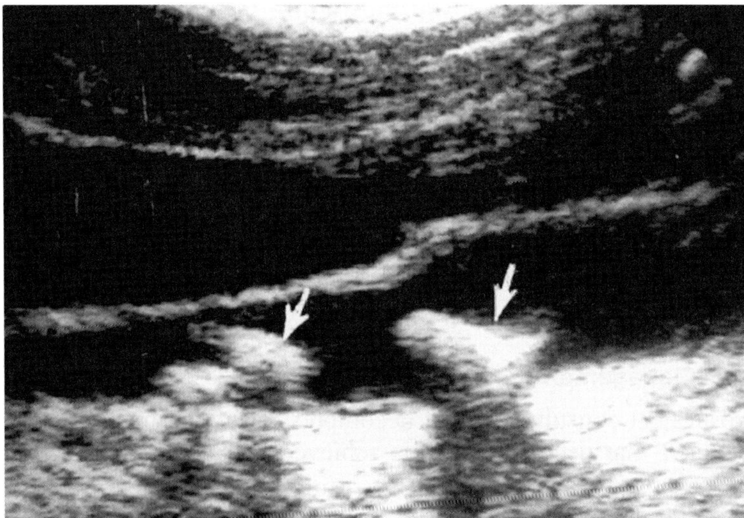

Figure 20-2. Doppler ultrasound of the carotid artery showing plaques. (*Reprinted with permission from McPhee SJ, Papadakis MA:* Current Medical Diagnosis and Treatment 2009. *48th ed. New York, NY: McGraw-Hill; 2009.*)

DON'T FORGET

If the patient is a candidate for thrombolytics, administer them as soon as possible. Make sure the family understands the risks.

DON'T FORGET

Admit all TIA patients for an expedited workup.

DON'T FORGET

Any patient with a history of cancer and signs or symptoms of radiculopathy needs an emergent MRI to rule out cord compression.

DON'T FORGET

The most sensitive finding for cord compression is post-void residual >100 mL.

DON'T FORGET

Notify the neurosurgeon immediately if you suspect cord compression. The sooner the patient is decompressed, the better the neurologic outcome.

  - Nitroglycerin: Drug of choice when angina or pulmonary edema is also present. 0.4 mg SL q5min or initial dose of 10-100 μg/min IV.
  - Sodium nitroprusside: Dose of 0.5-10 μg/kg/min.

Complications

- Natural progression of strokes may lead to increased intracranial pressure (ICP) and mental status deterioration.
- Symptomatic intracranial hemorrhage or other types of bleeding may result from tPA administration. Monitor the patient closely and discontinue the tPA immediately if any adverse reactions are noted.

Disposition

- Admit to a neurologic intensive care unit (ICU) for frequent neuro checks and monitoring.

SPINAL CORD COMPRESSION

Cauda equina syndrome is a serious complication of lumbar disc disease. It results from compression of several nerve roots in the cauda, from disc herniation, mass lesion, fracture with hematoma, or infection. Presenting with back pain, leg pain, loss of sensation in the saddle distribution, bowel and bladder retention (or incontinence), cauda equina syndrome must be diagnosed immediately and surgically decompressed to prevent permanent disability.

Additional History and Physical Examination

- Recent trauma.
- Recent back surgeries.
- History of cancer.
- Diabetes.
- Intravenous (IV) drug abuse.
- Thorough neurologic examination.
  - Saddle anesthesia.
  - Rectal tone.
  - Motor/sensory deficits.
  - Postvoid residual (>100 mL is abnormal).

Review Initial Results

- Basic labs: Rule out other metabolic causes of weakness.
- Blood cultures: Positive in >60% of epidural abscess.
- Plain films: Usually unhelpful when the diagnosis of cord compression is suspected. A negative film does not rule out disease.
- MRI: A spinal survey should be obtained for any patient with suspected cauda equina syndrome. A common mistake is to only order a focused lumbar MRI, but the whole spine should be imaged to rule out disease in the cervical and thoracic areas.

Definitive Management

- Neurosurgical consult: Surgical decompression is the mainstay of therapy. The sooner that decompression is achieved, the better the functional outcome for the patient.
- High-dose corticosteroids: Consider in conjunction with the neurosurgeon. Optimal dosing has not been established, but for patients with severe paralysis/paresis at onset, steroids have been shown to improve function.
- Radiation therapy: In the setting of primary cancer or metastatic lesions causing compression, emergent radiation oncology consultation and radiation therapy can reduce tumor burden and improve neurologic function.

Complications

- The most significant complication from cord compression is loss of function from a delay in diagnosis or surgical decompression.
- High-dose steroids may have significant side effects and are therefore still considered controversial.

Disposition

- Admit to a neurosurgical ICU.

GUILLAIN-BARRÉ SYNDROME

GBS usually occurs as a post-viral illness, especially after gastroenteritis, but can also occur infrequently after administration of the influenza vaccine. It presents as an ascending motor paralysis that peaks after about 2 weeks then resolves. Paralysis usually starts in the legs and progresses to absent deep tendon reflexes as well. Care is primarily supportive.

DON'T FORGET

Absent deep tendon reflexes is a classic finding in GBS.

Additional History and Physical Examination

- Recent viral illness.
- Recent immunizations.
- Absent deep tendon reflexes.
- Motor weakness/paralysis initially in legs greater than arms.
- Sensory examination will usually be normal.

Review Initial Results

- Basic labs: Rule out other metabolic causes.
- CT head: Rule out other intracranial lesions.
- LP: CSF classically shows an elevated protein with normal glucose and WBCs ("cytoalbuminologic dissociation").

Definitive Management

- Airway management: GBS may progress to respiratory failure, so be prepared to intubate.
- Cardiac monitoring: Autonomic dysfunction is common.
- Consider intravenous immunoglobulin (IVIG) for early or severe cases.

Complications

- An overdistended bladder can rupture or cause severe autonomic dysfunction if not addressed.
- Patients with GBS usually recover without lasting deficits.

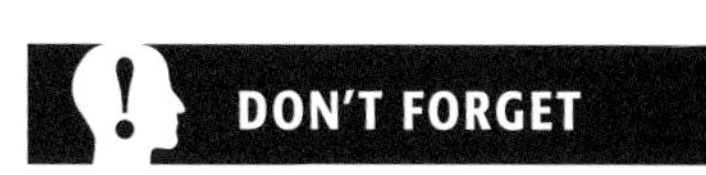

Cytoalbuminologic dissociation is classic for GBS.

Disposition

- Obtain emergent neurology consultation.
- Admit to an ICU for intensive monitoring.

MYASTHENIA GRAVIS

- MG is an autoimmune disease that attacks the acetylcholine receptors at the neuromuscular junctions. It occurs more commonly and earlier in women than in men (peak at teens—20's for women and >60 in men). Patients will present with generalized weakness with a predisposition for the proximal muscle groups: facial and bulbar muscles. In fact, ptosis and diplopia are the most common symptoms and may be the initial complaint in some patients.

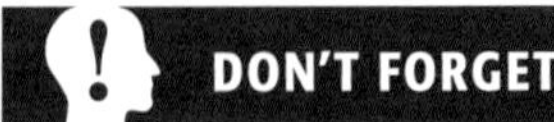

Monitor patients with MG very closely for signs of impending respiratory failure.

The thymus is found to be abnormal in 75% of patients, and thymectomy improves symptoms in the majority of patients.

- The most important aspect of MG is a life-threatening condition referred to as a *myasthenic crisis*. Muscle weakness may progress to involve the diaphragm and may progress to respiratory failure. Patients with shortness of breath with MG should be monitored extremely carefully for signs of impending respiratory failure.

Additional History and Physical Examination

- Family history of autoimmune disorders.
- Symptoms worse in evening or with continued use.
- Previous intubations.
- Dyspnea.
- Diplopia.
- Altered mental status.

Review Initial Results

- Basic labs, urine drug screen, thyroid studies: Rule out other metabolic causes of weakness.
- ABG: Evaluate respiratory status.
- CT head: Rule out intracranial lesions.
- Tensilon test: Improvement of symptoms after administration of edrophonium is diagnostic.
- Ice pack test: Application of ice pack to eyelids can improve ptosis in MG patients.
- Obtain negative inspiratory force and vital capacity values to follow objective parameters of respiratory status.

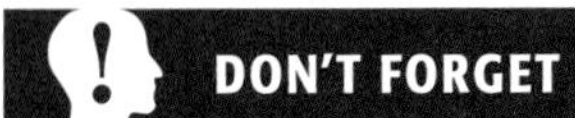

Interpret the ABG carefully in the setting of MG exacerbation. Subtle changes in CO_2 may actually indicate severe respiratory distress.

Definitive Management

- Airway management: Consider BiPAP or intubation for even the mildest of cases as respiratory failure can progress quickly.
- Neostigmine: 0.5-2 mg IV/SQ.
- Consider high-dose steroids in severe MG exacerbations.
- Avoid all drugs that can exacerbate crisis!
  - This includes fluoroquinolones, beta-blockers, and depolarizing agents.
  - On test day, ask pharmacy about possible interactions if you are unsure about a drug.
- Possible plasmapheresis or IVIG after discussion with neurology.

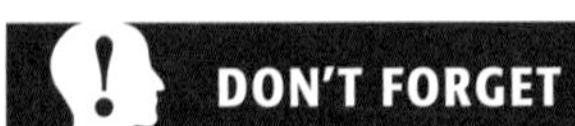

Avoid drugs that can exacerbate MG crisis! Ask the pharmacist if there are any questions about medications.

Disposition

- Neurology consult.
- ICU admission for all but the most stable MG patients.

WINNING STRATEGIES

- Focus on the details of the history including exact time of onset and progression to help narrow the differential and treatment plan.
- Clearly delineate the precise onset time if available to properly identify thrombolytic candidates.
- If the patient is a tPA candidate, aggressively manage the BP to <185/110 mm Hg. If the patient is not a tPA candidate, then the BP can be as high as 220/120 mm Hg without treatment.
- If the patient is a candidate for thrombolytics, administer them as soon as possible. Make sure the family understands the risks as well.

- On test day, admit all TIA patients for an expedited workup.
- Any patient with a history of cancer and signs or symptoms of radiculopathy needs an emergent MRI to rule out cord compression.
- The most sensitive finding for cord compression is postvoid residual >100 mL.
- Notify the neurosurgeon immediately if you suspect cord compression. The sooner the patient is decompressed, the better the neurologic outcome.
- Absent deep tendon reflexes is a classic finding in GBS.
- Cytoalbuminologic dissociation is classic for GBS.
- Monitor patients with MG very closely for signs of impending respiratory failure.
- Interpret the ABG carefully in the setting of MG exacerbation. Subtle changes in CO_2 may actually indicate severe respiratory distress.
- Avoid drugs that can exacerbate MG crisis! Ask the pharmacist if there are any questions about medications.

CHAPTER 21

Seizure

Janis Tupesis and John Dayton

INITIAL ASSESSMENT

- Initial focus on ABCs.
  - Is the airway patent?
  - Is the patient breathing without assistance?
  - Is there spontaneous cardiac activity? Are they perfusing well?
- Is the patient actively seizing on presentation?
- If so, what needs to be done immediately to break patient's seizure?

INITIAL HISTORY AND PHYSICAL EXAMINATION

History

- Evaluation of seizure
  - Prodrome: Was there abnormal eye movement, lip smacking, or facial movement?
  - Aura: Did the patient complain of any typical auras before event happened?
  - Length: How long did the seizure last?
  - Level of consciousness during the event: Was the patient awake and responsive during event?
  - Associated trauma: Was the seizure triggered by a fall? Did the seizure cause injuries?
  - Level of consciousness after the event: Was there a postictal period? How long did that last?
  - Did the patient return to their normal baseline after the seizure?
- Past Medical History
  - Prior seizure history
    - If so, how well controlled are their seizures?
    - What anti-epileptic medication do they take?
    - Have they had any recent changes to their medication doses or started other medications?
  - Any recent fever or infection?
  - Access to any medication—prescription or otherwise?
  - Any recent trauma?
  - Is the patient pregnant?

Physical Examination

- Vital signs, including pulse oximetry
- Head eyes, ears, nose, and throat (HEENT)
  - Evidence of head trauma?
  - Pupils: Check for reactivity, afferent and efferent defects, extraocular movements, and nystagmus.
  - Fundoscopy: Disk margins and hemorrhages
  - Tympanic membranes (TMs): Evaluate for blood and cerebrospinal fluid (CSF).
  - Pharynx: Is there intraoral trauma?
  - Neck: Evaluate for meningismus with Kernig and Brudzinski sign?
- Chest
  - Trachea midline?
  - Equal breath sounds?
  - Rales, rhonchi, wheezes?
- Cardiovascular (CV)
  - Rhythm?
  - Murmurs, rubs, gallops?
  - Equal pulses?
  - Good perfusion?
- Abdomen
  - Distended?

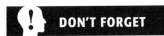

DON'T FORGET

On test day, the patient will have

- Metabolic derangements (usually hyponatremia)
- Intracranial mass or bleeding
- Meningitis
- Eclampsia
- Alcohol withdrawal/DTs
- Status epilepticus

DON'T FORGET

Stop the seizure first. Make diagnosis second.

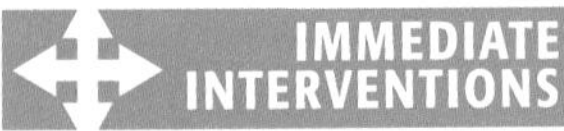

IMMEDIATE INTERVENTIONS

- **Stop the seizure!** If you have IV access, give IV lorazepam. If not, give IM midazolam or PR diazepam.
- IV, largest possible. Blood should be drawn at this time for laboratory studies.
- Supplemental oxygen via NC or NRB to keep oxygen saturation >95%.
- Cardiac monitor.

Thoughts in Early Management

- Is airway controlled? If not, control it.
- Do I need to call neurosurgery?
- How fast do I need to get the CT scanner?
- Is the patient stable enough to go the scanner without monitoring?
- Pregnancy status?

- Tender?
- Gravid?
- Evidence of bleeding?
- Extremities
  - Capillary refill
  - Warmth
  - Cyanosis
  - Edema
- Neuro
  - Motor
  - Sensory
  - Reflexes
  - Cranial nerves
  - Gait

DON'T FORGET

Pearls on clinical examination

- Look for signs of external trauma.
- Look at the tongue. Tongue laceration = seizure.
- Do a complete neurologic examination.

DIFFERENTIAL DIAGNOSIS

- Generalized seizure disorders: Seizures are divided into simple seizures, complex partial seizures, and those which are partial and evolve into generalized seizures. In simple seizures, there is no alteration of consciousness. In complex partial and generalized seizures, consciousness is impaired.
- Status epilepticus: Status epilepticus is defined as a seizure lasting >5 minutes or two or more seizures without recovery of consciousness/return to baseline in between the seizures. It includes both partial and generalized seizures.
- Meningitis: An infection of the meninges generally occurs as a complication of bacteremia, but can extend from primary infections of the sinuses or inner ear. These are much less common since widespread administration of pneumococcal and meningococcal vaccines. Varied presentations including headache, seizures, lethargy, and neck stiffness.
- Metabolic derangements: The most common metabolic derangements that will cause seizures in adults will be hyponatremia and hypoglycemia, though other derangements can also occur.
- Alcohol withdrawal/delirium tremens (DTs): Commonly seen 48-72 hours after ingestion of alcohol. Only an estimated 5% of alcoholics will develop DTs, but this is potentially life threatening with mortality approaching 35%, if untreated.
- Eclampsia: See Chap. 27, "Special Population: Pregnant Patients," for more detail.
- Head trauma: Traumatic head injury and multisystem trauma can be a cause of seizure. Causes include blunt head injury with postconcussive syndrome, traumatic subarachnoid hemorrhage (SAH), and epidural and subdural hematomas (SDHs).

DON'T FORGET

History is key!

- Circumstances
- Length of event?
- Loss of consciousness?
- Aura?
- Abnormal motor?
- Eye movements?
- Incontinence?
- Fever
- New medications in house?
- History of seizures?

GENERALIZED SEIZURE DISORDERS

Additional History and Physical Examination Findings

- Fever, central nervous system (CNS) infection, and epilepsy account for >75% of cases.
- Look for stigmata of seizure like head trauma and oral lacerations.
- Classification:
  - Generalized seizures
    - Convulsive: Tonic-clonic seizures
    - Nonconvulsive: Absence seizures
  - Partial seizures
    - Simple: Consciousness not impaired
    - Complex: Consciousness impaired

DON'T FORGET

Use a tool like GCS or AVPU to assess (and reassess) a patient's responsiveness to stimuli and level of consciousness.

Glasgow Coma Scale

Behavior	Response	Score
Eye Opening	Spontaneously	4
	To speech	3
	To pain	2
	No response	1
Verbal Response	A&Ox3	5
	Confused	4
	Inappropriate words	3
	Incomprehensible sounds	2
	No response	1
Motor Response	Obeys commands	6
	Localizes pain	5
	Withdraws from pain	4
	Decorticate flexion	3
	Decerebrate extension	2
	No response	1

AVPU: This tool is used to measure a patient's level of responsiveness to various stimuli

A = **A**lert

V= **V**oice

P = **P**ain

U = **U**nresponsive

DON'T FORGET

Know what medications you can give without an IV.

- Midazolam (Versed) can be given IM, intranasal, or via the buccal route. Midazolam is the only benzodiazepine that has equivalent onset and duration when given either IM or IV.
- Diazepam (Valium) can be given PR or IM

Review Initial Results

- Complete blood count (CBC): Evaluate infectious processes.
- Chemistries: Evaluate for electrolyte abnormalities, particularly for hypoglycemia and hyponatremia.
- Medication levels: Noncompliance with antiepileptic medication is the most common cause of seizure in adult.
- Neuroimaging: Non-contrast head computed tomography (CT)
  - Trauma
  - Suspicion of mass lesion
  - New onset seizure

Management

- ABCs: As with every patient, make sure that the patient has a patent airway, is breathing, and has good peripheral perfusion.
- Treat seizure.
  - Benzodiazepines
    - Lorazepam: Preferred first-line treatment for patients with IV access
    - Midazolam: Intravenous, intramuscular, intranasal, or buccal.
    - Diazepam: Intravenous, rectal suppository.
  - Phenytoin or fosphenytoin
    - Stabilizes sodium and calcium channels.
    - 20 mg/kg of either one, though fosphenytoin is preferred.
  - Valproic acid
    - Loading dose of 25-40 mg/kg
  - Barbiturates
    - Enhancement of gamma-aminobutyric acid (GABA) inhibition of neuronal firing
    - Causes sedation and reduces BP and respiratory rate (RR).
    - 20 mg/kg

Complications

- Depends on pathology of seizure.
- Todd paralysis: Post-seizure focal weakness that resolves within 48 hours.

Disposition

- Dependent on the etiology of the seizure.
- Workup includes lab work, neuroimaging, +/–electroencephalogram (EEG) for suspected status epilepticus.
- Typically, a patient with a single new-onset seizure with a negative workup can go home with neurology follow-up. However, most cases during the Oral Boards exam will require admission.
- Further treatment with antiepileptics and admission is determined by etiology:
  - Eclampsia: Obstetric (OB) admission, magnesium drip to prevent seizure, hydralazine for diastolic BP >105, supplemental oxygen, and delivery if still unstable
  - Febrile seizure: Infectious workup

STATUS EPILEPTICUS

Additional History and Physical Examination Findings

- Defined as a seizure lasting >5 minutes or recurrent seizures without recovery of consciousness between them.
- Occurs in about 50,000 people a year, with highest incidence in children aged <2 years of age and in those aged >60 years.

- Etiologies are generally divided into quarters:
  - 25% idiopathic
  - 25% febrile
  - 25% chronic (already has seizure disorder)
  - 25% acute symptomatic (trauma, metabolic, toxic, infectious)

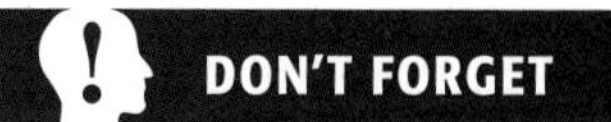

If seizures not breaking, consider using:

- Glucose: amp D50 for hypoglycemia
- Naloxone: 0.1 mg/kg for possible narcotic overdose
- Thiamine: 100 mg for possible deficiency
- Pyridoxine: 50-100 mg for functional or iatrogenic deficiency
- Antibiotics: Early institution if meningitis is suspected

Review Initial Results

- CBC: Evaluate for infectious processes.
- Chemistries: Evaluate for glucose and electrolyte abnormalities:
  - Hypoglycemia and hyponatremia are the most common causes.
  - Hypomagnesemia and hypocalcemia can also cause seizures.
  - In renal failure patients, uremia can cause myoclonic seizures.
- Toxicology screen: withdrawal states can cause seizure.
- Neuroimaging: Non-contrast head CT.
  - Trauma
  - Suspicion of mass lesion
  - New-onset seizure without fever

Management

- ABCs: Especially important in status epilepticus. Can expand to "A through F"
  - A = Airway control: Position patient.
  - B = Breathing control: Prepare to ventilate if needed.
  - C = Circulation control: Establish IV access early.
  - D = Disability: Evidence of trauma? Reversible cause like hypoglycemia?
  - E = Expose and examine patient. Evidence of trauma, infection or substance abuse?
  - F = Family: get history.
- Treatment of seizure: Drugs (Table 21-1: Treatment of Status Epilepticus)

Table 21-1. Treatment of Status Epilepticus

	Lorazepam	Midazolam	Diazepam	(Fos) Pheny-toin	Valproic acid	Levetira-cetam	Propofol	Pheno-barbital
Dose	0.1 mg/kg	10 mg IM; 0.15 mg/kg IV 10 mg Buccal or Intranasal	0.15mg/kg IV; 0.5 mg/kg PR	20 mg/kg	30 mg/kg	30 mg/kg IV	20 mg/kg	1-2 mg/kg
Route	Route: IV	IV, IM, Buccal, Intranasal	IV, PR	IV	IV	IV	IV	IV
Onset of action	5-10 min	3-5 min	1-3 min IV; 5 minutes PR	30-60 minutes	3-5 minutes	2 days	5 minutes	45 seconds

Recommended treatment:

1. Use a benzodiazepine to stop the seizure.
2. Use a non-benzodiazepine to prevent future seizure: (fos)phenytoin, valproic acid, or levetiracetam.
3. For persistent seizure, use a midazolam or propofol drip.
4. For persistent seizure, use a phenobarbital drip.

DON'T FORGET

Antibiotic coverage for meningitis depends on age

- <1 month: Ampicillin and Cefotaxime
- 1 month-50 years: Cover *Streptococcus pneumoniae* and *Neisseria meningitidis* with vancomycin and ceftriaxone.
- >50 years: Add ampicillin to *cover Listeria.*
- Consider steroids in adults

DON'T FORGET

Know how to evaluate LP results!

- High WBC count with predominance of polymorphonuclear leukocytes (PMNLs) = bacterial meningitis.
- High opening pressure (>180 mmH20), low CSF glucose and elevated CSF protein = bacterial meningitis.
- Normal WBC count with lymphocyte predominance = viral meningitis.
- If nothing fits = think tuberculous or fungal meningitis.

Complications

- Inability to control seizures
- Airway compromise from decreased mental status
- Hyperpyrexia
- Metabolic acidosis from prolonged seizure activity and increased lactic acid

Disposition

- Admit patient to either Intensive Care Unit or step-down unit.

MENINGITIS

Additional History and Physical Examination Findings

- Mortality of untreated bacterial meningitis approaches 100%.
- Risk Factors
  - Recent vaccinations, infection or surgery
  - Recent travel or patient from developing country
  - Daycare exposure
- History
  - Headaches?
  - Head trauma?

Review Initial Results

- Lab tests
  - CBC with differential
  - Platelet count
  - Blood cultures: Preferably two from two different sights
  - Serum electrolytes
  - Coagulation studies: Can be grossly elevated in patients who are septic or acutely ill
  - Bacterial antigen tests
- CSF analysis
  - Cell count: Characteristic findings include elevated WBC count with a neutrophilic predominance.
  - Glucose: Low
  - Protein: Normal to high
  - Gram stain

Management

- ABCs: As with every patient, make sure that the patient has a patent airway, is breathing, and has good peripheral perfusion.
- Early institution of bactericidal antibiotic therapy guided by age.
  - 18-50 years: Coverage for *Streptococcus pneumoniae, Neisseria meningitidis* by vancomycin and ceftriaxone.
  - >50 years: Add ampicillin to cover Listeria.
- Steroids
  - Adjuvant therapy to prevent neurologic sequelae like hearing loss and neurologic deficits.
  - Best evidence for preventing sequelae in Pneumococcal meningitis.
  - Dexamethasone: Give 15-20 minutes before antibiotics as
    - 0.15 mg/kg every 6 hours for 4 days, or
    - 0.4 mg/kg every 12 hours for 4 days

Complications

- Neurologic sequelae include vision loss, hearing loss, decreased mental functioning, higher rates of mental retardation, learning disabilities, and delayed psychosocial development.

Disposition

- Admit to intensive care unit (ICU) with strict isolation precautions.

METABOLIC ABNORMALITIES

Additional History and Physical Examination Findings

- Hyponatremia
  - Syndrome of inappropriate secretion of antidiuretic hormone (SIADH) and severe dehydration are common causes.
  - Also common in elderly patient with inadequate per os (PO) fluids intake.
- Hypoglycemia
  - History of diabetes mellitus (DM).
  - Ingestion of hypoglycemic medications.
  - Consider toxic ingestions and suicide attempts.
- Pyridoxine/B6 deficiency
  - Seen in patients on INH therapy for TB

Review Initial Results

- Electrolytes: Pay close attention to glucose and sodium levels.
- Pyridoxine level (as inpatient): Empiric treatment if on isoniazid (INH) therapy.
- CT head: Check for mass lesions or bleed.

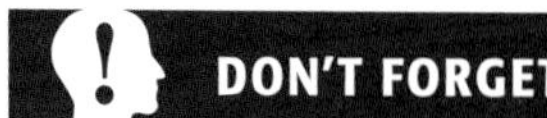

The most common metabolic abnormalities are electrolyte abnormalities!

Always check:

- Glucose
- Sodium

Management

- Replace electrolytes appropriately.
  - For symptomatic hyponatremia, give 100 mL of 3% saline over 10 minutes.
- Correct glucose, if low.
- Consider empiric B_6 administration.

Disposition

- For first, single seizure and negative workup in otherwise healthy adult, discharge home without medications for Neuro follow up and EEG as outpatient. However, almost all single oral board cases will require admission.
- For seizures due to medication noncompliance, load or give the first dose of antiepileptic medications, and discharge home after short observation period.
- Consider ICU admission for seizures caused by hyponatremia and status epilepticus for frequent neurologic checks and observation.

ALCOHOL WITHDRAWAL/DTS

Additional History and Physical Examination Findings

- Extent of alcohol use (can also occur with barbiturate abuse)
- History of previous DTs
- Anxiety?
- Tremulousness?
- Palpitations?

Review Initial Results

- Patients can present with DTs at any level of cthyl alcohol (EtOH) intoxication.
- Check glucose, sodium, and other electrolytes for source of seizure.
- CT head: Rule out SDHs or other intracranial pathology.

Management

- ABCs.
- Benzodiazepines are the first-line treatment, and very high doses may be required to control seizures.
  - Ativan: Best penetration across the blood-brain barrier
  - Valium: Two active metabolites
  - Librium: Very long-acting oral agent
- Barbiturates are second-line treatment, and act on GABA receptors (similar to alcohol and benzodiazepines).
  - Phenobarbital
  - Pentobarbital: Extremely sedating, so patient will need to be intubated before administration.
- Other medications to consider: Levels are frequently low in alcoholics due to poor diet and replacements are found in "banana bag" preparations.
  - Thiamine, Folate (and other vitamins)
  - Magnesium

Disposition

- Admit all patients with DTs from alcohol withdrawal to the ICU for frequent neurologic checks, IV benzodiazepines, and monitoring.

ECLAMPSIA

Eclampsia: See Chap. 27, "Special Population: Pregnant Patients," for more detail.

HEAD TRAUMA

Additional History and Physical Examination Findings

- Trauma is the leading cause of death from ages 1 to 44.
- Greater than 50% of head injury patients have permanent neurologic deficits.
- Injury is divided into primary and secondary injury.
  - Primary: Injury that occurs at the time of impact, either through direct trauma or acceleration/deceleration injuries.
  - Secondary: Result from response to initial injury. Can include hypotension, hypoxia, hypoperfusion, and hypercapnia. Can also include delayed injury of inflammation, microcirculatory damage, etc.

Review Initial Results

- Evaluation of trauma can be differentiated by neuroimaging.
- Normal head CT:
  - Concussion: Transient Loss of consciousness (LOC) as a result of head trauma. Patients often have normal head CT and normal neurologic examination. Usually a retrospective diagnosis.
  - Contusion: "Bruising" of brain tissue. Often with initially normal head CT. Patients can have delayed deterioration secondary to swelling or late developing hematomas.
  - Diffuse axonal injury: Results from acceleration/deceleration injuries. Though not seen on CT, magnetic resonance imaging (MRI) is diagnostic. Prognosis for full recovery is often poor.
- Abnormal head CT:
  - Skull fracture: Can be linear, comminuted, or depressed. Best seen on head CT. CSF leak merits further exploration by neurosurgeon. Also consult neurosurgeon for depression greater than one thickness of bone in depressed skull fracture.

- Basilar skull fracture: Usually caused by blow to back or side of the head. CSF otorrhea is early sign. Later manifestation seen with Battle sign and raccoon eyes.
- SAH: Blood in subarachnoid space is usually caused by disruption of small vessels in cerebral cortex. Blood typically collects along the falx cerebri or tentorium on CT (see Figure 21-1A).
- SDH: Blood between the cortex and the dura mater usually caused by tearing of the bridging veins. This is usually associated with severe parenchymal injuries and seen in elderly and alcoholic patients. Causes crescent-shaped blood on CT (see Figure 21-1B).
- Epidural hematoma (EDH): Blood in the epidural space between the skull and the dura mater is usually caused by tearing of middle meningeal artery. Initial LOC followed by lucid interval followed by rapid deterioration. Requires emergent neurosurgical evaluation. Causes lenticular (lens-shaped) blood on CT (see Figure 21-1C).

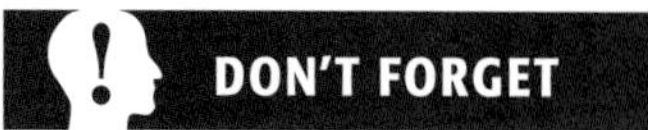

DON'T FORGET

Know how to differentiate bleeds on CT!

- Subarachnoid hemorrhage: Blood in cisterns, outlines gyri/sulci (Figure 21-1A)
- SDH: Hyperdense (white), crescent-shaped mass along the inner table of the skull (Figure 21-1B)
- Epidural hematoma: Extra-axial, smoothly marginated, lenticular, or biconvex blood collection (Figure 21-1C)
- Normal appearing CTs: concussion, early brain contusion, and diffuse axonal injury.

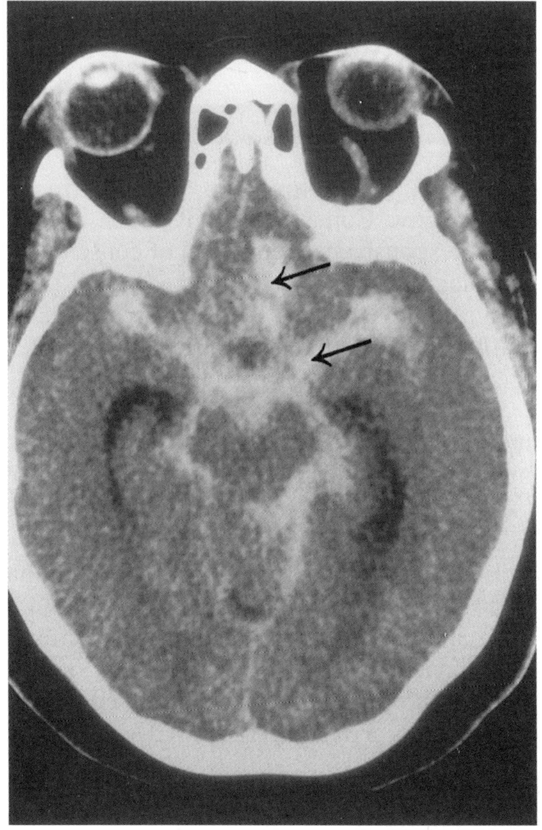

Figure 21-1. **(A)** A CT scan taken from a patient with an acute subarachnoid hemorrhage (SAH). Note the higher density in the suprasellar area and region outlining the midbrain. **(B)** Subdural hematoma (SDH) seen in non-contrast CT image in a middle-aged patient following a fall. **(C)** Epidural hematoma (EDH), crescentic, extra-axial, hemorrhagic collection layers over the right lateral convexity (*arrows*). There is associated mass effect on the adjacent brain parenchyma, with effacement of the cortical gyri, compression of the right lateral ventricle, and shift of the midline structures to the left. (*[A] Reproduced with permission from Pearlman MD, Tintinalli JE, Dyne PL.* Obstetric and Gynecologic Emergencies: Diagnosis and Management. *New York, NY: McGraw-Hill; 2009. [B, C] Reproduced with permission from Chen MY, Pope TL, Ott DJ.* Basic Radiology. *New York, NY: McGraw-Hill; 2004.*)

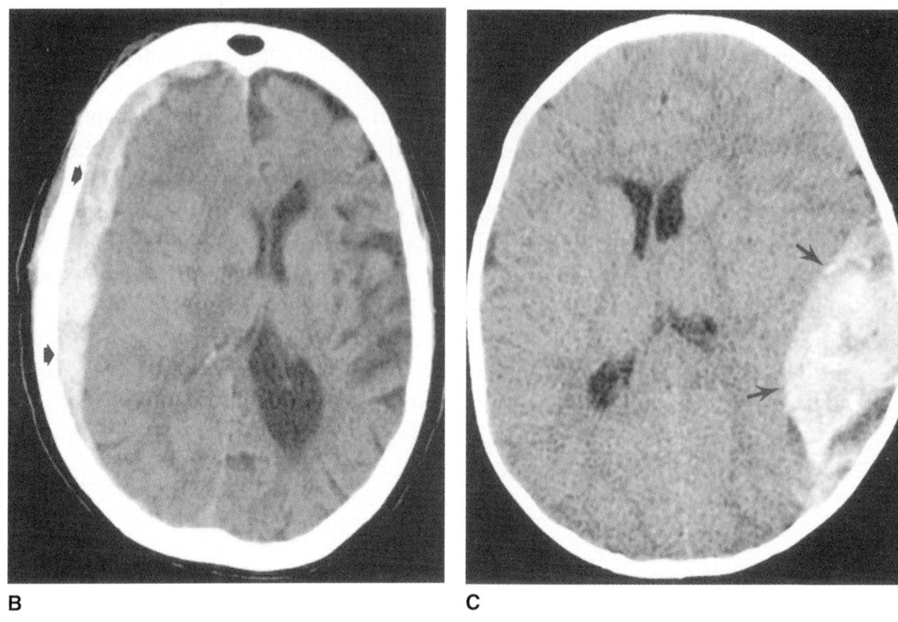

Figure 21-1. *(Continued.)*

MANAGEMENT

- Early evaluation of neurologic status.
- Use a tool like Glasgow Coma Scale (GCS) or AVPU to assess (and reassess) a patient's responsiveness and level of consciousness.
  - If GCS <8, consider intubation.
  - AVPU = Airway, Voice, Pain, and Unresponsive
  - There is a modified GCS score for pediatric patients.
- Early neurosurgical consultation for basilar skull fracture, SAH, SDH, and EDH.
  - Use IV Dilantin (phenytoin) for seizure prophylaxis for large bleeds.
  - Discuss mannitol or hyperventilation for increased intracranial pressure (ICP).

Disposition

- If patient has no LOC and has a normal neurologic examination, patient can be observed and discharged.
- If patient has LOC and/or has an abnormal neurologic examination, patient merits neuroimaging and admission.
- If patient has obvious head injury, patient needs immediate neuroimaging, neurosurgery consultation, and admission to ICU.

WINNING STRATEGIES

- Stop the seizure first, make the diagnosis second.
- Do a complete neurologic examination.
- History is the key.
- Know your GCS.
- Know what anti-seizure medications you can give without an IV.
- Initiate antibiotics early for suspected meningitis.
- Know how to interpret lumbar puncture (LP) results.
- Give 3% normal saline (NS) for symptomatic hyponatremia.
- Patients may require repeat very high doses of benzodiazepines and/or barbiturates to control DTs.
- Be able to identify common head bleeds on CT scan.
- Consider prophylactic Dilantin (phenytoin) administration for significant intracranial trauma.

CHAPTER 22

Eye Problems

Mária Némethy and David S. Howes

DON'T FORGET

For every patient with an eye complaint, consider

- Painful conditions:
  - Acute angle-closure glaucoma
  - Endophthalmitis
  - Anterior uveitis (iritis)
  - Corneal ulcer
- Painless condition:
  - Central retinal artery occlusion (CRAO)

Other vision-threatening conditions can include

- Painful conditions:
  - Optic neuritis
  - Chemical burns
  - Herpetic conjunctivitis
  - Temporal arteritis
- Painless conditions:
  - Retinal detachment
  - Central retinal vein occlusion (CRVO)
  - Vitreous hemorrhage
- Also consider other neurologic etiologies, such as stroke or migraine.

INITIAL ASSESSMENT

- Vital signs
- Visual acuity
- Focus on general appearance, age, comorbid conditions, associated symptoms.
- Consider diagnoses that pose immediate threat to vision.
- Initiate immediate interventions and obtain ophthalmologic consultation.

INITIAL HISTORY AND PHYSICAL EXAMINATION

History

- History of the present illness (HPI)
  - Onset (acute or chronic) and duration
  - Location (unilateral versus bilateral)
  - Frequency
  - Change in vision (monocular or binocular diplopia, flashes of light, floaters, halos, partial or complete blindness)
  - Painful (sharp, throbbing, foreign body sensation) versus painless condition
  - Exacerbating or relieving factors (eg, pain increases with eye movements or light)
  - Associated symptoms (tearing, photophobia, vomiting, headache)
- Past medical history (PMHx)
  - Contact lens use
  - Hypertension
  - Atherosclerotic disease
  - Hypercoagulable states
  - Recent or past history of trauma or surgery, collagen vascular disease, rheumatologic diseases, vasculitis, infectious diseases
- Medications
- Allergies
  - History of past tetanus immunization
- Family History (collagen vascular diseases, rheumatologic diseases, vasculitis, autoimmune diseases)

Physical Examination

- Vital signs
- Vision evaluation
  - Visual acuity (corrected with glasses or pin hole, hand movement detection, light detection, visual field defect)
  - Visual fields/confrontation
- Eye examination (it is best to think of the eye examination as going from outside structures to inside)
  - Orbital rim, eyelid (evert upper eyelid to assess for foreign body), conjunctiva (eg, redness, edema), sclera, cornea (eg, cloudy), iris, pupil (eg, size, shape, direct and consensual reactivity, afferent pupillary defect), extraocular movements (eg, observe for diplopia)
  - Fundoscopic examination (eg, red reflex, opacities, optic disc, retina, macula)
  - Slit lamp examination (eg, look for fluorescein uptake, anterior chamber for cells and flare, hyphema and hypopyon)
  - Intraocular pressure measurement (normal intraocular pressure is 10-20 mm Hg)
- Head, eyes, ears, nose, and throat (HEENT): Tender temporal arteries, cranial nerve deficits
- Neck: Bruits

- Cardiovascular: Irregularly irregular rhythm, murmur
- Neurologic: Cranial nerve or other sensory/motor/coordination deficits

DIFFERENTIAL DIAGNOSIS

- Acute angle-closure glaucoma
  - Increased intraocular pressure caused by overproduction of aqueous humor or decreased aqueous outflow. The result can damage the optic nerve and lead to eventual blindness.
  - Patients present with complaints such as severe eye pain, red eye, colored halos around lights (caused by corneal edema), and photophobia (Fig. 22-1).
  - However, eye pain may not be the presenting symptom. Nausea, vomiting, abdominal pain, and headache all can be presenting complaints of a patient with acute angle-closure glaucoma.
  - The goal of medical therapy is to lower intraocular pressure by blocking aqueous humor production, reducing vitreous volume, and facilitating aqueous outflow.
- Endophthalmitis
  - Infectious or noninfectious inflammation within the anterior or posterior segment or both. May be associated with ocular surgery, trauma, foreign body or other local infections, such as sinusitis or otitis media.
  - Patients typically present with severe eye pain.
  - Management includes hospitalization and emergent ophthalmologic consultation for intravitreal antibiotic therapy.
- Anterior uveitis (iritis)
  - Inflammation localized to the anterior chamber, iris, ciliary body, and anterior vitreous (Fig. 22-2A). It can be associated with infectious or systemic inflammatory processes such as juvenile rheumatoid arthritis, ankylosing spondylitis, Reiter syndrome, tuberculosis, syphilis, herpes simplex virus (HSV), and lymphoma.
  - Patients present with a painful red eye (initially perilimbic then diffuse), severe photophobia, miosis, and alteration of vision. A topical anesthetic will not arrest the pain. Slit lamp examination will demonstrate cells and flare in the anterior chamber (Fig. 22-2B).

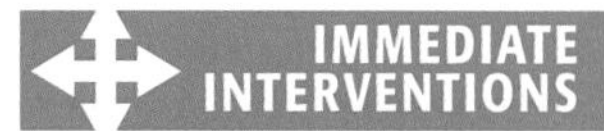

IMMEDIATE INTERVENTIONS

- Assess visual acuity.
- Consider immediate vision-threatening diagnoses.
- Address pain.
- When in doubt, obtain ophthalmologic consultation.

NOTE: Do not measure intraocular pressure if you suspect a ruptured globe.

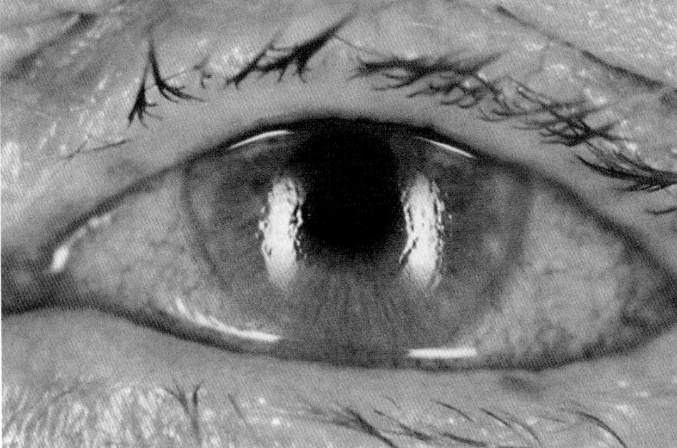

Figure 22-1. Acute angle-closure glaucoma. The cornea is edematous, manifest by the indistinctness of the iris markings and the irregular corneal light reflex. Conjunctival hyperemia is also present. (*Reprinted with permission from Knoop KJ, Stack LB, Storrow AB.* Atlas of Emergency Medicine. *2nd ed. New York, NY: McGraw-Hill; 2002.*)

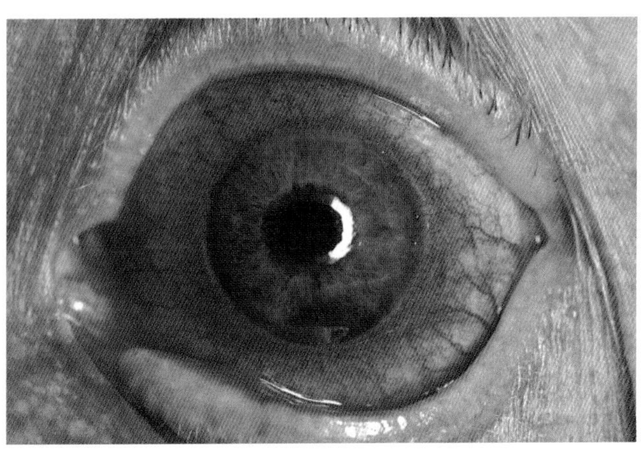

A

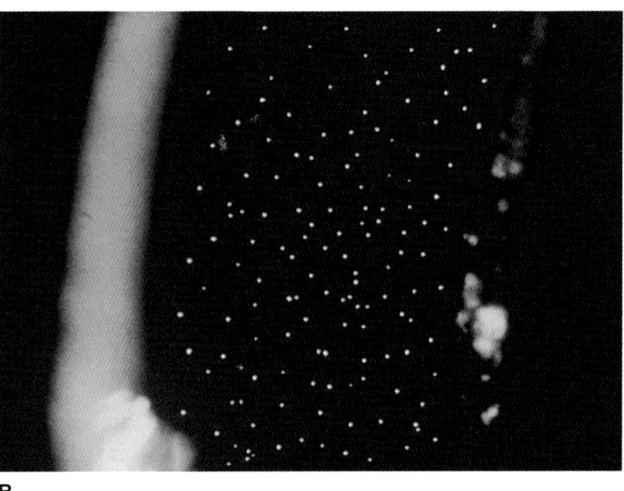

B

Figure 22-2. (**A**) **Anterior uveitis.** Marked conjunctival injection and perilimbal hyperemia ("ciliary flush") are seen in this patient with recurrent iritis. *(Reprinted with permission from Knoop KJ, Stack LB, Storrow AB.* Atlas of Emergency Medicine. *2nd ed. New York, NY: McGraw-Hill; 2002.)* (**B**) **Anterior chamber cells.** Cells in the anterior chamber are a sign of inflammation or bleeding and appear similar to particles of dust in a sunbeam. They are best seen with a narrow slit lamp beam directed obliquely across the anterior chamber. *(Reprinted with permission from Spalton DJ, Hitchings RA, Hunter PA [eds].* Atlas of Clinical Ophthalmology. *2nd ed. London, UK: Mosby-Wolfe Limited; 1994.)*

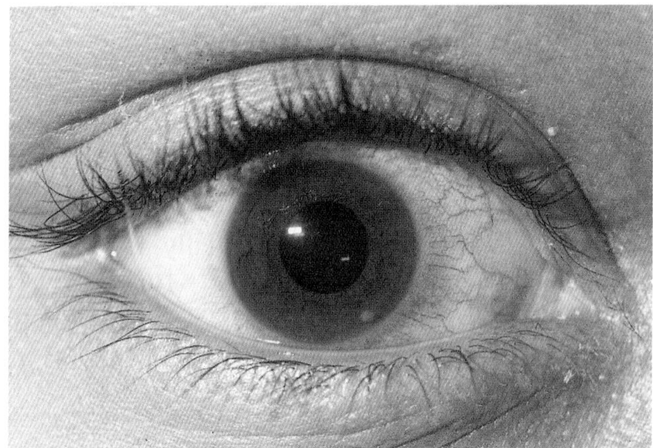

Figure 22-3. Corneal ulcer. An elliptical ulcer at 5 o'clock near the periphery is seen. This location is atypical for a bacterial ulcer. The patient presented with painful red eyes and normal uncorrected vision, but was a new wearer of soft contact lenses (for cosmesis). Bilateral corneal ulcers were diagnosed, which cleared after treatment with topical ciprofloxacin. The impressive ciliary flush is pathognomonic for corneal (versus conjunctival) pathology. *(Reprinted with permission from Knoop KJ, Stack LB, Storrow AB.* Atlas of Emergency Medicine. *2nd ed. New York, NY: McGraw-Hill; 2002.)*

- Corneal ulcer
  - Infection involving multiple layers of the cornea. Violation of the corneal epithelium allows invasion to the underlying stroma (Fig. 22-3).
  - Most often seen in extended wear contact lens users, especially those who sleep with their contact lenses. It can also be a complication of Bell palsy caused by incomplete lid closure and inadequate lubrication.

  - The presenting complaint is eye pain, and on examination there will be uptake of the fluorescein stain. Aggressive treatment is necessary to prevent scarring and permanent vision loss.
- Central retinal artery occlusion
  - Patients present with sudden, severe, persistent, painless, monocular loss of vision. They tend to be older with comorbidities and risk factors for embolic disease. Women are affected more often than men.
  - Rapid evaluation by an ophthalmologist is essential especially if symptoms are less than a few hours old. Irreversible retinal damage occurs within 2 hours, but treatment should be initiated in any patient presenting within 24 hours of symptom onset.
  - The goal of medical therapy is to lower intraocular pressure and increase retinal perfusion and oxygen delivery to ischemic tissues.

Optic Neuritis

- Most common cause of acute optic nerve-related vision loss in 20-40 age range. More common in women. Associated with multiple sclerosis.
- Often have eye pain with movement. Afferent pupillary defect may be present. Optic disc may be edematous or normal. May require magnetic resonance imaging (MRI) to diagnose.
- Ophthalmology consult to discuss treatment. Intravenous (IV) steroids for treatment.

Chemical Injury

- IRRIGATE FIRST. Do not delay irrigation to assess visual acuity! Apply topical anesthesia, then Morgan lens to affected eye(s) to rapidly deliver 1-2 L normal saline. Use litmus paper for pH testing; irrigate until pH range 7.5-8.
- Alkali burns are usually more severe because alkali penetrate deeper than acids. After irrigation, assess for corneal clouding and epithelial defects.
- Treatment: cycloplegics; erythromycin ointment; ophthalmology consult.

Herpes Zoster Ophthalmicus

- Ocular involvement of shingles on trigeminal nerve distribution. Always check for ophthalmic involvement if Hutchinson sign is present on tip of nose.
- Look for pseudodendrites on fluorescein staining (no epithelial erosion, as opposed to epithelial defects of dendrites seen in HSV).
- Treatment: antibiotic ointment; steroid drops; cycloplegics; pain control. Consider admission for IV acyclovir.

Orbital Cellulitis (Postseptal Cellulitis)

- Infection deep to the orbital septum; can be life-threatening.
- Physical examination findings: pain with extraocular movement (can help distinguish from preseptal/periorbital cellulitis); impaired extraocular muscles (EOM); proptosis; fever. Decreased visual acuity is a late finding.
- Orbital and sinus computed tomography (CTs) should be obtained.
- Requires admission for IV antibiotics.

Retinal Detachment/Vitreous Detachment

- Retinal: perception of dark veil or curtain descending; monocular vision loss.
- Vitreous: floaters, flashers (monocular).
- Can be diagnosed using bedside ultrasound. Ophthalmology consult (Fig. 22-4).

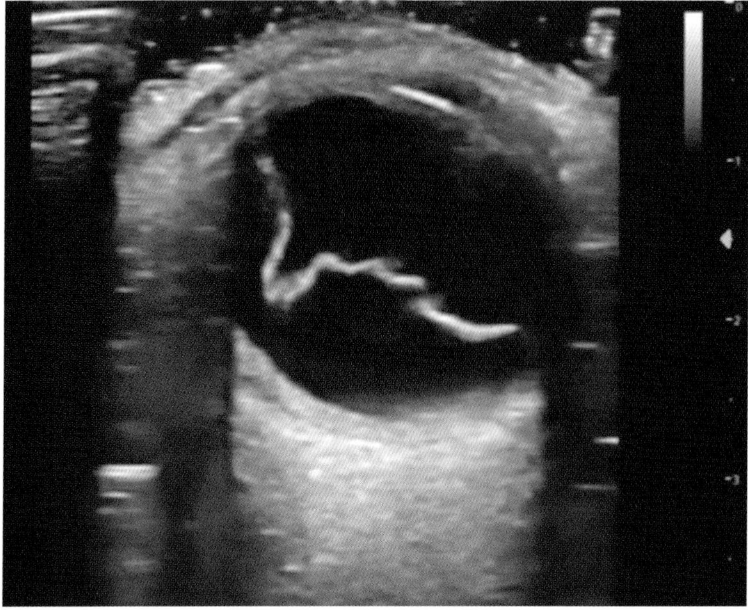

Figure 22-4. Retinal detachment. Seen as a hyperechoic membrane in the posterior aspect of the globe (arrow). (*Used with permission from Patrick M. Ockerse, MD.*)

DON'T FORGET

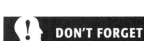

DDx Summary:

Painful:

- Acute angle-closure glaucoma: Red eye associated with vomiting and headache
- Endophthalmitis: Red eye after trauma or procedure
- Anterior uveitis (iritis): Red eye, miotic pupil with consensual photophobia, and associated infectious or systemic inflammatory processes
- Corneal ulcer: Red eye in a contact lens wearer with positive fluorescein uptake
- Optic neuritis: Eye pain with movement; associated with multiple sclerosis
- Chemical injury: Irrigate first, and copiously. Check pH. Alkali injuries worse.
- Herpes ophthalmicus: Hutchinson sign; pseudodendrites on fluorescein stain.
- Orbital cellulitis: Pain with extraocular movement, fever

Painless:

- Central retinal artery occlusion: Sudden, severe, persistent, monocular loss of vision. Retinal pallor and cherry red spot.
- Central retinal vein occlusion: Rapid, variable, monocular loss of vision. Blood and thunder fundus.
- Retinal detachment: dark veil or curtain; monocular visual field cut
- Vitreous detachment: spots, floaters

Central Retinal Vein Occlusion

- Painless, variable, rapid, monocular vision loss. Patients often with history of hypertension or vasculitis.
- "Blood and thunder" fundus (compare with pallor of CRAO). Contralateral fundus often normal.
- Treatment: consider aspirin; ophthalmology referral.

ACUTE ANGLE-CLOSURE GLAUCOMA

Additional History and Physical Examinations Findings

- Patients are typically aged >50.
- Onset typically after pupil dilation (entering a dark room, anticholinergic medications, mydriatic agents, intranasal cocaine into eye).
- Present with acute, sudden onset, severe unilateral eye pain
- Blurry vision
- Rainbow-colored halos around lights caused by corneal edema
- May often complain of unilateral headache and photophobia.
- Abdominal pain, nausea and vomiting, and malaise can be associated symptoms.
- Decreased visual acuity.
- Injected conjunctiva with a perilimbal flush and cloudy cornea (see Fig. 22-1).
- A nonreactive mid-dilated pupil.
- Shallow anterior chamber.
- Intraocular pressure >20 mm Hg; typically >30.
- Symptoms >48 hours may result in permanent loss of vision.

Review Initial Results

- Mid-dilated and nonreactive pupil with increased intraocular pressure establishes the diagnosis.

Risk Stratification: Management Priorities

- Time of onset of symptoms is important.
- Immediate ophthalmology consultation
- Rapid and aggressive reduction of intraocular pressure is achieved by:
  - Decreasing aqueous humor production
  - Reducing vitreous volume
  - Facilitating aqueous humor outflow

Definitive Management

- Place the patient in the supine position to move the lens posterior.
- Carbonic anhydrase inhibitor:
  - Decrease aqueous humor production
  - Acetazolamide: 500 mg IV q12h or 500 mg PO q6h
- Topical beta-blockers:
  - Decrease aqueous humor production
  - Timolol solution: 0.5%, 1-2 drops q10-15min for three doses, then 1 drop q12h
- Topical miotics:
  - Increase aqueous humor outflow
  - Pilocarpine: 2%, 1 drop q30min until the pupil is constricted, then 1 drop q6h
- Hyperosmotic agents:
  - Reducing vitreous volume
  - Mannitol: 20%, 1-2 g/kg IV over 30-60 minutes

Frequent Reassessment

- Recheck intraocular pressure hourly.

Disposition

- Per ophthalmology consultant

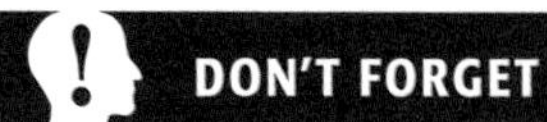

DON'T FORGET

Patients may present with headache, nausea, and vomiting without specific eye complaints. Perform an eye examination or you may miss the diagnosis.

A nonreactive mid-dilated pupil and increased intraocular pressure confirm the diagnosis.

Rapid intervention is the key!

Initial treatment consists of acetazolamide, timolol, pilocarpine, and mannitol.

Acute angle-closure glaucoma is an ophthalmologic emergency and immediate ophthalmology consultation is warranted.

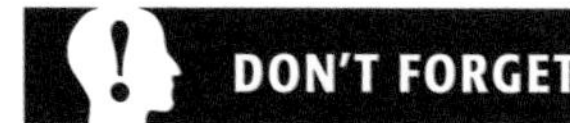

DON'T FORGET

For the purpose of oral boards, if you cannot remember the proper medication(s) or dosage(s), it is acceptable to say, "I will look it up in a reference."

ENDOPHTHALMITIS

Additional History and Physical Examination Findings

- History of sinusitis, orbital cellulitis, ocular surgery, trauma, or injury suspicious for occult intraocular foreign body
- Decreased visual acuity
- Unilateral deep ocular pain (worse with eye movement)
- Proptosis
- Photophobia, headache
- Corneal edema, redness, hypopyon
- May see preseptal cellulitis with erythema and edema

Review Initial Results

- Can perform a CT scan of the orbit looking for deep infection (eg, abscess)

Risk Stratification: Management Priorities

- Immediate ophthalmology consultation
- IV antibiotics with vancomycin 1 g and ceftriaxone 1 g

Definitive Management

- Ophthalmology consultation for admission, intravenous and intravitreal antibiotics

DON'T FORGET

Severe pain, especially with eye movement, redness, proptosis in a patient after ocular surgery or trauma, highly suggests endophthalmitis.

Look in the anterior chamber for the hypopyon.

Do not delay IV antibiotic therapy in these patients.

Obtain immediate ophthalmology consultation and plan on admission.

Complications

- Often requires numerous antibiotic regimens
- Recurrence; may result in permanent loss of vision and possible enucleation

Disposition

- Admission

ANTERIOR UVEITIS (IRITIS)

Additional History and Physical Examination Findings

- Patient may have symptoms associated with infectious, rheumatologic, or autoimmune disorders.
- Can be associated with ocular trauma
- Gradual onset of unilateral, deep eye pain
- Severe and consensual photophobia
- Blurry vision, decreased visual acuity
- Pain with accommodation
- Red eye (perilimbal and then diffuse) with excessive tearing (see Fig. 22-2A)
- Miotic and poorly reactive pupil
- Cornea can be clear to hazy
- Slit lamp examination reveals cells and flare in the anterior chamber (see Fig. 22-2B).
- Low intraocular pressure
- Topical anesthetics will not significantly alleviate the pain associated with uveitis.

Review Initial Results

- May need complete blood count (CBC), erythrocyte sedimentation rate (ESR), rapid plasma reagin (RPR), anti-nuclear antibody (ANA), purified protein derivative (PPD), and chest x-ray (CXR) for investigation of associated systemic illness.

Risk Stratification: Management Priorities

- Ophthalmologist consultation
- Initiating workup for possible associated systemic disease

Definitive Management

- In conjunction with the ophthalmologist, topical corticosteroids and cycloplegics are often prescribed to reduce the amount of scarring.

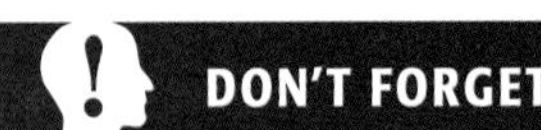

Look for consensual photophobia with cells and flare in the anterior chamber to make the diagnosis.

Do not forget autoimmune and infectious disorders associated with anterior uveitis (iritis).

Topical anesthetics will not significantly alleviate the pain associated with anterior uveitis (iritis).

Complications

- Posterior synechiae
- Glaucoma
- Neovascularization

Disposition

- May require admission for workup and management of associated medical condition.
- If stable, workup for the etiology may be performed as outpatient with prompt ophthalmology follow-up.

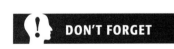

CORNEAL ULCER

Additional History and Physical Examination Findings

- History of contact lens use, specifically extended-wear lenses.
- History of trauma.
- Severe eye pain, redness, tearing, photophobia.
- Fluorescein examination shows staining of the epithelium.
- Corneal haziness noted at the border of ulcer.
- Hypopyon may be present (Fig. 22-5).

Review Initial Results

- Diagnosis is made by direct visualization.

Risk Stratification: Management Priorities

- Topical antibiotic therapy with early ophthalmology referral

Definitive Management

- Topical antibiotic therapy:
  - Sulfacetamide if no contacts
  - Ciprofloxacin or ofloxacin 1-2 drops q1h to cover pseudomonas in contact wearers
  - Cycloplegics (eg, cyclopentolate) with ophthalmology consultation
- No patching as this increases risk of worsening infection and perforation

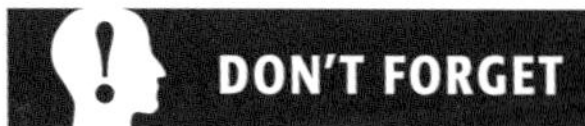

DON'T FORGET

Remember to ask all patients about contact lens use and perform fluorescein examination.

Consult ophthalmologist early in the course of management.

Do not patch the affected eye as this increases risk of worsening infection.

Complications

- Perforation of the cornea with permanent visual loss

Disposition

- These patients may be sent home.
- Follow-up with an ophthalmologist within 12-24 hours.

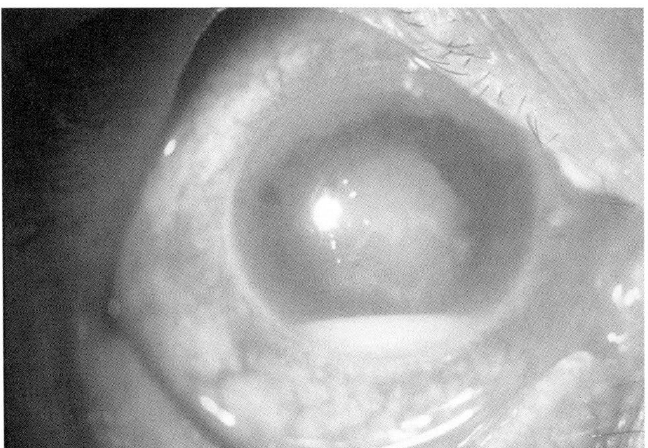

Figure 22-5. Corneal ulcer with hypopyon. The ulcer is seen as a shaggy, white corneal infiltrate surrounding the borders of the epithelial defect. The hypopyon represents the accumulation of white cells layering out in the lower one-sixth of the anterior chamber. (*Reprinted with permission from Tintinalli JE, Kelen GD, Stapczynski JS, et al.* Emergency Medicine: A Comprehensive Study Guide. *6th ed. New York, NY: McGraw-Hill; 2004.*)

CENTRAL RETINAL ARTERY OCCLUSION

Additional History and Physical Examination Findings

- History of hypertension, diabetes, cardiac valvular disease, atrial fibrillation, embolic stroke, carotid atherosclerosis, collagen vascular disease, vasculitis (temporal arteritis), sickle cell anemia
- Sudden, severe, persistent, painless monocular loss of vision
- Variable visual acuity (counting fingers, light perception only, complete blindness)
- Afferent pupillary defect (no consensual pupillary constriction with swinging flashlight test)
- Pale fundus caused by retinal edema (Fig. 22-6)
- "Cherry red spot" (non-edematous fovea)
- "Boxcar" appearance of retinal vessels (sign of severe obstruction)
- Narrow and irregular retinal arterioles
- Temporal tenderness, jaw claudication, bruits, irregularly irregular cardiac rhythm, and other manifestations of systemic diseases associated with CRAO.
- Permanent damage can ensue if vision loss persists for >2 hours.

Review Initial Results

- As indicated medically, patient may require
  - ESR
  - CBC
  - Glucose
  - Coagulation studies,
  - Lipid panel,
  - Blood cultures
  - Electrocardiogram (ECG)
  - Carotid ultrasound, echocardiogram
  - CT scan of the head
  - MRI and/or MRA of the head and neck

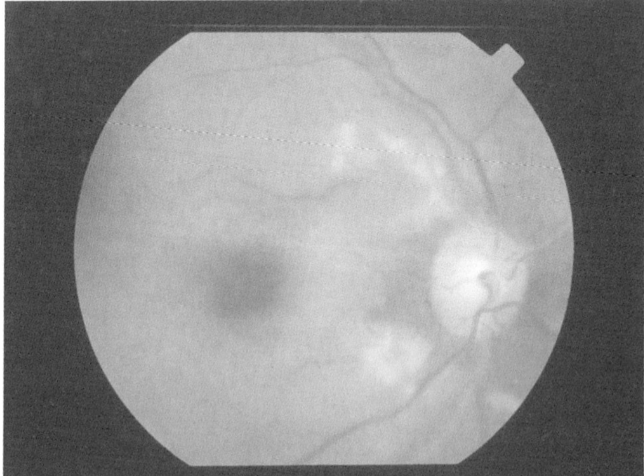

Figure 22-6. Central retinal artery occlusion. Note macular "cherry red spot" and retinal pallor between macula and disc. The retinal veins appear normal size, but the arteries are barely visible and are attenuated. (*Reprinted with permission from Tintinalli JE, Kelen GD, Stapczynski JS, et al.* Emergency Medicine: A Comprehensive Study Guide. *6th ed. New York, NY: McGraw-Hill; 2004.*)

Risk Stratification: Management Priorities

- Rapid evaluation by an ophthalmologist is essential especially if symptoms are less than few hours old (patient may require surgical decompression, eg, anterior chamber paracentesis).
- The goal is to lower intraocular pressure, increase retinal perfusion, and oxygen delivery to ischemic tissues.

Definitive Management

- Ocular digital massage to globe may be repeated several times as a rapid attempt to dislodge the clot in a pattern of 10 seconds on and off.
- Rebreathing CO_2 in an attempt to vasodilate retinal arterioles by breathing in a paper bag 10-15 minutes each hour.
- Can use agents that decrease the intraocular pressure:
  - Acetazolamide: 500 mg IV or 500 mg PO once
  - Timolol solution: 0.5%, one drop bid

Complications

- Irreversible retinal damage occurs within 2 hours, but treatment should be initiated in any patient presenting within 24 hours of symptom onset.

Disposition

- Often admitted for a complete systemic workup, especially if comorbid conditions are present

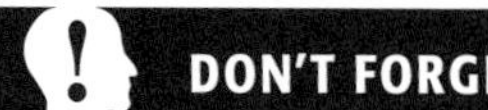

Sudden, severe, persistent, painless, monocular loss of vision should make you suspect CRAO.

CRAO may be associated with temporal arteritis.

Remember pale fundus and "cherry red spot" equals CRAO.

The goal of medical therapy is to lower intraocular pressure and increase retinal perfusion and oxygen delivery to ischemic tissues.

Rapid evaluation by an ophthalmologist is essential especially if symptoms are less than a few hours old.

WINNING STRATEGIES

- Every patient with eye pain has either:
  - Acute angle-closure glaucoma
  - Endophthalmitis/orbital cellulitis
  - Anterior uveitis (iritis)
  - Corneal ulcer or Herpes ophthalmicus
  - Chemical injury
  - Optic neuritis
- Consider acute angle-closure glaucoma if presented with a painful red eye associated with vomiting and headache.
  - You may be presented with a patient complaining of headache and nausea and vomiting without eye complaints. Perform an eye examination or you will miss the diagnosis of acute angle-closure glaucoma.
  - A red eye with a nonreactive mid-dilated pupil and increased intraocular pressure gives you the diagnosis of acute angle-closure glaucoma.
  - Acute angle-closure glaucoma is an ophthalmologic emergency and requires immediate consultation and rapid treatment with acetazolamide, timolol, pilocarpine, and mannitol.
- Suspect endophthalmitis if presented with a painful red eye after trauma or ocular procedure.
  - Obtain immediate ophthalmology consultation and do not delay intravenous antibiotic therapy in patients with endophthalmitis.
- Suspect anterior uveitis (iritis) if presented with a painful red eye and miotic pupil with consensual photophobia associated with infectious or systemic inflammatory symptoms.
  - Look for the consensual photophobia and cells and flare on slit lamp examination to make the diagnosis of anterior uveitis (iritis).
  - Do not forget the autoimmune or infectious disorders associated with anterior uveitis (iritis).
  - Topical anesthetics will not significantly alleviate the pain of anterior uveitis (iritis)—as opposed to a corneal ulcer or abrasion.

- Suspect corneal ulcer if presented with a painful red eye in a patient who wears contact lens and slit lamp examination reveals positive fluorescein uptake.
- Consider CRAO in a patient presenting with painless loss of vision.
  - Rapid evaluation of CRAO by an ophthalmologist is essential especially if symptoms are less than a few hours old.
- Remember pale fundus and "cherry red spot" equals CRAO. "Blood and thunder" fundus equals CRVO.
- Retinal detachment associated with "descending curtain."
- Vitreous detachment associated with "floaters."

THE BOTTOM LINE

- Everyone with eye complaints needs assessment of visual acuity.
- Construct the differential diagnosis in painful and painless conditions.
- When in doubt, obtain ophthalmology consultation.

CHAPTER 23

Rash and Skin Complaints

David Howes and Christopher Gee

INITIAL ASSESSMENT

- Focus on ABCs. Keep immediate life-threats in mind first and start treatment Stat.
- Ask for a full set of vitals with every patient including pulse, BP, respirations, temp, O_2 sat, glucose, finger stick hemoglobin.
- Large-bore IV, O_2, monitor, and airway equipment to the bedside for every patient.
- Draw full set of labs and hold for orders.

Case-Specific Recommendations

- Assess immediately whether the airway is swollen or in danger of obstruction. If airway issues are present, stabilize immediately with aggressive airway management.
- Shock with rash or skin swelling suggests life-threatening anaphylaxis or infection.

IMMEDIATE INTERVENTIONS

- Ill-appearing (abnormal vital signs, shock, airway involvement)
- IV.
- Oxygen.
- Monitor.
- Send blood for CBC, lytes, type and cross.
- Aggressive fluid resuscitation.
- Assess the need for emergent airway.
- Well-appearing (normal vital signs, no airway involvement).
- Defer diagnostic and therapeutic interventions until after completion of H+P.

INITIAL HISTORY AND PHYSICAL EXAMINATION

History

- History of the present illness (HPI)
  - Onset: When did it begin? Was it related to any activity, medication, event, or ingestion?
  - Distribution: Diffuse or localized? Symmetric? Involving the trunk or extremities?
  - Duration/extension: Getting better or worse?
  - Exacerbation/relief: Any attempts to treat prior to arrival?
  - Associated symptoms: Itchy? Airway swelling, stridor, change in voice, difficulty swallowing? Fever? Headache? Pain?
- Past medical history (PMHx)
  - Comorbidities
  - Similar reactions in the past
  - Medications: New medications, change in medications, use of angiotensin-converting enzyme (ACE) inhibitors or sulfa drugs.
  - Allergies: Drug allergies? Environmental allergies?

Physical Examination

- General appearance: Is the patient oriented, appropriate?
- Vital signs
  - Blood pressure: Shock is concerning and suggestive of anaphylaxis, severe dehydration, or infection.
  - Tachypnea: May require urgent airway management.
  - Tachycardia: May be the only initial sign of impending problems.
- Skin
  - Rash
    - Purpuric
    - Diffuse
    - Involving mucosal surfaces (eyes, mouth)
  - Swelling: Oral, facial, pharyngeal
  - Lesions
- Head, eyes, ears, nose, and throat (HEENT): Voice changes, intraoral swelling, mucosal erosions or sloughing?
- Neck: Supple? Stridor?

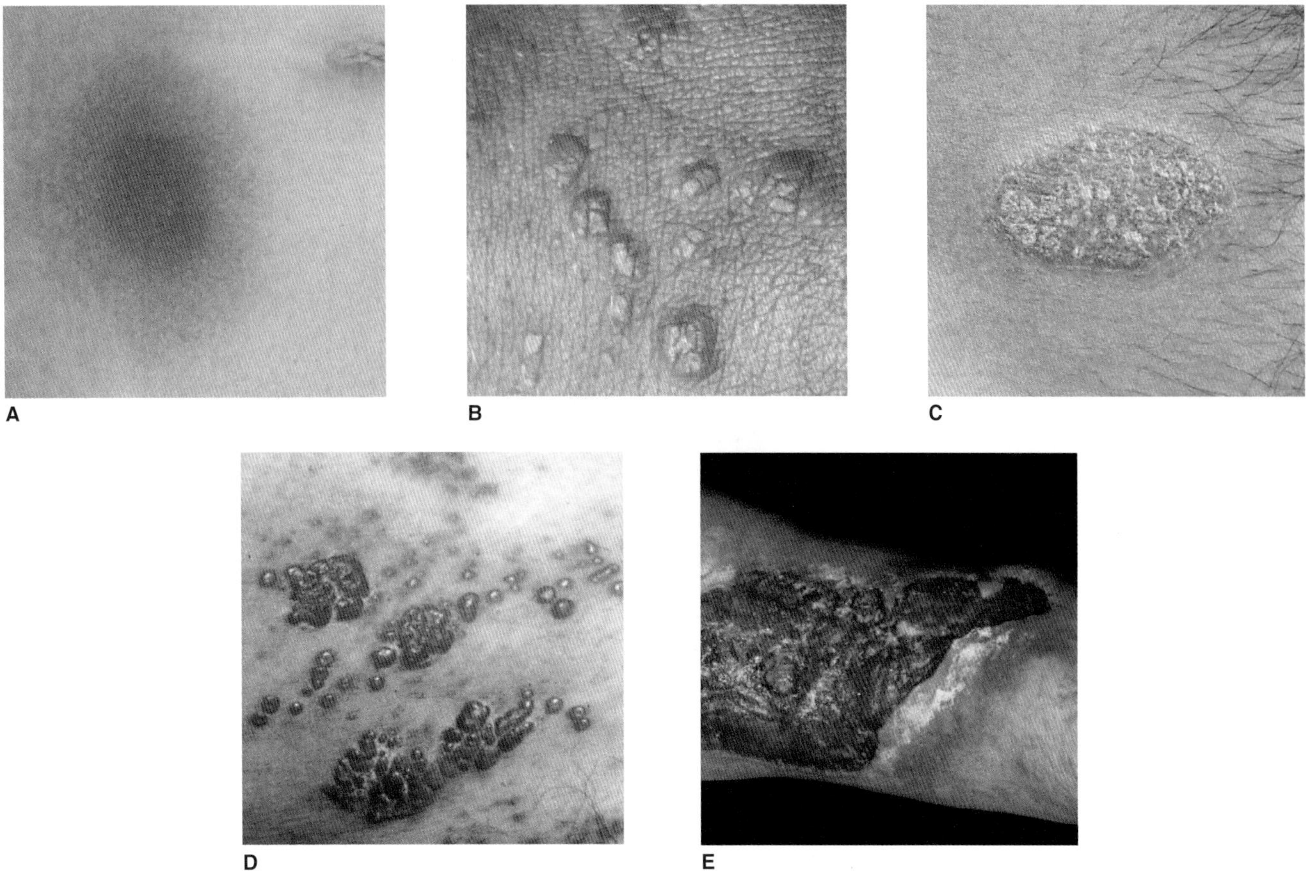

Figure 23-1. **(A)** Macules (<1 cm) and patches (>1 cm). **(B)** Papules. **(C)** Plaque. **(D)** Vesicles/bullae. **(E)** Ulcer. (*Reproduced with permission from Wolff K, Johnson RA.* Fitzpatrick's Color Atlas and Synopsis of Clinical Dermatology. *6th ed. New York: McGraw-Hill, NY; 2009.*)

- Chest: Breath sounds equal, crackles, wheezes, rubs?
- Cardiovascular (CV): Murmurs, rubs, gallops? Peripheral pulses symmetric?
- Extremities: Cyanosis, edema?
- Neuro: Motor, sensory, deep tendon reflex (DTR) symmetric?

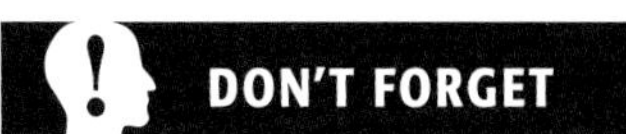

DON'T FORGET

Terms used to describe rash (Fig. 23-1)

- Macular: Flat, <1 cm
- Patchy: Flat, >1 cm
- Papular: Raised, <1 cm
- Plaque: Raised, >1 cm
- Vesicle: Fluid-filled blister, <1 cm
- Bulla: Blister, >1 cm
- Ulceration: Erosion into dermis or deeper

DIFFERENTIAL DIAGNOSIS

- Urticaria/angioedema
  - Referring to a mild allergic reaction confined to the superficial skin, urticaria appears as red plaques with central clearing. Will often move around.
  - Angioedema refers to an allergic reaction involving the deeper tissues. It is characterized by painless, nonpruritic swelling of the face, lips, oropharynx, larynx, or distal extremities (Fig. 23-2).
  - Acquired angioedema, in contrast to hereditary angioedema, occurs in association with urticaria and as a reaction to stimuli such as foods, drugs (especially ACE inhibitors), insect bites, inhalants, or system disease. Swelling can be severe and can last for hours to days. Airway compromise, with difficulty swallowing, swelling, and voice changes, is a feared complication.
  - Both urticaria and angioedema can progress to severe anaphylaxis.

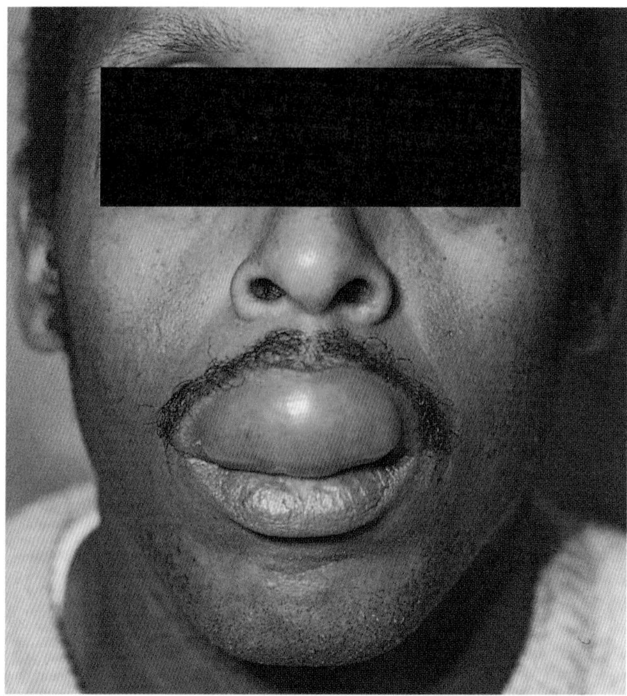

Figure 23-2. Angioedema. ACE inhibitor-induced angioedema of the upper lip in a man who had been taking an ACE inhibitor for 2 years. The patient had no previous episodes. (*Reproduced with permission from Knoop KJ, Stack LB, Storrow AB.* Atlas of Emergency Medicine. *2nd ed. New York*, NY*: McGraw-Hill; 2002.*)

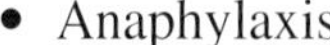

- Anaphylaxis
  - A severe, systemic allergic reaction characterized by hypotension, airway swelling and obstruction, and severe bronchospasm.
  - Anaphylaxis can be rapidly fatal and must be treated aggressively.
- Erythema multiforme (EM)
  - EM major includes three major syndromes: EM minor, Stevens-Johnson syndrome (SJS) and toxic epidermal necrolysis (TEN) (Fig. 23-3).
  - Often secondary to medication exposure, EM major is frequently severe, progressive, and potentially fatal.
- Meningococcemia
  - Referring to severe sepsis and meningitis caused by *Neisseria meningitidis*, a gram-negative coccus, meningococcemia often presents with a characteristic purpuric rash (Fig. 23-4).
  - Meningococcemia is discussed further in Chap. 32.
- Necrotizing infections
  - Severe, life-threatening infections of the skin and soft tissues, necrotizing infections are discussed in detail in Chap. 7.
- Rocky Mountain spotted fever (RMSF)
  - Having the highest incidence in children, RMSF usually presents with high fever, rash (classically petechiae on wrists), headache, and gastrointestinal (GI) symptoms (Fig. 23-5). The diagnosis must be considered and treated early in any ill-appearing child with rash and fever. RMSF is discussed further in Chap. 32.

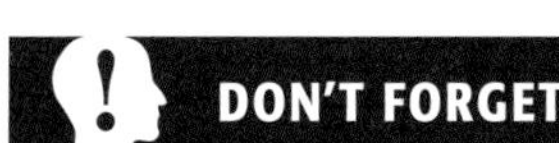

DON'T FORGET

DDx Summary

- Allergic reactions
  - Urticaria
  - Angioedema
  - Anaphylaxis
  - EM major
- Diffuse rash with fever
  - Meningococcemia
  - RMSF
- Localized rash with fever
  - Cellulitis
  - Necrotizing infections

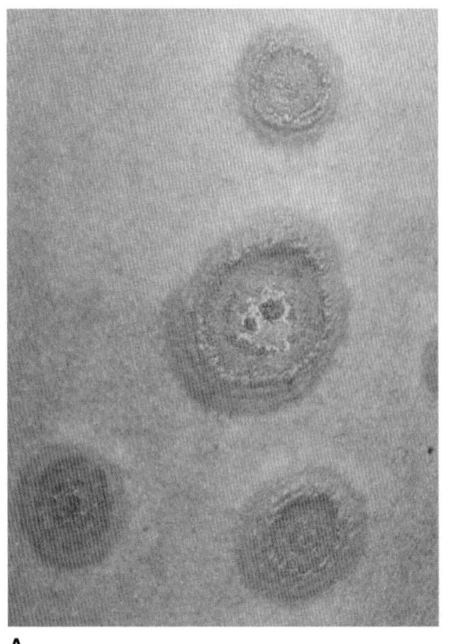

A

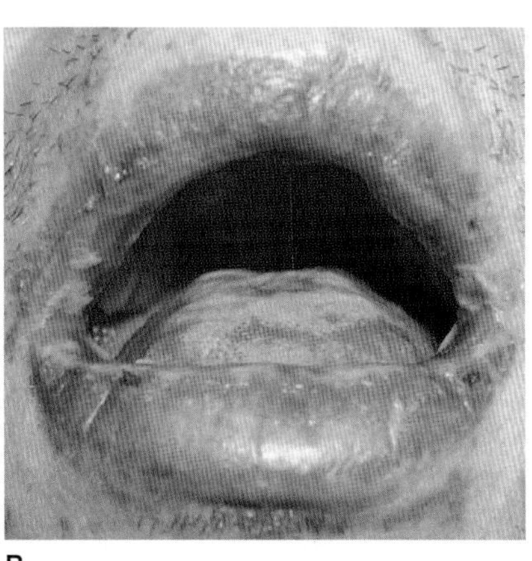

B

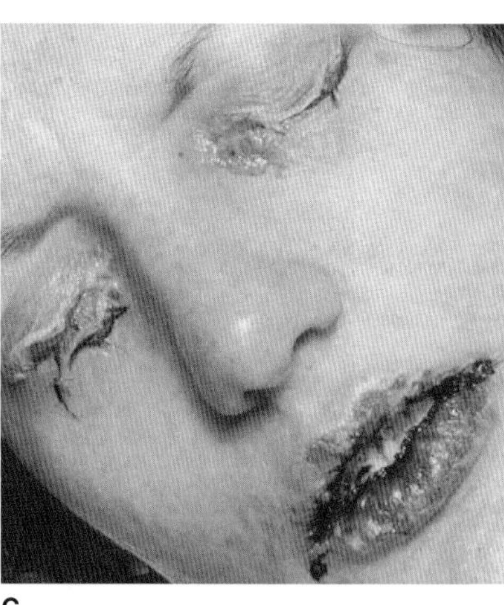

C

Figure 23-3. (**A**) **Multiple concentric vesicular rings** (herpes iris of Bateman). This pattern may be more frequent in *Mycoplasma pneumoniae*–related cases of **erythema multiforme** major. (**B**) **Stevens-Johnson syndrome.** A young man with mycoplasma pneumonia. Note the erosive lesions on the skin and mucosal surfaces. (**C**) **Toxic epidermal necrolysis.** Massive erosions covered by crusts on the lips. Note also shedding of eyelashes. (*Reproduced with permission from Wolff K, Johnson RA.* Fitzpatrick's Color Atlas and Synopsis of Clinical Dermatology. *6th ed. New York, NY: McGraw-Hill; 2009.*)

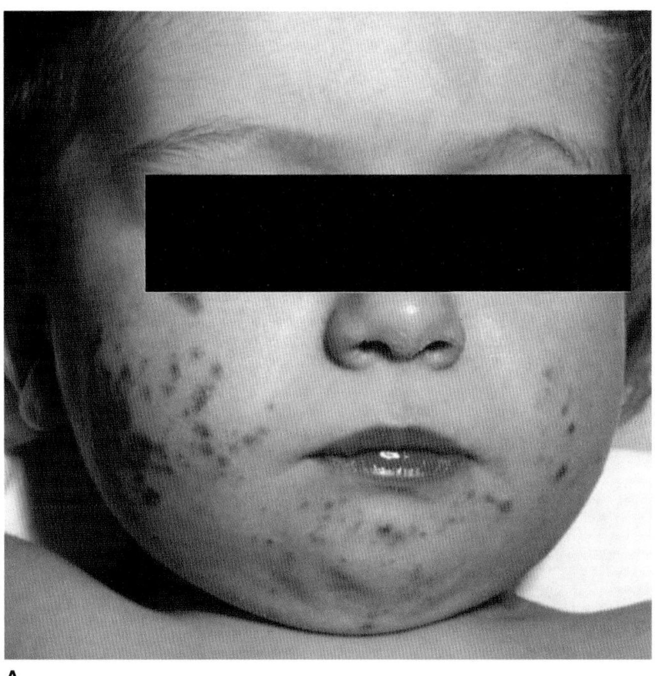

A

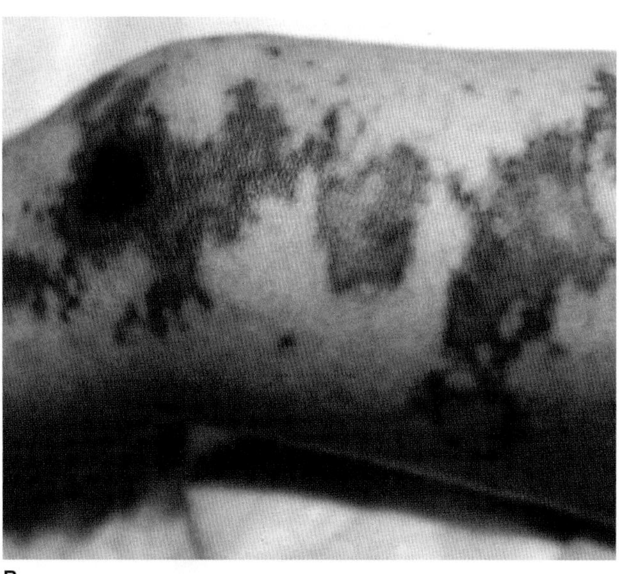

B

Figure 23-4. (**A**) **Acute meningococcemia: early exanthem.** Discrete, pink-to-purple macules and papules, as well as purpura on the face of this young child. These lesions represent early disseminated intravascular coagulation with its cutaneous manifestation, purpura fulminans. (**B**) **Acute meningococcemia: purpura fulminans.** Maplike, gray-to-black areas of cutaneous infarction of the leg in a child with *N meningitidis* meningitis and disseminated intravascular coagulation with purpura fulminans. (*Reproduced with permission from Wolff K, Johnson RA.* Fitzpatrick's Color Atlas and Synopsis of Clinical Dermatology. *6th ed. New York, NY: McGraw-Hill; 2009.*)

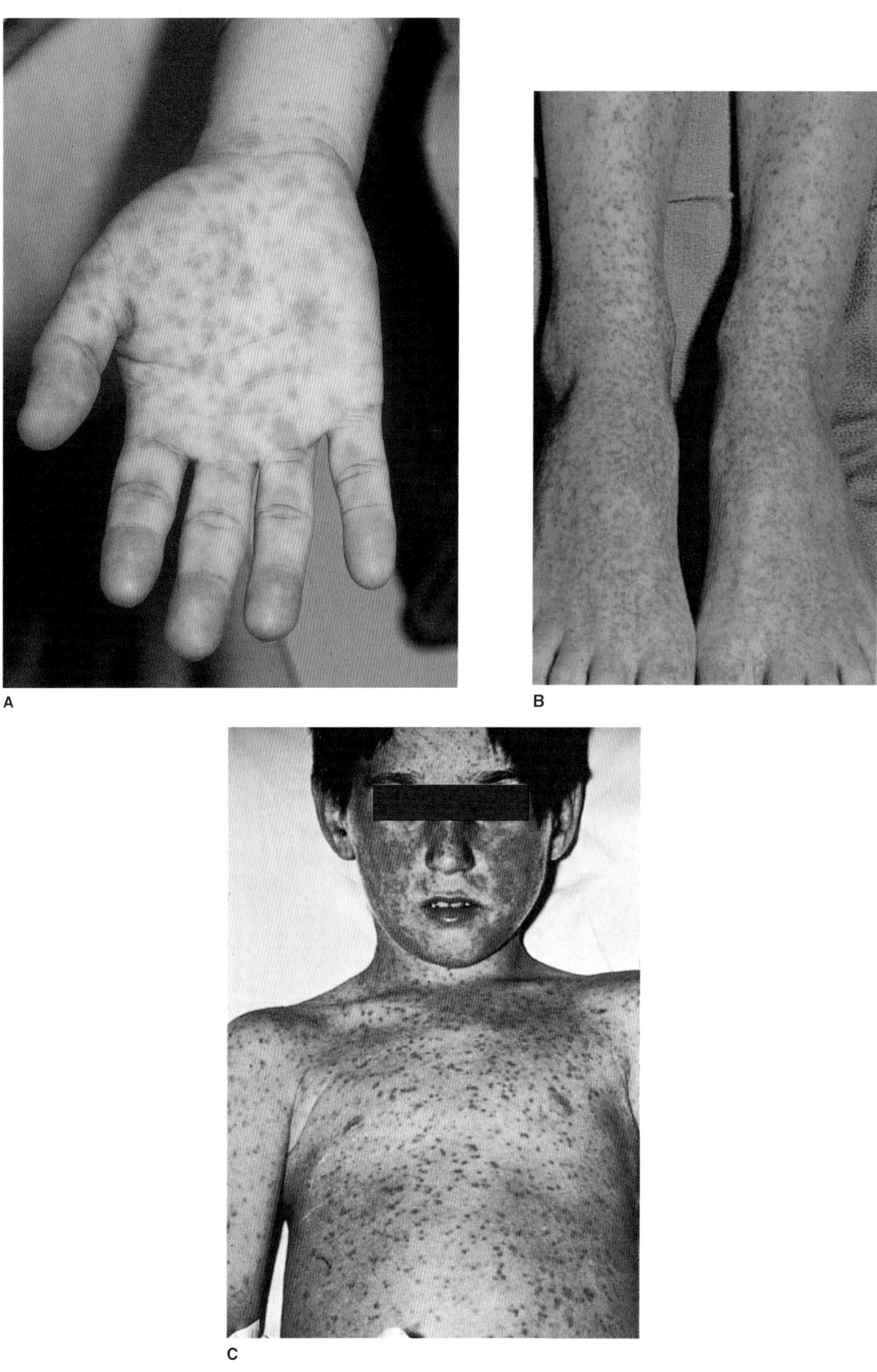

Figure 23-5. Rocky Mountain spotted fever. Erythematous macular lesions usually starting on hands, feet and ankles evolve into a petechial rash that spreads centrally. (*[A] Reproduced with permission from Knoop KJ, Stack LB, Storrow AB:* Atlas of Emergency Medicine, *2nd ed. New York, NY: McGraw-Hill, 2002. [B, C] Reproduced with permission from Wolff K, Johnson RA.* Fitzpatrick's Color Atlas and Synopsis of Clinical Dermatology. *6th ed. New York*, NY*: McGraw-Hill; 2009.*)

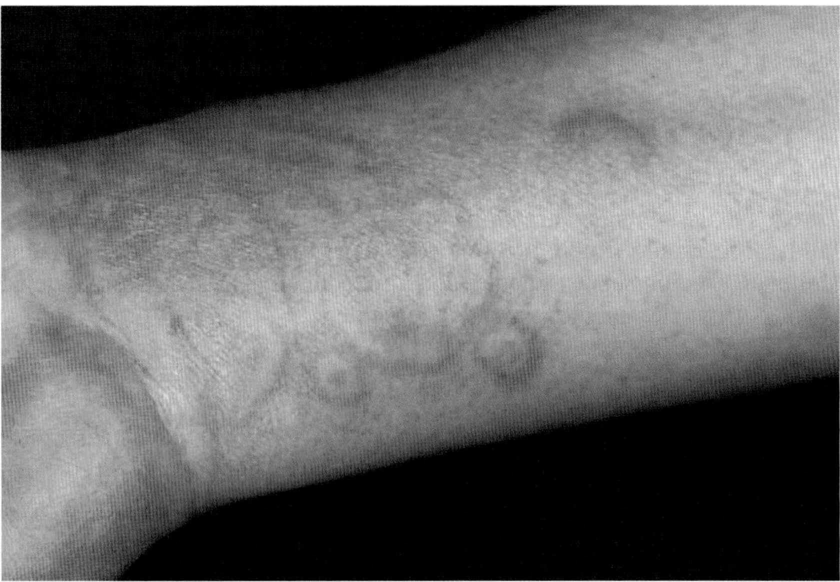

Figure 23-6. Urticaria. Wheals with white to light-pink color centrally and peripheral erythema in a close-up view. These are the classic lesions of urticaria. It is characteristic that they are transient and highly pruritic. (*Reproduced with permission from Wolff K, Johnson RA.* Fitzpatrick's Color Atlas and Synopsis of Clinical Dermatology. *6th ed. New York, NY: McGraw-Hill; 2009.*)

URTICARIA/ANGIOEDEMA

Additional History and Physical Examination Findings (Fig. 23-6)

- Urticaria
  - Pruritic, edematous, erythematous raised wheals or papules.
  - Central clearing frequently present.
  - Lesions blanch with pressure.
  - Etiologic agents are extremely numerous.
  - Food and drugs are the most common cause.
  - Urticaria may accompany more serious reactions including angioedema and anaphylaxis. Assess for vital sign instability, edema of deeper tissues, and airway edema.
- Angioedema
  - Swelling of the deep dermis or submucosal tissues due to vascular leakage. Often occurs in lips, eyes, face but can also occur in other areas like Airway or GI tract.
  - Drugs and food are the most common causes.
  - Angioedema secondary to ACE inhibitor use is common and potentially life-threatening.
  - Angioedema may occur months or even years after initial use.
  - Symptoms commonly last up to 24 hours.

Review Initial Results

- Ask for complete vital signs including pulse oximetry.
- Assess for signs of potential airway compromise, including stridor, voice change, swelling of pharynx, and swelling of the tongue or lips. Patients with evidence of airway involvement must be treated emergently and cannot be left alone until the airway is secure.
- Do not allow unstable patients to leave the emergency department (ED).

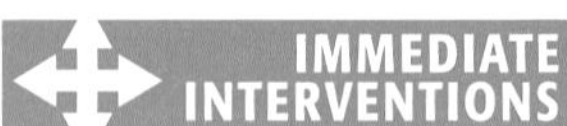

A patient with simple urticaria is unlikely on the oral board examination. Expect decompensation with angioedema or anaphylaxis!

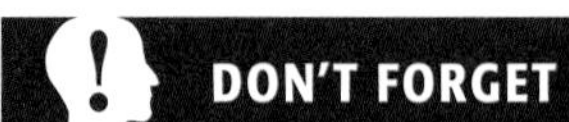

- IV, O_2, monitor, advanced airway equipment to the bedside.
- Remove exposure to allergic agent (if possible).
- Reassess and prepare to control airway.

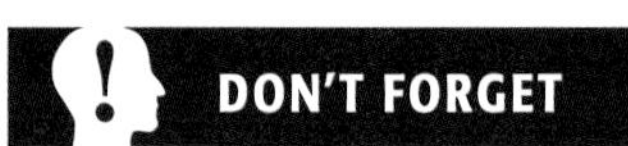

All patients with any airway involvement (stridor, voice change, inability to control secretions) get risk stratification with laryngoscopy.

DON'T FORGET

If you need to control the airway, employ the difficult airway algorithm. Call ENT and anesthesia early.

Risk Stratification

- Assessment based on presence of edema, potential involvement of airway.
- All patients with potential airway involvement need definitive risk stratification with direct visualization of the larynx and vocal cords. Fiber-optic laryngoscopy is the procedure of choice to evaluate for airway compromise. If the suspicion for airway involvement is high, preparations to intubate the patient should be made at the time of laryngoscopy.
- Mild: Urticaria alone with no angioedema or signs of airway involvement.
- Moderate: The presence of angioedema without signs of airway involvement.
- Severe: Angioedema with airway involvement.

Definitive Management

- Mild or moderate
  - H1 blocker
    - Diphenhydramine 50 mg PO/IV q4-6h
    - Loratadine 10 mg QD
  - H2 blocker
    - Cimetidine 300 mg PO
    - Ranitidine 150 mg PO
  - Steroids
    - Prednisone 60 mg PO
    - Decadron 10 mg IV
  - Long period of observation in the ED versus admission to ensure no progression of edema or involvement of airway
- Severe
  - Intravenous (IV), oxygen, monitor
  - IV medications
    - Epinephrine 0.3 mL of 1:1000 solution IM.
    - H1 blocker: Diphenhydramine 50 mg IV.
    - H2 blocker: Famotidine 20 mg IV.
    - Steroids: Decadron 10 mg IV or methylprednisone 125 mg IV.
    - Consider cryoprecipitate if hereditary angioedema is suspected.
  - Airway control
    - Employ predicted difficult airway algorithm (see Chap. 2).
    - Do not use rapid sequence induction (RSI).
    - Consider awake laryngoscopy or fiber-optic laryngoscopy.
    - Call ear, nose, and throat (ENT) and anesthesia early.
    - Prep patient and equipment for cricothyroidotomy.

Disposition

- Mild: Patients without progression may be discharged home with oral H1 blocker, H2 blocker, epinephrine pen, and 5-day course of oral steroids.
- Moderate: Patients with significant airway swelling of the tongue, lips, posterior pharynx, who do not require intubation for airway control, may still require admission for observation. Patients with angioedema secondary to ACE inhibitors should be admitted for close observation. Patients with involvement of the lips, tongue, or posterior pharynx should be watched in the intensive care unit (ICU).
- Severe: Intubated patients with severe angioedema must be admitted to the ICU.

ANAPHYLAXIS

Additional History and Physical Examination Findings

- Frequently caused by reactions to medications (ie, penicillin, non-steroidal anti-inflammatory drug [NSAIDs]), foods (ie, peanuts, shellfish), bee stings, or iodinated contrast media. When taking the history, try to identify the etiologic agent.

- Anaphylaxis occurs on repeat exposure to a foreign substance to which the patient was previously sensitized.
- Onset of symptoms typically occurs within 30 minutes of exposure, but may be immediate. Symptoms typically last up to 4 hours. In a small percentage of patients, symptoms recur within 24 hours despite complete resolution.
- Variable presentations range from minor urticaria to life-threatening shock and airway obstruction. Seemingly minor presentations of allergic reaction may develop into anaphylaxis.
- Common symptoms:
  - 90% of patients have urticaria or angioedema presenting with rash, swelling, itching, or tingling of the skin.
  - Laryngeal edema presenting with hoarseness, dysphagia, lump in throat, or complete airway obstruction is the most common cause of death.
  - Bronchospasm with wheezing and tightness is common.
  - Refractory hypotension presenting with syncope, dizziness, or altered mental status is the second most common cause of death.
  - GI symptoms of cramping, diarrhea, and vomiting are also common.

Review Initial Results

- Ask for complete vital signs including pulse oximetry and pay attention to the blood pressure.
- Assess for signs of airway compromise, including stridor, voice change, and pharyngeal, lip, or tongue swelling. Patients with evidence of airway involvement must be treated emergently and cannot be left alone until the airway is secure.

RISK STRATIFICATION

- All patients with anaphylaxis are emergent and require immediate attention.

Definitive Management

- Immediate IV, oxygen, monitor and advanced airway equipment to the bedside.
- Remove antigen, delay absorption.
- Epinephrine 0.3 mL of 1:1000 solution IM.
  - Indicated in all patients with anaphylaxis.
  - Do not withhold in patients >50 years or with cardiac history as benefits outweigh risks in severe anaphylaxis.
- Control airway
  - Albuterol aerosol
  - Consider IV epinephrine if airway compromise is imminent.
  - Definitive airway
    - Employ predicted difficult airway algorithm.
    - Do not use RSI.
    - Fiber-optic intubation if rapidly available and skilled provider.
    - Awake laryngoscopy.
    - Cricothyroidotomy.
    - Call ENT and anesthesia early.
- Treat hypotension.
  - Normal saline (NS) bolus (1 L), may repeat
  - Trendelenburg position
  - Dopamine infusion 5-20 μg/kg/min
  - IV epinephrine
- Consider IV epinephrine in patients with impending airway collapse or refractory hypotension.
  - Add 1 amp of epinephrine (1:10000) to 1 L of NS and start the drip at 1 μg/min.

DON'T FORGET

Anaphylaxis is frequently rapid and life-threatening.

For anaphylaxis, use epinephrine IM first.

Make an IV epinephrine drip quickly by adding 1 amp of 1:10,000 epinephrine (1 mg) to 1 L of NS and running the drip at 1 μg/min. Hypotension may be resistant. Aggressive fluid hydration and pressors are keys.

On test day, have a low threshold to admit patients.

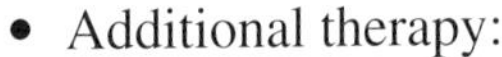

- Additional therapy:
  - H1 blocker
    - Diphenhydramine 50 mg PO/IV q4-6h
    - Loratadine 10 mg QD
  - H2 blocker
    - Cimetidine 300 mg PO
    - Ranitidine 150 mg PO
  - Steroids
    - Prednisone 60 mg PO
    - Decadron 10 mg IV

Disposition

- Complete, immediate resolution of symptoms: observe in ED for 2-4 hours then discharge with prednisone, diphenhydramine, and cimetidine.
- Patients with life-threatening anaphylaxis with hypotension or airway involvement should be admitted. Patients with good response to therapy may be managed on the floor, whereas unstable patients with severe symptoms require the ICU.

ERYTHEMA MULTIFORME

Additional History and Physical Examination Findings

- EM major usually begins with symptoms of fever, malaise, and myalgias.
- The classic lesion of EM is the target lesion with a central gray bulla surrounded by erythematous rings (see Fig. 23-3A). Multiple types of lesions may present simultaneously. EM minor refers to classic lesions involving less than 10% of body area.
- Further on the spectrum of severity, SJS refers to the presence of EM, constitutional symptoms, and the involvement of at least two mucosal surfaces (see Fig. 23-3B). Erosive lesions appear on oral mucosa, genital mucosa, and ocular mucosa. Patients with SJS are ill appearing. SJS usually does not cause widespread denuding of skin.
- TEN is the most severe form of EM. Skin involvement is initially diffuse, hot, and red. Subsequently, blisters and large areas of denuded skin develop involving 30% of body surface area. Oral and conjunctival mucosal involvement, erosion, and sloughing are common (see Fig. 23-3C).
- SJS and TEN usually occur in adults and are usually precipitated by drugs such as phenytoin, sulfas, penicillins, and NSAIDs. Viral infections from herpes, influenza, hepatitis, and mycoplasma infections are also known precipitants.

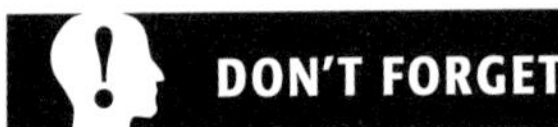

DON'T FORGET

Patients with SJS and TEN die from fluid loss and infections just like burn patients.

Review Initial Results

- Ask for complete vital signs including pulse oximetry and pay attention to the blood pressure.

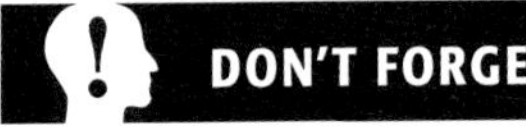

DON'T FORGET

Nikolsky sign is positive in TEN. Skin cleaves at the dermoepidermal junction leaving behind denuded dermis.

Risk Stratification

- EM: Patients with EM minor usually do well and are not severely ill.
- SJS: Patients with mild cases of SJS often do very well and can be managed as outpatients. More serious cases require hospitalization.
- TEN: The mortality of TEN is very high, approaching 50%. High-risk patients must be managed aggressively, often in the ICU or in a burn unit.

Definitive Management and Disposition

- EM minor
  - Consult with dermatologist.
  - Discontinue causative agent.

  - Treat infectious causes.
  - Most patients may be discharged home with close follow-up.
- SJS
  - Consult with dermatologist.
  - Discontinue causative agent.
  - Treat infectious etiologies if found.
  - IV fluid per Parkland formula.
  - Systemic steroids: prednisone, methylprednisolone, or dexamethasone
  - Local wound care with clean sterile dressings.
  - Consult ophthalmologist for ocular lesions.
  - Admit to hospital.
- TEN
  - IV fluid resuscitation per Parkland formula
  - Foley catheter to monitor urine output
  - Local wound care with clean sterile dressings
  - Consult with dermatologist.
  - Discontinue causative agent.
  - Consult ophthalmologist for ocular lesions.
  - Do not use systemic steroids.
  - Admit to ICU or burn unit.

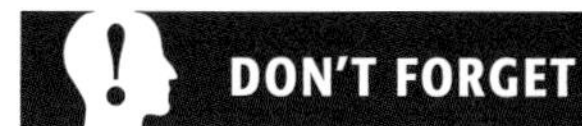

Parkland formula: 24-hour fluid requirement = 4 mL/Kg/% BSA burned. Administer as LR with ½ of total amount in the first 8 hours and remainder over the next 16 hours.

Complications (for SJS and TEN)

- Dehydration
- Infection
- Corneal ulceration and blindness
- Death is usually caused by fulminant sepsis and occurs in up to 30% of patients with TEN.

WINNING STRATEGIES

- On test day, treat allergic reactions aggressively. Chances are the patient will have life-threatening anaphylaxis or angioedema.
- All patients with signs of airway compromise get laryngoscopy (either direct or fiber-optic).
- All patients with glottic or supraglottic swelling get definitive airway control.
- Treat TEN patients like burn patients.

CHAPTER 24

Acid–Base Derangements

Tara Sheets and Tyson Pillow

- Acid–base derangements usually present as part of the full picture of disease and can help the candidate narrow the differential and guide therapy. Several conditions should alert the candidate to possible acid–base derangements: kidney disease, liver disease, endocrine disorders, ingestions, altered mental status (AMS), shock, respiratory distress, etc.
- Acid–base homeostasis is maintained primarily by the respiratory and renal systems. Acidosis results from a gain in acid or loss of bicarbonate. Conversely, alkalosis results from a gain in bicarbonate or loss of acid.
- There are four processes that contribute to the overall status of the patient: respiratory acidosis, respiratory alkalosis, metabolic acidosis, and metabolic alkalosis. The overall acid–base balance of the body is referred to as either acidemic or alkalemic.
- Once a primary derangement has shifted the acid–base status, compensatory mechanisms begin to restore the pH to normal. While the respiratory system responds within minutes, the renal system takes hours to days to fully compensate.
- Compensation can never return the pH to normal, so consider mixed disorders if a normal pH occurs on laboratory results. Consider normal pH to be 7.4 (range 7.6-7.44). Normal bicarbonate and Pco_2 are 24 and 40, respectively, when the patient's baseline is not known.

DON'T FORGET

-emia refers to the overall acid–base balance of the body, while *-osis* refers to the individual processes that contribute to the whole.

STEPWISE APPROACH TO ACID–BASE INTERPRETATION

Determine the Overall Acid–Base Status

1. If pH is ≤7.35, an acidemia is present. If the pH is ≥7.45, an alkalemia is present.

Determine the Primary Acid–Base Disorder

1. If pH indicates acidemia, look at bicarbonate (use this first) and Pco_2
   A. If bicarbonate is low, there is a primary metabolic acidosis.
      I. Calculate the anion gap.
         a. AG = Sodium – chloride – bicarbonate.
         b. If AG <15, then there is a non-gap acidosis.
         c. If AG >15, there is an anion gap acidosis.
      II. Determine if respiratory response is appropriate.
         a. In an acute disorder (<24 hours), fall in bicarb = fall in Pco_2 (as long as bicarb >8).
         b. In a disorder >24 hours, expected Pco_2 calculated with Winter's formula: $\text{Pco}_2 = [1.5(\text{bicarb}) + 8] +/- 2$.
         c. If decrease in Pco_2 is greater than expected, then there is a concomitant respiratory alkalosis.
         d. If decrease in Pco_2 is less than expected, then there is a concomitant respiratory acidosis.
   B. If the bicarbonate is high and the Pco_2 is high, there is a primary respiratory acidosis.
2. **If pH indicates alkalemia, then again look at bicarbonate and Pco_2.**
   A. High bicarbonate indicates primary metabolic alkalosis.
   B. Low Pco_2 indicates primary respiratory alkalosis.

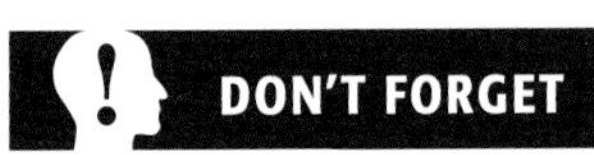

Always analyze acid–base problems in a stepwise fashion to identify all contributing disorders.

RESPIRATORY ACIDOSIS

- Frequently, this is a precursor to respiratory failure. The differential diagnosis includes asthma, chronic obstructive pulmonary disease (COPD), toxic ingestions, central nervous system (CNS) disease, trauma, etc.
- Acidosis also further depresses mental status and respiratory rate.
- Pulse oximeter readings can be misleading, especially if the patient is on supplemental oxygen, as Pco_2 elevations may occur before desaturation.

DON'T FORGET

Beware the patient who has a high respiratory rate with respiratory acidosis! This indicates very poor ventilatory status and impending respiratory failure.

Treat the underlying disorder and support ventilation as necessary.

RESPIRATORY ALKALOSIS

- This diagnosis can be a difficult one, as it is difficult to distinguish the patient who is simply anxious from those with pulmonary embolism, diabetic ketoacidosis (DKA), hypoxia, toxic ingestions, etc.
- As with respiratory acidosis, treat the underlying disorder. Consider anxiety only as a diagnosis of exclusion.

METABOLIC ACIDOSIS

DON'T FORGET

The patient who presents with combined respiratory alkalosis, metabolic alkalosis, and high anion gap acidosis has ASA overdose until proven otherwise.

- Acidosis can have several effects on the body including nausea, vomiting, pain, muscle weakness, breathing changes, AMS, depression of cardiac activity, and vasoconstriction.

Anion Gap Acidosis: MUDPILES

Methanol, Metformin

Uremia

DKA

Paraldehyde, **P**aracetamol

Iron, Isoniazid, Isopropyl Alcohol

Lactic acidosis

Ethanol, **E**thylene glycol

Salicylates, **S**tarvation (ketoacidosis)

Non-Anion Gap Acidosis: USED CARP

Ureterenterostomy

Small bowel fistulas

Extra chloride

Diarrhea

Carbonic anhydrase inhibitors

Adrenal insufficiency

Renal tubular acidosis

Pancreatic fistula, Parenteral nutrition

- Treat underlying cause and optimize tissue perfusion. In extreme circumstances, bicarbonate therapy should be considered (pH <6.9, bicarbonate <4 mEq/L) but this is very controversial.

METABOLIC ALKALOSIS

- Causes of metabolic alkalosis include dehydration, vomiting, excessive diuresis, mineralocorticoids and hypokalemia. Vomiting and excessive diuresis are the most common. Potassium loss and hypochloremia often accompany the metabolic alkalosis.
- Treat the underlying cause and administer intravenous fluids to correct dehydration.

WINNING STRATEGIES

- Use a stepwise approach to interpret acid–base status.
- Treat the underlying disorder. Rapid correction of the acid–base derangement is usually unnecessary.
- Always calculate an anion gap when metabolic acidosis is present.
- Remember MUDPILES and USED CARP.
- Beware the patient who has a high respiratory rate with respiratory acidosis! This indicates very poor ventilatory status and impending respiratory failure.

SECTION 4

SPECIAL POPULATIONS

CHAPTER 25

Trauma Patients

Robert Preston and John Dayton

INITIAL TRAUMA ASSESSMENT AND RESUSCITATION

Activate trauma team: Institutional guidelines should be observed based on reported injuries and mechanism of injury.

- Transition patient from portable emergency medical services (EMS) monitors to trauma bay equipment.
- Begin Primary Survey for unstable patients.
- Obtain focused trauma history.
- Begin Secondary Survey in stable patients.

Primary Survey

- A: Airway maintenance and cervical spine precautions
  - Maintain stabilization of cervical spine with a hard collar.
  - Clear oropharynx of blood, mucus, or any foreign bodies.
    - Intubate for airway compromise, imminent obstruction, or Glasgow Coma Scale (GCS) ≤8.
    - Perform cricothyrotomy if intubation fails or if it is unlikely to be successful (swelling, severe facial fractures).
- B: Breathing and ventilation
  - Inspect chest wall and diaphragmatic region for symmetry and injury.
  - Auscultate for bilateral breath sounds.
    - Perform needle decompression immediately for tension pneumothorax (do not wait for chest x-ray [CXR]).
    - Perform tube thoracostomy for unstable patients with pneumothorax and/or hemothroax.
    - Perform resuscitative thoracotomy and internal cardiac massage for patients with penetrating trauma with previously witnessed cardiac activity, but now unresponsive hypotension.
- C: Circulation and hemorrhage control
  - Assess blood pressure, heart rate, and search for evidence of bleeding.
  - Control identified bleeding with direct pressure.
    - Insert two large-bore intravenous (IV) lines and immediately bolus 2 L of normal saline.
    - Use blood products with major bleeding and if symptoms persist despite 2 L bolus of normal saline.
- D: Disability and neurologic status
  - Assess pupil size and reaction to light.
  - Assess level of consciousness with GCS (Table 25-1).
  - Note any gross neurologic deficits.
    - If GCS ≤8 and patient not yet intubated, proceed with intubation and then restart Primary Survey.
- E: Exposure and environmental control
  - Completely undress the patient and assess for injury.
  - Keep patient warm (blankets, warmed IV fluid).
- F: Focused assessment with sonography for trauma (FAST)
  - Perform in trauma patients to assess for pericardial effusion or intraperitoneal bleeding.

Focused Trauma History

- AMPLE
  - Allergies
  - Medications currently used
  - Past medical history, surgeries, and pregnancy
  - Last meal
  - Events/environment

IMMEDIATE INTERVENTIONS

- Oxygenate via NRB or nasal cannula if not intubated.
- Perform jaw thrust and chin lift with any sign of airway obstruction.
- Maintain C-spine immobilization with assistance if collar must be removed.
- Establish two large-bore IV access with blood draw for lab orders.
- Obtain ECG or cardiac monitor with rhythm strip.
- If ventilation and circulation become rapidly compromised (especially after intubation), consider pneumothorax.

DON'T FORGET

On test day, your patient *will* have a major traumatic injury with **multiple** injuries

Stabilize all life-threatening injuries before proceeding to the next step of your survey.

Frequently request repeat vital signs, especially after any intervention.

DON'T FORGET

- Some medicines can profoundly alter the response to trauma response (beta-blockers, blood thinners).
- Ask about DM as hypoglycemia may be cause of AMS.
- Obtain medical history through EMTs, family members, friends, medical alert bracelet, patient records, and via phone consult with PMD.

Table 25-1. Glasgow Coma Scale

Behavior	Response	Score
Eye opening	Spontaneously	4
	To speech	3
	To pain	2
	No response	1
Verbal response	A&Ox3	5
	Confused	4
	Inappropriate words	3
	Incomprehensible sounds	2
	No response	1
Motor response	Obeys commands	6
	Localizes pain	5
	Withdraws from pain	4
	Decorticate flexion	3
	Decerebrate extension	2
	No response	1

Secondary Survey

- Perform a thorough, systematic head-to-toe evaluation to find and treat additional injuries.
- Perform only after Primary Survey is *complete*, life-threatening injuries are stabilized, and resuscitation has commenced.

Physical Examination

- Vital signs: Repeat frequently—especially after any intervention.
- Neurologic: Reassess GCS, pupil size and response, and check motor strength, and sensation of extremities.
- Head, eyes, ears, nose, and throat (HEENT): Evaluate scalp for potential bleeding and facial bones for stability (airway compromise may not be immediate).
- Neck: Confirm presence of C-collar (emergency medical technicians [EMTs] often forget on exam day) or exchange soft for hard collars. Ensure trachea is midline, palpate for crepitus, and auscultate for bruits.
- Chest: Inspect anterior and posterior chest for deformities, lacerations, abrasions, and other markers of trauma such as a seat-belt sign. Palpate chest wall for rib fractures. Auscultate heart and lungs.
- Abdomen: Inspect for distension and palpate for rebound or guarding.
- Genitals/perineum/rectum: Examine for contusions, hematomas, lacerations, and urethral bleeding.

DON'T FORGET

- In context of bleeding or visible lacerations, obtain tetanus status or administer empirically if patient is unable to respond or recall.
- Perform a rectal examination prior to placing a Foley to test for high-riding prostate.
- Treat pain early and repeat as indicated.

- Musculoskeletal: Inspect for contusion or deformity and check skin for open fractures. Palpate all bony surfaces for tenderness, check range of motion, and check pelvic stability.
- Spine: Log-roll patient maintaining C-spine immobilization. Note deformity of spine and palpate for tenderness. Assess rectal tone and for presence of gross blood.

Imaging

- X-rays of chest and pelvis
- C-spine x-ray unless computed tomography (CT) will be performed.

SYSTEM-BASED APPROACH TO THE TRAUMA PATIENT: HEAD INJURIES

History

- Injuries to scalp, skull, brain, and blood vessels.
- Mechanism of injury (blunt vs penetrating).
- GCS
  - May be difficult to determine if level of consciousness is related to hypotension, traumatic brain injury, or alcohol/drug intoxication.
  - GCS 14-15: Mild head injury.
  - GCS 9-13: Moderate head injury.
  - GCS ≤8: Severe head injury.

Examination

- Scalp laceration may be obvious as these can bleed profusely.
- Discern open versus closed skull fractures.
  - May be evident on digital exploration of a scalp wound.
  - Fractures are described according to shape, location, and if there is skull depression (linear, stellate, comminuted, depressed, compound, basilar).
- Signs of basilar skull fracture
  - Hemotympanum
  - Battle sign (retroauricular ecchymosis)
  - Raccoon eyes (periorbital ecchymosis)
- Check for cerebrospinal fluid (CSF) leak from nose or ear
- Evaluate for focal neurologic deficits

Imaging

- Plain x-rays have only limited utility.
- Perform early head CT based on mechanism, mental status change, and injury and should be evaluated for skull and intracranial lesions.
- CT angiogram (CTA) if vascular neck injuries are suspected (fractured vertebral or carotid foramina).
- Magnetic resonance imaging (MRI) not usually used in for head trauma.

Diagnosis

- Alcohol level and drug screen complement altered mental status (AMS) workup.
- Concussions are a clinical diagnosis in setting of normal imaging after transient loss of consciousness.
- Epidural hematoma (Fig. 25-1A)
  - Classic presentation is patient with an initial loss of consciousness, followed by a "lucid interval," and then a decreased level of consciousness that can lead to coma and death.
  - Biconvex, lentiform appearance on head CT.
  - Account for <1% of intracranial lesions, but common board case.

- Subdural hematoma (Fig. 25-1B)
  - Acute: Crescent-shaped, hyperdense (bright) lesion
  - Chronic: Can have delayed presentation with hypodense lesion—especially in elderly and alcoholic patients
- Subarachnoid hemorrhage (Fig. 25-1C)
  - Patient may be mildly lethargic to full coma
  - Hyperdense, linear areas often in characteristic locations (Sylvian fissure)
- Cerebral contusions and intracerebral hematoma
  - Distinction between contusion and intracerebral hematoma is ill-defined.
  - Bleeding of brain tissue mostly in frontal and temporal lobes.
  - Classically caused by blunt trauma.
  - Presentation can be delayed due to slow progression of bleed.
  - 20% are not evident until repeat CT.
- Diffuse axonal injury
  - Classically caused by disruption of axons during rapid acceleration or deceleration (auto accidents, abuse in pediatric patients, etc).
  - Loss of grey/white differentiation.
  - Easier to diagnose on MRI.

DON'T FORGET

- Involve neurosurgery early and transport patients if no neurosurgery is available.
- On CT, evaluate for mass effect and shift.
- Consider further intracranial bleeding if the neurologic status deteriorates.

Management

- General measures
  - The use of sedatives and pain medications must be balanced with the need for frequent neuro reevaluation.

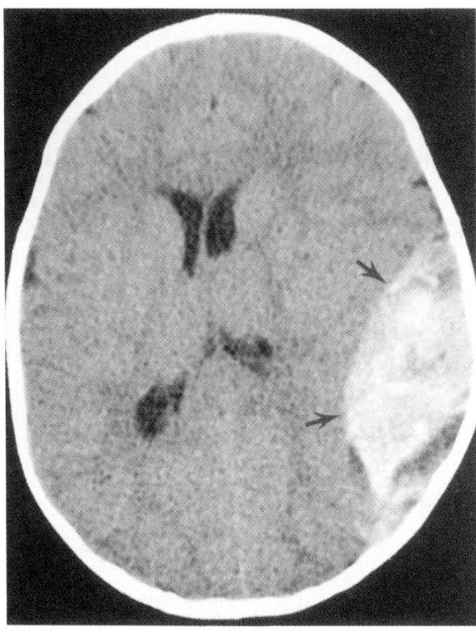
A

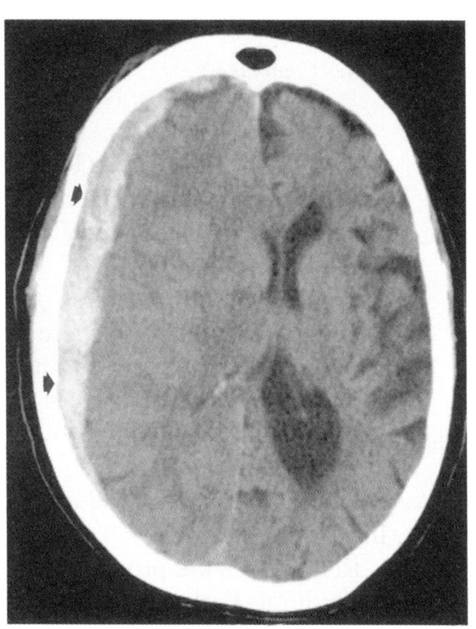
B

Figure 25-1. **(A)** Epidural hematoma (EDH), crescentic, extra-axial hemorrhagic collection layers over the right lateral convexity (arrows). There is associated mass effect on the adjacent brain parenchyma, with effacement of the cortical gyri, compression of the right lateral ventricle, and shift of the midline structures to the left. **(B)** Subdural hematoma (SDH) seen in non-contrast CT image in a middle-aged patient following a fall. **(C)** A CT scan taken from a patient with an acute subarachnoid hemorrhage (SAH). Note the higher density in the suprasellar area and region outlining the midbrain. (*[A,B]: Reproduced with permission from Chen MY, Pope TL, Ott DJ.* Basic Radiology. *New York, NY: McGraw-Hill; 2004. [C]: Reproduced with permission from Pearlman MD, Tintinalli JE, Dyne PL.* Obstetric and Gynecologic Emergencies: Diagnosis and Management. *New York, NY: McGraw-Hill; 2009.*)

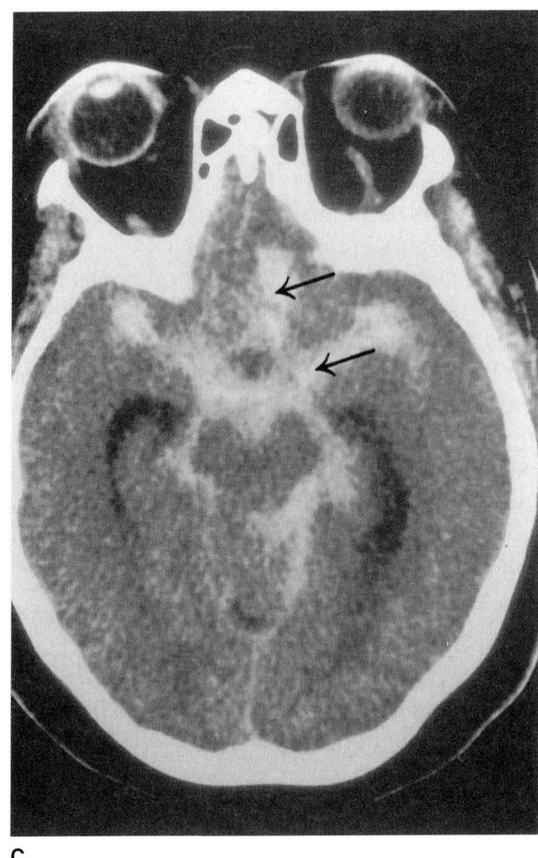

Figure 25-1. (*Continued.*)

- In mild head injury (GCS 14-15) it may be possible to avoid sedatives and narcotic pain medication entirely.
- Check for C-spine injury with any significant head injury.

- Scalp lacerations
  - Staple or running sutures prior to leaving trauma bay.
  - Blood loss can be severe leading to potential for deterioration during diagnostic workup due to hemorrhagic shock.
  - Give tetanus, as indicated.
- Skull fractures
  - Surgical intervention required for skull depression >5 mm, gross contamination, dural tears, and underlying hematomas.
- Intracranial lesions
  - Require seizure prophylaxis.
  - Epidural: Early burr hole associated with a favorable prognosis.
  - Subdural: Neurosurgical intervention required with mass effect and neurologic impairment.
  - Subarachnoid: May require intracerebral pressure monitoring if GCS <8.
- Concussions
  - Short-term observation (2-4 hours) is appropriate.
  - Advise patients to expect postconcussive syndrome involving headache and nausea.
  - Advise to avoid contact sports until cleared by a primary care physician.
- Contusions and intracerebral hematoma
  - Seizure prophylaxis.
  - Repeat head CT at 6-hour interval and STAT for any acute deterioration.
- Diffuse axonal injury
  - Trauma can cause prolonged posttraumatic mental status changes or coma.

- Deeply comatose patients may persist in this state.
- Often associated with decortication or decerebration and can cause severe disability.
- May have autonomic dysfunction—hypertension, hyperhidrosis, hyperpyrexia.
- May coexist with hypoxic brain injury and the two can't be easily differentiated.
- Management goals involve blood pressure (BP) management and control of intracranial pressure (ICP).

- Elevated ICPs
  - Provide low stimulation environment
  - Pharmacology
    - Maintain adequate sedation and pain control regimen.
    - Mannitol.
    - Hypertonic saline.
  - Ventilator
    - Maintain carbon dioxide (CO_2) around 35%.
    - Avoid repeated hyperventilatory episodes as this can precipitate acute lung injury.

DON'T FORGET

- ABCs should be checked early and often as head injury sequelae will be worsened by failure to address airway and fluid resuscitation.
- Be aggressive with fluid resuscitation.
- If neurologic status deteriorates, check vitals, treat hypotension, check blood sugar, and repeat CT scan if no other source is found.
- Every effort should be made to enhance cerebral perfusion and blood flow by reducing elevated ICP, maintaining normal intravascular volume and MAP, and restoring normal oxygenation and normocapnia.
- Perform a FAST or DPL in the ED, CT scanner, or the OR, so they do not delay neurosurgery.

Disposition

- Mild head injury
  - Observe and perform serial neurologic evaluations if unable to perform CT, if patient has significant alcohol and/or drug intoxication, or if there is no reliable companion at home.
  - Have a low threshold for admitting head injury patients on exam day.
- Moderate head injury
  - Admit for observation if symptoms don't resolve completely.
  - Perform frequent neurologic checks to evaluate for continued bleed.
- Severe head injury
  - Involve neurosurgery early.
  - Transfer to appropriate facility if neurosurgery unavailable.
  - Admit to neurosurgical or surgical intensive care unit (ICU).

MAXILLOFACIAL INJURIES

History

- Frequent association with airway compromise, head injury, cervical spinal injury, and severe multisystem trauma.
- Airway obstruction can result from hemorrhage, hematoma, aspiration, and displacement of bony structures (flail mandible).
  - Use jaw thrust and suction to relieve the obstruction.
  - If unsuccessful, then intubate or perform cricothyrotomy.
- After the airway is secured, the patient should be assessed for ongoing bleeding from the oropharynx.
- Most common fractures involve the nasal bone, zygoma, or mandible.
  - Facial fractures can lead to significant hemorrhage from the maxillary and palatine arteries (branches of the external carotid artery).
  - Orbital blowout fractures have a high association with ocular injury (up to 45%).

DON'T FORGET

During the Primary Survey, evaluation of the maxillofacial region is limited to evaluation and control of the airway and control of significant ongoing bleeding. All other diagnostic measures are of secondary importance and should not be undertaken until the patient is stable.

Examination

- Signs of facial fracture include asymmetry, step-offs, pain on palpation or movement, crepitus, trismus, malocclusion, diplopia, extraocular muscle movement abnormality, CSF leak, ecchymosis, hematoma, cheek anesthesia, and blood in the external auditory canal.

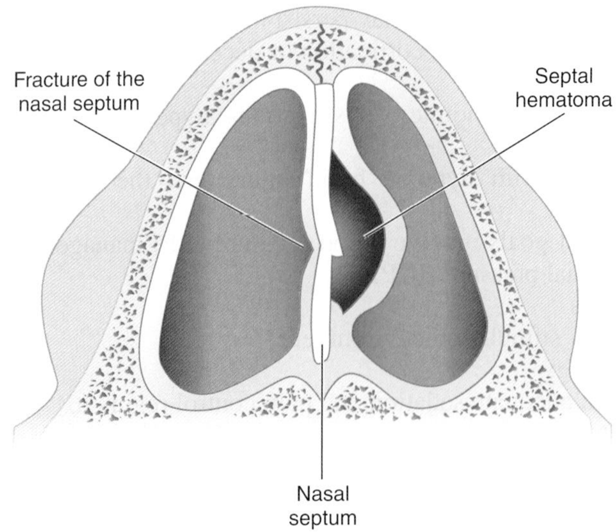

Figure 25-2. Graphic depiction of nasal septal hematoma. (*Reproduced with permission from Schwartz DT.* Emergency Radiology: Case Studies. *New York, NY: McGraw-Hill; 2008.*)

- Check for septal hematomas with nasal fractures (Fig. 25-2) as blood supply can be compromised.

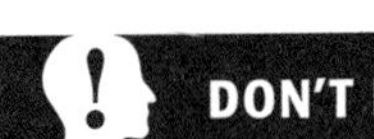

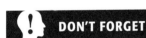

DON'T FORGET

- When you find a mandibular fracture, look for a concomitant fracture.
- Sublingual/buccal ecchymosis is pathognomonic for a mandibular fracture.
- When you diagnosis an orbital fracture, rule out globe injury.

Diagnosis

- Direct eye trauma may be associated with retrobulbar hematoma and globe rupture.
- Nasal bone films are indicated only for isolated nasal bony injury with obvious displacement.
- Panorex mandibular films are useful, but may not be available.
- Facial bone CT with reconstruction is preferred over plain films.
  - This study is time-consuming and may be deferred in major trauma patients initially.
  - As the mandible is C-shaped, more than one-half of fractures have a concomitant fracture.
- Le Fort fractures of the mid-face:
  - Le Fort I fractures are horizontal and go through the maxilla, making the upper row of teeth mobile.
  - Le Fort II fractures are pyramidal and separate the nasomaxillary segment from the zygoma and orbits, making the central face mobile.
  - Le Fort III fractures create a craniofacial dissociation with a fracture that involves the nasal bridge and extending to the orbits, separating the skull and facial bones, making the face mobile.
  - There is a strong association between Le Fort II and III fractures and airway compromise, intracranial injury, CSF leak, and C-spine injury.

Management

- Control bleeding by packing and pressure, but angiography and embolization may be necessary.
- Use antibiotics for all open fractures.
- Mandibular fractures:
  - Soft diet for 4 weeks and close follow-up recommended if fracture does not involve malocclusion, is closed, and involves the condylar, subcondylar, or coronoid process.

  - Intermaxillary fixation for 6 weeks with abnormal occlusion and with condylar or subcondylar fractures.
  - Open fractures involving occlusal surfaces with contiguous intraoral lacerations require admission for surgery and IV antibiotics.
  - Open reduction with internal fixation (ORIF) is required for displaced mandibular fractures and symphysis fractures.
- Eye trauma:
  - Check for globe rupture by using a Seidel test (fluorescein streaming from area on eye).
  - Cover the affected eye with a metal shield to prevent further damage.
  - If proptosis is suspected, measure the intraocular pressure and be prepared to perform a lateral canthotomy.
- Orbital blowout fractures
  - Ophthalmology consultation indicated for orbital injury.
  - Use antibiotics if fractures are open or if sinus is involved.
  - Surgery is required for diplopia (persists >2 weeks), enophthalmos, or large fractures with herniation.
- Zygomatic fracture
  - No treatment required for nondisplaced zygomatic fractures.
  - Use antibiotics for open fractures or with sinus involvement.
  - ORIF is required for open fracture, deformity, displacement, enophthalmos, diplopia, and dystopia.
    - Surgery may be delayed 1-3 days to allow swelling to subside.
- Maxillary fracture
  - Emergency department (ED) management consists of airway protection and bleeding control with pressure, nasal packing, or reduction as necessary.
  - Use antibiotics for all maxillary fractures.
  - Isolated maxillary fractures are treated with intermaxillary fixation.
  - Le Fort II or III fractures require ORIF as soon as possible.
- Nasal fracture
  - Minimal displacement requires no treatment.
  - Antibiotics are indicated for open fractures or if nasal packing is placed.
  - Attempt reduction for gross deformities. Definitive repair can be delayed for 3 days to 6 weeks.
- Upper facial fracture
  - Antibiotics for all.
  - Obtain immediate consult for ORIF.

DON'T FORGET

- Although airway management may not be required during Primary Survey, continue to reevaluate the airway for bleeding and airway compromise.
- Evaluate and treat eye trauma aggressively to prevent irreversible vision loss.
- Rule out globe injury with orbital blowout fractures.
- If your patient has a zygomatic fracture, check for superior orbital fissure syndrome by evaluating cranial nerves III, IV, and VI, and checking for a fixed and dilated pupil, upper lid ptosis, ophthalmoplegia, and hypoesthesia of the zygomatic branch of the fifth nerve.
- Maxillary fractures are associated with increased risk for retropharyngeal hematoma.

Disposition

- Most patients with closed, nondisplaced, and isolated facial fractures can be discharged home for follow-up for outpatient operative repair after a discussion with the consultant.
- Patients with open or displaced facial fractures should receive antibiotics and be admitted for operative repair.
- In patients with significant multisystem trauma, the patient may be admitted because of their other injuries, but you should speak with a consultant about any facial fractures that need to be addressed during hospitalization.

VASCULAR NECK TRAUMA

History

- Any injury above the clavicle requires evaluation for C-spine injury.
- Blunt trauma patients require C-spine immobilization.
- In cases of isolated penetrating trauma, routine c-collar use is deferred because of the risk of airway obstruction due to large or enlarging neck hematomas.

- Early definitive airway control is the top priority in cases of major neck injuries.
    - The airway can be obstructed as a result of direct injury to the larynx or trachea, expanding hematoma within the neck, or bleeding into the airway.
    - Progressive bleeding or swelling may make endotracheal intubation difficult. Be prepared to describe to the examiner how you would perform a cricothyroidotomy (surgical airway).
    - Penetrating wounds may present an immediate life threat because of airway compromise and/or hemorrhage.

Examination

- Anatomy:
    - The anterior triangle contains large vessels, the trachea, and the esophagus deep to the platysma.
    - The anterior and posterior triangles are divided by the sternocleidomastoid.
    - Three zones of the neck (Fig. 25-3):
        - Zone 1 extends from the sternal notch to the cricoid cartilage, and injury to this zone has the highest mortality due to the presence of great vessels and the difficult surgical approach.
        - Zone 2 extends from the cricoid cartilage to the angle of the mandible.
        - Zone 3 extends from the angle of the mandible to the base of the skull.
- "Hard" clinical signs are more often associated with significant vascular injury and include active bleeding or unexplained shock; hematomas that are expanding or pulsatile; significantly diminished (or absent) pulses; bruit.
- "Soft" signs are merely suggestive of vascular injury and include stable hematoma, slow bleeding, or mild shock.
- Aerodigestive injury may be suspected by air movement through the wound with breathing, crepitance, or subcutaneous emphysema in the neck, voice change, dysphagia, odynophagia, respiratory distress, or massive hemoptysis.

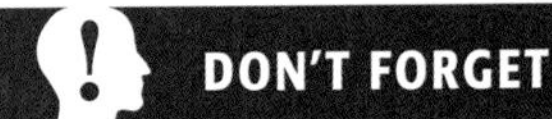

- An initially patent airway may become compromised a short time later.
- Zone 2 injuries require operative management.
- Zone 1 and 3 injuries require angiography and esophagram.

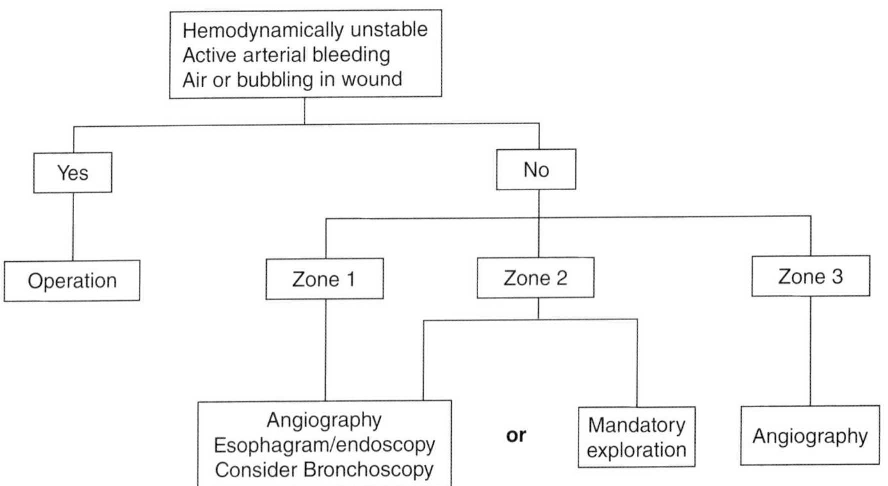

Figure 25-3. Zones of the neck. (*Reproduced with permission from Tintinalli JE, Kelen GD, Stapczynski JS, et al.* Emergency Medicine: A Comprehensive Study Guide. *6th ed. New York, NY: McGraw-Hill; 2004.*)

Diagnosis

- Plain film CXR and C-spine imaging for fractures, foreign bodies, hemopneumothorax, subcutaneous emphysema, and hematomas.
- CTA for vascular or laryngotracheal injuries.
  - Presence of contrast-medium extravasation, nonvisualization of vascular structures, or free air in the tissue planes suggests injury.
- Diagnostic angiography still has utility following inconclusive CTAs or in cases of shotgun injuries (multiple pellets).
- Esophagram in cases of penetrating trauma with associated signs/symptoms suggesting injury.
- Endoscopy (esophagoscopy, upper endoscopy, bronchoscopy) for patients with suspicious signs/symptoms.

Management

- Airway management is your first priority.
- Clinical indications for immediate surgery and deferred imaging:
  - All Zone 2 injuries.
  - Zone 1 and 3 injuries in an unstable patient.
  - Vascular concerns: Expanding hematoma, external hemorrhage, or decreased carotid pulse.
  - Airway concerns: Stridor, hoarseness, dysphonia, hemoptysis, and subcutaneous air.
  - Digestive concerns: Dysphagia or odynophagia, subcutaneous air, or blood in oropharynx.
  - Neurologic concerns: Lateralized neurologic deficit consistent with injury or altered state of consciousness not caused by head injury.
- Bony injuries mandate neurosurgical/orthopedic consultation.

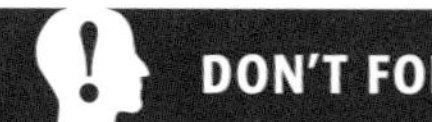

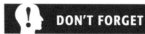

DON'T FORGET

- Bleeding and swelling can progressive rapidly and can complicate intubation via direct laryngoscopy.
- Have adjunct airway tools immediately available and "dual setup" for emergency cricothyroidotomy should be considered.

Disposition

- Patients with nonoperative lesions should be admitted for further evaluation such with bronchoscopy, endoscopy, and/or esophagography.
- Patients with significant penetrating injury should be admitted to the hospital to monitor the airway for further swelling or bleeding over time.
- Patients requiring operative management need specialty consultation and admission for operative management.

THORACIC TRAUMA

History

- Address this rapidly! Chest trauma is a significant cause of mortality, and many deaths could be prevented with prompt diagnosis and treatment.
- Prevent hypoxia with intubation, needle decompression, and tube thoracostomy during the Primary Survey.
- Rib fractures are the most common thoracic cage injury.
- Fractures of the scapula, first or second rib, or of the sternum suggest significant injury, and associated injuries should be suspected.
- Deceleration injuries (high-speed impact, falls from height) increase the likelihood of aortic injury.
- Penetrating transmediastinal injuries place heart, great vessels, tracheobronchial tree, and aerodigestive structures at risk.

Examination

- Airway injury
  - Check for stridor, change in voice quality, and a palpable defect of the sternoclavicular joint.

DON'T FORGET

- Subtle signs of chest injury or hypoxia include increased respiratory rate and change in breathing pattern. Cyanosis may be a late finding.
- Tension pneumothorax and cardiac tamponade can both present with chest pain, hypotension, and jugular vein distention (JVD). However, the two can be differentiated by the presence or absence of lung sounds.

- Pulmonary
  - Consider and treat tension pneumothoraces in patients with chest pain, air hunger, respiratory distress, tachycardia, hypotension, tracheal deviation, unilateral absence of breath sounds, and neck vein distension.
  - Evaluate for diaphragmatic injury by checking for bowel sounds on lung auscultation.
- Chest wall
  - Consider rib fractures with crepitus and increased rib mobility.
    - Evaluate for associated injuries such as pneumothorax and damage to underlying vascular structures.
  - Immediately address large chest wall defects (holes larger than two-thirds the diameter of the trachea) with three-way occlusive dressings.
- Cardiovascular
  - Neck vein distension may be a sign of cardiac tamponade, tension pneumothorax, or traumatic diaphragmatic injury.

Diagnosis

- Electrocardiogram (ECG)
  - Cardiac tamponade may cause electric alternans.
  - Blunt trauma and myocardial contusion can cause premature ventricular contractions (PVCs), atrial fibrillation, and conduction delays.
- CXR
  - This is included in the Secondary Survey.
  - Findings that may indicate aortic injury include the following (Fig. 25-4A):
    - Widened mediastinum
    - Obliteration of the aortic knob
    - Deviation of the trachea to the right
    - Obliteration of the space between the pulmonary artery and the aorta
    - Depression of the left main stem bronchus
    - Deviation of the esophagus or nasogastric (NG) tube to the right
    - Widened paratracheal stripe
    - Widened paraspinal interfaces
    - Presence of a pleural or apical cap, left hemothorax, and fractures of the first or second rib or scapula (Fig. 25-4B).
  - Check for findings indicative of diaphragmatic injury (lower rib fractures, pleural effusion, elevated hemi diaphragm, intrathoracic abdominal viscera, or an NG tube above the diaphragm) as this can cause bowel strangulation and pulmonary compromise.
- Extended FAST (EFAST)
  - This includes evaluation for cardiac tamponade (pericardial fluid) and pneumothorax (absence of lung slide) in addition to traditional FAST.
- CT
  - May be indicated based on mechanism of injury, evidence from physical examination, or suspicious findings on CXR.
  - Systematically evaluates bony structures (sternoclavicular joint, rib fractures, and flail chests), lung fields (contusion, aspiration, hemo- or pneumothorax, tracheal deviation), diaphragm for rupture (bowel, stomach, or termination of NG tube in chest), and vascular structures (widened mediastinum or tamponade) for injury.
  - CT with IV contrast can be utilized in stable when there is concern for aortic injury or injury to other great vessels.
  - Unstable patients should go to the operating room (OR) instead of CT.
- Evaluate patients with mediastinal wounds for vascular, tracheobronchial, esophageal, and spinal injuries. This may include CT, ultrasound, angiography, esophagography (with water-soluble contrast), and bronchoscopy as indicated.

DON'T FORGET

- Evaluation for tension pneumothorax should be performed during the Primary Survey and be repeated with any change in vital signs, breathing pattern, or with any decompensation (especially after intubation).
- If cardiothoracic surgery is unavailable, stabilize and transfer patients with concern for aortic injury.

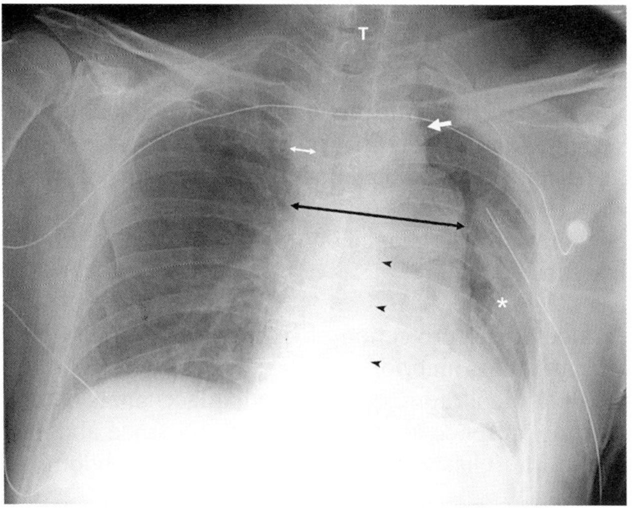

A

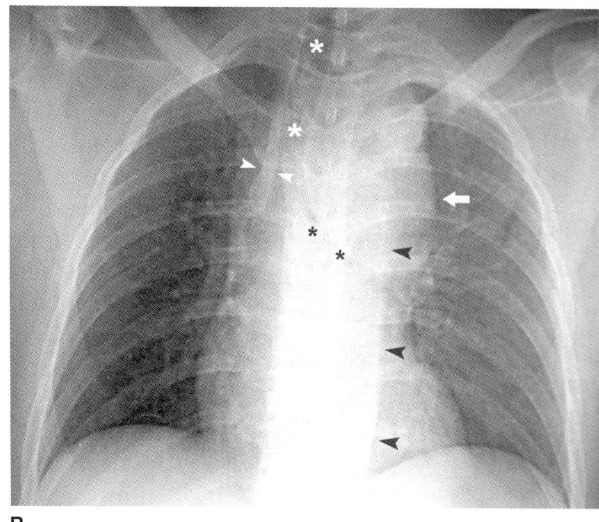

B

Figure 25-4. (**A**). The chest radiograph revealed marked widening of the mediastinum (11 cm) (*black double-headed arrow*). There are three other signs of hemomediastinum: abnormal contour above the aortic knob (*white arrow*), wide right paratracheal stripe (20 mm) (*white double-headed arrow*), and displaced left paraspinal line (*arrowheads*). The trachea (T) is displaced to the left because of rotated positioning of the patient. Opacification of the left lung is caused by pulmonary contusion (*asterisk*). (**B**) Definite signs of hemomediastinum in a patient with aortic injury. The mediastinum is widened and the aortic knob is distorted by surrounding blood (*arrow*). Mediastinal blood causes widening of the **right paratracheal stripe** (*white arrowheads*) and displacement of the **left paraspinal line** (*black arrowheads*), which extends up to the aortic knob. The **trachea** is displaced to the right (*white asterisks*) and the left mainstem bronchus is displaced inferiorly (*black asterisks*). This is caused by blood surrounding the aorta. The faint shadow of the SVC is visible to the right of the paratracheal stripe. (*Reproduced with permission from Schwartz DT.* Emergency Radiology: Case Studies. *New York, NY: McGraw-Hill; 2008.*)

- ○ Diagnostic peritoneal lavage (DPL) or laparoscopy can exclude diaphragm injury in high-risk patients as CT scans cannot reliably exclude diaphragmatic injury.

Management

- The patient's airway is your priority.
- Reduce a sternoclavicular joint fracture or dislocation by extending the shoulders, grasping the clavicle with a clamp, and manually reducing the fracture.
  - ○ If successful, the reduction is usually stable.
- Pneumo- and hemothorax
  - ○ For suspected tension pneumothorax, place a large-bore needle into the second intercostal space in the midclavicular line.
  - ○ Place a chest tube in the fifth intercostal space just anterior to the midaxillary line to allow lung reexpansion and evacuation of air and/or blood.
  - ○ Avoid progression from stable to tension pneumothorax by chest tube thoracostomy.
  - ○ Connect the chest tube to suction immediately and assess for large air leaks. Air leaks could represent equipment problem or tracheobronchial tree injury.
  - ○ Consult CT surgery if one chest tube is insufficient to expand the lung in setting of a very large leak.
  - ○ Massive hemothorax (>1500 mL) requires simultaneous fluid resuscitation and chest tube placement with at least a 36-French size tube.
  - ○ Check for large chest wall defects or contiguous rib fractures.

- Perform a thoracotomy only on victims of penetrating trauma who were observed to have vital signs entering the ED but then became apneic and pulseless in the ED.
  - This is contraindicated in patients with obvious nonsurvivable injuries, patients who have been apneic and pulseless since arrival, and in patients who received >15 minutes of prehospital cardiopulmonary resuscitation (CPR).
- Open chest wound
  - Use a flutter valve (occlusive dressing taped on three sides with fourth left open to vent) and chest tube.
- Diaphragmatic injury
  - More common on left side due to protection of right by liver, and right is rarely clinically significant unless anterior.
  - If a laceration of the left diaphragm is suspected, place an NG tube prior to CXR and look for presence above the diaphragm since abdominal viscera may herniate into chest due to the positive intra-abdominal pressure.
- Myocardial contusion
  - Patients with severe chest trauma are at risk for myocardial injury and should be monitored for dysrhythmias.
  - Troponin may be elevated, and it is useful to follow trends.
  - Repeat cardiac ultrasound frequently to check for development of tamponade.
  - Pericardiocentesis is a temporary treatment for cardiac tamponade in this setting and requires further intervention (pericardial window).

DON'T FORGET

- Don't wait for a CXR if you are concerned about tension pneumothorax as this is a clinical diagnosis. Perform immediate needle decompression using a 10 gauge, 7.5 cm armored angiocatheter.
- Initial hemothorax of >1500 mL or a continued blood loss of 200 mL/h for 2-4 hours warrants consideration of thoracotomy.
- A simple pneumothorax should not be ignored or overlooked as it can progress to a tension pneumothorax. Repeat a CXR whenever the patient condition changes.
- Have a high clinical suspicion for diaphragm injuries.

Disposition

- Admit patients with myocardial contusion. They are at risk for sudden dysrhythmias and should be monitored for the first 24 hours.
- Patients with mediastinal injury require surgical intervention by CT surgery.
- Any patient with significant thoracic trauma should be admitted to the hospital as pulmonary distress caused by inadequate ventilation or pulmonary contusion can cause significant morbidity and mortality.

ABDOMINAL TRAUMA

Figure 25-5 shows zones of the abdomen.

History

- Blunt trauma
  - May cause crushing or rupture of viscus, laceration of liver and spleen, and peritonitis.
  - Evaluate the patient for splenic and liver lacerations and also for retroperitoneal hematomas.
  - Mechanism of injury can be used to anticipate type of injury.
  - For motor vehicle collisions (MVCs), obtain history of the crash including patient seat, speed of vehicle, type of collision, restraint and air bag use, and status of other passengers.
- Penetrating trauma
  - Gunshot wounds (GSWs) and stab wounds typically injure by laceration or cutting.
  - High-velocity rifles can also cause injuries from bullet fragment movement.
  - Obtain history including time of injury, type of weapon, distance from assailant, number of shots or stab wounds, and amount of blood at scene.

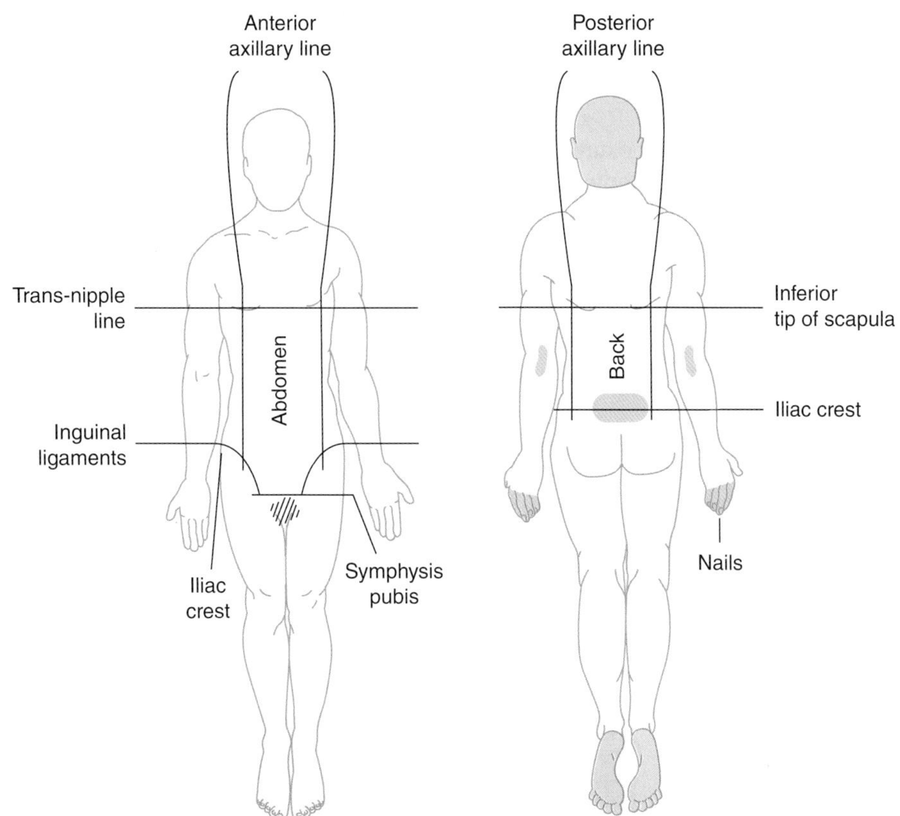

Figure 25-5. The anterior abdomen includes area between the trans-nipple line superiorly, inguinal ligaments and symphysis pubis inferiorly, and the anterior axillary lines laterally. The flank is between the anterior and posterior axillary lines from the sixth intercostal space to the iliac crest. The back is defined as the area located posterior to the posterior axillary lines from the tip of the scapulae to the iliac crests. These areas are outlined in the figure above. (*Modified from Wolff K, Johnson RA.* Fitzpatrick's Color Atlas and Synopsis of Clinical Dermatology. *6th ed. New York, NY: McGraw-Hill; 2009.*)

Examination

- Areas for evaluation:
  - Anterior abdomen: Area between the trans-nipple line superiorly, inguinal ligaments and symphysis pubis inferiorly, and the anterior axillary lines laterally
  - Back: Area located posterior to the posterior axillary lines from the tip of the scapulae to the iliac crests.
  - Flank: Area between the anterior and posterior axillary lines from the sixth intercostal space to the iliac crest.
- Assessment may be impaired by alcohol intoxication, drugs, or injuries to the brain, spine, or adjacent areas.
- With MVC, look for "seat-belt sign" across abdomen which may indicate bowel injury.
- In penetrating trauma, note the location, shape, and size of any wounds.

Diagnosis

- Laboratory
  - Complete blood count (CBC) to evaluate blood loss.
  - Type and cross if you anticipate blood transfusion.
  - Pregnancy test.
  - Alcohol and drug screen.

- X-ray
  - CXR to look for free air and diaphragmatic rupture.
  - Pelvis x-ray to evaluate for pelvic fractures.
- FAST (Fig. 25-6)
  - Rapid, reliable, repeatable test for bleeding.
  - A positive FAST shows internal bleeding, but a negative FAST does not rule out internal bleeding.
    - A better tool to "rule-in" than "rule-out"
  - EFAST also includes thoracic views to check for pneumothorax and pericardial tamponade.
- DPL
  - Perform when FAST is unavailable or nondiagostic, or when CT is unavailable.
  - Useful in diagnosing diaphragmatic injury which is frequently missed on CT and may cause substantial morbidity and mortality.
  - In blunt abdominal trauma, a positive test (and indication for operative management) is an initial aspirate of more than 5 cc of blood or 100,000 red blood cells (RBCs)/mm^3 or more.

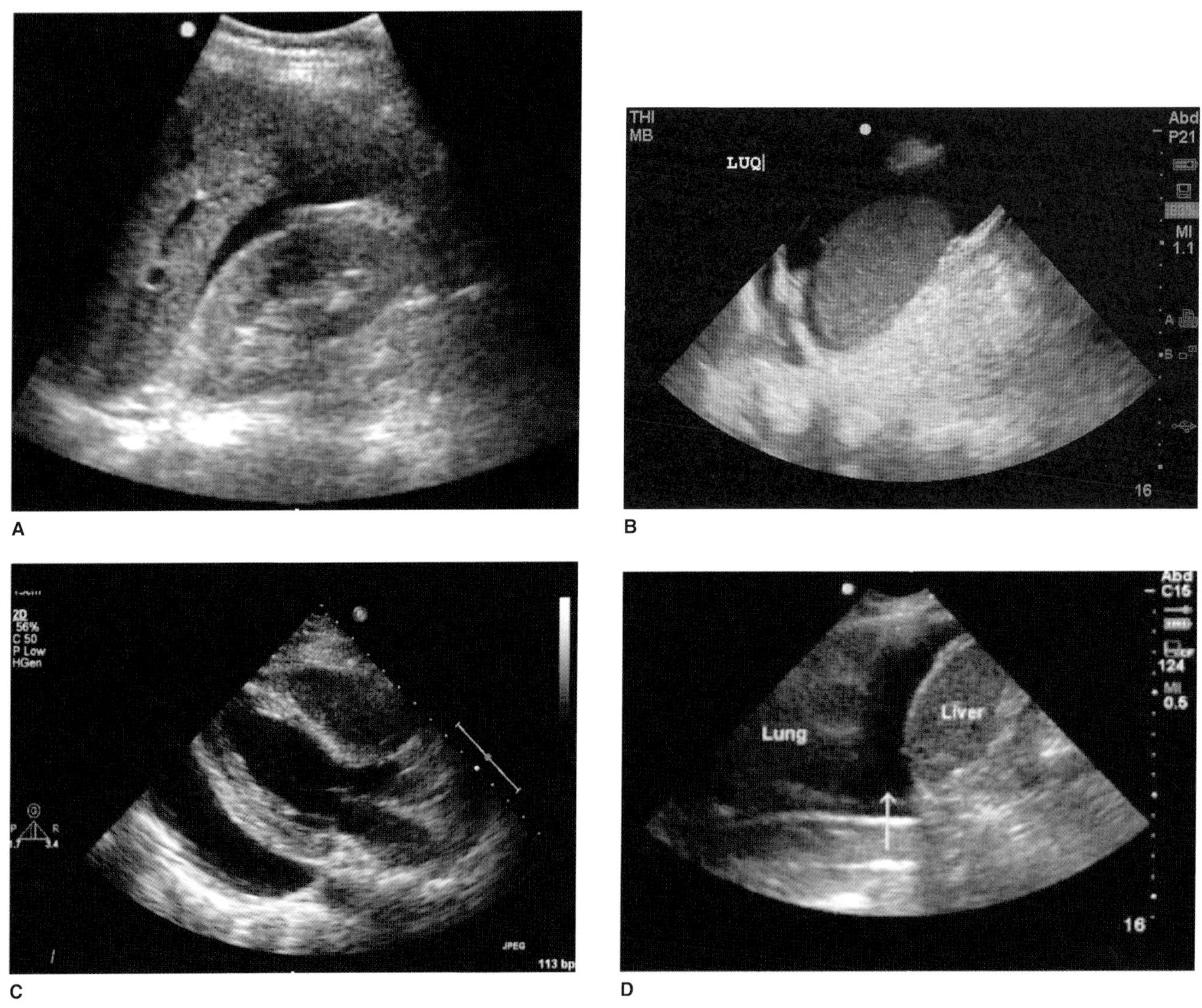

Figure 25-6. These EFAST images show positive findings. (**A**) In the RUQ view, fluid is present in between the liver and right kidney. (**B**) In the LUQ view, fluid is present between the spleen and left kidney. (**C**) In this parasternal cardiac view, fluid is present in the pericardiac sac, concerning for pericardiac efffusion. (**D**) In this thoracic view, fluid is present above the diaphragm and at the base of the lung, concerning for hemothroax. (*Used with permission from Patrick M. Ockerse, MD.*)

- In penetrating trauma, a positive test is indicated by 5000-10,000 RBCs/mm^3.
- Urethrography
  - If examination suggests possible urethral injury, perform a retrograde urethrogram (RUG).
- CT scan
  - Perform only if patient is stable.
  - Retroperitoneal injuries missed on FAST and undetected on DPL can be seen with CT.
  - The need for contrast is debatable and use is institution-specific.

DON'T FORGET

- Hypotensive patients should get a FAST or DPL, but they are too unstable for CT.
- Do not allow unstable patients to leave the ED for radiologic studies. Perform definitive diagnostic tests in the ED under close monitoring.

Management

- Resuscitation
  - Use NS or lactated Ringer (LR) to correct hypotension.
  - Initiate transfusion if hypotension persists despite crystalloids.
    - Some institutions use a "massive transfusion" protocol
- GSWs to abdomen require operative intervention as incidence of significant intraperitoneal injury approaches 90%. Hemodynamic instability mandates operative intervention.
- Stab wounds
  - Approximately two-thirds cause peritoneal violation of which half will require surgery.
  - If there is suspicion that a penetrating wound is superficial, obtain surgical consult to explore the wound and determine operative need.
- Indications for operative intervention and prompt surgical consultation:
  - Peritonitis.
  - Free air, retroperitoneal air, or rupture of the hemi diaphragm after blunt trauma.
  - CT demonstrating ruptured intestine, bladder injury, renal pedicle injury, or severe visceral parenchymal injury after blunt or penetrating trauma.
  - Blunt trauma with a positive FAST or DPL.
  - Blunt trauma with hypotension and clinical evidence of intraperitoneal bleeding.
  - Penetrating abdominal injury and hypotension.
  - Penetrating trauma and bleeding from stomach, rectum, or genitourinary tract.
  - GSW traversing the peritoneal retroperitoneal cavity.
  - Evisceration.

DON'T FORGET

- Any hemodynamically unstable patient with a GSW or stab wound to the abdomen, or with peritonitis, requires immediate operative intervention.
- Injuries to the liver, spleen, or kidneys that result in shock, hemodynamic instability, or evidence of continued bleeding are indications for immediate operative intervention.

Disposition

- Stabilize and transfer the patient if resources are not locally available.
- Admit patient with operative concerns to surgery.
- Admit patients with stable isolated solid organ injuries for observation and reevaluation after consultation with surgery.

SPINAL TRAUMA

History

- Falls from height (>15 feet) have a high incidence of spinal injury.
- High index of suspicion for spine injury in setting of neurologic deficits and multiple injuries.
- Approximately 55% of spinal injuries are cervical, 15% thoracic, 15% at the thoracolumbar junction, and 15% are lumbosacral.
- Approximately 5% of head injury patients have an associated spinal injury and 25% of spine injury patients have an associated head injury.

- The spinal column is generally conceptualized as having three columns. Injuries involving only one column are stable and injuries involving 2 or 3 columns are unstable:
  - The anterior spinal ligament and the anterior walls of the vertebral bodies.
  - The posterior spinal ligament and posterior walls of the vertebral bodies.
  - The posterior elements of the vertebral column.

Examination

- Sensory level: The most caudal spinal cord segment with normal sensory function to both sides.
- Motor level: The most caudal spinal cord segment with at least 3/5 strength.
- Bony level: Level at which the vertebral body injury results in damage to the cord.
- Incomplete spinal injury
  - Any loss of sensation (including position sense) or voluntary movement in the lower extremities
  - Sacral sparing (perianal sensation), voluntary anal sphincter contraction, or voluntary toe flexion
- Central cord syndrome
  - Caused by hyperextension injury in a patient with cervical spondylosis.
  - Disproportionately greater loss of motor in the upper extremities versus the lower with varying degrees of sensory loss.
  - Recovery occurs with lower extremity motor first, bladder function second, and proximal upper extremities and hands last.
- Anterior cord syndrome
  - Caused by injury to the anterior spinal artery and has a poor prognosis for return of function.
  - Results in loss of anterolateral pathway resulting in paraplegia, sensory loss, and loss pain and temperature sensation.
  - Posterior column function (position sense, vibration, and deep pressure) is preserved.
- Brown-Séquard syndrome
  - Hemisection of the cord which results in ipsilateral loss of motor function and position sense and contralateral loss of sensation.
  - Rare in the pure form and usually results in some recovery unless caused by direct penetrating injury.
- Neurogenic shock
  - Loss of vasomotor tone and caused by loss of sympathetic innervation to the heart leading to vasodilatation of visceral and lower extremity blood vessels, pooling of blood, and hypotension.

DON'T FORGET

- The physical examination in the potential spinal cord patient should include a thorough neurologic examination with attention to both motor and sensory functions for all major nerve roots and testing for anal sphincter tone, anal wink, and bulbocavernosus reflex.

Diagnosis

- Cervical spine x-rays are indicated for all trauma patients who have midline neck pain or tenderness to palpation, neurologic deficits referable to the cervical spine, an altered level of consciousness, or who are suspected of being intoxicated.
  - A complete C-spine series includes a lateral, open mouth, and anteroposterior (AP) view. Oblique views can be useful to visualize the facets, and a CT should be obtained if there is any question of fracture and stability.
  - A lateral film that includes all seven cervical vertebral bodies and the first thoracic should be obtained.
  - Pulling down on the shoulders or a swimmer's view may be necessary in order to see all vertebral bodies. If all seven vertebrae are not visualized, a swimmer's view should be obtained.
  - Assess the C-spine film for bony deformity, fractures of the vertebral body or processes, loss of alignment of the posterior aspect of the

vertebral bodies, increased distances between the spinous processes at any level, narrowing of the vertebral canal, or increased prevertebral soft tissue space (>5 mm at C-3).

- Evaluation and exclusion of spinal injury can be deferred in the presence of systemic instability and if the patient has been adequately immobilized.
  - If the patient is comatose or has a depressed level of consciousness, they can remain immobilized until sufficient and adequate x-rays can be obtained to exclude significant spinal injury.
- Approximately, 10% of patients with a C-spine fracture have a second, noncontiguous vertebral spinal fracture, so have a low threshold for imaging the rest of the spine, especially in comatose patients.
- If screening radiographs are normal, but the patient has continued pain or risk of ligamentous injuries, flexion-extension films should be obtained.
- AP and lateral thoracolumbar spine films should be obtained in patients who have spine pain or palpation tenderness, neurologic deficits, an altered level of consciousness, or are suspected of being intoxicated.
- Obtain MRI if there are neurologic deficits and to detect soft tissue compressive lesions such as a spinal epidural hematoma or traumatic herniated disc, which cannot be detected on plain films.

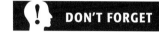

DON'T FORGET

High-cervical injuries can result in acute ventilatory decompensation caused by loss of phrenic nerve and intercostal muscle function. These patients should be intubated early.

Management

- Immobilize the neck to avoid damage caused by excessive manipulation or inadequate immobilization.
- Use a backboard only as transportation device.
  - Leaving a patient on a backboard for an extended period of time can result in serious decubitus ulcers.
  - The patient should be removed from the backboard within 2 hours.
- Presence of paraplegia or quadriplegia is presumptive evidence of spinal instability.
  - May be due to atlanto-occipital dislocation or craniocervical disruption that results from severe flexion and distraction.
  - Ensure spinal immobilization.
- Atlas (C-1) fractures (Fig. 25-7).
  - The most common form is a burst fracture of the ring, or Jefferson fracture, resulting from an axial load.
  - This is best appreciated on an odontoid, or open mouth, view.
  - Although usually not associated with spinal cord injury, the fracture is unstable and should be immobilized.

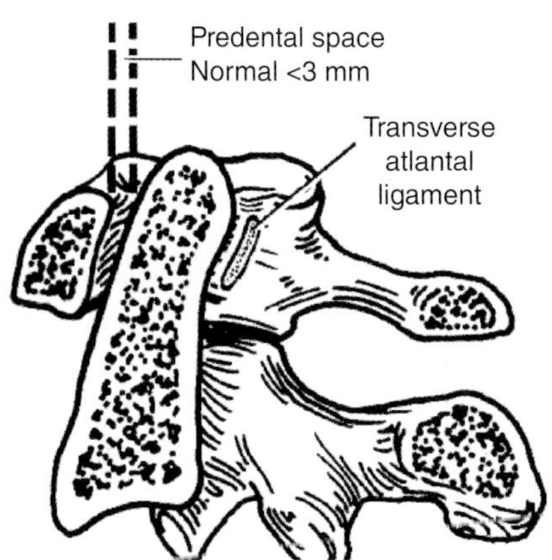

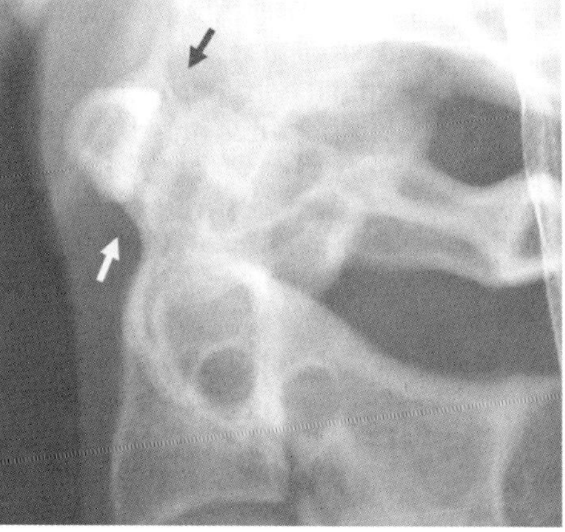

Figure 25-7. A common clinical scenario, causing an axial loading injury to the cervical spine—a dive head-first into a shallow body of water. (*Reproduced with permission from Schwartz DT.* Emergency Radiology: Case Studies. *New York, NY: McGraw-Hill; 2008.*)

- Atlas (C-1) rotary subluxation.
  - Usually seen in children and appears as persistent rotation of the head.
  - On the x-ray, the odontoid is not equidistant from the two lateral masses, and the patient should be immobilized without trying to overcome the rotation.
- Axis (C-2) odontoid fracture.
  - Best appreciated on lateral and odontoid (open mouth) views or CT scan.
  - Type 1 is a fracture through the tip.
  - Type 2 occurs through the base of the dens and is the most common.
    - In children age 6 or younger the epiphysis may be mistakenly called a type 2 fracture.
  - Type 3 fractures occur at the base and extend into the body of the axis.
- Hangman's (C2) fracture
  - Fracture through the posterior elements of C2 is called a hangman's fracture and result from an extension injury. This requires immobilization.
- Unstable C-spine fractures
  - Can be remembered with the mnemonic "Jefferson Bit Off a Hangman's Thumb."
    - Jefferson's fracture of C1
    - Bilateral facet fracture/dislocation
    - Odontoid type II and III
    - Any fracture/dislocation, including atlanto-axial dislocation and atlanto-occipital dislocation
    - Hangman's fracture of C2
    - Teardrop fractures
  - Burst and chance fractures are also unstable and almost always require internal fixation.
  - Surgery also indicated for restoration of spinal canal anatomy, removal of foreign bodies, and to remove any bone, disc, or hematoma that is compressing the cord.
  - Simple compression fractures are usually stable and often treated with a rigid brace.
  - Surgical therapy is indicated for neurogenic shock.
- When in doubt, leave the collar on until further evaluation can be obtained.
- Administer IV fluids in the patient with suspected spinal injury.
  - Persistent hypotension associated with bradycardia may require vasopressors.
  - Significant bradycardia can be treated with atropine.
  - Avoid overzealous fluid administration which can lead to pulmonary edema.

DON'T FORGET

- Neurogenic shock should be considered if a patient has no active hemorrhage but continues to be hypotensive despite crystalloid.
- As little can be done to repair the spinal cord in the ED, focus your attention on making a diagnosis, preserving function, and appropriate consultation.

Disposition

- Admit unstable fractures to neurosurgery or orthopedic surgery.
- ICU admission may be required to achieve therapeutic blood pressure to optimize spinal cord perfusion.
- Some stable fractures may be followed as an outpatient.

PELVIC TRAUMA

History

- Type of injury is dependent on mechanism.
- Unexplained hypotension may be the only initial indication of pelvic injury.
- There are four patterns of force that cause pelvic fractures:
  1. AP compression
  2. Lateral compression
  3. Vertical shear
  4. Complex (combination) pattern

- Motorcycle crashes, pedestrian–vehicle collisions, direct crush injuries, and falls from a height >12 feet are associated with a force vector that opens the pelvic ring and can tear the pelvic venous plexus, causing severe hemorrhage.
  - These fractures are frequently unstable and associated with ligamentous disruption and sacroiliac or sacral fracture.
  - Hemorrhage occurs rapidly and major venous injury must be identified early
    - Bleeding can be retroperitoneal.
- MVCs, on the other hand, are more commonly associated with a lateral force that rotates the hemipelvis internally (lateral compression) without putting tension on the vascular system.
  - This type of injury is more commonly associated with bladder and/or urethral trauma and is unlikely to result in severe hemorrhage.

DON'T FORGET

- Fractures involving the posterior ring are associated with more complications and a higher bleeding risk, requiring more fluid for resuscitation.
- Urethral injuries manifest as blood at the meatus, urethral bleeding, and inability to void with distended bladder.
- Do not place a Foley catheter if the patient has an unstable pelvic fracture, blood at the meatus, or a high-riding prostate. These patients require a RUG.

Examination

- Check for progressive flank, scrotal, or perianal swelling and bruising.
- Open fractures around the pelvis, a high-riding prostate, blood at the meatus, and mechanical instability are all signs of an unstable pelvic ring fracture.
- Manual manipulation ("pelvic rock") should be performed only once during the initial evaluation to assess for pelvic stability.
- Leg-length discrepancy or rotational deformity without an extremity fracture can indicate an unstable pelvic ring injury.

Diagnosis

- Obtain an AP x-ray of the pelvis.
- Inlet and outlet views may further delineate the injuries.
- Obtain a CT of the pelvis if the patient is stable and you have concern for pelvic injury.

Management

- Use an external compression device (either commercially produced or a bed sheet will suffice) to compress the area and tamponade blood loss.
  - Use for all pelvic fractures except isolated pelvic wing fractures.
- Longitudinal traction on the extremities and internal rotation of the lower limbs may support and stabilize the pelvis and decrease the traction on the pelvic veins.
- Some fractures require operative repair.
  - Open book fractures require external fixation.
  - Posterior fractures with involvement of the sacroiliac joint are frequently associated with arterial bleeding and require embolization.
- Hemodynamically stable patients with a pelvic fracture should be scrutinized for other injuries via CT.
- Hemodynamically unstable patients with a pelvic fracture must first have other significant thoracic or abdominal bleeding sources evaluated and managed.
  - If bleeding is restricted to the pelvis, management options include embolization or surgical pelvic fixation at the discretion of the trauma surgeon.

DON'T FORGET

- Initial management is mainly directed at control of hemorrhage which can be accomplished by external fixation, commercially prepared pelvic compression devices (such as Pneumatic AntiShock Garments [PASG]) or a sheet wrapped around the pelvis.
- Stable patients with pelvic fracture should have an abdomen and pelvis CT to evaluate potential intra-abdominal and pelvic injuries.
- Some pelvic fractures can cause retroperitoneal bleeding and will have a negative FAST examination. These patients will require operative management.

Disposition

- Operative repair by an orthopedic and trauma surgeon is necessary for the hemodynamically unstable patient.
- Control of venous bleeding may be obtained with embolization by interventional radiology if the patient is deemed stable enough for the procedure.

MUSCULOSKELETAL TRAUMA

History

- Consider the mechanism of injury to assess for potential injuries.
  - For example, if involved in an MVC was the patient wearing a seatbelt, ejected, and what is the damage pattern to car?
  - Was there the potential for crush injury? If so, what was the weight of the object and length of time of crush injury?
- Find out what care was provided before arrival to ED.
  - Was there reduction or splinting at the scene?
  - What kind of dressings applied at the scene?
  - Was there any change in limb function, perfusion, or neurologic status after immobilization?
- Consider compartment syndrome risk factors.
  - Most common with crush injuries, tibial and forearm fractures, injuries immobilized in a tight dressing or cast, localized and prolonged external pressure to an extremity, burns, and exercise (CrossFit).
- Obtain history of with closed fist injury
  - Did the patient punch someone in the mouth?
  - Are there lacerations?

Examination

- Evaluate for deformity, warm joints, ligamentous injury, and check neurovascular status during Secondary Survey.
- Assess the skin for discoloration, open wounds, and bruising.
- Evaluate the 5 Ps of compartment syndrome
  - Pain out of proportion
  - Pallor
  - Paresthesia in the nerve distribution
  - Paralysis
  - Pulselessness
    - *Paralysis* and *pulselessness* are late findings (diagnosis ideally made prior to their development).
- Evaluate closed fist injuries.
  - Inspect for contamination, tendon injury, and vascular compromise.
  - Inspect for rotational deformity. With all metacarpophalangeal joints (MCPs) and proximal interphalangeal joints (PIPs) flexed at 90°, and all distal interphalangeal joints (DIPs) at 180°, all fingers should point to the same spot at the wrist.
  - Check two-point discrimination, tendon function and strength with both active and passive range of motion.

DON'T FORGET

- Neurovascular deficits are often mistaken for extremity injuries.
- A palpable distal pulse is present until late stages of compartment syndrome.
- It is important to examine compartments at risk, especially if the patient has an altered sensorium or is unable to respond to pain.
- Remember to use antibiotics and check the MCP joint capsule if you are concerned about "fight bite."

Diagnosis

- Evaluate for lower extremity arterial injury with an ankle brachial index (ABI) of <0.9.
- Confirm Doppler signals if pulses are not palpable in any affected extremity.
- Obtain imaging for any swollen, contused, lacerated, or tender bony surface.
- Obtain CTA in patients with a history or examination concerning for knee dislocation as these injuries are associated with high rates of associated vascular injury.
- Check for compartment syndrome by measuring the compartment pressures with Stryker ™ device. Pressures >35-45 mm Hg suggest decreased capillary blood flow and are indicative of compartment syndrome.

Management

- Vascular injury requires prompt assessment and intervention.
- Dislocations and fractures should be reduced and/or splinted immediately.
  - Evaluate neurovascular status before and after reduction.
- Arterial bleeding
  - Place direct pressure.
  - A pneumatic tourniquet should only be considered for uncontrolled hemorrhage as a life-saving measure.
  - Use aggressive fluid resuscitation.
  - Obtain early surgical consultation for limb-threatening bleeding.
- Arterial injury
  - Obtain arteriography or ultrasound to assess for vascular injury in hemodynamically stable patients with an ABI <0.9.
  - Obtain early surgical consultation when peripheral pulses are absent and there is concern for vascular injury.
- Fractures
  - Obtain x-rays, orthopedic consultation, and reduce fractures during the Secondary Survey after the trauma patient has been stabilized and more serious injuries have been addressed.
  - Reduce and splint open fractures; give antibiotics and update tetanus.
  - Reduce closed fractures immediately if there is evidence of neurovascular compromise or skin tenting.
- Compartment syndrome
  - Make the diagnosis early as delayed diagnosis causes greater damage.
  - Remove any constricting dressings, casts, or splints.
  - Consult orthopedics to perform fasciotomy as definitive treatment.
- Boxer's fractures (Fig. 25-8)
  - Open wounds over the MCP joint are concerning for "fight bite"
    - Irrigate these wounds and use an antibiotic such as Augmentin that covers oral and skin flora.

DON'T FORGET

- Don't forget antibiotics, tetanus, and pain control.
- Increased pain should warrant a reassessment of neurovascular status.
- Reassess neurovascular status before and after reduction and splinting.
- Reduce any digital rotational deformity because even small amounts of rotation in finger extension can cause disabling rotation in flexion and pseudo-clawing, involving MCP hyperextension and PIP flexion.

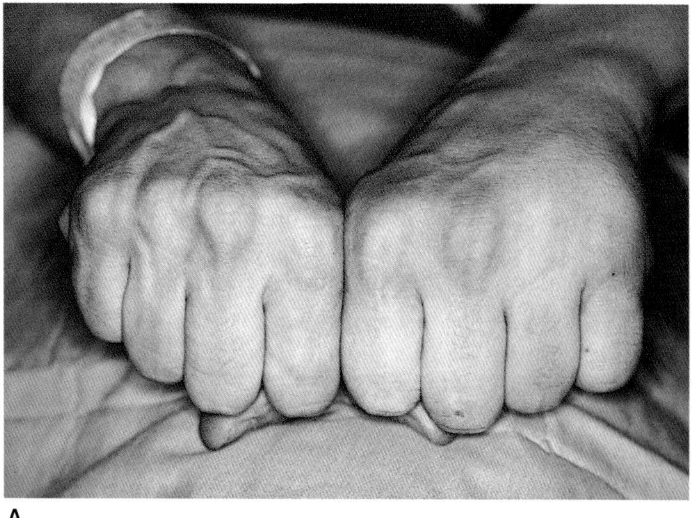

A

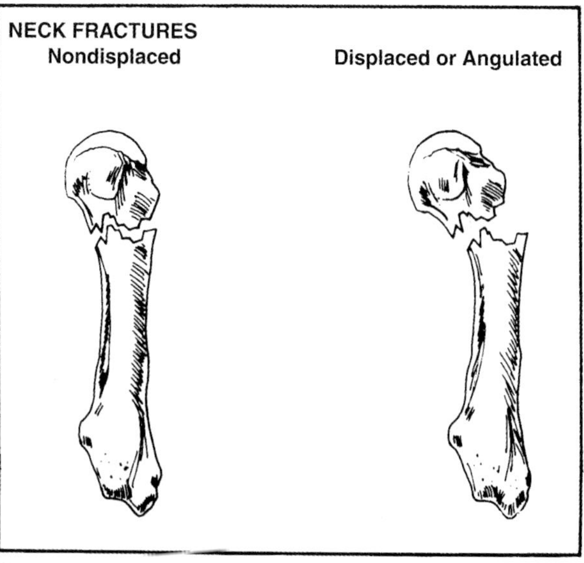

B

Figure 25-8. Boxer's fracture. (**A**) This boxer's fracture occurred when the patient punched a wall with his hand. There is loss of the "knuckle" when the dorsum of the hand is examined, especially noticeable when the patient makes a fist. (**B**) Metacarpal fractures—neck. (*[A]: Reproduced with permission from Knoop KJ, Stack LB, Storrow AB.* Atlas of Emergency Medicine. *2nd ed. New York, NY: McGraw-Hill; 2002. [B]: Reproduced with permission from Simon RR, Sherman SC, Koenigsknecht SJ.* Emergency Orthopedics: The Extremities. *5th ed. New York, NY: McGraw-Hill; 2007.*)

- Reduce any digital rotational deformity or metacarpal angulation of more than10° in the index finger, 20° in the middle finger, and 30° in the ring finger.

Disposition

- Closed, isolated fractures, without evidence of neurovascular compromise, can be splinted and treated as an outpatient.
- Open fractures and injuries involving neurovascular deficit require consultation and admission.
- Patients with possible arterial injury may require admission for serial physical examination and evaluation with color flow, duplex, Doppler ultrasonography.
- Admit patients with compartment syndrome to the ICU after fasciotomy.
- Even stable patients with signs of infection or joint space involvement may require admission for IV antibiotics and surgical evaluation.

WINNING STRATEGIES

- Identify yourself.
- Ask the patient his/her name.
- Ask about the mechanism for injury.
  - If the patient is unable to answer, ask EMTs, family member, or others for additional history.
  - If the patient responds appropriately that confirms a patent airway, sufficient air reserve to permit speech, and a clear sensorium.
- Perform a Primary Survey and address concerns as you find them.
- Your Secondary Survey should include a complete history and head to toe physical examination.
  - Reassess the ABCDEs and ensure vital signs are returning to normal.
- Avoid missing injuries by doing the following:
  - Obtain history of mechanism and have a high index of suspicion.
  - Reevaluate the patient frequently.
    - When the patient's status changes, repeat the Primary Survey and recheck vital signs after any intervention.
  - Check for a pneumothorax, diaphragm injury, pelvic fractures, compartment injuries, and address airway management.
  - Don't stop investigating when you've discovered the first injury. Trauma cases usually involve several injuries.
  - Don't begin the Secondary Survey until you have completed the Primary Survey and stabilized the patient by addressing any immediate concerns.
  - Call the surgeon early for any cases requiring operative management or potential hospital transfer.
  - Make sure all trauma patients get tetanus updates, antibiotics for open fractures, and perform accuchecks early.

THE BOTTOM LINE

- You will have a trauma case.
- It will likely be straightforward if you start with Primary Survey, perform any necessary interventions, and complete the entire Secondary Survey.
- Mistakes are usually related to omission. Don't forget to ask about the patients back, genitals, skin, and extremities.
- Repeat the Primary Survey with any change in status.
- Recheck vital signs frequently and after every intervention.

CHAPTER 26

Burn Patients

Michael Paddock and James Ahn

DON'T FORGET

Evaluate airway to determine if immediate intervention is needed, be cognizant that intubation will become more difficult as the edema in an involved airway increases.

IMMEDIATE INTERVENTIONS

- Intubation if airway is compromised.
- Large-bore IV access for fluid hydration.
- Supplemental oxygen.
- Place on monitor, especially for electrical burns.
- Administer pain medications.

DON'T FORGET

All burn patients should be evaluated as multiple trauma patients and all possible injuries should be investigated.

DON'T FORGET

Early airway intervention by endotracheal intubation or surgical airway may be necessary if airway edema, erythema, singed nasal hairs, or carbonaceous sputum is visualized on primary examination.

DON'T FORGET

Significant inhalation injuries may have no external signs of burn or heat exposure.

INITIAL ASSESSMENT

- Focus on airway, breathing, and circulation (ABCs) and keep immediate life threats in mind first.
- Ask for a full set of vitals with every patient including pulse, blood pressure (BP), respirations, temperature, oxygen saturation (O_2 sat), glucose, finger stick hemoglobin (Hgb)
- Large-bore IV × 2, O_2, monitor in every patient.
- Draw labs and hold for orders.

Case-Specific Recommendations

- Immediate assessment of hemodynamic status and fluid resuscitation
- Early and aggressive administration of pain medications

INITIAL HISTORY AND PHYSICAL EXAMINATION

- History of present illness (HPI)
  - How was the patient burned (mechanism of injury)?
  - Length of time exposed
  - Any treatment in the field (eg, irrigation or decontamination)
  - Syncope
  - Estimated time since incident
  - Mechanism of injury to determine if patient is at risk for other traumatic injuries
- Past medical history (PMHx)
  - Immunocompromised?
  - Cardiac disease
- Medications
- Allergies
- Tetanus status
- Physical examination
  - A complete set of vital signs should be obtained
  - Head, eyes, ears, nose, and throat (HEENT) examination: Singed eyebrows, eyelashes, or facial hair? Carbonaceous sputum? Airway swelling? Eye involvement? Tongue or lip swelling? Periorbital burns?
  - Chest: Tachycardia?
  - Lungs: Wheezing? Equal breath sounds? Good air movement?
  - Abdominal: Pain?
  - Extremity: Cap refill, cyanosis?
  - Rectal: Gross blood?
  - Neuro: Alteration in mental status?
  - Skin: Exit wounds? Percentage of body area involved?
  - Estimation of total body surface area (TBSA) burned:
    - Rule of nines assumes adult body proportions (Fig. 26-1)
      - Head and neck: 9%
      - Anterior chest: 9%
      - Posterior chest: 9%
      - Anterior abdomen: 9%
      - Posterior abdomen (w/buttocks): 9%
      - Each upper extremity: 9%
      - Each thigh: 9%
      - Each leg and foot: 9%
      - Genitals: 1%
      - Palmar surface of hand: 1%

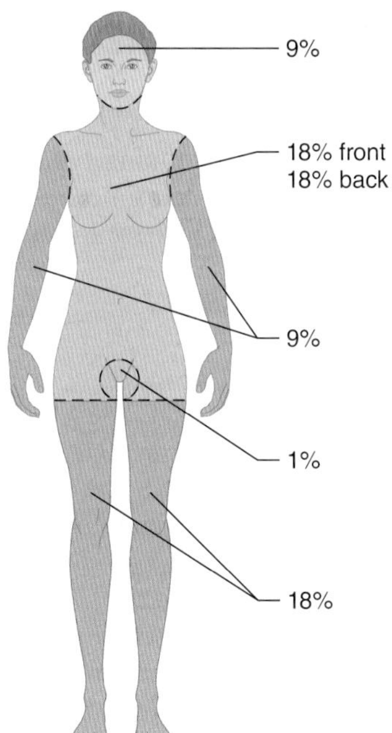

Figure 26-1. Adult and pediatric rule of nines. (*Tintinalli JE, Stapczynski JS, Ma OJ, Yealy DM, Meckler GD, Cline DM. Tintinalli's* Emergency Medicine: A Comprehensive Study Guide. *8th ed. New York, NY: McGraw-Hill Education, 2016. Figure 216-2.*)

DIFFERENTIAL DIAGNOSIS

- Younger children are at a higher risk for serious injury from burns and almost one-fifth of burns in this age group involve abuse or neglect.
- Skin burns are categorized into the depth of injury, depending on the layers of tissue involved.
  - *Superficial-thickness* (first-degree) burns involve only the epidermis (erythema and pain).
  - *Partial-thickness* (second-degree) burns involve both the epidermis and the dermis (erythema, blisters, and bulla—painful).
  - *Full-thickness* (third-degree) burns involve destruction of the epidermis, dermis, and dermal appendages (white in appearance and insensate).
- Burns can be produced from various types of exposures and although the general treatment is the same, each can produce specific injuries that need to be evaluated and treated.
  - *Electrical:* A burn that results from exposure to an electrical source. It can range from high-voltage exposures such as lightning or high-voltage electrical lines to low-voltage exposures that usually occur at home. Electrical exposures account for approximately 2%-3% of all burns seen in children and 3%-4% of admissions.
  - *Chemical:* A burn that results from exposure to a chemical source which is usually alkali or acidic. The majority of chemical exposures are from household cleaning products.
  - *Thermal:* A burn that results when energy is applied to tissue at a faster rate than it can be dissipated and thus causes injury. The heat can result from various sources including water, oil, steam, gas, fire, radiation (sunburn), or any liquid.
    - Patients with thermal burns often have other concurrent injuries such as inhalation injuries, carbon monoxide poisoning, and blunt trauma.

ELECTRICAL BURN

Additional History and Physical Examination Findings

- A thorough history is imperative, including type of voltage, current, length of exposure to the electrical current, and time since incident.
- Physics of injury (Ohm law I = V/R) where I = current (amps), V = voltage, and R = resistance.
- *Voltage* (V): Low: <600 V, high: >600 V
  - High-tension lines: 100,000 V
  - Homes: 110 V/240 V (220 V in Europe)
  - Lightning: >1,000,000 V
  - High-voltage exposures may leave an exit burn after the current transverses through the body.
- *Resistance* (R) is the tendency of a material to resist the flow of current (ohms) and high resistance tissues impede current flow and convert more energy to heat causing increased damage.
  - Bone > fat > tendons > skin > muscle > blood > nerves
  - Water greatly reduces resistance and can increase the current to the victim and increase damage (eg, electrocution from being in a bathtub or in the rain).
- *Current* (I) is the flow of electrons per second as measured by amperes. There are two types of current:
  - *Direct current (DC)*
    - Flows in only one direction (single-muscle contraction)
    - Lightning/high-voltage
  - *Alternating current (AC)*
    - Standardized frequency of 60 Hz (tetany)
    - Household and office appliances
  - Although AC current is more dangerous because this current can cause muscle tetany, which does not allow the victim to release the electrical source.
- Most high-voltage sources are DC and this usually throws the victim from the source (see Table 26-1).

Review Initial Results

- Electrocardiogram (ECG) and place on monitor to look for arrhythmias.
- Chemistry to look for electrolyte abnormalities (especially hyperkalemia associated with cell death).

Table 26-1. Currents and Physical Response to Contact

CURRENT		PHYSICAL RESPONSE
1 mA		Tingling sensation
4-9 mA		Average "let go" current
16 mA		Maximum "let go" current
16-20 mA		Tetany of skeletal muscle
50-100 mA	causes	Ventricular fibrillation
>2 A	causes	Asystole
15-30 A	found in	Households appliances
>200,000 A	found in	Lightning

DON'T FORGET

Electrical injuries are the type most often associated with significant blunt trauma and internal injuries.

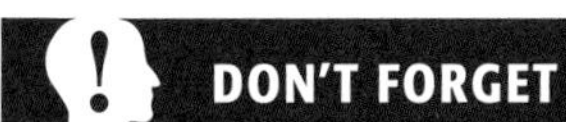

DON'T FORGET

One type of burn does not exclude others (eg, electrical fire) and other traumatic injuries should always be suspected in burn patients, especially when a good history cannot be elicited.

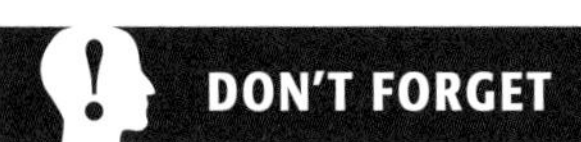

DON'T FORGET

Exposure to high voltages (such as lightning) carries morbidity 5-10 times that of low-voltage exposures.

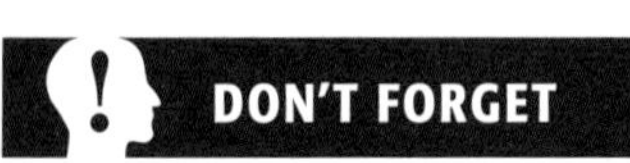

DON'T FORGET

Skin is the major source of resistance in electrical injuries (high resistance = thermal injury).

- Blood urea nitrogen (BUN) and creatinine for renal function.
- Creatinine kinase (CPK) to rule out rhabdomyolysis.
- Urine to look for myoglobin.
- Cardiac enzymes if abnormal ECG or arrhythmias.

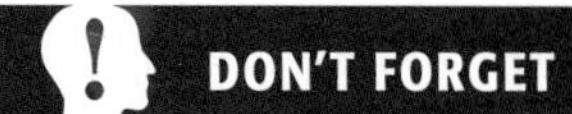

Young children are extremely vulnerable because of their thin skin. They often bite on electrical cords and the moist mucous membranes, and saliva reduces resistance.

Risk Stratification: Management Priorities

- External burn injuries are not a good indicator of internal injuries. Internal injuries may be greater as high resistance levels of bone and fat may cause high transfer of thermal heat and necrosis of internal structures.

Cardiac

- Up to one-third of electrical injuries may have a cardiac component.
- Low-voltage AC current is more likely to cause ventricular fibrillation and is the most common cause of death.
- DC and high-voltage AC current are more likely to cause asystole but circulation may return spontaneously.
- Patients with arrhythmias, loss of consciousness (LOC), or cardiac arrest or chest pain should be admitted for cardiac monitoring.

Neuro

- LOC occurs in up to 50% of patients with high-voltage injuries but is usually transient.
- Peripheral nerve damage is common and can manifest as parasthesias or weakness.

Skin

- Electrical burns can result in partial-thickness burns, full-thickness burns, or deep tissue burns.
  - *Low voltage*: This usually results in typical thermal burns that can be partial or full thickness depending on the exposure. These burns should be treated as normal thermal burns.
  - *High voltage*: This can cause both cutaneous thermal burns as well as deep tissue necrosis. High-voltage burns can also result from arc burns that occur when the electricity flashes over the body.
  - *Lightning*: This usually causes only superficial cutaneous burns and rarely involves the deep tissues because the short duration and extremely high voltages cause flashovers arcs.

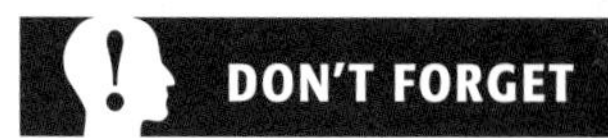

AC current is three times more deadly than DC current.

Definitive Management

- ABCs.
  - Intubate early if altered mental status or oral/airway involvement.
- IVF resuscitation generally accepted is to give a 20 mL/kg bolus, and then administer fluid to keep a good urine output (UOP).
- Pain management is imperative.
- Patients with high-voltage injuries including lightning strikes should be placed on a monitor in addition to receiving an ECG.
- Cutaneous burns should be cleaned and covered with antibiotic dressings (mafenide acetate or sulfadiazine silver).
- Escharotomy needs to be performed if there is neurovascular compromise present secondary to compartment syndrome from circumferential burns.
- Supplemental oxygen.
- Tetanus if needed.

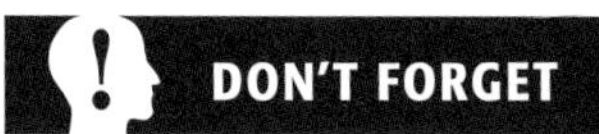

If mental status does not improve, patient should undergo a CT to rule out bleed from a traumatic injury.

Frequent Reassessment

- Reassess UOP to determine if fluid resuscitation is sufficient.
- Reassess pain scale and need for additional pain medications.

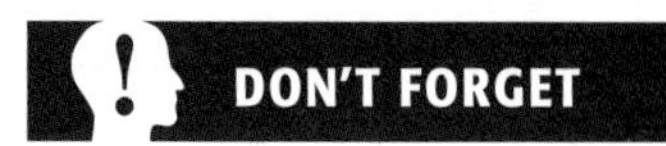

Patients exposed to high voltage or lightning are more likely to be thrown and are susceptible to blast injuries.

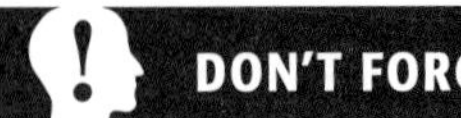

DON'T FORGET

The rule of nines or other fluid resuscitation formulas cannot be used in electrical burns to determine fluid resuscitation needs because skin burns can underestimate the amount of total body involvement.

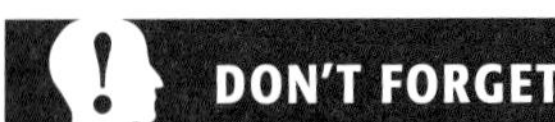

DON'T FORGET

With large-volume fluid resuscitation, LR is the fluid of choice as it does not cause the metabolic acidosis seen with NS.

- Reassess mental status in high-voltage injuries.
- Reassess extremity injuries for developing compartment syndrome.

Complications

- Arrhythmias secondary to cardiac involvement.
- Respiratory failure secondary to direct central nervous system (CNS) injury from lightning strikes or from muscle tetany in lower-voltage injuries.
- Infections secondary to skin burns.
- Cataracts in cases of lightning strikes.
- Rhabdomyolysis.
- Sepsis.

Disposition

- Admit all patients with the following:
  - LOC or mental status changes.
  - Cardiac arrhythmias, chest pain, abnormal ECG, or cardiac arrest.
  - Significant skin burns.
  - Myoglobinuria.
  - Other significant traumatic injuries.

CHEMICAL BURN

Additional History and Physical Examination Findings

- Obtaining a complete history of the events surrounding the injury is essential for proper treatment.
  - *Offending agent*
    - Composition (solid, liquid, aerosol)
    - Acid or alkali
    - Concentration
  - *Exposure*
    - Inhalation
    - Cutaneous
    - Ocular
    - Gastrointestinal
  - *Duration of exposure and volume of agent*
  - *Events associated with the burn*
    - Explosion
    - Fall
    - Trauma
- Was any decontamination performed prior to presentation?
- Dysphagia, stridor, wheezing, drooling, or dyspnea on examination?
- Acids: Some common agents include
  - *Sulfuric acid*: Used for household cleaners, automobile battery fluid, and industrial manufacturing.
  - *Nitric acid*: Used for engraving, metal refining, and industrial manufacturing.
  - *Hydrofluoric acid*: Used for rust, removers, tire cleaners, and tile cleaners.
  - *Hydrochloric acid*: Commonly found in toilet, bowl cleaners, metal cleaners, dye manufacturing, metal refining, plumbing applications, and laboratory chemicals.
  - *Phosphoric acid*: Found in metal cleaners, rust proofing, disinfectants, and detergents.
  - *Acetic acid*: Commonly found in printing, dyes, disinfectants, and hair wave neutralizers. Dilute acetic acid is also the main ingredient in vinegar.
  - *Formic acid*: Commonly found in airplane glue.

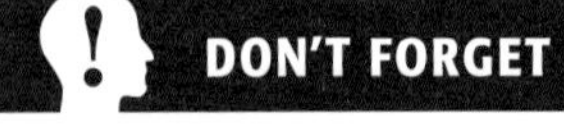

DON'T FORGET

Acids denature proteins and cause a coagulation necrosis that can limit the spread of further tissue destruction.

- Alkali (Bases): Some common agents include:
  - *Sodium or potassium hydroxide*: Found in drain and oven cleaners.
  - *Sodium or calcium hypochlorite*: Found in household bleach or pool chlorination systems.
  - *Calcium hydroxide*: Found in cement, mortar, or plaster.
  - *Potassium hydroxide*: Found in denture cleaners.
  - *Sodium carbonate*: Found in dishwashing or clothing detergents.
  - *Potassium hydroxide*: Found in toilet cleaners (lye).

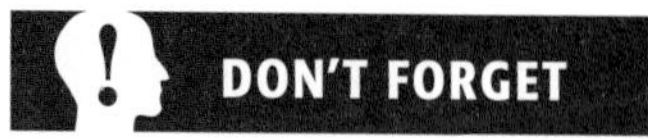

Always be sure chemical burns have been irrigated—retained chemicals may still be burning internal tissue.

Review Initial Results

- Chemistry to look for electrolyte abnormalities (especially hyperkalemia caused by cell death).
- BUN and creatinine for renal function.
- Calcium (hypocalcemia) in burns with hydrofluoric acid.
- CPK to rule out rhabdomyolysis.
- Urine to look for myoglobin.
- Chest x-ray (CXR) should be obtained if ingestion or suspicion of airway involvement, but is usually normal.

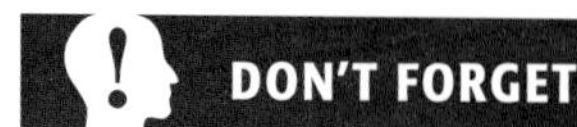

Bases also denature proteins but cause a liquefaction necrosis that can potentially cause a more severe injury than acids.

Risk Stratification: Management Priorities

- The strength of acid and bases are measured on the logarithmic pH scale, which ranges from 1 (strongly acidic) to 14 (strongly base) with 7 being neutral.
- Caustic ingestions are at a high risk for airway compromise.
- Ocular exposures can produce significant morbidity.

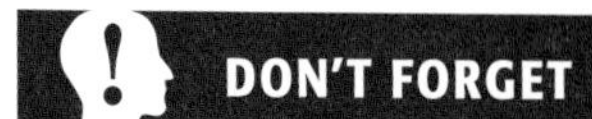

Chemical burns generally are not fatal with a mortality rate of <1% (around 20 deaths per year).

Definitive Management

- ABCs.
- Aggressively secure the airway in a chemical ingestion when the patient is excessively drooling, stridulous, or shows other signs of airway compromise.
- Decontamination (remove clothing, jewelry, shoes).
- Copious irrigation of affected sites (ocular rinse if eye involvement).
- IVF resuscitation: Estimate based on TBSA involved (see "Thermal Burn").
- Endoscopy for ingestions or suspected airway involvement.
- Pain management is imperative.
- Supplemental oxygen.
- Escharotomy needs to be performed if there is neurovascular compromise present secondary to compartment syndrome from circumferential burns.
- Debride loose, necrotic skin, broken, or infected blisters.
- Tetanus if needed.
- Hydrofluoric acid burns require special consideration and treatment because of the fluoride exposure.
  - While hydrofluoric acid burns can initially be irrigated like any other chemical exposure, calcium will be needed to treat hydrofluoric acid burns.
  - Topical calcium or magnesium gels for the superficial burns and intra-arterial injections of calcium for the deeper burns suffered from hydrofluoric acid.

Frequent Reassessment

- Continuous monitoring of the patient's vital signs.
- Reassess UOP to determine if fluid resuscitation is sufficient.
- Reassess pain scale and need for additional pain medications.
- Reassess airway in patients with possible ingestion or inhalation injury.

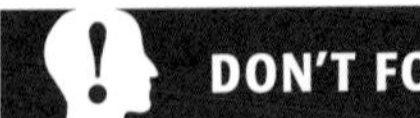

DON'T FORGET

Decontamination must not put the patient or health care providers at further risk of exposure. Prevent runoff of irrigation running into exposed tissue.

Complications

- Stricture formation in esophageal burns.
- Corneal opacification in ocular burns.
- Sepsis.
- Airway edema and respiratory distress if there are inhalational injuries.

Disposition

- All patients with a potentially chemical airway burn should be admitted for observation and endoscopy.
- Significant skin burns.
- Other significant traumatic injuries.

THERMAL BURN

Additional History and Physical Examination Findings

- Death rates are highest among children (<5 years) and the elderly (>65 years).
- A thorough history is crucial to determine the extent of other injuries.
  - Blast injury: Assess for blunt trauma.
  - Closed spaces: Assess for inhalation injury.
  - Fire: Assess for carbon monoxide and cyanide poisoning.
- Scald injuries are common in children and often result from cooking accidents.
- Children <4 years account for 50% of all pediatric burns.
- Consider child abuse in all pediatric burns; these are components to the history and physical examination that should raise suspicion:
  - Multiple stories or inconsistent description of accident.
  - Injury claimed to be unwitnessed.
  - Injury incompatible with development or abilities of the child.
  - Pattern burns that suggest contact with an object.
  - Cigarette burns.
  - Stocking, glove, or circumferential burns.
  - Burns to genitalia or perineum.
  - Burns consistent with dipping (both feet and hands or buttocks).

DON'T FORGET

Always consider child abuse when a child presents with a thermal burn of any type.

Review Initial Results

- Arterial blood gas (ABG) with lactate, carboxyhemoglobin, and cyanide levels to screen for carbon monoxide and cyanide poisoning.
- Type and cross.
- Electrolytes.
- Hgb/hematocrit.
- Coagulation profile.
- CXR if inhalation injury suspected.
- Computed tomography (CT), x-rays, ultrasound for blunt trauma workup as indicated.

DON'T FORGET

Look for and rule out blunt traumatic injury in all combustion-type accidents.

Risk Stratification: Management Priorities

- Suspect if inhalation injury if:
  - Enclosed space.
  - LOC or AMS.
  - Drug or ethyl alcohol (EtOH) abuse.
  - Facial burns.
  - Carbonaceous sputum.

Definitive Management

- ABCs.
- Supplemental oxygen.

- Wound care with ample pain management.
  - Gently cleanse with water.
  - Debride nonviable tissue and ruptured blisters.
  - Leave noninfected blisters intact.
  - Tetanus.
  - Apply antimicrobial agent.
  - Cool the wound with towels moistened with normal saline (NS).
- IVF resuscitation.
- *Parkland formula*: 2-4 mL of lactated ringer (LR) or NS per kilogram per body surface area (BSA)% burned. One-half is given in the first 8 hours after the burn (not from presentation to the department) and the remaining over the next 16 hours.
- Foley catheter placement for monitoring UOP if using *Parkland formula.*
- Pain management is imperative.
- Cutaneous burns should be cleaned and covered with antibiotic dressings (mafenide acetate or sulfadiazine silver).
- Escharotomy needs to be performed if there is neurovascular compromise present secondary to compartment syndrome from circumferential burns.

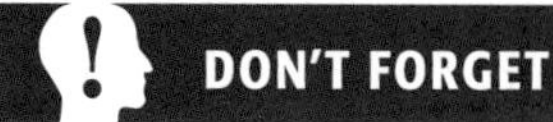

Maintain UOP of at least 1.0 mL/kg/h in adults and 1.0-1.5 mL/kg/h in children of <30 kg.

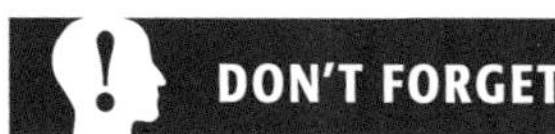

Patients with inhalation burns may need even more fluid (up to 50% added to their BSA calculated) because of intrapulmonary damage and fluid loss. The goal is not following the formula but appropriate UOP.

Frequent Reassessment

- Continuous monitoring of the patient's vital signs.
- Reassess UOP to determine if fluid resuscitation is sufficient.
- Reassess pain scale and need for additional pain medications.
- Reassess airway in patients with possible ingestion or inhalation injury.

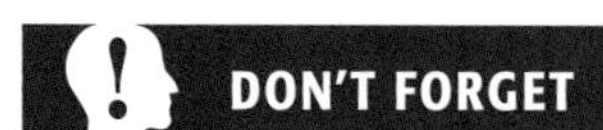

Consult plastic surgery or a burn specialist for your admitted patient.

Complications

- Scarring.
- Cosmetic deformity.
- Adult respiratory distress syndrome (ARDS).
- Sepsis.

Disposition

- Admission criteria:
  - Partial-thickness burns involving >10%-20% of BSA in adults not involving critical areas.
  - Partial-thickness burns involving >5%-10% of BSA in children and the elderly not involving critical areas.
  - Suspicion of child abuse.
  - Patients are unable to care for their wounds in as an outpatient.
- Criteria to transfer to a burn unit (per American Burn Association):
  - Partial-thickness burn covering >20% of TBSA in any person.
  - Partial-thickness burn covering >10% of TBSA in children and the elderly (>50 years).
  - Full-thickness burn covering >5% of TBSA in any patient.
  - Second- or third-degree burns involving critical areas (face, hands, feet, perineum, genitalia, major joints, circumferential burns of chest, or extremities).
  - Inhalation injury.
  - Electrical burns.
  - Severe burns complicated by coexisting trauma.
  - Preexisting disease that could complicate management of burn injury.
  - Chemical burns.
  - Children with severe burns.
- Prior to transfer ensure the following:
  - Airway is stable or intubate if indicated.
  - IVF resuscitation is started.
  - Large-bore IV access.

WINNING STRATEGIES

- Always focus on the ABCs and volume resuscitation in all burn patients.
- Obtain an extensive history from emergency medical services (EMS) and family to determine the type of burn and the potential for associated high-risk injuries.
- Aggressive and early airway interventions.
- Immediate IV access for fluid resuscitation.
- Pain medications early and often as needed.
- Start fluid resuscitation early and maintain based on UOP.
- Suspect and look for additional trauma injuries in all burn patients.
- In electrical exposures, do not use surface area of burns to gauge severity because superficial burns underestimate the total amount of tissue destruction.
- All burn patients should receive a tetanus booster or toxoid based on their prior immunization history.
- Look for indications of child abuse in pediatric burns.
- Transfer severe extensive burns or burns to critical areas.
- Suspect carbon monoxide or cyanide toxicity in patients with thermal burns resulting from fires.

CHAPTER 27

Pregnant Patients

Mohammad Subeh and David Howes

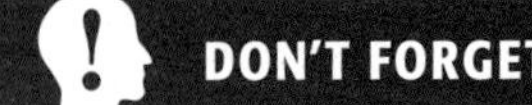

On test day, all women of childbearing age are pregnant.

INITIAL ASSESSMENT

- Focus on ABCs. Keep immediate life threats in mind first.
- Ask for a full set of vitals with every patient including pulse, BP, respirations, temp, O_2 sat, glucose.
- Large-bore IV × 2, O_2, monitor in every patient.
- Draw labs and hold for orders.

IMMEDIATE INTERVENTIONS

- Get stat urinary pregnancy tests on all women.
- Get the date of LMP.

Case-Specific Recommendations

- Focus on the last menstrual period (LMP), number of prior pregnancies.
- Identify unstable patients with immediate life threats.
  - Hypertension/hypotension
  - Vaginal bleeding/hemorrhage
  - Pre-eclampsia/eclampsia/subarachnoid hemorrhage (SAH)

INITIAL HISTORY AND PHYSICAL EXAMINATION

IMMEDIATE INTERVENTIONS

- Abnormal vital signs
  - Cardiac monitor.
  - Rhythm strip.
  - Establish 18-gauge IV.
  - Start 0.9% NS at KVO.
  - Draw blood for labs.
- Hypotensive or tachycardic
  - Bolus 1-L NS.
  - Monitor vitals frequently.
  - Type and cross for blood
- FAST: Obtain as soon as possible.

Do pelvic examination early except in third-trimester vaginal bleeding.

History

- History of the present illness (HPI)
  - LMP
  - Abdominal pain
  - Vaginal bleeding/discharge
  - Prenatal care (including previous ultrasounds [US])
  - Dysuria
  - Fever, vomiting, neurologic symptoms
  - History of fertility agents/drugs
  - Fetal movement
- Past medical hisory (PMHx)
  - Prior pregnancies/complications
  - History of sexually transmitted diseases (STDs)
- Medications
- Allergies

Physical Examination (Physical Examination Tips)

- Vital signs (VS) + check fetal heart tones.
- Head, eyes, ears, nose, and throat (HEENT): Symptoms of dehydration, anemia—mucous membranes, conjunctiva.
- Chest: Breath sounds equal, crackles, wheezes, rubs?
- Cardiovascular (CV): Murmurs, rubs, gallops? Peripheral pulses symmetric?
- Abdomen: Tender? Does gestational age correlate with fundal height?
- Pelvic: os open/closed, bleeding, uterus size, adnexal examination, cervical examination, signs of infection?
- Extremities: Cyanosis, edema?
- Neuro: Motor, sensory, DTR symmetric?

DON'T FORGET

Pregnant patients will have

- Ectopic pregnancy
- Placental abruption
- Placenta previa
- Pre-eclampsia/eclampsia/HELLP syndrome

DIFFERENTIAL DIAGNOSIS/COMMON EMERGENCY PRESENTATIONS OF PREGNANCY

Life-Threatening (Likely to Be on Oral Board Examination)

- Ectopic pregnancy: An ectopic pregnancy occurs when a fertilized ovum implants at a site other than the endometrial lining of the uterus. Clinical features of ectopic pregnancy include abdominal pain and vaginal bleeding. Many patients present within 4-8 weeks of their LMP. Patients can present with minimal symptoms to complete hypovolemic shock. Adnexal masses are commonly not felt on examination in the emergency department (ED). A good history should be focused to look for risk factors: previous tubal pregnancy or surgery, pelvic inflammatory disease, endometriosis, smoking, history of STD/IUD, fertility agents taken (increasing risk for heterotopic pregnancy). Because the physical examination is usually non-diagnostic in these patients, pelvic US should be done expeditiously.

- Placenta previa: Placenta previa is the implantation of the placenta over the cervical os. Incidence is increased with multi-parity and prior cesarean section. The patient presents with painless bright-red bleeding. Defer pelvic examination until the US has been completed to prevent increased placental bleeding or hemorrhage.
- Placental abruption: Placental abruption is the premature separation of the normally implanted placenta from the uterine wall, which can occur spontaneously (more common) or as the result of trauma to the abdomen. Risk factors should be identified: hypertension, increased maternal age, multi-parity, smoking, cocaine use, trauma, and previous abruptions. Abruption can be complete, partial, or concealed. The bleeding can be minimal or severe, depending on the size of the abruption. Patients will present with bleeding, abdominal pain, back pain, uterine tenderness, and uterine irritability. Fetal distress, hypotension, and disseminated intravascular coagulation (DIC) can develop.
- Pre-eclampsia: This condition fits the triad of hypertension (a BP 140/90 mm Hg or greater, a 20-mm Hg rise in the systolic or 10-mm Hg rise in the diastolic blood pressure), pathologic edema, and proteinuria.
- Eclampsia: Eclampsia describes the condition of pre-eclampsia with the presence of seizures or neurologic changes. Seizures are defined as *eclamptic* if they occur from the twentieth week of gestation to 7 days after delivery but have been reported as late as 26 days after delivery. The definitive treatment of seizures is expeditious delivery of the fetus. This diagnosis should be made as early as possible to prompt emergent OB consultation.
- Acute appendicitis: Acute appendicitis is a difficult diagnosis to make on a pregnant patient. The patient's pain will commonly be referred to the upper abdomen. The presence of fever, leukocytosis, and anorexia are non-diagnostic, and the differential includes ectopic pregnancy, UTI, acute cholecystitis, and tubo-ovarian abscess. Early consultation with OB and surgery is recommended, as well as US for imaging.

DON'T FORGET

Professionalism points! Tell patients before you do the pelvic examination and US and reassure them of what your concerns are.

Third-trimester vaginal bleeders should have emergent trans-abdominal ultrasounds before pelvic examination.

Third-trimester vaginal bleeding:
Painless = placenta previa
Painful = placental abruption

Must have confirmatory US to discharge patients with abortion or retained cyst from ED with close OB follow-up.

Patients with history of HTN are at risk for pre-eclampsia/eclampsia. Call OB on these patients and treat with antihypertensive medication. Patients with eclampsia need emergent OB consultation and prompt delivery of fetus.

Other Causes (Less Likely to Be on Oral Board Examination)

- Spontaneous abortion: Women who present with abdominal pain and vaginal bleeding in the first trimester of pregnancy must be evaluated to rule out an ectopic pregnancy. If an intrauterine pregnancy (IUP) is confirmed and if the adnexa and uterus are healthy with no free pelvic fluid, the patient's diagnosis is usually a threatened abortion or a spontaneous miscarriage. Abortions can be classified as threatened, complete, incomplete, or missed.
- Retained corpus luteum cyst: Retained corpus luteal cysts that have not degenerated can create pelvic pain during a normal pregnancy. These cysts should be identified on pelvic US after IUP is confirmed and treated as outpatient with OB consultation.
- UTI/pyelonephritis: Genitourinary tract infections are common during pregnancy. Pregnant women with UTI are at increased risk for pyelonephritis and hydronephrosis, which puts the patient's fetus at risk for preterm labor and low birth weight.
- Hyperemesis gravidarum: Hyperemesis gravidarum presents as nausea and vomiting in the first trimester of pregnancy, which puts patients at risk for significant volume depletion. These patients will respond to intravenous (IV) fluids and should be screened for infection. Patients with hyperemesis gravidarum should not have abdominal pain. The presence of pain is a sign of comorbidity and should be investigated further.

DON'T FORGET

For pregnant patients with UTI or pyelonephritis: Treat with antibiotics early, have low threshold for admission and consider renal US for patients who are being admitted or have complicated presentation.

DON'T FORGET

Hyperemesis patients should not have abdominal pain; this should be worked up.

DON'T FORGET

Assume all pregnant patients have an ectopic pregnancy until proven otherwise.

Goal is to confirm IUP ASAP, check bedside ultrasound (<16 weeks) or FHTs (>16 weeks)— role out ectopic pregnancy.

If you are ruling out an ectopic, keep your patient NPO and establish IV access.

Do not let unstable patients be discharged home.

Patients in shock will probably need blood, order it early, get the US at the bedside and call the OB consult stat.

Order type-specific blood for patients who are anemic that are being evaluated for ectopic pregnancy.

Give RhoGAM to Rh-negative pregnant patients with vaginal bleeding.

ECTOPIC PREGNANCY (FIG. 27-1)

Additional History and Physical Examination Findings

- Patients with history of fertility agents, prior pelvic surgery, smoking, prior ectopic, and STD/PID have an increased risk.
- Many patients have *no* risk factors.
- Classically, patients will present with a history of late or delayed menses, abdominal and/or pelvic pain and cramping, vaginal bleeding, shoulder pain, and faintness/weakness.
- Patients may not have vaginal bleeding on examination.
- Presentations can vary dramatically; abdominal pain may be minimal or severe. Some patients will present with no vaginal bleeding; some patients will present in shock while others have normal vital signs.
- Shoulder pain is suggestive of peritoneal free fluid.
- Frequently, adnexal masses may not be palpable.
- Pregnant patients who present with UTI or vomiting that have pain should be ruled out for ectopic pregnancy.
- Treat patients for pain if they are uncomfortable.
- Order initial blood tests: Stat urine pregnancy test, serum beta quantitative hCG, pelvic US, urinalysis (UA), type and screen, and complete blood count (CBC).
- All patients who are being ruled out for ectopic pregnancy should have an IV placed (even if vitals are stable!) to ensure access in the event of emergency resuscitation.
- Be sure to reassure patient during the course of the examination as this is a sensitive manner.

Review Initial Results

- US: Review the US carefully looking for gestational sac and IUP, look at adnexa carefully, and look for free fluid.
  - Is the US diagnostic of an IUP? If so, is there cardiac activity?
    - If yes, rule out adnexal mass or free fluid. If the patient has pain and/or tenderness, consider other diagnoses: appendicitis, cholecystitis.

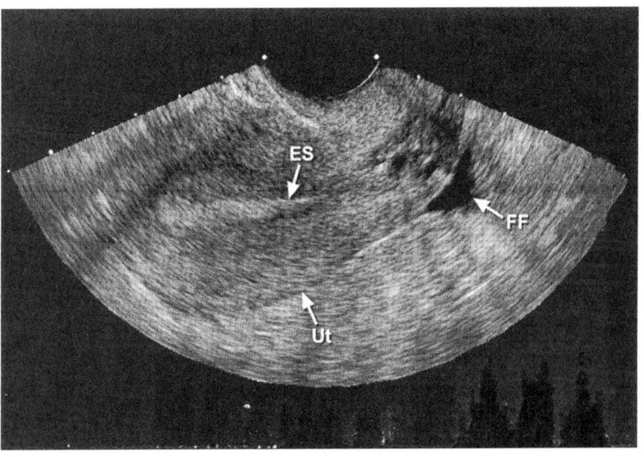

A

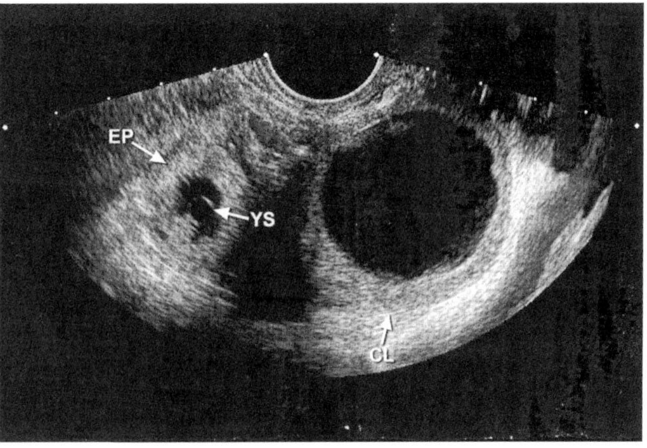

B

Figure 27-1. These images are from a vaginal sonogram of an ectopic pregnancy. (**A**) The empty uterus (Ut) is seen with an endometrial stripe (ES) and no intrauterine pregnancy (IUP). A small amount of free fluid (FF) is seen in the posterior cul-de-sac. (**B**) In this image the tubal ectopic pregnancy (EP) with its yolk sac (YS) is seen along with a corpus luteum (CL) cyst. (*Reprinted with permission from Cunningham FG, Leveno KL, Bloom SL, et al.* Williams Obstetrics. *22nd ed. New York, NY: McGraw-Hill; 2005.*)

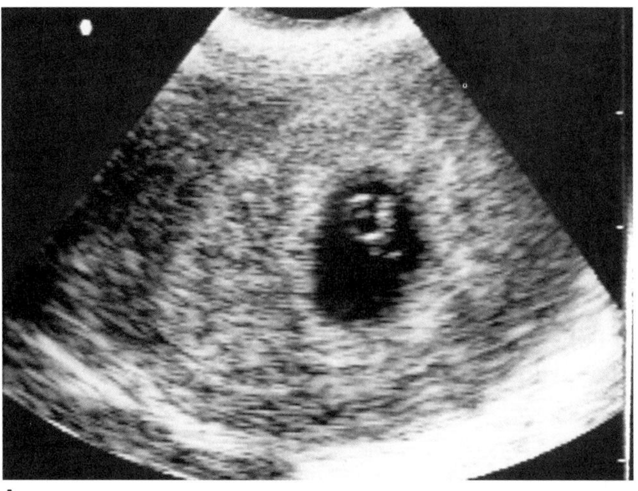

A

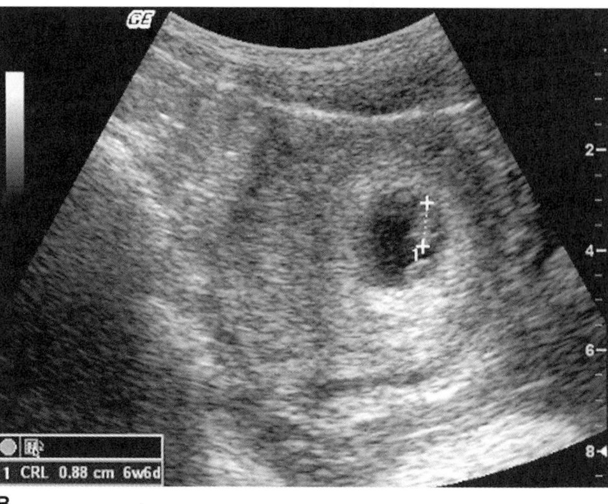

B

Figure 27-2. Small embryo and yolk sac within an intrauterine gestational sac. (**A**) The 5-mm embryo is positioned along the right side of the yolk sac in this image and cardiac pulsations were visible during real-time sonography. Transvaginal image at 7.5 MHz. (*Courtesy of James Mateer, MD.*) (**B**) Embryonic pole is separated from the yolk sac and measures 6 weeks + 6 days via crown rump length. (**I**) Transabdominal longitudinal view with empty bladder. (*Courtesy of Hennepin County Medical Center.*) (*Reproduced with permission from Ma OJ, Mateer JR, Blaivas M.* Emergency Ultrasound. *2nd ed. New York, NY: McGraw-Hill; 2008.*)

    - If no, call OB stat for emergent consultation of patient with suspected ectopic pregnancy and continue resuscitation.
  - Does the quantitative hCG result correlate with the US findings?
    - *Beta*-hCG (BhCG): Check serum levels on all pregnant patients; level doubles roughly every 2 days.
    - Level of 1500-2000 U/L should show signs of IUP on trans-vaginal US.
  - Do US findings correlate with estimated gestational age by LMP?
    - Gestational sac seen at 4.5 weeks
    - Yolk sac seen at 5.5 weeks
    - Fetal pole seen at 6 weeks
    - Cardiac activity seen at 6 weeks (Fig. 27-2)
- Check CBC. Expect that any anemia found is secondary to acute hemorrhagic loss.
- Check type and screen; an Rh-negative mother who is bleeding should receive RhoGAM, 300 µg IM. Rh-negative patient with first trimester miscarriage should receive RhoGAM 50 µg IM.
- Check UA to r/o infection.
- Send vaginal and cervical cultures if the history and physical examination reveal concerns for STDs.

Definitive Management

- Stabilization and resuscitation, normal saline or blood products as clinically indicated.
- Pain control:
  - Morphine sulfate 2-4 mg IV q15min or Dilaudid 1 mg IV q15min are good choices with close monitoring of VS.
  - Avoid non-steroidal anti-inflammatory drugs (NSAIDs).
- Keep patients at NPO.
- Call OB for surgical consultation, admission, or discharge planning.
- Insist that the OB consultant comes to the department if your patient is unstable. Unstable patients must go to the OR for definitive care.

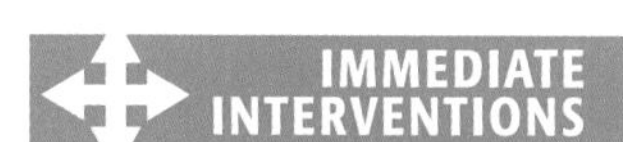

- IV access, two large-bore with fluid resuscitation.
- Patient and fetal monitoring
- Order CBC, electrolytes, LFTs, coags, type and cross, hCG.
- US: Trans-abdominal and trans-vaginal
- Call OB consult early.

Frequent Reassessment

- Repeat vital signs q15min. State this request in all patients who present with unstable vital signs and are receiving blood products or vasoactive medications.
- Keep the patient and her family (if she agrees) aware of the workup and decision-making progress.

Complications

- Hypovolemic shock
  - Institute wide open IVFs, blood products.
  - Consult OB immediately to arrange surgical assessment.

Disposition

- No IUP and signs of shock or abnormal US
  - Admit to OB/take to surgery.
  - Ensure that the patient is seen in a timely manner.
- No IUP and patient with persistent symptoms or concerning US findings
  - Admit to OB.
  - Ensure that the patient is seen in a timely manner.
- No IUP and HCG <1,500 with no concerning symptoms, US report, or lab findings
  - Consult OB for discharge planning.
  - Repeat beta quant in 48 hours.
  - Clear discharge instructions to patient.
- No IUP and HCG>1,500
  - Discuss case with OB, consider admission.
- IUP and persistent pain
  - Patients who have an IUP should be evaluated for threatened, complete, or incomplete abortion based on their US findings, symptoms, and patency of the cervical os.
  - Patients who have an IUP and have persistent pain should be evaluated for appendicitis, genitourinary infection, or cholecystitis.

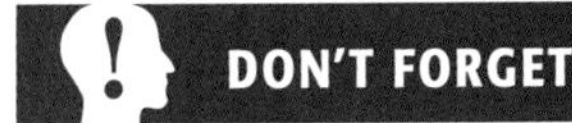

No BhCG level will completely rule out ectopic pregnancy!

When a pelvic mass or free fluid is seen with an empty uterus, the diagnosis of ectopic pregnancy is highly likely. The presence of a yolk sac, fetal pole, or cardiac activity within an intrauterine gestational sac confirms the presence of an IUP.

Visualization of a gestational sac alone should not be relied upon to make the diagnosis of an early IUP unless a double decidual sign is clearly seen.

PLACENTA PREVIA

Additional History and Physical Examination Findings

- Patients will present with painless, bright red vaginal bleeding after 28 weeks.
- Distinguish this complication from the bloody show, which is passage of a very small amount of bright-red blood mixed with mucus at the onset of labor.
- Abdominal palpation should be performed to assess fundal height, contractions, and tenderness of the uterus.
- Common risk factors: Prior previa, first subsequent pregnancy following a cesarean delivery, multiparity, advanced maternal age, multiple gestations, and smoking.
- Physical examination: Profuse hemorrhage, hypotension, tachycardia, soft and non-tender uterus, normal fetal heart tones (usually).
- Defer vaginal and rectal examinations until patient has had ultrasound or to OB consultant.

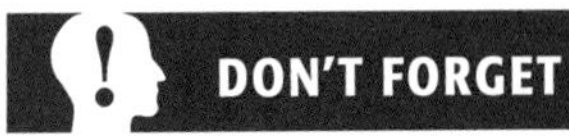

Stable patients, who are tender, have persistent pain and indeterminate US findings should be admitted for observation.

Review Initial Result

- Ultrasound: Abdominal ultrasounds should be performed on a stat basis to determine the lie of the placenta.

  - Total placenta previa occurs when the internal cervical os is completely covered by the placenta.
  - Partial placenta previa occurs when the internal os is partially covered by the placenta.
  - Marginal placenta previa occurs when the placenta is at the margin of the internal os.
  - Low-lying placenta previa occurs when the placenta is implanted in the lower uterine segment. In this variation, the edge of the placenta is near but not at the internal os.
- CBC: Order early and serially.
- Type and cross for at least 4 U PRBC.
- Prothrombin time (PT)/partial thromboplastin time (PTT), fibrinogen, fibrin split products, chem-7.
- Continuous fetal monitoring.

Risk Stratification: Management Priorities

- Consider differential diagnosis—normal labor, uterine rupture, vasa previa, placental abruption, and bloody show.

Definitive Management

- Keep mother on oxygen and cardiac monitor.
- Resuscitation
  - Establish large-bore IV access.
  - Aggressive resuscitation with NS boluses to correct hypotension.
  - Initiate transfusion with PRBCs if patient is in shock.
  - Position patient on her left side. This improves venous return via the IVC.
- Early ultrasound imaging and OB consultation.
- Use fresh frozen plasma (FFP) for DIC.

Further Diagnostic Considerations

- Screen all patients for DIC, HELLP syndrome.
- Examine patients carefully for other bleeding.
- Consider giving steroids in consultation with OB to patients with gestation <37 weeks to promote fetal lung development.

Disposition

- Stable patients are admitted to labor floor for continuous monitoring.
- Unstable patients are admitted to the operating room (OR) with OB ready to perform possible C-section.
- When consulting physician for admission, insist that s/he immediately sees the patient in the ED.

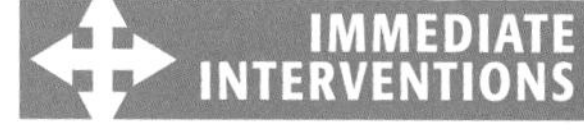

IMMEDIATE INTERVENTIONS

- IV access, two large bores with fluid resuscitation.
- Patient and fetal monitoring.
- Order CBC, electrolytes, LFTs, coags, type and cross.
- US: Transabdominal and transvaginal.
- Call OB; consult early.
- Give RhoGAM to RH-negative pregnant patients with vaginal bleeding.

PLACENTAL ABRUPTION

Additional History and Physical Examination Findings

- Painful vaginal bleeding, abrupt in onset, is the most frequent symptom.
- Up to 20% of patients may not present with bleeding.
- Abdominal or back pain and uterine tenderness are common.
- Fetal distress is seen in up to 60% of presentations.
- Patients may have abnormal uterine contractions or premature labor.
- Major risk factors include maternal hypertension (most common cause), maternal trauma, smoking, alcohol, cocaine use, advanced maternal age, a short umbilical cord, or retro-placental fibromyoma.

DON'T FORGET

Placenta previa is one of the leading causes of vaginal bleeding in the second and third trimesters.

Placenta previa is defined as the implantation of the placenta over or near the internal os of the cervix.

- Physical examination will be variable and usually correlates with the extent of separation (partial versus complete tears). Patients may present in varying forms of shock, uterine tetany, coagulopathy, and fetal distress.
- Half of cases present with mild, minimal, or no vaginal bleeding, a slightly tender uterus, normal maternal vital signs, and no fetal distress.

Risk Stratification: Management Priorities

- Resuscitation of the mother and fetus is critical as this diagnosis carries significant morbidity and mortality to the mother and fetus.
- Maternal complications include hemorrhagic shock, coagulopathy/DIC, uterine rupture, renal failure, and ischemic necrosis of distal organs secondary to shock.
- Fetal complications include hypoxia, anemia, growth retardation, central nervous system (CNS) anomalies, and fetal death.

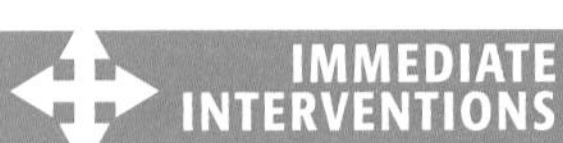

Obtain OB consultation ASAP and order a bedside ultrasound before you do a pelvic examination.

Repeat VS frequently and use continuous fetal heart monitoring.

Obtain a thorough history to identify if mother is the victim of domestic violence. If she is, then consult social services and consider other trauma.

Patients seen on examination day will present with classic signs and symptoms.

Definitive Management

- Attention to resuscitation and continuous monitoring is vital.
- Patients should be placed in the left lateral decubitus position.
- An amniotomy may be performed by the OB consultant.
- Immediate delivery of the fetus by cesarean delivery is indicated if the mother or fetus becomes unstable.
- Look for signs of DIC and coagulopathy and treat with FFP; these patients should be considered for emergent delivery.

Further Diagnostic Considerations

- In patients with suspected placental abruption induced by abdominal trauma, consider C-spine immobilization and further imaging and testing based on the history and physical examination. Additional consultation with a trauma surgeon and social services should be sought on examination day.
- Patients with abnormal neurological examinations should be evaluated closely for coagulopathy. Consider neuroimaging if the patient is stable.

IMMEDIATE INTERVENTIONS

- Two large-bore IVs.
- Fluid resuscitation and blood transfusion if necessary.
- Pain control with IV narcotics.
- *Immediate* OB consult.
- Administer supplemental O_2.
- Monitor urine output.
- Stat bedside ultrasound.
- Continuous fetal cardiac monitoring.
- Continuous maternal cardiac monitoring.
- Labs: CBC, T+C for 4 U, coags, lytes, DIC panel.

Disposition

- All stable patients that have symptoms and findings of placental abruption should be admitted to the L&D unit for continuous maternal and fetal monitoring.
- Fetal distress and maternal instability are indications for emergent delivery.

PRE-ECLAMPSIA/ECLAMPSIA/HELLP SYNDROME

Additional History and Physical Examination Findings

- Patients often present with edema, headache, visual changes, shortness of breath, decreased urine output, mental status changes, abdominal pain, and seizures.
- Patients with HELLP syndrome will have right upper quadrant (RUQ) pain, nausea, and vomiting.
- Physical examination will vary depending on the severity of the patient's illness. Findings can include papilledema, generalized edema, cerebrovascular accident (CVA) symptoms, abdominal tenderness, seizure activity, coma, ankle clonus, hyper-reflexia, and tremulousness. Some patients will have pulmonary edema, which will present as tachycardia, tachypnea, and rales. Patients who have HELLP syndrome may have petechiae.

Review Initial Results

- The CBC may reveal anemia because of the microangiopathic hemolytic anemia and dilution of pregnancy, and thrombocytopenia (platelet count <100,000 mm3) because of HELLP syndrome.

- The serum creatinine may be elevated because of decreased intravascular volume and a decreased glomerular filtration rate.
- LFTs may be elevated because of HELLP syndrome.
- Check a coagulation profile PT/PTT, fibrin split products, and fibrinogen levels to evaluate for associated disseminated intravascular coagulopathy (DIC).
- UA will show proteinuria.
- Chest x-ray (CXR) may show non-cardiogenic pulmonary edema, a normal-sized heart with bilateral infiltrates.
- Consider a head CT in patients with neurologic deficits, coma, or coagulopathy. The head CT may show intracranial hemorrhage or acute CVA.

DON'T FORGET

Pre-eclampsia = proteinuria, hypertension, and edema.

Eclampsia = pre-eclampsia + seizures or neurologic changes.

HELLP = hemolysis (microangiopathic hemolytic anemia), elevated liver-enzyme levels, and low platelet count leading to eclampsia.

Risk Stratification: Management Priorities

- Stabilize airway.
- Continuous maternal and fetal monitoring.
- Treat hypertension and seizures.
- Immediate OB consultation.
- Complications include intracranial bleeding, pancreatitis, renal failure, liver failure, pulmonary edema, and coagulopathy.

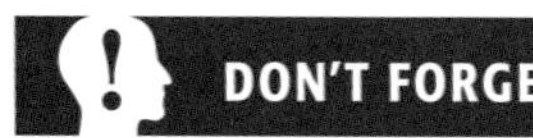

DON'T FORGET

All seizing women of childbearing age are eclamptic until proven otherwise!

Definitive Management

- Airway protection.
- Treat hypertension
  - Hydralazine: 5-10 mg IV, can repeat q20-30min
  - Labetolol: 20-40 mg IV, can repeat q15min up to max dose of 300 mg IV
- Seizure prophylaxis
  - Magnesium sulfate for seizures or severe hyper-reflexia, bolus is 4-6 g (20% solution) IV over 5-10 minutes, then drip at 1-3 g/h.
- FFP, blood products
- Rapid OB consult
- Prepare for delivery.

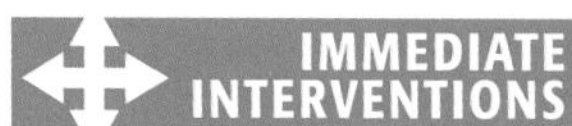

IMMEDIATE INTERVENTIONS

- High-flow mask oxygen.
- Two large-bore IVs.
- Maternal and fetal monitoring.
- Send CBC, BMP, LFTs, PT/PTT, fibrinogen, fibrin split products, CXR, and head CT as indicated.
- Order continuous cardiac monitoring for mother.
- Order serial Mg and Cr levels, and perform neuro examinations assessing for clonus on patients you are treating with Mg.

Calcium gluconate is used for magnesium toxicity.

Disposition

- For patient with mild pre-eclampsia, discharge with close follow-up instructions and OB consultation.
- May also admit patients with pre-eclampsia and proteinuria for observation.
- Patients with severe pre-eclampsia and pregnancy >36 weeks should be admitted and treated with magnesium sulfate.
- Immediate delivery is indicated if patient has altered mental status, coagulopathy, uncontrolled hypertension (HTN), fetal distress, or renal disease.
- Definitive treatment of eclampsia is delivery.

WINNING STRATEGIES

- All women of childbearing age are pregnant until proven otherwise.
- Mother is patient number 1, fetus is patient number 2.
- Immediate interventions in all unstable patients include oxygen, cardiac monitor with rhythm strip, IV, and immediate fetal monitoring. Place the mother in the left lateral decubitus position.
- Stabilize life-threats by employing early airway management, aggressive resuscitation, and expedient diagnostic testing and consultation.
- Any signs of fetal distress should prompt OB consultation and delivery.
- Insist that the OB physician come in to see unstable patients.
- Ask the nurse to tell you the vitals of mother and fetus frequently (every 5 minutes).

DON'T FORGET

Only stable patients may leave the ED for pelvic ultrasound.

- Unstable patients not responding to IV fluids need blood transfusion. Remember to warm blood products and ask for a rapid infuser.
- Perform complete examinations on all patients. Do not neglect the neurologic, extremity, and skin examinations.
- Consider domestic violence on all pregnant patients.
- Be sensitive to patient and family, you will win professionalism points!
- Confirm ED ultrasounds with "official" ultrasounds.
- Treat patient's pain and use medications that are safe in pregnancy.

THE BOTTOM LINE

- Pregnant patients on examination day will need OB consult, will likely be admitted, and require an immediate intervention.

CHAPTER 28

The Dialysis Patient

Philip Bossart and H. Megan French

DON'T FORGET

Every dialysis patient has hyperkalemia and/or fluid overload until proven otherwise.

Look for issues requiring emergent dialysis. Use the mnemonic AEIOU to remember them:

- Acidosis (metabolic)
- Electrolyte abnormalities
- Ingestions (toxic)
- Overload (fluids)
- Uremia

INITIAL ASSESSMENT

- Focus on general appearance, time of the last dialysis, type of dialysis (hemodialysis or peritoneal), vital signs (VS), evidence of fluid overload, presence of abdominal pain, and mental status.
- Identify unstable patients with immediate life-threats:
  - Cardiac dysrhythmias
  - Acute myocardial infarction (AMI)
  - Hypotension/sepsis
  - Pulmonary edema.
  - Pericardial tamponade.
- Be aware of indications for emergent dialysis: AEIOU (metabolic **A**cidosis, severe **E**lectrolyte imbalance, toxic **I**ngestions, fluid **O**verload, **U**remia) and get a nephrologist on the phone to dialyze patient immediately if any of these indications exist.

INITIAL HISTORY AND PHYSICAL EXAMINATION

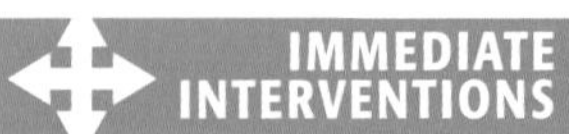

IMMEDIATE INTERVENTIONS

- Oxygen via NC or NRB to maintain O_2 >92%
- Consider NIPPV or intubation early if unable to maintain adequate oxygenation.
- Cardiac monitor with rhythm strip
- Repeat BP every 5 minutes.
- If hypertensive with SOB, consider NTG
- Give fluids only if hypotensive
- Hep-lock (heparin IV Lock) 18-gauge or 0.9% at KVO and draw blood for laboratory studies.
- ECG
- For SIRS, consider small boluses of crystalloid, early abx, and look at dialysis access for infection.

History

- History of the present illness (HPI)
- Past medical hisory (PMHx)
  - Cause of end-stage renal disease (ESRD)
  - History of coronoary artery disease (CAD)
  - Hypertension (HTN), diabetes mellitus (DM)
  - Congestive heart failure (CHF)
  - Medications
  - Allergies
  - Types of dialysis:
    - Hemodialysis
    - Peritoneal dialysis
- Obtain dialysis history including schedule, any missed sessions or complications, and most recent dialysis.
- Ask about any weakness, chest pain, shortness of breath (SOB), N/V/D, and neurologic complaints.
- Ask about their dry weight (for Hodgkin's disease [HD] patients)
- Do they produce urine?

Physical Examination

- VS: Fever? Hypertension? Hypotension? Tachycardia? Hypoxia? Tachypnea?
- Neck: Jugular venous distention (JVD)?
- Chest: Crackles? (suggests volume overload or infection) Accessory muscle use? (suggests respiratory distress and need for intervention such as intubation)
- Cardiovascular (CV): Are there signs of heart failure? Murmurs? Pericardial friction rubs? Muffled or distant heart sounds? Is the vascular access site tender to palpation or bleeding? Is there a bruit or thrill to suggest vascular site is functional?
- Abdomen: Does the patient have any abdominal tenderness? Any evidence of peritonitis such as rebound, guarding, or decreased bowel sounds? If the patient has peritoneal dialysis, does the peritoneal catheter site look erythematous, purulent, and tender to palpation or other indications of infection?
- Derm: Any diaphoresis? Does the vascular access site look erythematous, purulent, or infected?
- Extremities: Edema or cyanosis?

DON'T FORGET

Almost any patient who missed dialysis will ultimately require dialysis as their final disposition.

A nephrologist must be called to arrange dialysis as soon as you confirm that there are no other life threatening complications present.

- Rectal examination: Melena? bright red blood per rectum (BRBPR)?
- Neurologic examination: Mental status? Evidence of peripheral neuropathy? Asterixis?

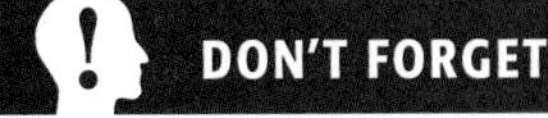

Look for signs of fluid overload, including JVD, crackles, pedal edema, and increased respiratory rate and work of breathing.

DIFFERENTIAL DIAGNOSIS

Missed Dialysis Patients

- Hyperkalemia
  - This is a significant problem in hemodialysis patients because 90%-95% of the daily potassium load is normally excreted through the kidneys.
  - Obtain a thorough history and an electrocardiogram (ECG) for dialysis patients who present with a vague chief complaint like "just not feeling right."
  - If history and ECG are concerning for hyperkalemia, do not wait for lab results to start treatment. These patients can develop dangerous arrhythmias (especially bradycardia, asystole and V. fib) (Fig. 28-1).
- Pericardial tamponade
  - Consider this diagnosis with physical findings of JVD and hypotension, ECG showing electrical alternans and/or low voltages, and a chest x-ray (CXR) showing an enlarged cardiac silhouette.
  - Use bedside ultrasound or a formal echocardiogram to confirm your suspicion. Right ventricular diastolic collapse confirms the diagnosis of tamponade.
  - Be sure to have a pericardiocentesis tray available at the bedside in case the patient decompensates (Fig. 28-2). Be able to describe to the examiner how you would perform an ultrasound-guided pericardiocentesis.
  - Contact a cardiothoracic surgeon early in the case if you are worried the patient will decompensate and for definitive management with a pericardial window surgery.

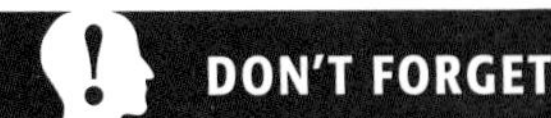

Any abdominal tenderness or altered mental status in a peritoneal dialysis patient is bacterial peritonitis until proven otherwise.

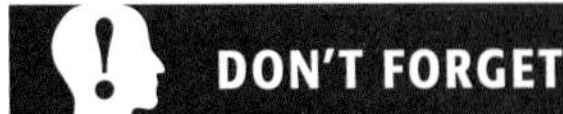

Any neurologic deficit in a dialysis patient should prompt further evaluation for cardiovascular or infectious etiology (though don't forget neuro). Uremia is a less likely cause on examination day.

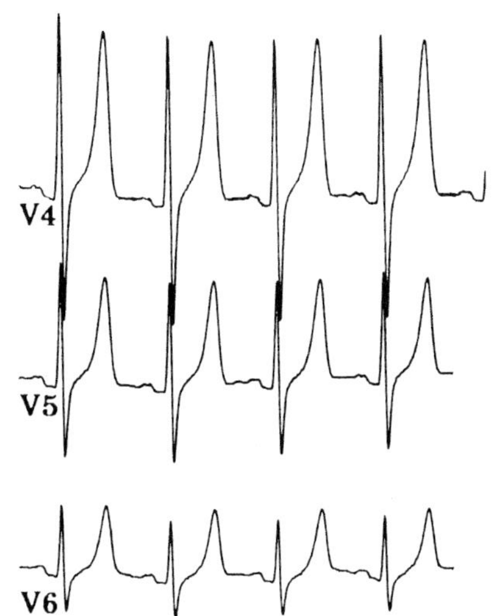

Figure 28-1. Electrocardiographic manifestations of early hyperkalemia. The slightly prolonged QRS complex is followed by a peaked T wave in all leads having a very narrow base. *([A] Reproduced with permission from Fuster V, O'Rourke RA, Walsh RA, Poole-Wilson P.* Hurst's The Heart. *12th ed. New York: McGraw-Hill; 2008.)*

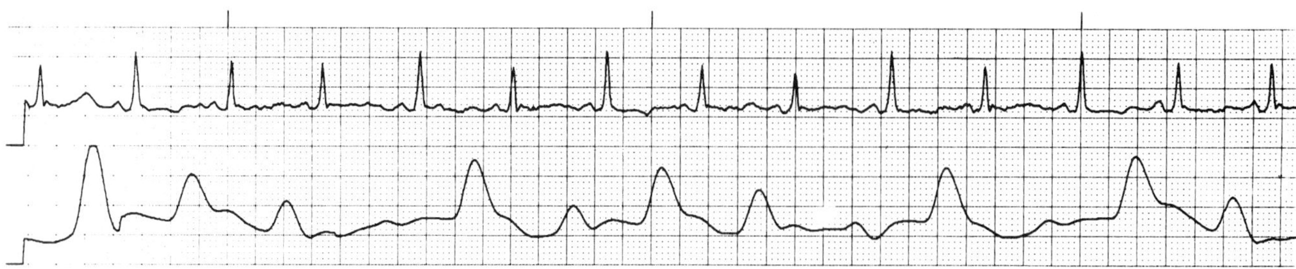

Figure 28-2. Electrical alternans (shown in this ECG) is the result of a pericardial effusion. (*Reprinted with permission from Tintinalli JE, Kelen GD, Stapczynski JS, et al.* Emergency Medicine: A Comprehensive Study Guide. *6th ed. New York, NY: McGraw-Hill; 2004.*)

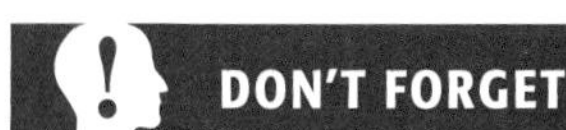

DON'T FORGET

Check a finger stick first to check for hypoglycemia as a cause of AMS!

- Volume overload
  - These patients will likely present complaining of SOB and have rales and peripheral edema on examination. Be sure to look at the ECG and CXR for other possible etiologies (ie, AMI, pneumonia, large pericardial effusion, flash/hypertensive pulmonary edema).
  - Acute coronary syndrome (ACS) is a common cause of death in ESRD patients, so make sure that pulmonary edema secondary to ACS remains high in your differential when treating these patients.

Recent Hemodialysis

- Bleeding from vascular access site or other bleeding complications
  - Renal failure patients may also have bleeding diathesis which increases the risk of bleeding complications such as subdural hematomas and gastrointestinal bleeding.
  - During hemodialysis, small amounts of intravenous heparin are used to prevent thrombosis at the vascular access site. If the patient is over heparinized, this could cause significant bleeding complications.

Common Problems of ESRD Patients

- Acute coronary syndrome
  - Because DM and HTN put patients at risk for both ESRD and ACS, be sure to consider ACS in your differential.
- Gastrointestinal bleeds
  - Common due to bleeding diathesis
- Infection
  - Renal failure patients are immunocompromised at baseline. HD patients have additional potential exposure to pathogens with each dialysis procedure.
  - Since dialysis patients have a very high mortality caused by infection and sepsis, be sure to consider this in your differential. Make sure to evaluate the vascular access site as a possible source if infection is suspected.
- Peritonitis
  - Consider this for all peritoneal dialysis patient with abdominal pain, SIRS, or AMS.
- Subdural hematoma
  - Consider this in your differential for AMS due to bleeding diathesis associated ESRD.

DON'T FORGET

Cardiac monitor and repeat ECGs are important in the management of hyperkalemia. Be sure to request follow-up ECGs or rhythm strips.

HYPERKALEMIA

Additional History and Physical Examination Findings

- The anuric patient who has missed dialysis is likely to be hyperkalemic.
- The classic symptoms are vague such as "weakness" or "general malaise."

- Suspect hyperkalemia for any patient in ventricular fibrillation or asystole with a history of ESRD on dialysis.

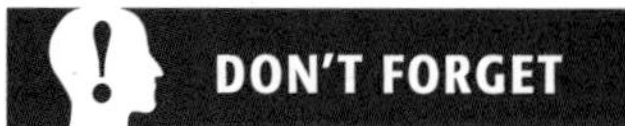

As soon as you find the patient to be hyperkalemic, get the nephrologist involved ASAP!

Review Initial Results

- ECG: Review the ECG carefully and promptly, even if it interrupts your H&P. Obtain an old ECG for comparison.
  - When reviewing the ECG, check for the following signs of hyperkalemia:
    - Peaked T waves
    - Absent P waves
    - Prolonged QRS duration
    - Conduction delays or arrhythmia
  - A completely normal ECG does not rule out hyperkalemia, but an abnormal EKG can lead you to the diagnosis earlier if any of the above is present.
  - Be certain to repeat the ECG after any intervention.
- CXR: Look for alternate causes of weakness or SOB (pulmonary edema, enlarged cardiac silhouette suggestive of pericardial effusion, pneumonia).
- Electrolytes: Be certain to ask for electrolytes. A potassium level of 6 mEq/L, or higher, should be considered dangerous and be treated.

Management Priorities

- Consult the nephrologist to discuss dialysis.
- Oxygen: Use nasal cannula or facemask for hypoxia.
- Cardiac monitor: Put the patient on a cardiac monitor and request that the nursing staff inform you of any dysrhythmias or changes immediately.
- Blood pressure: Instruct the nursing staff to obtain q5min blood pressure readings.
- Medication:
  - Calcium: 10 mL of 10% calcium gluconate (or calcium chloride if the patient is unstable) IV over 10 minutes. Monitor the ECG carefully while giving and repeat in 5-10 minutes if there is no improvement on the ECG. Onset of action is in 1 to 3 minutes and lasts for 30 to 60 minutes. This stabilizes the cardiac cell membranes. (Calcium chloride provides three times the calcium dose per equal volume.)
  - Insulin: IV dose of 10 U of regular insulin along with an IV bolus of dextrose (25-100 g as a 50% solution). Onset of action is in 10 to 20 minutes and lasts for about 2 hours. Make sure to recheck glucose. This forces K back into cells.
  - Albuterol: Nebulized albuterol via face mask can be utilized for alert and intubated patients. Onset of action is 20 minutes and lasts 2 hours. This forces K back into cells.
  - Bicarbonate: 50 mg/1 amp IVP over 5 mins can be given and repeated once. This is not as effective as measures listed above. Perhaps most useful in severely acidotic patients.
  - Loop diuretics: If the patient makes urine, consider an IV bolus of furosemide to aid potassium excretion.
  - If hypovolemia from over dialysis or dehydration (N/V/D) are present, judicious use of small volume fluid boluses may be indicated.
  - Repeat calcium, insulin, and beta-agonists for any recurring signs or symptoms of hyperkalemia (EKG changes or conduction blocks).

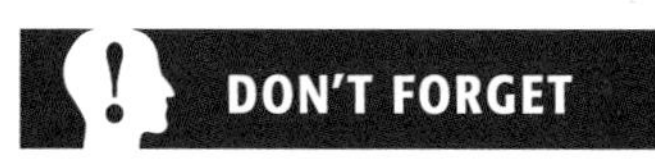

All hyperkalemic patients need to be on a cardiac monitor! Ask to be given a rhythm strip after each treatment given.

Definitive Management

- Dialysis is the definitive management for these patients. These patients need dialysis as quickly as possible.

Frequent Reassessment

- Continue to ask your examiner for repeat VS, cardiac rhythm strips, or ECGs to follow the patient's progress.

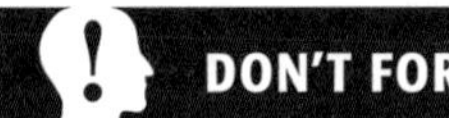

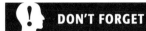

DON'T FORGET

No hyperkalemic patients go home after treatment on examination day.

Complications

- Ventricular fibrillation, pulseless electrical activity (PEA), or asystole
  - Initiate advanced cardiac life support (ACLS) protocols where indicated.

Disposition

- Stable appearing patient: Dialysis unit
- Recent cardiac event or hemodynamically unstable: critical care unit (CCU) or intensive care unit (ICU) with bedside dialysis arranged

DON'T FORGET

If you have to intubate a dialysis patient, only use non-depolarizing neuromuscular blockers, do not use succinylcholine!

Remember Beck's triad

- JVD
- Hypotension
- Muffled heart sounds

PERICARDIAL TAMPONADE

Additional History and Physical Examination Findings

- The classic presentation involves progressive dyspnea and/or weakness. The patient may complain of chest pain or unexplained fever consistent with a history of pericarditis or myopericarditis (>20% of uremic patients have clinical evidence of pericarditis).
- Vital signs:
  - BP: Usually hypotensive; a narrow pulse pressure should be present in tamponade. Pulsus paradoxus may be present.
  - HR: Usually tachycardic
- Cardiovascular
  - Look for distended neck veins.
  - A coarse friction rub is indicative of pericarditis (ask specifically about this).
  - Distant and muffled heart sounds are indicative of a pericardial effusion.

DON'T FORGET

Ask for a bedside ultrasound if you suspect a pericardial effusion or cardiac tamponade.

Review Initial Results

- ECG
  - Electrical alternans and low voltages are concerning for pericardial effusion.
- CXR
- A water bottle-shaped heart and cardiomegaly are concerning for a pericardial effusion.

DON'T FORGET

If you suspect a pericardial effusion or cardiac tamponade, be sure to get a pericardiocentesis tray placed at the bedside in case the patient deteriorates!

Management Priorities

- Bedside ultrasound (Fig. 28-3) to look for a large pericardial effusion and possible right ventricular diastolic collapse.
- Have a pericardiocentesis tray at the bedside and be prepared to perform emergency pericardiocentesis if the patient crashes. Be able to describe the steps of the pericardiocentesis procedure.
- Consult the cardiovascular surgeon early for definitive management with pericardial window surgery.
- Maintain oxygenation.
- Maintain blood pressure, using fluid challenges until the diagnosis can be established and fixed.
- Keep patient on a bedside cardiac monitor and request that you be informed of any changes.
- Do not allow patient to be transported to echo lab, request bedside echo so the patient can be closely monitored.

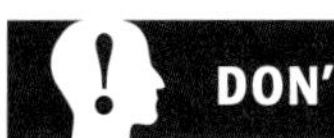

DON'T FORGET

If you suspect a cardiac tamponade, call CT surgery immediately!

Definitive Management

- Immediate pericardiocentesis and definitive pericardial window if patient has tamponade

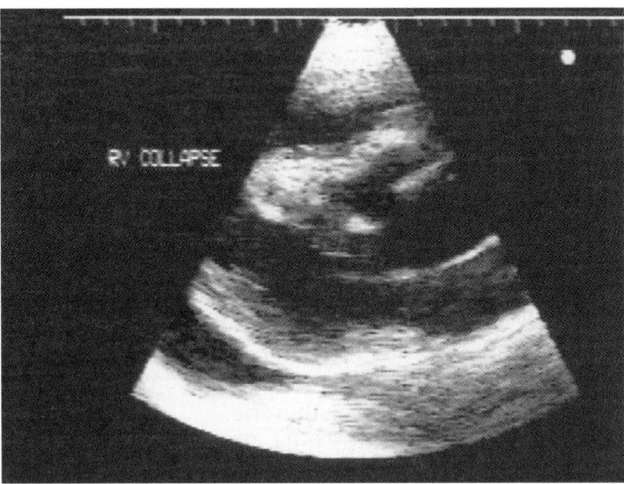

Figure 28-3. This ultrasound shows a fluid-filled pericardium and collapse of the right ventricle. This is evidence of pericardial tamponade. (*Reprinted with permission from Ma OJ, Mateer JR, Blaivas M.* Emergency Ultrasound. *2nd ed. New York, NY: McGraw-Hill; 2008.*)

Complications

- PEA: Caused by complete cardiac tamponade.
  - Be prepared to perform an emergent pericardiocentesis.

Disposition

- CCU if patient appears well for definitive management with CT surgeon.
- Operating room (OR) for pericardial window after ultrasound-guided pericardiocentesis if patient is unable to tolerate a delay in definitive management.

VOLUME OVERLOAD

Additional History and Physical Examination Findings

- Classically, the most frequent complaint is of progressive dyspnea.
- Investigate other potential causes of SOB such as AMI and cardiac tamponade with an ECG and CXR.
- Ask about recent weight gain—specifically for >5 pounds above "dry weight."
- Listen for rales on chest examination.

Review Initial Results

- CXR
  - "Bat-wing" perihilar infiltrates are consistent with pulmonary edema.
  - Check for other potential causes of dyspnea like pneumonia.
- ECG
  - Check for arrhythmia and for ACS as potential etiology of pulmonary edema.
- Cardiac biomarkers
  - Check for alternate causes of pulmonary edema, like ACS.
- Electrolytes (including Mg and P)
  - Ensure that asymptomatic hyperkalemia is not missed.

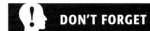

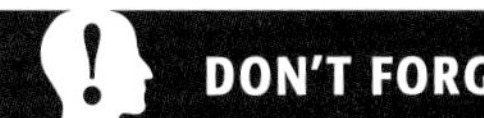

Recent weight gain and SOB in a dialysis patient is diagnostic of fluid overload.

Additional Management Priorities for Volume Overload

- NIPPV
- Nitrates
- Lasix
- Dialysis
- Consider afterload reduction (ACE-I, hydralazine).

Management Priorities

- Maintain oxygenation via high-flow oxygen by face mask in a sitting position.
- If the patient is still mentating, consider BiPAP therapy as a bridge to dialysis.
- Consult nephrologist to arrange dialysis ASAP.
- Reduce preload and afterload.
  - Nitrates: Sublingual nitroglycerin (0.4 mg q5min) or transdermal nitroglycerin (0.4 mg/h) can be used as a bridge if there is difficulty establishing IV nitroglycerin immediately (start at 20 μg/min and titrate q5min upward by 10-20 μg/min). Some advocate even higher doses such as starting at 50-100 ug/min and rapidly titrating to 200-400 ug/min.
  - Afterload reduction: Hydralazine (5 mg IV q5-10min) or ACE-I.
  - Furosemide: IV furosemide if the patient has any residual renal function, as this may have some utility as a diuretic.
  - Consider phlebotomy if all else fails. There is literature to support that even small volumes of blood removed (1-1.5 U) is safe and efficacious.

Definitive Management

- Dialysis is the definitive management.

Complications

- Respiratory failure
  - This may necessitate intubation.
  - Use vecuronium or rocuronium instead of succinylcholine if you are concerned about hyperkalemia.

Disposition

- Stable patient: Dialysis suite and admission for observation
- Unstable patient: Bedside dialysis in the ICU under care of an intensivist and nephrologist

BLEEDING FROM VASCULAR ACCESS SITE

Additional History and Physical Examination Findings

- Classically, the patient received dialysis earlier in the day.
- Check the patient for any evidence of significant hemorrhage: hypotension, tachycardia, pale conjunctiva, delayed capillary refill, etc.
- Check the access site for evidence of patency (check for thrill) and check for any significant wound or injury to area.
- Check PT/PTT to rule out coagulopathy.

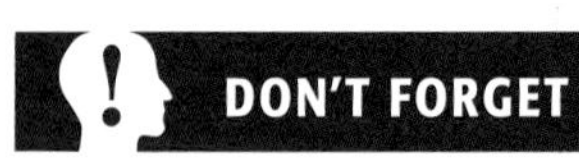

Consult vascular surgery early if there is bleeding from the graft site or vascular access site.

Review Initial Results

- Complete blood count (CBC)
  - Compare with prior CBCs and obtain a 4-hour CBC to ensure no significant hemorrhage.

Management Priorities

- Stop bleeding with application of non-occlusive pressure and/or fingertip point pressure.
- Consult vascular surgery for further evaluation.

Definitive Management

- Stop the bleeding with application of non-occlusive pressure.

Complications

- Thrombosis of the access site can occur when too much pressure is applied to the site.

Disposition

- Stable patient with no significant drop in hemoglobin or hematocrit from baseline after 4 hours and appropriate consultation with vascular surgery can go home.
- Patients with hemodynamic instability should be admitted to the ICU under vascular surgery.
- Patients with evidence of thrombosis to vascular access site, prolonged bleeding, or drop in hemoglobin (Hgb) or hematocrit (Hct) from baseline should be observed in the hospital.

WINNING STRATEGIES

- Every dialysis patient has hyperkalemia, ACS, pericardial effusion, and/or fluid overload until proven otherwise.
- Immediate interventions for all dialysis patients include oxygen, cardiac monitor with rhythm strip, ECG, and a hep-locked IV with a rainbow of labs.
- Obtain a CXR to check for evidence of pulmonary edema and/or significant pericardial effusion.
- Stabilize life-threats with airway management, aggressive treatment, and pericardiocentesis as necessary.
- Use Non-Invasive Positive Pressure Ventilation (NIPPV) early for dialysis patients with acute SOB.
- For intubations, use a non-depolarizing agent, like rocuronium, instead of succinylcholine, unless potassium is known.
- Call the nephrologist early for dialysis.
- Call the CT surgeon early for cardiac tamponade.
- Recheck the ECG in hyperkalemic patients after any intervention or with any change in status.
- You cannot repeat VS too often.

THE BOTTOM LINE

- ECG for dialysis patients to check for pericardial effusion or hyperkalemia
- CXR for dialysis patients to check for pulmonary edema or cardiomegaly consistent with pericardial effusion.
- Treat suspected hyperkalemia early and aggressively.

CHAPTER 29

Emergencies in Sickle Cell Patients

Seth Trueger and James Ahn

INITIAL ASSESSMENT

- Focus on ABCs in order to assess for immediate life-threats.
- Ask for a full set of vitals with every patient including pulse, BP, respirations, temperature, oxygen saturation, and glucose.
- Large-bore IV × 2, O_2, monitor in every patient.
- If not provided, be sure to ask for oxygen saturation.
- Draw labs and hold for orders.

Case-Specific Recommendations

- Focus on pain location, duration, and if typical of past pain crises.
- Identify sick patients with attention to acute chest syndrome, anemia, and sepsis.

DON'T FORGET

Always look for life-threatening causes of pain crisis in patients with sickle cell.

- Acute chest syndrome
- Sepsis
- Aplastic crisis

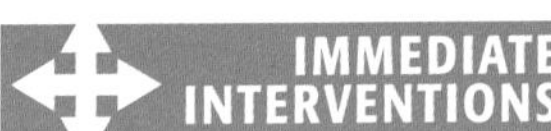

IMMEDIATE INTERVENTIONS

- Oxygen: high flow reservoir facemask.
- Large-bore IV access for fluid hydration and possible transfusion.
- Send blood for CBC with differential, reticulocyte count, electrolytes, and blood type and cultures.
- Analgesia.
- CXR.

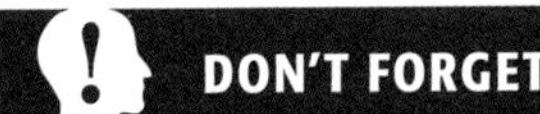

DON'T FORGET

In severe anemia, placing the patient high flow reservoir facemask, even with >95% saturation on room air, is equivalent to transfusing 1-1.5 U of blood!

INITIAL HISTORY AND PHYSICAL EXAMINATION

- History of the present illness (HPI)
  - Fever.
  - Onset of symptoms.
  - Location of pain.
  - Precipitating events (infection, dehydration).
  - Analgesia (what has been used and what usually works).
  - How does this episode differ from prior attacks?
  - Ask every patient with sickle cell disease about potential acute chest syndrome symptoms: chest pain, shortness of breath, cough/ upper respiratory infection (URI) symptoms, and fever.
- Past medical history (PMHx)
  - Type of disease (SS, SC, thalassemia)?
  - Asplenia or splenectomy?
  - Prior infections/acute chest?
  - Prior transfusions?
- Medications
  - Penicillin (PCN) prophylaxis (children).
  - Folic acid.
  - Analgesics.
- Allergies
  - Especially to antibiotics and pain medications.
- Immunizations
  - Pneumococcal vaccine.
  - Influenza vaccine.
  - Meningococcal vaccine.

Physical Examination

- Vital signs (VS) including temperature and oxygen saturation.
- Head, eyes, ears, nose, and throat (HEENT): Jaundice? Dehydration? Pale conjunctivae?
- Neck: Nuchal rigidity?
- Chest: Breath sounds? Rales? Wheezing? Dullness to percussion?
- Abd: Pain, hepatosplenomegaly? Right upper quadrant tenderness?
- Genitourinary (GU): Priapism?
- Back: Cerebrovascular accident (CVA) tenderness?
- Extremity: Cap refill, cyanosis?
- Neuro: Alteration in mental status?

DIFFERENTIAL DIAGNOSIS

- Sickle cell anemia (SCA)
  - Patients with SCA have two abnormal hemoglobin genes; hallmarks of SCA are paroxysmal pain crises.
  - While pain crises form the majority of emergency department (ED) presentations in patients with sickle cell, SCA leads to significant morbidity.
  - People with only one sickle cell gene (sickle cell trait) usually are asymptomatic and do not suffer the same pain crises and complications.
- Acute chest syndrome
  - Acute chest syndrome is a life-threatening complication of sickle cell disease usually caused by infection or vaso-occlusion of the pulmonary vasculature causing infarcts, which manifests as a new pulmonary infiltrate.
  - Acute chest syndrome has a high mortality rate (2%-14%), particularly if untreated, and is clinically indistinguishable from pneumonia.
- Sepsis
  - Sepsis is the leading cause of death in sickle cell patients. Sickle cell patients are susceptible to numerous different strains of bacteria, and infections can arise from various organ systems, including HEENT, pulmonary, gastrointestinal (GI), GU, and central nervous system (CNS).
- Aplastic crisis
  - Usually the production of red blood cells (RBCs) can compensate for the increased destruction of blood cells in the circulation. A dramatic drop in RBC production, often as a result of infection, can cause a severe anemia without the ability to replenish blood mass.
- Splenic sequestration
  - Acute trapping of RBCs in the small vasculature of the spleen causes painful splenomegaly and anemia, and can progress to circulatory collapse.

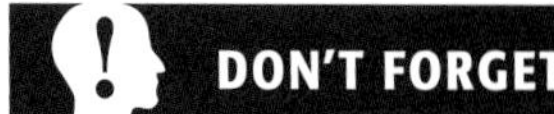

Patients with sickle cell disease will often have more than one problem. Don't forget to dose (and re-dose) analgesics in patients with acute chest syndrome, sepsis, or aplastic crisis.

Don't forget to look for sepsis in patients with acute chest syndrome or aplastic crisis, and vice versa!

ACUTE CHEST SYNDROME

Additional History and Physical Examination Findings

- Classically presents with fever, cough, dyspnea, chest pain, wheezing, and hemoptysis.
- Young children are more likely to present with complaints of fever and cough.
- Hemoptysis, productive cough, and chest pain are more common in older patients.
- Rales and dullness to percussion are the most common physical examination findings.
- Clinically this is indistinguishable from pneumonia.

Review Initial Results

- Chest radiograph: Infiltrate (Fig. 29-1)
- Elevated whited blood cells (WBC)
- Hemoglobin level to assess degree of anemia
- Elevated reticulocyte count
- Majority of patients are hypoxemic (oxygen saturation <90% or Pao_2 <80 mm Hg)

Risk Stratification: Management Priorities

- Can reoccur in patients with previous history of acute chest syndrome.
- Occurs more frequently in homozygous disease (SS) and less frequently in SC disease.

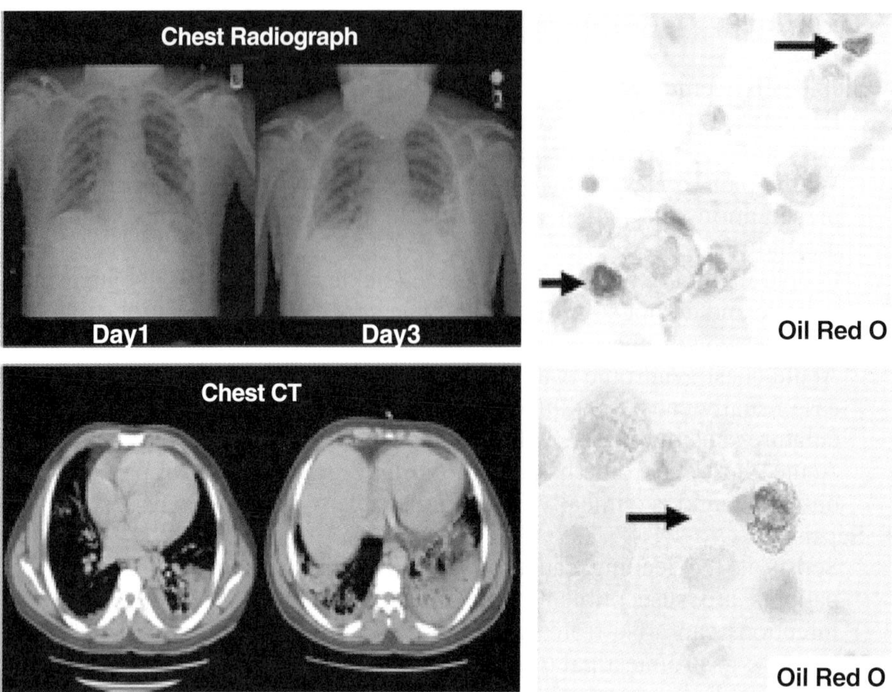

Figure 29-1. Acute chest syndrome of sickle cell disease. A 27-year-old male with sickle cell disease presented with fever, shortness of breath, and vaso-occlusive crisis with left chest wall pain. A chest radiograph on day 3, initially normal on day 1, demonstrates the development of a bilateral lower lobe infiltrate and bilateral pulmonary volume loss. (*Reprinted with permission from Hall JB, Schmidt GA, Wood LDH.* Principles of Critical Care. *3rd ed. New York*, NY: *McGraw-Hill; 2005.*)

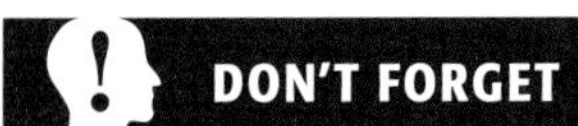

Patients with ACS can have a normal lung examination.

A new pulmonary infiltrate is necessary for diagnosis of acute chest syndrome.

Type and cross sick patients for possible transfusion/exchange transfusions.

Early identification and aggressive treatment can reduce mortality.

Antibiotics should be given early because infection is a common etiology of ACS and is difficult to differentiate in initial workup.

Frequent reassessment is needed because patient's condition can deteriorate rapidly.

- Children are more likely to develop acute chest syndrome but less likely to die from it.
- Acute chest syndrome is the second leading cause of death in sickle cell patients.
- As many as half of the cases of acute chest syndrome may not be diagnosed until days after the initial symptoms.

Definitive Management

- Treatment is largely supportive.
- Emergent exchange transfusion is the treatment of choice:
  - Often not started early enough.
  - Call a hematology/oncology consultant early.
  - Obtain central access.
  - Type and cross blood.
- Transfuse if severely anemic or if exchange transfusion is not immediately available.
- Empiric antibiotic therapy for bacterial pneumonia
  - Ceftriaxone 1 g IV + azithromycin 500 mg IV or
  - Levofloxacin 500 mg IV
- Supplemental oxygen, only if patient is hypoxic.
- Splinting may worsen lung pathology and may be reduced by adequate pain control.
- Hydration must be undertaken cautiously because acute chest syndrome patients are often susceptible to pulmonary edema and hydration can worsen the underlying pathology. Only hydrate if hypovolemic!

Frequent Reassessment

- Patients often need repeat doses of analgesics.
- Ensure patient is not heading toward impending respiratory failure.

Complications

- Respiratory failure
  - Mechanical ventilatory support.
- Shock
- Anemia: Transfusion of packed red blood cells (PRBC) may be necessary to support oxygen-carrying capacity in hypoxic and anemic patients.

Disposition

- All patients diagnosed with acute chest syndrome should be admitted to the intensive care unit (ICU).

SEPSIS

Additional History and Physical Examination Findings

- Patients with sickle cell disease are especially susceptible to infections from encapsulated organisms because of absent or decreased splenic function (*Staphylococcus, Pneumococcus, Haemophilus influenzae,* and *Salmonella*).
- Increased risk of cholecystitis.
- Children younger than the age of 5 should be on PCN prophylaxis to reduce chance of pneumococcal infections.
- Confirm that immunizations are up-to-date.
- VS: hypotension and tachycardia.
- Signs of poor perfusion: Cold clammy skin, diaphoresis, fever, altered mental status, tender abdomen.

REVIEW INITIAL RESULTS

- Chest x-ray (CXR): Pneumonia.
- Complete blood count (CBC): Elevated WBC (bandemia).
- Urinalysis: Urinary tract infection (UTI)/pyelonephritis.
- Arterial blood gas (ABG): Acidosis, respiratory status.
- Computed tomography (CT)/lumbar puncture (LP): Suspected meningitis.
- X-ray radiography (XR) and erythrocyte sedimentation rate (ESR) or C-reactive protein (CRP) for suspected osteomyelitis.

Risk Stratification: Management Priorities

- Sepsis/infection is the major cause of mortality in sickle cell patients.
- Encapsulated organisms are the major causes of sepsis in young children (*Neisseria meningitis*, *Streptococcus pneumoniae*, and *H influenzae*).
- Pneumococcal sepsis is 30-100 times more common in sickle cell patients than in the normal population.
- By the age of 2, 50% of sickle cell patients have functional asplenia.
- Stabilization and early identification of the source of infection should be a priority.
- Early administration of antibiotics and IV fluids.

Definitive Management

- Largely revolves around supportive measures and antibiotics.
  - Early, broad-spectrum antibiotic administration is imperative.
  - Fluid resuscitation.
  - Vasopressors if needed.

- Mechanical ventilation for respiratory failure.
- Blood, urine, and cerebrospinal fluid (CSF) cultures for definitive diagnosis infection.
- Ultrasound if suspicion for cholecystitis.

Frequent Reassessment

- Frequent reassessment is needed because patient's condition can rapidly deteriorate.

DON'T FORGET

A complete workup for source of infection is indicated in all febrile sickle cell patients.

Streptococcus pneumoniae is the most common cause of pneumonia in sickle cell patients.

Treat sickle cell patients as immunocompromised.

Complications

- Respiratory failure
  - Mechanical ventilatory support.
- Shock
- Anemia: Transfusion of PRBC may be necessary to support oxygen-carrying capacity in hypoxic and anemic patients.

Disposition

- All sickle cell patients with sepsis should be admitted and may need intensive care management—all are admitted to the ICU on examination day.

APLASTIC CRISIS

- Patients with sickle cell disease are prone to bone marrow suppression, which, in conjunction with, increased peripheral destruction of abnormal cells, can lead to a profound anemia.

DON'T FORGET

A reticulocyte count should usually be elevated in a patient with sickle cell disease in crisis—a "normal" value is abnormal.

Additional History and Physical Examination Findings

- Rule out sources of hemorrhage.
- A base line hemoglobin level from previous visits is helpful.
- Signs of anemia include pallor, tachycardia, hypotension, dyspnea, and alteration of mental status.

Review Initial Results

- CBC for anemia.
- Reticulocyte count should be elevated; low or normal is inappropriate with sickle cell disease.

DON'T FORGET

A hemoglobin of <6-7 g/dL, a drop in hemoglobin of >2 g/dL, or a reticulocyte count of <5% are very concerning for aplastic crisis.

Risk Stratification: Management Priorities

- Shock should be treated immediately when volume resuscitation and transfusions are indicated.
- Search for underlying infection and sepsis.
- Admit for supportive care until bone marrow function is reestablished.

SPLENIC SEQUESTRATION

- Patients with sickle cell disease may acutely trap RBCs in the spleen's small vasculature leading to painful splenomegaly and anemia and may progress to circulatory collapse, particularly children who still have functioning spleens.

Additional History and Physical Examination Findings

- History of prior splenic sequestration—this will recur in up to 50% of cases.
- Left upper quadrant tenderness or splenomegaly.
- Signs of anemia include pallor, tachycardia, hypotension, dyspnea, and alteration of mental status.

Review Initial Results

- CBC for anemia.
- Persistently elevated reticulocyte count.

Risk Stratification: Management Priorities

- Shock should be treated immediately with transfusion.
- Search for underlying infection and sepsis.
- Consider surgical consultation for splenomegaly.
- Admit to the ICU for close monitoring and supportive care as mortality rates approach 15%.

WINNING STRATEGIES

- Look for life-threatening complications of sickle cell disease.
- CXR should be obtained in all sickle cell patients with a fever, or any potential acute chest syndrome signs or symptoms: chest pain, shortness of breath, cough/URI symptoms, crackles, rales, tachypnea or hypoxia.
- If not provided, be sure to ask for oxygen saturation!
- All febrile patients with sickle cell should be evaluated comprehensively for a source of infection and receive empiric antibiotics.
- Admit all patients with suspicion of acute chest syndrome even with a normal initial CXR because of the often delayed diagnosis and potentially rapidly fulminant course.
- All sickle cell patients presenting to the ED should have a mild anemia and an elevated reticulocyte count. Worsened anemia or "normal" reticulocyte counts are signs of serious disease.

CHAPTER 30

Bleeding Disorders

Seth Trueger and James Ahn

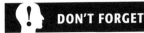

DON'T FORGET

All patients with active bleeding get two large-bore IVs or a central line.

IMMEDIATE INTERVENTIONS

- Intubation if airway is compromised or altered mental status (AMS)
- Large-bore IV access for fluid hydration or transfusion of blood products
- Supplemental oxygen
- Place on monitor
- Type and crossmatch for blood products.

DON'T FORGET

Place all patients with severe anemia on 100% NRB even if their O_2 saturations are 100% with room air or nasal cannula.

DON'T FORGET

Many patients with hemorrhagic shock won't be tachycardic; for example, certain common medications such as beta-blockers and calcium channel blockers will mask the tachycardic response. This may also be seen in patients with pacemakers or intrinsic heart disease, advanced age and even young, previously healthy patients. "Normal vitals signs" does not always mean a stable patient.

INITIAL ASSESSMENT

- Focus on ABCs. Keep immediate life threats in mind first.
- Ask for a full set of vitals with every patient, including pulse, blood pressure (BP), respirations, temperature, oxygen saturation, and glucose.
- Large-bore IV × 2, O_2, monitor in every patient.
- Draw labs and hold for orders.

Case-Specific Recommendations

- Immediate assessment of hemodynamic status and fluid resuscitation.

INITIAL HISTORY AND PHYSICAL EXAMINATION

- History of the present illness (HPI)
  - Onset of symptoms.
  - History of bleeding disorders.
  - Hematemesis, hematochezia, melena.
  - Bruising with trivial trauma or easy bleeding (eg, while brushing teeth).
  - Any other signs of active bleeding.
  - History of transfusions.
  - Familial history of bleeding.
  - Recent or remote trauma.
- Past medical history (PMHx)
  - History of bleeding disorders?
  - Blood type?
  - Prior transfusions?
  - History of factor replacement?
  - History of cancer?
  - History of liver disease?
  - Adverse reactions with prior transfusions?
- Family history
  - Familial history of bleeding disorders?
- Medications
  - Warfarin (Coumadin).
  - Heparin/enoxaparin (Lovenox).
  - Aspirin.
  - Antiplatelet drugs.
  - Novel oral anticoagulants (NOACs: dabigatran, apixaban, rivaroxiban).
  - Beta-blockers/calcium channel blockers.
- Allergies
- Physical examination
  - Vital signs (VS)
  - Head, eyes, ears, nose, and throat (HEENT): Jaundice? Dehydration? Pale conjunctivae or tongue? Gum bleeding? Nose bleeding?
  - Chest: Tachycardia? Murmurs?
  - Abd: Pain, hepatosplenomegaly? Rebound or guarding?
  - Extremity: Cap refill, cyanosis, cool extremities?
  - Rectal: Melena or hematochezia? Occult blood?
  - Skin: Petechiae? Bruising? Hemarthrosis?
  - Genitourinary (GU): Hematuria?
  - Neuro: Alteration in mental status? Headache?

DIFFERENTIAL DIAGNOSIS

- Acquired bleeding disorders
  - Inhibition of the coagulation cascade, increased fibrinolysis, clotting factor deficiencies, or thrombocytopenia can all be forms of acquired

bleeding disorders. The most common causes are warfarin, heparin, and aspirin toxicities, as well as liver failure.
  - Warfarin inhibits the production of vitamin K–dependent clotting factors by the liver and has a narrow therapeutic window. Adverse events from warfarin and insulin are the most common adverse medication events seen in the emergency department (ED).
  - Warfarin increases the risk of bleeding caused by the interruption of the coagulation cascade. Heparin (unfractionated, or low-molecular-weight heparin) causes the inactivation of thrombin from the common coagulation pathway.
  - Other newer antiocoagulants (sometimes called NOACs) work directly at specific clotting factors. Dabigitran (Pradaxa) is a direct thrombin (factor IIa) inhibitor. Rivaroxaban (Xarelto) and apixaban (Eliquis) inhibit factor Xa.
  - Advanced liver failure impairs the ability to produce clotting factors and can lead to massive hemorrhages.
  - Many cancers, especially those of the marrow, may cause thrombocytopenia.
  - Aspirin also inhibits platelet function and promotes bleeding for up to 7-10 days after use; uremia may also impair platelet function.
  - Other causes of thrombocytopenia to be aware of include the following: idiopathic thrombocytopenic purpura (ITP), thrombotic thrombocytopenic purpura (TTP), hemolytic-uremic syndrome (HUS), and disseminated intravascular coagulation (DIC).
- Hereditary bleeding disorders
  - Hemophilia A and B diseases are hereditary sex-linked recessive bleeding disorders caused by a deficiency in the coagulation cascade factors VIII and IX (Christmas disease), respectively.
  - von Willebrand disease (VWD) is an autosomal dominant deficiency of factor VII and von Willebrand factor (VWF). It is the most common bleeding disorder. VWF is essential for platelet adhesion, and patients with this disorder have bleeding consistent with platelet deficiencies.

DON'T FORGET

Thrombocytopenia and platelet function disorders generally present with easy bruising, epistaxis, gingival bleeding, hematuria, and GI bleeding, while coagulation deficiencies typically present with deep intramuscular hematomas, hemarthrosis, or retroperitoneal bleeding.

DON'T FORGET

DDX Summary

May be difficult to determine the etiology of bleeding disorder.

- A thorough history and physical examination is crucial in diagnosing a bleeding disorder.
- CBC, peripheral smear, PT/PTT/INR, reticulocyte count to help determine the type of bleeding disorder.
- Blood for type and cross or type and screen of packed red blood cells and blood products such as FFP, cryoprecipitate, or specific factors as needed for hemorrhage leading to shock.

ACQUIRED BLEEDING DISORDERS

Additional History and Physical Examination Findings

- History of anticoagulant use?
- History of nonsteroidal anti-inflammatory drug (NSAID) use?
- History of atrial fibrillation, prosthetic valves, stroke, severe cardiomyopathy, deep vein thrombosis, pulmonary embolism, congestive heart failure, or end-stage renal disease?
- Recent changes in diet or medications can affect warfarin therapy?
- Melena, hematochezia, hematemesis, epistaxis?
- History of previous bleeding episode, peptic ulcer disease, chronic alcohol use, or cirrhosis?
- Signs of liver failure, including jaundice, ascites, spider angiomata, and palmar erythema?
- Signs of sepsis or DIC?
- On dialysis?

DON'T FORGET

Always ask about indications for anticoagulation therapy in patients with a suspected bleeding disorder.

Review Initial Results

- Hemoglobin level to assess degree of anemia
- Prothrombin time (PT)/partial thromboplastin time (PTT) and INR
- Platelets
  - Liver function tests
  - Lectate dehydrogenase (LDH) and haptoglobin to assess for hemolysis
  - Lactic acid or serum base excess to help assess for shock
  - Peripheral smear may help identify the cause of the bleeding disorder.

DON'T FORGET

TTP classically presents with fever, anemia, renal failure, thrombocytopenia, and neurologic symptoms.

DON'T FORGET

Patients with end-stage renal disease may not realize that they may receive regular boluses of heparin with dialysis.

DON'T FORGET

Thrombocytopenia occurs in about 10% of patients receiving heparin.

DON'T FORGET

PT and INR prolongation are most commonly associated with warfarin, while PTT prolongation is associated with heparin exposure. However, high levels of either drug can produce abnormalities of both. DOACs may cause abnormalities in either PT/INR or PTT, but testing is not reliable for DOACs.

DON'T FORGET

In patients with severe bleeding, initial focus should be on assessment of hemodynamic status and volume resuscitation.

DON'T FORGET

The need for FFP, factor replacement, vitamin K, or protamine sulfate use should be balanced by the indications for anticoagulation therapy in stable patients.

Risk Stratification: Management Priorities

- Definitive management is dependent on etiology of the bleeding disorder.
- Administer fresh frozen plasma (FFP) or prothrombin complex concentrate (particularly in patients at risk for fluid overload), with vitamin K (warfarin toxicity), or protamine sulfate (heparin toxicity) in patients with active life-threatening bleeding.
- Patients with cardiac symptoms and bleeding should be transfused immediately.
- Central line placement should be in a compressible site if patient is at risk for uncontrolled bleeding.
- May need to transfuse with blood products prior to invasive procedures, such as lumbar puncture, if the patient is at high risk for bleeding from minor trauma.
- Have a low threshold for imaging coagulopathic patients, as they are subject to intracranial hemorrhage with trivial trauma, and spontaneous bleeding (eg, hemarthrosis, retroperitoneal hemorrhage).

Definitive Management

- ABCs.
- IVF resuscitation if hypotensive and blood not immediately available.
- Supplemental oxygen.
- Type and cross for transfusions of blood products if needed.
- The effects of heparin can be reversed with protamine sulfate; enoxaparin (Lovenox) is partially reversed by protamine.
- The effects of warfarin can be reversed with FFP or prothrombin complex concentrate, plus vitamin K, if life-threatening bleeding is present.
- There are no options to definitively reverse NOACs; prothrombin complex concentrate is likely the best option.
- Transfuse platelets in severe thrombocytopenia, and consider desmopressin (DDAVP) for patients with life-threatening bleeding and impaired platelet function, including dialysis patients.
- Treat suspected TTP with plasma exchange, and patients with ITP should get corticosteroids and likely intravenous immunoglobin (IVIG) in consultation with hematology.

Frequent Reassessment

- Continuous monitoring of the patient's VS is imperative.
- Repeat hemoglobin to assess stability of patient with brisk bleeding.

Complications

- Cardiovascular collapse caused by volume loss.
- Respiratory failure secondary to aspiration of blood.
- Hepatic encephalopathy in liver failure patients.

Disposition

- All patients with a known bleeding disorder and active bleeding should be admitted.
- All patients with hemodynamic instability or brisk bleeding should be admitted to an intensive care setting.

HEREDITARY BLEEDING DISORDERS

Additional History and Physical Examination Findings

- Bleeding from hemophilia A or B is characterized by deep intramuscular hematomas, hemarthroses (especially weight-bearing joints), or muscle pain but can occur anywhere.

- Hemophiliacs are at risk for bleeding from minor trauma or spontaneous bleeding.
- Bleeding from VWD presents with mucocutaneous bleeding including epistaxis, menorrhagia, and GI bleeding.
- History of HIV/AIDS or viral hepatitis?
- History of previous bleeding episodes?
- History of excessive bleeding after minor surgery, dental extractions, or minor lacerations or wounds?

Review Initial Results

- Hemoglobin level to assess degree of anemia/bleeding.
- PT/PTT and INR and bleeding time.
  - In hemophilia patients, the PT normal, activated partial thromboplastin time (aPTT) elevated, and bleeding time normal.
  - In VWD, PT normal, aPTT elevated, and bleeding time elevated.
- Factor VIII (hemophilia A) and factor IX (hemophilia B) levels.
- Normal hemostasis in hemophilia A patients requires about 25% factor VIII activity.

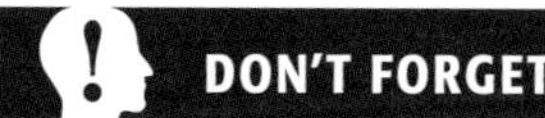

HIV/AIDS and viral hepatitis are common in the hemophiliac population as a result of recurrent transfusions. HIV/AIDS is a leading cause of death in hemophiliacs.

Risk Stratification: Management Priorities

- Immediate life-threatening bleeding occurs in the oropharynx (occludes airway) and central nervous system (CNS).
- If CNS bleeding is suspected, replace factor immediately, even before the patient goes for a computed tomography (CT) scan.
- It is important to note that signs of bleeding may not occur for days after an initial trauma and even trivial trauma can result in life-threatening bleeding in coagulopathic patients.
- Patients receiving multiple transfusions of blood products are at risk for volume overload.

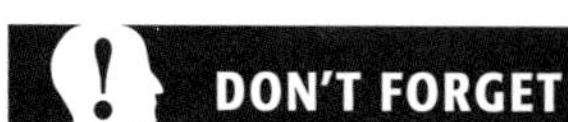

Must perform a comprehensive physical examination, including HEENT, skin, and neurologic to rule out spontaneous bleeding.

Definitive Management

- ABCs.
- Fluid resuscitation if anemic or bleeding.
- Factor replacement for hemophilia A.
- Factor VIII: Amount dependent on risk for severity of disease and each unit of factor VIII per kilogram will increase the activity level by about 2%.
- *Mild* (soft tissue bleeding, epistaxis, gingival bleeding) should transfuse to level >30% or 15-18 U/kg.
- DDAVP: an alternative to factor VIII replacement in mild hemophilia patients and will raise the factor VIII activity by 2-3 times transiently.
- *Moderate* (GU/gastrointestinal (GI) bleeding, hemarthrosis, CNS trauma without bleeding) should transfuse to level >50% or 25 U/kg.
- *Severe* (CNS bleeding, major trauma or surgery) should transfuse to level >90% or 50 U/kg.
  - FFP or prothrombin complex concentrate if factor VIII not available.
  - Cryoprecipitate if factor VIII not available; contains about half the factor VIII activity as FFP and 10% of the volume.
- Factor replacement for hemophilia B
  - Factor IX: Each unit of factor IX given per kilogram will increase the activity level by about 1%.
  - *Mild* should transfuse to level >20% or 20 U/kg.
  - *Moderate* should transfuse to level >25% or 25 U/kg.
  - *Severe* should transfuse to level >50% or 50 U/kg.
  - FFP or prothrombin complex concentrate if factor IX not available; each unit of FFP will raise the factor IX level by about 3%.

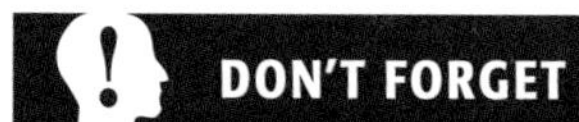

In mild hemophilia both the PT and aPTT can be normal.

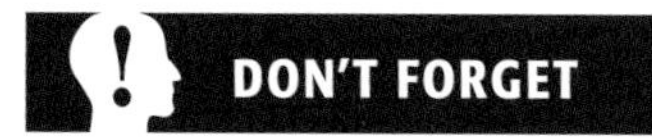

Spontaneous bleeding can occur at factor VIII levels <5%.

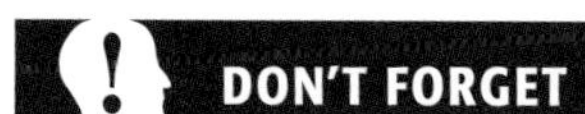

Bleeding that potentially affects the airway and CNS bleeding are indications for immediate factor replacement.

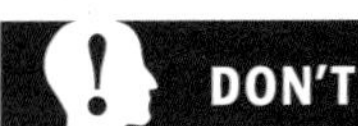

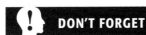

DON'T FORGET

Headache or neurologic complaints in hemophilia patients is an indication for immediate factor transfusion.

FFP contains 1 U/mL of each clotting factor. Cryoprecipitate contains 80 U of factor VIIIC and 80 U of VWF, fibrinogen, and factor XIII.

- Treatment of VWD by type
  - DDAVP can be used with mild bleeding in patients with type I VWD, the most common type.
  - Factor VIII concentrates with large amounts of VWF are the treatment of choice for types II and III VWD—the rare types.
  - Cryoprecipitate is effective for all types of VWD.
  - FFP may by used for all types of VWD.
- Transfuse if severely anemic (<7 g/dL) or unstable VS; also transfuse cardiac patients if hemoglobin <9 g/dL.
- Supplemental oxygen.

Frequent Reassessment

- Continuous monitoring of the patient's VS is imperative.
- Repeat hemoglobin to assess stability of patient with brisk bleeding.
- Reassess mental status, especially in patients with CNS complaints.

Complications

- Volume overload caused by large volume of transfusions.
- Risk of viral transmission (hepatitis, HIV) secondary to contaminated blood products.
- Joint deformity secondary to recurrent or chronic hemarthroses.

Disposition

- All patients with active bleeding should be admitted for factor levels and observation for delayed bleeding.
- All patients with hemodynamic instability or brisk bleeding should be admitted to an intensive care setting.

WINNING STRATEGIES

- A thorough history must be elicited because bleeding disorders can result from many different causes, including medication overdoses or interactions, diet changes, liver disease, or hereditary diseases.
- All patients with life-threatening bleeding and anticoagulation toxicity should be aggressively treated with FFP, prothrombin complex concentrate, or reversal agents (vitamin K or protamine sulfate as indicated). There are no options to definitively reverse DOACs. Prothrombin complex concentrate is likely the best option.
- Do not discount remote trauma as precipitating a bleeding event as onset can be slow.
- All hemophilia patients with CNS complaints (headache, AMS) should receive factor replacement immediately even prior to CT scan.
- Assume all patients with abnormal bleeding are unstable.

CHAPTER 31

Psychiatric Emergencies

Mária Némethy and David Howes

INITIAL ASSESSMENT

- Establish patient and staff safety (violent/agitated patient).
- Focus on vital signs (VS), general appearance, recent illnesses, comorbid diseases (eg, diabetes, liver disease).
- Look for overdose/toxidromes and traumatic injuries (either self-inflicted or inflicted by others).

INITIAL HISTORY AND PHYSICAL EXAMINATION

History

- History of the present illness (HPI)
  - Assess whether symptoms are an acute change from baseline or chronic in nature with an acute exacerbation.
  - Symptom onset (eg, rapid or gradual)?
  - History of similar episodes?
  - Exacerbating or complicating circumstances?
  - History of assault or trauma?
  - Suicidal or homicidal ideation or intent?
  - • Drug overdose?
- Past medical histor (PMHx)
  - Medical and psychiatric histories?
  - History of suicidal ideation and/or attempts?
  - History of overdose?
- Current medications
- Allergies
- Review of systems and social history
  - Suicidal/homicidal ideations?
  - Feeling of guilt or hopelessness?
  - Increased or decreased weight?
  - Energy loss?
  - Concentration problems?
  - Sleep irregularities?
  - Loss of job?
  - Divorce or marital problems?

DON'T FORGET

Every patient with a psychiatric complaint must be evaluated for a possible etiology of organic disease, especially >40 years old.

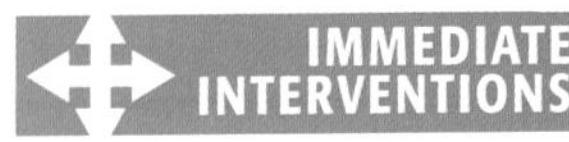

IMMEDIATE INTERVENTIONS

- Note the vital signs.
- Ensure patient's safety.
- Search for medical conditions that could have caused or exacerbated current symptoms.
- Stabilize medical conditions (eg, hypothermia, rhabdomyolysis, withdrawal, respiratory depression).
- Look for suicide attempt, overdose/toxidromes, and traumatic injuries.
- Always consider hypoglycemia, hypercarbia, and hypoxia in an uncooperative patient.

Fever and tachycardia may indicate thyroid storm.

Physical Examination

- VS, including pulse oximetry.
- If indicated, spot glucose check.
- Always perform a full physical examination, specifically:
  - Head, eyes, ears, nose, and throat (HEENT): Look for pupil size and reactivity, signs of trauma.
  - Respiratory/cardiovascular: Look for tachypnea and tachycardia.
  - Skin (eg, absence or presence of sweating as evidence of a toxidrome, ecchymosis).
  - Perform a thorough neurologic examination.

DIFFERENTIAL DIAGNOSIS (DDX)

After ruling out organic etiologies, in a psychiatric patient consider the following differential diagnosis:

- Depression: Mood disorders affect 10%-15% of the general population at some point in their lifetime. Depression with substance abuse and suicidal ideation/attempt often brings these patients to the emergency department (ED).

- Psychosis: Patients present with gross distortion or disorganization of affect, a diminished capacity to recognize reality, or decreased ability to communicate and relate to others in a way that meets the demands of everyday life. Be alert for possibility of psychosis from drug ingestion.
- Sexual assault: There are many legal definitions for sexual assault and these definitions vary from state to state. The incidence is dramatically underreported. Victims are often reluctant to undergo a sexual assault examination and evaluation, for fear of being blamed for the event, fear of retaliation, and embarrassment. The sexual assault response team should be notified as soon as possible when evaluating a patient with suspected sexual assault.

DON'T FORGET

Always assess for suicide risk and attempts. Look for toxidromes and evaluate for toxic ingestions.

DEPRESSION/SUICIDE

Additional History and Physical Examination Findings

- Multiple medical conditions and medical interventions can be related to depression as an associated symptom or complication.
- May or may not give a history of depression.
- May also have a chronic medical condition that is complicated by a depressed mood (eg, cancer).
- Older males without a support system are at the highest risk for successful suicide attempts.
- Overall, young females are at the highest risk for suicide attempts.
- Genetic predisposition; elicit family history of depression and suicide attempts.
- Patients often have multiple somatic complaints.
- Often have had multiple evaluations for chronic pain, weakness, malaise, and headache.
- Pediatric patients may present with change in baseline school and social functioning or with substance abuse.
- Medications and medication changes can be associated with depression.
- Diagnostic criteria include >2 weeks of depressed mood with >5 of the following criteria:
  - Low self-esteem.
  - Loss of interest, anhedonia.
  - Fatigue, decreased energy.
  - Appetite change.
  - Sleep problems.
  - Decreased attention.
  - Irritability.
  - Psychomotor agitation or retardation.
  - Feelings of guilt or worthlessness.
  - Difficulty with concentration.
  - Suicidal thoughts with or without a plan.
- Assess suicide risk (eg, previous attempts, having a plan, means to implement plan, etc.).
- Investigate for potential drug overdose.
- Look for trauma/sequelae of suicide attempt.

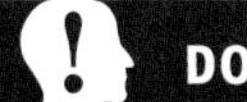

DON'T FORGET

Older single males without a support system are at a high risk for suicide.

DON'T FORGET

Young females are also at a high risk for suicide attempts.

DON'T FORGET

Pediatric patients may present with change in baseline school and social functioning or with substance abuse.

DON'T FORGET

Multiple medical conditions and medical interventions can be related to depression as an associated symptom or complication.

Review Initial Results

- As indicated by the history and physical examination:
  - Laboratory evaluation for electrolyte imbalances, anemia, thyroid disease, liver disease, and blood alcohol level.
  - Specific drug levels (eg, acetaminophen, salicylate).
  - Toxicology screen.
  - Always check a urine pregnancy in women of childbearing age.

DON'T FORGET

Patient may need involuntary admission because of danger to self and to others or grave disability.

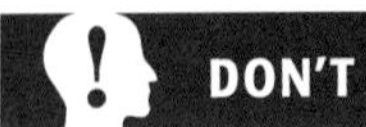

DON'T FORGET

Depression, schizophrenia and substance abuse increase suicide risk.

Risk Stratification: Management Priorities

- Ensuring patients' safety is paramount.
- Stabilization and evaluation of concurrent medical illnesses.
- Determination of suicide attempt and/or drug overdose.

Definitive Management

- Diagnosis and stabilization of associated medical complaints.
- Severity of symptoms and associated debilitation are important to ascertain as these determine disposition.
- Suicidal thoughts must be taken seriously and a patient's access to lethal means needs to be determined.
- Consultation with psychiatry for evaluation and admission.
- Patient may need involuntary admission because of a danger to self, others, or grave disability.

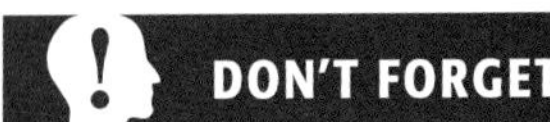

DON'T FORGET

Many drug ingestions can cause transient psychosis (methamphetamines, cocaine, spice) and/or may lower threshold (schrizophrenia).

Complications

- Coexisting medical diagnoses, suicide attempts, overdose, no access for follow-up, and unsafe living and social environment can complicate the evaluation and disposition of a depressed patient.

Disposition

- Medical or psychiatric admission as indicated.

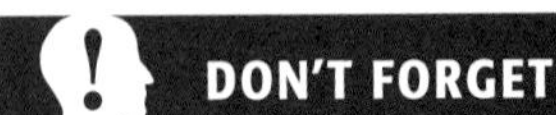

DON'T FORGET

Consider brain imaging when organic etiology suspected.

PSYCHOSIS

Additional History and Physical Examination Findings

- Age, onset of symptoms, family history, premorbid functioning can be used to aid in the determination of organic versus functional psychosis.
  - Age >40 years with no family history of psychiatric diagnoses and high premorbid level of functioning are more likely associated with an organic or medical etiology of psychosis.
  - Age <40 years with a gradual, progressive worsening of symptoms and a family history of psychiatric disorders are typically associated with a functional psychosis.
- Hallucinations in functional psychosis tend to be auditory and patients are often concerned about what the voices are saying but not about hearing voices.
- Nonauditory hallucinations (visual, olfactory, tactile) suggest a medical etiology.
- Patients may have an undiagnosed underlying illness (eg, human immunodeficiency virus [HIV]). A detailed physical examination is essential.
- Note the VS. Look for autonomic disturbances (eg, elevated or decreased blood pressure, tachycardia, tachypnea, fever).
- On examination, look for diaphoresis, pupil abnormalities, gait disturbances, focal neurologic deficits, incontinence, fluctuating level of consciousness, orientation, and disturbance of attention.

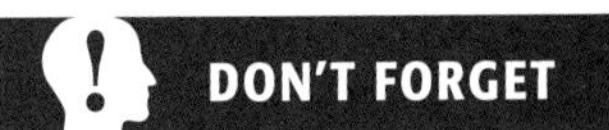

DON'T FORGET

Age <40 years with a gradual, progressive worsening of symptoms, and a family history of psychiatric disorders are typically associated with a functional psychosis.

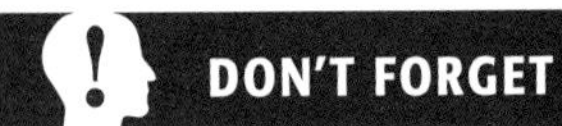

DON'T FORGET

Hallucinations in functional psychosis tend to be auditory.

Review Initial Results

- Search for associated medical conditions.
- As indicated, laboratory and radiographic tests can include complete blood count (CBC), electrolytes, liver function tests, thyroid studies, creatinine phosphokinase (CPK), urinalysis (UA), urine pregnancy test, toxicology screen, drug levels (eg, aspirin, acetaminophen), alcohol level, electrocardiogram (ECG), rapid plasma reagin (RPR), human immunodeficienc virus (HIV), and computed tomography (CT) scan of head.

Risk Stratification: Management Priorities

- Protect the patient and the ED staff as indicated.
- Determine the need for restraints (chemical and/or physical) and initiate medical/psychiatric hold as indicated.
- Look for and initiate therapy for potentially life-threatening conditions (eg, hyperthermia, rhabdomyolysis, aspirin/acetaminophen overdose, withdrawal, respiratory depression).

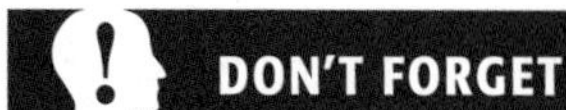

DON'T FORGET

Do not overlook any abnormal vital signs. They may be the key to a toxidrome.

Definitive Management

- Diagnosis and management of acute medical issues
- Admission to the appropriate service (medical versus psychiatric)

Frequent Reassessment

- These patients need close observation for potential decompensation or complications associated with chemical and physical restraints.

Complications

- Abuse, injury, toxic ingestions, and chronic disability complicate the long-term management of psychotic patients.

Disposition

- The psychotic patient may need medical or psychiatric admission for protection, diagnosis, and further treatment.

SEXUAL ASSAULT

Additional History and Physical Examination Findings

- Pertinent assault history
  - Who was the assailant? How many assailants, descriptive features, age, identity if known?
  - What happened? Actual or attempted oral, anal, vaginal penetration? With what? Foreign objects? Was there ejaculation? Was a condom used?
  - When?
    - Emergency contraception and forensic evidence are most useful within 72 hours of assault.
  - Where? Evidence found at the location may be useful.
  - Suspicion of drug-facilitated assault? Amnesia, waking with clothing removed, waking with genital or pelvic soreness.
  - Douche, shower, change of clothing?
    - Such actions may result in loss of evidence.
- PMHx
  - Last menstrual period, birth control method?
  - Last consensual intercourse?
  - Medical history, medications, allergies?
  - Prior sexual assault?
- Physical examination
  - General physical examination should be performed with careful documentation of physical injuries with wounds, bruises, abrasions, and lacerations detailed on a body map.
  - Specifically examine the wrists, breasts, neck, thighs, buttocks, and genital areas for injury.
  - Detailed examination of the vagina and anus/rectum with a speculum and anoscope are performed in conjunction with the sexual assault response team.
  - Use prepackaged special sexual assault examination and specimen kit.

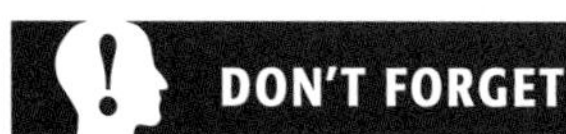

DON'T FORGET

Report sexual assault to law enforcement as soon as possible.

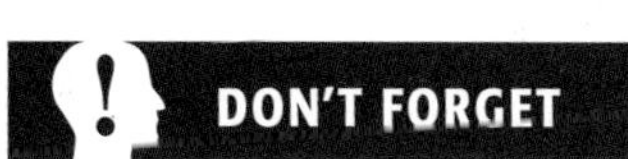

DON'T FORGET

General physical examination should be performed with careful documentation of physical injuries with wounds, bruises, abrasions, and lacerations detailed on a body map.

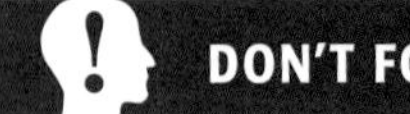

DON'T FORGET

Put clothing in dry paper bags and seal them. Do not wash or modify any potential evidence.

  - Informed consent must be obtained in order to perform the evidentiary examination.
  - The "chain of evidence" must be maintained.
  - Patients should be reminded that collection of evidence does not mandate that they seek prosecution, but that vital evidence will be lost if the examination is delayed or not performed.
  - Put clothing in dry paper bags and seal them.
  - Do not wash or modify any potential evidence as it is important to preserve evidence.

Review Initial Results

- Urine pregnancy test.
- If indicated, possible laboratory tests can include CBC, electrolytes, urinalysis, toxicology screen, drug levels (eg, aspirin, acetaminophen), alcohol level, HIV test, ECG.
- If indicated, cultures (vaginal, anal, penile swaps for gonorrhea and chlamydia), wet mount for fungus, clue cells, Trichomonas vaginalis, and sperm.
- Radiographic tests as indicated by history and physical examination (eg, head CT if head trauma).

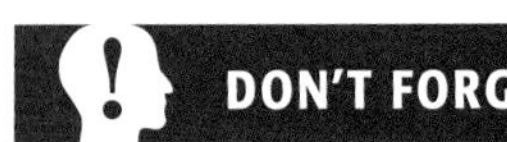

DON'T FORGET

If indicated, offer pregnancy and STD prophylaxis.

Risk Stratification: Management Priorities

- Treatment of physical injuries.
- Psychological support.
- If indicated, offer pregnancy prophylaxis:
  - Emergency contraception methods are most effective if initiated within 72 hours after intercourse (reported efficacy ~80%):
    - Plan B (levonorgestrel 0.75 mg): One tablet PO as soon as possible within 72 hours of intercourse; then one tablet PO 12 hours later or 1.5 mg PO x 1 within 72 hours.
    - Preven EC (100 μg ethinyl estradiol and 0.5 mg levonorgestrel per dose of two tablets): Two tablets PO as soon as possible within 72 hours of intercourse; then two tablets PO 12 hours later.
- If indicated, offer sexually transmitted disease (STD) prophylaxis:
  - Gonorrhea: Ceftriaxone 125 mg IM in a single dose.
  - Chlamydia: Azithromycin 1 g PO in a single dose.
  - Trichomoniasis: Metronidazole 2 g PO in a single dose.
  - Bacterial vaginosis: Metronidazole 500 mg PO bid for 7 days.
  - Hepatitis B: Hepatitis B vaccine if never immunized.
  - HIV prophylaxis: Offered based on risk of transmission.

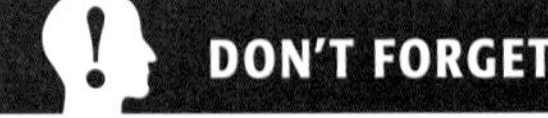

DON'T FORGET

Emergency contraception and forensic evidence are most useful within 72 hours of assault.

Definitive Management

- Physical injuries and medical issues need consultation, admission, and treatment as indicated.
- Sexual assault response teams often have follow-up plans and psychiatric interventions as a part of their evaluation and treatment.
- Report sexual assault to law enforcement as soon as possible.
- Involve family and friends in the care of the patient.

Complications

- Injuries, STDs, unwanted pregnancy, and prolonged psychological trauma all complicate the care of the assault patient.

Disposition

- As indicated by the associated injuries and medical issues.
- Patient safety is paramount.

WINNING STRATEGIES

- Every patient with a psychiatric complaint must be evaluated for a possible organic etiology of disease.
- In your differential diagnosis, consider delirium, psychosis, depression, drug use, and sexual assault.
- Don't overlook any abnormal VS; these may be the key to the diagnosis (eg, toxidrome).
- Physical and chemical restraints may need to be used to protect the patient and staff.
- Psychotic patients have a gross distortion of reality, affect, and communication.
- Hallucinations in functional psychosis tend to be auditory.
- Patients who have been sexually assaulted may not be forthcoming with this information.
- Patients may need involuntary admission because of a danger to self, others or grave disability.
- Remember to address all complicating medical issues, injuries, and the need for follow-up and treatment.
- When available, use the expertise of the sexual assault response team.
- If indicated, offer pregnancy and STD prophylaxis.

THE BOTTOM LINE

- Look for toxidromes; investigate possible drug overdose and suicide attempt.
- Initiate therapy for potentially life-threatening conditions (eg, hyperthermia, rhabdomyolysis, withdrawal, respiratory depression).
- Protect the patient and the ED staff as indicated; determine the need for restraint (chemical and/or physical).
- As indicated, involve law enforcement, the sexual assault response team, and/or psychiatry as soon as possible.

SECTION 5

PEDIATRIC PATIENTS

CHAPTER 32

Pediatric Fever

Lindsey Caley, John Dayton, and Matthew Steimle

INITIAL ASSESSMENT

- Focus on age, vital signs (VS) (including rectal temperature), and general appearance. Are they toxic-appearing, well-appearing, or ill-appearing?
- Identify unstable patients with immediate life threats.
  - Sepsis
  - Shock
  - Meningitis

INITIAL HISTORY AND PHYSICAL EXAMINATION

History

- History of present illness (HPI)
  - Fever history: Onset, how measured, highest temperature, were antipyretics given, and when was the last dose?
  - Associated symptoms
    - General: Are they irritable, consolable, lethargic? Are symptoms continuous or sporadic?
    - Head, eyes, ears, nose, and throat (HEENT) examination: Ear pain or discharge, throat pain, trouble swallowing?
    - Respiratory: Cough, rhinorrhea, trouble breathing?
    - Gastrointestinal (GI): Vomiting, diarrhea, abdominal pain?
    - Urinary: Dysuria, frequency, urgency?
    - Skin: Rash? Any warm joints?
  - Any known exposure to illness (family members, daycare, etc)?
  - Any recent travel?
- Past medical history (PMHx)
  - Birth history: Prematurity, delivery complications such as premature rupture of membranes? Any maternal concerns such as sexually transmitted infection (STI) or group B Strep?
  - Chronic medical conditions: Sickle cell disease, cancer, immunocompromised status?
  - Prior illnesses/hospitalizations?
  - Immunizations: Are they up-to-date with vaccines?
- Medications: Any recent antibiotics or vaccinations?
- Allergies

Physical Examination

- VS: Including blood pressure (BP) and rectal temperature. On exam day, any missing VS are usually abnormal.
- General: Is the child alert or lethargic? Interested in surroundings? Consolable or irritable? Happy and playful?
- HEENT: Is the anterior fontanelle flat, depressed, or bulging? Are there tears with crying? Are mucous membranes moist? Is the oropharynx erythematous with exudates? Are the tympanic membranes red or bulging and are landmarks discernible? Are the conjunctivae clear? Is there nasal discharge?
- Neck: Is there nuchal rigidity? Are cervical nodes enlarged and tender?
- Lungs: Are breath sounds equal? Are there crackles, wheezes, rales, stridor, or grunting? Is there nasal flaring or retractions?
- Cardiovascular (CV): Are heart sounds regular? Murmurs, gallops, or rubs? What is the capillary refill?
- Abdomen/genitourinary (Abd/GU): Are bowel sounds present? Is there tenderness on palpation? In neonates does the umbilicus look clean and dry? Is there any erythema or swelling of the penis or scrotum?
- Extremities (Ext): Are there any warm or swollen joints? Is there full range of motion (ROM)? Does the child limp?
- Skin: Does it appear mottled? Is there a rash and where is it located?

DON'T FORGET

On exam day, the patient will have

- Meningitis/encephalitis
- Kawasaki disease
- Rocky Mountain spotted fever
- Sepsis especially if 0-90 days of life
- Osteomyelitis/septic arthritis
- Occult pneumonia
- Occult bacteremia

DON'T FORGET

All children younger than 3 months with fever have a serious bacterial infection until proven otherwise.

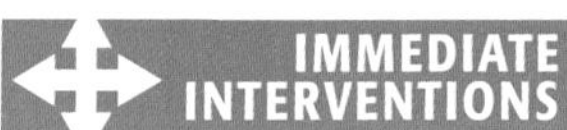

IMMEDIATE INTERVENTIONS

- Address ABCs.
- Cardiac monitor and supplemental O_2 for kids who are toxic-appearing or in shock.
- IV with rapid 0.9% NS bolus (20 cc/kg) for kids with severe dehydration or poor perfusion. Obtain bloodwork and cultures for future lab orders.
- Order antibiotics for any child who is possibly septic or meningitic within the first 30 minutes of arrival.

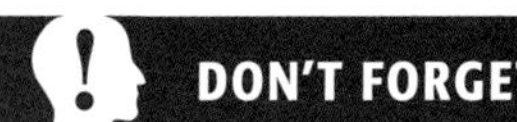

DON'T FORGET

Toxic-appearing = lethargic, weak cry, little interest in environment, poor perfusion, hypo- or hyperventilating, hypo-or hypertonia

DIFFERENTIAL DIAGNOSIS

The differential diagnosis for fever in the pediatric patient is extensive.

- Fever of unknown etiology: The risk of a serious occult infection rises with the degree of fever. Although most patients seen in the emergency department (ED) will likely have an underlying viral infection, serious occult bacterial infections must be ruled out first. All toxic-appearing children, regardless of age or degree of temperature, get a full septic workup and admission for appropriate intravenous (IV) antibiotic therapy until culture results are known. In otherwise well-appearing children, the diagnostic and therapeutic approach varies by age.
- Occult bacteremia: This refers to bacteria found on blood culture in an otherwise well-appearing child with no obvious source of infection. In infants >2 months, *Streptococcus pneumoniae* is the predominant agent involved. In infants <2 months, organisms primarily responsible include *Escherichia coli*, group B *Streptococcus*, and *Listeria*.
- Pneumonia: In febrile children >3 months, a chest x-ray (CXR) should be considered when the fever is ≥39°C (102.2°F) and the physical examination reveals tachypnea with or without associated fever, nasal flaring, retractions, crackles, rales, decreased breath sounds, or grunting. Obtain a CXR in children <3 months for any symptoms indicative of pulmonary disease such as tachypnea without fever, decreased breath sounds, rales, wheezing, grunting, stridor, nasal flaring, retractions, or cough.
- Urinary tract infection (UTI): In infants and young children, symptoms may be nonspecific and include vomiting, diarrhea, and/or irritability. Urine should be obtained by transurethral catheterization as this method has the lowest risk of contamination. Urinalysis (UA) and culture are part of the septic workup and should also be obtained in infants/children at risk for UTI with no other apparent source for fever. This includes any child with a history of UTIs as well as females <2 years, uncircumcised males <1 year, and circumcised males <6 months and with a fever of 39°C (102.2°F) or higher.
- Meningitis: A lumbar puncture (LP) should be performed on all febrile patients <28 days old, on patients <90 days old who are ill-appearing or who have abnormal labs, and in all patients with meningismus. In neonates, consider group B Strep, *Listeria*, and *E coli*. In infants >3 months, *S pneumoniae* and *Neisseria meningitides* are primarily responsible. From 1 to 3 months, there is some overlap of organisms. Viral sources of meningitis, such as enterovirus and herpes simplex virus (HSV), should also be considered.
- Clinically identifiable source of fever: Your goal is to rule out life-threatening entities. This category can be further subdivided into diseases associated with a rash and diseases associated with joint pain.
- Fever and rash: Although most children will have a viral infection, other etiologies which require urgent treatment must first be considered. The following are "can't miss" diseases—both in real life and on test day:
    - Meningococcemia refers to an invasive infectious disease caused by the gram-negative diplococcus *N meningitides*. Symptoms of fever, malaise, and rash can begin abruptly and progress rapidly to disseminated intravascular coagulation (DIC), CV collapse, and death. The rash may initially be maculopapular. A generalized petechial rash and/or purpura develop as the disease progresses. Palms and soles are frequently involved. Most cases occur in children <5 years with a peak incidence in the <6-month age group. The mortality rate is 10%. Transmission occurs via respiratory droplets, so all close contacts (family members, school contacts, etc) must receive chemoprophylaxis.
    - Rocky Mountain spotted fever (RMSF) is a rickettsial disease transmitted by the bite of an infected tick. RMSF results in a systemic small vessel vasculitis. Usually seen between April and September, fever is present in nearly all patients and may precede other symptoms by a week or more. A rash usually appears on the fourth day of illness and usually starts on the extremities (including palms and soles) and spreads centrally to the

DON'T FORGET

Fever is defined as a *rectal* temperature of 38°C (100.4°F) or higher. Keep in mind that rectal temp ≤36°C (96.8°F) can also be associated with SBI in infants. In the newborn the child may present with hypothermia, hypothermic infant <36 usually require a full septic workup.

DON'T FORGET

- Vomiting and diarrhea must be present for a diagnosis of acute gastroenteritis.
- The patient must have had two doses of Hib vaccine (scheduled for 2 and 4 months) to be considered at low risk for *Haemophilus influenzae* type b.

DON'T FORGET

Rectal temperature is considered the most accurate. Do not accept any other method of measurement on exam day.

DON'T FORGET

Febrile infants with bulging fontanelles have meningitis until proven otherwise.

DON'T FORGET

DDx Summary

- All toxic-appearing children and those suspected of having meningitis get a full septic workup and admission for IV antibiotics regardless of age or temp. The child that is in septic shock or respiratory failure or requiring intubation may have his lumbar puncture postponed until they get more stabilized. But aggressive IVF and early antibiotics should be given.
- Fever with rash
  - Meningococcemia
  - RMSF
  - KD
  - Cellulitis
- Fever with joint pain
  - Osteomyelitis
  - Septic arthritis

trunk. Mortality rate of 3%-7% in treated patients and increases to 30%-70% when the diagnosis and subsequent treatment are delayed.

- Kawasaki disease (KD) is a systemic vasculitic disease of unknown etiology. Most cases occur in children <5 years, with a peak incidence between 18 and 24 months. Although seen year round, the highest incidence is in the late winter/spring months. KD involves most organ systems, but long-term prognosis is primarily determined by coronary artery involvement. Coronary artery aneurysms develop in up to 25% of untreated patients and predispose the patient to subsequent rupture, stenosis, and myocardial infarction (MI). Major clinical findings are fever >5 days without other explanation, conjunctivitis, cervical adenopathy (usually one large node), mucus membrane changes (strawberry tongue or cracked lips), and rash (may be polymorphic but is classically desquamating).

- Cellulitis is a skin infection involving the dermal and subcutaneous layers. Common regions affected in children include the extremities, perianal area, and periorbital/orbital area. Simple cellulitis usually results from a break in the skin and is caused by *Staphylococcus aureus* or Strep (group A or B). *Pasteurella multocida* is prevalent following cat and dog bites. Periorbital cellulitis is limited to the preseptal portion of the eye. It has decreased in incidence since the advent of the *H influenzae* vaccine. Orbital cellulitis can occur as a complication of sinusitis and represents a true emergency.
- Fever and joint pain: Clinically evident causes of fever can also involve joints and can represent both benign and severe etiologies.
  - Osteomyelitis is a bone infection most commonly caused by *S aureus*. Other organisms to consider include group B Strep in neonates, *Salmonella* in children with sickle cell disease, and *Pseudomonas aeruginosa* in children with a puncture wound of the foot. This can be due to hematogenous spread of an infection or as a result of direct infection from a local source of trauma.
  - Septic arthritis is a joint infection most commonly caused by *S aureus*. Other organisms to consider include group B Strep in neonates and *Neisseria gonorrhea* in sexually active adolescents. See Chap. 36 for further information.

FEVER OF UNKNOWN ETIOLOGY: 0-1-MONTH AGE GROUP

Additional History and Physical Examination Findings

- Birth history: Any pre- or postnatal complications including prematurity, premature rupture of membranes, maternal fever, ventilator support, STI, and group B Strep status of mother.
- Any temperature ≥38°C (100.4°F) or ≤36°C (96.8°F) is significant in this age group and requires evaluation for serious bacterial infection (SBI).
- Determine if the patient is toxic-appearing.
- During physical examination, look for focus of infection.
  - Anterior fontanelle may be bulging in the case of meningitis or depressed if the patient is dehydrated.
  - Check the umbilical area for redness and foul-smelling discharge (omphalitis).
  - Skin: Check for jaundice and for a vesicular rash that could indicate infection with HSV.

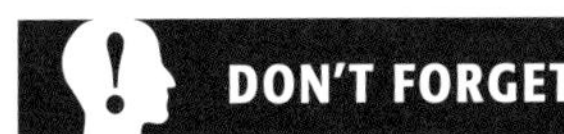

DON'T FORGET

The introduction of the pneumococcal vaccine has significantly reduced the occurrence of occult bacteremia from pneumococcus. Even one dose is highly protective.

Review Initial Results

- Complete blood count (CBC) with differential (diff): Although frequently obtained, this adds limited value to the workup as the lack of an elevated white blood cell (WBC) count will not likely change your management.
- UA: WBC ≥ 5/HPF, positive nitrites, positive leukocyte esterase, or bacteriuria are suggestive of UTI. However, a negative UA does not rule out UTI in this age group. If an infant is <90 days old, obtain a urine culture. A UA

concerning for UTI should prompt consideration of an LP due to the concern of bacterial seeding in this age group.

- Cerebrospinal fluid (CSF): Findings suggestive of bacterial meningitis include a low glucose level (<40 mg/dL), an elevated protein level (>150-170 mg/dL in neonates), and an elevated WBC (>500/mm^3 with up to 22 WBC/mm^3 is normal in neonates). Gram stain is only significant if positive.
- CXR (if obtained): Look for focal infiltrates.

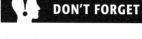

DON'T FORGET

Full septic workup includes cultures of blood, urine, and CSF.

Risk Stratification: Management Priorities

- Strategies used to determine which infants are at low risk for SBI (Rochester and Philadelphia criteria) miss a significant number of neonates <1 month with serious illness and are therefore unreliable in this age group.
- All febrile infants in this age group are admitted for IV antibiotic therapy until culture results return.
- Infants who are toxic-appearing, or are suspected of having meningitis, should have antibiotics started within 30 minutes of arrival, regardless of whether an LP has been performed.

DON'T FORGET

Physical examinations are unreliable in excluding SBI in this age group. Often no meningismus is seen in infants.

Definitive Management

- Empiric IV antibiotic therapy includes:
  - Ampicillin 25-50 mg/kg/dose and either gentamicin 2.5 mg/kg/dose or cefotaxime 50 mg/kg/dose.
  - Consider adding acyclovir if HSV infection is considered or if infant is <14 days old.

Frequent Reassessment

- Toxic-appearing patients and patients in shock require frequent reassessment of vitals and hydration status.

Disposition

- Admission for empiric antibiotic therapy pending culture results.
- Toxic-appearing infants or infants with meningitis are admitted to the pediatric intensive care unit (PICU).
- Well-appearing infants are admitted to the pediatric floor.

1-3-MONTH AGE GROUP

Additional History and Physical Examination Findings

- Birth history: Any pre- or postnatal complications including prematurity, premature rupture of membranes, maternal fever, ventilator support, STI, and group B Strep status of mother.
- Temperatures ≥38°C (100.4°F) are significant in this age group and require a high suspicion for SBI.
- Determine if the infant is toxic-appearing.
- On physical examination, look for signs of infection.
  - Anterior fontanelle may be bulging (Fig. 32-1) in the case of meningitis or depressed if the patient is dehydrated.
  - Neck: Check for nuchal rigidity (can be very unreliable in this age group, so maintain a high index of suspicion).
  - Skin: Look for rashes. Petechial rash and/or purpura are seen with meningococcemia.

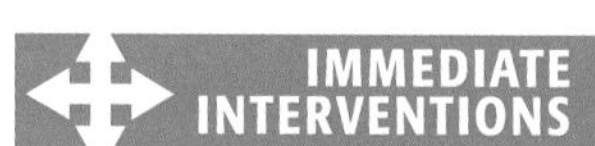

- 100% O_2 and consider intubation if obtunded.
- IV with fluid resuscitation as needed using 0.9 NS boluses (20 cc/kg).
- Order CBC with diff, blood culture, UA, urine culture (by catheterization), CSF studies (cell count, glucose, protein, Gram stain, and culture).
- Order CXR if patient is having respiratory symptoms and stool study with diarrhea.

Review Initial Results

- CBC with diff: Children with WBC counts ≥15,000 or a bandemia have a higher risk of bacteremia and LP should be considered.

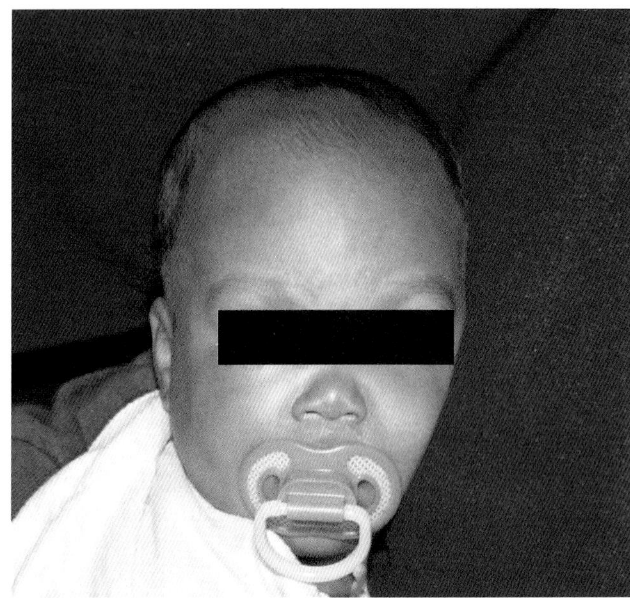

Figure 32-1. The anterior fontanelle is normally open in infants (it usually closes between 9 and 18 months), and is pulsatile and slightly depressed in an infant in an upright position. The anterior fontanelle may appear full in an infant lying in a supine position or during crying. A bulging anterior fontanelle suggests increased ICP from any etiology (eg, meningitis, tumor, hydrocephalus). *(Reproduced with permission from Shah BR, Lucchesi M.* Atlas of Pediatric Emergency Medicine. *New York, NY: McGraw-Hill; 2006).*

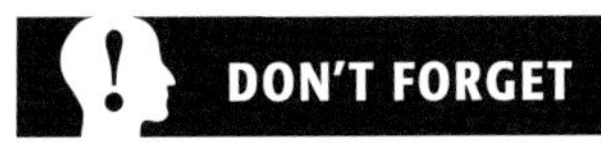

DON'T FORGET

Meningeal signs are also unreliable in this age group.

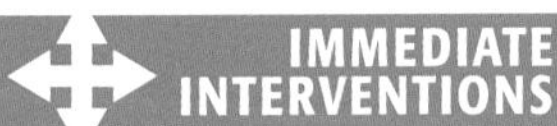

IMMEDIATE INTERVENTIONS

Toxic-appearing/meningismic, any age

- Full septic workup

Well-appearing with fever <28 days

- Full septic workup

Well-appearing, 29-90 days

- CBC/diff
- UA and urine culture
- Blood culture
- LP with meningismus, if toxic-appearing, with leukocytosis, positive UA, or if planning to discharge home on empiric antibiotics
- CXR if clinically indicated

- UA: WBC ≥ 5/HPF, positive nitrates, positive leukocyte esterase, or bacteriuria are considered suggestive of a UTI. However, a negative UA does not rule out UTI in this age group. Obtain a urine culture. A UA concerning for UTI should prompt consideration of an LP due to the concern of bacterial seeding in this age group.
- CSF: Findings suggestive of bacterial meningitis include a low glucose level (<40 mg/dL), an elevated protein level (>100 mg/Dl), and a WBC count >9 WBC/microL); Gram stain is only significant if positive.
- CXR (if obtained): Look for focal infiltrates.

Risk Stratification: Management Priorities

Several strategies have been offered to manage febrile infants in this age group by determining which infants are at low risk for SBI based on several different criteria (Table 32-1).

- Philadelphia criteria
  - Low-risk patients were sent home with no antibiotics but close follow-up.
  - Higher-risk patients were hospitalized and given empiric antibiotics pending culture results. The sensitivity for identifying patients with SBI was 98% and the specificity was 42%.
- Rochester criteria
  - Low-risk patients were sent home with no antibiotics but close follow-up.
  - Higher-risk patients were admitted for empiric antibiotic therapy. The sensitivity of these criteria was 92% with a specificity of 50%.

Table 32-1. Philadelphia and Rochester Criteria for Identifying Low-Risk Infants

	Philadelphia Criteria for Low Risk	Rochester Criteria for Low Risk
Age	29-60 d	≤60 d
Temperature	≥38.2°C (100.7°F)	≥38°C (100.4°F)
Appearance	Well-appearing with normal PE	Well-appearing with no focal infection and previously healthy (term infants, no perinatal antimicrobial therapy, not hospitalized longer than the mother)
White blood cell count	<15,000/mm^3	≥5000 and ≤15,000/mm^3
Band neutrophil ratio	<0.2	Absolute band count <1500/mm^3
Urinalysis	WBC <10/HPF Negative urine Gram stain	WBC ≤10/HPF
CSF	WBC <8/mm^3 Negative Gram stain	
Chest x-ray (if obtained)	Negative	
Stool (if obtained)	No blood and few or no WBCs on smear	WBC ≤5/HPF

Further Diagnostic Considerations

- Infants who are toxic-appearing, in shock, or suspected of having meningitis should have a full septic workup.
- For 1-28 days and well-appearing, most algorithms include a full septic workup.
- For 29-90 days and well-appearing, the approach is more controversial.
  - CBC, blood culture, UA, and urine cultures should be obtained.
  - Whether an LP needs to be performed is a matter of clinical acumen. For purposes of the oral board exam, if the patient has any signs of toxicity or meningitis, perform an LP. Do not place the patient on empiric antibiotics if an LP is not performed. A well-appearing febrile infant >28 days with negative labs may be discharged home without antibiotics if they have next day follow-up and have a reliable caregiver. Consider calling their primary care physician (PCP) to assure they have an appointment made.
  - Toxic-appearing infants and patients in shock require frequent reassessment of vitals and hydration status.

Definitive Management

- Toxic-appearing infants receive admission and empiric IV antibiotics.
  - 1-28 days of age receive ampicillin *plus* cefotaxime (not ceftriaxone) or gentamicin.
  - 29-90 days of age receive cefotaxime or ceftriaxone and vancomycin for cases of meningitis.
  - Antibiotics need to be ordered within 30 minutes of arrival.
    - Treatment should not be delayed for LP or while waiting for lab results to return.
- Well-appearing infants:
  - 1-28 days of age

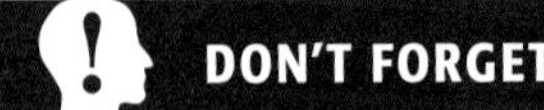
DON'T FORGET

When deciding whether or not to discharge on empiric antibiotics, consider the pros and cons.

Pros

- Prevent progression of bacteremia to more SBI.

Cons

- May perpetuate antibiotic resistance.
- Risk of allergic reactions.

- If the preliminary examination or lab values indicate a possible SBI, then the patients should be admitted for IV antibiotics (ampicillin plus cefotaxime or gentamicin) until culture results are known.
- Patients can be admitted for observation pending results of cultures, particularly if follow-up cannot be guaranteed.

- 29-90 days of age
  - Patients can be admitted for observation pending results of cultures, particularly if follow-up cannot be guaranteed.
  - Patients with reliable follow-up can be discharged with or without empiric antibiotics, (if they are to receive outpatient antibiotics they require negative preliminary LP results).
  - If the UA is suggestive for a UTI, discharge on cefdinir if looks well, not vomiting, and follow-up is reliable. Otherwise admit for IV ceftriaxone and hydration. It is generally advised to admit children <2 months with UTI.

Infant is ≤28 days with fever of ≥38 on single rectal temperature (or a reliable history of fever) or ill-appearing or concern for HSV or premature <37 weeks with underlying medical condition
Yes
No
Full Septic Workup
• CBC w diff
• Blood culture
• UA with culture
• CSF with culture
• CXR (if clinically indicated)
• Viral studies
Any positive or abnormal result
Limited Testing
• CBC w diff
• Blood culture
• UA with culture
• Consider viral studies
Positive Results/High Risk
• UA positive for LE, nitrites, bacteria, >10 WBCS/hpf
• CBC: WBC <5000 or >15,000
• CBC: Bandemia (absolute count > 1,500)
• ≤28 days of age, prematurity, or underlying condition
Abnormal CSF
• 1-28 days: >18 WBCs
• 29-90 days: >9 WBCs
• Grossly bloody tap: >10,000 RBCs
High Risk OR Abnormal CSF
Normal results
Low Risk
No treatment OR Antibiotics (perform LP first)

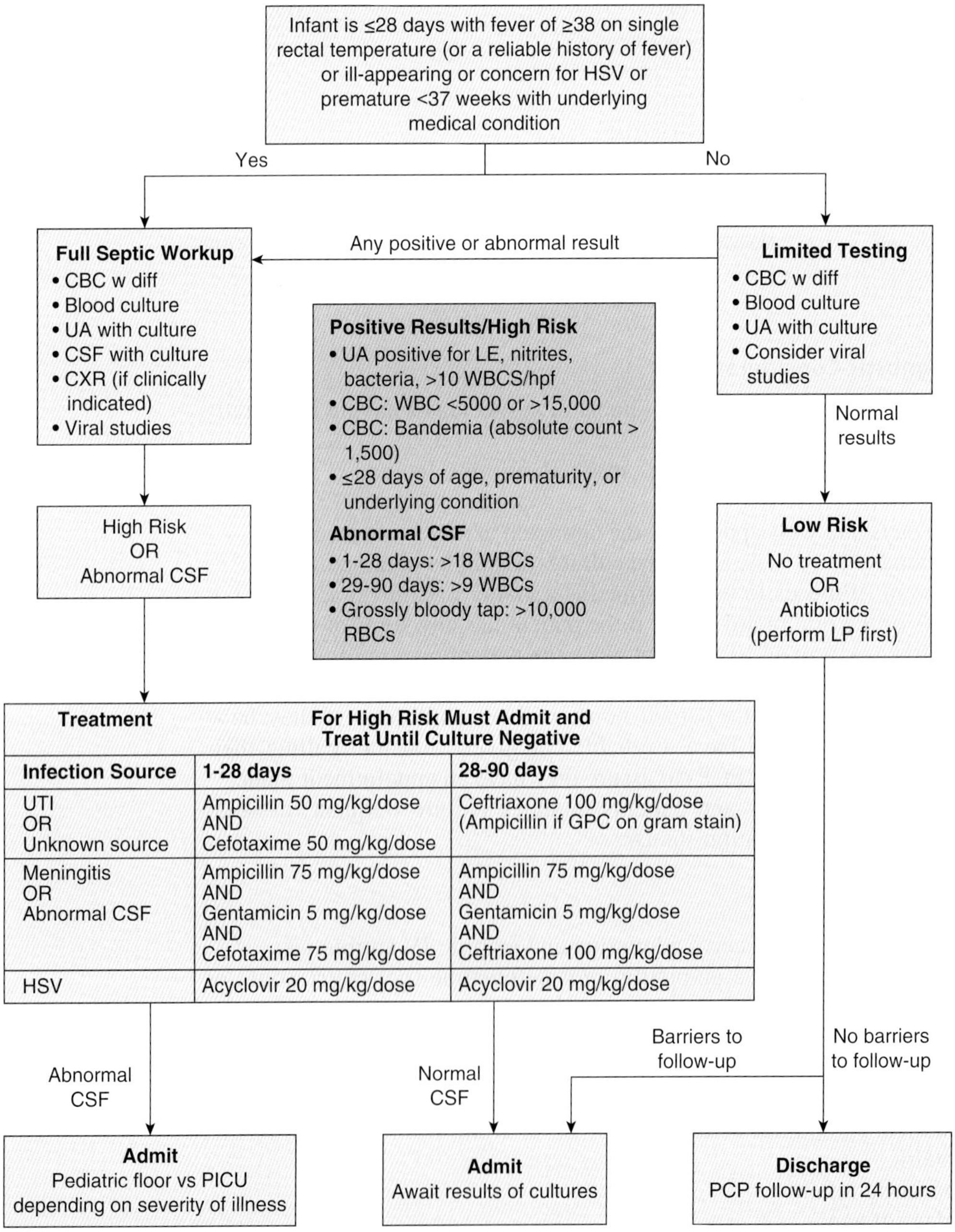

Treatment	For High Risk Must Admit and Treat Until Culture Negative	
Infection Source	**1-28 days**	**28-90 days**
UTI OR Unknown source	Ampicillin 50 mg/kg/dose AND Cefotaxime 50 mg/kg/dose	Ceftriaxone 100 mg/kg/dose (Ampicillin if GPC on gram stain)
Meningitis OR Abnormal CSF	Ampicillin 75 mg/kg/dose AND Gentamicin 5 mg/kg/dose AND Cefotaxime 75 mg/kg/dose	Ampicillin 75 mg/kg/dose AND Gentamicin 5 mg/kg/dose AND Ceftriaxone 100 mg/kg/dose
HSV	Acyclovir 20 mg/kg/dose	Acyclovir 20 mg/kg/dose

Abnormal CSF
Normal CSF
Barriers to follow-up
No barriers to follow-up
Admit
Pediatric floor vs PICU depending on severity of illness
Admit
Await results of cultures
Discharge
PCP follow-up in 24 hours

Figure 32-2. Febrile infant algorithm.

3-36-MONTH AGE GROUP

Additional History and Physical Examination Findings

- Fevers ≥39°C (102.2°F) are associated with a higher risk of a serious occult bacterial infection, though most will still be viral in origin.
- Your goal is to identify children who may have meningitis and who appear toxic.
  - Fever and altered mental status is meningitis until proven otherwise.
  - Look for nuchal rigidity as the reliability of Kernig and Brudzinski signs increase with ages. Absence of meningeal signs does not necessarily rule out meningitis.
  - Check fontanelle: Bulging may represent increased intracranial pressure (ICP) secondary to meningitis.
  - Perform a baseline neurologic examination if meningitis is in the differential.
  - Look for rashes: Purpura or petechiae below the nipple line are seen with meningococcemia. (See Table 32-2.)

Review Initial Results

- CBC with diff: High WBC counts (≥15,000/mm^3) have been shown to occur more frequently with bacterial infections than viral; however, the specificity and sensitivity are low.
- UA (if obtained): WBC ≥5/HPF, positive nitrates, positive leukocyte esterase, or Gram stain positive for bacteria are considered suggestive of a UTI. A negative UA does not rule out UTI in this age group. Urine culture is recommended in children 3-24 months. A UA positive for a UTI should prompt consideration of an LP due to concern of bacterial seeding in this age group.
- CXR (if obtained): Look for focal infiltrates.
- CSF (if obtained): Findings suggestive of bacterial meningitis include a low glucose level (<40 mg/dL), an elevated protein level (>100 mg/Dl), and a WBC count >9 WBC/microL); Gram stain is only significant if positive.

Further Diagnostic Considerations

- Infants who are toxic-appearing, in shock, or suspected of having meningitis should have a full septic workup (Fig. 32-2).
- For infants who are well-appearing, with no focus for infection by examination, check the following:
  - UA and urine culture by catheterization if in high-risk category.
  - CBC with diff and blood culture
    - Option 1: Send blood culture of all children in this age group with fevers ≥39°C (102.2°F). Only send for CBC if the result would influence your decision on whether or not to start empiric antibiotics.
    - Option 2: Send CBC with diff. Only send blood culture if WBC count is ≥15000/mm^3.
    - Option 3: No blood tests done.

Definitive Management

- Toxic-appearing or meningitic infants receive empiric IV cefotaxime or ceftriaxone.
  - Add vancomycin if patient has meningitis.
  - Treatment is not delayed for LP or other labs to return.
  - LP may be deferred if patient is too unstable.
- Well-appearing infants:
  - Admit for observation pending results of cultures, particularly if follow-up cannot be guaranteed.

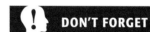

DON'T FORGET

Temperatures of 39°C (102.2°F) or higher are considered significant in this age group.

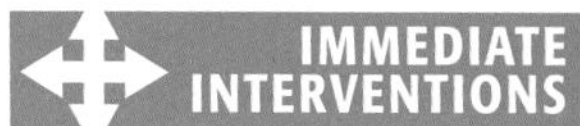

IMMEDIATE INTERVENTIONS

Toxic-appearing/meningeal

- Full septic workup

Well-appearing

- CBC with diff (optional)
- UA and urine culture if patient is in high risk category for UTI. (Urine culture recommended in children between ages 3 and 24 months.)
- Blood culture (optional)
- CXR with respiratory symptoms

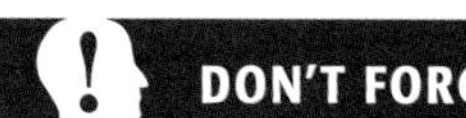

DON'T FORGET

Patients considered at high risk for UTI include those with prior history of UTI, females <2 years, uncircumcised males <1 years, and circumcised males <6 months.

- Patients with reliable follow-up can be discharged with or without empiric antibiotics.
- If the UA is suggestive for a UTI:
  - Discharge on cefdinir if not vomiting and follow-up is reliable.
  - Otherwise admit for IV ceftriaxone and hydration.

Frequent Reassessment

- Toxic-appearing infants and patients in shock require frequent reassessment of vitals and hydration status.

Complications

- Patients with occult bacteremia can progress to an SBI (ie, meningitis, osteomyelitis) if untreated.
- Pyelonephritis that remains undiagnosed and untreated for >5 days has an increased risk of causing renal scarring.

Disposition

- Toxic-appearing or meningitic infants are admitted to the PICU for appropriate IV antibiotic therapy.
- Well-appearing infants without focus for fever by examination or lab may be discharged with or without empiric antibiotics and follow-up in 24 hours.
- UTI.
  - Looks well and no vomiting: Discharge on cefdinir.
  - Otherwise: Admit for IV antibiotics and hydration.

FEVER ASSOCIATED WITH RASH

Table 32-2. Febrile Illnesses and Rashes

Illness	Rash
Meningococcemia	Maculopapular rash progresses to petechiae and purpura
Cellulitis	Erythematous, warm lesions with sharply demarcated borders
Rocky Mountain spotted fever	Papules appear first over palms and soles and spread to trunk
Kawasaki disease	Involvement of mucous membranes, maculopapular rash over trunk, and desquamation of fingers at 2 weeks

MENINGOCOCCEMIA

Additional History and Physical Examination Findings

- Typically, present with a history of sudden onset of fevers, rash, and lethargy.
- May have vomiting.
- Older children may report headaches or myalgias.
- Most children are septic-appearing on presentation with lethargy, poor perfusion, and hypo- or hyperventilating.
- May show signs of shock.

- Early (compensated/normotensive) shock: Poor perfusion, tachycardia, normal blood pressure
- Late (decompensated/hypotensive) shock: Tachycardia → bradycardia, hypotension

- Skin (see Fig. 32-3).
  - Initially may have a maculopapular rash which becomes petechial and/or purpuric as the illness progresses.
  - Purpura fulminans: Large areas of cutaneous hemorrhage and necrosis associated with DIC; presence indicates a poor prognosis
- If DIC is present, may have bleeding at needlestick sites or from the oral mucosa.

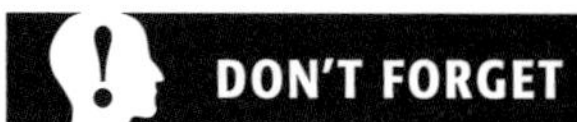

DON'T FORGET

Fever with purpura or petechiae below the nipple line is meningococcemia until proven otherwise.

Review Initial Results

- CBC with diff: WBC usually elevated (>15,000/HPF) with a left shift.
- Elevated prothrombin time (PT), partial thromboplastin time (PTT), and thrombocytopenia seen with DIC.
- CSF (if performed): Findings consistent with concurrent meningitis. Gram stain showing gram-negative diplococci is diagnostic.

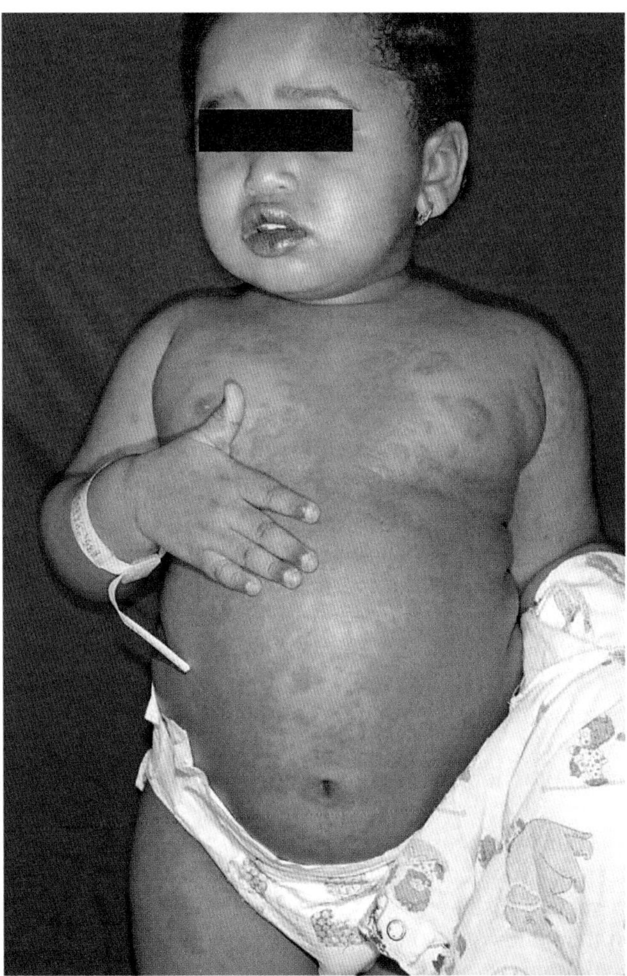

Figure 32-3. A 3-year-old child with a history of high fever of 6 days' duration associated with diffuse erythematous maculopapular rash, red lips, and bilateral conjunctival injection. *(Reproduced with permission from Shah BR, Lucchesi M.* Atlas of Pediatric Emergency Medicine. *New York, NY: McGraw-Hill; 2006.)*

IMMEDIATE INTERVENTIONS

- Toxic-appearing or in shock
- 100% O_2 via nonrebreather and consider intubation if obtunded.
- IV with fluid resuscitation, as needed, using 0.9% NS boluses (20 cc/kg).
- Order CBC with diff, platelets, PT, PTT, blood culture, CSF studies (cell count, protein, glucose, Gram stain, and culture).
- If patient is unstable, LP can be deferred.
- Order antibiotics to run ASAP regardless of whether LP has been or will be performed.

Risk Stratification: Management Priorities

- Any patient suspected of having meningococcemia must be placed on respiratory isolation.
- Antibiotics must be started immediately (goal is within 30 minutes of presentation).

Definitive Management

- Antibiotics: Cefotaxime 100 mg/kg/d divided QID or ceftriaxone 100 mg/kg/d IV plus vancomycin if patient has meningitis and organism has not been identified by Gram stain.
- Circulatory support
  - IV 0.9% NS boluses of 20 cc/kg until perfusion improves (may require >60 cc/kg).
  - Consider inotropic support if patient continues to show signs of shock despite fluid resuscitation.
- Treatment of DIC
  - Vitamin K.
  - Fresh frozen plasma (FFP) 8-12 mg/kg every 12 hours.
  - Consider platelet transfusion.

Complications

- Septic shock, DIC, meningitis, pericarditis, Waterhouse–Friderichsen syndrome (bilateral adrenal hemorrhage), gangrene of an extremity requiring amputation, death.

Disposition

- Admission to PICU for IV antibiotics and treatment of shock and DIC.

ROCKY MOUNTAIN SPOTTED FEVER

Additional History and Physical Examination Findings

- Onset 1-2 weeks following tick bite that patient may or may not remember.
- Travel history: Although seen throughout the United States, highest incidence is in southeastern and southern states.
- Symptoms typically start abruptly, though some cases have a more insidious onset.
- Almost all patients have fever, but this may precede other symptoms by a week.
- Other common symptoms include frontal headache, myalgias, nausea, vomiting, and anorexia.
- Malaise and photophobia.
- Rash
  - Appears around the fourth day of illness.
  - Initial lesions may be pinkish papules before progressing to the more classic petechial rash.
  - Starts on the hands and soles and spreads within hours to the trunk.
- Splenomegaly may be present.

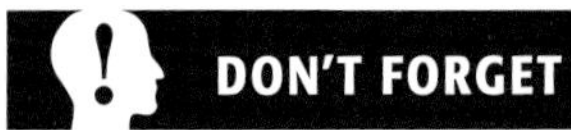

DON'T FORGET

Do not rely on a history of tick bite to make the diagnosis.

Review Initial Results

- CBC: WBC usually normal; may reveal anemia with low platelets
- Electrolytes: May have hyponatremia
- Electrocardiogram (ECG) for rhythm abnormalities

Risk Stratification: Management Priorities

- Highest incidence occurs during April through September.
- Treatment must be initiated presumptively as delays in waiting for titers can result in significant morbidity and mortality.

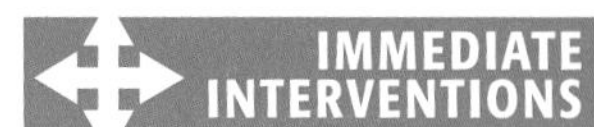

- Order CBC, platelets, electrolytes, ECG.
- Send acute titer: Definitive diagnosis rests on acute and convalescent blood titers showing a fourfold change.

Definitive Management

- Antibiotics
  - Doxycycline in children >8 years and children of any age with moderate to severe disease; 1.5 mg/kg/dose bid PO or IV.
  - Chloramphenicol in children <8 years with mild disease because of the risk of teeth staining seen with tetracyclines; 75 mg/kg/d divided every 6 hours PO or IV.

Complications

- Delay in treatment may result in DIC, shock, encephalopathy, GI bleeding, or myocarditis.
- Mortality rates.
  - In treated patients: 3%-7%
  - When diagnosis is delayed: 30%-70%

Disposition

- Admit patients with moderate to severe disease for IV antibiotics.
- Discharge patients with mild disease on oral antibiotics if close follow-up can be assured.

KAWASAKI DISEASE

Additional History and Physical Examination Findings

- For the diagnosis of "classic disease" patients must have a 5-day history of fevers of 38-41°C (100.4-105.8°F) plus four of the following:
  - Mucous membrane changes
    - Cracked, red lips
    - Strawberry tongue
    - Pharyngeal erythema
  - Bilateral conjunctival injection without discharge
  - Polymorphous, erythematous rash primarily over the trunk which can be morbilliform or maculopapular.
  - Extremity changes
    - Peripheral edema
    - Erythema of hands and feet
    - Desquamation of fingers, palms, and/or soles (usually occurs 2 weeks after the start of illness) (Fig. 32-4).
  - Unilateral cervical lymphadenopathy ≥1.5 cm
- "Atypical" KD occurs when classic criteria are not met.
- More common in children <1 year.
- Fever and rash are typically present.
- Other symptoms include irritability, abdominal pain, arthralgias, headache, and cough.
- Patients may have meningeal signs, jaundice, or hepatomegaly on examination.

Review Initial Results

- CBC with diff: Elevated WBC with left shift is common. Anemia and thrombocytosis may also be seen.

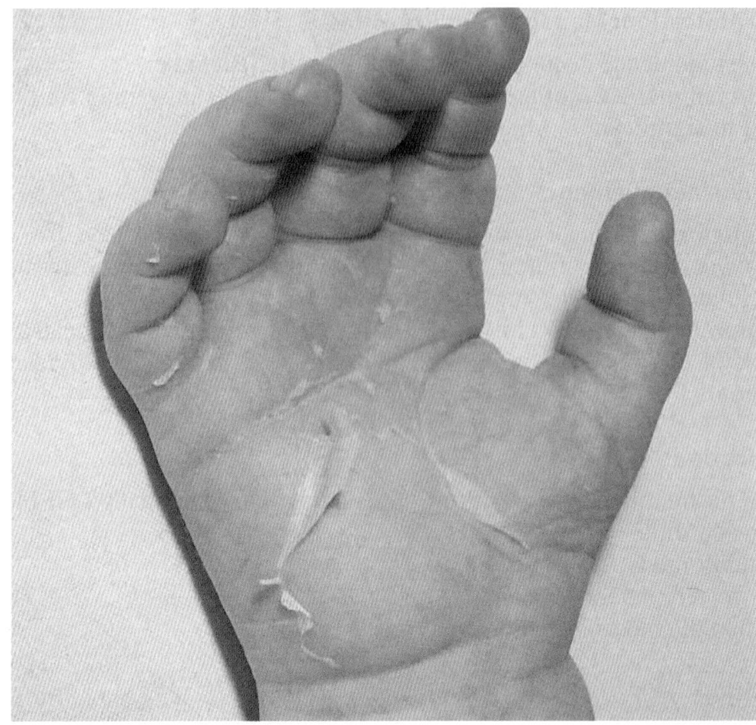

Figure 32-4. Kawasaki disease. Shedding of the epidermis on the palm of this child 10 days after the acute illness. *(Reprinted with permission from Wolff K, Johnson RA.* Fitzpatrick's Color Atlas and Synopsis of Clinical Dermatology. *6th ed. New York, NY: McGraw-Hill; 2009.)*

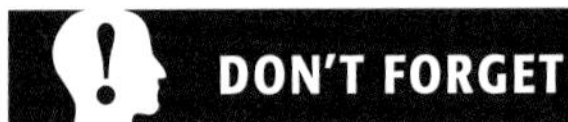

DON'T FORGET

Must rule out KD in any patient with ≥5 days of fever.

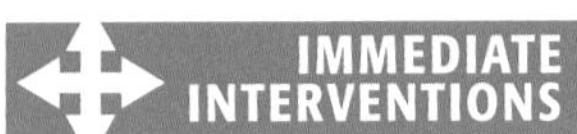

IMMEDIATE INTERVENTIONS

- CBC with diff, platelets
- ESR or CRP
- UA
- LFTs
- ECG
- CXR
- Arrange echo and cardiology consult

- Erythrocyte sedimentation rate (ESR), C-reactive protein (CRP): Elevated.
- UA: Sterile pyuria may be seen try to get a noncatheterized urine.
- Liver function tests (LFTs): Elevated transaminases and bilirubin may be seen.
- ECG: May have nonspecific ST-T wave changes or low voltage. Check ECG if having chest pain for signs of an acute MI.
- CXR: May show infiltrates or an enlarged heart.

Risk Stratification: Management Priorities

- Patients at highest risk for coronary artery aneurysms
  - Males
  - Age <1 year or >8 years
  - Fever >10-day duration
  - Low hemoglobin
  - Thrombocytopenia

Definitive Treatment

- Intravenous immunoglobulin (IVIG): 2 g/kg over 6-12 hours.
- High-dose acetylsalicylic acid (ASA): 80 mg/kg/d divided QID; dose is reduced once patient is afebrile for 4-5 days.
- Cardiology consult for echo to determine presence of coronary artery involvement.
- Treat acute MI as would for adults.

Complications

- Myocarditis: Most common cause of death in the acute phase.
- Coronary artery aneurysm rupture: Common cause of death in the subacute phase.

- Acute MI: Common cause of death in the subacute phase and most common cause of death in the convalescent phase.

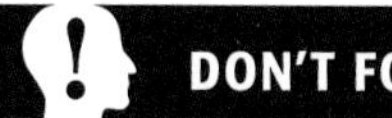

No lab test is diagnostic of KD.

Disposition

- Admission to hospital for IVIG, high-dose aspirin therapy, and echocardiogram.
- PICU admission for patients with abnormal ECGs, large coronary artery aneurysms, or acute MI.

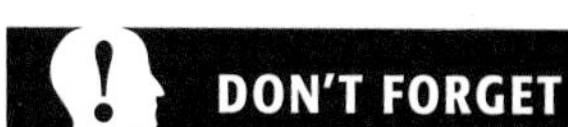

Early institution of IVIG decreases risk of coronary artery aneurysm.

CELLULITIS

Additional History and Physical Examination Findings

- May have systemic symptoms including fever, malaise, and chills.
- Infected areas are usually erythematous, edematous, warm, and tender.
- Lesions have irregular, but sharply demarcated, borders.
- Lesions may also develop vesicles, ulcers, or abscesses.
- May have regional lymphadenopathy and lymphangitis.
- Specific sites.
  - Perianal cellulitis: Well-defined area of erythema extending from the anus; associated symptoms include pain on defecation, blood-streaked stools, and pruritus.
  - Periorbital cellulitis: Unilateral lid swelling, erythema, and tenderness; normal eye movements; no proptosis or pain with eye movement; may have some conjunctival injection.
  - Orbital cellulitis: Unilateral periorbital swelling and erythema, eye pain with movement, ophthalmoplegia, proptosis, visual disturbances, usually also have a history consistent with sinusitis (headache, rhinorrhea, boggy nasal mucosa), usually ill-appearing, and may have conjunctival injection.

Review Initial Results

- CBC with diff: May be normal or show an increased WBC count with left shift.
- Computed tomography (CT) of facial bones/orbits with concern for orbital cellulitis.

DON'T FORGET

Swelling with periorbital cellulitis may be so severe that it is indistinguishable from orbital cellulitis due to limited examination. Treat as orbital cellulitis until the CT proves otherwise.

Definitive Management

- Antibiotics
  - Uncomplicated cellulitis: Oral augmentin, first- and second-generation cephalosporins, azithromycin, clindamycin, or dicloxacillin
  - Ill-appearing: IV cefazolin
  - Perianal cellulitis: Oral penicillin or erythromycin
  - Periorbital cellulitis
    - Not toxic-appearing, reliable follow-up: Clindamycin or trimethoprim-sulfamethoxazole plus one of the following: Amoxicillin, amoxicillin-clavulanic acid, cefpodoxime, or cefdinir. If discharged home needs follow-up examination in 24-48 hours.
    - Ill-appearing, systemic symptoms (eg, high fevers) or <1 year admit and treat per orbital cellulitis guidelines.
  - Orbital cellulitis.
    - IV vancomycin plus one of the following: ampicillin-sulbactam, pipericillin-tazobactam, ceftriaxone, or cefotaxime. Metronidazole can be added for anaerobic coverage.
    - Ophthalmology consult.
- Warm compresses to affected area

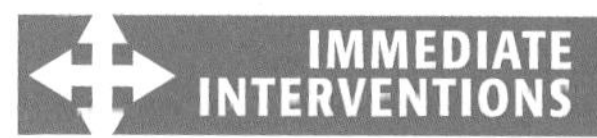

- Unless the patient is septic-appearing, labs are unnecessary in patients with simple cellulitis.
- Obtain blood culture in ill-appearing children.

Complications

- Local spread may lead to osteomyelitis, septic arthritis.
- Hematogenous spread may lead to meningitis, endocarditis.
- Sepsis.
- Orbital cellulitis may also result in blindness, cavernous sinus thrombosis, brain abscess, orbital/subperiosteal abscess and death.

Disposition

- Orbital cellulitis: Admit all for IV antibiotics.
- Periorbital cellulitis: Discharge if well-appearing with follow-up in 24 hours, otherwise admit for IV antibiotics.
- Uncomplicated cellulitis: Discharge on oral antibiotics with follow-up in 24 hours.
- Ill-appearing: Admit for IV antibiotics.

FEVER WITH JOINT PAIN

OSTEOMYELITIS

Additional History and Physical Examination Findings

- Neonates are frequently afebrile.
- In younger children/infants symptoms may be nonspecific and include fever, irritability, limp, or refusal to use affected limb.
- In older children, obtain a history of pain over infected bone.
  - May have other systemic symptoms including chills, malaise, nausea, and vomiting.
  - On examination, may have localized warmth, erythema, induration, and may have tenderness over infected bone.

Review Initial Results

- CBC with diff: Usually have an increased WBC with left shift.
- ESR, CRP are usually elevated.
- Plain films: Changes pathognomonic for osteomyelitis usually take 10-14 days to appear and include soft tissue swelling, periosteal changes, and lytic lesions secondary to bone demineralization. A normal film does not rule out osteomyelitis.

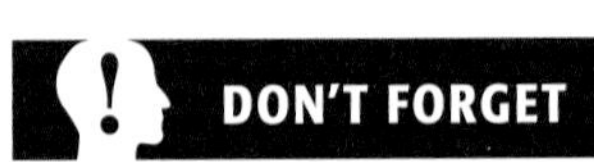

Limp and fever is osteomyelitis or septic hip until proven otherwise.

Further Diagnostic Considerations

- Bone scan to diagnose
  - More accurate than plain films early in disease, however, can still be falsely negative in first 1-2 day.

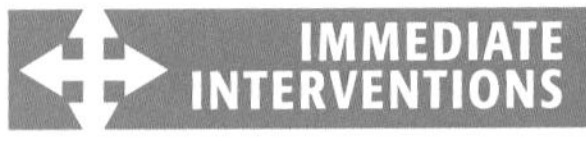

- CBC with diff
- ESR or CRP
- Plain films
- Blood cultures

Definitive Management

- IV antibiotics
  - Osteomyelitis: Penicillinase-resistant penicillin (nafcillin, oxacillin, methicillin) plus third-generation cephalosporin
  - Sickle cell patients: Third-generation cephalosporin
  - Foot following puncture wound: Ceftazidime

Complications

- Chronic osteomyelitis.
- Sepsis.
- Pathologic fractures.
- Septic arthritis.
- Shortened extremity if the epiphysis is involved.

Disposition

- Admit for IV antibiotics.
- Ortho consult to aspirate bone for culture.

Other Sources of Fever with Joint Pain

- Toxic/transient synovitis
- Septic arthritis
- These topics are covered in Chaps. 15 (adults) and 36 (pediatrics).

WINNING STRATEGIES

- Ask about immunizations. If they are not up-to-date, they are susceptible to other organisms (in particular *H influenzae*).
- Full septic workup includes CBC with diff, blood culture, UA with urine culture, and CSF.
- Hypothermia (temp ≤36°C [96.8°F]) in an infant should be treated as though the patient is septic.
- All toxic-appearing children get a full septic workup and admission for IV antibiotics, regardless of age or degree of temperature.
- All infants (0-1 month) get a full septic workup and admission for IV antibiotics when temperature is >38°C (100.4°F).
- Do not rely on meningeal signs to exclude meningitis in infants and young toddlers.
- Bulging fontanelles in febrile infants signify meningitis until proven otherwise.
- Fever and mental status change is meningitis or encephalitis until proven otherwise.
- Do not delay antibiotics in children who are suspected of having meningitis. Start within 30 minutes of arrival.
- Do not send children <3 months home on antibiotics unless an LP has been done.
- Obtain UA and urine cultures by transurethral catheterization. Get urine studies on all children with fevers ≥39°C (102.2°F) and without other source on exam who are at risk for UTI defined by prior history of UTI, females <2 years, uncircumcised males <1 years, and circumcised males <6 months.
- All febrile children with purpura or a petechial rash extending below the nipple line are presumed to have meningococcemia until proven otherwise.
- Do not rely on history of tick bite to diagnose RMSF.
- Consider KD in any patient with rash and at least a 5-day history of fever.
- Orbital cellulitis requires orbit and sinus CT and ophthalmology consult.
- Fever and limp is osteomyelitis or septic arthritis until proven otherwise.
- If an IV cannot be obtained on a child, do not forget to use an intraosseous (IO).

THE BOTTOM LINE

- Full septic workup and admission for IV antibiotics if toxic-appearing and/or ≤1 month.
- Full septic workup if 1-3 months, but may consider discharge if deemed at low risk for SBI.
- Febrile with purpura or petechiae below the nipple line = meningococcemia.
- Febrile with petechiae that started on hands and feet and spread centrally = RMSF.
- Febrile for at least 5 days with polymorphous rash = KD.
- Orbital cellulitis requires sinus/orbit CT.
- Febrile with limp = osteomyelitis or septic arthritis.

CHAPTER 33

Pediatric Shortness of Breath

Lindsey Caley, John Dayton, and Matthew Steimle

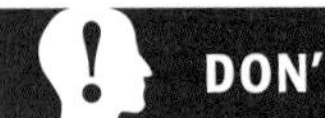

DON'T FORGET

On exam day, every child will be sick with an age-related cardiorespiratory diagnosis:

- Congenital heart disease
- Brief resolved unexplained event (BRUE) formerly known as apparent life-threatening event (ALTE)
- Bronchiolitis
- Croup
- Bacterial tracheitis
- Asthma
- Foreign body

INITIAL ASSESSMENT

- Immediate assessment of the sick patient and attention to airway, breathing, and circulation (ABCs).
- The initial evaluation and management of sick children is similar to that of adults; perform a rapid cardiopulmonary assessment and attention to the ABCs.
- Focus on age-related issues.
- History
- Physical examination
- Identify unstable patients with immediate life threats.
  - Central apnea
  - Airway obstruction
  - Respiratory failure
  - Decompensated congenital heart disease
- Rapidly identify available diagnostic or therapeutic interventions that will immediately aid your management.
- Know when to ask for help: Identify patients requiring consultation or transfer to higher level of care.

INITIAL HISTORY AND PHYSICAL EXAMINATION

- From-the-door assessment: Are they awake, playful, distressed, crying, unresponsive, limp, mottled, blue, ashen?
- Focus on age-related issues. Many conditions are age-specific.
- Developmental stages make some conditions more or less likely, eg, foreign body (FB) aspiration, toxic ingestion.
- History
  - Always ask about duration of symptoms, events surrounding onset of symptoms, rapidity of onset, and home treatments tried.
  - Identify associated symptoms (eg, cough, congestion, fever, etc) and ask about difficulty feeding, and work of breathing (WOB).
  - Ask if the child was born at term and note any history of respiratory issues in the past.
- Physical examination
  - Obtain a full set of vital signs, including temperature, blood pressure (BP), heart rate, respiratory rate, and pulse oximetry. Correlate with age (Table 33-1).
  - Level of consciousness. Alert? Interactive? Playful? Listless? Lethargic? Unresponsive?
  - Head, eyes, ears, nose, and throat (HEENT) examination for significant rhinorrhea, congestion, or FB.
    - Mouth
      - Check the mucus membranes for hydration status.
      - Identify pooling secretions or excessive drooling.
      - Carefully assess the posterior oropharynx for any evidence of FB.
    - Ears
      - Tympanic membranes (TMs): Look for erythema, bulging, purulence, and movement on otoscopy.
    - Neck
      - Check for midline trachea, and marked tracheal tenderness.
    - Chest
      - Note any increased WOB, accessory muscle use, retractions between ribs or sternal notch, belly breathing, or head bobbing.
      - Listen for rales, rhonchi, wheezes or stridor. Assess for diminished breath sounds, asymmetry, or prolonged expiration.

- Cardiovascular (CV)
  - Identify the rate and rhythm and any murmurs, rubs, or gallops.
  - Check pulses and capillary refill to assess perfusion.
- Abdomen
  - Identify any tenderness or distension.
  - Palpated the liver and spleen for enlargement.
- Extremities
  - Capillary refill
  - Warmth
  - Cyanosis/mottling
  - Edema
- Neuro
  - Check for age-appropriate strength, tone, gait, and reflexes.

- Identify rapidly available diagnostic or therapeutic interventions that will aid your immediate management of the child.
  - Laboratory or radiographic studies: Chest x-ray (CXR), arterial blood gas (ABG)/CG8, electrocardiogram (ECG)
  - Pharmacotherapy: Inhaled adrenergic agents (albuterol, epinephrine), corticosteroids, antibiotics
  - Titrate oxygen to maintain SPO_2 >88% may need noninvasive positive pressure ventilation (NIPPV) or high-flow nasal cannula (HFNC)
  - Suction
- Know when to ask for help: Identify patients requiring consultation or transfer to a higher level of care.
  - It may be apparent very early that you require consulting services and/or transfer to a higher level of care. Begin coordination as soon as possible in tandem with stabilization, evaluation, and management of the patient.

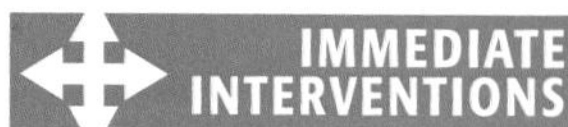

- Oxygen per nonrebreather mask, or high-flow nasal cannula.
- Cardiopulmonary monitor.
- Pulse oximeter.
- IV 0.9% NS KVO or 20 cc/kg bolus depending on perfusion and hydration status.
- CXR: To differentiate respiratory from cardiac causes.
- Search for FB.

Table 33-1. Normal Vital Signs by Age

AGE	HR (PER MINUTE)	RR (BREATHS/MIN)
Newborn to 3 months	90-205	30-60
3 months to 2 years	90-180	24-40
2-5 years	80-140	20-34
5-10 years	60-120	18-25
>10 years	50-100	12-20

Definition of Hypotension by Systolic Blood Pressure

AGE	SYSTOLIC BLOOD PRESSURE (MM HG)
Neonates	60-84
Infants	72-104
Children 1-10 years	72-120
Children >10 years	102-131

DIFFERENTIAL DIAGNOSIS

- Congenital cardiac abnormalities
  - Most congenital heart defects, particularly the cyanotic lesions, are diagnosed in the newborn nursery or neonatal intensive care unit (NICU). There are several notable exceptions, however, that may present in the emergency department (ED). They are due primarily to the normal transition from fetal to newborn circulation during which two main changes occur—the ductus arteriosus closes, and the resistance pattern shifts from high to low in the pulmonary circuit and low to high in the systemic circuit (Table 33-2).
  - The three possible physiologic results that may occur in the decompensating congenital heart patient include cyanosis, shock, and congestive heart failure. Tetralogy of Fallot, hypoplastic left heart (HLH), and coarctation of the aorta are the most common congenital heart lesions likely to present in acute life-threatening decompensation in the ED.
  - Although congenital heart lesions require an echocardiogram and a cardiologist for definitive diagnosis, a good physical examination can reveal the most important telltale clues. Performing a hyperoxia challenge may be useful in distinguishing cardiac from pulmonary causes of cyanosis, as pulmonary conditions generally improve with hyperoxia.
- Asthma
  - Asthma is one of the most common diagnoses for all patients in all settings. For the pediatric patient it is generally ranked as the diagnosis with the highest frequency of both total ED visits, as well as number of hospitalizations and pediatric intensive care unit (PICU) admissions.
  - Management has been standardized by means of a variety of clinical scoring measures and national treatment recommendation guidelines. Although the treatment should be swift and aggressive, not all asthmatics require intubation, and in fact intubation is an outcome clearly to be avoided due to its increased morbidity. In addition to inhaled beta-agonists, standards require multidose ipratropium and early corticosteroids. NIPPV is just as helpful in children as in adults and is a good consideration, as well as other adjunct agents such as magnesium sulfate. Additionally, increasing preload by giving 20-60 mL/kg normal saline (NS) can be very helpful in status asthmaticus.

Table 33-2. Pathophysiologic Characteristics Associated with the Most Common Congenital Heart Defects Presenting in the Emergency Department

Congenital Heart Defect	Critical Change in Fetal Circulation	Physiologic Result	Clinical Presentation
Hypoplastic left heart Coarctation of the aorta Critical aortic stenosis	PDA closure	Loss of ductal-dependent systemic blood flow	Shock
Tetralogy of Fallot Transposition great vessels Pulmonary stenosis	PDA closure	Loss of ductal- dependent pulmonary blood flow	Cyanosis
Patent ductus arteriosus Ventriculoseptal defect Tricuspid atresia	Shifts in resistance (↓PVR, ↑SVR)	Left-to-right shunting	Congestive heart failure

PDA, patent ductus arteriosus; PVR, pulmonary vascular resistance; SVR, systemic vascular resistance.

- Bronchiolitis
  - Bronchiolitis is a ubiquitous disease that all children are exposed to and will acquire by the age of 2 years. It is a seasonal disease presenting almost exclusively during the winter months from November to March.
  - It is generally a relatively benign respiratory illness requiring only supportive treatment. But there are several notable exceptions.
  - Infants <2 months old or significant prematurity, and those with comorbidity (particularly congenital heart or lung disease), are particularly at risk.
- Pediatric FBs
  - Children in the 1-4-year age range are at particular risk for FB aspiration. The FBs may become lodged anywhere in the aerodigestive tract.
  - Infants are at particular risk for FBs that are too big to swallow or aspirate yet become trapped in the vallecular region and cause a ball-valve airway obstruction. Objects that are smaller may be aspirated into the airway or lungs and cause predominance of true respiratory symptoms, or into the upper esophagus causing drooling, cough, stridor, etc.
  - A portable chest radiograph should rapidly identify the location of the FB in the majority of cases. Figure 33-1 shows three common locations of esophageal FBs.
- Croup
  - Croup is another very common viral respiratory illness seen in children (6 months to 3 years). In its milder form, children often do not present to the ED and just have cough managed at home symptomatically. At worst, they can have severe swelling and complete airway obstruction. The disease is seasonal with peaks during the fall and spring.

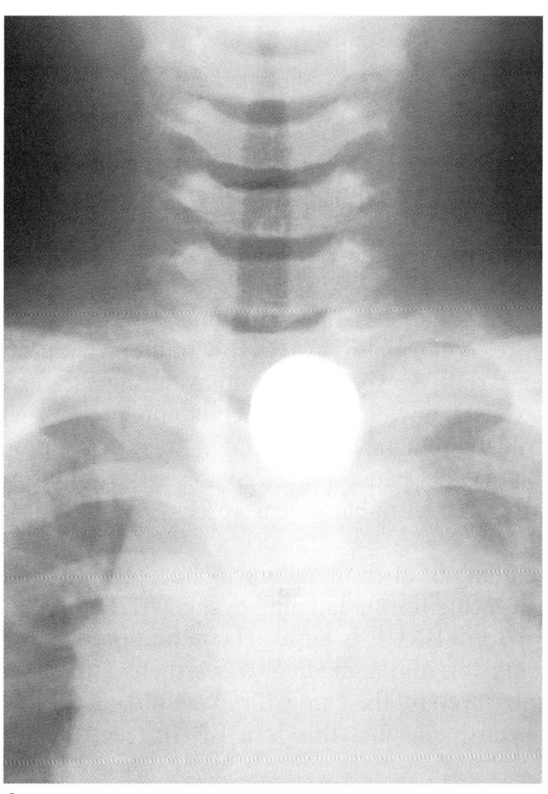

A

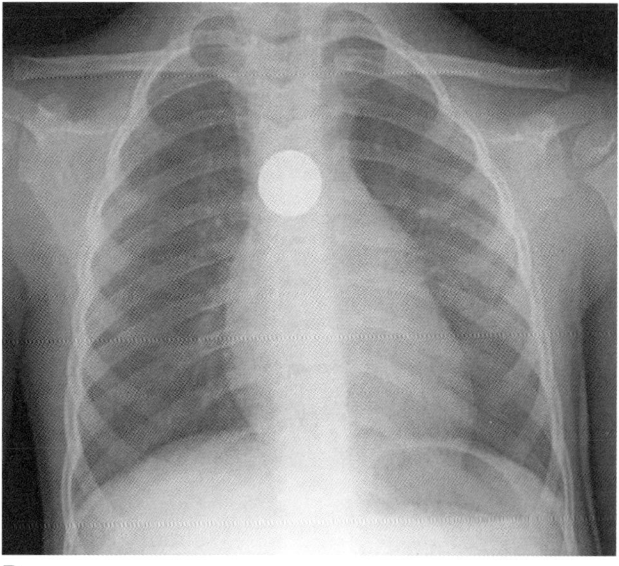

B

Figure 33-1. The three common locations of esophageal foreign bodies: (**A**) *Proximal esophagus* at the cricopharyngeus muscle or upper esophageal sphincter at the thoracic inlet (defined as the area between the clavicles on a chest x-ray) is the *most common location of entrapment*. (**B**) *Mid-esophagus* at the level of the aortic arch (the aortic arch and carina overlap the esophagus). (**C**) *Distal esophagus* just proximal to the gastroesophageal junction. (*Reproduced with permission from Shah BR, Lucchesi M.* Atlas of Pediatric Emergency Medicine. *New York, NY: McGraw-Hill; 2006.*)

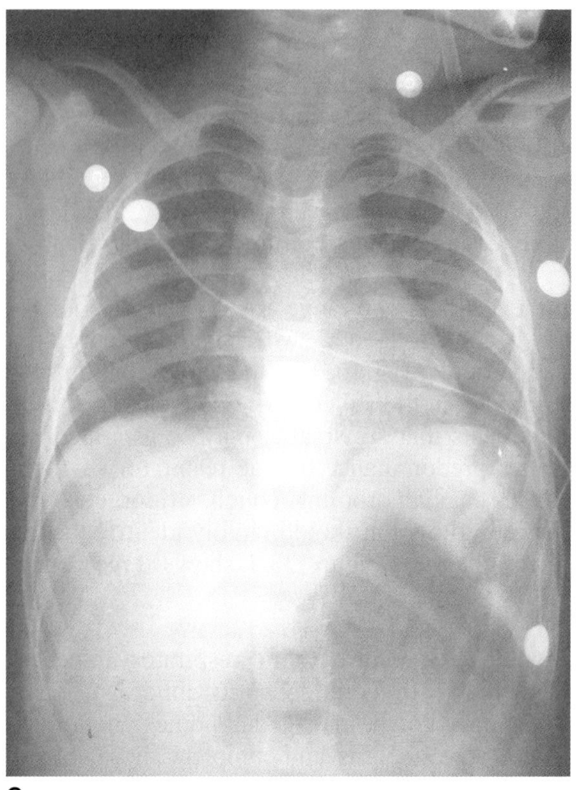

C

Figure 33-1. (*Continued.*)

- There is a very classic presentation. Parents are woken suddenly by a loud barking cough and what appears to be severe stridor. They take the child "out into the cool night air" and to the ED. By the time of arrival, the child is better.
- All children should receive single-dose dexamethasone, but racemic epinephrine is only indicated for those with stridor at rest.
- Children with classic croup (age, season, symptoms, and response to treatment) do not require confirmatory x-rays. Children with atypical features—wrong age, wrong season, presentation during the day, no response to therapy, toxic or unwell appearance, temperature >39°C, marked tracheal tenderness, reluctance to cough—require additional workup and consideration of other causes, most notably FB aspiration and other infectious causes such as retropharyngeal abscess, epiglottitis, and tracheitis.

- Acute events in infancy including brief resolved unexplained events (BRUE) in infancy formerly known as acute life-threatening events (ALTEs)
  - The differential diagnosis for a BRUE is large. The definition of a BRUE is when a patient presents for initial medical assessment after a brief, resolved event that was observed by the caregiver in a child <1 year old.
  - Once the decision has been made that this is a BRUE, then you must stratify risk.
    - Is the patient well-appearing or ill-appearing (abnormal vital signs, additional symptoms: cough, respiratory distress, fever, etc)? If the latter it is not a BRUE.
    - Clinician must characterize the event as sudden, brief, and now resolved of one or more of the following: Cyanosis or pallor; absent,

decreased, or irregular breathing; marked change in tone (hyper- or hypotonia; altered responsiveness. If the event can be described by gastroesophageal reflux (GER) or feeding difficulties or airway abnormality, then not a BRUE.
    - Perform appropriate history and physical examination. If no explanation found by history and physical examination then it is a BRUE.
  - Risk stratification of low-risk BRUE: Age >60 days; born ≥32 weeks' gestation and corrected age ≥45 weeks; no cardiopulmonary resuscitation (CPR) by trained medical provider; event lasted <1 minute; first event. For low-risk BRUE should not perform excessive workup may consider pertussis testing and 12-lead ECG, should briefly monitor patients with continuous pulse oximetry and serial observations.
  - Higher-risk BRUE: More thorough evaluation required for social, feeding, or respiratory problems, or for family history of sudden cardiac death. This often includes a full sepsis evaluation with a lumbar puncture (LP) and antibiotics. It also includes consideration of nonaccidental trauma and a possible computed tomography (CT) scan.

DON'T FORGET

DDx Summary

- History and physical examination give greatest information as most are age-related diagnoses.
- CXR can provide important clues.
- Hyperoxia test may be helpful to distinguish cardiac from pulmonary cause of cyanosis.
- Infants with warning signs should be admitted to the hospital for observation, and additional evaluation performed as guided by the history and physical examination.
- CT head and skeletal survey are indicated if suspect nonaccidental trauma.

CONGENITAL CARDIAC ABNORMALITIES

Additional History and Physical Examination Findings

- Determine how long the symptoms have been present—sudden versus gradual, and associated symptoms such as fever, vomiting.
- Tetralogy of Fallot (TOF) hypercyanotic spells come on suddenly with crying or pain and often have occurred previously.
- Other cardiac causes, however, may be gradual and are associated with gradual pallor, feeding intolerance (sweating during feeding, pulling off to "catch their breath"), and lethargy (hypoplastic left heart, coarctation).
- Infectious causes are usually more gradual in onset and may be associated with fever and cough.
- Focused examination of the ABCs provides important clues. Is the airway patent? Stridor or any upper airway problems? Breathing comfortably or is there excess WOB? Circulation and cardiac examination. Is the heart on the left side of the chest? Is there a murmur? What is the perfusion like? Are the pulses symmetric? What are the 4-point BPs?
- Shock with symmetric decreased pulses/perfusion indicates the possibility of hypoplastic left heart syndrome (HLHS).
- Shock with asymmetric pulses/perfusion/BPs raises the suspicion for coarctation.
- The presence of the murmur may not immediately identify the lesion, but it should raise your suspicion that a cardiac problem rather than a primary respiratory problem is present.

Review Initial Results

- Determine the infant's response to oxygen. Was there a significant change toward normal or near normal? If so, it is not a fixed cardiac lesion. If not, then chances are that it is—freely mixing cardiac lesions such as TOF do not correct with supplemental oxygen.
- Portable CXR: Provides a huge amount of information—cardiac location, size, aortic arch, lung parenchyma (Fig. 33-2).
- ECG: This is a nonspecific indicator of cardiac decompensation, but can be helpful for establishing the cause of congestive heart failure such as cardiac arrhythmia or myocardial ischemia.

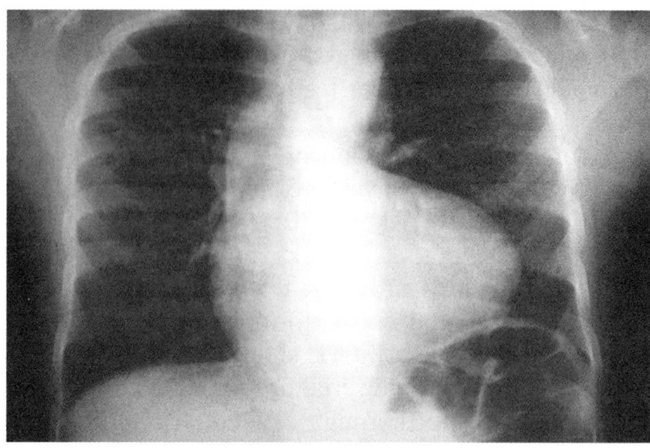

Figure 33-2. A typical boot-shaped heart (uplifted apex due to the RV enlargement associated with concavity of the upper left heart border due to a small or absent main pulmonary artery segment). There are also decreased pulmonary vascular markings. *(Reproduced with permission from Shah BR, Lucchesi M.* Atlas of Pediatric Emergency Medicine. *New York, NY: McGraw-Hill; 2006.)*

 **DON'T FORGET**

Cyanotic, gray neonates in the first week of life, afebrile, and not wheezing are decompensated until proven otherwise.

 **DON'T FORGET**

Differentiating the most common congenital heart diseases (CHDs) to present in the ED and appropriate management requires only physical examination skills—whether or not they are severely cyanotic (TOF), shock with symmetric pulses (HLH), or shock with asymmetric pulses (coarctation).

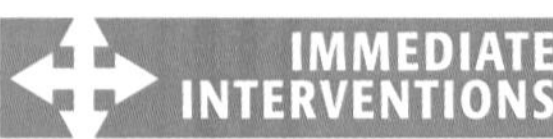

IMMEDIATE INTERVENTIONS

If the possibility of HLH is present, then consider prostaglandin (Alprostadil) in consultation with a pediatric cardiologist. It maintains patency or reopens a closing ductus arteriosus.

Risk Stratification: Management Priorities

- Infants or children with TOF may present during an acute hypercyanotic episode otherwise known as a "tet spell." The priorities are to calm the child, alleviate pain, and reverse the flow and cyanosis.
- In infants with coarctation and/or critical aortic stenosis, obtaining IV access for medications and correcting acidosis is essential. These patients may require intubation.

Definitive Management

- IV, oxygen, and monitoring.
- Fluid bolus of 5-10 ml/kg of NS in patients with suspected congenital heart disease.
- For TOF: Morphine 0.1 mg/kg for pain and vasodilation, and to reverse the shunt and decrease hypercyanotic state. Use the knee-to-chest position.
- For HLH or aortic coarctation: Initiate prostaglandin E1 to keep the ductus arteriosus open. Consult with a pediatric cardiologist for this.

Frequent Reassessment

- Children with known TOF can sometimes be managed without an IV by being given oral fluids (which on its own can sometimes initiate or worsen a spell)—calm, soothe, relax, knee-chest position.
- Frequent reassessments should be performed—continuous pulse oximetry mandatory.
- ABGs not necessary unless progresses to respiratory failure requiring intubation.

Complications

- Respiratory failure, shock, altered mental status from prolonged cyanosis and lactic acidosis

Disposition

- Requires emergent consultation with pediatric cardiology and transfer to a tertiary care center

ASTHMA

Additional History and Physical Examination Findings

- Identify what has been done prior to arrival: Number of treatments, spacing, severity, response.
- Identify triggers.
- What is the child's risk for short-term morbidity or mortality? Ever been in the PICU, intubated, worst ever episode? Number of admissions? Steroids?
- Physical examination of the chest should focus on respiratory rate, effort, excursion, symmetry, air entry, and breath sounds. Palpate the chest for subcutaneous emphysema that might indicate a pneumothorax.
- Presence and degree of retractions is an important indicator of WOB effort. The ability of the child to speak in full sentences versus single words also indicates severity.
- In younger children nasal flaring and grunting are important signs of severe respiratory distress.

Review Initial Results

- Pulse oximetry is usually sufficient to guide most matters related to oxygenation.
- For severe cases—eg, possible respiratory failure, tiring out—an ABG should be obtained to evaluate P_{CO_2} and pH.
- CXR should be obtained for any history of fever or asymmetric breath sounds (pneumothorax or pneumonia).
- No other labs usually needed.

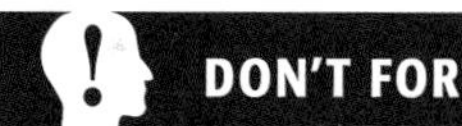

DON'T FORGET

If it is going to be asthma, then it will be severe asthma. Otherwise it will be wheezing with some other cause in the differential in a child—FB, allergic reaction, etc.

Risk Stratification: Management Priorities

- Patients with a history of previous intensive care unit (ICU) admission or intubation are at highest risk for morbidity or mortality—so-called "fatality prone asthmatics."
- Patients who describe this as being their worst episode are also at higher risk.
- Patients who have been on good control at home and were already maximizing care (q4h nebs and oral steroids, in addition to inhaled steroids and leukotriene inhibitor) are also at increased risk of severity.

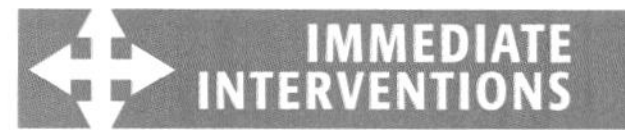

IMMEDIATE INTERVENTIONS

Consider BiPAP to reduce the WOB and potentially obviate the need for intubation.

Definitive Management

- IV, O2, monitor
- Continuous, or multiple repeated inhaled beta-2 agonist bronchodilator (albuterol)
- Multidose ipratropium bromide
- Oral/IV corticosteroid 2 mg/kg, or oral dexamethasone 0.6 mg/kg max 16 mg.
- If in the severe category and/or had already maximized therapy prior to arriving, then need to consider other adjuvant therapies, such as magnesium sulfate, heliox, and BiPAP, additionally giving IV fluids can help increase cardiac preload which is especially helpful if intubation is needed.

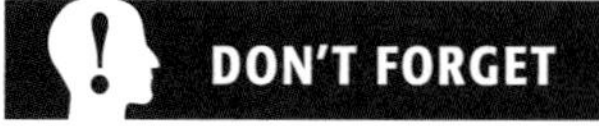

DON'T FORGET

Monitor for deterioration, tiring, and potential need for intubation.

Frequent Reassessment

- Requires frequent reassessment and essentially continuous albuterol inhalation therapy until wheezing is controlled.
- Continuous cardiopulmonary and pulse oximetry monitoring.

Complications

- Respiratory failure
- Pneumothorax, pneumopericardium

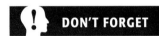

DON'T FORGET

In the event that RSI needs to be performed, ketamine is an excellent choice. Do not forget to use atropine.

Disposition

- If the child responds to one or two series of treatments (1-2 hours of continuous), there is good follow-up and understanding, the child can be discharged with steroids.
- Still wheezing or requiring oxygen, needs to be admitted.
- Severe distress requires admission—floor versus ICU.

BRONCHIOLITIS

Additional History and Physical Examination Findings

- First ever episode of wheezing during the appropriate months of November to March.
- Usually between ages 3 and 12 months.
- Physical examination reveals classic coarse wheezing in all lung fields. Sounds worse than the child looks—"happy wheezer."
- Usually present when the disease process is at its worst—day 3 or 4; usually some mild upper respiratory tract infection (URTI) symptoms and low-grade fever. Post-tussive vomiting is not uncommon.
- Age and comorbidity (prematurity, congenital heart, or lung disease) are important historical features.

Review Initial Results

- CXR is not usually required, but if obtained may show nonspecific perihilar cuffing with perhaps diffuse mild increased interstitial markings. There should not be a discrete focal infiltrate.
- Well-appearing, fully immunized infants generally do not require any labs.

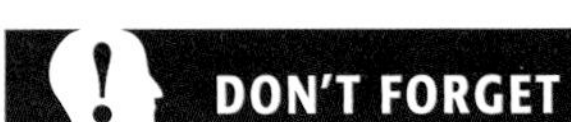

Classic presentation—first time wheezing in an infant.

Risk Stratification: Management Priorities

- Infants <6-8 weeks old are at risk for central apnea.
- Congenital heart or lung disease is a major risk factor.

Definitive Management

- The majority with mild disease require nothing.
- Severe cases may benefit from a trial of inhalation therapy (otherwise, not recommended). Controversy remains as to whether a pure beta-2 agonist (albuterol) or mixed alpha and beta (epinephrine) is preferred, but either are reasonable choices.
- If dehydration is present decreased oral intake and decreased wet diapers consider IVF, and checking a capillary blood gas.
- Glucocorticoids are not recommended in children without an associated history of asthma and first-time wheezers.
- In infants with respiratory distress (nasal flaring, grunting, retracting, hypoxia) use high-flow nasal cannula and escalate to continuous positive airway pressure/bi-level positive air pressure (CPAP/BiPAP) as needed. Severe disease may require intubation.
- Secondary infection has been well documented. In such cases blood and urine should be obtained and the infant started on broad-spectrum antibiotics. Ceftriaxone 50 mg/kg is a reasonable choice.

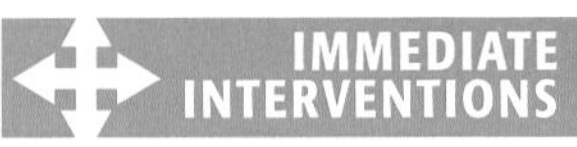

- Supplemental oxygen and nasal suctioning.
- Try albuterol or epinephrine if severe, highly controversial.
- Support breathing with HFNC or BiPAP.
- If febrile or toxic, do sepsis labs and give ceftriaxone.

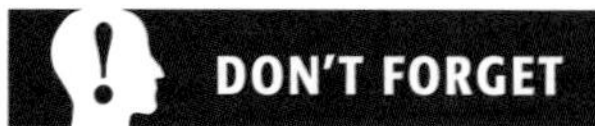

These infants can tire out or decompensate rapidly. Be prepared to intubate. Do not forget to use atropine.

Frequent Reassessment

- Continuous cardiopulmonary and pulse oximetry.
- These infants require very frequent repeat examinations and rechecks to determine response to inhalation therapy and the need for repeat dosing.

Complications

- Respiratory failure
  - Dehydration, inability to eat secondary to increased WOB.
- Secondary infection

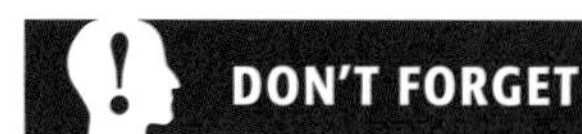

Know the admission criteria for bronchiolitis.

Disposition

- General considerations/indications for admission:
  - Age <6 weeks
  - Hypoxemia (generally SPo_2 <90%-92% on room air, however, should be assessed in conjunction with the overall WOB and comorbidities)
  - Poor feeding
  - Excessively high WOB
  - Congenital heart disease
  - Comorbidities
  - Social reasons

PEDIATRIC FOREIGN BODIES

Additional History and Physical Examination Findings

- Most cases should be relatively rapid in onset and/or give a history of some type of ingestion. Ask about any older siblings in the home who may play with and/or leave small objects on the floor.
- Exceptions are the stridor, cough, or wheeze of indeterminate origin without any coexisting symptoms that would otherwise suggest an infection.
- HEENT examination should focus on the ability to handle secretions and the presence of drooling or stridor.
- Chest examination should focus on the WOB, presence of adventitial sounds, and symmetry. Asymmetric sounds would suggest the possibility of an FB.
- In general the rest of the examination should be normal, and there should be no alterations in perfusion.
- The other very common, but not life-threatening location is in the esophagus. When located high at the thoracic inlet, patients may have drooling, cough, or stridor. Lower locations—at the carina or lower esophageal sphincter—are usually relatively asymptomatic. All esophageal FBs require removal so as to eliminate the possibility of perforation. Once they have made it into the stomach, however, no further treatment is necessary.
- Beware the button battery. These require immediate surgical consultation and removal if in the esophagus or distal to the esophagus and symptomatic.

Review Initial Results

- CXR often will reveal the FB as most often they are radiopaque, and most go up high enough into the pharynx to also view a high FB. When in doubt, the request for soft tissue (ST) of the neck and CXR can be made.
- When specifically evaluating for FB, there are special views to obtain, particularly when the possibility of a radiolucent FB exists (food).
- The purpose is to look for asymmetry. The best views are R and L lateral decubitus views. You are looking for alterations in the filling of the lungs and therefore the variable radiolucency of the lungs. Essentially you are looking for air trapping and its consequences. You may also see mediastinal shift, but that is only more severe cases.

DON'T FORGET

- Stridor or nonspecific choking/respiratory distress may be the presentation. Know that in the 12-36-month age group FB is a likely cause—particularly when sudden onset and without any premonitory symptoms.
- Know the key findings to look for on R and L lateral decubitus CXR—asymmetry and the hallmarks of air-trapping—altered lucency and volumes ± mediastinal shift.
- These children may suddenly go from respiratory distress awake and moving air to apnea—know pediatric BLS techniques and protocols.

Risk Stratification: Management Priorities

- Management priorities are the usual ABCs.
- Symptomatic patients require appropriate testing and referral for removal.

Definitive Management

- Requires removal: Usually in the operating room (OR) either by pediatric surgery, GI, or pulmonary, depending on the location and the local practices of the subspecialty services.

Frequent Reassessment

- Continuous cardiopulmonary and pulse oximetry monitoring.
- Requires frequent reevaluation to ensure that the FB is not moving and airway obstruction or respiratory failure is not developing.

Complications

- Airway obstruction
- Esophageal perforation
- Respiratory failure

Disposition

- Those requiring surgical removal usually are admitted as a 23-hour observation.

CROUP

Additional History and Physical Examination Findings

- Classic history of loud barking cough in the middle of the night that awakens parents and then gets much better on the trip to the ED.
- Occurs during classic months of fall and spring.
- Usually ages 6 months to 3 years.
- Classic loud barking cough and intermittent stridor with agitation or crying; usually nontoxic in appearance with mild to moderate fever; often has a mild URTI prodrome with cough, congestion, runny nose.
- Need to document general appearance, presence of drooling, stridor at rest.
- Generally lungs clear and no wheeze or respiratory distress.

Review Initial Results

- Classic croup as described with correct age, season, presentation, and response to therapy requires no diagnostic x-ray to "verify" diagnosis.
- Atypical cases that are the wrong age, season, or presentation, or do not respond to therapy do require further evaluation and consideration of an extended differential (FB, retropharyngeal abscess, epiglottitis, bacterial tracheitis).
- ST neck: Evaluate the appearance of the epiglottis and the retropharyngeal space.
- CT neck if concerned to rule out retropharyngeal abscess.

Risk Stratification: Management Priorities

- Children with craniofacial abnormalities are at higher risk of airway obstruction.
- Children with previous or recurrent history are also at higher risk.

Definitive Management

- All children presenting to the ED with croup, even if their symptoms have for the most part resolved, should receive corticosteroids—in the form of single-dose dexamethasone—either PO or IM.
- 0.5 cc nebulized racemic epinephrine is indicated for stridor at rest. It may be repeated up to every half hour if needed. There is the potential for patients to "rebound" back to their initial presentation. So, even though all patients will have a very good response, they should all be watched in the ED for several hours prior to being sent home. The exact number of hours varies from two to four following a single treatment prior to discharge.

Frequent Reassessment

- All children receiving racemic epinephrine should be closely monitored for recurrence of symptoms with a minimum pulse oximetry.

Complications

- Airway obstruction

Disposition

- Most patients can be safely discharged after dexamethasone alone and anticipatory guidance regarding the disease process—the loud barking will periodically recur during the next couple of days and may be worse at night. The "cool night air" is actually a very good therapy—put on your coats and go for a walk around the block.
- Admission should be considered for patients requiring two or more racemic epinephrine nebs.
- Children with craniofacial abnormalities.
- Severe stridor at rest, hypoxemia, persistent respiratory distress.
- Other comorbid conditions, social reasons.

DON'T FORGET

- Classic croup presentation most likely.
- All kids get single-dose dexamethasone—can be oral or IM.
- Racemic epinephrine should be given to patients with stridor at rest.
- Know the differentiating points for croup and epiglottitis, FB, retropharyngeal abscess, and bacterial tracheitis—essentially all are history and physical examination findings, with some confirmatory radiographic findings.

ACUTE EVENTS IN INFANCY INCLUDING BRIEF RESOLVED UNEXPLAINED EVENTS (BRUE)

Additional History and Physical Examination Findings

- The term BRUE should be used instead of ALTE whenever possible (ie, when episodes are brief, resolved, and unexplained). For events that do not fit the definition of BRUE, guidelines encourage the use of event characteristics rather than the term "ALTE" to describe the event.
- BRUE is not a specific diagnosis but a description of a sudden, brief, and now resolved episode in an infant that includes one or more of the following:
  - Cyanosis or pallor
  - Absent, decreased, or irregular breathing
  - Marked change in tone (hyper- or hypotonia)
  - Altered level of responsiveness
- The term should only be applied when the infant is asymptomatic on presentation, and when there is no explanation for the episode after a focused history and physical examination.
- The estimated duration of the event is usually <1 minute (and typically <20-30 seconds). Then you must risk stratify low-risk BRUE versus higher-risk BRUE.
- Low risk BRUE
  - Age >60 days
  - Gestational age ≥32 weeks and postconceptional age ≥45 weeks
  - Occurrence of only one BRUE (no prior BRUE, and BRUE did not occur in clusters)
  - Duration of BRUE <1 MINUTE

  - No cardiopulmonary resuscitation (CPR) by a trained medical provider was required
  - No concerning historical features
  - No concerning physical examination findings
- It is important to identify warning signs that increase the likelihood that the acute event is medically significant and may have a pathologic cause, infants with these signs should be admitted to the hospital for observation with cardiorespiratory monitoring, with specific evaluation guided by the history as outlined below.
  - Toxic appearing at time of evaluation, lethargy, unexplained recurrent vomiting, or respiratory distress.
  - Significant physiologic compromise during the event, sustained cyanosis, or sustained loss of consciousness.
  - Bruising or evidence of trauma.
  - History of prior events in this patient, especially in the past 24 hours.
  - History or clinically significant events or unexpected death in a sibling.
  - History of suspicion of child maltreatment.
  - Dysmorphic features, congenital anomalies, and/or syndromes.

Definitive Management

- Low-risk BRUE infants who are asymptomatic and have no concerning features identified on history and physical examination, require little intervention, the following steps are recommended:
  - Educate caregivers about BRUEs and the low risk for infants with these characteristics.
  - Offer resources for training in CPR.
  - Engage in shared decision-making about further evaluation and disposition.
  - Arrange for a follow-up medical check with a medical provider within 24 hours to identify infants with evolving medical concerns that would require further evaluation and treatment.
- Optional steps:
  - A brief period of in-hospital observation 1-4 hours with continuous pulse oximetry and serial observations.
  - 12 lead ECG with attention to QT interval.
  - Testing for pertussis (especially for infants with suggestive symptoms). Respiratory virus testing such as respiratory syncytial virus (RSV), is reasonable if rapid testing is available, but this testing is not required.
  - Educate family that there is no known association between low-risk BRUE and sudden infant death syndrome (SIDS). Teach family about sleeping infant in supine position with face free and in a safe sleeping environment, and eliminating any exposure to tobacco smoke.
- The management of higher-risk BRUE is not yet known and require additional evaluation as guided by the history and physical examination, these children will likely require admission and further observation.
- Infants with warning signs indicating that the event was medically significant should be admitted to the hospital for observation, and additional evaluation performed and guided by the history and physical examination.

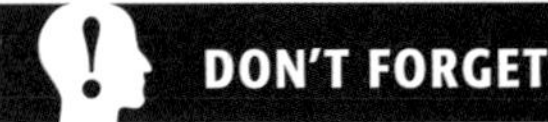

Be able to elicit the history and physical examination key features from the parent. They will guide whether this is a low-risk BRUE or higher-risk BRUE or if warning signs are present.

Review Initial Results

- Have to make an initial determination: Is this a low-risk BRUE or a higher-risk BRUE? Does this infant have any warning signs? (Table 33-3)
- If low-risk BRUE: Consider obtaining pertussis, RSV, or a viral respiratory testing if rapid. Consider ECG with attention to the QT interval; observe 1-4 hours in the ED.
- If higher-risk BRUE or warning signs present: Will require additional evaluation performed and guided by history and physical examination, and will require hospital admission for further observation.

Table 33-3. Differential Diagnosis of ALTE

Cardiovascular	Congenital heart disease Dysrhythmia Prolonged QT syndrome Shock
Infectious diseases	Sepsis Respiratory syncytial virus Pertussis Meningitis, encephalitis Pneumonia Infantile botulism
Central nervous system	Seizures Structural lesions, tumors, cysts Hydrocephalus Congenital central hypoventilation syndrome
Miscellaneous	Gastroesophageal refluxdisease Non-accidental trauma Poisoning Munchausen by proxy syndrome Metabolic disorders

Risk Stratification: Management Priorities

- Low-risk BRUE
  - Age >60 days
  - Born ≥32 weeks gestation and corrected gestational age ≥45 weeks.
  - No CPR by trained medical provider
  - Event <1 minute
  - First and only event

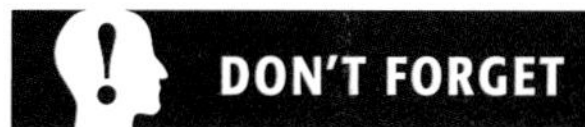

Respiratory viruses are notorious causes of central apnea—respiratory syncytial virus (RSV) and pertussis. Swabs or cultures should be sent.

Definitive Management

- Definitive management is determined by risk stratification:
  - Infants with warning signs admit, workup guided by history and physical exam
  - High-risk BRUE likely admit, workup guided by history and physical exam
  - Low-risk BRUE may discharge home with shared decision making; consider ECG, pertussis testing and observation with continuous pulse oximetry and serial observations

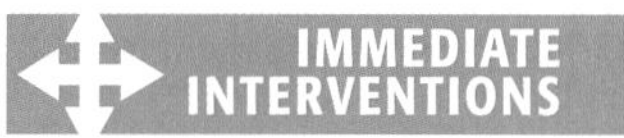

If the possibility of seizures is considered, then lorazepam or other anticonvulsant can be considered.

Frequent Reassessment

- These infants require continuous cardiopulmonary and pulse oximetry monitoring as they may be at risk for apnea, as guided by which type of BRUE.
- Frequent reassessments should be performed to evaluate for subtle seizures, ongoing shock, or other decompensation.

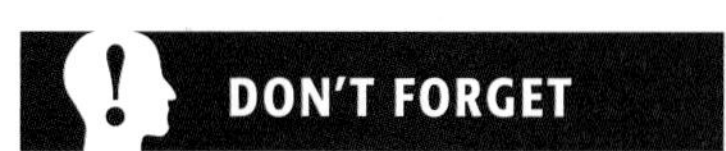

Continuous monitoring and frequent reassessments

Complications

- Apnea
- Aspiration

- Respiratory failure
- Shock
- Seizure

Disposition

- Admit high-risk BRUE patients. Consult Pediatrician about disposition for low-risk BRUE patients. At ABEM General, have a low threshold for involving consults and admitting patients.

WINNING STRATEGIES

- Every child will be sick with an age-related cardiorespiratory diagnosis.
- Give high-flow oxygen per nonrebreather mask—**not** "blow by."
- The most useful information you will obtain will be from the history and physical examination, and not from testing.
- Of those diagnostic studies performed, CXR is the most useful to differentiate respiratory from cardiac causes, and to identify FBs.
- When evaluating children with stridor and looking at a ST neck film, identify the epiglottis (normal or abnormal) and evaluate the retropharyngeal space (normal or abnormal).
- Cyanotic, gray neonates in the first week of life, afebrile, and not wheezing are decompensated congenital heart disease until proven otherwise.
- If it is going to be asthma, then it is going to be severe asthma. Otherwise it will be wheezing with some other cause—FB, allergic reaction.
- For severe asthma, consider BiPAP to reduce the WOB and potentially obviate the need for intubation.
- Monitor all kids for deterioration, tiring, and the potential need for intubation.
- If rapid sequence induction (RSI) is needed, ketamine is an excellent choice. Do not forget atropine.
- Many of the respiratory viral illnesses have strong seasonal components—RSV, bronchiolitis, croup.
- Know the treatment options for severe bronchiolitis—albuterol, frequent suctioning, O_2, positive pressure ventilation including high flow nasal cannula and BiPAP.
- Know the admission criteria for infants with bronchiolitis.
- Know the DDx for stridor or nonspecific choking/respiratory distress. Know also that in the 12-36-month age group FB is a likely cause—particularly when sudden onset and without any premonitory symptoms.
- In cases of FB aspiration, know the key findings to look for on R and L lateral decubitus CXR—asymmetry and the hallmarks of air-trapping—altered lucency and volumes ± mediastinal shift.
- Know basic pediatric CPR guidelines—kids with FB may go from moving air to apnea rapidly.
- All kids with croup get single-dose dexamethasone; know the criteria for racemic epinephrine (stridor at rest).
- Be able to identify acute events in infancy specifically low-risk BRUE versus higher-risk BRUE versus warning signs. Know the management and disposition of the above.

THE BOTTOM LINE

- Age of the patient dictates likely diagnosis and ultimate workup and management.
- History and physical examination usually provide more information than test results.
- Subtle but important clues are provided in the mental status, vital signs, and overall WOB of the patient.

CHAPTER 34

Pediatric Sore Throat

Janis Tupesis and Matthew Steimle

INITIAL ASSESSMENT

- Initially, focus on airway, breathing, and circulation (ABCs).
  - Is the child's airway patent?
  - Are they sitting upright or in a tripod position?
  - Is the child's breathing labored or fast?
  - What is the patient's heart rate?
  - What is the patient's blood pressure?
  - Are they perfusing well or do they appear mottled?
- If any of the ABCs are unstable, what needs to be done emergently?
  - Airway: Open the airway (head tilt chin lift, jaw thrust) if they are not doing it on their own or they are obtunded.
  - Breathing: Give them oxygen if needed or medication to decrease edema (steroid, antihistamine)
  - Circulation: Do they need intravenous fluid (IVF)?

INITIAL HISTORY AND PHYSICAL EXAMINATION

History

- Has the patient been complaining of sore throat? Have them describe symptoms if they are able. Is their throat itchy, swollen, can they swallow liquids or solids, does it hurt to touch the neck midline, lateral, inside, can they move their neck?
- How long have patient's symptoms been present? Does it hurt constantly or only in the morning after they have been sleeping, do they have nasal congestion, does it feel better the longer they are awake suggesting a postnasal drip? What makes it feel better or worse? Do they have a cough, are they reluctant to cough?
- Has the patient had a fever?
- Have the parents noticed a change in their voice (eg, hoarse, muffled, quiet)?
- Has the patient had sick contacts?
- Has the patient been complaining of other somatic complaints, such as
  - Headache
  - Abdominal pain/vomiting
  - Anorexia
  - Chills
  - Malaise

> **DON'T FORGET**
>
> On exam day, every pediatric sore throat has either
>
> Bacterial pharyngitis,
>
> Bacterial tracheitis,
>
> Epiglottitis,
>
> Mononucleosis or
>
> Retropharyngeal abscess

Past Medical History

- Prior history of sore throat/strep infection or recurrent ear infections?
- Ever been hospitalized before?
- Prior history of "atypical" infections?
- Underlying medical problems? Immunosuppression?
- Normal developmental milestones?
- Immunizations up to date?
- Reluctance to cough?

> **DON'T FORGET**
>
> Every sore throat is a potential airway problem until proven otherwise!

Physical Examination

- Vital signs, including pulse oximetry
- General appearance: Toxic, unwell, well-appearing
- Head, eyes, ears, nose, and throat (HEENT) examination: Marked tracheal tenderness with palpation
  - Check the mucus membranes for hydration status
  - Evaluation of voice (ie, muffled, clear hoarse)

  - Dentition
  - Identify pooling secretions or excessive drooling
- Carefully assess the posterior oropharynx for
  - Pharyngeal edema/erythema
  - Enlarged tonsils (remember, children have large tonsils at baseline)
  - Tonsillar exudates
  - Soft palate petechiae
  - Uvular deviation
  - Vesicles on the soft or hard palate
  - Vesicles on the tongue, gingiva, lips
- Ears
  - Tympanic membranes (TMs): Erythema, bulging, purulence, and no movement on pneumatic otoscopy
- Neck
  - Lymphadenopathy: Anterior cervical, submandibular, and posterior auricular
  - Range of motion (eg, refusal to look a certain direction)
- Chest
  - Rales, rhonchi, or wheezes
  - Any evidence of consolidation: Ablation of breath sounds, egophony, etc.
- Cardiovascular (CV)
  - Rate and rhythm
  - Murmurs, rubs, gallops
  - Check pulses and capillary refill to assess perfusion
- Abdomen
  - Identify any tenderness or distension
  - Palpate the liver and spleen
- Extremities
  - Capillary refill
  - Warmth
  - Cyanosis/mottling
  - Edema
- Neuro
  - Check for age-appropriate strength, tone, gait, and reflexes.

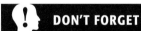

IMMEDIATE INTERVENTIONS

- Large-bore IV (size will vary with age of child) and blood draw
- Supplemental oxygen via blow-by, NC or NRB to keep oxygen saturation >95%.
- Cardiac monitor.
- Keep patient in a position of comfort.

DIFFERENTIAL DIAGNOSIS

- Acute bacterial pharyngitis
  - Approximately 10% of all pediatric visits to health-care providers are for evaluation of pharyngitis. Of these, anywhere between 25% and 50% will have group-A β-hemolytic *Streptococcus* (GABHS). It occurs in all age groups, but has the greatest incidence in children between the ages of 5 and 18 years. The male to female ratio is 1:1.
  - This infection usually presents with typical triad of fever, sore throat, and lymphadenopathy. Other common signs and symptoms include exposure to known carriers, malaise, chills, anorexia, abdominal pain, vomiting, and headache.
  - The physical examination shows enlarged tonsils with ± exudates, pharyngeal erythema and edema, cervical and submandibular lymphadenopathy, and possible petechiae on the soft palate.
  - Diagnosis is made with a physical examination and either rapid strep test or throat culture. Treatment is with antibiotic therapy treating all likely pathogens.
- Acute viral pharyngitis
  - This is the most common cause of acute pharyngitis in children < 2 years old. It is often difficult to differentiate from acute bacterial pharyngitis

DON'T FORGET

No single element in the history or physical examination is sensitive or specific enough to exclude the diagnosis of strep pharyngitis!

Important to treat!

Antibiotic treatment of GABHS pharyngitis prevents rheumatic fever and suppurative complications.
Shortens the course of disease.
Reduces transmission to contacts.
Does not prevent post-streptococcal glomerulonephritis.

DON'T FORGET

In the absence of cough, rhinorrhea, and conjunctivitis = think bacterial instead of viral cause for pharyngitis!

DON'T FORGET

The clinical presentation of bacterial tracheitis is very similar to croup discussed in Chap. 33. Bacterial tracheitis presents with symptoms of stridor, fever, marked tracheal tenderness and reluctance to cough, and toxicity generally worsening over a 3-7 day period, Racemic epinephrine and steroids are generally not effective, and many patients will require intubation and surgical debridement of the membranous tracheal exudates.

as both clinical entities often present with similar symptoms. One should look for other stigmata of viral illness including conjunctivitis, rhinorrhea, and cough.

- Epiglottitis
  - This is a severe, life-threatening inflammation of the supraglottic structures, most often the epiglottis. It was predominantly a disease of children but the incidence has drastically decreased since the advent of the Hib vaccine in 1985. It is now seen more often in adults. The cause is primarily bacterial and viral infections, although it can also be due to direct thermal injury and/or direct trauma. The most common pathogen was *Haemophilus influenzae* type B. More common pathogens are now non-typable *H influenzae*, *H parainfluenzae, Streptococcus pneumoniae, Staphylococcus aureus,* and GABHS.
- Mononucleosis
  - Infectious mononucleosis is a clinical syndrome in which the patient is infected with Epstein-Barr virus. Constellation of symptoms includes fever, lymphadenopathy, and pharyngitis—it is difficult to distinguish from acute bacterial pharyngitis. Other symptoms may include splenomegaly, hepatomegaly, periorbital edema, and jaundice.
- Retropharyngeal abscess
  - This is an infection of the potential retropharyngeal space which is most common in children <5 years. Symptoms include fever, dysphagia, drooling, odynophagia, reluctance of the child to move the neck, stiff neck, and occasionally some element of respiratory distress from inflammation of the airway. It is usually polymicrobial in origin.
  - Diagnosis is made clinically, with lateral neck radiograph to investigate for widening of the upper cervical prevertebral tissues. Computed tomography is confirmatory. Management includes IV antibiotics and sometimes, surgical drainage.
- Diphtheria
  - This is an infection of the posterior oropharynx and upper airways with the gram-positive rod, *Corynebacterium diphtheria*. It has an incubation period of 2-5 days, followed by fever, malaise, sore throat, hoarseness, and dysphagia. The bacteria produce toxin which inhibits protein synthesis. Prior to routine immunization, 100,000-200,000 cases were reported annually. Now it is exceedingly rare.

ACUTE BACTERIAL PHARYNGITIS

Additional History and Physical Examination Findings

- The classic presentation is sore throat, fever, tonsillar edema and exudates, and lymphadenopathy.
- Children will often have associated headache, abdominal pain, and vomiting.
- Alternate chief complaints that suggest a different etiology are sneezing, rhinorrhea, and cough (viral pharyngitis); conjunctivitis (adenovirus infections); significant cervical or generalized adenopathy and hepatosplenomegaly (mononucleosis); and vesicular lesions (herpes and enterovirus infections).

Review Initial Results

- The standard of care for the diagnosis of acute bacterial pharyngitis is a throat culture.
- To maximize accuracy, tonsils and posterior pharyngeal wall should be swabbed.

- Throat culture takes about 24 hours, so rapid antigen testing is a useful alternative in the emergency department (ED).
- Rapid antigen testing is 95%-100% specific, but the sensitivity can be as low as 70%.
- Patients with positive tests should be treated with appropriate antibiotics. Those with negative rapid tests should be treated with supportive care while awaiting the culture result. If the patient has unreliable follow-up or barriers to care, they may be treated presumptively.

Definitive Management

- The treatment for acute bacterial pharyngitis is antibiotic therapy. Acceptable regimens include:
  - Penicillin: Either penicillin G benzathine 1.2 million units (if >27 kg) IM once or penicillin VK, 250 mg per dose for children and 500 mg per dose for adolescents, PO bid/tid × 10 days.
  - Amoxicillin has no advantage to PCN, but offers a better taste in the liquid preparation. Dose is 25 mg/kg PO bid × 10 days
  - Erythromycin: Primarily used for penicillin-allergic patients. Dose is 10 mg/kg PO qid × 10 days.
  - Cephalosporins: Many can be used including cefuroxime (Ceftin), cefixime (Suprax), cefpodoxime (Vantin), cefditoren (Spectracef), and cephalexin.
- Recent studies show that systemic steroids can be used as an adjuvant therapy to decrease length of symptoms and decrease discomfort.
  - Dexamethasone, 0.6 mg/kg with a maximum dose of 10 mg, given one time PO.
- Acetaminophen and ibuprofen are helpful for symptomatic treatment.

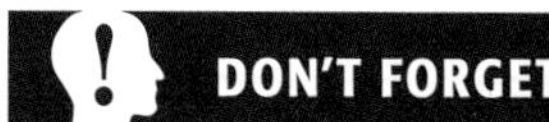

Strep validation score: Use it to guide therapy!

Symptoms	*Points*
Fever	1
No cough	1
Exudates	1
+ nodes	1
Age	*Points*
3-15	1
15-45	0
≥45	−1

Points:

−1 to 0: Strep ruled out (2%)

1-3: Rapid antigen test and treat accordingly (46%)

3-5: Probable strep pharyngitis, consider empiric antibiotics (52%)

Complications

- If patient has documented GABHS, the following complications need to be considered:
  - Rheumatic fever: Rare complication with annual incidence of 2-14 cases per 100,000. Should be suspected if patient has had documented GABHS infection and presents with joint pain and swelling, subcutaneous nodules, abnormal movements (chorea), and/or heart murmur. Diagnosed with elevated erythrocyte sedimentation rate (ESR) and antistreptolysin-O titer (ASO).
  - Glomerulonephritis: Rare complication of post-strep infection—presenting with hematuria, proteinuria, and edema. Also have elevated ASO.
  - Scarlet fever: Punctate, erythematous exanthem that is found on the neck, axilla → more predominantly at the skin folds. Other findings include pharyngeal edema, exudative pharyngitis, and a bright red tongue (strawberry tongue).
  - Peritonsillar abscess: Progression of localized infection to include tissues of the posterior oropharynx with a fluctuant peritonsillar mass. Occurs in <1% of patients treated with antibiotics. Treatment is incision and drainage in the emergency room (ER) or the ENT clinic.

DON'T FORGET

Reasons to treat children with GAS

- Earlier symptomatic response. Shortens the course of disease.
- Prevents suppurative complications: Otitis, sinusitis, peritonsillar abscess formation.
- Prevents nonsuppurative complications: Rheumatic fever. Glomerulonephritis is not prevented by treatment.
- Prevents transmission within families and school settings (reduces transmission to contacts).

Disposition

- Not tolerating oral fluids: Admit to hospital for parenteral antibiotics. Usually a very small percentage of children. Even if patients are dehydrated and require IVFs—if they are able to tolerate liquids as an outpatient, they can be safely discharged.
- Tolerating oral intake: Discharge home with antibiotic therapy, supportive care, and follow-up with primary care pediatrician.

DON'T FORGET

Use clinical history to help diagnose viral pharyngitis.

- Sick contacts
- Cough
- Low-grade fever
- Malaise
- Hoarseness
- Coryza
- Conjunctivitis

ACUTE VIRAL PHARYNGITIS

Additional History and Physical Examination Findings

- Most common type of pharyngitis in both children and adults.
- Viral pharyngitis usually associated with conjunctivitis, sneezing, cough, and rhinorrhea.
- Many etiologies. Correlate with seasonal outbreaks. Most common include:
  - Rhinovirus: The "common cold."
  - Adenovirus: Infection manifests as pharyngitis, tonsillitis, and pharyngo-conjunctival fever. No real distinguishing traits that separate it from other viral infections.
  - Parainfluenza virus: "Croup" clinical syndrome.
  - Coxsackie virus: Causes herpangina with small vesicles in the posterior oropharynx.
  - Herpes simplex virus (HSV): Fever, severe discomfort, cervical lymphadenopathy. Approximately 10% will have characteristic ulcerative lesion on their lip.
  - Echovirus.
  - Epstein-Barr virus: Will be discussed in section on Mononucleosis.
  - Cytomegalovirus.
- Children with viral pharyngitis can present with atypical symptoms including vomiting, abdominal pain, diarrhea, and dyspnea.

Review Initial Results

- Clinical diagnosis: No reliable lab test to diagnose or characterize viral pharyngitis.

Definitive Management

- The treatment for acute viral pharyngitis is supportive.
- Need to ensure that patient can tolerate oral hydration.
- Antipyretics.
  - Ibuprofen at 10 mg/kg/dose PO q6h
  - Acetaminophen at 15 mg/kg/dose PO q4h
- For patients with herpangina:
  - Maalox/benadryl mixed 1:1
  - Dosed on benadryl component of 1.25 mg/kg/dose PO—used as swish and swallow q6h prn

Complications

- Rare to have complications from acute viral pharyngitis. Some may include
  - Secondary bacterial infection; most commonly transforms to bacterial pharyngitis or otitis media
  - Dehydration
  - Rhinitis
  - Sinusitis
  - Pneumonia

EPIGLOTTITIS

Additional History and Physical Examination Findings

- Bacterial infection of the supraglottic structure, epiglottis, and adjacent tissues. It was formerly caused by *H influenzae* type B, but now it is more likely due to other pathogens.
- Be sure to confirm immunization status.

- Clinical presentation: Abrupt onset and rapid progression of fever, stridor, severe sore throat, dysphagia, muffled voice "hot potato voice," difficulty handling oral secretions, refusal to lie down, "sniffing position," anxiety anterior neck pain at the hyoid, marked retractions and labored breathing indicate impending respiratory failure.
- Duration of illness before presentation is <24 hours and frequently <12 hours.
- May present with erythematous mucosa and pooling secretions in the oropharynx. Do NOT use a tongue depressor.

DON'T FORGET

The 3Ds of epiglottitis: Dysphagia, distress, drooling.

Review Initial Results

- Fever between 38.0 and 40.0°C is almost universal.
- Leukocytosis with white blood cell (WBC) commonly over 20,000 (generally do NOT obtain lab work until a secure airway is obtained).
- "Left shift" with increase in immature forms of neutrophils and bands.
- Imaging.
  - X-rays of the lateral neck: Classic appearance of enlarged epiglottis protruding from the anterior wall of the hypopharynx ("thumb sign") (Fig. 34-1).

DON'T FORGET

Epiglottitis is an airway emergency. Act quickly and definitively!

- Early recognition
- Early airway control if needed
- Early imaging
- Early antibiotics
- Early consultation with ENT/surgery

Definitive Management

- Two main keys to the treatment of epiglottitis are definitive airway management and the early institution of antibiotic therapy.
- Airway management
  - Put patient in position of comfort.
  - Reduce stimulation and keep the child calm (eg, do not start IV, parents hold blow-by oxygen).
  - Establish airway as soon as possible. Should typically be done in the operating room (OR) under a controlled setting.
  - Nasopharyngeal intubation is method of choice, preferably with fiberoptic guidance.
  - Tracheostomy is reserved for inability to intubate secondary to severe epiglottic edema.

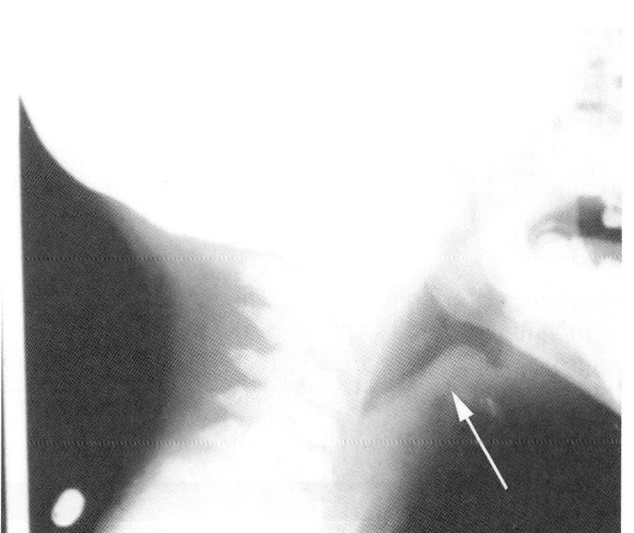

Figure 34-1. Lateral neck view of a child with epiglottitis. *(Reproduced with permission from Tintinalli JE, Kelen GD, Stapczynski JS, et al.* Emergency Medicine: A Comprehensive Study Guide. *6th ed. New York, NY: McGraw-Hill; 2004.)*

- Antibiotic therapy
  - Should be geared toward covering staph, strep, and pneumococci.
  - Empiric therapy should be started as soon as possible. Regimens could include a third-generation cephalosporin, such as Ceftriaxone or Cefotaxime plus an anti-staphylcoccal agent (vancomycin or clindamycin).

DON'T FORGET

Early imaging, early airway—ideally established in the OR—and early antibiotics

Complications

- Airway compromise
- Disseminated infection: Bacteremia, sepsis, local invasion

Disposition

- Admit patient to intensive care unit (ICU) or ICU stepdown setting.

MONONUCLEOSIS

Additional History and Physical Examination Findings

- Immunopathologic syndrome that occurs in response to a patient's infection with Epstein-Barr virus.
- Infection activates lymphoid tissue in the posterior oropharynx—leading to the characteristic lymphoid hyperplasia.
- The most symptomatic patients are typically between 15 and 25 years old.
- Classic presentation is usually with malaise, fever, pharyngitis (often exudative), and cervical lymphadenopathy (involvement of axillary, and inguinal nodes is common).
- Other possible clinical findings: Splenomegaly, hepatomegaly, periorbital edema, diffuse maculopapular rash.

Review Initial Results

- Fever, usually not exceeding 102°C.
- Leukocytosis, usually between 10,000 and 20,000 with a lymphocytic predominance (often >50%).
- Increased liver function tests are found in 80% of patients.
- Positive heterophile antibody test.
- Monospot assay.

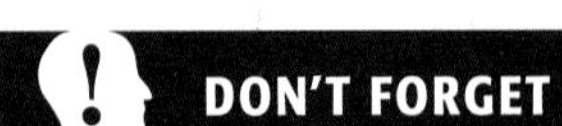

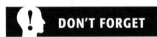

Morbidity and mortality come from the following complications:

- GI: Splenic rupture. Keep patients out of contact sports, aggressive physical activity.
- Neuro: Meningitis, encephalitis, Guillain-Barré syndrome.
- ENT: Airway obstruction due to massive posterior pharyngeal edema

Definitive Management

- Primarily supportive.
- Primary treatment is antipyretics and analgesics.
- If patient has gross pharyngeal edema, may benefit from short course of oral steroids. Prednisone 2 mg/kg for 3 days, then tapered off over 5-7 days.

Complications

- Airway compromise: Very rare finding. Thought to occur in 1 in 1000 cases from severe inflammation and swelling of the tonsils.
- Splenic rupture: Usually from trauma (can be mild) to enlarged, infected spleen. Occurs more often in males. Educate regarding avoidance of contact sports and potential trauma.

RETROPHARYNGEAL ABSCESS

Additional History and Physical Examination Findings

- Infection of the retropharyngeal space in the neck. The potential space extends to the level of the second thoracic vertebrae.
- Most commonly affects children between the ages of 2 and 4.

- Typically presents as sore throat, intense dysphagia, drooling, reluctance to move neck, and ± respiratory distress (stridor).
- May see swelling to one or both sides of the neck. May rarely see swelling to the posterior oropharynx. Inability to turn their neck side to side, or to look up is suspicious for RPA. A stiff neck is suspicious for RPA.

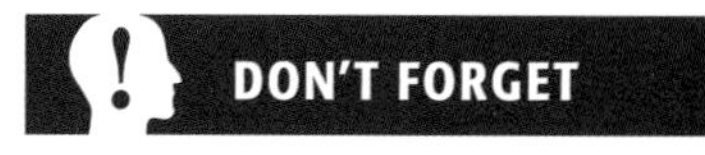

Think retropharyngeal abscess if there is history of running with something in mouth. Sharp objects can puncture posterior oropharynx and introduce bacteria.

Review Initial Results

- Soft tissue of the neck: Considered widened and pathologic if it is >7 mm at C2 or 14 mm at C6 (Fig. 34-2).
- CT scan of the neck: Diagnostic modality of choice. Can differentiate between cellulitis and frank abscess.

Definitive Management

- Treatment is surgical drainage and antibiotic therapy.
- Surgery: Incision and drainage of abscess in a controlled environment with complete airway control—preferably the OR.
- Antibiotic therapy: Broad coverage due to polymicrobial nature of infections. Common pathogens include group A strep, *S aureus,* and anaerobes. Commonly used antibiotics include:
  - Ampicillin/sulbactam 200 mg/kg/d IV divided qid
  - Clindamycin 30 mg/kg/d IV divided tid

Complications

- Airway compromise.
- Extension of infections into mediastinal structures: Potential space extends into upper thorax.
- Pneumonia.
- Sepsis.

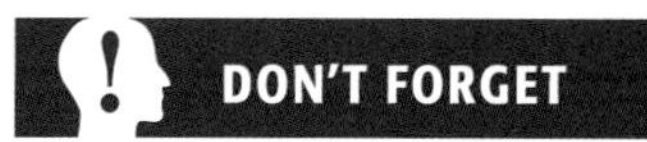

As with other pharyngeal infections, *think early airway, early consult, and early antibiotics.*

Disposition

- All patients with retropharyngeal abscess (RPA) must be admitted and managed in consultation with ENT. Particular attention must be paid to the maintenance of the airway. Initial therapy depends on the severity of respiratory distress and likelihood of drainable fluid based upon CT findings.

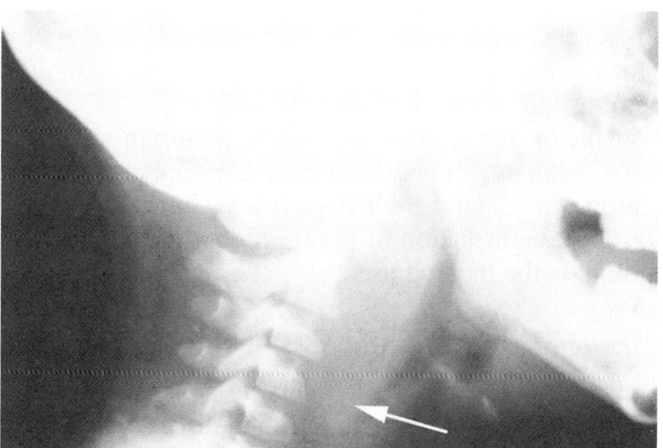

Figure 34-2. Lateral neck view of a child with retropharyngeal abscess and widened retropharyngeal space. (*Reproduced with permission from Tintinalli JE, Kelen GD, Stapczynski JS, et al.* Emergency Medicine: A Comprehensive Study Guide. *6th ed. New York, NY: McGraw-Hill; 2004.*)

- Empiric antibiotics should be initiated as soon as possible including coverage for *S aureus* and methicillin-resistant *Staphylococcus aureus* (MRSA) if appropriate, and respiratory anaerobes. Immediate surgical drainage is necessary for patients with airway compromise.
- Complications of RPA are potentially fatal. Infections can spread from the retropharyngeal space to other deep neck spaces, to adjacent structures and to the bloodstream.

DIPHTHERIA

Additional History and Physical Examination Findings

- Infection with the gram-positive rod *Corynebacterium diphtheria.*
- Cases are rare now due to the vaccine. Be sure to confirm the patient's immunization history.
- Incubation period of 2-5 days, followed by:
  - Fever and chills
  - Malaise
  - Sore throat
  - Hoarseness and dysphagia
  - Cervical edema and lymphadenopathy
- Physical examination reveals lesions in the posterior oropharynx that appear as punched out ulcerations with gray membranes at the margins (pseudomembrane).
  - May be observed on the palate, pharynx, epiglottitis, larynx, or trachea. The diphthertic membrane is usually gray and adheres tightly to the underlying tissue.
- May have cutaneous lesions, nonhealing sores, or shallow ulcers with a dirty gray membrane.

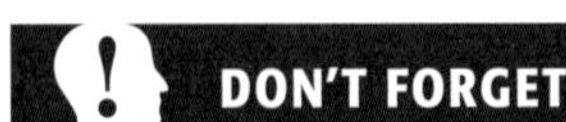

Think of diphtheria in patients who have questionable immunization history. Absorption and dissemination of the diphtheria toxin can lead to damage of the heart and nervous system.

Review Initial Results

- No quick diagnostic modality; must have a high index of suspicion and thorough clinical examination.
- Gram stain: Aerobic, club-shaped, gram + rod
- Definitive diagnosis: Requires culture of *C diphtheriae* from the respiratory tract secretions or cutaneous lesions and a positive toxin assay.
  - Culture should be obtained from the throat and nose including a portion of the membrane and material beneath the membrane. Special culture media are needed; ask the microbiology lab to plate on appropriate media.
  - Testing for toxin production must be performed to differentiate toxigenic from nontoxigenic strains of *C diphtheriae.*
- If clinical suspicion for diphtheria is high, antitoxin should be considered and discussed with infectious disease or the Centers for Disease Control and Prevention (CDC) or health department, and should be administered promptly prior to confirmation of toxin production, which may take several days depending on the method used.

Definitive Management

- Most important treatment is isolation, airway control, antibiotic therapy, and consideration of diphtheria antitoxin. (Antitoxin can induce serum sickness.) Antitoxin is not commercially available in the United States, but may be obtained from the CDC which also provides telephone consultation. Call them for guidance with antitoxin, American Academy of Pediatrics (AAP) recommends treatment for pharyngeal/laryngeal disease and nasopharyngeal disease.
- Isolation: Throughout therapy. Respiratory droplet precautions for respiratory tract infections and contact precautions for cutaneous disease.

- Early airway control: For severe disease and possible removal of adherent of tracheobronchial membranes.
- Antibiotic therapy:
  - Erythromycin 20-50 mg/kg/d IV divided bid
- Consult infectious disease or CDC (1-404-639-2889) for antitoxin guidelines as the dosage and route depend on the extent and duration of the disease.
- Follow-up cultures should be performed at 24-48 hours and 2 weeks following infection to ensure eradication of the organism. Isolation should be continued until two consecutive cultures taken at least 24 hours apart are negative. Patients will need diphtheria toxoid immunization during their convalescence since natural infection does not induce immunity.

Frequent Reassessment

- Infections mandate inpatient admission and IV antibiotics.
- Culture all suspected cases.
- Close contacts need to be identified, cultured, and considered for antimicrobial prophylaxis.
- Contact national and local health departments to report disease outbreak.

Complications

- Pneumonia and respiratory failure
- Cardiac complications
  - Myocarditis
  - Heart blocks and other dysrhythmias
  - Patients should be monitored with serial ECGs and measurement of cardiac enzymes that reflect the intensity of myocardial damage.
- Sepsis
- Cranial and peripheral neuropathies
  - Neurologic status should also be monitored carefully.

Disposition

- Patients must be admitted to the hospital.
- Stable patients may be admitted to the floor.
- Patients with airway compromise or sepsis must be admitted to the ICU.

WINNING STRATEGIES

- Every sore throat is a potential airway problem until proven otherwise! Get early consults, early antibiotics, and early intubation if needed.
- No single element in the history or physical examination is sensitive or specific enough to exclude the diagnosis of strep pharyngitis—use both the rapid strep test and the strep validation score to guide your treatment.
- Epiglottitis is a true airway emergency—keep the child calm, treat with early antibiotics, and airway management—preferably in the OR.
- Be sure your discharge instructions in mononucleosis include stopping contact sports to avoid splenic rupture.
- Think of diphtheria in patients with an unknown or incomplete immunization history.

CHAPTER 35

Pediatric Abdominal Pain

Lindsey Caley, John Dayton, and Matthew Steimle

DON'T FORGET

On exam day, every child presenting with abdominal pain has a surgical emergency until proven otherwise. The exception to this rule is the child with DKA.

IMMEDIATE INTERVENTIONS

- Address ABCs
- Cardiac monitor and supplemental O_2 for kids in shock
- IV with rapid NS bolus (20 cc/kg) for kids with severe dehydration or shock
- NPO status
- hCG for all menstruating females

DON'T FORGET

- Sudden onset of pain is typically associated with perforation, volvulus, or torsion.
- Slow onset is usually related to appendicitis.
- Intermittent, colicky pain can be related to intussusception.

DON'T FORGET

- When abdominal pain comes before vomiting it is more likely to be of a surgical origin.

DON'T FORGET

- For children in shock, use fluid boluses to treat hypotension, and intubate when obtunded. If concern for surgical emergency make them NPO.

INITIAL ASSESSMENT

- Focus on age, gender, vital signs (VS), and general appearance. Is the child happy, playful, crying, writhing, lying still, lethargic, withdrawn?
- Identify unstable patients with immediate life threats:
  - Hypovolemic shock due to severe dehydration or trauma.
  - Septic shock due to surgical abdomen.

INITIAL HISTORY AND PHYSICAL EXAMINATION

History

- History of present illness (HPI)
  - Any fevers?
  - What is the character of the pain?
  - Onset of symptoms: When did they start? Was the onset sudden or insidious?
  - Pain: Location, radiation, and migration? Is pain episodic or constant? Are there aggravating or relieving factors?
  - Any similar episodes in the past?
  - Vomiting: Any bright red blood or coffee-ground material? Was the emesis bilious? Did vomiting start before or after the pain began?
  - Stools: How frequent? What is the consistency? Is there mucous or blood? Has the patient had flatus?
  - Urination: When was the last urination/wet diaper? Is there dysuria, frequency or urgency? How many wet diapers in the past 24 hours?
- Past medical history (PMHx)
  - Birth history: Birth weight, gestational age, complications pre- and postnatal infections, vaginal delivery or Cesarean section, prenatal care
  - Chronic medical problems
  - Immunizations
  - Prior surgeries
  - Menstrual and sexual histories in adolescents
- Medications
- Allergies

Physical Examination

- VS: Include temperature and blood pressure
- Head, eyes, ears, nose, and throat (HEENT) examination: Check for sunken fontanelle, sunken eyes, tears, dry mucous membranes.
- Lungs: Check for equal sounds, crackles, rales, and wheezing. Assess for tachypnea and overall work of breathing.
- Cardiovascular (CV): Check pulses (are they strong, weak, or absent peripherally) and capillary refill.
- Abdomen: Listen for bowel sounds. Palpate and note tenderness, guarding, rebound pain, or distension. Assess for peritoneal signs with a heel tap or asking them to jump up and down.
- Rectal: Feel for masses and look for grossly bloody stool.
- Genitourinary (GU): Check for hernias, scrotal pain/swelling.
- Neuro: Assess their level consciousness.

DIFFERENTIAL DIAGNOSIS

- Pyloric stenosis
  - Hypertrophy of the pylorus causes gastric outlet obstruction.
  - This is the most common cause of gastrointestinal (GI) obstruction in infancy.

- Rarely occurs before 1 week of age or later than 5 months of age, (symptoms usually begin between 3 and 5 weeks of life.).
- More likely to occur in the child of an affected parent (particularly mothers). Males (particularly firstborns) are affected four times more frequently than females.

- Intussusception
  - Involves telescoping of a segment of proximal intestine into adjacent distal intestine leading to bowel obstruction and vascular compromise.
  - The majority are ileocolic, although ileoileal and colocolic invaginations may also occur.
  - In younger children, the "lead point" is usually a hypertrophied Peyer patch following a viral infection.
  - Older children are more likely to have an identifiable lead point (ie, lymphoma, ileal duplication, polyp, or Meckel diverticulum).
  - Henoch-Schönlein purpura (HSP) is associated with intussusception and is characterized by a purpuric rash generally seen over the buttocks and legs.
  - Males are affected twice as often as females.
- Midgut volvulus
  - Congenital malrotation of the midgut results in abnormal attachment to the mesentery, causing the small intestine to twist around the mesenteric stalk.
  - Compression of bowel leads to obstruction and compression of the superior mesenteric artery leads to ischemia.
  - More than half of cases present during the first month of life.
  - Males are more commonly affected than females.
- Testicular torsion
  - Can be caused by trauma or congenital abnormality.
  - Result of congenital abnormality in which the testicle is inadequately anchored to the scrotum ("Bell clapper deformity"). The testicle is predisposed to rotate on itself causing compression to the spermatic cord and vessels causing vascular compromise and can lead to infarction as early as 6 hours after onset.
  - Bell clapper deformity is typically bilateral, although usually only one testicle will torse at a time.
  - Bimodal peak incidence occurs during puberty (12-15 years) and also during the first year of life.
- Appendicitis
  - Obstruction of the lumen of the appendix causes distension and inflammation.
  - Most common surgical emergency in children and can occur at any age.
  - Very difficult diagnosis in younger children, leading to a high rate of perforation before diagnosis. Among patients <2 years old, 70%-94% are perforated before diagnosis. As a result, these patients typically present with signs of peritonitis or sepsis.

INFANTILE HYPERTROPHIC PYLORIC STENOSIS

Additional History and Physical Examination Findings

- The classic presentation is a 3 to 6-week-old infant with nonbilious, postprandial, projectile vomiting.
- Vomiting increases in frequency and forcefulness.
- Vomiting may be blood-streaked if mucosal tear has occurred.
- Initially, infants will still be hungry after vomiting, but eventually lose interest in feeding as they become progressively dehydrated.
  - Premature infants with infantile hypertrophic pyloric stenosis (IHPS) may have less forceful vomiting, and they may not display hunger.

DON'T FORGET

- Assess hydration status if anorexic or vomiting.

DON'T FORGET

- Lethargic and withdrawn = shock
- Lying still with knees flexed = peritoneal irritation
- Crying/moaning and unable to lie still = colicky pain

DON'T FORGET

- Observing reaction of patient to jostling bed is a good way to assess for peritoneal irritation.

DON'T FORGET

DDx Summary

Most common surgical causes of abdominal pain/vomiting by age

- Neonate: Necrotizing enterocolitis, volvulus, pyloric stenosis, testicular torsion
- 2 months to 2 years: Intussusception, incarcerated hernia
- 2 years to 5 years: Appendicitis, intussusception
- 5 years to 12 years: Appendicitis, perforated ulcer
- Adolescence: Appendicitis, testicular or ovarian torsion, ectopic pregnancy

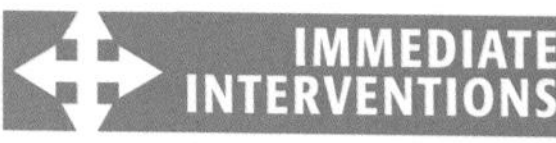

- IV access for fluid resuscitation and labs
- NPO
- Order lytes, glucose
- With obstruction concern, NG tube to decompress the stomach and reduce the risk of aspiration

- May be a history of pyloric stenosis in one of the parents.
- Will show poor weight gain or even weight loss.
- Examination may reveal palpable "olive" in upper abdomen, jaundice, or peristaltic waves moving left to right across upper abdomen. These, however, are rare findings.
- Examination more likely to show varying degrees of dehydration, depending on duration of symptoms at time of presentation.

Review Initial Results

- Electrolytes: Persistent vomiting may cause both hypoglycemia and a hypokalemic, hypochloremic metabolic alkalosis. Normal results do not exclude the diagnosis.

Risk Stratification: Management Priorities

- Intravenous fluid (IVF)
  - Correct dehydration and hypovolemic shock with 20 cc/kg boluses of normal saline (NS) until volume deficit is corrected (tachycardia resolves and patient urinates).
- If hypokalemic, place on cardiac monitor, check electrocardiogram (ECG), and add potassium supplementation to IVF.
- If "olive" is palpated, consult a surgeon as there is no need for further diagnostic tests.
- If diagnosis is in doubt, order radiographic study.

Further Diagnostic Considerations

- Abdominal ultrasound
  - Study of choice
  - Will demonstrate thickened pyloric muscle wall (>3 mm) and elongated pyloric canal >14 mm (remember π 3.14) (Fig. 35-1).
- Barium swallow
  - Order if abdominal ultrasound is not available or not diagnostic.

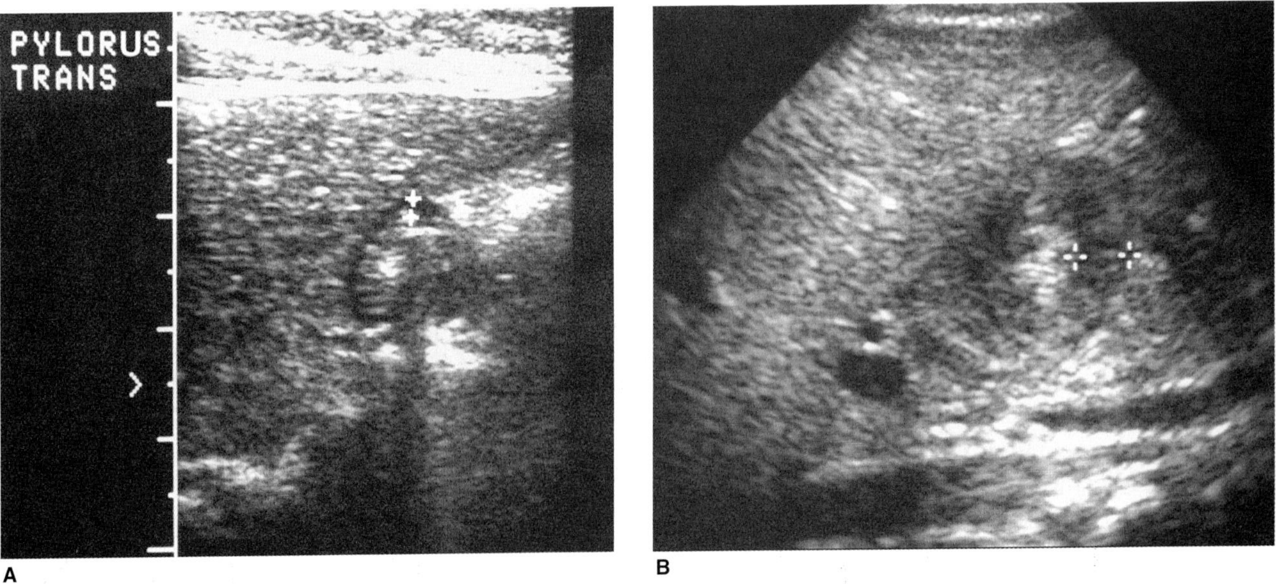

Figure 35-1. Ultrasound: (**A**) Normal pylorus in cross section. The muscle wall thickness was measured as 1.5 mm. (**B**) Transverse view of pyloric stenosis. The muscle wall thickness was measured at 4.7 mm. *(Reproduced with permission from Ma OJ, Mateer JR, Blaivas M.* Emergency Ultrasound. *2nd ed. New York, NY: McGraw-Hill; 2008.)*

- Will show either the "string sign" representing passage of contrast through narrowed, elongated pylorus or show complete gastric outlet obstruction.
- After study, remove contrast via nasogastric (NG) tube to suction to prevent aspiration of dye.

DON'T FORGET

- Patients with pyloric stenosis do not typically present with abdominal pain, so this is an important surgical entity to consider in infants with vomiting.

Definitive Management

- Consult surgeon for pyloromyotomy.

Frequent Reassessment

- If patient presented with dehydration or shock, or if patient continues to vomit in the emergency department (ED), give 20 cc/kg NS boluses and reassess vitals frequently.

DON'T FORGET

- The "olive" is best palpated with an empty stomach and relaxed abdominal muscles.
- Palpate immediately after vomiting or after NG suction.

Complications

- Hypokalemic, hypochloremic metabolic alkalosis
- Hypoglycemia
- Hypovolemic shock

Disposition

- Admit for surgery.
- Pediatric intensive care unit (PICU) if patient remains unstable after fluid boluses or has severe hypokalemia.

DON'T FORGET

- Because pyloric stenosis is not considered a surgical emergency, patients can be stabilized before going to OR.

INTUSSUSCEPTION

Additional History and Physical Examination Findings

- Classic presentation is a 6 to 36 month-old infant (also classically 2 months to 2 years) who is experiencing episodes of sudden, severe, crampy abdominal pain that resolve spontaneously.
- 75% are "idiopathic" although some of these may be caused by viral infections.
- 25% are caused by an underlying condition which creates a pathologic lead point, most commonly a Meckel diverticulum.
- All three symptoms of the "classic triad" actually only occur in about 15% of patients:
  - Intermittent, severe, colicky abdominal pain
  - Palpable sausage-shaped abdominal mass
  - Currant jelly stools
- Episodes are characterized by inconsolable crying and drawing the knees up to the abdomen.
- Early in the course of disease, infants may appear normal between episodes.
- As the disease progresses, the painful episodes increase in frequency and duration. The patient will become more lethargic between episodes. Patient will also begin to vomit. Emesis may become bilious. May present with only lethargy or altered consciousness.
- Low-grade fever may be present.
- May show varying degrees of dehydration or shock depending on progression of disease at time of presentation.
- Abdominal examination
  - Usually presents with abdominal tenderness.
  - May have abdominal distension and bowel sounds may be decreased due to ileus.
  - Right upper quadrant (RUQ) mass/fullness may be palpated (usually described as "sausage-shaped").

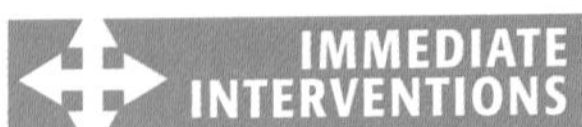

IMMEDIATE INTERVENTIONS

- IV access for fluid resuscitation and labs.
- NPO.
- NG tube to reduce the risk of aspiration.
- Order BMP and CBC. These may not have any clinical value unless patient has been vomiting, but most surgeons will expect these labs.
- Order abdominal x-rays (left lateral decubitus and abdominal series).

DON'T FORGET

- Very important to get surgical consult early. Do not let patient go for an enema without one.

DON'T FORGET

- Only two symptoms of the "classic triad" are present in 70% of intussusception cases.
- Ask caregivers to demonstrate what these episodes look like without leading them into the description.
- Neurologic symptoms may actually predominate in which case presentation will be related to lethargy, generalized weakness, and possibly even seizures.

- Rectal: Very important as most patients (all on exam day) will have guaiac positive stools.
  - Bloody, mucoid stools ("currant jelly") typically occur later in the course and indicate bowel ischemia.

Review Initial Results

- Electrolytes: Persistent vomiting may cause a hypokalemic, hypochloremic metabolic alkalosis.
- Hypoglycemia may be present.
- Abdominal x-rays: Although initially unremarkable, may eventually show signs of intestinal obstruction with dilated loops of bowel and paucity of gas distally. Findings more specific for intussusception include mass in the RUQ and lack of right lower quadrant (RLQ) air (Fig. 35-2).

Risk Stratification: Management Priorities

- IVF
  - Treat hypovolemic shock and dehydration with 20 cc/kg boluses of NS until stable and improved perfusion.
- Consult surgeon
  - Although intussusception is frequently reduced by a radiographic procedure, surgeons still need to be consulted very early in the process in case of complications and unsuccessful reductions.
- Use triple antibiotic coverage if patient is ill-appearing or if perforation or peritonitis is present.
  - Ampicillin, gentamicin, and clindamycin

Further Diagnostic Considerations

- Contrast enema is the gold standard for diagnosing intussusception and is frequently therapeutic as well.

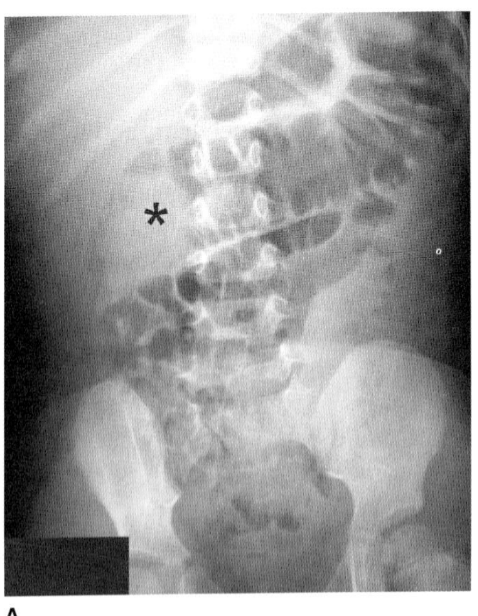

A

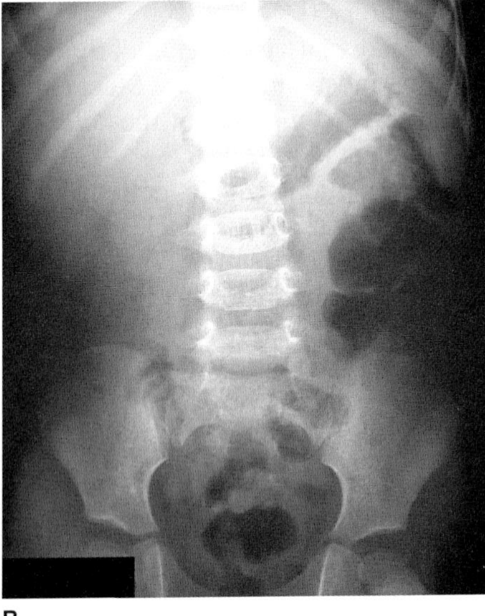

B

Figure 35-2. Intussusception. (**A**) The crescent-shaped head of the intussusceptum is seen as an intraluminal mass in the gas-filled transverse colon (asterisk). (**B**) The initial radiograph may be nonspecific. However, the right side of the abdomen is gasless, a finding suggestive of intussusception. *(Reproduced with permission from Schwartz DT.* Emergency Radiology: Case Studies. *New York, NY: McGraw-Hill; 2008.)*

- Air enema has the advantage of causing no further problems should the bowel perforate during the procedure.
- The disadvantage is that it is a poor contrast medium and may miss lead-point masses which would be an indication for surgery.
- Barium enema is a good contrast medium and is better for visualizing lead-point masses, if present. The disadvantage is that it may cause a chemical peritonitis if perforation occurs during the procedure.
- Both are absolutely contraindicated if there is evidence of perforation, peritonitis, sepsis, or shock.

- Ultrasound
  - Used in some centers to identify intussusception and lead-point mass if present.
  - Accuracy is operator-dependent.
  - Advantage is that it is not invasive and can be used when enema is contraindicated.
  - Disadvantage is that it is not therapeutic. However, it can identify lead points.
- Computed tomography (CT)
  - Can identify intussusception and other possible etiologies of pain.

Definitive Management

- Reduction by air or barium enema
- Surgical correction if enema reduction is contraindicated, if bowel perforates during enema, or if reduction is unsuccessful.

Frequent Reassessment

- Reassess vitals and urine output, and give NS boluses as needed.

Complications

- 7%-10% recurrence rate following radiological reduction, particularly if reduced within the first 24 hours
- Bowel necrosis resulting in perforation and peritonitis
- Hypovolemic or septic shock
- GI bleeding
- Death

Disposition

- Admit for observation following successful reduction.
- Admit to operating room (OR) if reduction by enema is unsuccessful or if bowel perforates.

MIDGUT VOLVULUS

Additional History and Physical Examination Findings

- Patients classically present between birth and 1 month of age with bilious vomiting and sudden onset of constant abdominal pain. Vomiting may not be bilious.
- Patient may have had self-resolving episodes of bilious vomiting before presentation which were not evaluated.
- The patient may present in shock if bowel is significantly compromised.
- Jaundice is present in about one-third of patients.
- Abdominal examination:
  - May reveal an abdominal mass representing a dilated loop of bowel.

DON'T FORGET

- Use contrast enema unless the patient has perforated, has peritonitis, is septic, or in shock.

DON'T FORGET

- "Never let the sun set on bilious vomiting." This is **never** normal in infants and requires immediate surgical consult, even if the patient is nontoxic appearing and diagnosis is not yet confirmed.

DON'T FORGET

- Bloody stools are associated with severely ischemic or gangrenous bowel.

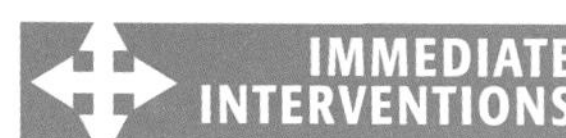
IMMEDIATE INTERVENTIONS

- Address ABCs if patient is in shock.
- Cardiac monitor
- Supplemental O_2
- IV for fluid resuscitation and lab draw.
- NPO
- NG tube to reduce the risk of aspiration
- Order plain abdominal x-rays (left lateral decubitus and abdominal series).
- Send CBC with diff, BMP and type and screen/cross

DON'T FORGET

- Diagnose by history and physical, and then obtain surgical consult.
- Further studies are only indicated if diagnosis is still in question.
- Consult the surgeon early! Surgical delays result in more extensive bowel damage and increased morbidity and mortality.

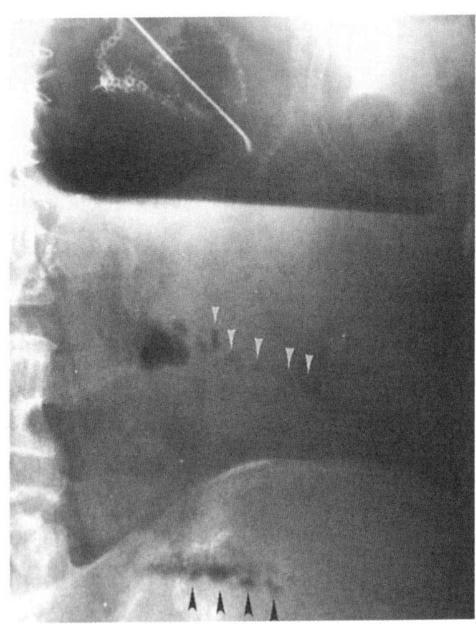

A

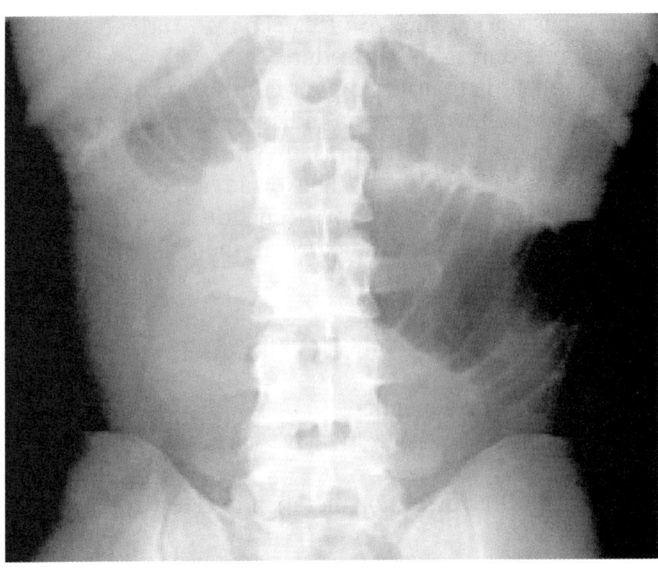

B

Figure 35-3. (**A**) Small bowel obstruction. Two rows of air bubbles (arrowheads) with fluid levels in the left mid-abdomen are indicative of mechanical obstruction in the small intestine. *(Reproduced with permission from Chen MY, Pope TL, Ott DJ.* Basic Radiology. *New York, NY: McGraw-Hill; 2004.)* (**B**) Markedly dilated small bowel in a mechanical small bowel obstruction can have a similar appearance to dilated large bowel, particularly the transverse colon. (*Reproduced with permission from Schwartz DT.* Emergency Radiology: Case Studies. *New York, NY: McGraw-Hill; 2008.)*

- There will likely be some abdominal distension and diffuse tenderness to palpation.
- Stools, if present on rectal examination, may be guaiac positive or grossly bloody.

Review Initial Results

- Abdominal x-ray (flat and upright): May show "double-bubble sign" representing dilated stomach and duodenum with no air distally (Fig. 35-3).
- Blood work: Generally only needed for pre-op purposes
  - Elevated white blood cell (WBC) (>20,000) likely with peritonitis

Risk Stratification: Management Priorities

- IVF
  - Treat dehydration and hypovolemic shock aggressively with 20 cc/kg boluses of NS until stable.
- Stat surgical consult is required if the patient is unstable or decompensating.
  - Do not delay surgical exploration with imaging studies if you have high clinical suspicion as this is a surgical emergency.
- If the patient is hemodynamically stable, obtain two-view plain abdominal radiographs. If perforation is present, resuscitate with fluids, provide empiric antibiotics to cover bowel flora, and consult with a pediatric surgeon to obtain emergency surgery.
- If the patient is stable with no perforation, obtain limited upper GI series with oral contrast, if intestinal malrotation present emergently consult with a pediatric surgeon, if study is negative consult with pediatric radiologist and surgeon for additional imaging or diagnostic laparoscopy.
- Use triple antibiotics coverage (ampicillin, gentamicin, clindamycin) for peritonitis or if patient is ill-appearing.

Further Diagnostic Considerations

- Upper GI contrast series is 96% sensitive.
- Barium swallow
  - Study of choice if diagnosis is still in question.
  - Will demonstrate abnormal location of ligament of Treitz, narrowing at site of obstruction, and twisting of the small bowel around the superior mesenteric artery.
  - Remove contrast via NG tube to suction following the study to prevent aspiration.
- Other options:
  - Abdominal x-ray my illustrate "double bubble" sign, but may be completely normal.
  - Ultrasound may show "whirlpool" sign of volvulus, dilated duodenum, and movement of distal duodenum from regular retromesenteric location.
  - CT with IV contrast is not first choice due to radiation exposure, but will show arterial compromise and bowel concerns.

Definitive Management

- Emergent surgical detorsion of volvulus and resection of infarcted bowel.

Frequent Reassessment

- Reassess VS and urine output, and give further 0.9 NS boluses as needed.

Complications

- Delay in presentation or diagnosis will result in bowel necrosis with subsequent perforation, peritonitis, electrolyte disturbances, shock (hypovolemic and septic), and possibly death.
- Short gut syndrome: Resection of a large amount of gangrenous bowel results in dependence on parenteral nutrition and other associated complications.

Disposition

- To OR for emergent surgery
- PICU bed following surgery

TESTICULAR TORSION

Additional History and Physical Examination Findings

- Patients classically present with a history of sudden onset of severe unilateral scrotal pain
  - This may occur upon awakening in the morning or after testicular trauma.
  - Might also present with intermittent symptoms due to intermittent torsion.
  - Atypical presentations with a chief complaint of lower abdominal pain are common.
- Approximately 40% of patients with testicular torsion report having recently experienced a similar episode of scrotal pain that resolved spontaneously.
- Systemic symptoms such as nausea/vomiting (50%) and fevers may also be reported.
- Abdominal examination
  - Relatively benign, even if the location of pain is the lower abdomen.
- GU examination
  - Diffuse tenderness over testicle with degree of swelling related to duration of torsion.
  - Testicle may have a horizontal lie to testicle.
  - Lack of cremasteric reflex occurs with testicular torsion but is not a reliable finding.

DON'T FORGET

- Patients presenting with an acute scrotum have testicular torsion until proven otherwise.
- Be careful with intermittent torsion, which can occur, presenting with sudden onset of acute and intermittent sharp testicular pain and scrotal swelling, with rapid resolution—be sure to obtain ultrasound and seek immediate follow-up within 7 days and return to ED if pain recurs sooner.

DON'T FORGET

Torsion vs Epididymitis

Torsion

- Sudden onset
- Fever in <20%
- Vomiting is common
- Sudden onset of pain
- Dysuria is rare

Epididymitis

- Average age is older (25 years)
- Fevers in up to 95%
- Vomiting is unusual
- Gradual onset with pain severity peaking in days
- Dysuria is common

DON'T FORGET

- **Never** leave out the GU examination on patients with abdominal pain.

Review Initial Results

- UA: Usually unremarkable in torsion (as opposed to epididymitis)

Risk Stratification: Management Priorities

- Consult urologist/surgeon early if testicular torsion is strongly suggested based on history and physical examination rather than performing imaging. The diagnoses of testicular torsion can be made clinically.
    - Urologist may take patient for exploratory surgery if history and physical are strongly suggestive of torsion.
    - If diagnosis is in doubt, order stat Doppler ultrasound to check blood flow.

Further Diagnostic Considerations

- Color-flow Doppler ultrasound (Fig. 35-4) is the study of choice because it is noninvasive and usually available.
    - Torsion causes decreased blood flow to the affected testicle when compared with unaffected side.
    - Limited value in infants due to normal low arterial flow to smaller testicles.
    - If testicle spontaneously detorses before study, may see near normal or even increased blood flow.
    - Nondiagnostic study is an indication for surgical exploration.
- Radionuclide scan is time-consuming when time is of the essence.

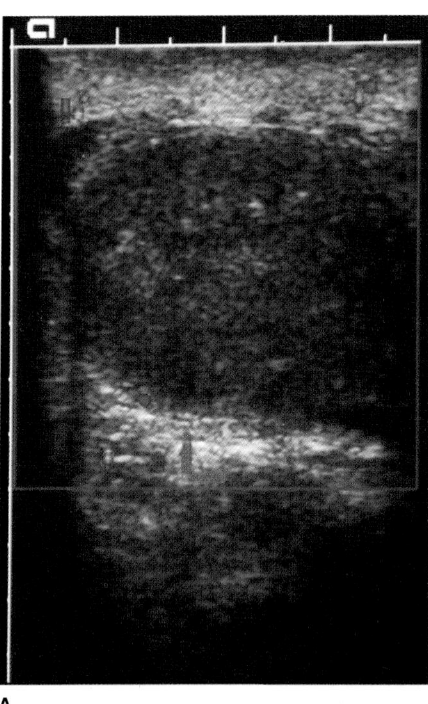

A

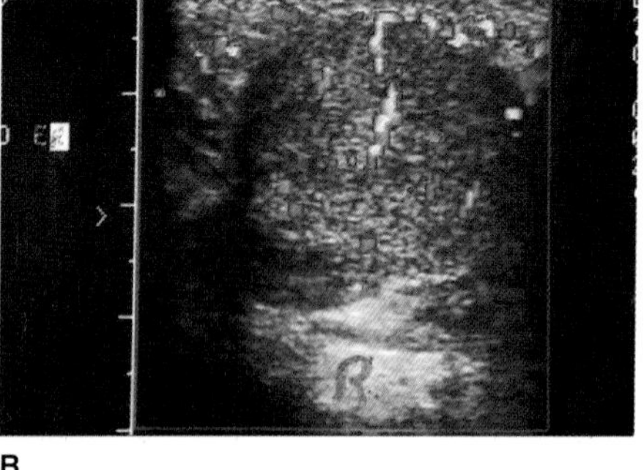

B

Figure 35-4. The left testis (**A**) is heterogeneous and hypoechoic and slightly enlarged compared to the right. The left epididymis is enlarged and heterogeneous. There is thickening of the overlying scrotal skin and soft tissues, along with a reactive left hydrocele. There is an absence of vascular flow in the parenchyma of the left testis with flow in the surrounding soft tissues. The right testis (**B**) demonstrates normal perfusion. *(Reproduced with permission from Shah BR, Lucchesi M.* Atlas of Pediatric Emergency Medicine. *New York, NY: McGraw-Hill; 2006.)*

Definitive Management

- Pain control with IV narcotic medication.
- Surgical detorsion and bilateral orchiopexy.
- There are no contraindications to attempting manual detorsion once the patient is diagnosed and set for surgery. Manual detorsion can be attempted if operative care is not rapidly available.
  - Treat with IV pain medication and sedation.
  - Testicles typically torse in a medial direction, so "open the book," one to two full 360° turns, until prompt relief of pain, lower position of the testis, and return of arterial flow on Doppler ultrasound. If no improvement, try rotating the testicle in the opposite direction (lateral to medial) one-third of torsed testicle may have lateral rotation.
  - Bedside detorsion is not a replacement for definitive surgical correction.

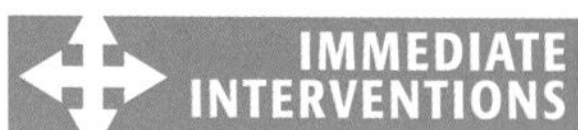

- NPO
- Obtain UA
- Scrotal ultrasound
- Stat urology consult.

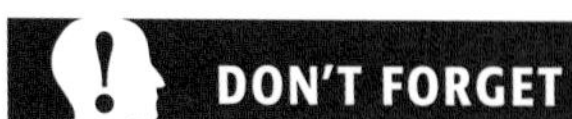

- Prolonged torsion causes increased ischemia.
- After 6 hours the rate of salvage is poor.

Complications

- Testicular atrophy
- Loss of spermatogenesis

Disposition

- To OR for detorsion and bilateral orchiopexy

APPENDICITIS

Additional History and Physical Examination Findings

- Classic presentation is history of constant, vague periumbilical pain which over time localizes to the RLQ with associated nausea, vomiting, anorexia, and low-grade fever.
- Pediatric pitfalls:
  - Younger children cannot verbalize the progression of symptoms and up to 95% of patients <2 years old will have perforated appendices before the diagnosis is made.
  - Anorexia is not always seen in children and patients may in fact be hungry.
  - Diarrhea is more common in children with appendicitis than in adults and can lead to confusion with acute gastroenteritis.
  - Temperature may be normal.
  - Children <5 years do not present classically have high index of suspicion.
- Observe patient position and movement before starting examination.
  - May have a limp or shuffling gait when walking.
  - Lying still with right hip flexed may be position of comfort.
- Abdominal examination.
  - Tender to palpation over McBurney point.
  - May have RLQ guarding or rebound.
  - Rovsing sign: Pain in RLQ with palpation in left lower quadrant (LLQ).
  - Decreased bowel sounds as an ileus develops.
  - Obturator sign: With the patient lying supine, flexion and internal rotation of the right hip will cause pain in the RLQ.
  - Psoas sign: With the patient lying on their left side, hyperextension of the right hip will cause pain in the RLQ.
- Classic abdominal findings may not be present if appendix is in a retrocecal or pelvic location.
  - Retrocecal location causes back or flank pain.
  - Pelvic location causes suprapubic pain.
- Rectal: May palpate mass or cause pain in the RLQ.

Review Initial Results

- Blood work
  - No lab tests should be relied on to diagnose appendicitis.
  - Typically obtain: Complete blood count (CBC) with differential, C-reactive protein (CRP), urinalysis (UA), and urine pregnancy
  - CBC: WBC may be increased with left shift, but as many as 10%-20% of patients will have normal WBC counts.
  - Human chorionic gonadotropin (hCG): If positive must also consider pregnancy-related emergencies such as ectopic pregnancy.
- UA: Usually unremarkable, however, may have a reactive pyuria.

Risk Stratification: Management Priorities

- Use a diagnostic approach guided by clinical impression of risk (low, moderate, or high). There are multiple validated clinical scoring systems that can be used for guidance.
- For high risk for acute appendicitis consult a surgeon prior to obtaining imaging studies.
- Low risk may be managed without imaging at the initial evaluation. They need very clear instruction regarding signs of appendicitis to prompt reevaluation, or if RLQ pain or tenderness is present they need reevaluation within 12-24 hours.
- Children with atypical, equivocal, or moderate likelihood for appendicitis warrant diagnostic imaging. Ultrasonography is the recommended initial imaging study.
- IVF
  - Treat hypovolemic shock and dehydration aggressively with 20 cc/kg boluses of NS until stable.
- Surgical consult: Obtain if history and physical are suggestive of appendicitis.
- Use broad-spectrum antibiotics (eg, cefoxitin, piperacillin and tazobactam, or ceftriaxone and metronidazole).
- Imaging studies: Order if diagnosis is uncertain following surgical consultation.

DON'T FORGET

- Fever and abdominal pain = appendicitis until proven otherwise.
- High fevers generally are seen only after perforation has occurred.
- Vomiting typically follows the onset of pain.
- For nonverbal children, check for anorexia by asking parents when last meal was eaten.
- Ask what patient's reaction is to jumping up and down. This may give you a good indication if peritoneal signs are present.

Further Diagnostic Considerations

- Ultrasound
  - Look for noncompressible appendix with diameter >6 mm.
  - May find appendicolith.
  - Accuracy of diagnosis is operator-dependent.
  - If appendicitis is found, call surgeon. If study is nondiagnostic, proceed with CT
- Abdominal CT
  - Use IV and oral or rectal contrast.
  - Visualizes inflamed appendix as well as complications.
  - Can rule out other causes of abdominal pain.

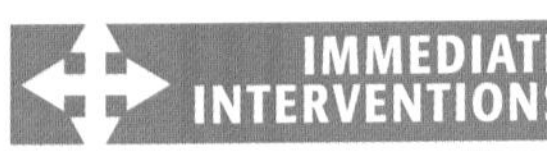

- Address ABCs.
- Establish IV for fluid resuscitation and lab draw.
- NPO
- NG tube if there is significant vomiting in order to reduce the risk of aspiration.
- Order CBC with diff, CRP, UA, and hCG in menstruating females.

Definitive Management

- Appendectomy
- Pain medication

Frequent Reassessment

- Perform serial abdominal examinations when diagnosis is in doubt to check progression of symptoms.
- If dehydrated, reassess status after fluid boluses and repeat as needed.

Complications

- Perforation can then lead to:
  - Phlegmon
  - Appendiceal abscess
  - Peritonitis
  - Septic shock
  - Pylephlebitis: Septic phlebitis of the portal veins

Disposition

- To OR for appendectomy

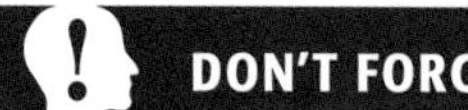

DON'T FORGET

- Abdominal x-rays should only be ordered if concerned about perforation.
- The Pediatric Appendicitis Score and Alvarado Score can help you identify low-, medium-, or high-risk patients, but should only be used as guidelines.

WINNING STRATEGIES

- The age and gender of the patient and the characteristics of the abdominal pain direct which differentials to consider. The physical examination should narrow the spectrum to a single surgical entity.
- Never wait for results of labs or radiographic studies on exam day to consult the surgeon when faced with a surgical emergency.
- Speak to primary caregivers (typically the parents) frequently. This shows your understanding of the pathology and represents easy points to get on exam day.
- For infants <1 year with apparent abdominal pain, you must rule out intussusception.
- In children >1 year, you must rule out appendicitis.
- For bilious emesis in infants, think midgut volvulus.
- Always do a GU examination when evaluating abdominal pain to check for hernias and testicular torsion.
- Pain due to peritonitis is exacerbated by motion, so these patients prefer to lie still.
- Pain associated with obstruction is usually colicky, associated with restlessness, and patients seem unable to find a comfortable position.
- Intermittent episodes of abdominal pain, with asymptomatic episodes in between, are intussusception until proven otherwise.
- Reassess, reassess, reassess.
- Plain abdominal x-rays are only useful when you suspect perforation or obstruction.
- Be generous with pain meds once examination is complete and diagnosis is made.
- Do not forget the rectal examination and guaiac.

THE BOTTOM LINE

- Episodic, severe abdominal pain and vomiting with plus guaiac or grossly bloody stools in infants = intussusception
- Sudden onset lower abdominal pain ± vomiting and unilateral scrotal tenderness = testicular torsion
- Sudden onset abdominal pain and bilious emesis in first month of life = midgut volvulus
- Gradually worsening, nonbilious, postprandial, projectile vomiting in 3 to 6-week-old patients = pyloric stenosis
- Periumbilical pain which localizes to the RLQ = appendicitis

CHAPTER 36

Pediatric Joint Pain

Christopher Gee and John Dayton

INITIAL ASSESSMENT

- Focus on the age and general appearance of the child. Certain conditions will be more or less likely depending on child's age and history.
- Identifying the child as toxic or ill-appearing is the most important initial distinction to make in these cases.
- Check the child's vital signs with this first look at the patient.

INITIAL HISTORY AND PHYSICAL EXAMINATION

- History of present illness (HPI)
  - Child's age? Onset of symptoms? Affected joint(s)? Duration? Radiation? Presence of swelling, erythema, or heat? Ability to bear weight? Position of joint at rest?
  - Any recent or current associated infectious/systemic symptoms including rash, fevers, upper respiratory infection (URI) symptoms (sx), gastrointestinal (GI) sx, or urinary sx?
  - Any history of remote or recent trauma?
  - Any risk factors for child abuse (babysitter, foster home)? Does the reported history correspond to the injury and is it age-appropriate?
  - Any recent sick contacts?
- Past medical history (PMHx)
  - Is the child immunocompromised? Is there a history of similar injury or complaints?
  - Has child had normal growth and development?
- Medications
  - Any immunosuppressants?
  - Has any medication helped the symptoms?
- Allergies
- Physical examination (PE)
  - Recheck the vital signs, especially if the child is toxic-appearing.
  - What is the activity level? Are they playful, lethargic, or refusing to walk?
  - What is the child's weight?
  - What is the child's hydration/perfusion status? Sunken fontanelle, dry mucous membranes, poor skin turgor, sluggish cap refill, skin cool or warm?
  - Head, eyes, ears, nose, and throat (HEENT) examination: Are there any localized findings (uveitis or conjunctivitis, retinal hemorrhages, hemotympanum)?
  - Chest: Any crackles, coarseness, areas of decreased sound?
  - Heart: Rubs, gallops, murmurs, tachycardia?
  - Abdomen: Any focal tenderness, guarding, masses?
  - Skin: Any rash, erythema or bruising of different ages?
  - Neurologic: Any altered sensorium? Are they moving all extremities? Is there normal strength and sensation?
  - Musculoskeletal examination: Are there one or multiple joints involved?
    - What is the position of the limb at rest?
    - Is the joint(s) erythematous and warm?
    - Is there point tenderness at or around the joint(s)?
    - Is there increased pain with passive or specific movements of the joint(s)?
    - Is the affected limb neurovascularly intact?
    - Is the child able to walk? Are they weight bearing? Is there a limp or ataxia?

DON'T FORGET

On exam day, a child with hip pain has either:

- Septic hip
- Legg-Calvé-Perthes (LCP) disease
- Slipped capital femoral epiphysis (SCFE)

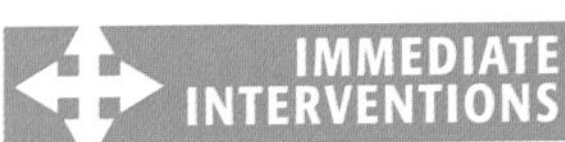

- IV, O_2, monitor, and airway equip to bedside if there is evidence of sepsis or major trauma
- IVF boluses as vitals dictate
- Analgesia after checking allergies

DIFFERENTIAL DIAGNOSIS

The following causes of pediatric joint pain are most likely to be tested on the oral boards. They are broken down by mechanical versus inflammatory causes of joint pain.

MECHANICAL CAUSES OF JOINT PAIN OR LIMPING

- Trauma with fracture, dislocation, or soft tissue injury
  - A mechanism of injury should be directly reported in the history.
  - Location of the injury, including any joint involvement, and neurovascular status dictate the need for subsequent interventions.
  - Oral board cases frequently involve multiple areas of trauma. Don't stop asking questions because you have identified one injury. Continue asking questions because there may be other injuries.
- Slipped capital femoral epiphysis (SCFE)
  - Epiphyseal portion of the femur literally shifts across the physis (looks like ice cream falling off a cone).
  - It typically occurs in overweight pubertal boys.
  - Children present with a limp and insidious unilateral or bilateral hip or knee pain.
  - Diagnosis with x-ray needs to be made as early as possible, as further slippage leads to permanent degenerative changes to the hip and avascular necrosis (AVN) of the femoral head.
- Legg-Calvé-Perthes (LCP) disease
  - Idiopathic AVN of the femoral head, thought to be related to interruption in vascular supply.
  - Occurs between ages 3 and 12 years and presents with insidious onset of pain in the hip or knee and an associated limp.
  - Treatment is observation, physical therapy, and activity modifications.
  - Occasionally, may be severe enough to require surgery.
  - Prognosis varies with age of onset and sphericity of femoral head. Children that are diagnosed when they are younger have a better prognosis.
- Apophysitis
  - An apophysis is a bony projection where a tendon inserts. In kids, there is a growth plate underneath this site. These areas become inflamed during periods of increased growth, persistent overuse (like in athletes), or can even be avulsed by the attached tendon.
  - This process is most commonly seen over the anterior tibial tubercle where the patellar tendon inserts (Osgood-Schlatter disease).
  - Other common sites for this condition include the calcaneal apophysitis (Sever disease) and the elbow medial epicondyle apophysis (Little League elbow).
  - Excellent prognosis with conservative treatment (rest).

SYSTEMIC/INFLAMMATORY CAUSES OF JOINT PAIN OR LIMPING

- Toxic/transient synovitis
  - Most common cause of hip pain in children.
  - Usually associated with previous viral URI or GI illness.
  - Insidious onset of groin or thigh pain.
  - Children appear nontoxic and have an excellent prognosis.
  - Diagnostic challenge to differentiate this condition from a septic joint or osteomyelitis.
- Septic arthritis
  - Children usually appear toxic, have a "hot joint," and require emergent joint arthrocentesis, orthopedic consult, antibiotics, and admission.
  - Even with early treatment, there is a risk of permanent damage which could precipitate early arthritis, nearby bone growth arrest, or nonunion of growth plates.
  - Joint infections may also be the nidus for severe sepsis presentations.

DON'T FORGET

The key to the case is to quickly decide if the problem is an **infectious/inflammatory** process or a **mechanical** issue. If an infectious/inflammatory process, the next concern should be whether it is a local or systemic issue.

- Rheumatologic etiologies
  - Rheumatologic conditions are infrequent, but should be included in your differential.
  - These typically present with subacute or chronic complaints that involve the joint and related area.
  - Juvenile idiopathic arthritis (JIA) is the most common pediatric rheumatologic process but is a diagnosis of exclusion and requires rheumatologic lab work and follow-up.
- Hematologic etiologies
  - Children with hemophilia or sickle cell disease present with bone and joint pain with associated limping.
  - Hemophiliacs present with hemarthrosis secondary to seemingly mild trauma and require emergent factor eight or nine replacement.
  - Children with sickle cell disease present in vaso-occlusive crisis with severe joint and bone pain that requires treatment with O_2, hydration, analgesics, and possibly blood transfusions.

COMMON FRACTURES AND DISLOCATIONS IN CHILDREN

DON'T FORGET

X-rays to diagnose mechanical injuries.

Additional History and Physical Examination

- Typically, a clear mechanism of injury can be determined and helps to focus your examination.
- When taking the history, determine whether the mechanism warrants a more extensive "trauma" workup and ask about associated injuries.
- A thorough distal neurovascular examination of any suspected traumatic injury must be conducted.
- Make sure the story matches the patient's injuries, as fractures and soft tissue injuries are the most common presentation of child abuse.
- Be sure to conduct a thorough hip examination with any patient presenting with knee pain, and vice versa, as there is a significant amount of referred pain between these areas.
- Children from a few months to 6 years of age may present with symptoms consistent with nursemaid's elbow. Classic story of axial traction of a pronated forearm (the child is picked up by the arm). The child will hold the arm close to the body with the forearm pronated and the elbow slightly flexed. Child won't use the arm. There may be some mild point tenderness over the radial head, but there should be no erythema or warmth.
- Treat nursemaid's with reduction (either hyperpronation or flexion technique) and observation until return of use.

DON'T FORGET

Always contact DCFS and the police if there is any concern of child abuse.

DON'T FORGET

Legg-Calvé-Perthes disease is usually found in patients between ages 3 and 12 years.

Review Initial Test Results

- X-rays
  - Image the area of concern as well as the joints above and below the injury.
  - Clavicle fractures are the most commonly seen fractures in pediatric patients. Determine which third of the clavicle is fractured and check for pneumothorax and neurovascular injury.
  - Supracondylar fractures of the elbow are common. The laxity of the child's ligaments allows hyperextension of the joint which makes it susceptible for this type of fracture.
    - Look for posterior fat pad along the distal portion of the humerus on lateral films as a sign of intra-articular blood and fracture (always abnormal). A small anterior fat pad that is not in the shape of a sail can be normal (Fig. 36-1).
  - Draw the anterior humeral line on lateral elbow x-ray to detect occult supracondylar fracture. This line goes along anterior cortex of humerus and through the joint. The line should pass through the middle one-third

DON'T FORGET

Blood work and joint aspiration are the mainstays of diagnosis of septic arthritis on test day.

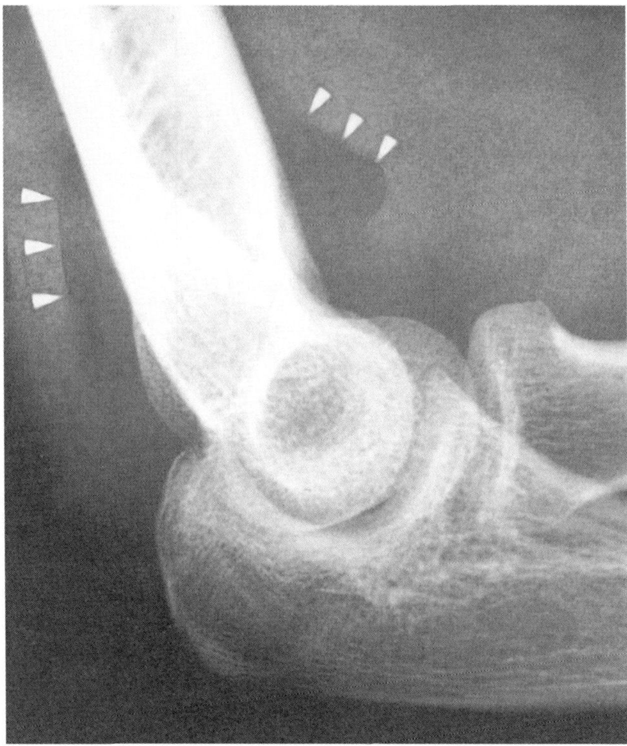

Figure 36-1. Anterior and posterior fat pads of the elbow (arrowheads). *(Reproduced with permission from Tintinalli JE, Kelen GD, Stapczynski JS, et al.* Emergency Medicine: A Comprehensive Study Guide. *6th ed. New York, NY: McGraw-Hill; 2004.)*

of the capitellum (Fig. 36-2). In a supracondylar fracture, the line will pass anterior to capitellum.

- Hip fractures usually occur as a result of trauma. Avulsion fractures can occur with extreme or sudden forceful movement.
- Avulsions of the greater trochanter are seen after falls with significant lateral rotation of the leg, or with forceful extension of the hip.
- Lesser trochanter avulsion fractures are seen with sudden, forceful hip flexion by the iliopsoas muscle group.

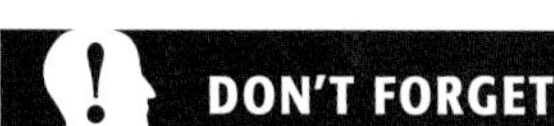

DON'T FORGET

Be aware that sickle cell patients may present with a limp for multiple reasons. The limp may be due to sickle crisis, ataxia secondary to a CVA, and/or joint infection secondary to encapsulated organisms that patients are susceptible to due to functional asplenia.

Definitive Management

- Pain control.
- Reduce and splint a fractured or dislocated extremity.
- Ensure intact neurovascular status after reduction and splint placement.
- Consult orthopedics for surgery or necessary follow-up.
- Supracondylar fractures are especially prone to neurovascular injury. If the hand of the affected limb is cold and gray, or if there is concern for neurologic injury, a reduction with gentle traction and realignment of fragments should be attempted. Further manipulations should be done in the operating room.
- Attempt reduction in any fracture where distal neurovascular status is compromised.
- If the fracture is open, administer tetanus if deficient, and antibiotics to cover for bacterial skin flora (usually a first-generation cephalosporin and an aminoglycoside), and place sterile saline or betadine-soaked gauze over the wound before splinting.

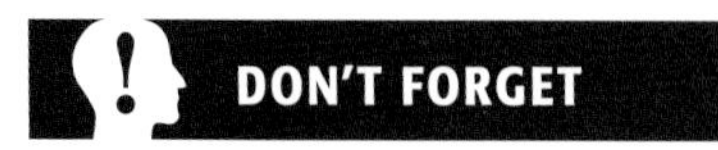

DON'T FORGET

Be aware of fractures associated with child abuse: Spiral femur fractures, fractures of varying ages, and bucket handle fractures.

DON'T FORGET

Be aware that hip pathology often presents only with knee pain. Get knee films with any hip pain and vice versa.

Knowing the order in which the ossification centers develop is important for diagnosing elbow fractures in children. Use the mnemonic "**C**ome **R**ub **M**y **T**ree **o**f **L**ove" to remember this sequence:

Capitellum	6-12 months
Radial head	4-5 years
Medial epicondyle	5-7 years
Trochlea	8-10 years
Olecranon	8-10 years
Lateral epicondyle	9-13 years

Particularly remember that the trochlea ossifies after the medial epicondyle. The medial epicondyle can avulse down into the joint and look like a trochlea.

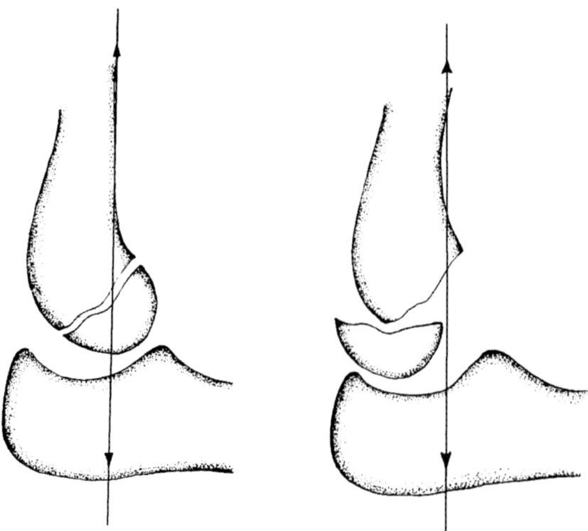

Figure 36-2. The anterior humeral line is a line drawn on the lateral radiograph along the anterior surface of the humerus through the elbow. Normally this line transects through the middle of the capitellum. With an extension fracture of the supracondylar region, this line will either transect the anterior third of the capitellum or pass entirely anterior to it. *(Reproduced with permission from Simon RR, Sherman SC, Koenigsknecht SJ.* Emergency Orthopedics: The Extremities. *5th ed. New York, NY: McGraw-Hill; 2007.)*

DON'T FORGET

Posterior fat pads and large, sail-shaped anterior ones represent an elbow effusion that is likely a supracondylar fracture on exam day (Fig. 36-1).

- Immobilize the affected bone, including the joint proximal and distal to the fracture. Use a fiberglass splint (Ortho-Glass), and not a circumferential plaster cast, with any acute fracture.
- Nursemaid's elbow should be reduced without radiographs. This condition is a subluxation of the radial head out of the annular ligament that holds it in the joint space. Reduce the radial head using one of the following techniques:
  - Place a thumb over the radial head and push down, while the other hand is used to supinate the forearm while flexing the elbow.
  - Place the thumb of one hand over the radial head, while the other hand is used to hyper-pronate the forearm. Studies have shown this hyperpronation technique to be significantly more effective.
    - When the radial head is reduced a click or give is usually felt.
    - The child should be observed until they use the affected arm (usually 10-15 minutes).

Frequent Reassessment

- If awaiting consult or transfer, the patient's neurovascular status must be reassessed every 30 minutes. This is important to remember during a "triple case."

Complications

- Compartment syndrome
  - Alert orthopedics about the possibility and request a stat evaluation.
  - Check compartment pressures. Pressures more than 30 mm Hg require fasciotomy.
- Neurovascular compromise
  - Attempt traction or reduction if an orthopedic consult is not available in 30 minutes or less.

- Clavicle fractures with any neurovascular compromise warrant stat thoracic and orthopedic surgery consults aimed at evaluating the great vessels and/or brachial plexus.

DON'T FORGET

Assess soft tissue firmness surrounding the break and remember the "Six Ps" (pain, pallor, paresthesias, paralysis, pulselessness, poikilothermia) of compartment syndrome.

Disposition

- Successful reduction of a nursemaid's elbow is indicated by a child using the arm. They can be discharged without immobilization, but give precautions on prevention.
- Clavicle fractures that are open, involve the medial third, cause neurovascular compromise, or tent the skin require orthopedic consult. Always evaluate for pneumothorax. Closed clavicle fractures, without neurovascular compromise or skin tenting, may be sent home after the arm is immobilized with a sling. Give pain medication.
- Supracondylar and hip fractures require orthopedic consultation.
- Any potential child abuse needs to be reported to Department of Child and Family Services and the child should be admitted.

DON'T FORGET

Be wary of patients who are continuously asking for pain meds on exam day. You need to rule out compartment syndrome in these patients—especially those with high-risk fractures such as tib/fib, forearm, and femur fractures.

SLIPPED CAPITAL FEMORAL EPIPHYSIS

Additional History and Examination Findings

- Classic case is obese African-American pre-teenager with limp, and presenting with either hip or knee pain.
- Risk factors include male gender, African-American ethnicity, obesity, previous hip joint infection, endocrine disorders, renal osteodystrophy, and radiation treatment nearby.
- Peak age of occurrence is between ages 11 and 13 years and in association with puberty.
- Patients describe an insidious, progressive pain, that is dull or aching and that classically presents more with knee than hip pain.
- Pain comes from the epiphysis of the femoral head slipping away from the physis. The greater the degree of slippage, the worse the pain.
- Children may complain of bilateral pain as SCFE occurs clinically in both hips in 25%-40% of patients.
- PE reveals a gait notable for the patient externally rotating the leg with flexion to keep the epiphysis of the femur in the acetabulum. At rest the child keeps the leg abducted and externally rotated.

Review Initial Results

- X-rays
  - Anteroposterior (AP), lateral, and frog leg views should be ordered (Fig. 36-3).
  - Slippage usually occurs posteriorly and inferiorly; therefore, the lateral view may be the first to show signs.
  - Early slippage can be detected by drawing "Klein lines." A line is drawn along the superior border of the femoral neck on AP view, and extended into the joint space. The line should pass through the superior portion of the femoral head with more than 20% of the head lying above it.
  - Comparison views can be helpful.
- Computed tomography (CT)/magnetic resonance imaging (MRI): Should be ordered with high clinical suspicion and a negative x-ray.

DON'T FORGET

Typically described as the epiphysis of the femoral head. It looks like a scoop of ice cream that is sliding off its cone.

Risk Stratification

- The greater the degree of slippage, the greater the risk of complications.
  - Short-term: AVN of the femoral head
  - Long-term: Nonunion, premature closure of the growth plate, degenerative changes, and early arthritis

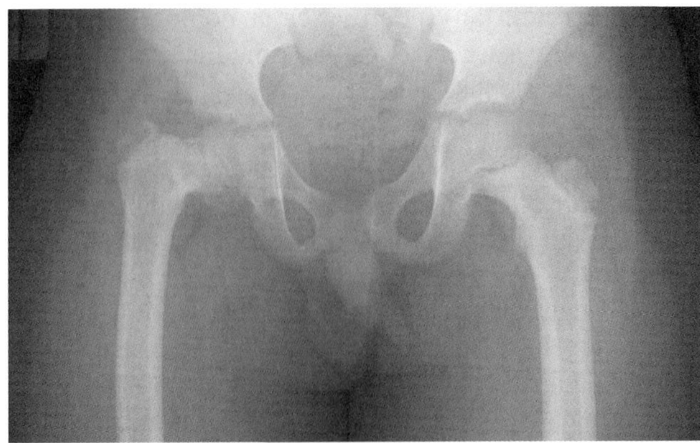

Figure 36-3. This x-ray shows an AP view of the pelvis with a slipped capital femoral epiphysis on the right. Note the obliteration of the epiphyseal plate and the more superior position of the femoral neck and greater trochanter (there is nearly a 90° angle formed by the femoral neck and the femoral shaft) in relationship to the left. *(Reproduced with permission from Shah BR, Lucchesi M.* Atlas of Pediatric Emergency Medicine. *New York, NY: McGraw-Hill; 2006.)*

Definitive Management

- Pain control.
- Child should be made nonweight bearing.
- Orthopedic consult.

Disposition

- Orthopedic consult, ideally in the emergency department (ED), or in clinic the next day if the child is kept nonweight bearing.

LEGG-CALVÉ-PERTHES DISEASE

Additional History and Physical Examination Findings

- The presenting age is younger than SCFE, ranging from 3 to 12 years with a peak at 6 years.
- It is an idiopathic AVN of the femoral head. Children at higher risk include those who are later in the birth order, have older parents, have low birth weight, and have attention deficit hyperactivity disorder (ADHD).
- Boys are affected more frequently than girls at a ratio of 3-5:1.
- Pain is insidious in onset and 15%-20% of children have bilateral complaints. Pain is usually in groin or proximal thigh.
- Child has had limp for 3-6 weeks. Activity worsens the limp. They have limited hip abduction on examination.

Review Initial Results

- AP, lateral, and frog leg views are the initial diagnostic modality of choice (Fig. 36-4).
- MRI can detect LCP earlier than plain films if suspicion is high.

Definitive Management

- Analgesia.

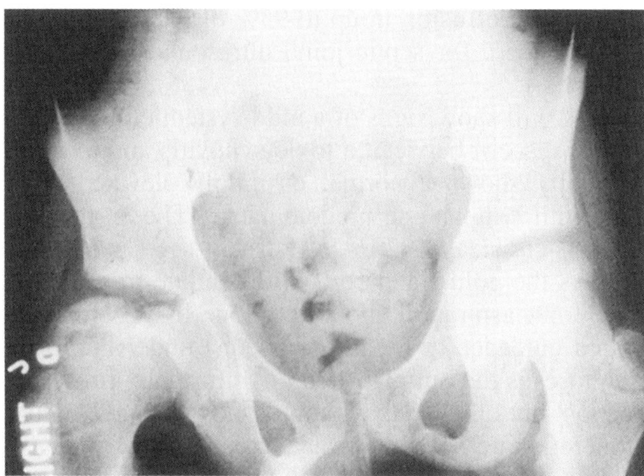

Figure 36-4. Legg-Calvé-Perthes disease. The right hip illustrates joint-space widening, reduced size of the ossific nucleus of the femoral head, and increased opacification of the femoral head. *(Reproduced with permission from Tintinalli JE, Kelen GD, Stapczynski JS, et al.* Emergency Medicine: A Comprehensive Study Guide. *6th ed. New York, NY: McGraw-Hill; 2004.)*

- Patient should be nonweight bearing.
- Orthopedics consult for possible abduction bracing or surgery.

Complications

- Minimal short-term complications include premature physeal arrest, irregular femoral head formation, and osteochondritis dessicans.
- Long term complications included degenerative joint disease (DJD) and early arthritis.
- Children tend to do very well and have return of good range of motion.

Disposition

- Patient may be followed up in the next 1-2 days with the orthopedist. The patient should be kept nonweight bearing with adequate outpatient analgesia.

TRANSIENT SYNOVITIS

Additional History and Physical Examination Findings

- Affects boys more often than girls.
- Patients typically range in age from 3 to 10 years.
- The patient will refuse any movement of the affected joint and may eventually refuse to bear weight entirely.
- The PE reveals a nontoxic-appearing child who may be in significant pain, especially with any manipulation of the affected joint.
- As the disease progresses, more fluid is produced within the joint causing increased pressure within the affected joint capsule. This causes more pain. In the hip, the patient holds the joint flexed, abducted slightly, and externally rotated as this maximizes the joint size and decreases pressure.

Review Initial Test Results

- X-rays reveal little change. A mild widening of the joint space may be observed in comparison views. With severe disease, the epiphysis may appear to be laterally shifted.

DON'T FORGET

- Transient synovitis:
  - Child is nontoxic.
  - Synovial fluid.
  - WBC <50,000.
  - PMNs <70%.
  - Clear or straw colored.
  - ESR <20.
- Septic arthritis:
  - Child is toxic.
  - Synovial fluid.
    - WBC >50,000.
    - PMNs >70%.
    - Turbid or cloudy.
  - ESR >>20.

- Ultrasound shows an effusion in up to 95% of patients with this condition. If there is any concern for septic joint, ultrasound should be used to help guide arthrocentesis.
- Laboratory work will show signs of a mild systemic inflammatory state, but can be useful to discern between a toxic synovitis and a septic joint. Toxic synovitis typically shows a normal or mildly elevated white blood cell (WBC) count with lymphocyte predominance. The erythrocyte sedimentation rate (ESR) is classically <20.
- Arthrocentesis is the gold standard to differentiate transient synovitis from a septic joint. Joint aspiration should be done by an emergency physician with ultrasound guidance or by an orthopedist under fluoroscopy. Absence of positive cultures is the only lab result that formally rules out the presence of joint infection, but other tests with the synovial fluid can help suggest the presence of infection until culture results are finalized.
  - Synovial fluid from transient synovitis is typical clear or yellow with <50,000 WBCs and <70% polymorphonuclear leukocytes (PMNs).

Definitive Management

- Once the diagnosis of transient synovitis is made, the primary treatment is pain control. First-line agents include nonsteroidal anti-inflammatory drugs (NSAIDs), followed by narcotics for breakthrough pain. The child may bear weight as tolerated. The parents may need significant reassurance.

Disposition

- Home with personal medical doctor (PMD) follow-up.

DON'T FORGET

On test day, every child gets arthrocentesis to distinguish between toxic synovitis and a septic joint.

SEPTIC ARTHRITIS

Additional History and Physical Examination Findings

- These children appear toxic and history will reveal significant systemic symptoms including fever, lethargy, irritability, poor feeding, nausea, and vomiting.
- Infants may not appear as toxic, but may display a range of symptoms including fever, poor feeding, refusal to move the affected limb, and severe irritability with diaper changes (movement of affected hip joint).
- Infection typically arises from hematogenous spread from a distant source. Direct spread from a nearby osteomyelitis is the second most common source of infection.
- Infections of the lower extremity are the most common, with the knee, hip, and ankle accounting for 80% of cases. The hip is the most commonly affected joint.

Review of Initial Tests

- X-rays show the same findings as for transient synovitis: Possible widening of joint space and epiphyseal shift.
- Serum laboratory typically reveals:
  - Elevated WBC with left shift.
  - Elevated ESR (usually >20 and >100 with a concomitant osteomyelitis).
- Ultrasound will reveal a joint effusion which should then be aspirated for synovial fluid analysis.
- Synovial laboratory tests typically reveal:
  - WBC >50,000
  - >70% PMNs
  - Decreased glucose and elevated lactate level
  - Classically appears turbid and purulent.

Risk Stratification

- Joint infection is an orthopedic and infectious emergency. The longer it takes to make the diagnosis, the more extensive the joint damage and the higher the risk for progressive systemic toxicity.

Definitive Management

- An orthopedist must evaluate the patient and arrange for drainage of the joint space emergently. This may be done via open irrigation and drainage or via percutaneous methods.
- Start empiric antibiotics as soon as there is a serious suspicion of a joint being infected. Different infectious agents are typically encountered at different ages, but there are two generic antibiotic regimens that can be used to empirically cover a pediatric patient:
    - Birth to 2 months: Most encountered bacteria are *Staphylococcus aureus* and group B strep. Cover with nafcillin and gentamicin.
    - Beyond 2 months: *Staph* is still frequently encountered as well as *Streptococcus pneumoniae* and *Streptococcus pyogenes, Haemophilus influenzae,* and *Neisseria gonorrhoeae*. Cover all ages with nafcillin and ceftriaxone. Add vancomycin if there is any possibility of methicillin-resistant *Staphylococcus aureus* (MRSA).
- Resuscitate the child as indicated by their level of systemic toxicity.

Disposition

- The child must be admitted after drainage of the joint. If the child is in shock or shows any hemodynamic instability, admit to the pediatric intensive care unit (PICU).

WINNING STRATEGIES

- Decide whether the pain is mechanical or inflammatory/infectious.
- Early IV, O_2, and monitor for any toxic-appearing child. Resuscitate while performing workup.
- Any child with joint pain suspected to be inflammatory/infectious in nature gets an arthrocentesis—no matter how good they look.
- Watch out for joint infections in immunocompromised patients. Treat more conservatively and with broader antibiotics.
- Immediate reduce fractures causing significant neurovascular compromise.
- Be vigilant about checking for compartment pressures. Pressures > than 30 mm Hg requires fasciotomy.
- Get comparison films in pediatric patients if you are unsure about pathology.

THE BOTTOM LINE

- On test day, joint pain in children will be either SCFE (teens), LCP (younger children), septic joint, transient synovitis, or possibly a nursemaid's elbow as a quick part of a triple.
- Decide whether the pain is mechanical or inflammatory and proceed accordingly.

CHAPTER 37

Pediatric Seizure

Michael A. Ward and Janis Tupesis

DON'T FORGET

On test day, the patient will have

- Metabolic derangements
- Intracranial mass or bleeding
- Child abuse
- Meningitis
- Status epilepticus

INITIAL ASSESSMENT

- Initially, focus on airway, breathing, and circulation (ABCs).
  - Is the child's airway patent? Is the airway controlled? If not, control it immediately.
  - Is the child breathing on their own?
  - Does the child have spontaneous cardiac activity? Are they perfusing well?
- Is the patient actively seizing when they present, and if so, what needs to be done immediately to break the patient's seizure?
- Do I need to call neurosurgery?
  - How fast does a computed tomography (CT) need to be done and is the patient safe to go to the scanner by themselves?

DON'T FORGET

Stop seizures first, make diagnosis second.

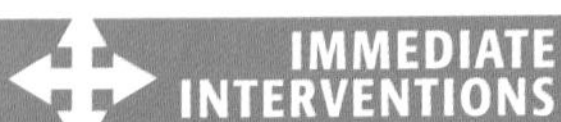

IMMEDIATE INTERVENTIONS

- **Stop the seizure.** If have IV, give IV meds. If not, can give IM, IO, PR, intranasal, or buccal.
- IV = largest possible. Blood should be drawn at this time for laboratory studies.
- Check a blood sugar.
- Supplemental oxygen via NC or NRB to keep oxygen saturation >95%.
- Cardiac monitor.
- Intubate if needed.

INITIAL HISTORY AND PHYSICAL EXAMINATION

History

- Evaluation of seizure itself
  - Prodrome: Was there abnormal eye movement, lip smacking, or facial movement?
  - Aura: Did the patient complain of any typical auras before event happened?
  - Length: How long did the seizure last?
  - What movements were observed—focal or generalized?
  - Level of consciousness during the event: Was the patient awake and aware during event? Was there bowel or bladder incontinence?
  - Associated trauma: Did they fall down? Was there any secondary trauma? Tongue biting?
  - Level of consciousness after the event: Was there a postictal period? How long did that last?
  - Did the patient return to their normal baseline after the seizure?
- Past medical history
  - Prior seizure history, including febrile seizures?
  - Fever? Vaccination history?
  - Access to any medication: Prescription or otherwise?
  - Trauma?
  - Normal developmental milestones?

Physical Examination

- Vital signs
- Head, eyes, ears, nose, and throat (HEENT) examination
  - Head trauma?
  - Pupils: Reactivity, afferent, and efferent defects. Extraocular movements, nystagmus, and hemorrhages?
  - Fundoscopy: Disk margins and hemorrhages?
  - Tympanic membranes (TMs): Evaluate for blood and cerebrospinal fluid (CSF)?
  - Mouth: Bites on tongue? Moist mucous membranes?
  - Neck: Evaluate for meningismus: Kernig sign? Brudzinski sign?
- Chest
  - Trachea midline?
  - Equal breath sounds?
  - Rales, rhonchi, wheezes?
- Cardiovascular (CV)
  - Rhythm?
  - Murmurs, rubs, gallops?

- Equal pulses?
- Good perfusion?

- Abdomen
  - Distended?
  - Tender?
  - Evidence of bleeding?
- Extremities
  - Capillary refill?
  - Warmth?
  - Cyanosis?
  - Edema?
- Neuro
  - Level of consciousness?
  - Motor?
  - Sensory?
  - Reflexes?
  - Cranial nerves?
  - Gait?

DON'T FORGET

- Look for signs of external trauma. Scalp laceration, scalp hematoma → may indicate other trauma.
- Look at the eyes. Retinal hemorrhages = abuse until proven otherwise.
- Look at the tongue. Tongue laceration = seizure.
- Do a complete neuro examination if possible.

DIFFERENTIAL DIAGNOSIS

Generalized or Focal Seizures

Seizures are generally divided into generalized and focal (partial) seizures.

Generalized seizures involve both hemispheres of the brain and subsequently, include full-body movements or atony. Absence seizures include sudden interruption of normal consciousness, which may include staring spells or poor responsiveness, and is a type of generalized seizure.

Focal seizures involve a localized part of the brain with the following classifications:

Simple partial = no alteration of consciousness.

Complex partial = alteration of consciousness.

Partial seizure evolving into a generalized seizure = initial focal movements followed by full-body involvement.

Status Epilepticus

Status epilepticus is defined as a single seizure lasting >5 minutes or two or more seizures without recovery of consciousness/return to baseline in-between the seizures. It includes both focal and generalized seizures.

Febrile Seizures

Febrile seizures are seizures that accompany fever without evidence of intracranial infection or any specific cause in children between ages 6 months and 5 years. They occur in 2%-5% of children, thus being the most common seizure disorder of childhood. Febrile seizures are classified into simple and complex:

Simple = generalized, <15 minutes in duration, and a short postictal period.

Complex = focal, >15 minutes, or recurrence within 24 hours.

Meningitis

Infection of the meninges. Generally occurs as a complication of bacteremia, but can primarily extend from infection of the sinuses or the inner ear.

DON'T FORGET

History is key.

- Circumstances?
- Length of event?
- LOC?
- Aura?
- Abnormal motor?
- Incontinence?
- Fever?
- New medications in house?
- Delayed milestones?
- History of seizures?

DON'T FORGET

Any seizing infant <3 months gets a full septic workup.

Metabolic Derangements

Inborn errors of metabolism that can cause seizures in the child include disorders of protein or carbohydrate metabolism, lysosomal storage disorders, fatty acid oxidation disorders, and mitochondrial/peroxisomal disorders. Acquired metabolic derangements that can cause seizures include derangements of glucose, sodium, potassium, calcium, and magnesium metabolism.

Trauma

Traumatic head injury and multi system trauma can be a cause of seizure in children. Causes include blunt head injury with post-concussive syndrome, traumatic subarachnoid hemorrhage, epidural hematoma, and subdural hematoma. Acute volume loss and secondary anoxia can be a cause of primary seizure in the child.

DON'T FORGET

Glasgow Coma Scale (Infant scale in parentheses)

Eyes

4 Open
3 Opens to verbal
2 Opens to pain
1 No response

Verbal

5 Oriented (smiles, tracks objects, interactive)
4 Disoriented (cries but consolable, not interactive)
3 Inappropriate words (inconsolable, moaning)
2 Incomprehensible sounds (inconsolable, agitated)
1 No response

Motor

6 Obeys commands
5 Localizes to painful stimulus
4 Flexion withdrawal
3 Decorticate (flexion)
2 Decerebrate (extension)
1 No response

Modifications for children

Verbal

- 2-5 years: ± using appropriate words
- 0-2 years: ± crying appropriately

GENERALIZED SEIZURE DISORDER

Additional History and Physical Examination Findings

- Up to 1% of pediatric patients seen in the emergency department will be evaluated for seizures.
- Fever, central nervous system (CNS) infection, and epilepsy account for >75% of cases.
- Look for stigmata of seizure: Head trauma, tongue biting, incontinence.
- Perform a careful examination to look for neurologic deficits.

Review Initial Results

- Complete blood count (CBC): Evaluate infectious processes.
- Chemistries: Evaluate for electrolyte abnormalities, including hypoglycemia and hyponatremia.
- Neuroimaging: Noncontrast head CT should be done for:
  - Trauma
  - Suspicion of mass lesion
  - <6 months where physical examination may be unreliable
  - New onset seizure without fever, unless well-appearing and discussed with a neurologist

Management

- ABCs: As with every patient, make sure that the patient is breathing, has a patent airway, and adequate perfusion.
- Treat seizure.
  - Benzodiazepines: First-line therapy (doses discussed in section "Status Epilepticus")
    - Midazolam: Intravenous (IV), intramuscular (IM), intranasal, or buccal
    - Diazepam: IV or rectal suppository
    - Lorazepam: IV or IM
  - Phenytoin or fosphenytoin
    - Second-line therapy for persistent seizures
  - Phenobarbital
  - Valproic acid: May be more effective in patients previously on valproic acid.
  - Levetiracetam (Keppra)

Complications

- Depends on etiology of seizure; will be discussed in each section specifically.

Disposition

- Simple febrile seizures and uncomplicated generalized seizures may be safe for discharge to home with scheduled follow-up.
- Typically, oral board cases will be more complicated and will require hospital admission.
- Typical workup of seizures includes lab work, neuroimaging, and electroencephalogram (EEG).
- Further treatment with antiepileptics and further follow-up is determined by inpatient workup.

STATUS EPILEPTICUS

Additional History and Physical Examination Findings

- Defined as a seizure lasting >5 minutes or recurrent seizures without recovery of consciousness or baseline mental status between them.
- Occurs in about 50,000 people a year—with highest incidence in children <2 years and those >60 years old
- Etiologies generally divided into quarters:
  - 25% idiopathic
  - 25% febrile
  - 25% chronic (already has seizure disorder)
  - 25% acute symptomatic (trauma, metabolic, toxic, or infectious)
- Mortality rate of children is 3%-6%.

Review Initial Results

- CBC: Evaluate for infectious processes.
- Chemistries: Evaluate for electrolyte abnormalities, including hypoglycemia and hyponatremia.
- Neuroimaging: Noncontrast head CT should be done for:
  - Trauma
  - Suspicion of mass lesion
  - New onset seizure without fever

Management

- ABCs: Especially important in status epilepticus. Can expand to "A through F"
  - A = Airway control.
  - B = Breathing control: Be ready to ventilate if needed.
  - C = Circulation control: Get IV early.
  - D = Disability: Trauma? Reversible cause (hypoglycemia)? **Treat seizure here.**
  - E = Expose and examine patient.
  - F = Family: Get history.
- Treatment of seizure: Medications
  - Benzodiazepines
    - Lorazepam. Dose: 0.05-0.1 mg/kg; route: IV, IM (poorly absorbed); onset of action: 5-10 minutes; half life: 13-15 hours.
    - Midazolam: Dose: 0.05-0.2 mg/kg; route: IV or IM; 0.2-0.3 mg/kg buccal or intranasal; onset of action: 3-5 minutes; half life: 2-6 hours.
    - Diazepam: Dose: 0.1-0.2 mg/kg IV; 0.5-1mg/kg PR per dose; route. IV, PR; onset of action: 1-3 minutes IV, 5 minutes PR; half life: 20-100 hours.
  - Phenytoin
    - Stabilizes sodium and calcium channels.
    - 18-20 mg/kg slow IV infusion; rate of 1 mg/kg/min.

DON'T FORGET

Know what medications you can give without an IV.

- Midazolam (Versed) can be given IM, intranasal, or via the buccal route.
- Midazolam is the only benzodiazepine that can be given IM with equivalent onset and duration as IV.
- Diazepam (Valium) can be given IM or PR.
- Lorazepam (Ativan) can be given IM.
- Fosphenytoin can be given IM.

DON'T FORGET

If seizures not breaking, consider prophylactic treatment (aka "fishing"):

- Glucose: 0.25-0.50 g/kg for hypoglycemia
- Naloxone: 0.1 mg/kg for possible narcotic overdose
- Thiamine: 100 mg for possible deficiency
- Pyridoxine: 50-100 mg for functional or iatrogenic deficiency
- Antibiotics: Early administration if meningitis is suspected

---

- Fosphenytoin (prodrug of phenytoin)
  - 18-20 mg PE/kg IV or IM; rate of 3 mg PE/kg/min.
- Phenobarbital
  - Barbituate = Enhancement of gamma-aminobutyric acid (GABA) inhibition of neuronal firing.
  - Loading dose: 20 mg/kg up to maximum of 600 mg IV; rate of 1 mg/kg/min.
- Valproic acid
  - Loaded in doses of 25-40 mg/kg.
  - Rate of 3-6 mg/kg/min.
- Levetiracetam
  - Loaded in doses of 20-30 mg/kg.

Complications

- Inability to control seizures.
- Airway compromise from decreased mental status.
- Hyperpyrexia.
- Metabolic acidosis from prolonged seizure activity and lactic acid release.
- Rhabdomyolysis.

Disposition

- Admit patient to either pediatric intensive care unit or step-down unit.

DON'T FORGET

Look for underlying cause of fever. Remember that common things are common.

- Otitis media
- Pharyngitis, including herpangina
- Viral illness
- Urinary tract infection
- Pulmonary infection
- Cellulitis

FEBRILE SEIZURES

Additional History and Physical Examination Findings

- Most common type of seizure in the pediatric patients.
- Definition: Occurs between the ages of 6 months and 5 years—associated with fever, but without evidence of intracranial infection or other cause.
- 2%-5% of children will have a febrile seizure before age of 5.
- Slight male predominance.
- Characteristic features (simple febrile seizure):
  - Associated with rapidly rising fever.
  - Last <5 minutes.
  - Are generalized (not focal).
  - Isolated, single event in a 24-hour period.
  - Short postictal period without postictal deficits.
  - Often family history of same is present.
  - EEG does not reveal epileptic activity.
- History of fever should be elucidated: Duration, exposure to illnesses, and history of vaccinations.
- On physical examination: Look for source of fever. Make sure to evaluate for otitis media, pharyngitis, and viral rashes.
- Complex febrile seizure = lasting >15 minutes, focal, or recurrence within 24 hours.

DON'T FORGET

Any febrile seizure in a child that starts with focal shaking, lasts >15 minutes, or recurs within 24 hours is a complex febrile seizure and should receive a full workup.

Review Initial Results

- There are no specific lab evaluations for febrile seizures but consider lumbar puncture (LP) in any child 12 months or less with a febrile seizure.
- Lab evaluation should be geared toward evaluation of underlying disease causing fever. Examples:
  - Urinalysis: Evaluation of urinary tract infection
  - Rapid strep test/pharyngeal swab: Evaluation for group A *Streptococcus pharyngitis*

- Patients with simple febrile seizures have similar rates of bacteremia, including meningitis, compared to those children with fever alone.

Management

- For simple febrile seizures:
  - Antipyretics.
  - If patient is actively seizing when presents to emergency department, measures to break seizure should be taken.
  - As always: ABCs first.
- For complex febrile seizure:
  - In addition to the treatment for simple febrile seizures, a full septic work-up (including LP and cultures) and neuroimaging is indicated.

Disposition

- Patients can typically be discharged home with careful follow-up after prolonged observation period in the emergency department.
- Patients should be awake, alert with a normal neurologic evaluation before they are discharged home.
- Inpatient admission should be considered for the following patients:
  - Complex febrile seizures
  - Unstable CV status.
  - Abnormal neurologic examination.
  - Inability to ensure adequate follow-up.
  - Inability to ensure safe home situation.

Complications

- Approximately 30% of patients with febrile seizure will have at least one recurrence.

MENINGITIS

Additional History and Physical Examination Findings

- Death or severe sequelae with untreated bacterial meningitis approaches 100%.
- Quick determination if seizure has occurred.
- Drug allergies?
- Recent vaccinations?
- Recent travel or exposure to any sick contacts?
- Recent infections?
- Recent head trauma or surgery?

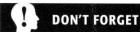

DON'T FORGET

Bug for different age groups

- <1 month: *Escherichia coli*, group B strep, and *Listeria monocytogenes.*
- 30-60 days: Group B strep (gram-negative decline in frequency).
- >1 month: *Streptococcus pneumoniae, Neisseria meningitides,* and *Haemophilus influenzae* (if not yet received vaccine).

Review Initial Results

- Lab tests
  - CBC with differential.
  - Platelet count.
  - Blood cultures: Preferably two from two different sites.
  - Serum electrolytes.
  - Coagulation studies: Can be grossly elevated in patients who are septic or acutely ill.
  - Bacterial antigen tests.
- Cerebrospinal fluid analysis
  - Should be sent for cell count and differential, glucose, protein, Gram stain, and culture.
  - Cell count: Characteristic findings include elevated white blood cell count with a neutrophilic predominance.

- Glucose: Low.
- Protein: Normal to high.
- Gram stain: Is positive in approximately 90% of children with pneumococcal meningitis and approximately 80% of children with meningococcal meningitis.

DON'T FORGET

Know how to evaluate LP results.

Hints:

- High WBC count with predominance of PMNs = think bacterial meningitis.
- Glucose <50% of serum glucose = think bacterial meningitis.
- WBC count <500/mm^3 with lymphocyte predominance = think viral meningitis.
- If nothing fits = think tuberculous or fungal meningitis.

Management

- ABCs: As with every patient, make sure that the patient is breathing, and has a patent airway and good peripheral perfusion.
- Early administration of bactericidal antibiotic therapy guided by age.
  - Newborn to 1 month: Ampicillin and cefotaxime or gentamicin.
  - 1 month-18 years: Ceftriaxone: 100 mg/kg/d, divided qid or bid, max 4 g/d and vancomycin 15-20 mg/kg IV q6h.
- Steroids
  - Adjuvant therapy to improve neurologic sequelae.
  - Best evidence for *H influenza* meningitis.
  - Dexamethasone
    - 0.15 mg/kg every 6 hours for 16 doses **or**
    - 0.4 mg/kg every 12 hours for 4 doses.

Complications

- Neurologic dysfunction including: Vision loss, hearing loss, and decreased mental functioning —with higher rates of cognitive delay, learning disabilities, and psychosocial development.

Disposition

- Admit to intensive care unit with strict isolation precautions.

METABOLIC ABNORMALITIES

Additional History and Physical Examination Findings

- Typically divided into acquired and inherited.
- Acquired
  - Hypoglycemia
    - Typically presents within the first day of life.
    - Can happen with ingestions of hypoglycemic medications.
  - Hypocalcemia
    - Typically happens between day 3 and 14 of life.
    - Multiple possible etiologies: Decreased albumin, decreased magnesium or phosphate, parathyroid hormone deficiency, and problems with vitamin D metabolism.
  - Pyridoxine/B_6 deficiency
    - Usually in breast-feeding children.
    - Due to low maternal pyridoxine levels leading to low levels in child.
    - Other causes: Malnutrition, decreased absorption, and liver disease.
- Inherited/inborn errors
  - Amino acid disorders
    - Phenylketonuria (PKU): Inability of body to utilize phenylalanine. Increasing levels lead to CNS problems with late development of cognitive delay and seizures.
    - Maple syrup urine (MSU) disease: Inability to utilize branch chain amino acids leucine, isoleucine, and valine. Accumulation of these amino acids leads to progressive encephalopathy and seizures.

- Urea cycle disorders
  - Defects in metabolism of nitrogen produced by catabolism of protein.
  - Any defect in any pathway or enzyme leads to pathologic features.
  - Progressive encephalopathy from ammonia accumulation—seizures.

DON'T FORGET

Most common metabolic abnormalities are electrolyte abnormalities.

Always check:

- Glucose
- Calcium
- Magnesium
- Phosphate
- Sodium

Review Initial Results

- Electrolytes: Pay close attention to glucose, sodium, calcium, magnesium, and phosphate levels.
- Pyridoxine level (as inpatient).
- Amino acid disorders (as inpatient):
  - PKU: Phenylalanine level.
  - MSU disease: Elevation of branch chain amino acids, alloisoleucine.
- Urea cycle disorders (as inpatient):
  - Elevations of specific enzymes in the urea cycle.
  - Ammonia level.

Management

- Replete electrolytes appropriately.
- As inpatient: Dietary modification for alteration of levels of amino acids, protein levels, etc.
- As inpatient: Genetic counseling for inherited disorders.

Disposition

- If simple electrolyte abnormality with simple, explainable cause: Patient may be discharged with appropriate follow-up with primary care pediatrician.
- If unable to evaluate cause, unable to follow-up, or unsure of home situation: Admit.
- All inborn errors of metabolism: Admit.

HEAD TRAUMA

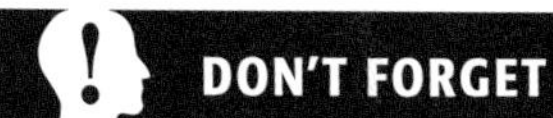

DON'T FORGET

If story does not fit, make sure to consider child abuse.

Additional History and Physical Examination Findings

- Trauma is leading cause of death in children >1 year old in the United States.
- Thought to occur in about 200/100,000 population each year.
- Mortality from head injury in children: Between 20% and 30%.
- Morbidity: Moderate head injury → 20% experience short-term memory problems; severe head injury → >50% experience permanent neurologic deficits.
- Children are more susceptible to head trauma due to: Cranium is a larger portion of total body surface area. There is a higher water content within the pediatric brain = softer and more prone to injury. The head is more dependent on ligamentous structures for stability.
- Usually injury divided into primary and secondary injuries
  - Primary: Injury that occurs at the time of impact—either through direct trauma or acceleration/deceleration injuries.
  - Secondary: Injury in response to initial injury. Can include hypotension, hypoxia, hypoperfusion, and hypercapnea. Can also include delayed injury of inflammation, microcirculatory damage, etc.

Review Initial Results

- Evaluation of trauma can be differentiated by neuroimaging.
- Normal head CT
  - Scalp injury: Superficial injury to scalp. Need to look for foreign bodies and underlying skull fractures.

  - Concussion: Transient loss of consciousness as a result of head trauma. Patients often have normal head CT and normal neurologic examination. Usually a retrospective diagnosis.
  - Contusion: "Bruising" of brain tissue. Often with a normal head CT. Can have delayed deterioration secondary to swelling or late developing hematomas.
  - Diffuse axonal injury: Results of acceleration/deceleration injuries. Due to density gradient of gray/white matter. Often not seen on CT. Magnetic resonance imaging (MRI) is diagnostic. Prognosis for full recovery is often poor.
- Abnormal head CT: (Fig. 37-1)
  - Skull fracture: Linear, comminuted, or depressed. Best seen on head CT. If have CSF leak—merits further exploration by neurosurgeon. If displaced by > one thickness of bone = depressed skull fracture and neurosurgical consultation.
  - Basilar skull fracture: Usually caused by blow to back of the head. Battle sign, raccoon eyes, or CSF otorrhea hint at diagnosis.
  - Epidural hematoma: Blood in the epidural space between the skull and the dura. Usually due to tearing of middle meningeal artery. Initial loss of consciousness (LOC) → lucid interval → rapid deterioration. Emergent neurosurgical evaluation. Lenticular (lens shaped) blood on CT.
  - Subdural hematoma: Blood between the cortex and the dura. Usually caused by tearing of the bridging veins. Usually associated with severe parenchymal injuries. Crescent-shaped blood on CT.

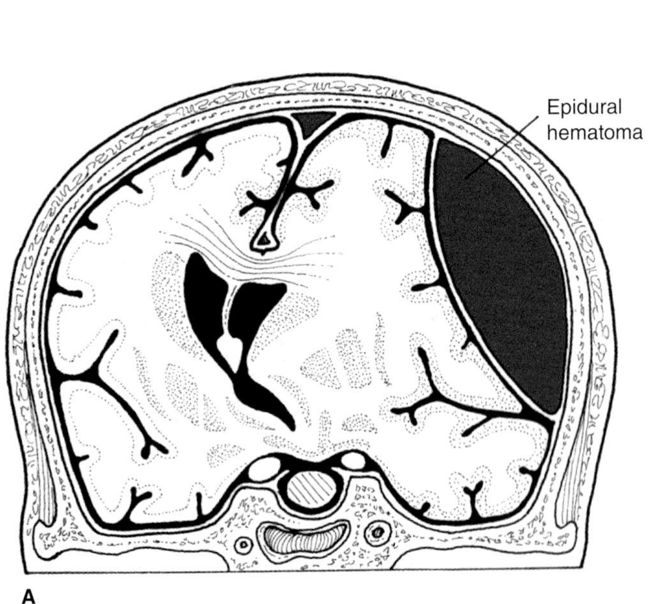

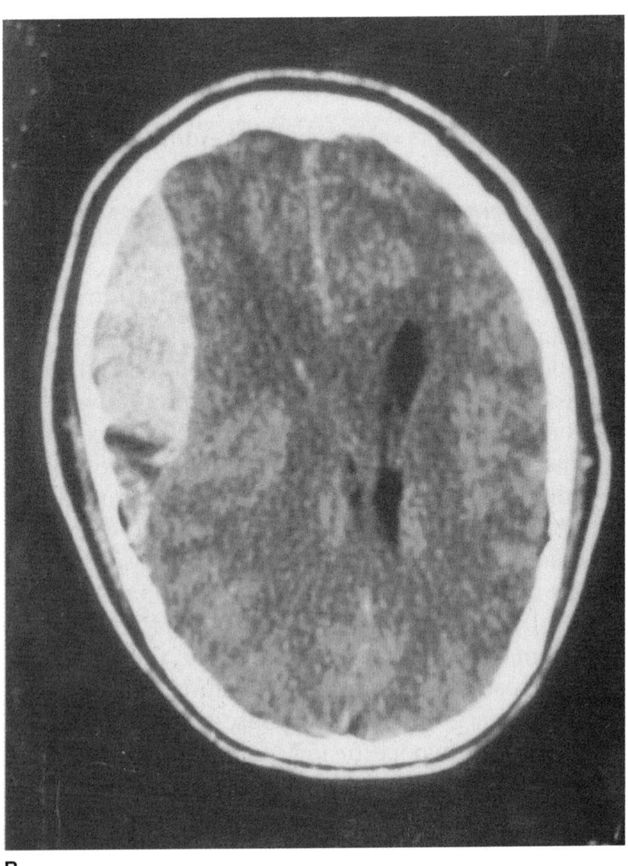

Figure 37-1. (**A**) Illustration of an epidural hematoma. (**B**) CT scan of an epidural hematoma. (**C**) Illustration of a subdural hematoma. (**D**) CT scan of a subdural hematoma. (**E**) Illustration of a subarachnoid hemorrhage. (**F**) CT scan of subarachnoid hemorrhage. *([A-D]: Reproduced with permission from Reichman RF, Simon RR.* Emergency Medicine Procedures. *New York, NY: McGraw-Hill; 2004. [E, F]: Reproduced with permission from Schwartz DT.* Emergency Radiology: Case Studies. *New York, NY; McGraw-Hill; 2008.)*

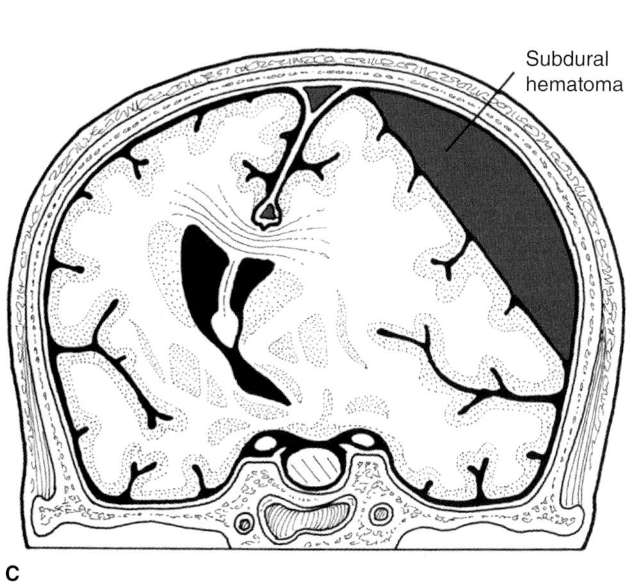
Subdural
hematoma

C

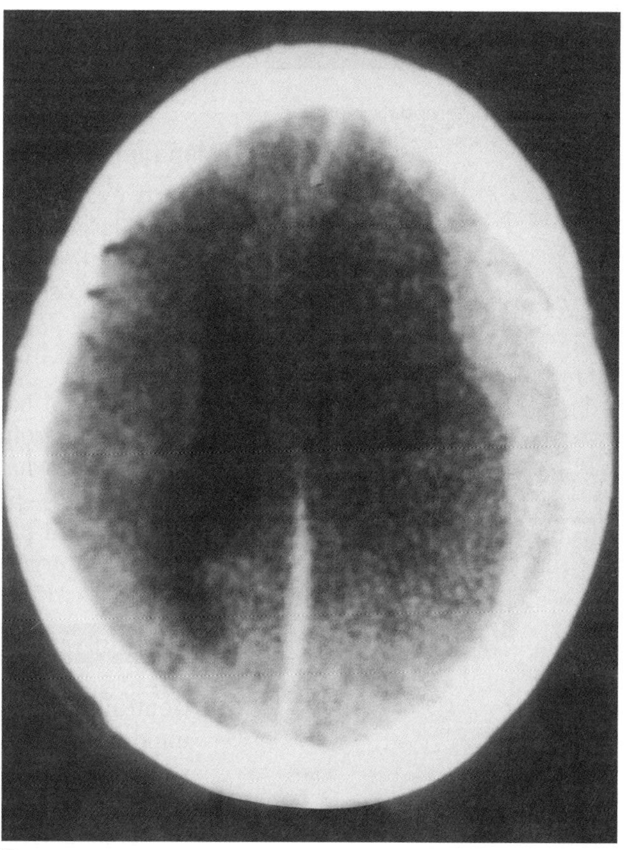

D

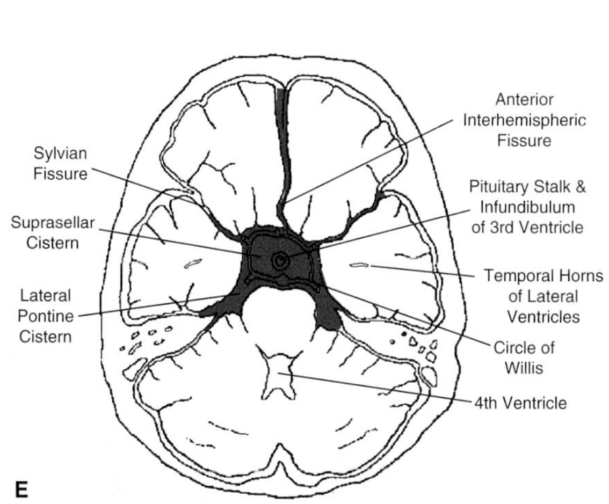
Anterior
Interhemispheric
Fissure
Sylvian
Fissure
Pituitary Stalk &
Infundibulum
of 3rd Ventricle
Suprasellar
Cistern
Temporal Horns
of Lateral
Ventricles
Lateral
Pontine
Cistern
Circle of
Willis
4th Ventricle

E

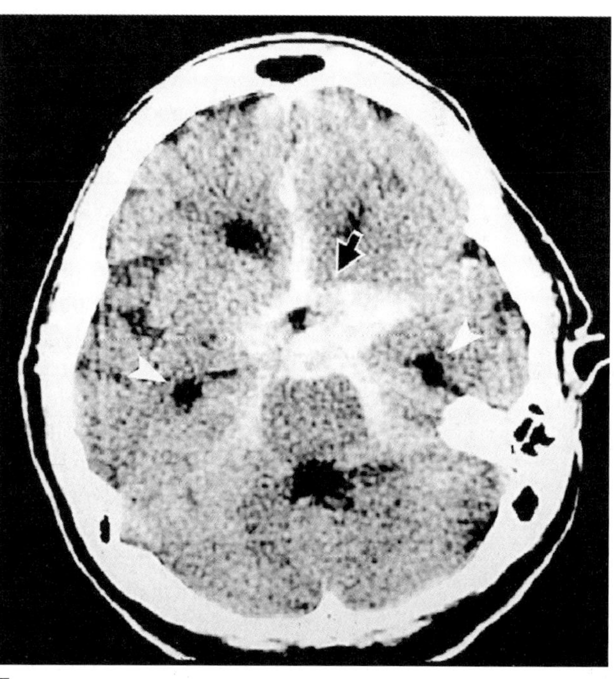

F

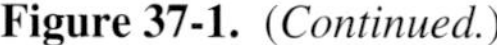

Figure 37-1. (*Continued.*)

DON'T FORGET

Know how to differentiate bleeds on CT.

- Subarachnoid hemorrhage: Blood in cisterns; outlines gyri/sulci.
- Subdural hematoma: Hyperdense (white) crescent-shaped mass along the inner table of the skull.
- Epidural hematoma: Extra-axial, smoothly marginated, lenticular, or biconvex blood formation.
- Diffuse axonal injury: Typically normal CT findings.

  - Subarachnoid hemorrhage: Blood in the subarachnoid space. Usually due to disruption of small vessels in cerebral cortex. Blood typically collects along the falx cerebri or tentorium on CT.

Management

- Early evaluation of neurologic status.
- Use Glasgow Coma Scale (GCS).
- If GCS <8, consider aggressive airway management.
- Early neurosurgical evaluation.

Disposition

- If the patient had no loss of consciousness, signs of skull fracture, and has a normal neurologic examination, patient may be observed and discharged.
- If the patient had loss of consciousness and/or has an abnormal neurologic examination—patient merits neuroimaging and admission.
- If the patient has obvious head injury, patient needs immediate neuroimaging, neurosurgery consultation, and admission to intensive care unit.

WINNING STRATEGIES

- Controlling the airway and stopping the seizure activity are the two most important steps. Do not proceed to any other diagnostic or management strategies until these two steps are accomplished.
- Look for signs of external trauma such as scalp laceration, hematomas, or retinal hemorrhages (indication of child abuse).
- Any seizing infant <3 months old gets a full septic workup no matter what.
- The new definition of status epilepticus is a single seizure lasting >5 minutes or two or more recurrent seizures without recovery of baseline consciousness between them.
- Midazolam (Versed) can be given IM, intranasally, or via the buccal route, and diazepam (Valium) can be given via the IM or PR route.
- Midazolam is the only benzodiazepine that can be given IM with equivalent onset and duration as IV.
- The definition of a simple febrile seizure is one that occurs in a child between 6 months and 5 years. They are associated with rapidly rising fever, last <15 minutes, are generalized (not focal) and isolated (a single event in 24-hour period), and resolve with no focal postictal deficits when the fever breaks.
- Any seizure in a child that starts with focal shaking and then generalizes is not a simple febrile seizure and should receive a full workup.
- Patients with simple febrile seizures can be discharged home with careful follow-up if they are awake and alert with a normal neurologic evaluation.
- Whenever you suspect meningitis, give empiric antibiotics and steroids at once. Do not wait for the CT or the LP results.
- In head trauma, if patient had no loss of consciousness, no evidence of skull fracture, and has a normal neurologic examination, patient can be observed and discharged. If patient had loss of consciousness and/or has an abnormal neurologic examination—patient merits neuroimaging and admission.

CHAPTER 38

Pediatric Trauma

Katie Tataris

DON'T FORGET

On test day, the patient will have

- Intracranial bleeding
- Splenic/liver laceration
- Bowel rupture
- Significant thoracic injuries
- Child abuse

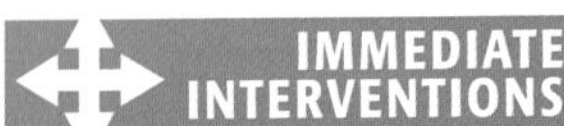

IMMEDIATE INTERVENTIONS

- IV
- O_2
- Cardiac monitor
- Immobilize on a backboard and with a C-collar
- Intubate for a GCS of <8 or severe respiratory distress

DON'T FORGET

Children have larger craniums relative to their bodies than adults. Young children/infants will require a pad or towel under their shoulder blades to ensure that the cervical spine is straight.

DON'T FORGET

All multiple trauma patients will be in shock—treat early.

DON'T FORGET

When establishing vascular access care must be taken to try and find sites away from fractured extremities, opposite the side of any penetrating injury, away from burn sites, and yet as proximal to the chest as possible.

INITIAL ASSESSMENT

- In cases of pediatric trauma, remember to start with your initial assessment and stabilize any life-threatening conditions before moving on. Keep a high index of suspicion for internal injury as pediatric patients have strong compensatory mechanisms when in shock.

IMMEDIATE ACTIONS

- Immobilization: Ensure any child who has experienced significant trauma is properly immobilized.
  - Rigid backboard or papoose.
  - Cervical collar.
- Ancillary staff activities: Ancillary members of the trauma team should ensure:
  - High-flow oxygen by mask even if the child does not appear hypoxic.
  - Monitors: Cardiac and pulse oximetry.
  - Vascular access preferably the largest possible and at least two in the following order of preferred locations/methods:
    - Peripheral intravenous (IVs) in the upper extremities.
    - Central venous catheter placed in the femoral vein.
    - Intraosseous access in the proximal tibia.
- Abbreviated history: The "AMPLE" history:
  - **A**llergies.
  - **M**edicines.
  - **P**ast medical history.
  - **L**ast meal.
  - **E**vents surrounding the patient's reason for presenting.
- Directed physical: The initial care of a trauma patient involves conducting the primary survey that follows the familiar ABCDEF pathway. As you move through this algorithm, any life-threatening condition should immediately be addressed before continuing on to the next phase of the survey.
- Airway: Assess for patency of the airway and the patient's ability to protect it.
  - Assess for presence of voice changes, stridor, or a gag reflex.
  - Clear mouth of foreign debris with suction or forceps if necessary.
  - Use jaw-thrust maneuver and manual in-line cervical stabilization when access to the oropharynx is needed.
  - Early intubation via rapid sequence intubation (RSI) protocol if patient is unable to maintain airway.
  - Prepare alternative airway equipment in the case of severe facial trauma.
  - Be aware of signs of possible laryngeal fracture and use alternative airway stabilization technique if present.
- Breathing: Assess for inadequate oxygenation or ventilation and possible etiologies of any problems that are detected.
  - Hemothorax/pneumothorax/hemopneumothorax
    - Decreased breath sounds.
    - Tension pneumothorax if increased pressure from accumulating extrapleural air is compromising blood flow (look for tracheal deviation!)
    - Immediate needle decompression followed by tube thoracostomy.
    - Check for bowel sounds as a sign of diaphragm herniation before chest tube placement.
  - Pulmonary contusion
    - Decreased breath sounds often at the point of any direct blow to the chest.
    - Most common serious chest injury in children.

- Intubate if compromised oxygenation or ventilation.
  - Flail chest
    - Paradoxical chest wall movements with respirations.
    - At least two rib fractures in at least three levels.
    - Intubate if compromised oxygenation or ventilation.
  - Sucking chest wounds
    - Open communication between pleural cavity and the extrathoracic environment.
    - Place a three-sided occlusive dressing to act as a one-way valve followed by chest tube on the affected side.
- Circulation: Hemorrhagic shock in a child is diagnosed as much by physical findings as by direct blood pressure measurements. Rapidly assess skin turgor, capillary refill, pulse quality, and overall alertness of the child as signs of hypovolemia. External hemorrhage should be controlled with direct pressure.
  - Cardiac tamponade
    - Beck's triad: Hypotension, jugular venous distention (JVD), muffled heart sounds.
    - Treat with fluid resuscitation followed by pericardiocentesis or pericardiotomy (pericardial window) if no response.
  - Loss of pulse: Witnessed traumatic arrest
    - Thoracotomy for penetrating trauma (consider for extraordinary cases of blunt trauma).
- Disability: This portion of the survey entails a brief but focused examination of the patient's neurologic status.
  - Depressed mental status: Calculate the Glasgow Coma Scale (GCS).
  - Localized neurologic injury.
    - Quickly assessed by noting some movement in response to noxious stimulus or voice command in all extremities.
    - Also note the presence of any posturing.
- Exposure: Fully undress the patient taking care to maintain spinal immobilization. The patient should be log-rolled to both sides to look for further signs of injury. It is convenient to perform a spine and rectal examination at this time.
- Family: Some include this as part of the primary survey for pediatric trauma patients. Involving the guardian in care, including having one in the room, can greatly ease a child's anxiety allowing care to proceed more efficiently. Early involvement allows the physician to obtain critical information and keeps the family informed of the patient's condition to help alleviate some of their anxiety.

DIFFERENTIAL DIAGNOSES AND CONSIDERATIONS: THE SECONDARY SURVEY

- Head trauma
  - Head trauma is the leading cause of morbidity and mortality among pediatric trauma patients. Traumatic brain injury must be considered in any child sustaining multiple traumas.
  - Pediatric brains reside in relatively large skulls, so they have more room to be jarred during traumatic injury. This predisposes them to more diffuse brain damage and therefore increased risk of generalized brain edema. Children are more prone to herniation and display quick and severe changes in neurologic function which, if not aggressively treated, lead to permanent brain damage and/or death.
  - Evaluating isolated head trauma is difficult, especially in younger patients, given barriers to communication and the variety of symptoms which children display secondary to minor trauma.

DON'T FORGET

Prehospital information is important to understanding the mechanism of injury and condition of the patient prior to arrival to the Emergency Department. Ask the paramedics for a report if the patient is transported by EMS.

DON'T FORGET

- Choosing pediatric ETT size: Age/4 + 4 = ETT size or the diameter of the patient's little finger (fifth digit) is approximately the same as the appropriate size ETT.
- ET tube depth is approximately 3 × the ETT size.
- Chest tube size at least 3 × the ETT size.

DON'T FORGET

Hypotension in the initial assessment should be treated with a 20 mL/kg isotonic fluid bolus, repeated as necessary and blood product transfusion of 10 mL/kg after fluid resuscitation.

DON'T FORGET

Miller blades only for patients <2 years.

DON'T FORGET

Pediatric chest tube placement fifth intercostal space, anterior axillary line.

DON'T FORGET

Patient requires OR thoracotomy if initial chest tube return is >15 cc/kg or chest tube drains >4 cc/kg/h.

- Neck trauma
  - Pediatric patients make up a very small percentage of spinal cord injury patients in the United States per year. However, the morbidity from these injuries makes their diagnosis imperative.
  - Diagnosis of C-spine and spinal cord injuries in the pediatric population is unique for several reasons. First, the younger pediatric population (age ≤8) have proportionately larger heads compared to their bodies. This along with their developing anatomy causes different injury patterns compared to adults. Next, undeveloped and unfused ossification centers make radiographic interpretation of the spine more difficult. Furthermore, these patients' softer bones, and increased ligamentous laxity predisposes them to a higher rate of isolated cord injury which may have a delayed but significant presentation.
- Chest trauma
  - Isolated chest trauma is rare in the pediatric trauma patient unless caused by penetrating injury
  - Because the pediatric rib cage is more pliable than that of adults, it can withstand greater forces without fracturing. However, this increased compliance allows greater transmission of the same forces internally that may have caused only external trauma in the adult. Recognizing significant chest trauma can be more difficult in this population and subsequently leads to delays in diagnosis.
- Abdominal trauma
  - Children are particularly susceptible to abdominal injury due to their relatively undeveloped abdominal musculature, paucity of fat, and compliant lower rib cage.
  - The abdominal examination is unreliable for pediatric patients in a trauma setting; therefore, any child with vague abdominal complaints or even those without complaints in the setting of a potentially significant mechanism should undergo diagnostic testing.

DON'T FORGET

Children do not show signs of lowered blood pressure until a much greater percentage of their blood volume has been lost as compared to adults.

DON'T FORGET

Do not forget to maintain the patient body temperature. Use warmed blankets, fluid, heat lamps to keep the patient normothermic.

HEAD TRAUMA

Additional History and Physical Examination

- Investigate details surrounding the event: Height of fall? Was the fall witnessed? Was there loss of consciousness (LOC)? How long did it last?
- If the patient was in a motor vehicle collision (MVC): How were they restrained? Location in the car? Speed of travel? Point of impact? Damage of the vehicle? Airbag deployment?
- Ask about nausea or vomiting, vision changes, focal neurologic complaints including paresthesias, somnolence, lethargy, or increased irritability.
- Inquire about seizure activity: How long did it last, was there focality, and how long after the event did it occur?
- Palpate the skull for any sign of depressed fractures, significant hematomas, and bulging of the fontanels.
- Reactivity and size of the pupils.
- Any step-offs of the orbital rim.
- Look for periorbital ecchymosis (raccoon eyes) or ecchymosis about the mastoids (Battle sign) as indication of basilar skull fracture.
- Palpate the face for crepitus as a sign of facial bone fractures.
- Look in the ears for hemotympanum or signs of CSF leak which indicate a possible basilar skull fracture.
- Examine the mouth and oropharynx for loose teeth, foreign bodies, and any mobility as a sign of possible Le Fort fractures.
- Reevaluate overall neurologic status including GCS.

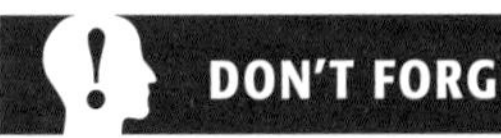

DON'T FORGET

Do not hyperventilate unless there are signs of herniation as prolonged hyperventilation may promote cerebral swelling. Also do not lower P_{CO_2} <30 as overly aggressive hyperventilation can compromise cerebral blood flow.

Review Initial Results

- The likelihood of significant traumatic brain injury (TBI) in the trauma setting is initially judged by patient's history and physical. If significant trauma is suspected, particularly if initial neurologic assessment reveals pediatric GCS <8 or there is a significant decline in neurologic status in serial examinations, definitive management should be employed prior to any further testing.

Definitive Management

- Maintain blood pressure, as hypotension increases mortality.
- High-flow oxygen as hypoxemia increases mortality.
- Intubate patients with significant TBI and optimize oxygenation. Premedication with lidocaine and a nondepolarizing paralytic should be used during RSI in an effort to blunt the rise in intracranial pressure (ICP) with endotracheal tube placement.
- Mannitol 0.25-1 g/kg for patients with evidence of impending herniation.
- Seizure prophylaxis for any patient with severe head injury. Phenytoin 15-20 mg/kg or the fosphenytoin equivalent is generally accepted.
- Prompt neurosurgical consultation.

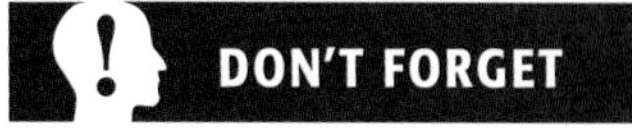

As opposed to adults, give mannitol as an infusion over 15 minutes in pediatric patients as IV boluses may cause an increase in ICP in the pediatric population.

Frequent Reassessment

- Frequent reassessment of overall neurologic status looking for any signs of deterioration is paramount.

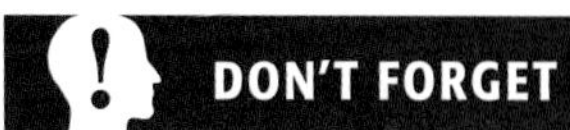

The younger the child, the higher the risk of intracranial injury. If there is any concern, obtain a head CT on test day.

Risk Stratification

- Any child involved in significant multiple system trauma requires thorough neurologic evaluation including computed tomography (CT) imaging.
- Risk stratifying pediatric patients with isolated head trauma is challenging. The following is a general approach to treating pediatric patients with isolated head injury:
  - Patients 0-2 years old are considered separately given the difficulty with communicating with this population.
    - Low-risk: Outpatient observation is for responsible adults with easy access to follow-up.
      - Trivial mechanism (falls <3 ft).
      - No LOC.
      - No focal neurologic signs or symptoms.
    - Medium- or high-risk: All the rest. Get a CT.
  - Patients >2 years old are easier to assess and consensus groups have suggested using a scoring system such as the GCS in conjunction with surrounding circumstances to dictate diagnostic workup.
    - Minor head trauma
      - GCS 14-15 at the time of presentation.
      - No focal neurologic deficits.
      - No evidence of skull fracture.
      - Includes patients with brief episodes of LOC.
      - Observation at home.
    - Moderate (GCS 9-13): CT scan
    - Severe (GCS 8 or less): CT scan

Further Diagnostic Testing

- CT scanning in children should be considered as described above.

Disposition

- Any child with multiple trauma and history of LOC should be observed at least overnight as an inpatient.

DON'T FORGET

- Anterior cord
  - Motor: Complete paralysis below the lesion
  - Sensation: Pain and temperature lost below lesion (fine touch, proprioception intact)
  - Etiology: Flexion injuries, direct compression
- Central cord
  - Motor: Worse in upper extremities > lower extremities
  - Sensation: Variable loss
  - Etiology: Hyperextension
- Brown-Séquard
  - Motor: Ipsilateral loss
  - Sensation: Contralateral pain + temperature loss; ipsilateral loss of fine touch + proprioception
  - Etiology: Hemisection of the cord

- Children who are low risk for intracranial injury do not require CT scan or who have a negative CT scan may be discharged with strict head injury instructions if the caregivers are reliable and health care access is ensured.

NECK TRAUMA

Additional History and Physical Examination

- Mechanism of injury.
- In MVCs and falls, obtain similar history as for head-injured patients.
- Neck pain location, radiation, and intensity.
- Any complaints of paresthesias, focal neurologic symptoms, problems with urination or defecation, or change in ability to ambulate.
- Any neck tenderness is helpful but difficult to elicit in younger, scared pediatric patients or those with altered mental status.
- Breathing pattern may be predominately via accessory or thoracic muscle use if there is a C3, C4, C5 lesion and the phrenic nerve is paralyzed. Be aware of potential hypoventilation.
- Any focality to the neurologic examination including discrepancies in strength or sensation (make sure to assess light touch as well as response to painful/noxious/pressure stimulus) and decreased rectal tone or priapism.
- Do a complete neurological examination including motor, sensation, reflexes, cerebellar, gait (if possible), and cranial nerves.
- Ensure the child is adequately immobilized with cervical collar and padding underneath the shoulder blades to ensure the C-spine in a neutral/straight position.

Review Initial Results

- Note neck pain or midline spine tenderness with neurological deficit in your trauma assessment. Keep a high index of suspicion for spinal injury in complex trauma patients.

Definitive Management

- Don't forget! Fluid resuscitation and/or pressors to maintain perfusion and minimize secondary damage to the cord.
- Neurogenic shock may cause or contribute to hypotension. However, in the multiple trauma patient hypovolemia must be presumed as the cause of hemodynamic instability. If volume resuscitation is not adequate to control blood pressure, and neurogenic shock is considered to be significantly contributing; add vasopressors to the treatment regimen.

Frequent Reassessment

- Imperative as some spinal cord injuries such as spinal cord injury without radiographic abnormality (SCIWORA) may have slow progression of symptoms that occur over hours to days.

Risk Stratification

- Is the cervical spine fracture stable or unstable? Consult neurosurgeon for all fractures even if deemed to be "stable."

Further Diagnostic Testing

- C-spine x-rays: There are several considerations to keep in mind when evaluating pediatric C-spine x-rays. Portable cervical spine x-rays are an option for unstable trauma patients.

- The atlanto-occipital junction of C7 on T1 needs to be completely visualized to adequately evaluate the C-spine.
- Keep in mind the appearance of ossification centers and ages at which they fuse.
- Pseudo-subluxation of C2-C3 is present in 40% of patients <7 years old. A smaller percentage of patients have it at the C3-C4 level.
- Predental space may be up to 5 mm in children ≤10 years old.
- Prevertebral swelling is present if the thickness of the soft tissue measures >75% of the diameter of its adjacent vertebral body.
- In children ≤8 years two-thirds of C-spine fractures involve C3 or above. Fracture patterns do not completely resemble those of adults (C5 and below) until age 16 (Fig. 38-1).
- SCIWORA accounts for between 25% and 75% of all pediatric spinal cord injuries in children <7 years.
  - In these cases, no abnormalities are found on x-ray or even CT.
  - Symptoms may be as subtle as paresthesias—usually upper extremity.
  - Further symptoms may be delayed up to days.
  - Significant long-term morbidity in many cases.
  - Magnetic resonance imaging (MRI) needed for formal analysis.

- CT imaging: CT imaging of the cervical spine provide a more complete picture of the vertebrae but the patient must be stable enough to leave the department. If there is concern for a fracture on x-ray, CTs can be used for further diagnosis.
- MRI: Provides evaluation of the spinal cord in patients with or without associated fracture. MRI is often delayed, however, secondary to more immediate resuscitative efforts.

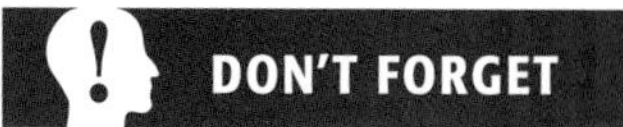

Spinal shock after a cord injury makes exact evaluation of the extent of injury difficult. In spinal shock the bulbocavernosal reflex is absent (increased anal sphincter tone with touching the scrotum or pulling on the Foley catheter). This is different from neurogenic shock which produces a characteristic bradycardia and hypotension.

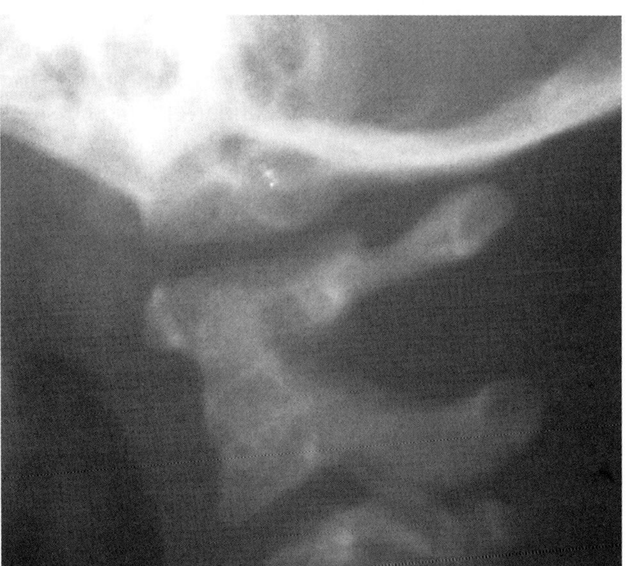

Figure 38-1. An x-ray of a young child brought in on a long board in a cervical collar after a motor vehicle collision. Note the alarming space between the base of the cranium and the cervical spine. This is a lateral cervical spine view that shows findings consistent with atlanto-occipital dislocation. An x-ray such as this mandates an emergent CT scan or MRI, which in this case was normal. This normal variant can be seen in young children due to the laxity of the cervical spine ligaments, in combination with an oversized cervical collar, resulting in slight axial traction. (*Reproduced with permission from Shah BR, Lucchesi M.* Atlas of Pediatric Emergency Medicine. *New York, NY: McGraw-Hill; 2006.*)

Disposition

- Any child with a significant trauma and focal neurologic complaint needs to have a thorough evaluation of their C-spine and spinal cord including MRI. Until these tests have been completed, the patient must remain immobilized with strict spinal precautions.

CHEST TRAUMA

DON'T FORGET

Think tension pneumothorax in any intubated patient with rapid unexplained decompensation with hypotension, deviated trachea, decreasing, or unequal breath sounds.

Additional History and Physical Examination

- The majority of significant blunt chest trauma results from MVCs, so ask about the circumstances surrounding the event, particularly method of restraint, airbag deployment, and speed at the time of impact.
- Shortness of breath, chest pain, and upper back pain are common complaints for patients with significant chest trauma.
- Lungs should be reexamined noting asymmetry or areas of diminished breath sounds. Cardiovascular assessment should include assessment of JVD and muffling of heart sounds.
- The chest wall examination should focus on crepitus, any significant bruising, paradoxical chest movement.
- Isolated injury to the chest from a sudden high-velocity strike from a helmet or hard object may cause the heart convert into a potentially life-threatening rhythm.

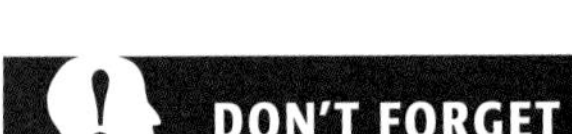

Do not forget to decompress the stomach. A child's respiratory function is extremely sensitive to expanding intra-abdominal volume.

Review Initial Results

- Chest x-ray (CXR) is often available quickly in a trauma evaluation. CXRs are usually supine and therefore differentiating between pneumothorax/hemothorax or both can be difficult. Generally, any pneumothorax >20% or significant hemothorax mandates placement of a chest tube. Because of the likelihood of a mixed process, a large caliber chest tube should be placed in a posterior position. Note to always insert a finder into the chest cavity to check for the presence of abdominal contents or lung tissue that may be adhering to the chest wall (Fig. 38-2).
- If the patient is intubated, any size pneumothorax mandates a chest tube.
- If no CXR is readily available, the clinician must rely on clinical signs of significant hemothorax or pneumothorax to dictate need for tube thoracostomy. Ultrasound can also be used.

Definitive Management

- High-flow oxygen is essential in all trauma patients, especially those with evidence of chest trauma.
- Aggressive airway management
  - Even if breathing is initially adequate, patients with significant chest trauma may experience progressive respiratory failure quickly due to pulmonary contusions, diaphragmatic injury, or flail chest. Reassess frequently.
- Fluid bolus 20 mL/kg for hypotensive patients.
- Early tube thoracostomy for hemo/pneumothorax.
- Pericardiocentesis or thoracotomy for patients with suspected cardiac tamponade.
- Thoracotomy is indicated for patients who have a pulse upon initial emergency department (ED) presentation, especially in the setting of penetrating chest trauma.
- The patient should be taken to the operating room (OR) if there is evidence of massive hemothorax, penetrating cardiac injury, diaphragmatic rupture, evidence of esophageal perforation, or injury to any significant vascular structures.

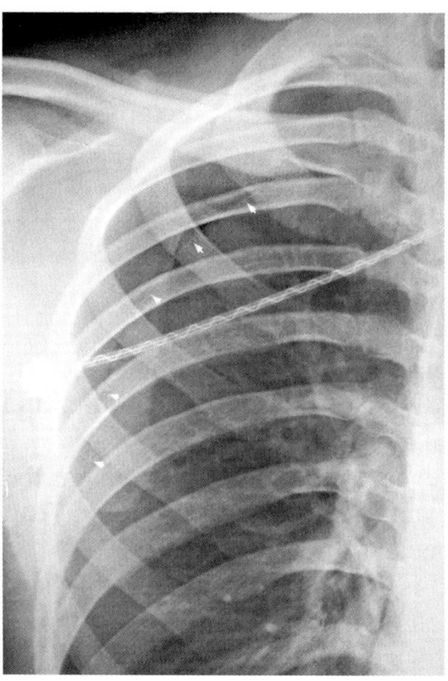
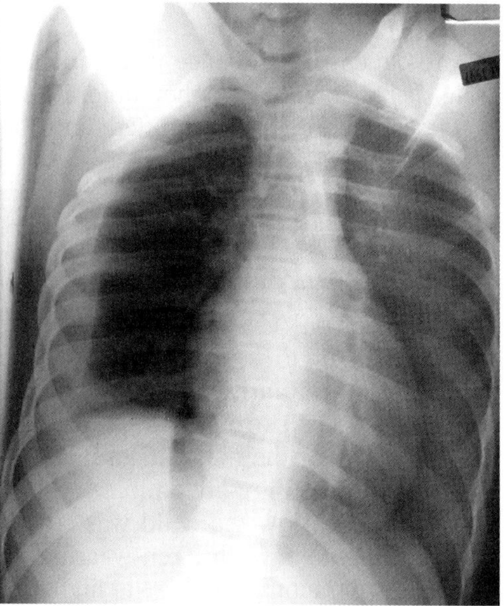

A B

Figure 38-2. (**A**) A pneumothorax can be seen along the right pleural margin, the side of the patient's chest pain (*arrowheads*). (**B**) Hemothorax seen on lateral decubitus view. *([A] Reproduced with permission from Schwartz DT.* Emergency Radiology: Case Studies. *New York, NY: McGraw-Hill; 2008. [B] Reproduced with permission from Shah BR, Lucchesi M.* Atlas of Pediatric Emergency Medicine. *New York, NY: McGraw-Hill; 2006.)*

Risk Stratification

- Children with rib fractures have a high likelihood of more extensive internal injury, most commonly pulmonary contusion.

Further Diagnostic Testing

- CXR is usually quickly available. Considerations when looking at the initial film include:
  - Evidence of hemopneumothorax such as layering of fluid in the hemothorax, air in the soft tissue structures, or deep sulcus signs.
  - Evidence of pulmonary contusion which may not be initially present.
  - Evidence of a "boot-shaped" or "water-bottle-shaped" cardiac silhouette as a sign of pericardial effusion.
  - Evidence of rib fractures.
  - Widened mediastinum as an indication of mediastinal hematoma or dissection.
  - Abdominal contents in the chest from a diaphragmatic herniation or rupture.
  - Free air under the diaphragm from a perforated hollow viscous.
  - Pneumomediastinum or pneumopericardium as evidence of perforated esophagus, larynx, or proximal respiratory tree.
- Recheck CXRs after performing a procedure. If pneumothorax or other injuries persist, consider placing more chest tubes.
- If time permits inspiratory and expiratory chest films may sometimes help delineate the presence of a pneumothorax.
- Chest CT is warranted in stable patients with significant chest trauma as it helps delineate the presence of internal injury.
- Diagnosis of mediastinal hematomas and aortic injuries can be done by chest CT or angiography.
- Electrocardiogram (ECG) and cardiac monitoring for anyone with significant anterior chest wall trauma.

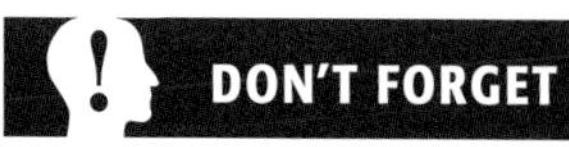

Chest CT is not a sensitive test for diaphragmatic injury.

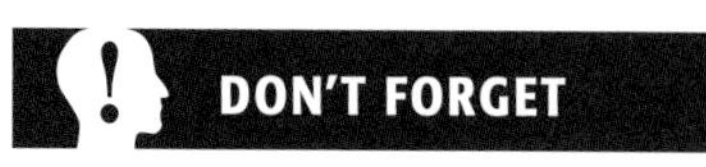

Blunt cardiac injury is relatively rare in the pediatric population. However, with significant anterior chest wall trauma or persistent pain, ECG and cardiac enzymes are warranted to look for signs of cardiac injury. If highly suspicion, consider echocardiography.

Disposition

- Any child with evidence of significant chest trauma (ie, significant ecchymosis, pneumothorax, hemothorax, ECG changes, cardiac ectopy, or rib fractures) needs to be admitted to the hospital.

ABDOMINAL TRAUMA

Additional History and Physical Examination

- Aside from MVCs, other leading causes of blunt abdominal injury include handle bar injuries from bicycles and child abuse in younger children, and sports-related injuries as children become older.
- Circumstances surrounding the traumatic event are important to gauge the significance of the mechanism of injury, even seemingly trivial trauma can cause injury to intra-abdominal organs, especially the solid organs.
- In particular, how the child was restrained is important as a small but significant number of children wearing lap belts will have small bowel injury or Chance fractures, and are at higher risk for diaphragmatic perforation.
- A history of vomiting or bloody stool may indicate bowel injury.
- The patient's abdomen should be examined for bruising, auscultated, and then palpated noting any signs of even vague tenderness. Pediatric patients, especially younger children will have a hard time localizing pain and tenderness, making findings unreliable for prediction of the actual source of injury.
- All patients should have a rectal examination looking for gross blood in their stool. In males, note should be made of prostatic position even though the rate of urethral injury is low in this population.

Review Initial Results

- As with most scenarios involving the trauma patient little information will be available past the initial history, physical and x-ray imaging of the chest or pelvis ("babygram" if the child is small enough). These films may reveal lower rib fractures as a sign of significant impact, pelvic fractures which may contribute to lower abdominal pain and hemodynamic instability, or free air as a sign of a perforated hollow viscous.

Definitive Management

- High-flow oxygen.
- Aggressive fluid resuscitation is essential to maintain adequate tissue perfusion.
- Transfusion of blood products as necessary.
- Definitive management will depend on the type of abdominal injury sustained by the patient. Bedside focused assessment with sonography for trauma (FAST) examination can diagnose free intraperitoneal fluid and a positive examination is indication for exploratory laparotomy in the OR. Ultrasound can be done quickly in the unstable patient.
- Pelvic fractures may need stabilization in the ED with a sheet or binder prior to angiography or surgical fixation.
- Indications for the OR include: A positive FAST examination, significant laceration to the liver or spleen, perforated bowel, and persistent hypotension. Consult with a trauma surgeon for definitive management.

Risk Stratification

- A child who remains hemodynamically unstable despite aggressive fluid resuscitation in the face of any significant history or signs of abdominal trauma should be taken to the OR for exploration.

- A child with multisystem trauma should have abdominal imaging with either FAST examination or a CT scan.

Further Diagnostic Testing

- CT scanning is the imaging modality of choice for hemodynamically stable pediatric patients. It is noninvasive, can image the retroperitoneum, and can diagnose intra-abdominal injury. Sensitivity is not as high for detection of hollow viscous and diaphragm injuries. There still may be a need for exploratory laparotomy if there is a large amount of intra-abdominal fluid for which there is no obvious source.
- Lab tests, particularly amylase and lipase, may be helpful in detecting pancreas or bowel injuries, both of which can be missed by imaging methods.

Disposition

- Given the unreliability of the physical examination in pediatric patients and the poor sensitivity for detecting certain intra-abdominal injury, any patient who experiences a significant abdominal trauma gets admitted to the hospital.
- Those with documented intra-abdominal injury but remain hemodynamically stable should be admitted to the hospital, ideally to the pediatric intensive care unit (PICU) setting.
- Again, any patient with abdominal trauma who remains hemodynamically unstable despite adequate resuscitative efforts needs to undergo an exploratory laparotomy.

GENITOURINARY TRAUMA

Because the kidneys are not as firmly attached in the pediatric patient's retroperitoneum, they are more susceptible to deceleration and shearing forces. Therefore, for any significant abdominal or multisystem trauma, renal injury must be considered. Lower genitourinary (GU) tract trauma is important to diagnose, as immediate urologic consult will be needed to evaluate the injury. Upper GU tract injury is important to diagnose as renal vascular injury may be a source of significant bleeding.

Additional History and Physical Examination

- Note any direct blows to the flank area.
- Look for flank tenderness or ecchymosis
- Ask about hematuria
- On examination, a perineal hematoma, high riding prostate or blood from the urethral meatus should prompt concern for lower GU tract injury.

Initial Review Results

- As part of the resuscitation process for major trauma, Foley catheter placement is indicated to accurately measure urine output. Any of the abovementioned signs of lower GU tract injury should stop placement of a Foley catheter until a retrograde urethrogram can be performed.
- The initial urine retrieved should be sent for urinalysis (UA) as later samples may be diluted from resuscitative efforts.

Risk Stratification

- Any severe multisystem trauma, especially involving the abdominal or flank areas, poses significant risk of injury to the kidneys.

- The presence of red blood cells (RBCs) >50/HPF of UA suggests significant risk of renal injury and mandates follow-up studies.
  - Further diagnostic interventions
  - Retrograde urethrogram for any signs of lower GU tract injury.
  - If extravasation of dye is noted, a Foley catheter cannot be placed as it may convert a partial urethral tear to a complete one. A suprapubic catheter should be placed instead.
  - Retrograde cystogram for any suspicion of bladder disruption
  - CT abdomen and pelvis with IV contrast is the preferred imaging modality to look for GU injury.

Disposition

- Any patient with evidence of significant GU trauma requires evaluation by a urologist.

CHILD ABUSE

There is a wide range of what constitutes abuse or neglect of children. Children who have suffered physical or sexual abuse constitute a special population of trauma patients. Be wary of misleading, incomplete, or minimized recounts of the injury making full evaluation of acute injuries more difficult.

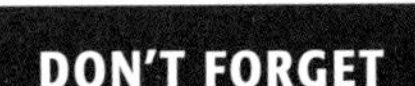

DON'T FORGET

Over half of all abused children are <3 years of age, and one-third are <6 months.

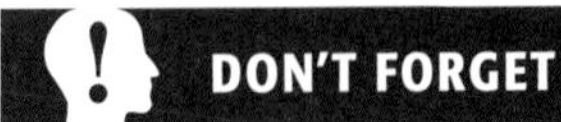

DON'T FORGET

Classic physical findings of abuse including burns in a stocking or glove distribution or burns that involve entire buttocks are consistent with the child being dipped in scalding water.

Additional History and Physical Examination

- Pay attention to injuries not consistent with the events reported to have caused them.
- Be wary of stories that keep changing.
- Look for signs of injuries of varying ages.
- Look for signs of neglect such as failure to thrive and poor hygiene.
- Look for signs that are characteristic of abuse: Burn marks inconsistent with splash patterns, burns consistent with the size of cigarettes or irons, or bruises in the shapes of hands, electrical cords, or belts.
- Look for behavioral clues: Children overly fearful of a parent, parents who refuse to let their spouse respond, or children who are acting out especially in an inappropriate manner.
- Infants need funduscopic examination to evaluate for retinal hemorrhage as a sign of repeated shaking.
- If sexual abuse is suspected, examine the genital area.
- Take cultures (GC/*Chlamydia*) of any potential area of contact. Conduct a sexual assault kit according to local practice guidelines.

Definitive Management

- Initial stabilization and resuscitation for any traumatic injury.
- If there is any suspicion of abuse, physicians are mandatory reporters. Contact Department of Children and Family Services (DCFS) and file a police report.
- Ensure that the patient has a safe environment if planning to discharge.

Diagnostic Testing

- As dictated by the severity of the patients presentation.
- Skeletal survey for infants.
  - Spiral fractures in young children, especially the femur, may be indicative of twisting injuries.
  - Metaphyseal chip fractures are common in child abuse.
  - Fractures of varying ages are evidence of possible abuse.

- Head CT if any concern for shaking injuries.
- Lab work for failure to thrive.

Disposition

- If no acute injuries, the child may be discharged only if appropriate follow-up has been arranged and the patient has an ensured safe destination.

NEAR DROWNING

Drowning is a significant cause of death in the pediatric population seen predominately in young children and then again in the teenage years. The pathophysiology is hypoxemia that leads to cardiac arrest. Additionally, traumatic comorbidities need to be ruled out (ie, diving accidents).

Additional History and Physical Examination

- How long was the patient submerged?
- Were there any witnesses, was there any trauma?
- What care was administered prehospital?
- Special attention should be paid to the patient's core temperature. If hypothermia is a concern, use a thermometer capable of measuring low temperatures.
- Look for signs of spinal cord injury and complete a full neurological examination.

Definitive Management

- Initial resuscitation of the patient stabilizing the ABCs.
- Cervical spine immobilization if there is any suspicion of trauma.
- If severe hypothermia is present (<32°C) aggressively rewarm the patient.
- Monitor the patient's respiratory status for worsening lung function as inflammation develops.

Risk Stratification

- Good prognostic indicators include shorter time of immersion, early prehospital treatment, cold temperature of water, quick return of vitals postarrest, and higher level of alertness.
- Poor indictors include prolonged immersion, prolonged resuscitative efforts, severe acidosis, and lower levels of alertness. Although patients who are alert, and not comatose, often have significant recoveries.

Further Diagnostic Testing

- Testing should proceed as dictated by the situation. If there was significant trauma then testing should be carried out as outlined above with special attention to head and C-spine injuries.
- Arterial blood gasses (ABGs) should be followed to monitor adequacy of respiratory efforts.
- No matter how good the patient looks they get a CXR, as any abnormal findings, no matter how small, portend a significant respiratory decline for the patient.

Disposition

- Can discharge home if the patient has a GCS of 15, a clear x-ray, normal respiratory status, appears well, and is without complaints, but only after a minimum 4-6-hour observation period as seemingly well patients can still have a post-immersion decompensation.

- Well-appearing patients with any abnormal findings on their x-rays need to be observed overnight.
- Any significantly ill patient or patient with concomitant traumatic injury needs to be admitted to an intensive care unit (ICU).

WINNING STRATEGIES

- Do not forget prehospital care—ask paramedics about the mechanism of injury, vitals, and treatment given prior to ED arrival. Apply a cervical collar if not already in place for neck pain and/or neurological deficit.
- Every trauma patient gets high-flow oxygen and cardiac monitor no matter how good they look.
- Be methodical.
- Treat the underlying condition or life threat as you find it on the primary survey.
- For head injuries, order a CT scan on exam day (even if the mechanism sounds insignificant).
- Aggressively treat severe head injuries. Frequent reassessments are key! Children are more prone to generalized edema after severe injury and can decompensate quickly from it.
- Pediatric patients have a unique pattern of C-spine injuries.
- MRIs for everyone with significant neurologic symptoms or signs even if there is no associated spine fracture—rule out SCIWORA.
- Be cautious of a child with rib fractures. It takes significantly more force to break pediatric ribs and they are likely associated with underlying injury.
- Watch for late respiratory decomposition near-drowning patients. Any respiratory finding or abnormal x-ray finding mandates admission for observation.
- Children do not localize abdominal pain. If any pain or tenderness, obtain CT imaging.
- Renal trauma is common in children. Look for it.

THE BOTTOM LINE

- Remember ABCDEF.
- Act quickly and decisively. As soon as you find it, treat it.
- No pediatric trauma patient goes home on exam day.

SECTION 6

THE CASES

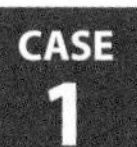

CASE 1 55 y/o Male With Chest Pain

Navneet Cheema and Rohit Gupta

INITIAL INFORMATION

Name: John Smith

Mode of arrival: Brought in by family

Age: 55 years

Gender: Male

VS: T 37.2°C, BP 150/90, HR 84, RR 16, O_2 sat: 96% on RA

CC: Left-sided substernal chest pain

PLAY OF THE CASE

C: "What do I see as I walk into the patient's room?"

E: "The patient is a well-nourished male, who appears in mild distress. He is diaphoretic and clutching his chest."

C: "Nurse, please place the patient on a cardiac monitor, show me a rhythm strip, begin O_2 via NC and titrate to keep O_2 sat above 97%, place an 18-gauge IV, begin NS at TKO, and draw blood for lab tests. Also, please obtain a stat 12-lead ECG and show it to me when it's ready."

E: "Those orders are being done. The rhythm strip shows an NSR in the 80s with occasional PVCs."

C: "Hello, Mr. Smith, I'm Dr. Payne. What brings you in to see us?"

E: "Doc, I have real bad pain in my chest. It started about 6 hours ago. I've never had a pain that was this bad before."

C: "Have you had chest pain before? Do you have any heart problems?"

E: "My doc says I have angina. I get chest pain once in a while if I'm shoveling snow or really exerting myself. I'm supposed to take nitroglycerin, but I haven't had to use it in a long time and I couldn't find it today."

C: "Does the chest pain feel like your typical pain?"

E: "Yes, except it's more severe and it's not going away."

C: "Do you feel SOB and are you nauseated or vomiting?"

E: "I'm SOB, but the oxygen is helping."

C: "What medical problems do you have?"

E: "High blood pressure and angina."

C: "What medications do you take?"

E: "Atenolol and aspirin."

C: "Do you have any allergies?"

E: "No."

E: "Your ECG is performed (Fig. C1-1)."

KEY QUESTION

Ask this open-ended question at the beginning of every case.

KEY ORDERS

Most of the patients you see during the exam will be unstable (or will become that way). Whenever confronted with an unstable patient this group of orders should be given.

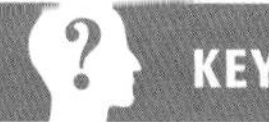

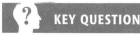

KEY QUESTION

Remember to ask about past medical history, medications, and allergies.

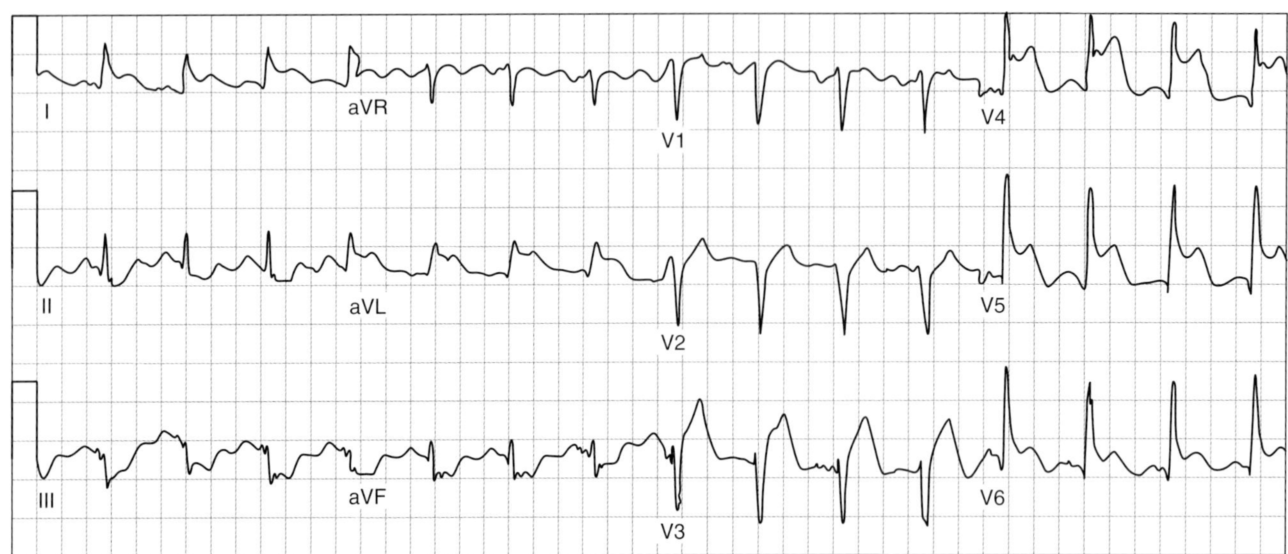

Figure C1-1. Initial ECG on presentation shows ST-segment elevation in the precordial leads, as well as I and aVL, indicative of acute anterolateral STEMI due to proximal left anterior descending (LAD) coronary artery occlusion. Note the reciprocal ST depression in the inferior leads. *(Reprinted with permission from Crawford MH.* Current Diagnosis and Treatment: Cardiology. *3rd ed. New York, NY: McGraw-Hill; 2009.)*

In this case recognizing that the patient is having an MI and initiating appropriate initial therapy with ASA, beta-blockade, and pain control is a critical action. This test-taker recognizes the MI, and starts some of the therapy appropriately.

C: "The patient is having an STEMI. Nurse, administer chewable aspirin, 162 mg. Give the patient nitroglycerin sublingual (SL) 0.4 mg q5min for ongoing chest pain. Please start a second IV. I would like to order the following tests: CBC, electrolytes, BUN/Cr, glucose, coags, and cardiac enzymes including troponin. I'd like to get the cardiologist paged."

E: "Those orders are being done."

C: "Mr. Smith your ECG shows that you are having a heart attack. It looks like it involves a significant portion of your heart. We are going to give you aggressive treatment to get you better. I need to ask you a few more questions. Have you had a heart attack before?"

E: "No."

C: "Have you had a stroke, bleeding in your brain, or a recent surgical procedure?"

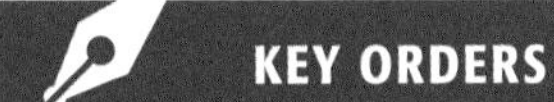

Remember to put parameters on your orders. ABEM General nurses will carry out all your orders without question.

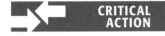

E: "No."

C: "Have you had any active bleeding, blood in your stool, or a history of peptic ulcer disease?"

E: "I did have a stomach ulcer that bled years ago. I had an operation, but that was 20 years ago. My chest is really hurting."

E: "The patient has been given three SL nitroglycerin with no improvement in pain."

C: "Administer morphine 4 mg IV. What is the patient's repeat BP?"

E: "130/80"

Here the test-taker completes the appropriate initial therapy.

C: "Administer metoprolol 5 mg IV, repeat the dose up to three times. Hold additional doses if the SBP drops below 100 mm Hg or a HR of 60 is reached."

E: "It is being done."

C: "How is your pain now?"

E: "I think it might be a little better."

C: "I'd like to examine the patient. Is the patient more comfortable? Is there cyanosis? Are the mucous membranes moist?"

E: "The patient appears more comfortable, there is no cyanosis and the mucous membranes are moist."

C: "Is there JVD or tracheal deviation?"

E: "No."

C: "What do I hear when I listen to the lungs and heart?"

E: "What are you looking for?"

C: "On the lung examination, I am listening for breath sounds, crackles, and wheezes. On the cardiac examination, I am listening for murmurs, rubs, and gallops. Also, are the peripheral pulses symmetric?"

E: "Breath sounds are present bilaterally, there are crackles at the bases. The heart examination is normal and the peripheral pulses are full."

C: "Are the bowel sounds present? Is there abdominal tenderness?"

E: "Bowel sounds are present and there is no tenderness."

C: "Rectal examination?"

E: "Normal tone, normal prostate, brown stool, guaiac negative."

C: "Extremities?"

E: "Normal."

C: "I would like to order a stat portable upright CXR. Is the cardiologist on the phone?"

E: "The radiograph is being taken. The cardiologist Dr. Hart is on the phone."

C: "Hello Dr. Hart, I am Dr. Payne. I have a 55 y/o male with chest pain. The ECG shows that he is having an anterior STEMI. I am trying to get him pain free and anticoagulating him. I would like you to come in for primary PCI."

E: "It's going to take me over 3 hours to get the cath lab activated."

C: "In that case, I'm going to give that patient tPA according to protocol. I'll need you to admit the patient to the CCU. Nurse, please administer heparin 5000 U bolus and then 1000 U/h."

E: "That is being done."

C: "After the heparin is started, administer tPA according to protocol."

E: "The heparin is given. The tPA is administered."

C: "Mr. Smith, how is your pain doing?"

E: "It's still there, but it's getting better Doc."

C: "I would like to get a repeat ECG and make arrangement for the patient to be admitted to the CCU."

E: "A bed is being arranged. The patient begins to complain about feeling dizzy."

C: "Recheck the patient's vital signs."

E: "Vital signs are now BP 90/60, HR 150."

C: "I would like to look at the rhythm strip and order a repeat 12-lead ECG."

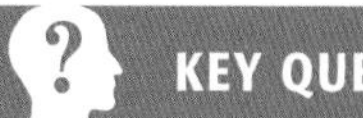

KEY QUESTION

Remember to reassess your patient frequently.

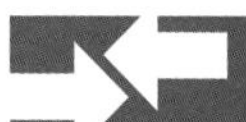

CRITICAL ACTION

There are two critical actions being taken here. First, the test taker is attempting to get definitive care for the patient by transferring him to a facility that has a cath lab. Recognizing that the time it would take to get to cath is too long, he elects to use tPA. Secondly, he is giving heparin for anticoagulation.

DON'T FORGET

When you do not know the dose of a medication off the top of your head, you can ask for it to be administered according to protocol or you can state that you will look it up or ask pharmacy to calculate it for you.

KEY QUESTION

Remember to reassess your patient frequently. This is a good strategy whenever you think you are close to done, or when you don't know what to do next. The answer will let you know if you are on the right track.

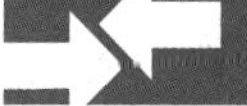

CRITICAL ACTION

On test day, almost no one will go home, and most people will go to the ICU. In this case, an active MI patient will go to the CCU.

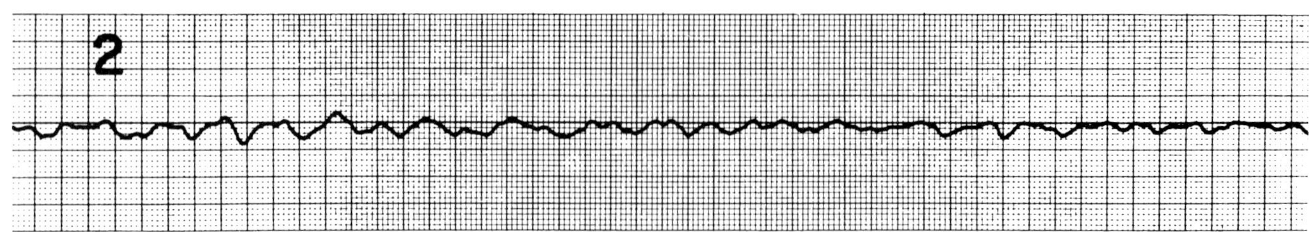

Figure C1-2. The ventricular complexes in this strip are rapid and irregular, consistent with ventricular fibrillation. *(Reprinted with permission from Tintinalli JE, Kelen GD, Stapczynski JS, et al.* Emergency Medicine: A Comprehensive Study Guide. *6th ed. New York, NY: McGraw-Hill; 2004.)*

E: "As the 12-lead ECG is completed, the patient loses consciousness."

C: "Does the patient have a pulse?"

E: "Yes, but it is weak."

C: "The rhythm strip shows ventricular fibrillation (Fig. C1-2). I will defibrillate the patient immediately at 200 J."

E: "The defibrillation is performed with no change in rhythm."

C: "I will defibrillate again at 300 J."

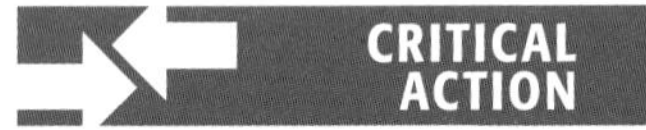

Intubating when a patient becomes unresponsive is a critical action.

Defibrillating and administering drugs to this patient in accordance with ACLS guidelines is a critical action.

E: "The defibrillation is performed with no change in rhythm."

C: "I'll defibrillate a third time at 360 J."

E: "There is no change in rhythm after the third cardioversion attempt and the patient no longer has a pulse."

C: "Start CPR. I will intubate the patient. Since the patient is unresponsive, I will not use any sedation or paralytics. Administer epinephrine 1 mg IV."

E: "The intubation is performed and the epinephrine is given."

C: "I will defibrillate the patient again at 360 J."

E: "After the fourth shock, the rhythm changes to the following (Fig. C1-3)."

C: "Is there a pulse or a blood pressure?"

E: "The pulse is 105, the blood pressure is 100/60."

C: "Administer amiodarone 150 mg IV over 10 minutes and then begin 1 mg/min drip."

E: "That is being done."

C: "What are the vital signs now?"

E: "BP 100/50, HR 95."

C: "I would like to get another 12-lead ECG (Fig. C1-4)."

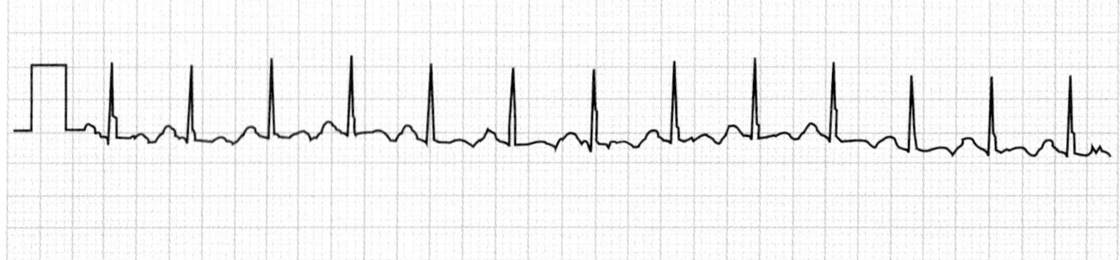

Figure C1-3. The rhythm strip shows sinus tachycardia. *(Reprinted with permission from Gomella LG, Haist SA.* Clinician's Pocket Reference. *11th ed. New York, NY: McGraw-Hill; 2007.)*

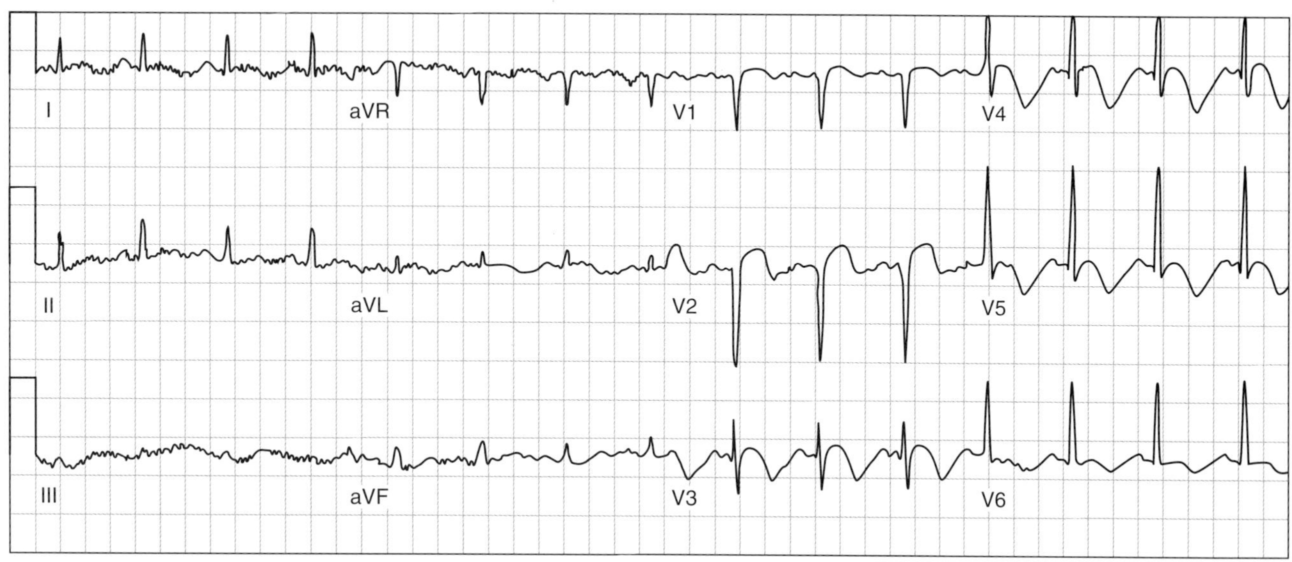

Figure C1-4. ECG changes in anterolateral STEMI. ECG after reperfusion therapy showing resolution of the anterolateral ST elevation and the reciprocal changes. Note the developing Q wave in V2. *(Reprinted with permission from Crawford MH.* Current Diagnosis and Treatment: Cardiology. *3rd ed. New York, NY: McGraw-Hill; 2009.)*

E: "Dr. Hart is on the phone from the CCU. He would like an update."

C: "Dr. Hart, Mr. Smith is quite ill. After administering heparin and tPA, the patient experienced a V Fib arrest. He was intubated and resuscitated, but required multiple defibrillations and initiation of amiodarone. Currently, his vital signs show a pulse of 95 and a BP of 100/50. His latest ECG shows that he is in a sinus rhythm with resolving ST-segment elevation."

E: "This case is now over."

CASE ASSESSMENT

Overall the candidate managed a difficult case extremely well. Throughout the encounter the candidate played the role of the physician well, issuing commands, addressing the patient, and moving through the case. At the start of the case, he saw that the patient was ill and instituted proper monitoring. He took an appropriate history and despite getting the electrocardiogram (ECG) with STEMI, he completed a thorough, directed physical examination that is specifically tailored for the chest pain patient. He accurately diagnosed the patient with an anterior ST-segment elevation MI and initiated therapy. Before lysing the patient, the candidate attempted to arrange percutaneous coronary intervention (PCI), which was not available, and likely will not be available on the actual oral examination. Notice that the candidate did not know the dose of tissue plasminogen activator (tPA) and asked that it be dosed according to protocol. For most medications this should be sufficient. All advanced cardiovascular life support (ACLS), pediatric advanced life support (PALS), neonatal advanced life support (NALS), and airway management drugs should be memorized, but other drugs can be looked up during the exam.

The candidate managed the myocardial infarction (MI) capably and absolutely met the standard of care. He instituted oxygen, aspirin, nitroglycerin, and morphine to alleviate pain as soon as he suspected cardiac ischemia. He administered an IV beta-blocker after ensuring that the patient was not in failure and after making the diagnosis of an acute coronary syndrome (ACS). Beta-blockers have been shown to decrease mortality and the risk of developing tachyarrhythmias in the setting of an MI. The candidate ordered a repeat ECG after administering thrombolytics, but the patient decompensated before getting it. If a repeat ECG after initiation of lytics shows persistent ST elevation, strong consideration should be given to transferring the patient for rescue angioplasty.

After decompensation, the candidate managed the resuscitation well. Initially, he diagnosed the cause of decompensation by requesting a rhythm strip. After seeing the ventricular fibrillation (V Fib) arrest, he immediately shocked the patient three times. When defibrillation failed, he started cardiopulmonary resuscitation (CPR), a step that is frequently forgotten, and then intubated the patient and administered epinephrine. After shocking the patient a fourth time, the rhythm converted. The candidate chose to manage the patient further with amiodarone to stabilize the rhythm. The examiner then led the case to closure by having the candidate update the patient's status to the admitting cardiologist.

The candidate managed this case well. As you are reviewing the case, do not worry if you would not have managed the case as efficiently. Remember the test requires each candidate to meet or exceed a national standard of care. Examinees do not need to provide perfect care.

Critical Actions

1. Diagnosis of anterior MI.
2. Pain control with appropriate medications for chest pain.
3. Administration of anticoagulation and tPA.
4. Three shocks for management of V Fib arrest.
5. Intubation
6. Admission to cardiac care unit (CCU).

Test Performance

1. *Data acquisition:* The candidate showed the ability to obtain more than an adequate history and physical examination in an efficient manner, as well as ordering appropriate tests to assist in diagnosis. Score = **7**
2. *Problem solving:* The candidate did an excellent job in problem solving and was able to quickly assimilate data from the patient encounter, interpret test results and synthesize information. Score = **8**
3. *Patient management:* The candidate made appropriate treatment decisions based on patient information and change in clinical status. This was done in a very efficient and timely manner. Score = **8**
4. *Resource utilization:* The candidate demonstrated very good use of resources with an efficient, cost-effective use of tests that did not compromise patient care. Score = **7**
5. *Health care provided (outcome):* The candidate did an excellent job of stabilizing the patient when the rhythm changed to ventricular fibrillation, quickly recognizing the change in patient status and effectively treating the dysrhythmia. Score = **8**
6. *Interpersonal relations and communication skills:* The candidate was able to engage in effective information exchange with both the patient and consultant. The candidate demonstrated appropriate professionalism conveying respect, compassion, and integrity. Score = **7**

7. *Comprehension of pathophysiology:* The candidate was able to articulate comprehension of the various ECG and rhythm strip findings in this case, specifically diagnosing the anterior MI and recognizing V Fib. Score = **8**
8. *Clinical competence (overall):* This candidate demonstrated a detailed and efficient investigatory and analytical approach to this case. Score = **8**

CASE 2 44 y/o Female With Headache

Navneet Cheema, Charles Maddow, James I. Syrett

INITIAL INFORMATION

Name: Ann Smith

Mode of arrival: Brought in by BLS ambulance

Age: 44 years

Gender: Female

VS: T 37.2°C, BP 160/90, HR 103, RR 24, O_2 sat: 99% on RA

CC: Headache

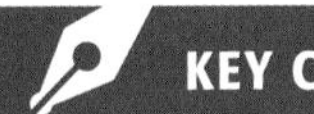

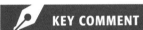

KEY QUESTION

Ask this open-ended question at the beginning of every case.

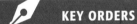

KEY COMMENT

This examinee will earn points for interaction with the family. This includes introducing themselves, reassuring the patient, and keeping the patient and family apprised of the test results and plan.

KEY ORDERS

Most of the patients you see during the exam will be unstable (or will become that way). Whenever confronted with an unstable patient this group of orders should be given.

KEY QUESTION

Remember to use the resources around you. If the patient cannot give you a good history, use family, witnesses, or the EMTs.

PLAY OF THE CASE

E: "Good morning, welcome to ABEM General. Do you have any questions?"

C: "No, thank you."

E: "OK. This is a single patient encounter. Here is the triage sheet for your patient."

C: "As I walk into the room what do I see, hear, or smell?"

E: "You see a well-nourished female on a bed, groaning with her eyes closed. Her husband is in the room as well. There are no unusual smells. She has vomited once."

C: "Ms. Smith, my name is Dr. Jones, I am going to speak to you in a minute, but I have to ask our nurses to do some things first."

E: "OK doctor, my head really hurts."

C: "Nurse, can you place this patient on the monitor, run a rhythm strip and show it to me, put her on 2 L NC oxygen, start a large-bore IV in the antecubital fossa, and draw off blood for labs. I will tell you in a minute what labs to send."

E: "All the things you have asked for are being done."

C: "Ms. Smith, what brings you to the hospital today?"

E: "Well doctor, I have been having headaches on and off for the last week but today I was shopping and I got a really bad one. I had to sit down and then I think I fainted. This headache is really bad."

C: "How did you get to hospital?"

E: "My husband called the ambulance and they brought me here."

C: "I would like to speak to your husband. Sir, what happened to your wife?"

E: "Well it is just as she said, this is not like her, she never gets headaches."

C: "How long did she lose consciousness for?"

E: "For about 2 minutes she just slumped over, when she came around, she said her headache was worse."

C: "Ms. Smith, how bad is your headache just now?"

E: "This is the worst headache of my life."

C: "I would like to give you some pain medicines for the headache, do you have any allergies?"

E: "No."

C: "Nurse, please give Ms. Smith 4 mg of morphine IV for pain and 4 mg of ondansetron IV for nausea and repeat her vital signs after they have been given."

E: "The drugs have been given, her BP is now 135/84 and pulse is 96."

C: "Ms. Smith, I have some more questions and then I would like to examine you. Other than the headache, have you noticed any other symptoms?"

E: "No, I am normally a healthy person, but I find the lights really bright to look at."

C: "Did you get any warning when this headache came on, did you see, hear, or smell anything funny?"

E: "No, the headache came on like someone hit my head and I think I vomited once."

C: "How is your pain after the medications?"

E: "It has taken the edge off, I feel a little better."

C: "Do you have any other health problems, allergies, or take any medications?"

E: "I take a multivitamin once a day, but nothing else."

C: "Does anything run in the family?"

E: "My mother died of a heart attack at 62."

C: "I would like to examine you now."

C: "What is the patient's general appearance? Is there respiratory distress or pallor?"

E: "She is a well-appearing 44-year-old of normal height and weight. There is no respiratory distress though she is slightly pale."

C: "Examining her HEENT what do I find?"

E: "What are you looking for?"

C: "Her pupils, eye movements, and funduscopic examination."

E: "Her pupils are 4 mm and reactive, eye movements are intact but you cannot visualize her fundi because she is photophobic."

C: "Examining her neck."

E: "What are you looking for?"

C: "Is her neck supple, are there any bruises, rashes, or marks?"

E: "Her neck is supple, there are no marks; however, she does wince when you move her head."

C: "Her chest examination?"

E: "Normal."

C: "Cardiovascular examination?"

E: "Normal."

C: "Abdominal examination?"

KEY ORDERS

You will be graded on how you treat your patient's pain. Do not forget to give analgesia when appropriate.

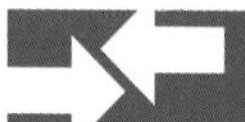

CRITICAL ACTION

This is a case of a sudden onset "worst headache of my life." One of the critical actions in this case is to do a full neuro examination including looking for photophobia and meningismus.

DON'T FORGET

If the examiner asks the candidate to be more specific about what elements of the examination they want, it normally indicates that there is something to be found. If the examiner dismisses a body system as normal it is not worth pursuing that system further.

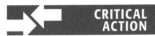

CRITICAL ACTION

Getting a stat head CT is a critical action in this case.

E: "What do you want to know?"

C: "Bowel sounds? Tenderness? Findings of peritonitis?"

E: "Active bowel sounds with no tenderness."

C: "Back and skin?"

E: "Normal, no rashes."

C: "Neurological examination?"

E: "What do you want to know specifically?"

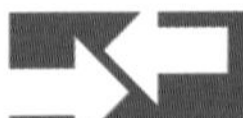

CRITICAL ACTION

There are two critical actions here. First, the examinee must treat (and prevent) hypertension. Secondly, he must contact neurosurgery immediately.

C: "Is the muscular strength, sensation, and DTRs symmetric? Are the facial muscles and sensation intact?"

E: "There are no focal neurologic findings and the cranial nerves are intact."

C: "Ms. Smith, I am concerned that your headache is due to possible bleeding in the brain area. Specifically, a condition known as subarachnoid hemorrhage. I am going to order a CT scan of your head."

E: "It sounds really bad, is this serious?"

C: "Yes it is, we need to make sure things don't get worse. If something shows up on your CT scan I will ask the neurosurgeons to see you; if the CT scan is normal we will still have to do a lumbar puncture to make sure nothing bad is going on."

E: "Neurosurgeons! Am I going to have an operation?"

KEY COMMENT

When you do not know the dose of a medication off the top of your head, you can ask for it to be administered according to protocol, you can state that you will look it up or ask pharmacy to calculate it for you.

C: "Sometimes people need an operation to fix this and sometimes a specially trained radiologist can fix it, but let's get the CT scan and find out what is going on." "I would like to order a stat head CT. Also can you send the following labs from the blood you drew: CBC, basic metabolic profile, and a coagulation profile? Also can you send a urine pregnancy test?"

E: "All of that is done, here is your CT scan of the head (Fig. C2-1)."

E: The nurse asks you what it shows?"

C: "The CT shows SAH."

C: "Please give the patient nicardipine and load her with phenytoin IV. Check her blood pressure every 15 minutes and if it starts to rise we will begin antihypertensive therapy. Please contact the neurosurgeon on call. I would also like to speak to Ms. Smith again."

KEY COMMENT

This examinee will earn high points for his interaction with the family. This includes introducing himself, reassuring the patient, and keeping the patient and family apprised of the test results and plan.

E: "What dose of nicardipine and phenytoin?"

C: "Please give phenytoin, a total of 20 mg/kg, by IV infusion over 30 minutes. I will look up the nicardipine dosage or consult the hospital pharmacist if not sure."

E: "OK, the drugs are being given."

C: "Ms. Smith, you do have a subarachnoid hemorrhage, a type of intracranial bleeding due to a rupture of a small artery. We are beginning treatment to protect your brain and to prevent seizure due to brain irritation. I am going to speak to the neurosurgeons now."

E: "Dr. Brain is on the phone."

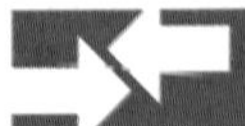

CRITICAL ACTION

Admitting this bleed to the ICU is a critical action in this case.

C: "Dr. Brain, this is Dr. Jones in the ED. I have a 44-year-old lady that presented with the worst headache of her life; she has a confirmed subarachnoid bleed on CT. We have loaded her with phenytoin, given nicardipine, and would like you to see her and admit her to the ICU."

E: "Dr. Brain will see her now, this concludes this case."

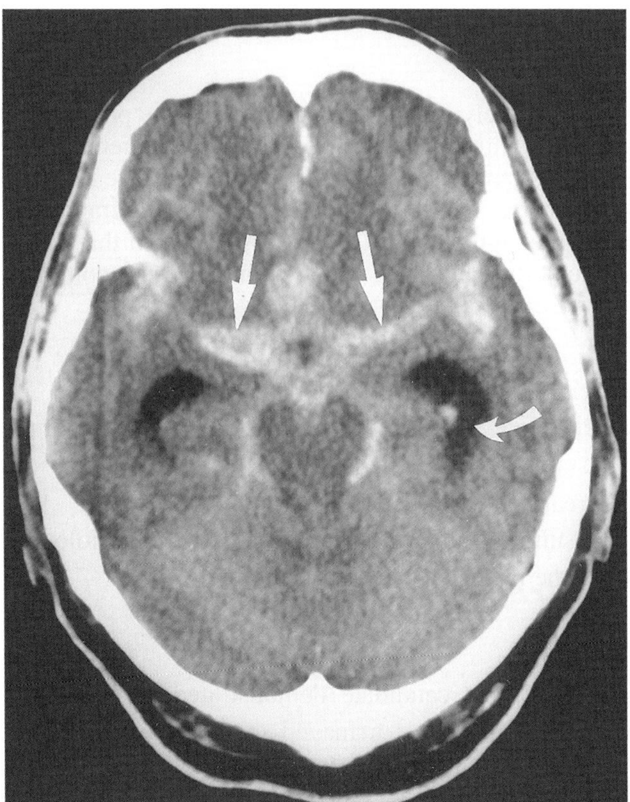

Figure C2-1. CT scan of head showing subarachnoid hemorrhage. *(Reprinted with permission from Tintinalli JE, Kelen GD, Stapczynski JS, et al.* Emergency Medicine: A Comprehensive Study Guide. *6th ed. New York, NY: McGraw-Hill; 2004.)*

CASE ASSESSMENT

Overall the candidate did very well in this case. The patient had no preexisting medical problems and this was an acute presentation. The sudden nature of the presentation with the recent onset of lesser headaches, along with the key words of "worst headache of my life," suggest the diagnosis of subarachnoid hemorrhage; though one may briefly consider migraine headache, the lack of prior history makes this much less likely. You will not be taking care of a typical migraine headache on the day of your exam.

The candidate also excelled in communication with the patient, remembering the important aspects of introduction to the patient and keeping the patient and family informed and updated about the progression in the case.

Some of the other highlights of the case and good learning points included the early use of analgesia after determining allergies and the use of pharmacy to determine the correct dose of less frequently used drugs. The candidate also demonstrated knowledge of the phenytoin dose without reference. Also the candidate asked for repeat vital signs following the morphine dose presumably trying to determine if the mild hypertension and tachycardia was due to pain or another pathology.

One point to note is during the examination component of the patient encounter. If the examiner asks the candidate to be more specific about what elements of the examination they want, it normally indicates that there is something to be found. If the examiner dismisses one body system as normal it is not worth pursuing that system further.

In all, this was a relatively straightforward case. Some potential complications that could have been introduced would include the patient being significantly hypertensive, the patient presenting with seizure or altered level of consciousness, or the patient having a negative computed tomography (CT) scan and requiring lumbar puncture—any of these may occur on the exam day and you should consider carefully how you would approach these complications!

Critical Actions

1. Suspicion of intracranial hemorrhage.
2. Thorough neurologic examination and checking for signs of meningismus.
3. Obtaining a stat head CT.
4. Aggressive treatment of hypertension when present.
5. Promptly consulting neurosurgery or interventional radiology.
6. Admission to the intensive care unit (ICU).

Test Performance

1. *Data acquisition:* The candidate demonstrated an efficient and focused approach to this case. They managed to find the important components of the history and examination while not being distracted by nonrelevant aspects. They also utilized additional sources of information, specifically involving the husband during the history. Score = **7**
2. *Problem solving:* The candidate used the contextual clues provided in the history very well, recognizing this as a "thunder-clap" headache that was concerning for subarachnoid hemorrhage (SAH). Score = **7**
3. *Patient management:* The candidate effectively treated the patient's pain in this case, recognizing the severity of the pain and the potential of a life-threatening illness requiring IV pain medications. Score = **7**
4. *Resource utilization:* Tests were appropriately ordered including labs and imaging that would help support the suspected SAH diagnosis. The candidate also could have considered a CT angiogram in addition to the plain CT. Score = **7**
5. *Health care provided (outcome):* The candidate immediately acted to treat the SAH ordering a calcium channel blocker and antiepileptics to prevent further morbidity. The appropriate consultant was also efficiently contacted. Score = **8**
6. *Interpersonal relations and communication skills:* The candidate interacted with the patient in a respectful and courteous manner. The patient was informed of the physicians' concerns throughout the case and there was no delay informing the patient of the CT results. The patient was reassured about her concerns while still communicating the severity of the illness. Score = **8**
7. *Comprehension of pathophysiology:* The candidate was able to demonstrate knowledge of the pathophysiology by explaining correctly to the patient the process of developing a SAH. Score = **7**
8. *Clinical competence (overall):* The candidate efficiently diagnosed a life-threatening illness while displaying compassion for the patient's pain and helping to reassure her by answering her questions. Score = **7**

CASE 3 20 y/o Male Pedestrian Struck by a Car

Navneet Cheema and Michael A. Gisondi

INITIAL INFORMATION

Name: Bill Smith

Mode of arrival: EMS

Age: 20 years

Gender: Male

VS: HR 110, RR 18, BP 126/92 (per EMS)

CC: Pedestrian struck by auto

PLAY OF THE CASE

E: "You are at a Level 2 trauma center with radiology services and subspecialty backup. You have two nurses, an ED technician, and an ED secretary. The paramedics arrive with a 20-year-old male pedestrian who was struck by an automobile."

C: "What do I see when I walk into the room?"

KEY QUESTION

Ask this open-ended question at the beginning of every case.

E: "The patient is a well-developed, well-nourished male in a cervical collar and on a backboard. He is yelling, appears uncomfortable, and has an obvious deformity of his left ankle. He has a peripheral antecubital IV placed by the paramedics, running normal saline."

C: "I will approach the paramedics regarding what happened. Nurse, please place the patient on a cardiac monitor and show me a rhythm strip, obtain pulse oximetry data, start another large-bore IV and save blood for labs, and place the patient on oxygen via 15-L mask."

KEY ORDERS

Most of the patients you see during the exam will be unstable (or will become that way). Whenever confronted with an unstable patient this group of orders should be given.

E: "Paramedic: Mr. Smith was running across a busy road when he was struck by a car going approximately 30-35 miles/h. He was on the ground about 20 ft from the car when we arrived; witnesses stated he was thrown on impact, but that he did not lose consciousness."

C: "Is the patient still yelling?"

E: "Yes."

C: "Airway is patent. I would like to examine the throat for signs of edema or tracheal deviation as well as crepitus."

E: "There is none."

C: "Sir, please take some deep breaths. What do I hear?"

E: "What are you listening for?"

C: "Are the breath sounds present and equal bilaterally?"

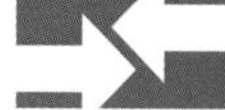

CRITICAL ACTION

Going through the ATLS primary and secondary survey correctly is a critical action in this case. The examinee assesses airway, breathing, and circulation first, and takes the correct action of initiating a fluid bolus in the hypotensive and tachycardic patient.

E: "Yes."

C: "Is there a palpable chest-wall deformity or crepitus?"

E: "There is not."

C: "I would like to palpate femoral and distal pulses as well as look for any signs of external or internal hemorrhage."

KEY ORDERS

The examinee should give analgesia at this point. Ignoring the patient's pain and questions will result in a lower score for interpersonal interaction.

KEY QUESTION

Always make sure that you get a complete set of vitals and/or labs. Any missing value will often be abnormal.

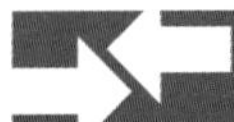

CRITICAL ACTION

The examinee has recognized that the patient is still hypotensive after a fluid bolus. Remember—in trauma all hypotension is hemorrhagic until proven otherwise. Having ruled out the extremities and the chest as a site of hemorrhage, the examinee now has to investigate bleeding into the pelvis or abdomen. Performing a FAST is a critical action in this case. The examinee is also preparing to initiate resuscitation with blood products.

KEY QUESTION

Remember to reassess your patient frequently. This patient is in shock. Another strategy would be to ask for vitals at 15-minute intervals, or to ask the nurse to apprise you of any change in vital signs. This puts the responsibility for reassessment back onto the examiner.

E: "What are you looking for?"

C: "Any obvious bleeding from wounds on the patient. I am also assessing for diaphoresis as well as cool or mottled skin, which may indicate inadequate perfusion."

E: "There are no other signs of external hemorrhage. His femoral pulses are weak and rapid, but equal. Radial pulses are thready bilaterally, as is his right dorsalis pedis pulse. There is no pulse palpable in the left dorsalis pedis. He is diaphoretic."

C: "Please give a bolus 2 L of NS; let me know when that is completed."

C: "Sir, can you wiggle your toes?"

E: "He can move his right toes, left toes are not moving."

E: "My leg is killing me, please help me, it hurts so bad!"

C: "What is his pupillary examination?"

E: "His eyes are open and his pupils are sluggishly reactive, 4 mm to 2 mm bilaterally."

C: "His GCS is 15."

C: "Nurse, I would like to undress the patient and log-roll him to examine his back. We will need the help of everyone in the room to prevent him from turning his neck and to protect his leg deformity."

E: "His back reveals abrasions over both shoulders."

C: "Nurse, please cover him with warm blankets. May I have a repeat set of vital signs?"

E: "The rhythm strip shows sinus tachycardia. Repeat vitals are BP 92/58, HR 120, RR 18, SPo_2 99% on 15-L mask."

C: "Temperature?"

E: "Oral temperature is 35.7°C (96.4°F)."

E: "Ow, my leg! My leg is killing me! Someone help me!"

C: "I would like a portable CXR and pelvis film. Please send blood for CBC, BMP, type and cross for 4 U of blood. I would like to perform a FAST examination."

E: "Please describe what you are looking for?"

C: "I am looking for evidence of free fluid in the abdomen, indicative of intra-abdominal trauma. I am looking in the splenorenal recess, in the hepatorenal recess, at the pericardium, and around the bladder."

E: "The pericardial and suprapubic windows are normal. There is free fluid noted in the hepatorenal and splenorenal recess."

E: "The 2 L of NS have infused."

C: "May I have another set of vitals please?"

E: "HR 120, RR 20, BP 88/56."

C: "Nurse, please prepare to transfuse 2 U of type O pRBCs via the rapid infuser. I will now place a cordis large-bore infuser IV line in the right groin. Please notify me when the blood is infused."

E: "Hey, what are you doing? That hurts!"

E: "The radiologist reports that the portable CXR and AP pelvis are normal."

C: "Sir, you were hit by a car and appear to have internal bleeding."

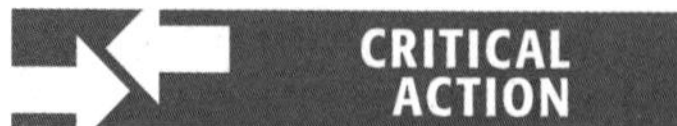

E: "My leg... which hospital am I in? Please call my girlfriend and tell her I'm fine."

C: "Sir, you might need an operation to repair your injuries. Are you allergic to any medications?"

E: "No."

C: "Do you take any medications every day or have any medical problems?"

E: "No."

C: "When was the last time you ate something?"

E: "I can't remember."

C: "Do you remember what happened?"

E: "The patient is now unresponsive and has vomited."

C: "I would like to orotracheally intubate the patient while the nurse maintains cervical immobilization. Is there a gag reflex?"

E: "Yes."

C: "Please suction the patient and apply cricoid pressure while giving him 15-L bag valve mask oxygen. Please administer lidocaine 100 mg IV, etomidate 30 mg IV, pancuronium 1 mg, then succinylcholine 100 mg IV. When the patient is relaxed, I will intubate with a 7.5 ETT."

E: "The patient has been intubated."

C: "Are the breath sounds symmetric? Is there color change with capnometry?"

E: "Yes."

C: "I would like the trauma surgeons paged."

E: "Doctor, the blood is infused."

C: "Repeat vitals please?"

E: "HR 110, BP 90/60, SPo_2 100%."

E: "Dr. Hatchet, the trauma surgeon, is on the phone."

C: "Dr. Hatchet, I have a hemodynamically unstable pedestrian struck by auto with abdominal free fluid visible on FAST examination. He needs to be taken for a laparotomy to identify and treat the cause of his bleeding."

E: "Yes, it sounds like he does need an operation. We'll be down to get him in a few minutes. How is his mental status?"

C: "He was initially alert and cooperative and had no evidence of serious head injury but he became less responsive and vomited, necessitating intubation with a neuro protection protocol. We will need to get neurosurgery involved in the ED or OR as he is too unstable for a trip to the radiology department."

E: "Fine, I will contact Dr. Brain to see if he wants to meet us here or in the OR."

C: "I would like to conduct a head to toe examination. Is there evidence of cranial injury? Tenderness, bogginess, deformity?"

E: "HEENT reveals tacky dry membranes, no lesions, atraumatic."

C: "Breath sounds still clear and symmetric? Is there evidence of chest wall deformity?"

E: "The chest rise is symmetric and there is no bruising or deformity. Breath sounds are equal bilaterally. There are no murmurs."

CRITICAL ACTION

The initiation of resuscitation with blood products after the initial 2 L of NS is a critical action.

KEY ORDERS

The examinee did not get consent, or discuss this procedure with the patient. At this juncture he should have explained to the patient what was going on, discussed the plan, and taken his consent for this invasive procedure.

KEY QUESTION

The examinee is getting an AMPLE history at this point—**A**llergies, **M**edications, **P**rior medical/surgical problems, **L**ast meal, and **E**vents (what happened?).

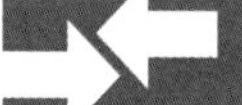

CRITICAL ACTION

Intubation of the unresponsive patient is a critical action. In order to get full credit for this action the examinee needs to use both in-line C-spine immobilization and a neuroprotective sedation strategy since an intracranial process cannot be excluded.

KEY ORDERS

Note that the candidate used a small dose of pancuronium to avoid the fasciculations associated with succinylcholine alone (vecuronium or rocuronium would also have been acceptable). Hyperventilation with BVM, premedication with lidocaine, and induction with paralysis are always preferable in these patients.

KEY QUESTION

Always confirm tube placement.

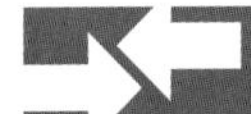

CRITICAL ACTION

Recognizing that the patient needs to go to the OR and getting the surgical team involved as soon as free fluid in the abdomen is conformed is a critical action in this case.

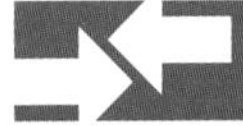

CRITICAL ACTION

At this point the examinee is completing the secondary survey, which completes the first critical action (doing a good primary and secondary survey in accordance with ATLS protocol). They have appropriately left management of the obviously broken leg until the primary survey (and the treatment of the ABC problems) has been completed.

C: "Is there abdominal distention, rigidity, bruising?"

E: "The abdomen is firm and slightly distended. There is an ecchymosis across the upper abdomen."

C: "Nurse, please place an orogastric tube to decompress the stomach."

C: "Pelvis? Is it stable on compression?"

E: "The pelvis is stable."

C: "Rectal? Prostate high riding?"

E: "Normal tone, no gross blood, prostate normal."

C: "Genitals? Is there blood at the meatus?"

E: "Normal male genitals, no blood at the urethral meatus."

C: "Nurse, please place a Foley catheter. While log-rolling the patient with spine immobilization, is there any bruising or other injuries?"

E: "No ecchymosis or additional abrasions to the back. There are no step-offs on examination of the spine."

C: "Extremities? Is there palpable deformity or laceration? What are the distal pulses like?"

E: "There is no deformity palpable in the upper extremities. The right lower extremity has abrasions over the knee and a right cordis catheter in place. His left foot is pale and cool, and the foot is rotated 90° laterally. There is tenting of the skin over the distal tibia."

C: "Is the patient at all arousable?"

E: "No."

C: "I will apply longitudinal traction and correct the deformity in an attempt to reduce his left ankle."

E: "His left ankle is no longer deformed."

C: "I would like to reexamine pulses in that foot."

E: "There is a thready pulse in the left DP, and the foot is regaining color."

C: "I would like a tech to splint the ankle in this position with an above the knee to foot posterior plaster mold. Please page orthopedics."

E: "Doctor, the patient's girlfriend and his mother is on the phone and would like to know what is going on."

C: "I will speak to the mother, she can relay the information to the girlfriend: 'Your son was struck by a car and is going to need surgery. He is stable. You should come to the hospital and we can talk more about what happened when you get here. Does he have any medical problems?'"

E: "No. I will be there as soon as I can."

E: "Orthopedics is present in the trauma room. They would like AP and lateral films of the left knee, left tib/fib, and left ankle."

C: "Those x-rays will delay the patient from getting to the operating room. His orthopedic injuries are not life threatening, and those x-rays may be obtained intra-operatively."

E: "The OR just called for the patient. The orthopedic surgeons will accompany the patient to the OR. The case is over."

CASE ASSESSMENT

This candidate managed a complicated case well. She immediately began to use the ATLS algorithm to assess her patient, moving from airway through exposure. Importantly, she addressed issues of hypotension and hypoperfusion as they were recognized. The thready, tachycardic pulse would indicate blood loss, and she appropriately utilized the trauma FAST examination to evaluate for intraperitoneal blood loss. Additionally, she frequently reassessed her patient, requesting vital signs after an intervention was completed. She succinctly communicated what she needed from her consultants, as well as gathered information from multiple sources such as the paramedics as well as the patient's mother.

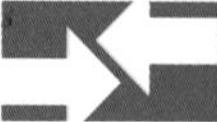

CRITICAL ACTION

Reducing this fracture in order to regain pulses and getting orthopedics involved for definitive management is a critical action. Although this fracture is not life threatening, because the pulses were absent it is limb threatening.

This candidate did skirt a couple of potential pitfalls. The first was deciding when to address the cold, pulseless foot noted in the primary survey. While the foot ischemia is unlikely to cause the immediate death of the patient, it would cause damage to his limb. It is important to remember, however, that the primary survey deals with the airway, breathing, and circulation (ABCs) and unless an extremity injury is causing an exsanguinating hemorrhage, it is better addressed during the secondary survey. In contrast, an apneic patient should be intubated prior to moving to the assessment of circulation or disability.

KEY ORDERS

Remember to observe HIPAA whenever possible. The examinee shared information with the next of kin, but not with the girlfriend.

A second potential snare occurred when this patient became unresponsive; the patient still had a gag, requiring the use of appropriate "neuroprotective" medications as part of the rapid sequence intubation (RSI) protocol, which the candidate accomplished in a straightforward manner. Note that the candidate used a small dose of pancuronium to avoid the fasciculations associated with succinylcholine alone. Hyperventilation with bag valve mask (BVM), premedication with lidocaine, and induction with paralysis is always preferable in these patients. The impaired mental status of a hypotensive, multiple trauma patient cannot be assumed to be due solely to hypovolemia; an intracranial process that cannot be categorically excluded must be assumed to be present and appropriate head injury premedication is then always warranted. The candidate provided for in-line immobilization of the cervical spine during intubation, however, in the absence of a paralytic agent, unexpected movements, jerking, gagging, or vomiting occur, thus it is imperative to be facile with RSI and the medications used in this procedure for both adults and children (both for one's practice and the ABEM oral exam!).

This scenario presented the candidate with the need to perform several major resuscitative procedures: RSI/orotracheal intubation, "FAST" ultrasound examination, ankle reduction, and central venous access. In this case, the candidate was asked to explain what she was looking for during the FAST examination. It would similarly be reasonable to expect to be asked what alternatives exist to FAST and how those might be performed. One should be able to and expect to explain how to intubate and how to obtain a surgical airway should intubation fail. Requests for descriptions of central venous cannulation and access (and its potential risks) are also fair game, as would be joint reduction. Other procedures commonly performed in trauma (chest tubes, pericardiocentesis, diagnostic perigoneal lavage [DPL]) should also be reviewed. The candidate must be able to discuss the appropriate indication and techniques for performing these common emergency procedures.

This case required intervention and expertise not available to the emergency physician in the trauma room. In this case, the candidate had the surgeon paged after the patient decompensated to the point of needing blood products and requiring intubation—several minutes after the FAST examination demonstrated free fluid in the abdomen. The principle is that a hypotensive patient without an externally exsanguinating injury and with free fluid in the abdomen on ultrasound will need emergent surgical evaluation (and most likely an exploratory laparotomy), therefore, the surgeon should have been paged earlier in the play of the case. This candidate appropriately paged orthopedics, and recognized that obtaining further films (per their request) would delay addressing the patient's life-threatening injury. As discussed earlier, this patient's mental status changes may have been due to hypovolemic shock but intracranial injury cannot be excluded. This patient is not stable enough to be taken out of the trauma room for a journey to the radiology department for a head computed tomography (CT) scan; consequently, it was appropriate to call neurosurgery and have them perform a baseline evaluation of the patient in the emergency department (ED) or in the operating room (OR) prior to induction of anesthesia—they may consider intraoperative placement of a bolt/intracranial pressure (ICP) monitor if needed.

Critical Actions

1. Appropriate advanced trauma life support (ATLS) primary and secondary survey. This is by the book and is a must!
2. Early surgical consultation.
3. Intubation while maintaining C-spine immobilization.
4. Reduction of ankle deformity.
5. Performing a FAST examination.
6. Use of blood products early on in the case.

Test Performance

1. *Data acquisition:* The candidate did a superb job obtaining an adequate history and physical examination. She was very logical in her approach to this multisystem trauma and articulate with nursing throughout the progression of the case. Score = **7**
2. *Problem solving:* The candidate acknowledged and addressed abnormal vital signs, quickly recognizing tachycardia and hypotension as likely hemorrhagic shock in a trauma patient. Score = **8**
3. *Patient management:* The candidate was excellent at prioritizing the patient's care, ensuring an unstable patient was not taken to CT and not allowing nonemergent x-rays (XRs) to delay addressing the life-threatening injuries in this trauma patient. Score = **7**
4. *Resource utilization:* The candidate demonstrated great use of resources in a cost-effective manner. The score could have been improved if the trauma surgeon was notified earlier in the case rather than after the patient became unstable requiring intubation. Score = **6**
5. *Health care provided (outcome):* The candidate efficiently stabilized this patient with intravenous fluids (IVFs) and then had an early transition to packed red blood cells (pRBCs). She also appropriately intubated the patient with a neuroprotective strategy once he decompensated. Score = **7**
6. *Interpersonal relations and communication skills:* This is the area the candidate needed the most improvement. She was able to effectively communicate with nursing and consultants; however, she did not consent the awake patient for an invasive central line or keep him apprised of the situation and test results. She also did not treat his pain or answer his questions

while he was awake. It is important to remember to explain all procedures, however briefly, to your patients. Score = **5**

7. *Comprehension of pathophysiology:* This candidate demonstrated an efficient investigatory and analytical approach to the clinical picture and effectively followed ATLS protocol. Score = **7**
8. *Clinical competence (overall):* The candidate had an organized, logical approach to this complicated patient. She was able to stabilize a multisystem trauma patient while maintaining focus and interacting well with her consults. Giving more frequent updates and treating his pain could have improved her communication skills with the patient. Score = **7**

CASE 4 A 24 y/o Female With Vaginal Bleeding

Navneet Cheema and Catherine Johnson

INITIAL INFORMATION

Name: Mia Jackson

Mode of arrival: Brought in by friend

Age: 24 years

Gender: Female

VS: BP 90/50, HR 112, RR 20, T 37.4°C, O_2 sat: 99%

CC: Vaginal bleeding

PLAY OF THE CASE

C: "What do I see when I walk in the room?"

E: "The patient is a young woman who is sitting on the edge of the bed with her legs crossed."

C: "Hello, I am Dr. Jones. Before I start our examination, I would like to ask your nurse to do a few things. Nurse, can you please start two large-bore IVs, 16 gauge preferred in the right and left antecubital fossae. Please infuse 1 L of 0.9 NS at a wide-open rate. Place her on 4-L N/C O_2 as well. After the bolus, please repeat her vital signs and let me know. Thank you, nurse. Ms. Jackson, what brings you in today?"

E: "I'm having a pretty heavy period and my cramping is worse than usual."

C: "When did the bleeding start?"

E: "Well, I really have been bleeding for almost 2 weeks now, it's just a lot heavier today."

C: "When was your last normal period?"

E: "About 7 weeks ago, usually I am really regular."

C: "Do you have any medical problems?"

E: "No, I'm healthy. I never have to go to the doctor."

C: "Are you sexually active?"

E: "Well, sometimes."

C: "With men, women, or both?"

E: "Just with men, I have a boyfriend; we just don't get to see each other much."

C: "Nurse, let's check a bedside pregnancy test. Has she had her bolus?"

E: "The bolus is in, the BP is 90/60, pulse 107. The pregnancy test is positive, doctor."

C: "OK, please send a type and screen, beta quantitative hCG, CBC, and bring in the ultrasound machine with a transvaginal probe. Please give her the second liter of 0.9 NS and ask the blood bank to type and cross for 4 U."

E: "OK, the labs are sent."

KEY QUESTION

Ask this open-ended question at the beginning of every case.

KEY ORDERS

Most of the patients you see during the exam will be unstable (or will become that way). This patient is hypotensive and tachycardic. Whenever confronted with an unstable patient this group of orders should be given. Notice how the examinee asked the examiner to reassess and report the patient's vital signs after the bolus. This places the responsibility on the examiner and relieves the examinee of having to remember to reassess—a good strategy!

CRITICAL ACTION

This patient is still hypotensive and tachycardic after 1 L of NS. Appropriate fluid resuscitation with fluids and blood products is a critical action in this case.

C: "Ms. Jackson, our test shows that you are pregnant. I am concerned that your bleeding may be a sign that the pregnancy may be developing in the wrong place. I will need to do some more tests and perform an ultrasound using a probe that we place in your vagina to get the best possible picture of what's going on so early in your pregnancy."

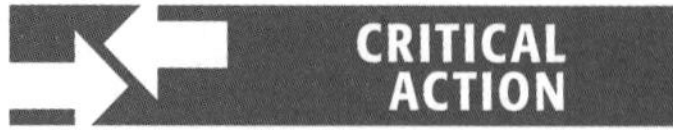

CRITICAL ACTION

Recognizing the possibility of an ectopic pregnancy and doing a US to confirm (or rule out) an IUP is a critical action in this case.

E: "OK, doctor."

C: "I need to know if you take any medications or have any allergies to medications. I also need to know the last time you ate."

E: "I just have been taking some ibuprofen for the cramping, and I had some toast about 3 hours ago. I'm allergic to penicillin."

C: "OK, I am going to take a closer look at you now. I will examine your head and neck. Any evidence of trauma?"

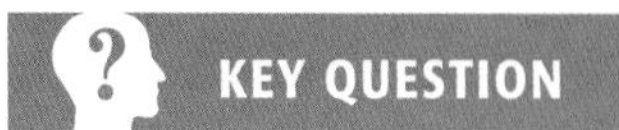

KEY QUESTION

Any patient who may need emergent surgery needs to answer the AMPLE questions—**A**llergies, **M**edications, **P**ast medical/surgical hx, **L**ast meal, and **E**vents (what happened).

E: "No, there is not."

C: "Are the pupils equal and reactive to light and accommodation bilateral? Are the cranial nerves intact?"

E: "The examination is normal for those findings."

C: "Is the neck supple?"

E: "Yes."

C: "I would like to examine the heart and lungs. Are the breath sounds clear and symmetric? Are there any murmurs, rubs, or gallops on the cardiac examination?"

E: "The lung examination is normal, the patient is tachycardic, no murmurs, rubs, or gallops."

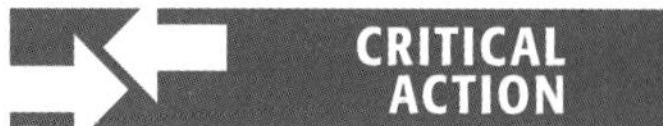

CRITICAL ACTION

Performing a through pelvic examination is a critical action in this case.

C: "Is the abdomen distended, tender to palpation? Are bowel sounds present on auscultation?"

E: "The abdomen is moderately distended and the bowel sounds are diminished. The abdomen is tender in the left lower quadrant."

C: "Is there guarding or signs of peritonitis?"

E: "There is voluntary guarding with mild rebound."

C: "I would like to perform a pelvic examination. Is there any blood in the vaginal vault?"

E: "Yes, there are some red clots in the vagina."

C: "On bimanual examination, is the cervix open or closed? Is the uterus tender or boggy? Are there adnexal masses or tenderness?"

E: "The cervix is open to fingertip and the uterus feels about 8 weeks gravid. There is fullness present on the left adnexa and the patient is very uncomfortable during the examination."

C: "I would like to perform a bedside transvaginal ultrasound examination at this time. Is there an intrauterine pregnancy? Is there free fluid?"

E: "Please interpret the image (Fig. C4-1)."

C: "Assuming that the structure in the right center of the image is the uterus, there is no obvious IUP. There is a mass seen in the adjacent adnexal region and there appears to be free fluid present."

C: "Nurse, please have the secretary call the OB doctor on call today while we finish our examination. Please have her call the lab to report the lab values and

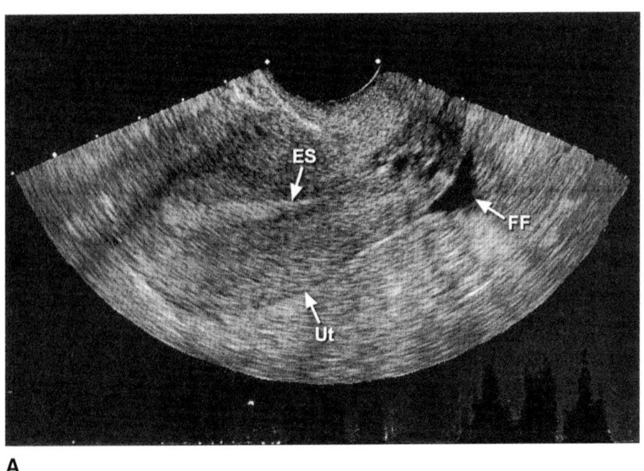

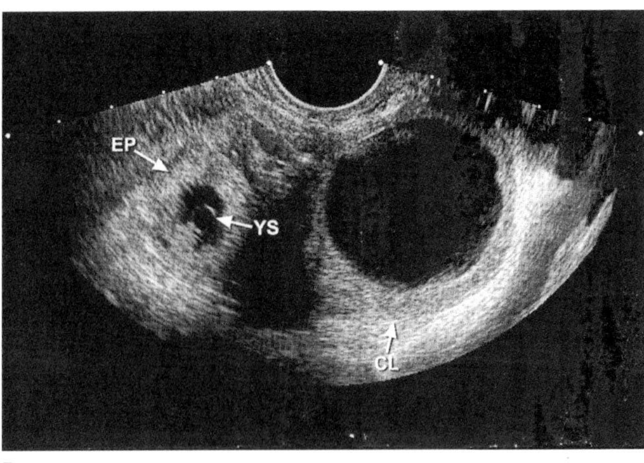

A B

Figure C4-1. Vaginal sonogram of an ectopic pregnancy. (A) The uterus (Ut) is seen with a normal endometrial stripe (ES). A small amount of free fluid (FF) is visible in the posterior cul-de-sac. (B) The tubal ectopic pregnancy (EP) with its yolk sac (YS) is seen along with a corpus luteum (CL) cyst. *(Reprinted with permission from Cunningham FG, Leveno KJ, Bloom SL, et al.* Williams Obstetrics. *22nd ed. New York, NY: McGraw-Hill. 2005.)*

CRITICAL ACTION

This patient is hypotensive and tachycardic and has an ectopic pregnancy until proven otherwise. The critical actions in this case are (1) contacting OB for definitive management and (2) understanding that treatment of an unstable patient should not be delayed (and the patient should certainly not be sent out of the ED except to the OR)!

ask the blood bank to bring a unit of type-specific blood. I would like to perform a rectal examination. Is the rectal tone normal? Is there blood in the stool?"

E: "The rectal tone is normal, the stool is brown and guaiac negative."

C: "I would like to examine the extremities. Is there any clubbing, cyanosis, or edema? Are the pulses and pressures equal and symmetric in all extremities?"

E: "There is no cyanosis, clubbing, or edema. Pulses are slightly diminished but symmetric in all extremities."

C: "Is the patient neurologically intact? Gait OK?"

E: "The patient has no sensory or motor deficits. When she tries to stand she complains of dizziness."

C: "That's OK, we don't have to test the gait if it is unsafe. Are there any bruises or the skin examination?"

E: "None present. Here are your laboratory studies:

CBC: WBC 12K, H/H 9/27.3, plt 212,000

UCG (from the lab): Positive

Quantitative hCG 2200

Type O positive

And Dr. Obewon is on the phone."

C: "What is her blood pressure now?"

E: "The blood pressure is 100/65."

C: "Hello, Dr. Obewon, this is Dr. Jones. I have a 24 y/o pregnant patient with a chief complaint of vaginal bleeding who presents at 7-8 weeks with hypotension, a very tender abdomen, and on ED bedside transvaginal US has no IUP and a mass in the left adnexa with free fluid. Her quant just came back at 2200. Her Hgb is 9. I would like you to see the patient."

E: "Send her for an official ultrasound and call me back."

C: "I'm sorry, Dr. Obewon, she is not stable to leave the department. I am very concerned that this patient has a ruptured ectopic pregnancy and I think we should continue our resuscitation in the ED until you are able to see the patient."

E: "All right, I'll be there in 10 minutes."

C: "Thank you for your willingness to see this patient promptly." "Ms. Jackson, I believe that it a very good thing that you came to the ED today. I am very concerned that your pregnancy has developed outside your womb and is causing internal bleeding; therefore, I have asked an OB specialist to come in and see you. You may need a blood transfusion and surgery. I will have the nurse help you call your family and we will give you some medication for pain just as soon as it is safe to do so. Right now your blood pressure is just a little too low for it. I don't want you to eat or drink anything while you are here, as you may need surgery. Do you have any questions?"

E: "No, doctor, thank you. I knew something was wrong. I'm glad I came in and you were able to help me. The case is now over."

CASE ASSESSMENT

The candidate handled the case extremely well. The candidate was aggressive with her resuscitation, an excellent patient advocate and very professional, and thoughtful of her patient and staff. The candidate quickly volume resuscitated the patient and got the history and laboratory tests she needed to establish priorities in managing the patient. The examiner gets a good sense of the candidate's ability to multitask and prioritize patient's needs.

The candidate performed all of the critical actions of this case and would have passed the case easily. The candidate picked up all of the "easy" points for professionalism and interpersonal skills by taking particular attention to the patient's need to be informed of treatment and procedures. The candidate is also sensitive to the patient's pain, which on some cases could even be a critical action. Always go for these points, on the exam and in real life; they are high yield.

The candidate was doing so well, the examiner created resistance to the OB consultant's responsiveness to the patient. The candidate's ability to advocate for his/her patient's condition will be tested. You will be tested on your ability to effectively communicate your clinical impressions and concerns to your consultants. If resistance is met, be persistent and do the right thing for the patient.

Critical Actions

1. Appreciate the possibility of ectopic pregnancy and perform a thorough abdominal and pelvic examination.
2. Perform a bedside transvaginal ultrasound to look for intrauterine pregnancy (IUP) or lack thereof. Also asking about the presence of free fluid or adnexal masses is important.
3. Volume resuscitation with normal saline (NS) and then blood.
4. Consult OB and insist on emergent response.

Test Performance

1. *Data acquisition:* The candidate was concise and organized. Score = **7**
2. *Problem solving:* The candidate gathered information in an organized approach, ordered labs and diagnostics appropriately, and made appropriate consultation and disposition. Score = **7**

3. *Patient management:* The candidate made appropriate treatment decisions very efficiently and advocated for her patient when the consultant was difficult. Score = **7**
4. *Resource utilization:* The candidate made good use of resources in a cost-effective manner. Score = **7**
5. *Health care provided (outcome):* The candidate stabilized the patient efficiently and effectively. Recognizing the need for IVFs early in the case and anticipating the need for blood products given the possibility of an ectopic pregnancy. Score = **7**
6. *Interpersonal relations and communication skills:* The candidate was respectful and effective in communications to staff, patient, and consultant. The candidate was very thoughtful of patient's need to be updated on her condition and her comfort. Score = **8**
7. *Comprehension of pathophysiology:* The candidate conveyed understanding of ectopic pregnancies and ordered appropriate tests. She could have gained more points by asking additional questions in the history that would have assessed for ectopic risk factors. Score = **7**
8. *Clinical competence (overall):* The candidate managed this case very well, quickly addressing abnormal vital signs, establishing the diagnosis early, and advocating for the consultant to evaluate the patient in the department. Score = **7**

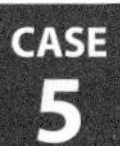

CASE 5 55 y/o Male With Mental Status Changes

Navneet Cheema and James W. Rhee

INITIAL INFORMATION

Name: Nat Key

Mode of arrival: Brought in by ambulance

Age: 55 years

Gender: Male

VS: BP 140/80, HR 110, RR 16, T 38.2°C, O_2 sat: 96% on RA

CC: Not waking up

PLAY OF THE CASE

C: "I walk in to the room and what do I see?"

KEY QUESTION

Ask this open-ended question at the beginning of every case.

E: "You see a middle-aged male lying in bed unresponsive with sonorous respirations. He appears well nourished, but slightly yellow."

C: "Hello Mr. Key."

E: "No response from the patient."

C: "Nurse, please start two 18-gauge IVs running NS and bolus 2 L, draw labs, place patient on a cardiac monitor, and place him on oxygen by NC at 2 L/min. I also want an ECG and stat fingerstick glucose on the patient. Let me know the result of the fingerstick as soon as it is available. Please administer thiamine 100 mg IV, naloxone 2 mg IV, and let me know if he has any response."

KEY ORDERS

Most of the patients you see during the exam will be unstable (or will become that way). Whenever confronted with an unstable patient this group of orders should be given. In this case, as the patient is unresponsive, the examinee has added on a "coma cocktail" of a rapid glucose check, naloxone, and thiamine.

E: "Your orders are being carried out. The patient's fingerstick glucose is 110, and the ECG shows sinus tachycardia and is otherwise normal."

C: "Does the patient still have sonorous respirations after the naloxone administration?"

E: "Yes."

C: "I will check his gag reflex."

E: "Patient has no gag reflex."

C: "I will intubate the patient without any medications as patient is unresponsive—I will use a number 4 curved laryngoscope blade and a 7.5 ET tube. Under direct visualization, I advance the ET tube past the vocal cords, inflate the cuff, and check end-tidal CO_2."

KEY ORDERS

The examinee has asked the examiner to tell them the results of tests as they come back. This is an excellent strategy as it relieves the examinee of the responsibility to remember to ask about test results and places that responsibility on the examiner instead.

E: "Done. Patient is now intubated with positive end-tidal CO_2 and is placed on the ventilator with normal ventilator settings for patient's weight."

C: "I want to talk to the paramedics."

E: "They are in the room."

C: "How did you find the patient?"

E: "We got the call from the patient's daughter because he was not waking up. When we got to the house, the patient was in his bed and unresponsive. So we

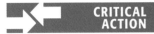

CRITICAL ACTION

Intubation of this unresponsive patient is a critical action.

KEY ORDERS

Memorize this phrasing to use for every intubation.

KEY QUESTION

Remember to use your resources to get a history on your patients. When they are unresponsive ask for family or EMS personnel.

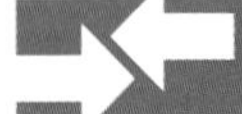

CRITICAL ACTION

There are three critical actions taking place at once at this point in the case. First, the examinee must recognize that the patient has the physical signs and symptoms of hepatic failure. Then, the examinee must combine that knowledge with the presence of empty pill bottles and realize that there is a possibility of overdose in this unresponsive patient—and that acetaminophen is a likely offending agent. Finally, after realizing this risk, they must treat with NAC. (The examinee is also sending off all the other appropriate labs to evaluate an ingestion.)

just scooped him up and brought him here. He had an empty pill bottle by his bed. We brought that too, but it has no label on it. The daughter is out in the waiting room."

C: "Nurse, would you please bring her into the room? And please send the blood that you drew for BMP, LFTs, PT/PTT, and CBC. I also want a tox screen, APAP level, ASA level, EtOH level, and ABG. I'm concerned that the patient overdosed on something. Considering he appears jaundiced, I will insert an NG tube and administer NAC at 140 mg/kg. I will order a non-contrast head CT head as well. Please place a Foley catheter prior to his going to CT."

E: "Yes doctor. Your orders are being carried out. The patient's daughter, Ms. Key, is now here."

C: "Ms. Key, your father is very ill. He was unresponsive when he got here and we needed to put him on a machine to breath for him. We are still evaluating him to figure out what is going on here. Do you have any idea what happened?"

E: "Geez doctor. I'm not sure. My dad has been kind of down recently. He just lost his job, and my mom just died last month from breast cancer. I was just with him 2 days ago and he was kind of down, but seemed fine physically."

C: "Does he have any medical problems?"

E: "No."

C: "Does he take any medications?"

E: "No."

C: "Does he have any allergies?"

E: "No."

C: "Does he drink alcohol?"

E: "Only occasionally."

C: "Has he tried to commit suicide in the past or have a history of depression?"

E: "No, but he has been talking about not being able to go on anymore with his life."

C: "Ms. Key, I'm concerned that he overdosed on something and need to make sure we are not missing anything. Do you know if he has eaten any herbs or taken any drugs or used any natural medicines?"

E: "Not that I know of."

C: "Thank you Ms. Key. I will finish examining your father now and do my best to help him."

E: "Thank you doctor. Please do everything that you can. He is the only family that I have left."

C: "I examine the patient's head—are there any signs of trauma?"

E: "No."

C: "Anything on eye examination?"

E: "What are you looking for?"

C: "Pupil size and reactivity, color of conjunctiva, any evidence of scleral icterus."

E: "His pupils are 3 mm symmetric and reactive. His conjunctivae are pink, and he's got obvious scleral icterus."

C: "I examine the mouth, what do I see?"

E: "Normal oropharynx and moist mucous membranes."

C: "I examine the patient's neck—supple?"

E: "Yes."

C: "I listen to the patient's heart and lungs."

E: "The patient is slightly tachycardic, and his lung examination is normal."

C: "I listen to his abdomen for bowel sound, palpate his abdomen for tenderness and masses."

E: "Bowel sound present, diffuse abdominal tenderness without rebound or guarding."

C: "Is his skin examination normal?"

E: "You notice jaundice."

C: "I check deep tendon reflexes, muscle tone, and plantar reflexes."

E: "All normal."

C: "Are any of his labs back?"

E: "His ABG is 7.2/40/100, Na 140, K 4.0, Cl 105, HCO_3 18, BUN 30, Cr 2.4, WBC 15, Hgb 10, Hct 30, Plt 170, AST 5000, ALT 5000, total bilirubin 4, INR 5, APAP level 50, ASA undetected, and the rest of the studies are normal."

KEY QUESTION

If you do not ask the examiner to tell you lab results as they come back (the most efficient way to get the information relayed to you), do not forget to ask about results. It may help to write down all the lab tests you order so that nothing gets dropped on exam day.

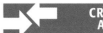

C: "Nurse, please arrange for a bed in the ICU. I want to talk to the ICU physician."

E: "Dr. Intense is on the phone."

C: "Hi Dr. Intense. I have a patient here, Mr. Key, who I'm afraid has overdosed on acetaminophen. It appears that he may have done this a couple of days ago and only now presents. He is now encephalopathic, coagulopathic, azotemic, and anemic. He fulfills King's College Criteria for possibly needing a liver transplant. Since arriving to the ED we have intubated him and given him a dose of NAC. We want to admit him to the ICU under your care—will you be able to call the transplant physician, or shall I?"

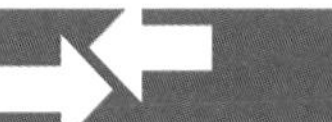

CRITICAL ACTION

Admitting this critically ill patient to the ICU is a critical action in this case.

E: "Send the patient up, I'll see him and I'll talk to the transplant physician. This case is over."

CASE ASSESSMENT

The candidate managed this case very well. Initially, the patient recognized that the patient's condition required prompt attention and administered a "coma" cocktail as well as addressing the patient's tachycardia with intravenous fluid (IVF). As the patient wasn't hypoglycemic and had no response to naloxone, the patient appropriately intubated the patient. In this scenario, it is okay that the candidate did not intubate the patient right away as the other interventions that he made may have obviated the need.

After initial stabilization procedures, the candidate was able to ascertain that the patient overdosed on some agent, and correctly surmised that the patient had taken at least an acetaminophen (APAP) overdose. Appropriately, N-acetylcysteine (NAC) was administered right away as the patient's jaundice provided evidence of hepatic dysfunction (as NAC has very few side effects but does have a finite window in which it is effective it can be administered before APAP levels come back). APAP toxicity should always be considered in a patient with hepatotoxicity from an overdose and treatment should be undertaken immediately as hepatotoxicity occurs after the ideal window of treatment. Only if the patient presents right after an overdose of APAP is there time to wait for an APAP level first before administering NAC.

The candidate finally gets to the physical examination and performs a perfunctory examination. He probably could have obtained a more detailed examination, but it is at least important that he did one. He did miss performing a rectal examination to detect blood—while not critical in this case, patients who present late from APAP toxicity can develop a significant coagulopathy resulting in gastrointestinal (GI) bleed. On exam day, as in real life, the physical examination may take a backseat to initial stabilization and other forms of data gathering—however, it is always a critical action, and must always be performed. It would have been easy in this case for the candidate to completely forget to do an examination, but he did touch on it.

The lab results are confirmatory and prognostic in this case. The patient demonstrates all of the risk factors for liver transplant—acidemia, coagulopathy, encephalopathy, and renal insufficiency. The APAP level is not important to assess for toxicity—we already know that the patient has it—also the time frame of ingestion is unknown so we would be unable to plot the result on the Rumack-Matthew nomogram. The APAP level in this scenario, however, is confirmatory—it demonstrates that he did take APAP at some time and in conjunction with the fulminant hepatic failure, confirms APAP-induced hepatotoxicity.

The candidate makes the correct dispositions and admits the patient to the intensive care unit (ICU) and makes sure that there will be a transplant surgery consult.

Critical Actions

1. Perform intubation.
2. Recognition of physical examination findings of hepatic dysfunction.
3. Diagnosis of APAP overdose.
4. Administration of NAC.
5. Admission to the ICU.

Test Performance

1. *Data acquisition:* This phase is adequate as the candidate shows the ability to obtain a history and performs a perfunctory physical examination. He orders all the appropriate tests to assist in diagnosis. He could have scored higher by performing a more complete physical examination. Score = **6**
2. *Problem solving:* The candidate is excellent at problem solving, as he is able to quickly assimilate data from the patient encounter, emergency medical services (EMS), the daughter, and test results to synthesize information, arrive at a diagnosis, and efficiently direct further management. Score = **8**
3. *Patient management:* The candidate had no delays in treatment, made appropriate treatment decisions based on the data available to him, his knowledge base, and clinical judgment. Score = **7**
4. *Resource utilization:* The candidate demonstrates very good use of resources with an efficient use of tests that did not compromise patient care. Score = **6**

5. *Health care provided (outcome):* The candidate was able to start the antidote in a timely manner in this case while awaiting lab confirmation and prognostication of the diagnosis. Score = **7**
6. *Interpersonal relations and communication skills:* The candidate was able to effectively communicate with both EMS and the daughter. He was professional, respectful, and demonstrated integrity and compassion. Score = **7**
7. *Comprehension of pathophysiology:* This candidate demonstrated a highly detailed and efficient investigatory and analytical approach to the clinical picture. He was able to demonstrate an understanding of acetaminophen overdoses, recognizing that if a patient presented with jaundice already they needed NAC as quickly as possible. He could have scored higher if he was able to articulate his thought process to the examiner. Score = **6**
8. *Clinical competence (overall):* This candidate efficiently stabilized a patient who needed intubation, used ancillary sources to collect information, and ordered the antidote in a timely fashion. Score = **7**

CASE 6 A 50 y/o Female With Syncope

Navneet Cheema and Marc Bellazzini

INITIAL INFORMATION

Name: Ann Smith

Mode of arrival: Brought by husband

Age: 50 years

Gender: Female

VS: T 37.2°C, BP 138/78, HR 76, RR 14, O_2 sat: 98% on RA

CC: Fainting

PLAY OF THE CASE

C: "What do I see as I walk into the patient's room?"

E: "The patient is a well-nourished female who is well appearing and in no acute distress."

C: "Hello, Ms. Smith, I'm Dr. Tors. What brings you in today?"

E: "Well, I was at the football game this afternoon and I passed out."

C: "Has anything like this happened to you before?"

E: "No, never. I feel just fine now."

C: "Have you been ill recently?"

E: "I am just getting over a sinus infection and really bad watery brown diarrhea that's going away now."

C: "Tell me how you felt immediately before you passed out."

E: "It was rather sudden. I was standing and felt very light-headed and then everything started getting dark and that's the last thing I remember before I passed out."

C: "Did you have any chest discomfort or headache before the event?"

E: "No."

C: "Who saw the event happen?"

E: "My husband was standing next to me."

C: "Mr. Smith, can you tell me what happened after your wife passed out."

E: "She just went limp and I caught her before she hit the floor. She was out for about 45 seconds to a minute. She woke up and she appeared to be just fine."

C: "Ms. Smith, do you have any medical problems?"

E: "No major medical problems, just some seasonal allergies and a recent sinus infection."

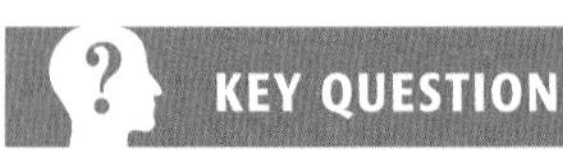

Ask this open-ended question at the beginning of every case.

C: "Do you have any allergies to medications?"

E: "No."

C: "What medications are you taking?"

E: "I have been taking some old seldane (Terfenadine) because I thought it may help with my sinus infection. The doctor put me on erythromycin last week and I have been taking that too."

C: "Thank you, Ms. Smith. I would like to do some tests to better define what may have caused your fainting."

C: "Nurse, please draw a basic metabolic profile with a magnesium level and start an IV line with an 18-gauge catheter running NS at a TKO rate. Please place the patient on the telemetry monitor and obtain a stat 12-lead ECG and show me the results when they are available."

C: "Nurse, please obtain orthostatic vital signs by placing the patient in a supine position for 5 minutes and measuring both pulse and blood pressure. Repeat this after the patient has been standing 3 minutes and advise me of the results."

E: "Doctor, the orthostatic vital signs are complete. There was an increase in heart rate by 15 and a drop in systolic blood pressure by 20 when the patient stood up."

C: "Ms. Smith, did you feel light-headed or dizzy when you were standing?"

E: "No."

E: "Doctor, the IV has been established and your labs submitted. The patient is hooked up to the telemetry monitor (Fig. C6-1)."

C: "Nurse, please administer a 500-cc NS bolus IV."

C: "I would like to perform the physical examination. What is the patient's general appearance?"

E: "The patient is well appearing and resting comfortably."

C: "Are the mucous membranes moist?"

E: "The mucous membranes appear moderately dry."

C: "Does the thyroid appear enlarged or nodular?"

E: "The thyroid examination is normal."

C: "Do I hear crackles on the patient's lung examination and is the respiratory rate normal?"

E: "There are no crackles; the lungs are clear and the respirations non-labored."

C: "Is the patient's jugular venous pressure normal?"

E: "The patient's jugular venous pressure is slightly decreased."

C: "Is there a regular rhythm on cardiac auscultation? Are there any murmurs? Are the pulses symmetrical?"

E: "The cardiac examination is normal. There are no murmurs and the rhythm is regular. The pulses are symmetrical."

C: "Are there any masses, pulsations, or tenderness on abdominal examination?"

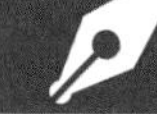

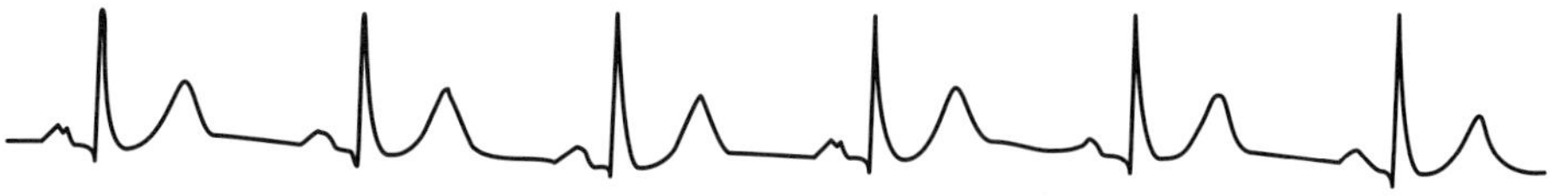

KEY ORDERS

Most of the patients you see during the exam will be unstable (or will become that way). Every unstable patient requires IV access (preferably two large-bore IVs), oxygen, and cardiac monitoring. In this case, as the patient appears stable with normal vitals the examinee delayed starting these orders until after they got a brief history. It could be argued, however, that syncope in any older person is cardiac until proven otherwise, and these orders should have been given before the history was taken.

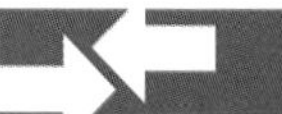

CRITICAL ACTION

Ordering an ECG in this older patient with syncope to screen for cardiac abnormalities (specifically a prolonged QT) is a critical action.

Figure C6-1. A rhythm strip showing normal sinus rhythm.

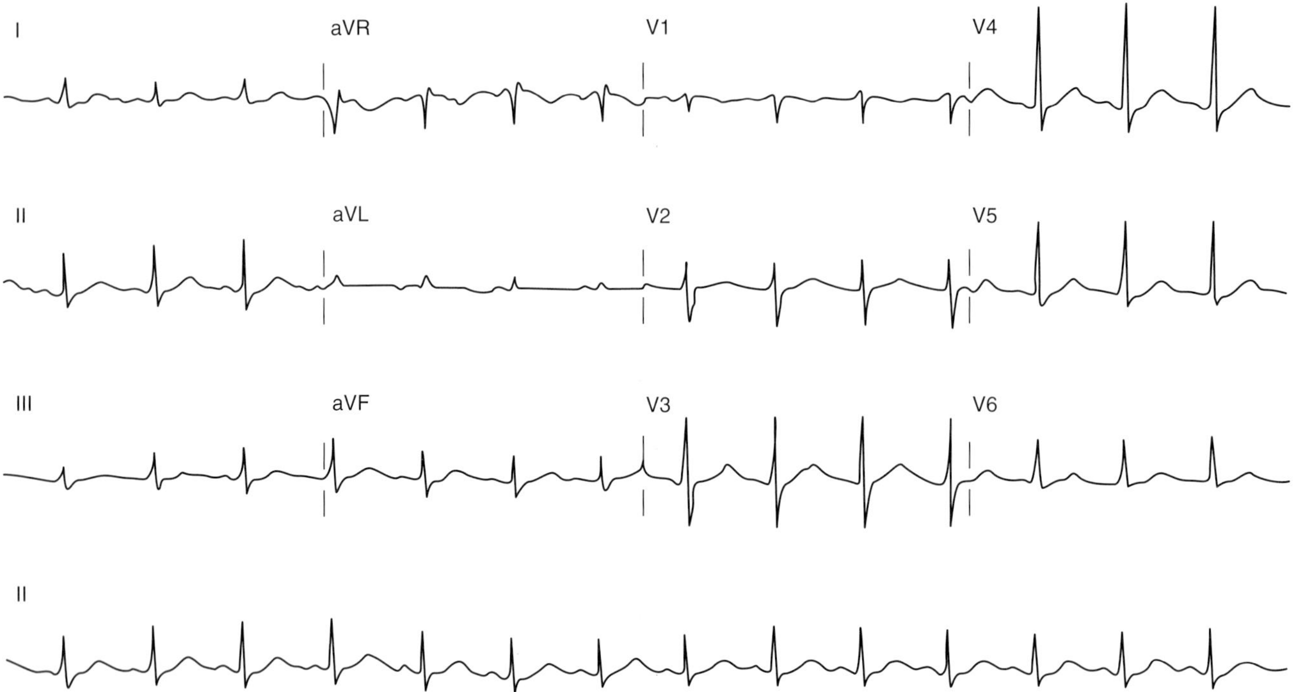

Figure C6-2. An ECG showing QT prolongation to about 500 milliseconds.

E: "No."

C: "Is there peripheral edema?"

E: "No."

C: "Is the patient's strength and sensation intact and equal in all extremities?"

E: "Yes."

E: "Your ECG is available for review (Fig. C6-2)."

C: "The ECG shows a normal sinus rhythm with QTc prolongation of approximately 500 milliseconds"

C: "Ms. Smith, I believe your fainting episode was caused by an adverse interaction between the medications you are taking. I would like to admit you to the hospital."

E: "Doctor, I don't feel very well. I feel very light-headed and. . ."

E: "Doctor, the patient's heart rhythm does not look right. Please take a look at the monitor (Fig. C6-3)."

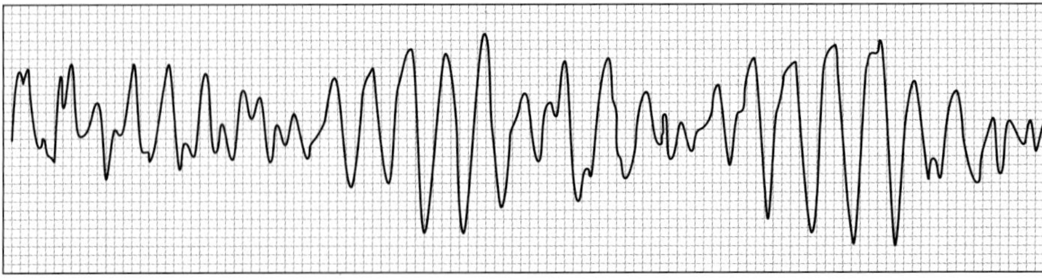

Figure C6-3. Rhythm strip showing torsades de pointes.

C: "Does the patient have a pulse?"

E: "No."

C: "The patient's rhythm is torsades de pointes. I am defibrillating at 360 J, then starting immediate CPR for 2 minutes and preparing for intubation."

E: "CPR is started."

C: "I will intubate the patient without paralytics or sedation with a 7.5 endotracheal tube since the patient is unresponsive and apneic."

E: "Intubation is successfully performed."

C: "After 2 minutes of CPR, I will recheck the pulse and rhythm."

E: "Patient still has no pulse and the rhythm is torsades de pointes."

E: "Doctor, the patient's labs are back. The only abnormality noted is a serum magnesium level of 1.2 mEq/L."

C: "I will administer 2 g of magnesium sulfate intravenously and defibrillate at 360 J, then continue CPR for 2 minutes."

E: "The shock is delivered and CPR is resumed."

E: "Magnesium has been administered."

E: "After the last round of CPR the telemetry monitor shows the following (Fig. C6-4)."

C: "The patient's rhythm has returned to normal sinus."

C: "Nurse, please repeat the vital signs."

E: "The patient's blood pressure is 122/68, HR 88, O_2 sat 99%. The patient is being manually ventilated at a rate of 14."

C: "Nurse, please get me the cardiology attending for the CCU on the phone."

E: "Dr. Heart is on the phone."

C: "Dr. Heart, this is Dr. Tors. I have an intubated 50-year-old female I would like to admit to the intensive care unit. She has experienced a syncopal episode and a cardiac arrest precipitated by torsades de pointes while in the emergency department. The patient has been taking terfenadine and erythromycin over the last week for a sinus infection. Her magnesium level was 1.2 mEq/L upon presentation. She was successfully converted back to sinus rhythm after two defibrillation attempts and the administration of 2 g of magnesium sulfate. Her vital signs are currently stable."

E: "Fine. Please send her to the CCU with a nurse and I will be happy to see her there."

E: "The case is now over."

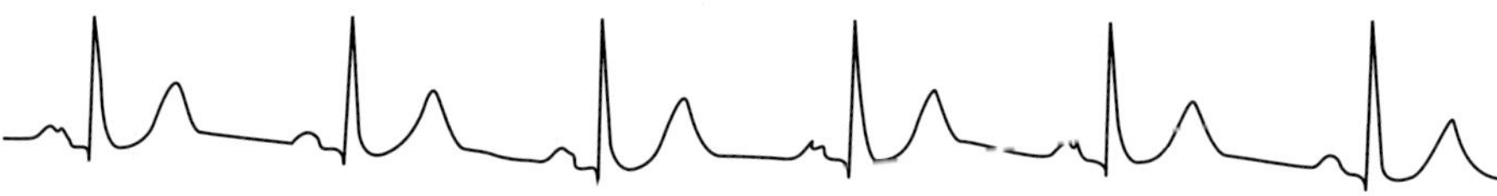

Figure C6-4. Rhythm strip showing normal sinus rhythm again.

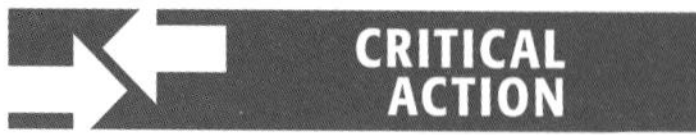

Recognizing that the patient's syncope is the result of torsades de points is the first of two critical actions at this point. Initiation of the appropriate treatment (CPR, intubation, defibrillation, and magnesium) is the second critical action.

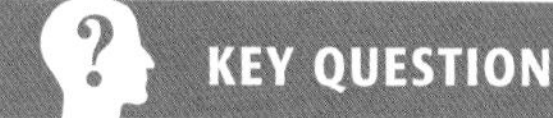

Remember to reassess your patient frequently. This is a good strategy whenever you think you are close to done, or when you don't know what to do next. The answer will let you know if you are on the right track.

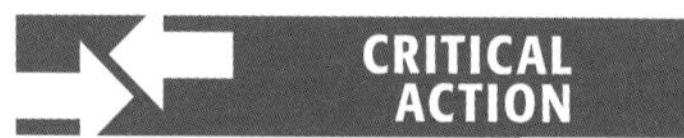

Admitting this patient to the CCU is a critical action in this case.

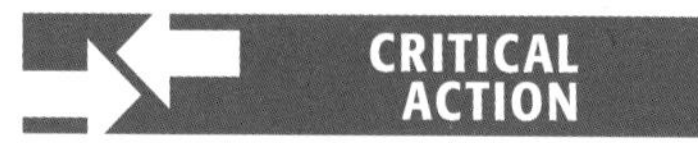

When the examinee presents this patient to the CCU they show that they knew that terfenadine and erythromycin are drugs, which can cause QT prolongation, thereby completing the initial critical action of recognizing that this syncope could be caused by torsades de pointes.

CASE ASSESSMENT

This case was managed according to the standard of care. The candidate identified the patient as having had a syncopal episode and sought historical clues that may have been associated with a life-threatening etiology such as chest discomfort seen in aortic dissection, acute coronary syndrome, or pulmonary embolism. There was no presence of headache or neurologic impairment to suggest a central venous system (CNS) etiology. The patient's rapid onset of light-headedness and tunnel vision suggested an acute decrease in cerebral perfusion possibly consistent with an arrhythmia. The patient's symptoms prior to the event did not suggest a reflex-mediated etiology nor was there evidence by bystanders to suggest seizure activity. Although the patient did have signs of dehydration and mild orthostatic changes in her vital signs the candidate correctly identified that her signs or symptoms were not reproduced when orthostatic vital signs were obtained.

The candidate also placed the patient on a cardiac monitor, established an IV, and supplied additional oxygen when a cardiac etiology and arrhythmia were suspected. The presence of diarrhea suggested a possible electrolyte abnormality and chemistries were appropriately sent to the lab. The combination of terfenadine and erythromycin placed the patient at risk for QT prolongation and torsades de pointes that the candidate identified on ECG and telemetry.

The patient went into cardiac arrest due to torsades de pointes and was promptly defibrillated and given magnesium intravenously. The patient was stabilized and sent to the intensive care unit (ICU) appropriately after discussion with the attending cardiologist.

Critical Actions

1. Diagnosis of syncope due to torsades de pointes.
2. Recognition of drug interactions causing QTc prolongation.
3. Defibrillation and administration of magnesium for torsades de pointes.
4. Admission to the cardiac care unit (CCU).

Test Performance

1. *Data acquisition:* The candidate showed the ability to obtain a more than adequate history and physical in an efficient manner, as well as ordering appropriate tests to assist in diagnosis. Score = **7**
2. *Problem solving:* The candidate did an excellent job problem solving, quickly assimilating data from the patient encounter, interpreting test results and synthesizing information to efficiently direct further management. Score = **7**
3. *Patient management:* The candidate made appropriate treatment decisions based on patient information and clinical course, quickly recognizing torsadess de pointes and appropriately treating it with defibrillation and magnesium. Score = **7**
4. *Resource utilization:* The candidate demonstrated very good use of resources with an efficient, cost-effective use of tests that did not compromise patient care. The candidate could have considered ordering a complete blood count (CBC) to evaluate for anemia as a cause for syncope. Score = **6**

5. *Health care provided (outcome):* The candidate had a systematic approach to the patient when she decompensated, clearly outlining a logical approach to her care. Score = **6**
6. *Interpersonal relations and communication skills:* The candidate engaged in effective information exchange with both patients and professional associates. Score = **6**
7. *Comprehension of pathophysiology:* The candidate demonstrated a detailed and efficient investigatory and analytical approach to syncope, systematically evaluating for the associated broad differential. Score = **8**
8. *Clinical competence (overall):* The candidate overall performed well on this case, recognizing life threats, prioritizing medical care, and communicating effectively with the patient. Score = **7**

CASE 7 35 y/o Male With Head Injury

Navneet Cheema and Michael A. Gisondi

INITIAL INFORMATION

Name: John Small

Mode of arrival: EMS

Age: 35 years

Gender: Male

VS: BP 140/70, HR 110, RR 16, T 36.5°C (97.8°F), O_2 sat: 95% on RA

CC: Fall from 12 ft

PLAY OF THE CASE

E: "You are at a Level 2 trauma center with radiology services and subspecialty backup. You have two nurses, an ED technician, and an ED secretary. The paramedics arrive with a 35-year-old male construction worker who fell approximately 12 ft off a ladder, landing against steel beams on the ground. The initial impact was to the right side of his head and thorax. According to coworkers, he had a loss of consciousness for about 2 minutes. He also has a right arm laceration. When the ambulance arrived, the patient was insisting that he was fine and was reluctant to come to the hospital. The paramedics were unable to obtain IV access as the patient was moving too much with each IV attempt."

C: "What do I see as I walk into the patient's room?"

E: "The patient is a well-nourished male, he is on a backboard, and has a cervical collar in place. He is moving all four extremities and loudly exclaiming that he needs to get back to work right now. He is complaining of head and arm pain."

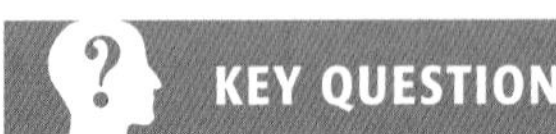

KEY QUESTION

Ask this open-ended question at the beginning of every case.

C: "Nurse, please place the patient on a monitor and provide a rhythm strip when available, and start two 16-guage antecubital IVs. Initiate mask O_2 at 15 L. Please draw basic trauma labs including CBC, metabolic panel, tox screen, and coags."

E: "Those orders are being done. The rhythm strip shows sinus tachycardia."

C: "To the patient: Hello, my name is Dr. Zen. I am going to be taking care of you today. Can you please tell me your name?"

KEY ORDERS

Most of the patients you see during the exam will be unstable (or will become that way). Every unstable patient requires IV access (preferably two large-bore IVs), oxygen, and cardiac monitoring (always request to see a rhythm strip). In this case, as the patient is in trauma, sending appropriate trauma labs is also appropriate at this time.

E: "My name is John Small. Hey, can you take this thing off my neck? I have a wedding today and I need to get out of here so I can get my dog ready to go to Paris."

C: "**Airway is intact**. The patient appears confused. Mr. Small, you are in a safe place and we are going to take good care of you here. Your job is to relax and let us do our job. How are his breath sounds?"

E: "Clear bilaterally."

C: "Is there equal chest expansion? Is there any palpable chest wall tenderness, paradoxical wall motion, deformity, or crepitus?"

E: "There is equal chest expansion, without signs of flail chest or crepitus."

C: "Heart tones and pulses in all extremities?"

E: "Tachycardia without murmurs, rubs, or gallops. Good bilateral radial and dorsalis pedis pulses."

C: "Pupils?"

E: "Pupils are equal, round, and reactive to light bilaterally."

C: "Mr. Small, can you wiggle your fingers and toes?"

E: "He moves his fingers and toes. The patient is complaining that his head hurts and is actively trying to sit up and take off his collar."

C: "His initial GCS is 14. He gets 4 points for spontaneous eye opening, 4 points for confused speech, and 6 points for following commands. Let's logroll the patient, making sure to use C-spine precautions. Anything remarkable on patient's back, eg, tenderness, bruises, or abrasions; Is his rectal tone good? Is there any blood or prostate abnormalities?"

E: "No step-offs or tenderness, good rectal tone, and no gross blood. Prostate non-tender."

C: "Sir, do you have any medical problems?"

E: "No, now let me go!"

C: "Do you have any allergies to medications?"

E: "Let me out of here!"

C: "The patient seems to be getting more confused. Can I get chest, pelvis and C-spine films please?"

E: "They will be done ASAP."

C: "What are the vital signs now?"

E: "HR 110, BP 90/60, RR 16, SPo_2 99% on 2-L NC."

C: "I am going to start my secondary survey while I have the nurses start a 2 L NS bolus, 1 L through each IV. Any facial instability, rhinorrhea, otorrhea, hemotympanum, or lesions in the mouth?"

E: "There is a cephalohematoma in the right temporal area. The nurse points out that your patient is becoming drowsy."

C: "I am palpating the extremities and looking for injuries there."

E: "There is a deformity and swelling of the right upper arm, about mid-shaft humerus. There is a large laceration on right forearm that is bleeding profusely."

C: "I will ask one of the nurses to wrap that area in kerlex and hold pressure. I am now auscultating, then I will palpate the abdomen. What do I hear and feel; Is there any tenderness?"

E: "There are active bowel sounds. The abdomen is soft."

C: "Mr. Small, does it hurt when I push on your belly?"

E: "Mr. Small is not answering you and he does not open his eyes to your voice."

C: "Given this patient's declining mental status, I am going to intubate him for airway protection." "Nurse, could you please give 20 mg etomidate and 150 mg succinylcholine." I will intubate using a 7.5 endotracheal tube. Do I have equal breath sounds and color change on the CO_2 detector?"

E: "Yes."

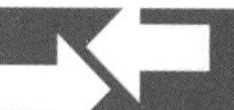

CRITICAL ACTION

In every trauma patient (or potential trauma patient) the correct application of the ATLS primary and secondary survey is a critical action. In this section the examinee is conducting their primary survey.

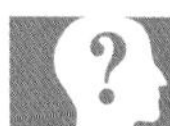

KEY QUESTION

The examinee is attempting to get an AMPLE history (Allergies, Medications, Prior medical/surgical problems, Last meal, and Events [what happened?]), which is appropriate. (It would also be appropriate to ask for EMTs or family at this point to help get the AMPLE history.)

KEY QUESTION

Remember to reassess your patient frequently—trauma patients can deteriorate rapidly.

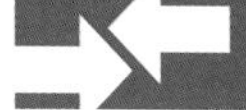

CRITICAL ACTION

In every trauma patient (or potential trauma patient) the correct application of the ATLS primary and secondary survey is a critical action. In the section the examinee is doing their secondary survey. A second critical action taking place at this time is fluid resuscitation for hypotension and tachycardia.

KEY QUESTION

Always remember to confirm tube placement.

CRITICAL ACTION

Intubation of the unresponsive patient is a critical action. In order to get full credit for this action the examinee should have to use both in-line C-spin immobilization and a neuroprotective sedation strategy since an intracranial process that cannot be excluded. (A neuroprotective strategy would include a defasciculating dose of pancuronium to avoid the fasciculations associated with succinylcholine alone (vecuronium or rocuronium are also acceptable.) Hyperventilation with BVM, premedication with lidocaine, and induction with paralysis are always preferable in these patients.

KEY QUESTION

Remember to reassess your patient frequently—trauma patients can deteriorate rapidly. In a patient with possible head injury the pupil examination should be reassessed with every vital sign check.

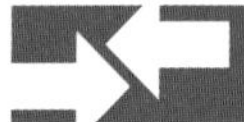

CRITICAL ACTION

Recognizing the signs and symptoms of herniation and treating with hyperventilation and mannitol are critical actions in this case.

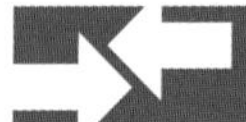

CRITICAL ACTION

Getting neurosurgery involved early is a critical action in this case.

C: "Please set up a ventilator to give 16 breaths/min SIMV, tidal volume of 500 with 50% FIO_2. Let's order a repeat portable CXR. What are the vitals now, after the 2 L of NS?"

E: "HR 80, BP 140/95."

C: "What is the pupil examination?"

E: "The right pupil is 8 mm and sluggishly reactive and the left pupil is reactive, 4 to 2 mm."

C: "I would like to start mannitol 1 g/kg IV. I am going to hyperventilate this patient to a PCO_2 of 30-35 mm Hg, as he is showing signs of herniation. I'll ask the nurse to get a neurosurgeon on the phone for an emergent consult."

E: "Neurosurgeon is on the phone. 'Hello, this is Dr. Braney. What is the problem?'"

C: "I have a 35-year-old man who fell from a ladder and landed on his right side and hit his head. He initially lost consciousness, then was lucid during transport. On arrival to the ED he had a GCS of 14, but then rapidly deteriorated. He is now unresponsive, with a dilated, poorly reactive right pupil suggesting herniation."

E: "Did you start mannitol?"

C: "Yes. He is intubated as well. I will get a head CT."

E: "I'll be there in 15 minutes."

C: "I would like to do a CT scan of the head. Let's also get one of the abdomen and pelvis, as we were unable to get a reliable examination secondary to decreased mental status. Although the bleeding laceration of the arm could account for a large blood loss, I would like to rule out an abdominal or pelvic bleed using CT."

E: "The CT is available for your review (Fig. C7-1). Please interpret the films."

C: "CT scan shows a right temporal bone fracture with underlying large epidural hematoma. There is mass effect to the degree that herniation is a concern."

E: "Thank you. The abdomen and pelvis CT scans are normal. The patient is now showing some decerebrate posturing."

C: "Neurosurgery will have to evacuate that epidural hematoma. I'll ask the nurse to notify the OR."

E: "She does so."

C: "Is the arm laceration still actively bleeding?"

E: "No. The nurse has applied a pressure dressing and the bleeding seems to have stopped. The patient still has good radial pulse in that arm."

C: "I would like to apply a splint to the presumed right humeral fracture. The surgeons can order films of the arm after the patient is out of the operating room."

E: "Done."

C: "I did not get to the GU portion of the secondary survey. Is there blood at the urethral meatus?"

E: "No."

C: "I will ask for a Foley catheter and nasogastric tube to be placed at this time."

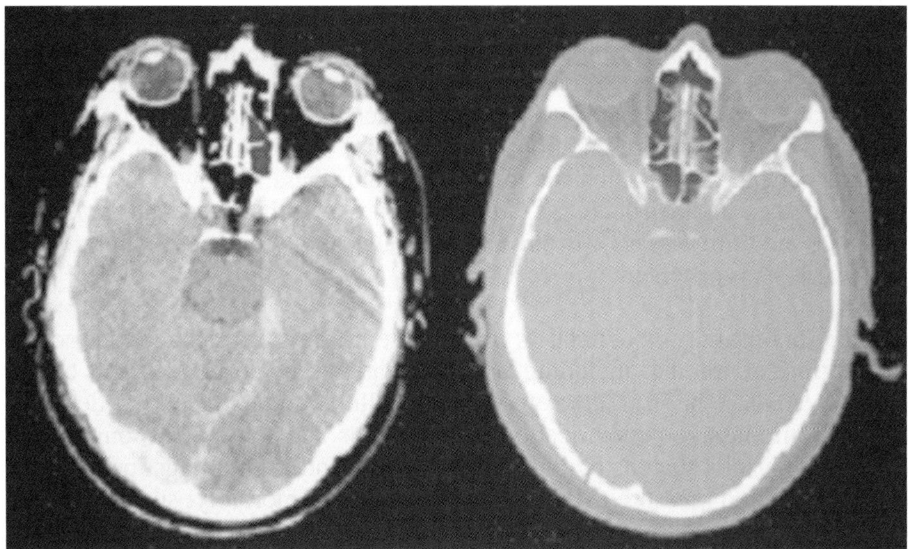

Figure C7-1. Epidural hematoma. CT of the head windowed for brain (left) and bone (right) shows an epidural hematoma resulting from an underlying occipital skull fracture. This injury was caused by a blow to the back of the head. Notice the classic lens-shaped hematoma. The brain window also shows a thin left tentorial subdural hematoma appearing as a white line running from the midline posteriorly and curving toward the left of the pons. *(Reprinted with permission from Doherty GM.* Current Surgical Diagnosis and Treatment. *12th ed. New York, NY: McGraw-Hill; 2006.)*

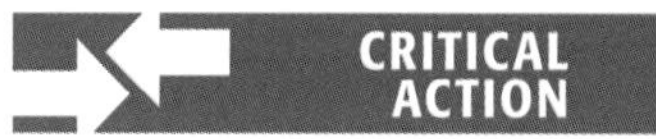

In every trauma patient (or potential trauma patient) the correct application of the ATLS primary and secondary survey is a critical action. In the section the examinee is finishing the secondary survey after stabilizing the patient as much as possible.

E: "The nurse places these for you."

C: "What is the pupil examination now?"

E: "It appears that the right pupil is approximately the size of the left. The patient is no longer showing posturing and neurosurgery is ready to take the patient."

C: "Good. I will notify the family and PMD of this patient at this time."

E: "The case is now over."

CASE ASSESSMENT

The candidate managed this difficult case very well. He introduced himself to the patient and gave direct orders to the nurses, including the initial intravenous (IV), oxygen, and monitor. As with many "real" patient encounters, the history was difficult to obtain from this uncooperative, head-injured patient, forcing the candidate to proceed with minimal background information. By following the advanced trauma life support (ATLS) protocol closely, he was less likely to miss any hidden injuries. He reassessed vital signs and patient condition frequently. In addition to the head injury, the candidate also identified and treated the left humerus fracture that the patient suffered during his fall. Patients with severe closed head injuries often will have important neck injury as well as frequent long bone or pelvic fracture.

The patient suffered an epidural hematoma, a collection of blood between the inner table of the skull and the dura. Epidural hematomas generally result from injury to the middle meningeal artery, though they can be caused by venous disruptions as well. They appear hyperdense, biconvex, ovoid, and lenticular when visualized using computed tomography (CT). The most common locations are in the temporal region or posterior fossa. These lesions tend to be unilateral and are associated with other intracranial pathology in up to 40% of cases. The classic presentation of an epidural hematoma is that of a head-injured patient with a transient loss of consciousness, followed by a "lucid interval," then another decrease in consciousness. Such a presentation is seen in about one-third of cases. If these injuries are rapidly diagnosed and treated, the prognosis is excellent.

Primary brain injury is defined as irreversible mechanical damage that occurs at the time of trauma, including brain lacerations, hemorrhages, and contusions. Secondary brain injury refers to intracellular and extracellular derangements from massive depolarization of brain cells and subsequent ionic shifts. Secondary insults such as hypotension, hypoxia, and anemia must be avoided. A systolic blood pressure (SBP) <90 almost doubles mortality; survivors often have a very poor neurologic outcome. When hypoxia is documented, the overall mortality of severe closed head trauma doubles. All current acute therapies for traumatic brain injury are directed at reversing or preventing further secondary injury. The candidate acted to maintain normal SBP by giving saline and prevented hypoxia by giving the patient supplemental oxygen.

This candidate did an excellent job of identifying and treating increased intracranial pressure (ICP), defined as ICP above 15 mm Hg. (Remember: cerebral perfusion pressure = mean arterial pressure – intracranial pressure [CPP = MAP–ICP].) Intracranial compensatory mechanisms can accommodate increases in volume of 50-100 cc (as from an epidural hematoma in this case). Beyond that level, even small changes in volume can result in dramatic increases in ICP. With the loss of autoregulation, massive cerebral vasodilatation occurs and edema worsens. If ICP rises to level of systemic circulation, CPP ceases and brain cell death occurs.

Methods to reduce ICP include hyperventilation, osmotic and diuretic agent use, and cerebrospinal fluid (CSF) drainage. Hyperventilation to CO_2 levels of 30-35 mm Hg will temporarily reduce ICP by promoting cerebral vasoconstriction. This usually lowers ICP by 25%. It is recommended for brief periods during acute resuscitation and only in patients with neurologic deterioration. In instances of deepening coma and unequal pupils, one may consider the use of mannitol (0.25-1 g/kg). This osmotic agent reduces brain volume and edema, taking effect in minutes. Mannitol also serves as a free radical scavenger. While barbiturates may also decrease ICP, they can promote systemic hypotension as well. The candidate was right not to use them in this case. There is no indication for steroids in the acutely brain-injured patient.

Patients with signs of herniation refractory to all other attempts to decrease ICP should be considered for placement of emergency burr holes. A brief description of the procedure from "The Occasional Burr Hole," by Keith MacLellan, MD, follows:

> *Use a sterilized penetrator, burr hole bits and braces for a formal two-stage entry through the cranium. If these are not available, use a 1/2-in steel drill bit (slightly smaller for a child). Shave and prep the area of entry. Make about a 3-cm incision vertically over the entry point through the skin, temporalis muscle, and periosteum. For an adult, drill two fingerbreadths above the top of the ear and two fingerbreadths anterior to the auditory canal. For a child, approximate that point. The goal is to be just above the roof of the zygoma and to avoid drilling into the orbit or into the temporal artery. Have cautery available. At*

this point, drill through the outer table of the skull with the penetrator. Then, if available, use the bit and brace in the tray to complete the skull penetration. Once through the skull, evacuate the hematoma with a soft suction tip and suture in a Penrose drain.

This particular patient had an uncal herniation from an expanding mass lesion. These are often associated with traumatic extra-axial hematomas in the lateral middle fossa of temporal lobe. As herniation begins, cranial nerve (CN) III is compressed resulting in anisocoria, ptosis, impaired extraocular movements, and a sluggish pupillary light reflex on the ipsilateral side of expanding mass lesion. Contralateral compression of CN III eventually occurs, as well as contralateral abnormal Babinski reflexes, followed by decerebrate posturing. Decorticate posturing is abnormal flexion of the upper extremities with extension of the lower extremities and implies injury above the midbrain. Decerebrate posturing is extension and adduction of arms, with extension and internal rotation of the legs, implying injury below midbrain. The latter carries a worse prognosis.

Intubation was a critical action for this case. The candidate recognized that the patient was deteriorating and would need to have a definitive airway established. Etomidate and succinylcholine were chosen for induction and paralysis, respectively. The candidate did not opt to use a defasciculating dose of a nondepolarizing agent. This decision was made because of the need for rapid airway protection, though some would argue that the 40 additional seconds taken to wait for a small dose of pancuronium (or similar agent) to be on board prior to giving the succinylcholine justifies giving it, especially as fasciculations have been shown to transiently increase ICP. The use of lidocaine in rapid sequence intubation of head-injured patients is indicated though clear benefit has not been shown and it does add time to the protocol.

Critical Actions

1. Identification of intracranial pathology.
2. Administration of appropriate volume resuscitation.
3. Intubation and mechanical ventilation (bonus points for mild hyperventilation).
4. Identification and discussion of treatment of brain herniation.
5. Neurosurgical consultation
6. Complete primary and secondary survey.

Test Performance

1. *Data acquisition:* This phase is superb as the candidate shows ability to obtain an adequate history and physical examination findings in an efficient, orderly manner that adhered to the primary and secondary surveys as outlined by ATLS. Score = **7**
2. *Problem solving:* The candidate is able to quickly assimilate data from the physical examination and synthesizes information to efficiently direct further management. Score = **8**
3. *Patient management:* This candidate demonstrated a highly detailed and efficient investigatory and analytical approach to the clinical picture. He recognized the deterioration of the patient's condition and quickly intervened with intubation. He would have gotten higher score if he had either premedicated the patient for intracranial hemorrhage (ICH) or verbalized why he was not doing this. Score = **6**

4. *Resource utilization:* The candidate demonstrates very good use of resources with an efficient, cost-effective use of tests that does not compromise patient care. He requests a C-spine x-ray (XR) along with his initial chest and pelvis XR. It could be argued that a CT C-spine would be a better test to request. Score = **6**
5. *Health care provided (outcome):* The candidate makes appropriate treatment decisions based on patient information and preferences, scientific evidence, and clinical judgment. Score = **7**
6. *Interpersonal relations and communication skills:* The candidate engages in effective information exchange with both patient and professional associates. The physician even remembers to contact family members and a primary physician. Score = **7**
7. *Comprehension of pathophysiology:* The candidate has an excellent understanding of the underlying pathophysiology in this case, repeating his pupil examination serially to monitor for signs of herniation. Score = **7**
8. *Clinical competence (overall):* The candidate had a very organized approach to this complex multisystem trauma. Score = **7**

CASE 8 70 y/o Female With Abdominal Pain

Navneet Cheema, Thomas J. Regan, and Aleksandr Gorenbeyn

INITIAL INFORMATION

Name: Mary Anderson

Mode of arrival: Brought in by EMS

Age: 70 years

Gender: Female

VS: T 37.2°C, BP 115/70, HR 60, RR 18

CC: Abdominal pain

PLAY OF THE CASE

C: "Is the EMS crew that brought the patient in still present in the ED?"

E: "Yes, they are."

C: "I would like them to remain in the ED until I can talk to them. As I walk into the patient's room, what do I see?"

E: "The patient is an elderly moderately obese female, who appears in mild distress. She is lying in the bed fully clothed."

C: "Nurse, please undress the patient and put her in a hospital gown. Also can you place the patient on a cardiac monitor, show me a rhythm strip, obtain a pulse ox and then begin O_2 via 2 L NC, and place an 18-gauge IV, begin NS at TKO, and draw blood for lab tests."

E: "Those orders are being done. The rhythm strip shows NSR in the 60s. The pulse ox is 97% on room air. The patient is now unclothed and lying on the hospital bed."

C: "Hello, Mrs. Anderson. I'm Dr. C. What brings you into the ED today?"

E: "Well, my husband called the ambulance because my stomach is hurting today."

C: "Nurse, is the patient's husband here in the ED?"

E: "Yes, he's standing outside in the hallway."

C: "Can you please bring him in?"

E: "The nurse brings the patient's husband into the room."

C: "I introduce myself to the husband and then continue to question the patient. Mrs. Anderson, what were you doing when you first experienced the abdominal pain today?"

E: "I was sitting in a chair about 1/2 hour ago watching TV with my husband. I tried getting out of the chair, and felt a severe, sharp pain in my stomach. I got really dizzy and nauseated and fell back into my chair."

C: "Did you pass out?"

E: "I don't think so, I really can't remember exactly."

C: "Mr. Anderson, did you notice if your spouse passed out?"

KEY QUESTION

Ask this open-ended question at the beginning of every case. Also, note how the examinee requested that the EMS personnel be on hand in case they require more information.

KEY ORDERS

Most of the patients you see during the exam will be unstable (or will become that way). Every unstable patient requires IV access (preferably two large-bore IVs), oxygen, and cardiac monitoring (always request to see a rhythm strip).

KEY QUESTION

Remember to always ask for past medical history, medications, allergies, and surgeries.

KEY QUESTION

Remember to use your resources—always ask to talk to EMS and/or family when you have a chance and the patient is stable.

KEY QUESTION

Remember to reassess your patient's vitals and pain frequently.

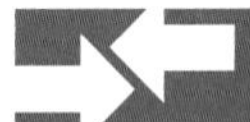

CRITICAL ACTION

The first critical action in this case is to demonstrate a strong suspicion for a ruptured AAA to rule out (or in) the most catastrophic life threats. This line of questioning in the physical examination (as well as palpation for pulsatile masses) meets that requirement.

E: "Yes, she did doctor. She was out for a good 10 seconds. That's when I called the ambulance."

C: "Mrs. Anderson, when you woke up, did you have any chest pain or shortness of breath?"

E: "I felt nauseated, but I didn't vomit. I didn't have any chest pain or shortness of breath."

C: "Was the abdominal pain still present?"

E: "Yes, it was still there."

C: "Did the pain radiate anywhere?"

E: "Yes, it seemed to radiate to my left lower back."

C: "Do you have any medical problems?"

E: "Yes, I have high blood pressure and I've had a kidney stone in the past."

C: "Did this feel like kidney stone pain to you?"

E: "No, this was different from my kidney stone pain in the past."

C: "Are you on any medications? Do you have any allergies?"

E: "Yes, I take atenolol, HCTZ, and an ASA. I have no allergies."

C: "I would like the nurse to repeat a set of vitals on this patient. I want blood sent to the lab for CBC, electrolytes, BUN/Cr, glucose, and coags. I'll need a urine dip and an ECG as well. While this is being done, I'd like to talk to the EMS team that brought the patient into the ED."

E: "They're right here, doctor."

C: "Hello, EMS crew. This patient that you brought in, I've heard her history of having abdominal pain and passing out. Can you add anything else to the story?"

E: "When we arrived at the scene, the patient was sitting in her chair and appeared diaphoretic and pale. Her initial vitals showed a HR 60 but BP 95/60. We put her in a supine position and repeated her vitals. Her blood pressure then improved to 115/70."

C: "Nurse, are the repeat vitals finished?"

E: "Yes, doctor. They are HR 62, BP 110/65, RR 18. Here is your ECG (Fig. C8-1)."

C: "Mrs. Anderson, has your abdominal pain gotten any better?"

E: "No, doctor. It's still there. It actually feels a little worse."

C: "I would now like to examine the patient. What do I hear when I examine the patient's heart and lungs?"

E: "They are normal."

C: "I would like to examine her abdomen."

E: "What are you looking for?"

C: "I am listening for bowel sounds or bruits, palpating for any pain, rebound, guarding, or pulsatile masses. I also want to see if I can palpate her aorta."

E: "The patient has hypoactive bowel sounds, no rebound, no guarding, and no bruits. She does have diffuse mild abdominal pain, but moderate pain when palpating her epigastric/supra-umbilical area. You are having a hard time palpating her aorta because of her body habitus."

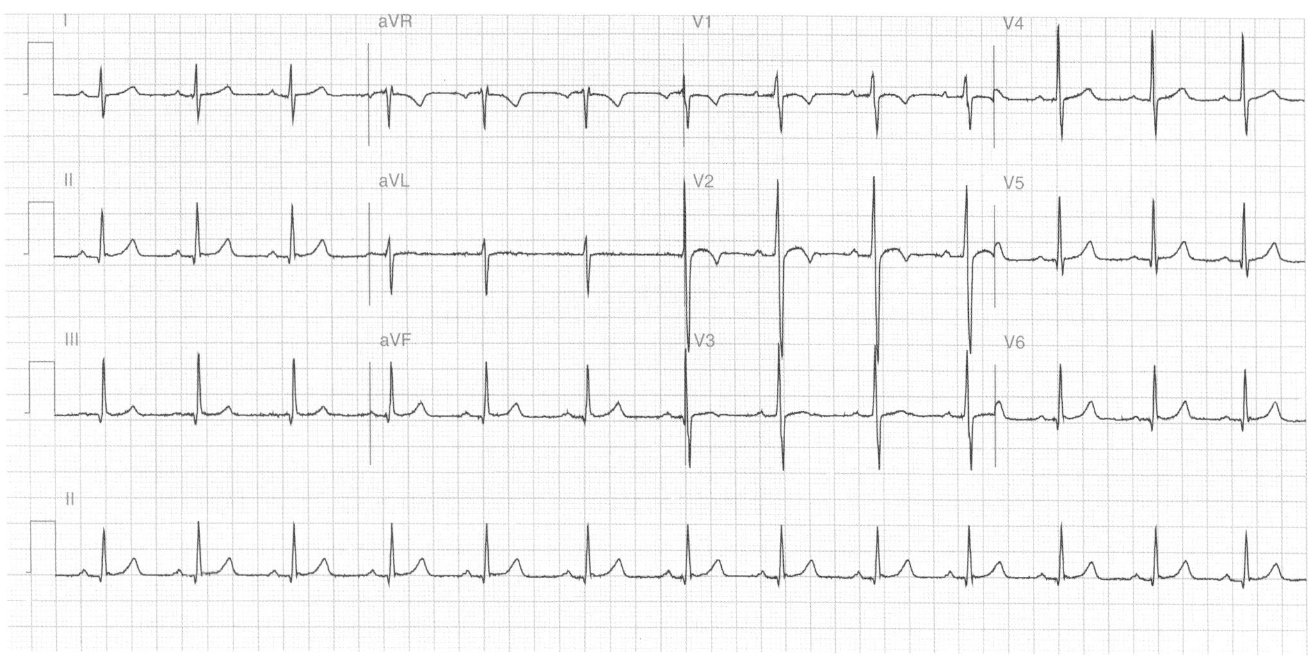

Figure C8-1. ECG with normal sinus rhythm in the 60s with left axis deviation, and voltage criteria consistent with LVH; no acute ST-T changes. *(Reproduced with permission from Fauci AS, Braunwald E, Kasper DL, et al.* Harrison's Principles of Internal Medicine. *17th ed. New York, NY: McGraw-Hill; 2008.)*

C: "I would like to examine her flank and back."

E: "They are normal."

C: "I would like to do a rectal examination."

E: "It is normal. Guaiac is negative."

C: "I'd like to examine her distal pulses."

E: "What are you looking for?"

C: "I'd like to examine the strength of her distal pulses and see if there is any pulse discrepancy between her upper and lower abdominal pulses."

E: "She has pulses all four extremities, although the femoral and DP pulses are only +1. Her radial pulses are both +2. There is no delay between her radial and femoral pulses."

C: "I would like the nurse to obtain a second 18-gauge IV, and to page the vascular surgeon. Please send off a type and screen as well. I would also like a repeat set of vitals please."

E: "This is done. Her repeat vitals: HR 60, BP 105/65, RR 18. I also have some of her lab work for you. Her UA is normal, her CBC is unremarkable with a Hgb of 11 and a Hct of 33."

C: "I'd like to have the patient type and crossed for 8 U PRBC. I'd like to give the patient a bolus of NS 1 L. I'd like a set of vitals on her every 5 minutes, and also after the bolus is completed. Has the vascular surgeon called back yet?"

E: "No, he hasn't, doctor. I will page him again."

C: "Mrs Anderson, I would like to do a quick ultrasound test of your abdomen. It may help me determine what is causing your pain. I'm also having the

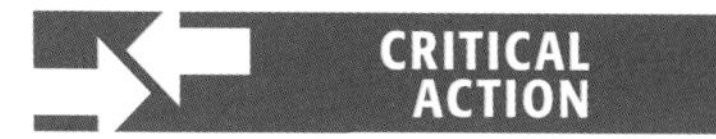

CRITICAL ACTION

Sending a T & C for 8-U PRBC on any potential vascular surgery case is a critical action, as is assuring that you have appropriate vascular access in case you should need to do volume resuscitation. Getting vascular surgery involved is the final critical action that takes place at this point.

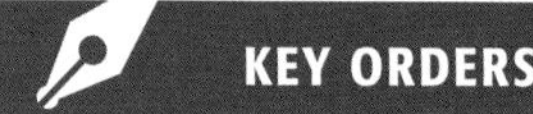

KEY ORDERS

Note how the examinee asks the examiner to give them updates on the vitals every 5 minutes. This places the responsibility for noticing any change in blood pressure or heart rate on the examiner, so that the examinee does not need to remember to reassess as often—a good strategy!

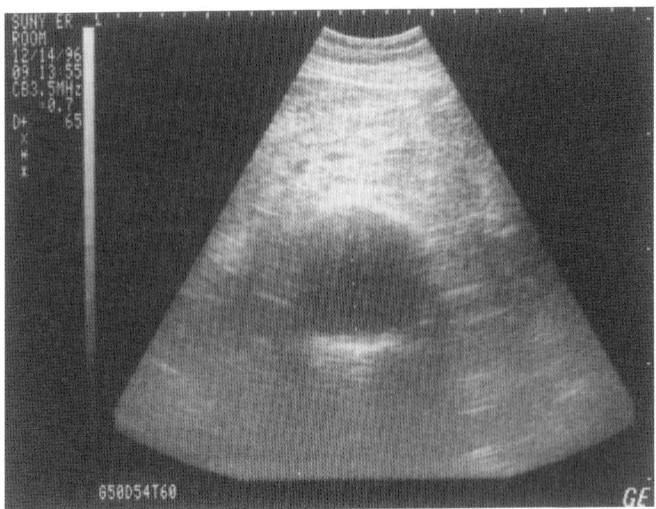

Figure C8-2. Transverse abdominal US showing a 6.5-cm aorta. *(Reprinted with permission from Tintinalli JE, Kelen GD, Stapczynski JS.* Emergency Medicine: A Comprehensive Study Guide. *6th ed. New York, NY: McGraw-Hill; 2004.)*

nurse give you some fluid in your vein. Your blood pressure seems to be a bit low and I'd like to bring it up a little."

E: "OK, doctor, whatever you say."

C: "I would like to perform a bedside ultrasound on this patient (Fig. C8-2)."

C: "Mrs. Anderson, this pain may be a result of the large artery in your body, the aorta, developing a weakness in its wall, and possibly developing a leak. It may be from something else, but at this time, my suspicions are quite high that it is in fact your aorta. I'm calling a vascular surgeon to come in and help me treat you."

E: "Is this serious doctor?"

C: "Yes, it is very serious, and there is a good chance you will need surgery to repair this. You can lose a lot of blood because of this problem, and therefore I'm going to have the nurse start administering some blood to you."

E: "Doctor, the vascular surgeon, Dr. Red, is on the phone."

C: "Hello, Dr. Red, this is Dr C. I have a 70-year-old woman with a history of hypertension who presents with sudden onset of abdominal pain radiating to the back with syncope. Here in the ED she has a steadily decreasing blood pressure, and a bedside ultrasound shows an enlarged 6.5-cm abdominal aorta."

E: "Did you see any free fluid?"

C: "No, but again, it was only a bedside ultrasound."

E: "Are you sure that's what this is? Maybe you should obtain a CT of the abdomen if you're not sure of your diagnosis."

C: "Actually, at this point, AAA is at the top of my list for a diagnosis. I've already ordered blood for her, and am bolusing her with NS. I don't think any further testing would be advisable, especially with her decreasing blood pressure. I'd be hesitant sending her out of the ED for tests. In fact, I'd only feel comfortable with her leaving the ED as a direct transfer to the OR."

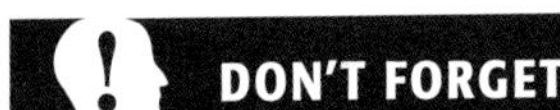

If the consultant is not answering a page, it is probably your examiner's way of telling you that something else needs to be done. In this case, the bedside US should be performed before talking to the vascular surgeon.

Remember to update the patient on their condition and the plan. This will earn you points for interpersonal interactions and professionalism.

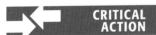

Understanding how unstable this patient is a critical action. The examinee shows this by starting fluid resuscitation early and refusing to let the patient leave the ED for non-bedside testing.

E: "Very well. I'll have my chief resident come down to prep her for the OR."

C: "Thank you. I would like to go and check on the patient again and obtain another set of vitals. I would like to tell the patient that I have spoken to the vascular surgeon and that she will be going to the OR. The surgeons will be coming down to talk with them in a few minutes. I would like to ask both the patient and her husband if they have any questions."

E: "This case is now over."

CASE ASSESSMENT

The candidate did an excellent job managing this particular patient. He was capable of multitasking throughout the progression of this case: Gathering information as he issued commands, keeping the patient well informed as the workup progressed, and constantly reassessing the status of the patient as the eventual life threat was revealed.

At the start of the case, the patient did not appear seriously ill; her relatively normal vitals perhaps influenced by her beta-blocker. An elderly patient with abdominal pain, especially radiating to the back, is concerning. This point was reinforced as the candidate utilized other sources (ie, husband and emergency medical services [EMS] crew) to obtain crucial bits of information (ie, syncope and initial hypotension) that facilitated the diagnosis of a rupturing abdominal aortic aneurysm (AAA), and influenced the manner of treatment and choice of diagnostic test. As the gravity of the diagnosis revealed itself, the intensity of intervention increased, as did the frequency of reassessment. When it was realized from the history and physical that a rupturing AAA was high on the differential, additional intravenous (IV) access, saline bolus, and blood products (minimum 8 U in a vascular case) were ordered in anticipation of the patients worsening status. Consultation was also initiated and took precedent over obtaining an imaging study. Calling the appropriate consult early is key, but notice that consultation communication was delayed until the candidate completed his diagnostic bedside testing. Remember—if the consultant is not answering a page, something else needs to be done.

After resuscitative measures were instituted, consultation obtained, and the imaging study completed, the candidate continued to update the patient on her disposition, as well as continued to reassess while the patient remained in the emergency department (ED).

The candidate managed this case well, and was particularly adept at using all available sources for data acquisition. Many important pieces of information can be obtained from sources other than the patient.

Critical Actions

1. Strong suspicion for a potentially ruptured AAA.
2. Large-bore IV access × 2 with fluid resuscitation.
3. Type and cross for blood—minimum of 8 U in all vascular cases!
4. Bedside diagnostic testing—patient is not to go to radiology department.
5. Early vascular/surgical consult.

Test Performance

1. *Data acquisition:* This phase was exceptional with the candidate using all sources available to obtain important details of the history. The candidate

promptly recognized the missing vital sign and asked for that information. The physical examination was focused, and helped confirm the candidate's suspicion of the presence of a life-threat. Score = **8**

2. *Problem solving:* The candidate was able to assimilate information from the history and physical as well as the lab data to direct his ongoing management of the patient. Score = **7**
3. *Patient management:* The candidate was able to accurately predict and prepare for probable impending resuscitation measures, increasing his level of clinical vigilance in accordance with the increasing possibility of a significant life-threat. Score = **8**
4. *Resource utilization:* This was effectively displayed by the candidate's efficient and cost-effective use of resources. They used the appropriate tests to arrive at the correct disposition. Score = **7**
5. *Health care provided (outcome):* The candidate was very adept at both the investigational and analytical aspects of this patient's clinical case. Score = **7**
6. *Interpersonal relations and communication skills:* The candidate constantly updates the patient and her husband on her diagnosis and eventual disposition. The candidate was also able to effectively convey the seriousness of the situation to the consultant, and ensure appropriate rapid intervention of the life threat. Score = **8**
7. *Comprehension of pathophysiology:* The candidate quickly recognized the potential for a patient with a ruptured abdominal aneurysm to deteriorate and quickly ordered IVFs and packed red blood cells (pRBCs). Score = **7**
8. *Clinical competence (overall):* This case was handled efficiently, utilizing all available sources of information to help make the diagnosis quickly. Score = **8**

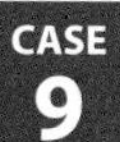

CASE 9 1 mo/o Male With Fever of Unknown Origin

Navneet Cheema and Kip Adrian

INITIAL INFORMATION

Name: Jayla Smith

Mode of arrival: Brought by family

Age: 1-month-old boy

VS: BP 50/25, HR 200, RR 80, O_2 sat: 95% RA

CC: Fever

PLAY OF THE CASE

C: "What do I see as I walk into the patient's room?"

KEY QUESTION

Ask this open-ended question at the beginning of every case.

E: "You see an infant being held by his mother. He appears limp and pale."

C: "Nurse, while I introduce myself to the family please measure a rectal temperature on the child and get his weight."

E: "Consider it done, doctor."

C: "Hello, my name is Dr. Coole. I was looking at your son's vital signs and noticed that he appears quite pale. I think we need to start an IV to begin and give Jayla some fluids. Is that OK with you?"

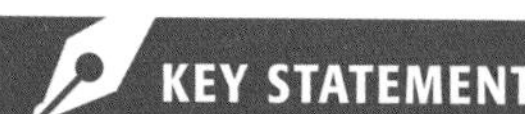

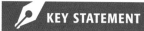

KEY STATEMENT

Remember to introduce yourself and discuss invasive actions with the patient/family.

E: "Hello, my name is Ms. Smith. Yes, that would be OK. Meanwhile, the nurse reports the rectal temperature is 38.5°C (101.4°F) and that the child weighs 4.5 kg."

C: "Nurse, this patient also needs a 22-gauge IV in the antecubital fossa. At the same time please draw blood for labs including blood cultures. The child will need 90-cc NS bolus as quickly as we can get that in. Please catheterize the child for urine. Send the blood for CBC, BMP, and blood cultures. Please administer acetaminophen 60 mg per rectum. Please let me know as soon as the bolus is complete and any lab tests are back."

KEY ORDERS

Most of the patients you see during the exam will be unstable (or will become that way). Every unstable patient requires IV access (in the pediatric population an 18-gauge IV is often not possible; if you are unsure of what IV size to request, you can ask for the "largest peripheral IV possible"), oxygen, and cardiac monitoring. In this case, as the patient appears septic, a fluid bolus, cultures, and antipyretics are also appropriate at this moment.

E: "The nurse goes to carry out the orders."

C: "Ms. Smith, how long has Jayla had the fever?"

E: "I think it started yesterday."

C: "Has Jayla been able to keep any fluids down?"

E: "Very little."

C: "Has Jayla been coughing, vomiting, or had any change in his bowel habits?"

E: "Yes, he has had a small cough. He has not been vomiting or had any change in his bowel habits, though."

C: "Is Jayla bringing anything up with the cough?"

E: "No, he has not."

C: "Has Jayla been sneezing or had any drainage from his nose?"

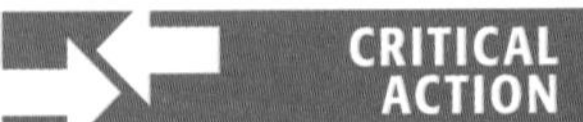

CRITICAL ACTION

Recognizing that this infant is critically ill and initiating immediate IV fluids are critical actions in this case.

KEY ORDERS

Note how the examinee asks for the examiner to give them updates when the orders and labs are complete. This places the responsibility for reassessment on the examiner, making it so that the examinee does not need to remember to reassess as often—a good strategy!

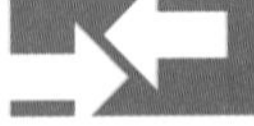

CRITICAL ACTION

Taking a good birth history that includes any risks of maternal infection is a critical action in this case.

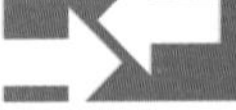

CRITICAL ACTION

Treating this potentially septic infant with empiric antibiotics is a critical action.

E: "No, he hasn't."

C: "Ms. Smith, was Jayla a full-term baby?"

E: "Yes, he was born at 39 weeks."

C: "Did Jayla have to stay in the hospital for any prolonged period as far as you know?"

E: "No, he stayed 2 days and then went home with me. They did give him some antibiotics at first as a precaution."

C: "Does Jayla have any allergies?"

E: "Not that I am aware of."

C: "When you were pregnant or in labor were you treated for any infections?"

E: "Yes, they had to give me some antibiotics because of a vaginal infection that possibly involved my womb."

C: "Nurse, please administer ampicillin 225 mg IV and Cefotaxime 225 mg IV."

E: "The nurse will carry out those orders immediately."

C: "Ms. Smith, do you have a history of herpes infections?"

E: "Yes, I have had herpes outbreaks, but only once in a great while. I didn't have any during my pregnancy." (The nurse reports that the initial fluid bolus is in and the VS include a BP 55/40, HR 176, RR 70.)

C: Please repeat the saline bolus, 90 cc, as quickly as possible. As I examine the child, is the anterior fontanel bulging or depressed?"

E: "The fontanel is firm to touch and slightly bulging."

C: "Are the child's mucous membranes dry appearing?"

E: "Yes."

C: "Are the pupils equal and reactive to light?"

E: "Yes, they remain equal."

C: "As I examine the rest of the head, is there any erythema or lesions of the oropharynx, pus behind the TMs, bulging of the TMs, rhinorrhea, or scleral icterus noted?"

E: "No, the rest of the HEENT examination appears normal, although you were unable to see the TMs."

C: "Are there any abnormal findings on the lung examination including decreased breath sounds, wheezing, or crackles?"

E: "The lungs sound normal."

C: "Is the heart in a regular rhythm, without any rubs or murmurs?"

E: "Yes."

C: "Is the abdomen soft, non-distended with bowel sounds?"

E: "Yes."

C: "Are there any rashes or obvious skin abnormalities?"

E: "No."

C: "What are the pulses and cap refill like?"

E: "The pulses are thready and weak, the skin is cool in the extremities, and the cap refill is approximately 3 seconds."

C: "Is the child crying with the examination or waking up? What is the child's muscle tone like?"

E: "The child whimpers slightly with the manipulation of the examination. The child has overall decreased tone but appears to be moving all extremities equally."

C: "Ms. Smith, fevers more than 38°C (100.4°F) in children Jayla's age are concerning for possibly serious infections. Jayla in particular appears to be very dehydrated from his fever and will need us to continue to give him IV fluids. Also, we need to rule out meningitis, which is an infection of the fluid that surrounds the brain and spinal cord, as a possible cause for Jayla being so sick. To do this we need to do a lumbar puncture. This procedure consists of placing a very small needle in Jayla's lower back to take a small amount of this spinal fluid to check for signs of infection. There are some small risks to doing this including introducing an infection into the fluid or causing a small amount of bleeding in the space around the spinal cord or its coverings, but overall, the risks of these occurring are very, very small. The procedure usually takes less than 10 minutes to perform. Also, we will send the blood that we drew for Jayla to the lab and take an x-ray to help us find out if Jayla does have a serious infection. Is this OK with you?"

E: "Ms. Smith agrees and a nurse takes her out of the room."

C: "I would like to perform a spinal tap on the patient."

E: "You do a spinal tap without apparent incident and collect 4 tubes of fluid that appears persistently cloudy and blood tinged."

C: "Nurse, please send the spinal fluid off for the following tests: tube 1 for cell count; tube 2 for Gram stain and culture; tube 3 for protein, glucose, and PCR testing for HSV; and tube 4 for cell count. Also, please give the patient acyclovir 90 mg IV, and vancomycin 65 mg IV. Thank you."

E: "Before sending off the fluid the nurse reports the second bolus of NS is completed and the vitals are as follows: T 37.4°C (99.4°F), HR 160, RR 60, BP 65/48, O_2 sat 97% on room air."

C: "Nurse, please also give another 90 cc bolus of NS as quickly as possible. Please let me know when it is finished along with repeat vital signs. Also, I would also like to speak to the patient's primary doctor and the PICU doctor, as well as request a PICU bed for Jayla."

E: "The first of the lab results are coming back as follows: CBC shows WBC 30.3, Hgb 14.5, Hct 44, platelets 330; BMP shows Na 138, K 5.0, Cl 108, CO_2 15, BUN 19, Cr 0.8, Glucose 85. The chest x-ray is normal."

C: "Ms. Smith, the lumbar puncture went very well. The fluid appeared as if it is infected and the cause of Jayla's fever. We gave him antibiotics for this when we first began the evaluation, but we will need to keep him in the hospital to continue to administer antibiotics and fluids through the IV if it is alright with you."

E: "Yes, whatever he needs to get better."

E: "Dr. Pediatron, the patient's primary physician, is on the phone."

C: "Hello Dr. Pediatron, this is Dr. Coole at ABEM General. I have Jayla Smith here. His mother brought him in with a fever and he appears to have meningitis. When he arrived he was very dehydrated. He is responding to fluids, but I think it would be best to at least observe him in the PICU overnight.

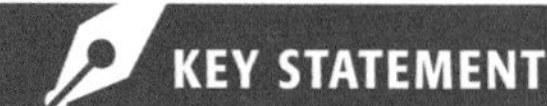

KEY STATEMENT

Remember to keep the patient (or in pediatric cases the family) updated about the lab results and the plan, and to get consent for any invasive procedures.

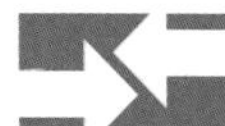

CRITICAL ACTION

Getting a LP on this patient with possible meningitis is a critical action. Although it is not a formal critical action, doing the rest of a septic workup is also appropriate.

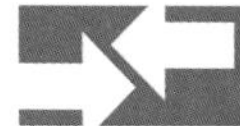

CRITICAL ACTION

Here the examinee completes the critical action of treating the patient with the appropriate antibiotics.

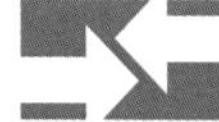

CRITICAL ACTION

There are two critical actions going on here—first, continued fluid resuscitation, and second, admission to the PICU.

KEY QUESTION

Remember to reassess your patient after every intervention to make sure you are on the right track.

Of note, his mother was treated for what is likely group B strep during her delivery so that may be the source of the infection. I also noticed there was blood in the spinal fluid that did not clear so I added acyclovir to the treatment regimen in case the infection is HSV related."

E: "That sounds fine. Thank you for the call."

E: "The nurse reports the second bolus is complete and the vital signs are as follows: T 37.5°C (99.6°F), HR 165, RR 60, BP 65/45, O_2 sat 98% on room air. Also, the PICU attending is on the phone."

C: "Nurse, please tell the PICU attending I will be with him momentarily. When I reexamine the child is he less lethargic? How are his pulses and cap refill? Is his tone improved?"

E: "The pulse is stronger with the cap refill brisk at approximately 2 seconds. The child's tone is improved and the nurse reports that he cried much more loudly when she was taking his last set of VS."

C: "Hello Dr. Picyou, this is Dr. Coole in the ER. There is 1-month-old male in the ER who presented severely dehydrated with a fever and likely meningitis. His mother was treated for group B strep during her delivery and the child has cloudy blood-tinged spinal fluid on LP. The child is responding to fluid therapy with increased tone and cry, and has received cefotaxime, ampicillin, vancomycin, and acyclovir here in the ER. Given the severity of the patient's dehydration, initial lethargy, and meningitis I would like him observed in the PICU."

E: "That sounds fine. Go ahead and send him upstairs."

E: "The Gram stain results are called up stat from the lab which reports the spinal fluid shows gram-positive bacteria in chains. The case is over."

CASE ASSESSMENT

The candidate efficiently handled a very straightforward case for a sick patient. The cases at ABEM General tend to be cases that test the fundamentals, and rarely will throw any completely unexpected curve balls at the candidate. With this in mind, the candidate needs to expeditiously proceed through the case making sure to nail down the basics.

This case presented a fever in a newborn, a common presentation in most emergency rooms (ERs). However, the child was exceptionally toxic and required immediate fluid resuscitation, in addition to moving through the usual steps of a septic workup. Failure to promptly administer fluid would have resulted in failure to pass the case and in the real world may have proved disastrous. Also, key to the case was continued reevaluation of the patient with attention toward whether he was improving. This child was in shock and had his status declined or not improved it would have possibly warranted intubation. The take home message is to always monitor the patient for response to interventions. Asking the nurse to report back when certain tasks are finished will help the candidate ensure reevaluation.

In addition to early fluids for the patient, early antibiotics for the patient are key to the case. As a rule begin therapeutic interventions as early as possible. Even though some institutions will try to perform a lumbar puncture (LP) prior to giving antibiotics, the rule of thumb is to treat as early as possible, especially when considering antibiotic therapy for meningitis. In this case there is a history that strongly suggests a group B strep infection. While the critical action in the case is to give the initial antibiotics (ampicillin and cefotaxime or gentamicin), the addition of vancomycin is appropriate and would help the candidate score higher for "style points" in the case. Also, the addition of acyclovir is appropriate in any toxic-appearing neonate with a fever, especially in the presence of a mother with known history of herpetic infection.

The candidate did well to keep the mother involved in the evolution of the case. Especially with pediatric patients, keeping the parents involved will help the treatment progress smoothly. Failure to communicate with the patients or their families will cause a deduction from communication points, and may even cause problems with characters in the case.

Critical Actions

1. Adequate IV fluid resuscitation.
2. Early antibiotic administration.
3. Obtaining appropriate birth history as well as history of maternal infection at birth (extra points for asking about maternal herpetic infection).
4. Performing a LP.
5. Admission to the pediatric intensive care unit (PICU).

Test Performance

1. *Data acquisition:* This phase is superb as the candidate shows the ability to obtain a more than adequate history and physical examination findings in an efficient manner, as well as ordering appropriate tests to assist in diagnosis. Score = **7**
2. *Problem solving:* The candidate is able to quickly assimilate data from the patient encounter and interprets test results and synthesizes information to direct further management. Score = **8**
3. *Patient management:* The candidate recognizes the need for early intravenous fluids (IVFs) and antibiotics in this ill-appearing child. Score = **7**
4. *Resource utilization:* The candidate demonstrates good use of resources with an efficient, cost-effective use of tests that does not compromise patient care. Score = **7**
5. *Health care provided (outcome):* The candidate asked appropriate questions to the mother helping to ensure his antimicrobial therapy was targeted and appropriate. Score = **7**
6. *Interpersonal relations and communication skills:* The candidate engaged in effective information exchange with the mother from the very beginning of the case asking for consent to place the IV. Score = **7**
7. *Comprehension of pathophysiology:* This candidate demonstrated a detailed and efficient investigatory and analytical approach to this sick child. Score = **7**
8. *Clinical competence (overall):* The candidate excelled in this case, quickly recognizing the severity of the child's illness and keeping the mother informed of his concerns. Score = **7**

CASE 10 6 y/o Female With Abdominal Pain

Navneet Cheema, Thomas J. Regan, and Aleksandr Gorenbeyn

INITIAL INFORMATION

Name: Golden Appy

Age: 6 years

Mode of arrival: Brought in by parents

Gender: Female

VS: T 37.7°C (99.9°F), BP 90/60, HR 110, RR 20, O_2 sat: 99% on RA

CC: Abdominal pain

PLAY OF THE CASE

C: "What do I see as I walk into the patient's room?"

E: "A little girl, appearing about 6 years of age, lying on the stretcher; she appears anxious. Her parents are standing beside the bed."

C: "Hello Golden, Mr. and Mrs. Appy, I am Dr. Lyme. How are you?"

E: "Child: My tummy hurts. Mother: She has complained about it since early this morning."

C: "Where in your stomach does it hurt, Golden?"

E: "All over."

C: "Have you been eating today?"

E: "Patient: No. Mother: She just ate a piece of toast this morning. She didn't touch her lunch."

C: "Has she vomited?"

E: "No."

C: "Has she been sick lately with any cold symptoms, sore throat, earache, or runny nose?"

E: "Oh, no. She's been quite healthy. She's rarely sick."

C: "Golden, can you tell me if anything else hurts you, like your back or legs?"

E: "I don't know. My tummy hurts."

C: "Did she have any bowel movements today? If so, were they normal?"

E: "She had one earlier this morning and it was normal."

C: "Has she been urinating today?"

E: "Yes, she has."

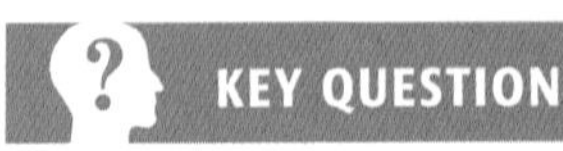

KEY QUESTION

Ask this open-ended question at the beginning of every case.

C: "Did you give her anything for pain at home?"

E: "No, I did not."

C: "Does she have any prior medical problems or surgeries?"

E: "No."

C: "Any medicines she takes regularly?"

E: "No."

C: "How about allergies?"

E: "She is allergic to amoxicillin. She took this for an ear infection a year ago, and she got hives."

C: "I would like to examine the patient. Is she in a hospital gown? How is her general appearance now? Is there respiratory distress? Is her color OK?"

E: "She is in a hospital gown. She appears slightly uncomfortable, but is now less anxious. Slightly pale but in no respiratory distress."

C: "Is she icteric? Are the mucous membranes moist? Is there tonsillar redness or exudates?"

E: "No icterus or tonsillar abnormalities; the mucous membranes are dry."

C: "Are the lungs clear? Are there any abnormal heart tones?"

E: "All normal."

C: "Are there any abnormal abdominal findings?"

E: "What would you like to know?"

C: "I would like to inspect her abdomen for appearance, particularly distention, listen for bowel sounds, and palpate for softness, masses, tenderness, guarding, or rebound tenderness."

E: "The abdomen is flat, soft, with bowel sounds present. The patient has some degree of voluntary guarding throughout and is tender peri-umbilically and bilaterally in the lower quadrants. No rebound tenderness is noted."

C: "I would like to do a rectal examination looking for masses or bleeding."

E: "It is normal with heme occult negative brown stool."

C: "Vascular examination of all extremities, including capillary refill?"

E: "Normal."

C: "Gross neurological examination?"

E: "Normal."

C: "Any skin rash, bruising, petechiae?"

E: "The mother asks: What do you think is wrong, doctor? She looks so uncomfortable."

C: "Well, I think she is a bit dehydrated and may need some IV fluid. I will need to order some blood tests and monitor her here in the ED for a while. This could be something as simple as stomach flu, but she may have something more serious like a bladder infection or appendicitis. It's too early to tell just yet."

E: "Will she go home?"

C: "She may, if she feels better and if her tests come out normal. Nurse, please start an IV on this patient, draw blood for labs and send CBC and electrolytes. Please give this patient a NS bolus at 20 cc/kg and obtain a UA. Please also repeat her vitals and report them back. Please also let me know about any changes in patient's condition."

E: "The orders are being done. Her vitals are T 37.7°C (100°F), BP 88/60, HR 112, RR 20. Doctor, she vomited twice in a row. Some liquid yellow stuff came up."

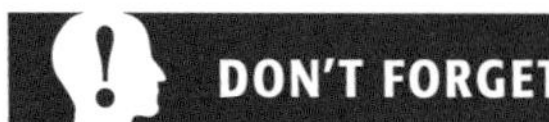

When the examiner states that an organ system is "normal" there is nothing more to look for on that part of the examination. If they state "what are you looking for" that means that there is a finding in that organ system that you should be looking for.

KEY ORDERS

Most of the patients you see during the exam will be unstable (or will become that way). Every unstable patient requires IV access (preferably two large-bore IVs), oxygen, and cardiac monitoring (always request to see a rhythm strip). In this case, giving IV fluids is also appropriate.

KEY ORDERS

Note how the examinee asks for the examiner to give them updates on the vitals and changes in the patient's condition. This places the responsibility for noticing any change in blood pressure or heart rate on the examiner, making it so that the examine does not need to remember to reassess as often—a good strategy!

 KEY QUESTION

Frequent reassessment of the patients is vital—in this case both vital signs and the patient's abdominal examination should be reassessed frequently.

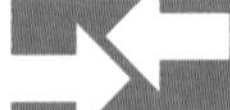 CRITICAL ACTION

There are two critical actions here—first, getting a surgeon involved, and second, treating the patient's pain.

 DON'T FORGET

While analgesia is not always a critical action, it will be in some cases. It is important to treat pain in all your patients.

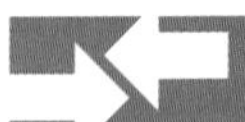 CRITICAL ACTION

Treating with the appropriate antibiotics and giving appropriate fluid resuscitation are both critical actions in this case.

 DON'T FORGET

When you do not know the dose of a medication off the top of your head, you can state that you will look it up or ask pharmacy to calculate it for you.

C: "I am back in the room. How does the patient look now?"

E: "More uncomfortable."

C: "I would like to reexamine her abdomen. Are there any changes from the previous examination? Is there localizing tenderness to the RLQ or elsewhere? Is there rebound tenderness?"

E: "She appears to be guarding more and her tenderness is localized to her right lower quadrant. She also has some localized rebound in the lower abdomen, right more than left. Some labs have returned, doctor, and the UA is normal."

C: "Golden seems to be developing signs of possible appendicitis. Nurse, please page a surgeon. I would also like to order an ultrasound of the abdomen and give the patient a dose of morphine for pain at 0.1 mg/kg IV."

E: "OK doctor, your orders are being done. Dr. Knife is busy in the OR and will call you back as soon as he is free. I have called in a tech to do an ultrasound. It will be an hour before she gets here."

C: "Can I have a new set of vitals on the patient?"

E: "Doctor, patient was crying in pain despite morphine and then vomited again and felt better. Her vitals now are T 38.8°C (102°F), HR 130, BP 80/55, RR 24."

C: "I would like to reexamine the patient's abdomen. What do I find now?"

E: "She is guarding, she is very tender in her lower abdominal quadrants, right greater than left. There is also now rebound tenderness in both lower quadrants."

C: "Golden may have ruptured her appendix. Let's give her another fluid bolus, repeat the dose of morphine and give her a dose of ceftriaxone and metronidazole. I will have to look up the exact dosing of these drugs."

E: "Mother: Is she going to be OK? Will you still need an ultrasound? Is the surgeon coming?"

C: "Mrs. Appy, I think you brought her here just in time. I think this is most likely appendicitis, and I think she might need surgery right away."

E: "Her blood work is back. Her WBC is 16,000. The rest of her CBC and Chem 7 are within normal limits."

E: "Dr. Knife is on the phone now."

C: "Dr. Knife, this is Dr. Lyme. I have a 6-year-old girl here who came in with nonspecific abdominal pain and anorexia and over last few hours progressed to fever, vomiting, RLQ abdominal pain and now has peritoneal signs. I suspect she has ruptured her appendix. Her white count is elevated at 16,000. I think she needs surgical intervention. I have given her a dose of antibiotics, both ceftriaxone and metronidazole."

E: "OK, I will be right down. This concludes this case."

CASE ASSESSMENT

This candidate managed this straightforward case very well. Appropriate history was taken and a likely differential was formulated. He tried to involve the patient in history telling to some extent, though given patient's young age, only limited information could be obtained. A good move was to ask the nurse to report any changes in the patient's condition. That allowed detecting the patients initial vomiting as well as changes in pain. The standard of care in diagnosis/management of appendicitis has been met. It includes clinical reexaminations while awaiting an ultrasound or a computed tomography (CT) in suspicious cases. Institution of pain control and antibiotics were satisfied once the diagnosis was made or when the patient developed peritoneal signs (as this patient did). Surgery was contacted early, but in the spirit of this an oral examination, only became available once surgical intervention was needed for certain.

KEY STATEMENT

Remember to always take a moment to keep the patient (and/or family) informed of lab results and pending procedures.

Critical Actions

1. Frequent reassessment of the abdominal examinations.
2. Initiate fluid resuscitation.
3. Judicious use of medications for pain relief.
4. Antibiotics to cover the gastrointestinal (GI) tract.
5. Surgical consult with emphasis on "selling" an acute appendicitis picture as most likely diagnosis.

CRITICAL ACTION

Admitting this patient to the OR is a critical action.

Test Performance

1. *Data acquisition:* The candidate did an outstanding job of data acquisition, especially serial abdominal examinations to detect changes in the patient condition. Score = **8**
2. *Problem solving:* Detailed and efficient investigation was displayed with good overall approach to the clinical picture. Score = **7**
3. *Patient management:* The candidate displayed strong clinical judgment with appropriate treatment decisions based upon available information and resources. Score = **7**
4. *Resource utilization:* The candidate had good use of resources, was cost-effective, and didn't compromise patient care. Score = **7**
5. *Health care provided (outcome):* The candidate appropriately escalated care as the patient's abdominal examination worsened. Score = **7**
6. *Interpersonal relations and communication skills:* Effective information exchange was demonstrated with the patient, the family, and the nurse. The explanations were clear and presented in a manner that was easily understandable. Score = **8**
7. *Comprehension of pathophysiology:* The candidate identified the most likely pathology early in the case and narrowed the differential effectively as more information as available. Score = **7**
8. *Clinical competence (overall):* The candidate did an excellent job managing a classic case of appendicitis and particularly excelled at data acquisition and communication. Score = **7**

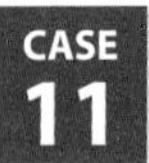

CASE 11 90 y/o Male With Headache

Navneet Cheema and Fiona Gallahue

INITIAL INFORMATION

Name: Noah Calhoun

Mode of arrival: Ambulance

Age: 90 years

Gender: Male

VS: T 37.8°C (100.1°F), BP 160/80, HR 106, RR 20, O_2 sat: 98% on RA

CC: Headache

PLAY OF THE CASE

C: "What do I see as I walk into the patient's room?"

E: "The patient is a well-nourished male, who appears uncomfortable, clutching his head while sitting upright on the stretcher."

C: "Hello, Mr. Calhoun, I'm Dr. C. What seems to be the matter today?"

E: "Hi doctor, I have a headache that won't go away. It's lasted for the past 12 hours and is getting worse."

C: "Can you tell me a little bit more about your headache—where do you feel it and have you ever had headaches before?"

E: "The headache is all over my head though may be worse along the front, I don't usually get headaches."

C: "Would you say this is the worst headache of your life?"

E: "Well, not exactly the worst but it's the most constant."

C: "Can you tell me how the headache began? Did it come on all of a sudden or more gradually?"

E: "More gradually."

C: "Do you see anything unusual with your headaches such as flashing lights or colors?"

E: "No, nothing like that."

C: "Have you been feeling generally ill? Have you noticed a fever, joint or muscle pains, any rashes, or anything else new?"

E: "I've been feeling hot sometimes and a little run down but I haven't taken my temperature to see if I have a fever. I haven't noticed any rashes, muscle or joint pains, or anything else unusual."

C: "Have you taken any medications to help with the pain?"

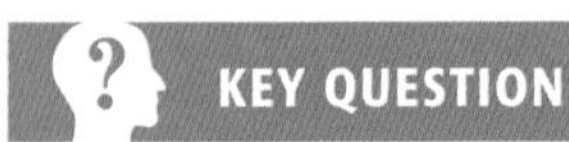

KEY QUESTION

Ask this open-ended question at the beginning of every case.

E: "I've been taking ibuprofen, but it doesn't seem to be helping."

C: "Have you had any recent travel anywhere outside of the country or been hiking recently."

E: "No, I really don't travel much and I haven't been hiking in years. Doc, I hate to ask, but could you please give me something for pain?"

C: "Certainly, but I'd like a little more information first, do you have any allergies?"

E: "None that I know of."

C: "Do you have any medical problems?"

E: "Diabetes, osteoarthritis, and high cholesterol."

C: "Do you take any medications including herbal medications or over-the-counter medications?"

E: "I take glipizide and simvastatin; I've also been taking ibuprofen for the headache."

C: "Do you have any family history of headaches? Any family history of migraines or aneurysms?"

E: "No."

C: "Do you use alcohol?"

E: "I drink a beer sometimes with my friends but not every night."

C: "Do you smoke or use any drugs?"

E: "No."

C: "Where do you live? Do you live alone?"

E: "No, I live in an assisted care facility since I have some trouble walking around these days."

C: "Do you have a doctor at this hospital?"

E: "Yes, Dr. Smith is my internist."

C: "Sir, I'd like to give you something for your pain now as well as get some blood from you to help me evaluate you. Nurse, I'd like to get the patient on oxygen at 2 L NC. I'd also like to put him on a cardiac monitor. I'd also like you to place an 18-gauge IV, give him 500 cc of NS, draw blood for CBC, electrolytes, PT/PTT, and a type and screen. I'd like a 12-lead ECG, a CXR, and a non-contrast head CT. I'd also like a rectal temperature on Mr. Calhoun and please let me know what the temperature is. Could you also please give Mr. Calhoun 30 mg of IV ketorolac? Thank you. Mr. Calhoun, I'd like to examine you now."

E: "OK."

C: "I'd like to examine the patient now. On HEENT, does he have any nuchal rigidity, moist mucous membranes, and any evidence of pharyngitis and see if he has papilledema on funduscopic examination?"

E: "He does have nuchal rigidity on examination, no papilledema, and an otherwise normal HEENT examination."

C: "Before I continue my examination, I'd like to place the patient on respiratory isolation in case he has bacterial meningitis."

E: "OK, that's been done. The nurse wants to let you know that the patient's rectal temperature is 103.5°F."

C: "Thank you, please give the patient 1 g of acetaminophen for his fever, would you also draw two sets of blood cultures and send a UA and urine culture. I'm going to continue with my examination now. What do I hear when I listen to his heart and his lungs?"

E: "The cardiac and pulmonary examinations are normal."

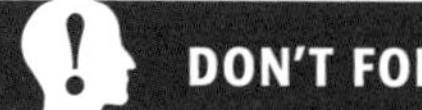

DON'T FORGET

While analgesia is not always a critical action, it will be in some cases. Err on the side of caution and treat pain in all your patients.

KEY ORDERS

Most of the patients you see during the exam will be unstable (or will become that way). Every patient requires IV access (preferably two large-bore IVs), oxygen, and cardiac monitoring (always request to see a rhythm strip). In this case, as the history has already been taken, getting labs and a head CT is also indicated.

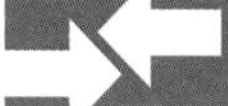

CRITICAL ACTION

Getting a head CT without contrast is a critical action in this elderly patient with a new headache.

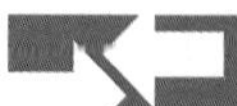

CRITICAL ACTION

Placing this patient with possible bacterial meningitis in isolation is a critical action.

C: "I'd like to do an abdominal examination."

E: "His abdominal examination is normal."

C: "I'd like to make sure he's completely undressed and examine his extremities and skin."

E: "He's undressed, what are you looking for?"

C: "I'd like to see if he has any petechiae, purpura, bruising, or joint swelling."

E: "His skin examination is normal. He has no joint swelling or bruising."

C: "I'd also like to look for a Kernig and Brudzinski sign."

E: "How would you do that?"

C: "I'd see if I could straighten the patient's leg to a position of full knee extension when the patient is lying supine with the hip flexed to a right angle to check for a Kernig sign. There are two Brudzinski signs so I'd check to see if the patient had either of them by seeing if the patient flexes at the hips when I flex the patient's neck or by seeing if the patient flexes the opposite hip when I try to flex the hip on one side."

E: "The patient has both Kernig and Brudzinski signs."

C: "OK, I'm really concerned that the patient may have bacterial meningitis now and I'd like to give the patient antibiotics to cover him for bacterial meningitis."

E: "What would you like to give the patient?"

C: "I'd like to give the patient ceftriaxone, vancomycin, as well as ampicillin to cover possible *Listeria*; I will give these medications at the standard doses as dictated by my pharmacy or by a pharmacopeia or PDR that I have available at ABEM General. I would also like to give this patient dexamethasone 10 mg IV with his antibiotics."

E: "That is being done. Radiology is ready to take your patient for his CT and x-ray."

C: "OK, but I'd like to make sure that he is wearing a mask and that full respiratory precautions are taken with him."

E: "That's being taken care of."

C: "Do I have his ECG here?"

E: "Yes, it's a normal ECG with sinus rhythm at a rate of 99, normal axis, no ST elevations or depressions."

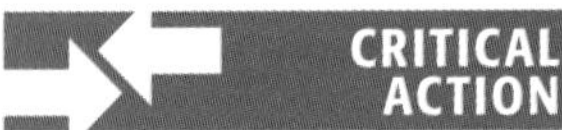

Giving this patient empiric antibiotics before sending him to CT is a critical action in this case.

C: "Are any of his laboratories back yet?"

E: (Shows candidate the laboratories for the patient):

CBC: WBC of 13,000, 75% neutrophils, 15% bands, H/H 13/39, plt 180

PT 12 (INR 1.0), PTT 28

BMP: Na 140, K 4.0, Cl 116, CO_2 18, BUN 18, Cr 1.2, Glu 230, Ca 8.9

UA: Normal

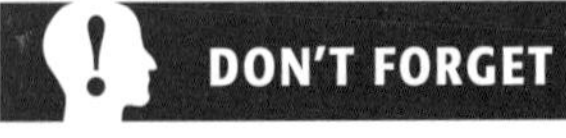

When you do not know the dose of a medication off the top of your head, you can state that you will look it up or ask pharmacy to calculate it for you.

C: "Is the patient back from radiology yet?"

E: "Yes."

C: "Do I have his head CT and CXR read?"

E: "His head CT is read as normal with age-related atrophy for age, his CXR is also normal."

C: "Has the patient received his antibiotics?"

E: "They're being given now."

C: "Mr. Calhoun, I'd like to do a lumbar puncture on you because I'm concerned that you may have meningitis and I'd like to be sure."

E: "What is a lumbar puncture and are there any risks involved?"

C: "I need to insert a needle into your back between your lumbar vertebrae in order to remove the fluid that surrounds the brain and check for evidence of infection. The risks involved are pain from the needle although I will give you numbing medicine to help prevent too much discomfort, bleeding from the needle site, and the possibility of introducing infection into the fluid from the skin."

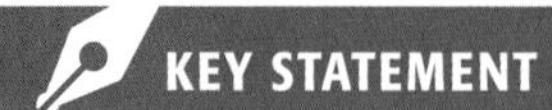

Informing the patient about test results, answering their questions, and getting informed consent are important to get full credit in the interpersonal relations and communication skills category.

E: "The patient agrees to the procedure."

C: "OK, I'm going to do a LP on the patient, what does the fluid look like?"

E: "It's turbid."

C: "I'm going to send the fluid for cells, glucose, protein, Gram stain, and culture."

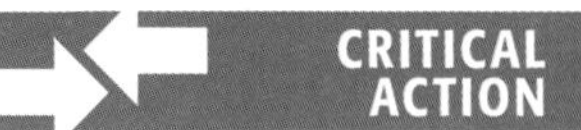

Getting a LP to rule out (or in) meningitis is a critical action in this case.

E: "That's done."

C: "I'm going to call Dr. Smith to admit him to the hospital."

E: "Dr. Smith is on the phone."

C: "Dr. Smith, this is Dr. C, I wanted to speak to you about your patient Noah Calhoun. He's a 90-year-old man who is complaining of a severe headache for the past 12 hours, he's febrile to 103.5°F here with nuchal rigidity and Kernig and Brudzinski signs. I gave him ceftriaxone, vancomycin, and ampicillin here. His CT head was normal and I performed a LP with cloudy fluid return consistent with bacterial meningitis. I believe he needs to be admitted to the hospital to an isolation room for probable bacterial meningitis."

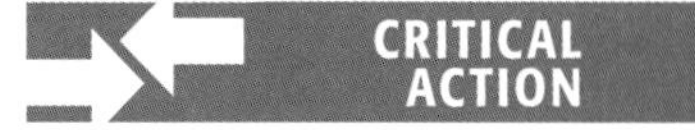

Admitting this patient to the hospital is a critical action in this case.

E: "That sounds like a reasonable plan, please admit him to my service, thank you. This case is now over."

CASE ASSESSMENT

Overall, the candidate did very well on this case. She was able to move through the case rapidly, getting a good history and physical once she determined the patient appeared not to need any stabilization of his airway, breathing, or circulation. She demonstrated her ability to narrow down the differential of headache fairly rapidly with a good history and physical. She was able to address the patient's concerns and communicate with the patient and nurse appropriately to address the patient's needs. She also demonstrated an ability to discuss the case concisely to another physician.

The candidate met the standard of care for treating meningitis by identifying it early, treating with intravenous (IV) antibiotics immediately and isolating the patient. Although she didn't know the doses of the antibiotics she needed, she demonstrated an ability to find the information, which is appropriate on exam day.

Notice that the case was over before the lumbar puncture (LP) results were returned. As long as the patient is being treated appropriately, do not worry if this happens. Often, the diagnosis is clear from the patient's presentation and a few additional historical or clinical factors. Not every single test needs to come back if the diagnosis is clear and the patient is receiving appropriate treatment.

There are potential debates about the best antibiotics to manage this patient given the emergence of *Listeria monocytogenes* in the elderly patients (although *Streptococcus pneumoniae* is still by far, the leading cause of bacterial meningitis in the over-60 age group). In the oral board examinations, there is no time to get stuck on these issues. If you are unsure of the appropriate antibiotics to give the patient, ask for an ID consultation or tell the examiners that you will check with your Sanford guide or any other infectious disease guide you may use clinically and move on! It is very important not to let yourself get stuck on anything and keep moving through the scenario.

There were a few minor areas where the candidate could have done better. She did not readdress the patient's pain after giving ketorolac to ensure the pain was adequately managed. The candidate also could have rechecked vital signs on the patient during the scenario to see if the initial abnormalities were improving. Lastly, the candidate should have checked a rectal temperature earlier since the patient was borderline febrile on the triage vital signs. These are common mistakes given the rapid pace of the oral board cases and would not significantly affect the candidate's overall score. Remember that examinees do not need to give perfect care in order to pass but need to demonstrate that they can follow the standard of care.

Critical Actions

1. Placing the patient in respiratory isolation.
2. Early antibiotic therapy for bacterial meningitis before the computed tomography (CT) scan.
3. Head CT scan to R/O space occupying lesion, eg, abscess.
4. LP if CT permits.
5. Admitting the patient.

Test Performance

1. *Data acquisition:* The candidate showed the ability to obtain an excellent history and physical examination as well as ordering appropriate tests to assist in diagnosis. Score = **7**
2. *Problem solving:* The candidate was able to synthesize data from the patient encounter and test results in order to direct management appropriately. Score = **8**
3. *Patient management:* The candidate initiated antibiotics and steroids early and obtained a CT scan prior to LP. Pain management could have improved as the patient was given ketorolac, but there was no reevaluation of his pain. Score = **7**
4. *Resource utilization:* The candidate demonstrated appropriate use of resources using the PDR in the department to look up appropriate medication dose and also demonstrated cost-effective care with targeted diagnostics. Score = **8**
5. *Health care provided (outcome):* There was early recognition of a life threat in this case, which allowed for expedited antibiotics and care for the patient. Score = **8**

6. *Interpersonal relations and communication skills:* The candidate demonstrated an excellent ability to exchange information with the patient, the nurse, and the private physician in this scenario. She was responsive to the patient's questions and concerns. Score = **8**
7. *Comprehension of pathophysiology:* The candidate demonstrated her knowledge of the most common causes of meningitis by ordering appropriate antibiotics, including *Listeria monocytogenes* coverage in this elderly patient. Score = **8**
8. *Clinical competence (overall):* This case was excellently managed with early diagnosis, efficient care, and effective patient communication. Score = **8**

CASE 12 50 y/o Female Dialysis Patient With Fever

Navneet Cheema and Fiona Gallahue

INITIAL INFORMATION

Name: Cynthia Cannon

Mode of arrival: Ambulance

Age: 50 years

Gender: Female

VS: T 39.4°C (103°F), BP 90/50, HR 120, RR 20, weight: 65 kg, O_2 sat: 97% on RA

CC: Fever

PLAY OF THE CASE

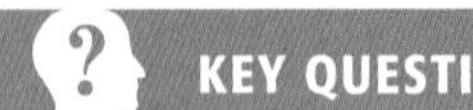

KEY QUESTION

Ask this open-ended question at the beginning of every case.

C: "What do I see when I come into the room?"

E: "The patient is sitting on the stretcher, appears comfortable but she is diaphoretic."

C: "Nurse, I'd like to have this patient on oxygen via NC at 2 L, I'd also like her placed on a cardiac monitor and to get a 12-lead ECG. I'd like to see the ECG or a rhythm strip as soon as it is available. I'd like you to place an 18-gauge IV, give the patient 250 cc bolus of NS and draw blood for CBC, electrolytes including Mg and phosphate, BUN, Cr, PT/PTT, and type and screen as well as two sets of blood cultures please. I'd like to check an ABG and a lactate on this patient. I'd also like to give her 1 g of acetaminophen if she has no allergies. Would you please repeat the vital signs after the NS bolus and let me know the results?"

KEY ORDERS

Most of the patients you see during the exam will be unstable (or will become that way). Every unstable patient requires IV access (preferably two large-bore IVs), oxygen, and cardiac monitoring (always request to see a rhythm strip). In this case, as the patient is hypotensive, tachycardic, and febrile, sepsis is high on your differential, and sending cultures, giving IVF and acetaminophen is also appropriate at this time.

E: "Those orders are being carried out. The ECG shows a sinus tachycardia at 115, normal axis, and normal QRS, ST segments, and T waves."

C: "Hello Ms. Cannon, I'm Dr. Macabeem, what brought you to the hospital today?"

E: "Well, I was at dialysis today and when they checked my temperature before I was leaving, they told me I had a fever and that I needed to come to the hospital so here I am."

C: "Did you finish your full dialysis?"

E: "Yes."

C: "How do you feel—have you been feeling ill, have you noticed any fevers at home?"

E: "I feel a little tired but otherwise OK and I haven't noticed any fevers before the dialysis center."

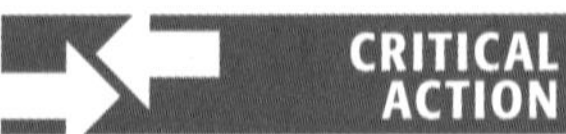

CRITICAL ACTION

Giving fluids to this hypotensive and febrile patient is a critical action.

C: "Do you get dialysis regularly?"

E: "Yes, I go every Monday, Wednesday, and Friday like clockwork, I haven't missed dialysis in a long time."

C: "Do you produce urine?"

E: "No."

C: "Have you had any shortness of breath, sore throat, or cough?"

E: "No."

C: "Have you had any abdominal pain, nausea, or vomiting?"

E: "No."

C: "Have you noticed any rashes?"

E: "No, not really."

C: "Any areas of tenderness on your body?"

E: "Well, my access site was a little more tender than usual when I was getting hemodialysis today." "The nurse would like to let you know that the patient's repeat BP is 100/60, HR 105, RR 18, T 37.7°C (100°F)."

C: "Thank you. Can you please give Ms. Cannon a repeat bolus of 250 cc of fluid if her lung sounds are normal? Do I have the results of my ABG and lactate level?"

E: "Her ABG is back, the lactate is pending."

ABG: pH 7.30, Po_2 120, Pco_2 40, BE −6, HCO_2 18, O_2 sat 98%

C: "Thank you. Ms. Cannon, do you have any medical problems besides kidney failure?"

E: "I have high blood pressure and anemia."

C: "Do you take any medications for your blood pressure?"

E: "I take atenolol, epoetin, and some vitamins that my doctor prescribed."

C: "Do you have any allergies to any medications?"

E: "No."

C: "Do you have a regular doctor?"

E: "Well, I have a kidney doctor, Dr. Smith and a vascular doctor who placed my access catheter, Dr. Cutter."

C: "Do you drink alcohol, smoke cigarettes, or use any drugs?"

E: "No." "Doctor, the nurse would like you to know that the patient has a BP of 110/70, HR 90, T 37.7°C (100.0°F), RR 18."

C: "Thank you. Nurse, I'd like to get a CXR on Ms. Cannon and give her 1 g of vancomycin and 80 mg of gentamicin after her blood cultures are drawn. Could we please give the patient another bolus, 250 cc of NS if her lungs sound clear? I'd also like to get Ms. Cannon's old records to find out all of her medications and a BP after the fluid bolus."

E: "Those orders are being carried out."

C: "Ms. Cannon, I'd like to examine you now."

E: "OK."

C: "What do I see on HEENT examination?"

E: "What are you looking for?"

C: "I'm looking for moist mucous membranes, pharyngeal erythema or exudates, evidence of an odontogenic infection, JVD, lymphadenopathy."

E: "She has moist mucous membranes, no pharyngeal erythema or exudates, no evidence of odontogenic infection, and no JVD; she does have anterior lymphadenopathy."

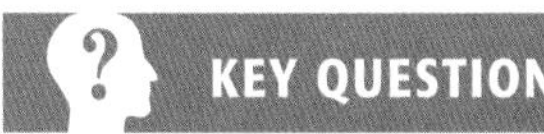

Remember to reassess your patient frequently—especially when they have unstable vital signs, or after a vasoactive intervention such as giving fluids or blood pressure meds.

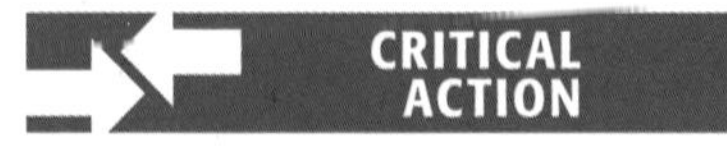

Giving antibiotics and continuing fluid resuscitation to this septic patient is a critical action in this case.

C: "What do I see on her chest examination?"

E: "What are you looking for?"

C: "I'd like to listen to her heart for evidence of a murmur, gallop, friction rub, and distant heart sounds and I'm listening to her lungs for any evidence of rales, rhonchi, or crackles."

E: "Her heart and lungs are normal."

C: "What is her abdominal examination like?"

E: "Normal, no tenderness, no rebound, normal bowel sounds."

C: "I'd like to do a rectal examination and look for any evidence of a perirectal abscess and guaiac the patient."

E: "Her rectal examination is normal, no evidence of a perirectal abscess, and she is guaiac negative with brown stool."

C: "What do I see when I look at her extremities, especially does she have an AV fistula?"

E: "Her extremities are normal with no clubbing, cyanosis, or edema and she does not have an AV fistula."

C: "What do I see on her dermatologic examination?"

E: "What are you looking for?"

C: "I'm looking for any rashes especially petechiae or purpura, I'm looking for any evidence of cellulitis, I'm looking for a vascular access catheter to see if there is any evidence of infection there."

E: "She has no petechiae or purpura; she does have a double lumen catheter located at the right third ICS, mid-clavicular line. There is surrounding erythema, warmth, and tenderness to palpation."

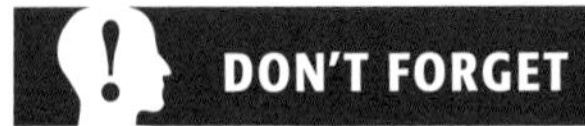

DON'T FORGET

When the examiner states that one part of the exam is "normal" that means that there is probably nothing important going on in that organ system. When they say, "What are you looking for?" that usually indicates that there is a finding that is relevant.

C: "Is there any fluctuance to the area?"

E: "No."

C: "First I'd like to remove the catheter and send the tip for culture, then I'd like to get her doctors, Dr. Smith and Dr. Cutter on the phone and I'd like to make sure that the patient has received her antibiotics. Do I have any of her laboratories, her CXR, or her old chart?"

E: "Here are her results, her old chart is unavailable and her repeat BP is 130/70."

CBC: WBC 15,300, 75% neutrophils, 15% bands, H/H 10/30, Platelets 260

PT 15 (INR 1.6), PTT 39

BMP: Na 140, K 4.0, Cl 106, CO_2 15, BUN 60, Cr 6.5, Glu 120, Ca 6.9,

Mg 2.8

PO_4 5.5

Lactate 4.3

CRITICAL ACTION

Doing a thorough history and physical to identify the source of infection (including UA in patients who make urine and a CXR) is a critical action in any septic patient.

CXR: No effusions or infiltrates seen, vascular access catheter visualized at the right subclavian vein.

E: "Dr. Smith is on the phone for you, Dr. Macabeem."

C: "Hello, Dr. Smith, this is Dr. Macabeem, I'd like to talk to you about your patient, Cynthia Cannon. She came in after receiving dialysis for evaluation of a fever to 39.4°C (103°F) here. She was tachycardic to 120 on triage, hypotensive with a BP of 90/50 initially which responded to three fluid boluses of 250 cc each. Her BP now is 130/70 with a HR of 105. She has no complaints indicating a source of infection except for tenderness around her dialysis catheter. On examination, she has evidence of a vascular access catheter infection with surrounding erythema, warmth, and tenderness to palpation. Her ECG was normal except for sinus tachycardia. Her labs show a white count of 15K with a left shift and anemia with a Hgb of 10 and a Hct of 30. We've drawn blood cultures and started the patient on vancomycin and gentamicin. I believe that she has a line infection with possible early sepsis. I removed the catheter and sent the tip for culture. I think she needs to be admitted for antibiotics, observation, and a new access catheter when the infection is clearing up. Although she seems to be getting better, I am worried about her hypotension initially as well as her elevated lactate and acidosis, I'd like to admit her to the ICU."

E: "I agree, please admit her to my service, her usual blood pressure is 150/80 so 130/70 is still low for her. Would you also notify her vascular surgeon, Dr. Cutter, so that he can see her as well?"

C: "Certainly."

E: "Dr. Cutter is on the phone for you, Dr. Macabeem."

C: "Hello Dr. Cutter, this is Dr. Macabeem. I am calling you for a consult regarding your patient, Cynthia Cannon. She came in with a fever today and appears to have a line infection with erythema, warmth, tenderness to the site. I've given her antibiotics, removed the line, and spoken to her primary doctor, Dr. Smith, who will admit her but we'd like for you to see and follow the patient as well."

E: "I'd be happy to, I'm currently in the OR, can I see her in 3 hours when I'm out?"

C: "Yes, that would be fine, thank you. I'd like to call the ICU consultant for this patient."

E: "Dr. Brown is on the line for you."

C: "Hello Dr. Brown, this is Dr. Macabeem. I have a patient of Dr. Smith's, a 50-year-old dialysis patient by the name of Cynthia Cannon. She has a history of ESRD and HTN. She came from dialysis today with a fever, hypotension, and evidence of a line infection. She has a metabolic acidosis with an elevated lactate. She's received three 250 cc boluses of NS, had the line removed and sent for culture, she also has blood cultures pending, and been started on vancomycin and gentamicin. I believe she needs to be observed in the ICU although she appears to be improving and is now normotensive at 130/70 which is still not her baseline BP of 150/80."

E: "That seems reasonable, I agree. Thank you. That concludes this case."

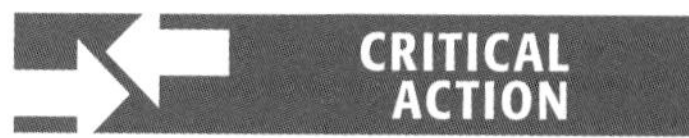

Admitting this septic patient to the ICU is a critical action.

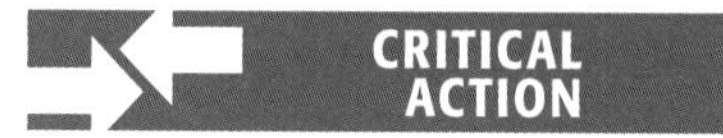

Getting vascular surgery involved for replacement of the patient's dialysis line is a critical action in this case.

CASE ASSESSMENT

Overall, the candidate managed this case extremely well. The candidate addressed the potentially life-threatening concerns quickly, cautiously treating the hypotension with fluids and asking for repeat vital signs and a directed physical examination after each intervention. While stabilizing this patient, she completed a very thorough history and physical examination appropriately given the potential for multiple reasons for the hypotension such as gastrointestinal (GI) bleed, sepsis, or overdialysis of the patient. The candidate came up with an appropriate assessment and plan after her history and physical. She was able to coordinate the PMD and the consultant appropriately to get the patient the necessary care.

Notice that the examiner often asked specifically what the candidate was looking for during the physical examination and did not offer additional information than what was requested. During the chest examination, the candidate did not ask for a superficial examination of the chest and so, only received an examination of the heart and lungs but not any information about the dialysis catheter present in the right chest. The candidate did not receive this information until the dermatologic examination when she specifically requested information about a dialysis catheter. If the examiner asks you what you are looking for specifically, try to be as comprehensive as possible with your verbal request for information since it is likely that there is an abnormality there.

Another issue in this scenario is that the candidate never tells the patient what her concerns are for the patient's health or why she is receiving antibiotics and requires admission. While the candidate will pass the scenario since she met standard of care in treating this patient, she might lose a few points on interpersonal relations and communication skills.

Critical Actions

1. Addressing the patient's hypotension appropriately with fluid resuscitation.
2. Appropriate history and physical to look for source of the infection—specifically looking for signs of a line infection.
3. Prompt IV antibiotics.
4. Admission to an intensive care unit (ICU) setting.
5. Obtaining a vascular surgery consult.

Test Performance

1. *Data acquisition:* The candidate showed the ability to obtain an excellent history and physical examination with attention to identifying a source for the patient's abnormal vital signs. Score = **8**
2. *Problem solving:* The candidate was able to assimilate data from the patient encounter and was able to interpret test results and synthesize information to direct further study. Score = **7**
3. *Patient management:* The candidate did an excellent job being appropriately cautious with intravenous fluids (IVFs) in a patient with end-stage renal disease (ESRD), being sure to reexamine for fluid overload prior to subsequent boluses. Score = **8**
4. *Resource utilization:* The candidate demonstrated appropriate use of resources and consultants. Score = **8**
5. *Health care provided (outcome):* The care provided was efficient, appropriate, and judicious. Score = **7**
6. *Interpersonal relations and communication skills:* The candidate interacted very well with the consultants, providing appropriate information to each to manage the case. She did not provide the patient with any details regarding her management, including her concern for sepsis and need for antibiotics and an ICU admission. Score = **6**
7. *Comprehension of pathophysiology:* The candidate had a clear approach to her care of a septic patient, which demonstrated her understanding of the underlying pathophysiology. Score = **7**
8. *Clinical competence (overall):* This case was managed very well with the early identification of a source of infection in a septic patient, appropriate IVF and antibiotic administration. The candidate could have improved her communications skills by updating the patient more frequently. Score = **7**

CASE 13 44 y/o Male With Hypotension

Navneet Cheema and Alan Kumar

INITIAL INFORMATION

Name: Rob Hart

Mode of arrival: Ambulance

Age: 44 years

Gender: Male

VS: T 37.2°C, BP 75/60, HR 110, RR 24, O_2 sat: 98% on RA

PLAY OF THE CASE

C: "What do I see as I walk into the patient's room?"

E: "The patient is a thin male who is resting quietly on the stretcher though he appears moderately short of breath."

C: "Have the nurse start a large-bore IV, draw and hold blood work for possible tests, place the patient on 2 L O_2 by NC, place him on a cardiac monitor, and get me a 12-lead ECG. Please start a 1 L NS IV bolus."

C: "Mr. Hart, what brings you to the ED today?"

E: "I have been feeling very weak today. I am undergoing chemotherapy for lung cancer and my last treatment was 2 days ago but I have never felt this weak with the past treatments."

C: "Are you eating OK? Any vomiting? Diarrhea?"

E: "Yeah, no problems eating or drinking. I have not been throwing up. The only thing I have noticed is that I'm getting really winded with any activity recently. I'm feeling short of breath just lying here."

C: "Is your shortness of breath worse when you lie flat?"

E: "No."

C: "Any fevers or cough?"

E: "No."

C: "Any chest pain?"

E: "No."

C: "Any leg pain or swelling?"

E: "No."

C: "Any other medical problems?"

E: "I've been pretty depressed since I found out I had this 4 months ago."

C: "What medications are you on?"

E: "Just a multivitamin a day."

C: "Any allergies to medications?"

E: "No allergies."

KEY QUESTION

Ask this open-ended question at the beginning of every case.

KEY ORDERS

Most of the patients you see during the exam will be unstable (or will become that way). Every unstable patient requires IV access (preferably two large-bore IVs), oxygen, and cardiac monitoring (and in most cases an ECG). In this case, as the patient is hypotensive, starting a fluid bolus is also appropriate at this time.

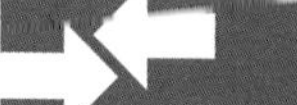

CRITICAL ACTION

Giving a bolus of IV fluids is a critical action in this hypotensive patient.

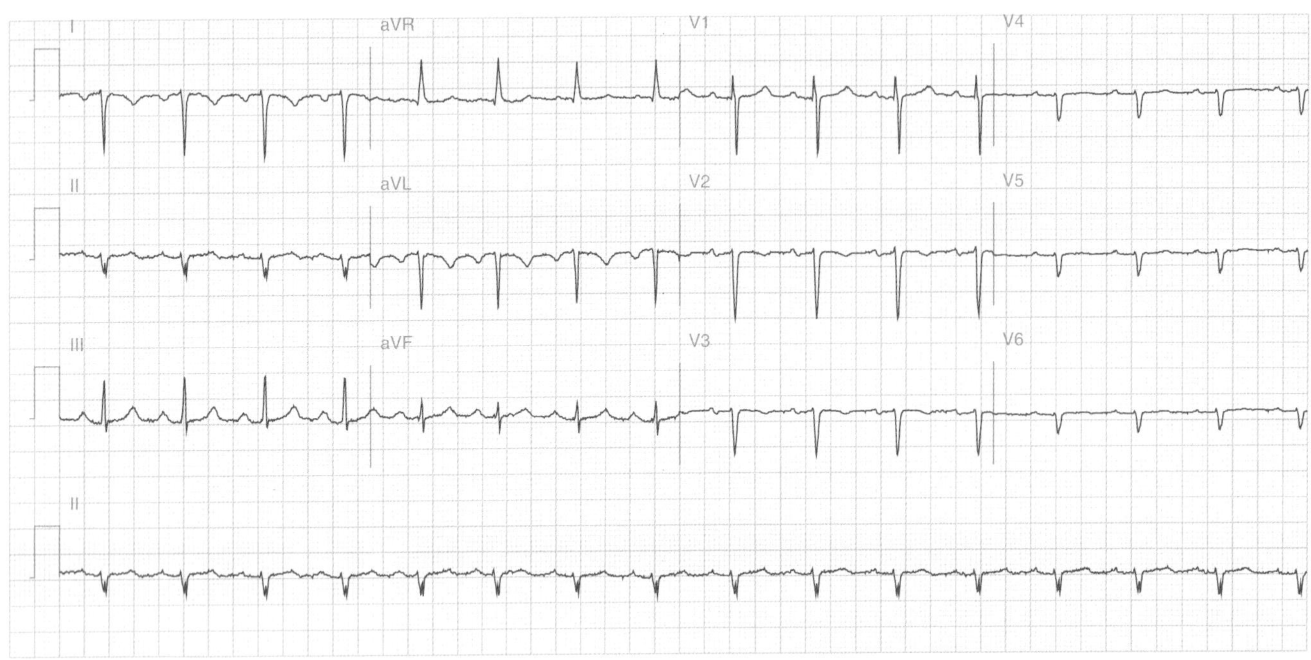

Figure C13-1. The ECG shows sinus tachycardia with low QRS voltages otherwise normal. *(Reprinted with permission from Fauci AS, Kasper DL, Braunwald E, et al.* Harrison's Principles of Internal Medicine. *17th ed. New York, NY: McGraw-Hill; 2008.)*

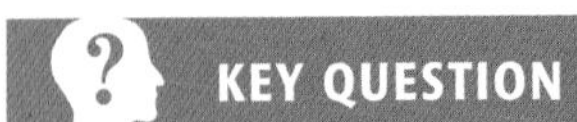

Remember to always ask your AMPLE questions on an unstable patient—**A**llergies, **M**edications, **P**ast medical history, **L**ast meal, and **E**vents (HPI).

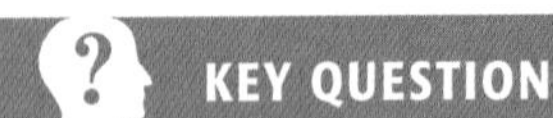

Remember to reassess your patient frequently—especially if they are unstable.

C: "I'd like to examine the patient."

E: "The nurse informs you the IV is started and the bolus is running. The patient is on the monitor, O_2 is started, and here is your ECG (Fig. C13-1)."

C: "I would like to order a stat portable chest x-ray. Please send off blood work for a chem-7, CBC, and PT/PTT."

C: "What are the repeat vital signs?"

E: "Vitals are unchanged."

C: "What is the HEENT examination?"

E: "Pupils are reactive, TMs are normal, and the oropharynx is clear with moist mucous membranes."

C: "How is the neck examination?"

E: "What would you like to know?"

C: "Is there JVD? Tracheal deviation? Is the neck supple? Is there lymphadenopathy?"

E: "There is no LAD or tracheal deviation. The neck is supple. Neck veins are distended."

C: "Lung examination?"

E: "Lungs are clear."

C: "Heart examination?"

E: "What would you like to know?"

C: "What is the rate? Are there any murmurs, rubs, or gallops? How are the heart sounds?"

E: "Tachycardic rate, no obvious murmurs, heart sounds are distant. Normal S_1, S_2."

C: "Abdominal examination?"

E: "The abdomen is soft, non-tender, non-distended. No organomegaly."

C: "Extremities?"

E: "Range of motion is normal, no joint swelling or tenderness, distal pulses are weak. There is no calf tenderness or swelling."

C: "Neuro examination?"

E: "The patient is awake and alert but is slow to answer questions. The rest of the neuro examination is non-focal."

C: "Do I have my chest x-ray yet?"

E: "The 1 L bolus of fluid has finished. Here is your CXR (Fig. C13-2)."

C: "What are the vital signs?"

E: "HR 105, BP 80/70, RR 24."

C: "I would like to perform a bedside ultrasound."

E: "The ultrasound machine is brought to bedside. What would you like to do?"

C: "I would like to take a look at the cardiac activity and pericardial space using the sub-xiphoid approach."

E: "The ultrasound reveals a large pericardial effusion."

C: "Please place the patient on high-flow O_2 via face mask, call the cardiologist on call, and ask for a CCU bed for this patient."

KEY QUESTION

Remember to reassess your patient frequently—especially after an intervention such as fluids or vasoactive medications.

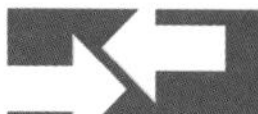

CRITICAL ACTION

Recognizing the possibility of cardiac tamponade and getting a bedside ultrasound is a critical action in this case.

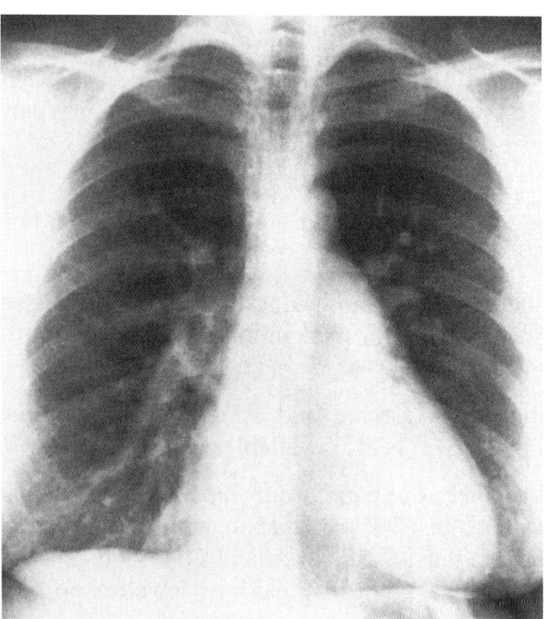

Figure C13-2. The Chest x-ray shows mild cardiomegaly and otherwise normal. *(Reprinted with permission from Chen MYM, Pope Jr. TL, Ott DJ.* Basic Radiology. *New York, NY: McGraw-Hill; 2004.)*

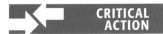

CRITICAL ACTION

There are two critical actions here: (1) calling cardiology for this pericardial effusion and (2) ordering a CCU bed as your disposition.

C: "Can you also call for a formal echocardiogram to be done? Continue the fluid at 500 cc/h of NS."

E: "The bed request is entered. The patient is wondering what is going on."

C: "Mr. Hart, you have developed fluid filling the sac that contains the heart and that is making it difficult for your heart to pump properly. I am going to talk to a cardiologist who might have to withdraw some of that fluid to make you feel better."

E: "That sounds dangerous, doc."

C: "It can be, but they usually do the procedure under the guidance of the ultrasound machine I just used which makes it a much safer procedure."

E: "Thanks, doc."

E: "The cardiologist is on the phone."

CRITICAL ACTION

Doing an emergent pericardiocentesis on this crashing patient is a critical action.

C: "Hello, This is Dr. C at ABEM General. I have a 44-year-old male with a lung cancer history who presents complaining of weakness with a noted blood pressure of 85/70 who on examination had distended neck veins and distant heart sounds. The ECG showed low voltages, the chest x-ray showed mild cardiomegaly, and a bedside ultrasound performed by myself shows a large pericardial effusion. I think the patient has cardiac tamponade and needs an urgent pericardiocentesis. I have put him in for an ICU bed."

E: "I'm on my way in."

E: "The nurse informs you that the patient is now unconscious and the BP has dropped to 50/40."

C: "Start fluids wide open and prepare for an emergent pericardiocentesis."

E: "What equipment will you need?"

C: "An 18-guage spinal needle attached to a 30-cc syringe, and the V-lead of the ECG machine attached to the needle."

DON'T FORGET

You will need to be able to describe emergent procedures such as chest tube, intubation, pericardiocentesis, etc. This is a good outline for how to describe a pericardiocentesis—memorize this.

E: "The equipment is ready. How will you proceed?"

C: "Insert the needle at a 45° angle 2 cm below and 1 cm to the left of the xiphoid process in the direction of the left shoulder of the patient and aspirate as I advance slowly looking for signs of acute injury pattern on the ECG machine. I advance until I see ST elevation on the ECG or I get blood in the syringe."

E: "You withdraw 25 cc of blood into the syringe and the patient's BP improves from 50/40 to 90/70."

C: "Remove the needle, keep monitoring the patient's vital signs. Please order a repeat chest x-ray looking for a pneumothorax or pleural effusion as a result of my procedure."

E: "The cardiologist has arrived and is asking for an update. Your post-procedure XR (Fig. C13-3) is also available."

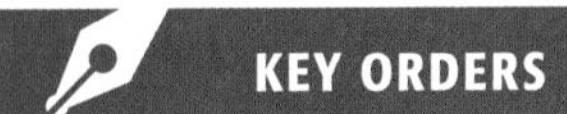

KEY ORDERS

Remember to order follow-up studies after any invasive procedure to check for complications.

C: "Since we last spoke, the patient decompensated and I had to perform an emergent pericardiocentesis. I was able to withdraw 25 cc of blood and the patient has improved but is still in critical condition. I am wondering if he might need a pericardial window. I have reviewed a post-pericardiocentesis XR, and it is normal, showing no pneumotherax."

E: "The cardiologist agrees to take the patient to the ICU where he will talk to the cardiac surgeon and monitor the patient further."

E: "The case is now over."

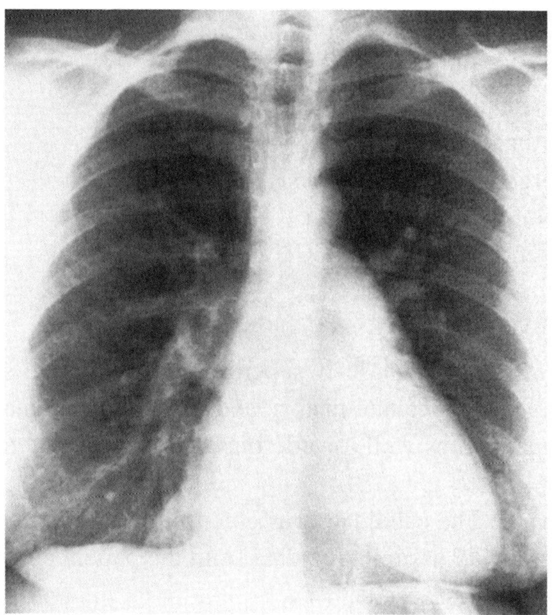

Figure C13-3. The Chest x-ray shows mild cardiomegaly and otherwise normal. *(Reprinted with permission from Chen MYM, Pope Jr TL, Ott DJ.* Basic Radiology. *New York, NY: McGraw-Hill; 2004.)*

CASE ASSESSMENT

Overall, the candidate managed the case very well. The systematic approach in getting an overview of the patient, instituting early therapy when he noted a low blood pressure, and getting a thorough history and physical all led to a straightforward handling of a case where the diagnosis could have been difficult to ascertain.

At the start of the case, the candidate started fluids in a patient noted to be hypotensive and gave orders to ensure proper monitoring throughout the case. The history and physical was very orderly and systematic which allowed him to ask questions directed at a differential diagnosis that encompassed the patient's past medical history and decide if this was more likely to be infectious, cardiac, or vascular in origin. Once the history did not bear out an obvious answer to the cause of the hypotension, a head-to-toe physical examination quickly led to findings of distended neck veins, muffled heart sounds, and no other obvious abnormalities. This allowed the candidate to use the ultrasound properly to come to the diagnosis of cardiac tamponade and direct the care properly. When the patient decompensated, the candidate quickly performed the proper procedure to alleviate the cardiac filling restriction. He then admitted the patient properly to the appropriate service and showed a deeper understanding of possible therapeutic options in mentioning the pericardial window.

The candidate managed this case well. As you are reviewing the case, do not worry if you would not have managed the case as efficiently. Remember the test requires each candidate to meet or exceed a national standard of care. Examinees do not need to provide perfect care.

Critical Actions

1. Administration of fluid bolus.
2. Perform bedside ultrasound.
3. Diagnose cardiac tamponade.
4. Perform emergent pericardiocentesis.
5. Consult cardiology.
6. Admit to the cardiac care unit (CCU).

Test Performance

1. *Data acquisition:* This phase is superb as the candidate shows ability to obtain a more than adequate history and physical examination findings in an efficient manner, as well as ordering appropriate tests to assist in diagnosis. Score = **7**
2. *Problem solving:* The candidate was able to arrive to a potentially difficult diagnosis by quickly assimilating data from the patient encounter and accurately interpreting test results. = **7**
3. *Patient management:* The candidate appropriately escalated care from intravenous fluids (IVFs) and a nonemergent pericardiocentesis to an emergent bedside pericardiocentesis when the patient deteriorated. Score = **8**
4. *Resource utilization:* The candidate demonstrates great use of resources in a cost-effective manner. Score = **7**
5. *Health care provided (outcome):* There was appropriate care delivered throughout all phases of this case, including early initiation of IVFs to a hypotensive patient. The candidate also was able to effectively outline the steps of a pericardiocentesis. Score = **8**
6. *Interpersonal relations and communication skills:* The candidate was able to engage in effective information exchange with both patients and professional associates. This score could have been improved if the candidate updated the patient prior to the examiner having to initiate an update. Score = **7**
7. *Comprehension of pathophysiology:* This candidate demonstrated excellent understanding of pathophysiology as evidenced by the ability to synthesize physical examination and ultrasound (US) findings to arrive at an accurate and timely diagnosis. Score = **7**
8. *Clinical competence (overall):* The candidate excelled in patient management, diagnosis, and understanding of the underlying pathophysiology in this case. Score = **8**

CASE 14 16 y/o Female With Mental Status Change

Navneet Cheema and James Rhee

INITIAL INFORMATION

Name: Tracy Klick

Mode of arrival: Brought in by ambulance with father

Age: 16 years

Gender: Female

VS: T 37.2°C, BP 86/60, HR 120, RR 12, Pulse ox 96% on RA

CC: Unarousable

PLAY OF THE CASE

C: "What do I see as I walk into the patient's room?"

E: "The patient is a well-nourished teenage female, who appears somnolent and is snoring. The patient's father is by the bedside. Patient then starts experiencing a generalized tonic-clonic seizure, which stops spontaneously after about 20 seconds. The patient is now unresponsive."

C: "Nurse, place the patient on a cardiac monitor, show me a rhythm strip, begin O_2 via NC and titrate to keep O_2 sats above 98%, place two 18-gauge IVs, begin NS and bolus 2 L of 0.9NS, and draw blood for lab tests. Please obtain a stat fingerstick glucose and let me know what it is as soon as possible. Also administer naloxone 2 mg IV as soon as the IV is established and let me know if there is any response."

E: "Done. The patient's fingerstick glucose is 90, the cardiac monitor shows a sinus tachycardia with a rate of 100 with some PVCs and the QRS width is slightly widened. There is no response to the naloxone administration."

C: "I open the patient's airway and check her gag reflex."

E: "The patient has no gag reflex."

C: "I will intubate the patient without any medications as patient appears unresponsive—I will use a number 4 curved laryngoscope blade and a 7.5 ET tube. Under direct visualization, I advance the ET tube past the vocal cords, inflate the cuff, and check end-tidal CO_2."

E: "Done. Patient is now intubated with positive end-tidal CO_2. What ventilator settings would you like?"

C: "How much does the patient weigh?"

E: "You estimate 60 kg."

C: "Please set the vent on SIMV with a tidal volume of 480, rate of 16, FIO_2 of 50%, PEEP of 5."

E: "Done. The patient is tolerating the ventilator well."

C: "Are the breath sounds symmetric?"

E: "Yes."

C: "Please send an arterial blood gas immediately."

KEY QUESTION

Ask this open-ended question at the beginning of every case.

KEY ORDERS

Most of the patients you see during the exam will be unstable (or will become that way). Every unstable patient requires IV access (preferably two large-bore IVs), oxygen, and cardiac monitoring (always request to see a rhythm strip). In this case, as the patient has altered mental status they should also get naloxone, and a fingerstick glucose.

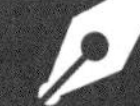

KEY ORDERS

Note how the examinee states that they want the O_2 titrated to keep sats about 98%. Always attach requirements to your orders that will place responsibility for your patient reassessment on the examiner. This is a good strategy.

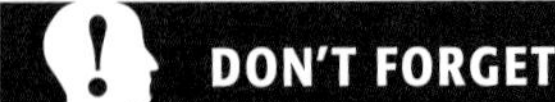

You will need to be able to describe emergent procedures such as chest tube, intubation, pericardiocentesis, etc. This is a good outline for how one describes an uncomplicated intubation—memorize this.

Intubating this unresponsive patient is a critical action.

There are two critical actions taking place here. First, the examinee has to notice the widening of the QRS complex, and realize that there may be ingestions at work. Second, they must test for multiple concomitant ingestions.

E: "It is sent."

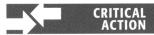

C: "Nurse, the widened QRS on the monitor has me concerned about a toxic ingestion. Can you order a stat ECG, a stat CXR, and send the blood for CBC, BMP, LFTs, EtOH, tox screen, ASA, APAP. I also want to order a UA, and pregnancy test. Also now that we have her airway secured, please insert a 36-Fr orogastric tube into her stomach and lavage with 300 cc of warm NS followed by administration of 75 g of activated charcoal. I want to talk to the father."

E: "Those orders are being done. The patient's father is in the room now."

C: "Mr. Klick, what happened?"

E: "Doc, I'm not sure. When I got home today, she was kind of sleepy, then all of a sudden she started shaking all over—it looked like a seizure. She has never had any problem like this before. It freaked me out. Anyway, she's been kind of moody lately after she broke up with her boyfriend a week ago, but she's always kind of moody. She sees a psychiatrist for this."

C: "What does she see the psychiatrist for?"

E: "Depression."

C: "Does she have any other medical problems?"

E: "No."

C: "What medications does she take?"

E: "Some sort of antidepressant."

C: "Does she have any allergies?"

E: "No."

E: "Your ECG is performed (Fig. C14-1)."

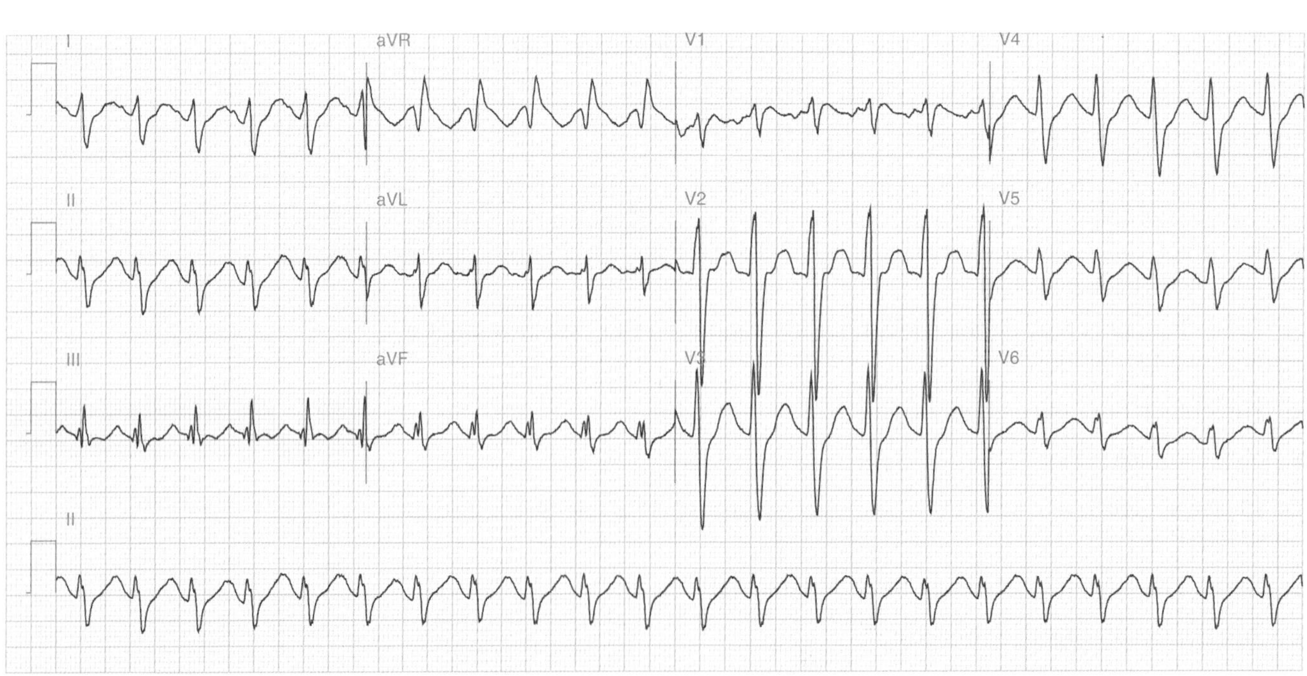

Figure C14-1. ECG which shows signs of TCA overdose (tachycardia, QRS wide, tall R wave in aVR). *(Reprinted with permission from Fauci AS, Braunwald E, Kasper DL, et al.* Harrison's Principles of Internal Medicine. *17th ed. New York, NY: McGraw-Hill; 2008)*

C: "The patient's QRS is wide and she has a large R wave in aVR. I'm concerned that she overdosed on a TCA. Nurse, please bolus one ampule of sodium bicarbonate and then repeat vitals and repeat ECG."

E: "Those orders are being done."

The ABG is available: pH 7.22, Pco_2 36, CO_2 14, BE −12

C: "Mr. Klick, I'm concerned that your daughter took an overdose of her antidepressants and that's why she had a seizure. Does she take any other medications or do any other drugs?"

E: "Not that I'm aware of."

C: "Has she ever tried to commit suicide before?"

E: "No."

C: "Nurse, do we have a repeat set of vitals?"

E: "Blood pressure has improved to 110/80, and her pulse is now 100. Here is her repeat ECG (Fig. C14-2)."

KEY ORDERS

Remember to order the appropriate XR to check for tube placement and/or complications from any invasive procedure you do.

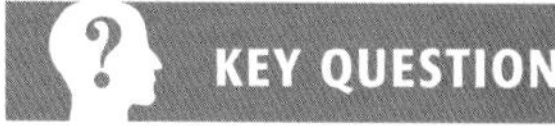

KEY QUESTION

Remember to use alternate sources of history if the patient is unresponsive.

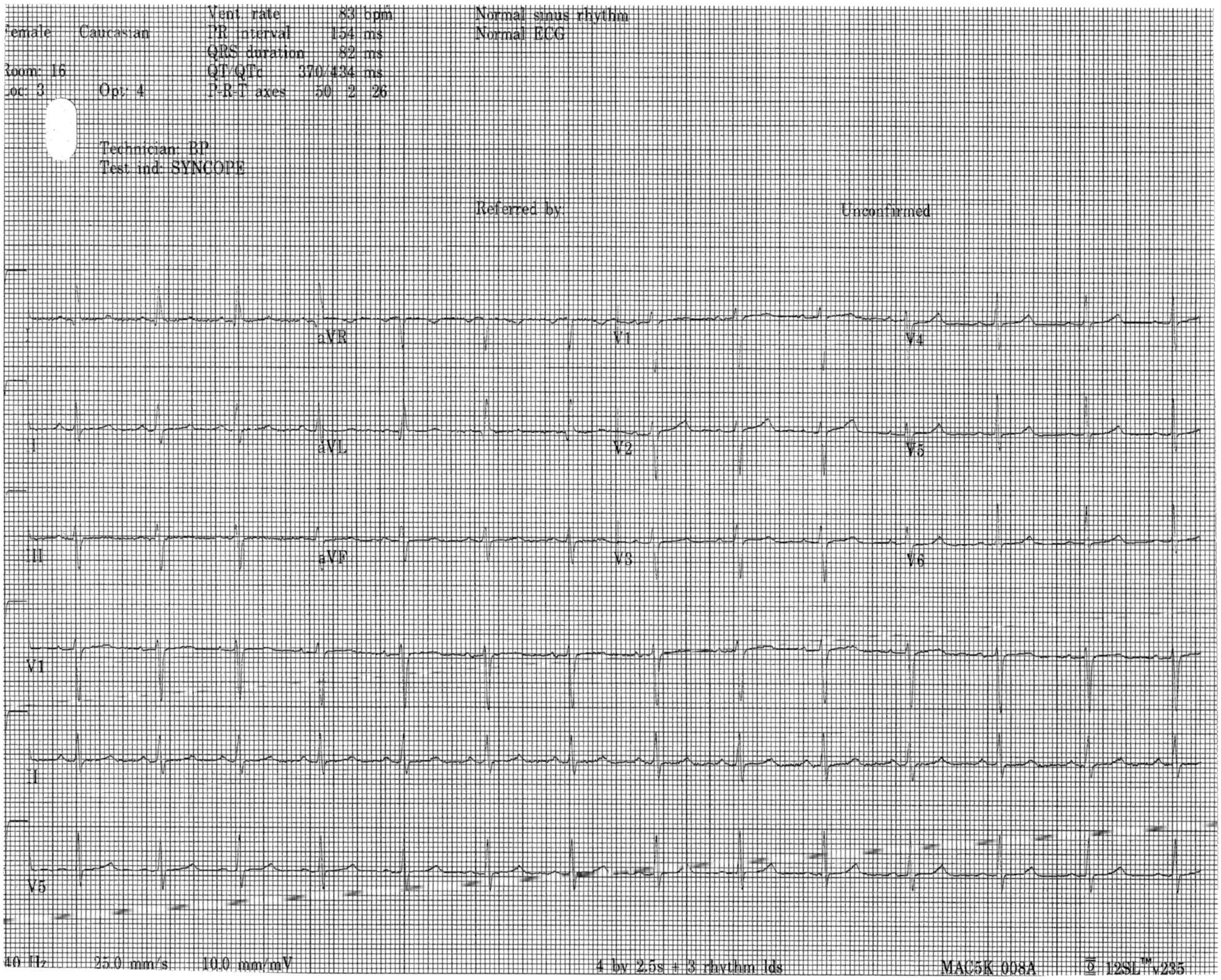

Figure C14-2. Normal ECG. *(Reprinted with permission from Stone CK, Humphries RL.* Current Diagnosis and Treatment: Emergency Medicine. *6th ed. New York, NY: McGraw-Hill; 2008.)*

There are two critical actions going on here: (1) recognizing the ECG and physical signs of a TCA overdose, and (2) giving sodium bicarbonate.

C: "Nurse, please continue to keep the patient on the cardiac monitor and alert me if there is any change. Also please call the ICU and arrange for a bed while I do a more thorough physical examination."

E: "Orders are being carried out."

C: "Is the patient responsive at all to verbal or painful stimuli?"

E: "Still unresponsive."

C: "Is there any evidence of trauma to the head? Any hemotympanum, Battle sign, or raccoon eyes?"

E: "None."

C: "Pupils size? Mucous membranes wet or dry? Oropharynx otherwise normal?"

E: "Pupils are 5 mm and symmetric and reactive. Mucous membranes are dry and you note a superficial laceration at the tip of the tongue. Endotracheal tube still in place."

C: "Is there JVD or tracheal deviation?"

E: "No."

C: "What do I hear when I listen to the lungs and heart?"

E: "What are you looking for?"

C: "On the lung examination, I am listening for breath sounds, crackles, and wheezes. On the cardiac examination, I am listening for murmurs, rubs, and gallops; also, are the peripheral pulses symmetric?"

E: "Breath sounds are present bilaterally, with no crackles or wheezes. The heart examination is slightly tachycardic and the peripheral pulses are full."

C: "Are the bowel sounds present? Is there abdominal tenderness or masses?"

E: "Bowel sounds are diminished; there is no tenderness or masses."

C: "Skin examination—is the patient flushed, warm, and dry?"

E: "Yes she is."

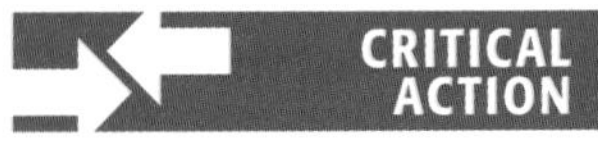

Admitting this overdose to the ICU is a critical action.

C: "I would like to check patient's DTRs and Babinski."

E: "DTRs are 2+ and symmetric and plantar response is downward."

C: "Nurse, do we have the pregnancy test back yet?"

E: "She is not pregnant. Because of her comatose state, we placed a Foley catheter—she had a liter of urine in her bladder."

C: "Do we have any other labs back on the patient?"

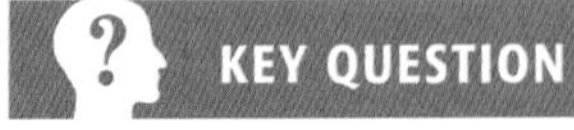

It is always better to tell the examiner to give you the lab results as they come back—this relieves you of the responsibility of remembering to ask for them, and places that responsibility on the examiner—a good strategy.

E: "The labs are back. They are the following:

CBC: Hgb 12.4, Hct 38, Plt 212,000

BMP: Na 136, K 5.7, Cl 100, CO_2 14, BUN 19, Cr 1.4, Glu 99, Ca 8.9

LFTs: wnl

ASA, APAP levels are negative.

Tox screen is pending.

EtOH level is 0.

CXR is normal with good positioning of the ET tube."

C: "Nurse, what are the patient's vital signs?"

E: "Same."

C: "In that case, I would like to order a stat non-infused head CT and talk to the ICU doctor."

E: "Dr. Intense is on the phone."

C: "Dr. Intense, I have a patient here who I suspect took a TCA overdose. She is on antidepressants for her underlying psychiatric condition and recently has been feeling depressed according to her father. She presented here after being unarousable at home. She subsequently had a generalized seizure here, which spontaneously resolved. Her ECG demonstrated a widened QRS interval with a prominent R wave in aVR. She also exhibits an anticholinergic toxidrome on physical examination. This is all consistent with a TCA overdose and we subsequently gave her an ampule of sodium bicarbonate, which resulted in normalization of the QRS complex on ECG. Other than a moderate acidosis, which may in part be due to recent seizure as well as her poisoning, the rest of her labs are normal and she has not had any more seizure activity. She will be getting a head CT to rule out an ICH; assuming that the CT is normal she needs to be admitted to the ICU under your care."

E: "Sounds good, I'll see her when she gets here. Case is over."

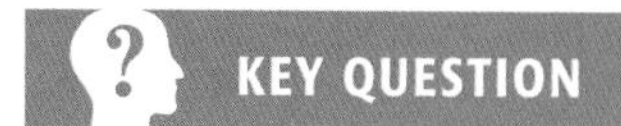

KEY QUESTION

Remember to reassess your patient frequently—especially if they are intubated.

CASE ASSESSMENT

The candidate managed this case very well. Initially, the patient recognized that the patient's condition required prompt attention and administered a "coma" cocktail as well as addressing patient's hypotension and tachycardia. As the patient wasn't hypoglycemic and had no response to naloxone, the candidate appropriately intubated the patient. In this scenario, it is okay that the candidate did not intubate the patient right away because the other interventions that he made may have obviated the need. It's always very embarrassing intubating an unresponsive patient only to find out that they were unresponsive due to hypoglycemia, which could have been readily corrected. Some would also argue that thiamine needed to be given as part of the "coma cocktail," but since the patient is young and appears well nourished, it is probably an intervention that can be skipped. If the patient appeared malnourished, then administration of thiamine may be warranted.

Once the patient's airway was secured, the candidate performed a gastric lavage followed by the administration of activated charcoal. It is unclear in this case whether the lavage and charcoal would have any effect, as we don't know when the patient took the mediations. We could argue that tricyclic antidepressants (TCAs) have inherent anticholinergic properties and subsequently delay gastric emptying, making this ingestion more amenable to these forms of gastric decontamination. Regardless, the decision to perform gastric lavage and administer activated charcoal fall well within the scope of standard of care and some might even consider this a critical action. However, the true critical action is securing the airway prior to performing gastric lavage and activated charcoal administration. If the patient seized while performing these maneuvers, the patient would have aspirated and may have died.

The initial widening on the cardiac rhythm strip tipped this candidate off to a possible toxic ingestion as the cause of the patient's current condition. Of course, if he had just talked to the father, as he later did, he would have found out that a toxic ingestion is very likely earlier. Once establishing that the patient had likely taken a TCA overdose, the candidate appropriately ordered an electrocardiogram (ECG) and evaluated the QRS interval. He again appropriately administered sodium bicarbonate to overcome the sodium channel blockade caused by the TCA overdose.

The candidate finally performs a physical examination and correctly identifies an anticholinergic toxidrome—mydriasis, altered mental status, tachycardia, urinary retention, and flushed, dry, warm skin. All of these symptoms are consistent with TCA toxicity as TCAs have some anticholinergic properties. He appropriately did not administer physostigmine for the anticholinergic toxidrome—although this wasn't really addressed in this case, if the nurse had prompted him and asked if it should be given, the correct answer would be no as this may cause a patient with TCA toxicity to become asystolic.

Critical Actions

1. Perform intubation.
2. Order ECG and recognize QRS widening.
3. Appreciate and articulate at some point in the case the idea of a toxidrome with anticholinergic properties; eventually specifically suspect a TCA overdose.
4. Administer sodium bicarbonate.
5. Does not administer physostigmine despite anticholinergic signs.
6. Check for concomitant ingestion.
7. Admit to the intensive care unit (ICU).

Test Performance

1. *Data acquisition:* This phase is excellent as the candidate shows ability to obtain a more than adequate history and physical examination findings in an efficient manner, as well as ordering appropriate tests to assist in diagnosis. Score = **7**
2. *Problem solving:* The candidate was able to obtain the history from other sources and use the findings on the ECG to help arrive at the correct diagnosis. Score = **8**
3. *Patient management:* The candidate delivered efficient and timely care with no delays in treatment. The coma cocktail was administered promptly and once there was no response, the candidate appropriately immediately proceeded to intubation. Score = **8**
4. *Resource utilization:* There was appropriate use of resources in this case that allowed for an efficient and timely diagnosis. Score = **7**
5. *Health care provided (outcome):* The candidate diagnosed a TCA overdose and appropriately treated the sodium channel blockade with sodium bicarbonate and avoided the use of physostigmine. Score = **8**
6. *Interpersonal relations and communication skills:* The candidate was thoughtful in his interactions with the family and effectively exchanged information with the consultant. Score = **7**
7. *Comprehension of pathophysiology:* The candidate demonstrated an excellent understanding of the signs and symptoms associated with TCA overdose as outlined in his presentation to the ICU physician. Score = **8**
8. *Clinical competence (overall):* This case was managed superbly utilizing all information available to efficiently and effectively arrive at the diagnosis of TCA overdose. Score = **8**

CASE 15 40 y/o Male With Chest Pain

Navneet Cheema and Mark P. Bogner

INITIAL INFORMATION

Name: John Smith

Mode of arrival: Ambulance

Age: 40 years

Gender: Male

VS: T 37.1°C, BP 192/110, HR 82, RR 20, O_2 sat: 96% on RA

CC: Severe chest pain

PLAY OF THE CASE

E: "It is 10:00 AM Monday morning and you are working a single coverage shift in a busy rural hospital ED with an annual volume of 18,000 ED visits. You have excellent nursing and ancillary staff to assist you. The hospital resources and medical staff are superb for this environment. The nearest tertiary care center is 18 minutes away by helicopter (each way), and is a 60-minute trip by ground ambulance."

C: "What do I see as I walk into the patient's room?"

E: "The patient appears his stated age, well kempt, and dressed in work boots, jeans, and heavy outdoor clothing. He is obviously very uncomfortable. He is diaphoretic and having trouble getting undressed."

C: "Hello Mr. Smith, I am Dr. Emergency. Can I help you with your coat? Nurse, please place the patient on a cardiac monitor and show me a rhythm strip when available. Let's start him on oxygen via NC at 4 L, place a 16-gauge IV with NS lock and draw blood for labs. We will need cardiac enzymes, including troponin, a CBC, electrolytes, BUN, creatinine, glucose, UA, and a BNP. Please obtain a stat ECG and hand it to me when it is done. Also, please get a stat bedside CXR."

E: "Your orders are being done. The patient's rhythm strip shows a sinus rate of 80 bpm."

C: "So Mr. Smith, the triage nurse tells me you are having chest pain . . . can you fill me in on the details?"

E: "It just hurts, doc. I've never had anything like this before."

C: "When did it start?"

E: "About an hour ago."

C: "What does it feel like?"

E: "It is hard to describe. It is just this terrible pain in my chest."

C: "What were you doing when it started?"

E: "Working."

C: "What kind of work do you do?"

KEY QUESTION

Ask this open-ended question at the beginning of every case.

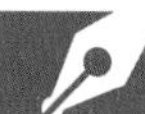

KEY ORDERS

Most of the patients you see during the exam will be unstable (or will become that way). Every unstable patient requires IV access (preferably two large-bore IVs), oxygen, and cardiac monitoring (and in most cases an ECG). In this case, as the patient has chest pain, sending cardiac labs and getting a stat portable chest XR is also appropriate at this time.

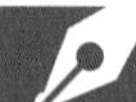

KEY ORDERS

When you order a test, always ask to be told the results when they come back. This places the responsibility for remembering to check the lab values on the examiner and relieves you of them—a good strategy.

E: "I own a general contracting company. We are building several big houses out on the west side of town. I was helping some of my subcontractors unload bundles of shingles when the pain hit me."

C: "Has the pain gotten better or worse since it started?"

E: "Not really, it is just there. The pain is very intense, and pretty much constant."

C: "Did it get any better with the oxygen or morphine the paramedics gave you?"

E: "Maybe a little."

C: "Show me where it hurts you the most."

E: "The patient points to his sternal area."

C: "Do you feel it anywhere else—such as your jaw, neck, shoulders, arms, back?"

E: "Well, it hurts right in the middle of my back, up high, but I figured that was from all the lifting. I do a lot of physical work and my back hurts more often than not."

C: "Is this pain in your back different than pain you have had before?"

E: "Yes it is. It feels like someone is tearing my back open with a hot knife."

C: "Did the back pain start at the same time as the chest pain?"

E: "Not exactly, it seemed to come on a bit later in the ambulance."

C: "I would like the nurse to obtain blood pressure readings in both of the patient's arms and report them to me."

E: "Here is the ECG for your review (Fig. C15-1)."

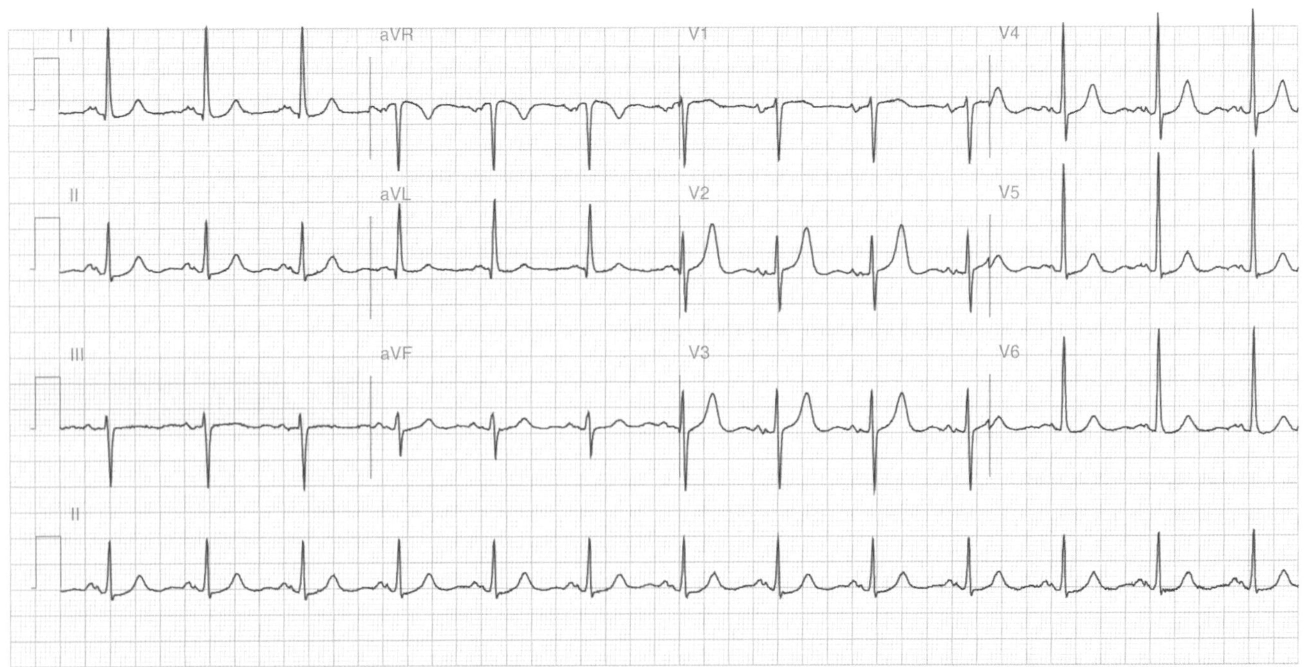

Figure C15-1. ECG with signs of LVH. *(Reprinted with permission from Fauci AS, Braunwald E, Kasper DL, et al.* Harrison's Principles of Internal Medicine. *17th ed. New York, NY: McGraw-Hill; 2008.)*

E: "BP in right arm is 192/110, left arm is 160/95."

C: "Nurse, please administer 20 mg IV labetalol and also 4 mg morphine IV."

C: "Mr. Smith, I am worried that you may have something called an aortic dissection, which is a tear in the wall of the main artery coming from your heart. We are going to be doing a lot of things here to get your blood pressure under control and to find out for sure what is going on. I have some more questions for you and will need to examine you in just a minute."

E: "Okay doc, whatever you say. Am I going to be OK? I have a wife and three small children at home that depend on me."

C: "These things are serious, but I am going to do everything in my power to make sure you are OK. You are young and strong and you are at the right place. I would say the odds are in your favor."

CRITICAL ACTION

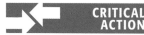

There are two critical actions here. First, the examinee has to recognize the possibility of aortic dissection from the history and physical. Second, the blood pressure must be controlled.

E: "Okay doc, what's next?"

C: "Other than the pain, is anything else troubling you?"

E: "I feel weak, nauseated, and light-headed."

C: "Did the pain come on suddenly or did it start off not so bad and then get worse?"

E: "It came out of nowhere and was terrible from the start. It has been pretty much the same ever since."

C: "Have you ever experienced similar pain while exerting yourself?"

E: "Never."

C: "Do you smoke?"

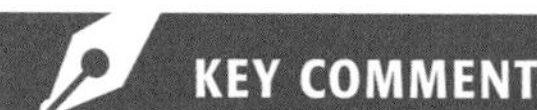

KEY COMMENT

You get points for professionalism and interpersonal interactions by responding to patient's concerns with empathy.

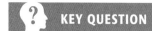

E: "Yes, about a pack a day."

C: "Do you drink alcohol?"

E: "Rarely, at occasional parties and during the holidays."

C: "Do you have any medical problems?"

E: "Not that I know of, I haven't seen a doctor for over 10 years."

C: "Have you ever had surgery?"

E: "When I was 29 I had open heart surgery to repair some kind of 'hole in my heart'—but I have been fine ever since."

KEY QUESTION

Remember to reassess your patient frequently—especially if they are unstable.

C: "Do you take any medications?"

E: "No."

C: "I would like to perform a physical examination."

E: "Go ahead with your examination."

C: "Is the patient getting any pain relief? How does he look now? And what are his current vitals please."

E: "He reports feeling a bit better. BP right 170/98, left 150/80. What do you mean when you ask 'how does he look?'"

C: "I'm sorry. Is he still pale, diaphoretic, and 'shocky' in appearance? Or is he appearing more comfortable, less pale, less diaphoretic?"

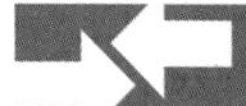

CRITICAL ACTION

Controlling the patient's pain is a critical action in this case.

E: "He looks somewhat better in all respects."

C: "Good, nurse, please administer 40 mg IV labetalol and 4 mg IV morphine."

E: "Done."

C: "Are there any significant findings on the patient's HEENT examination?"

E: "No."

C: "How about his neck?"

E: "What are you looking for?"

C: "Tracheal deviation, JVD, subcutaneous emphysema, swelling or hematoma formation."

E: "Neck examination is normal."

C: "When I auscultate his chest, do I hear wheezing, rales, rhonchi, diminished or asymmetrical breath sounds? Also, is there any chest tenderness or deformity?"

E: "Chest examination is normal aside from well-healed median-sternotomy scar."

C: "On the cardiac examination, is his PMI displaced, are S_1 and S_2 clear, are there any murmurs, rubs, or gallops?"

E: "Cardiac examination is normal."

C: "When I examine his abdomen, do I palpate any masses, pulsatile or otherwise, tenderness, guarding, rebound? Are bowel sounds normal?"

E: "Abdominal examination is normal."

C: "In the extremities, are there any pulse deficits or asymmetries, deformities, swelling, or edema?"

E: "His right radial pulse is palpably stronger than the left. Lower extremity pulses are intact and symmetrical, but also seem a bit weak. Extremities are otherwise normal."

C: "Please call cardiology and the echo lab. I would like a stat bedside transesophageal echocardiogram. Please also have the cardiothoracic surgeon paged."

C: "Continuing my examination, is there occult or gross blood in the stool on the rectal examination?"

E: "No."

C: "Any neurologic deficits."

E: "Be specific."

C: "Is there any difference in strength between right and left arms, legs? Are there any cranial nerve deficits? Are there any gross sensory deficits, particularly unilateral loss or altered sensation? His mental status can be stated as grossly normal from the history session."

E: "No deficits."

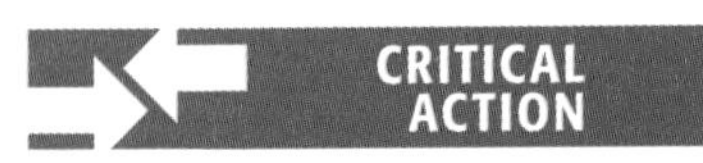

Consulting the appropriate specialist is always a critical action.

E: "The CXR is available for your review (Fig. C15-2). Please interpret the film."

C: "The mediastinum is widened consistent with a thoracic aortic dissection. I see no evidence of effusion or apical capping, thus rupture has probably not occurred at this point."

E: "The local cardiologists are all in the middle of cardiac catheterization procedures. TEE cannot be performed. You are practicing at a busy community hospital in a suburban setting. The nearest cardiothoracic surgeon is 20 miles away."

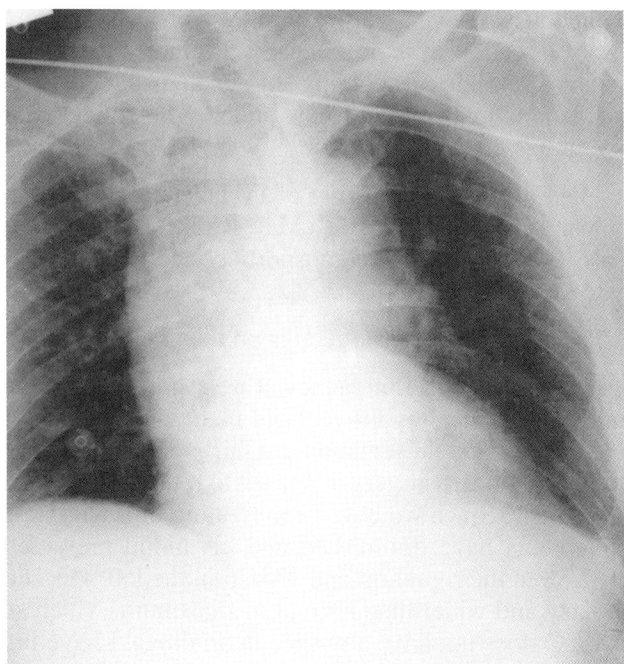

Figure C15-2. CXR with widened mediastinum. *(Reprinted with permission from Hall JB, Schmidt GA, Wood LDH.* Principles of Critical Care. *3rd ed. New York, NY: McGraw-Hill; 2005.)*

C: "May I speak to the radiologist on call to explore my options?"

E: "This is Dr. Rads. What's going on?"

C: "I have a patient who I suspect is likely to have an acute thoracic aortic dissection. His CXR is supportive of the diagnosis. As TEE is not available at this time, I would like to get a CT angiogram; the patient is hypertensive, which we are treating, but has otherwise remained stable."

E: "That sounds like a fine approach; I will let the techs know that the patient will be coming over shortly."

C: "Great."

C: "Nurse, please get in touch with the nearest tertiary care center cardiothoracic surgeon on call, and please contact the nearest aeromedical helicopter transport service. Let me know when they are on the phone."

E: "All that is being done."

C: "I would like another set of vitals now, please. And have we reached the helicopter transport service and/or the cardiothoracic surgeon? Are labs back? Can the patient go to CT scan now?"

E: "BP right 162/88, left 138/75. The following lab results are available:"

CBC: WBC 10,000, 65 PMNs, 8 bands; H/H 14/42; platelets 345,000

PT 12 (INR 1.1), PTT 34

BMP: Na 142, K 4.5, Cl 106, CO_2 19, BUN 13, Cr 1.2, Glucose 134, Ca 9.7

CPK 121, MB 3.4, Troponin <0.05

BNP 150

UA unremarkable

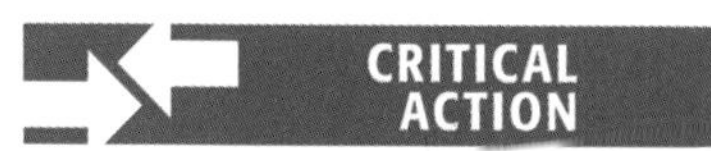

Admitting the patient to the appropriate level of care is always a critical action. In some cases—that may mean transfer to a tertiary care center.

E: "The helicopter service is just returning from another transport. They can launch in our direction in approximately 5 minutes, flight time to get here is approximately 10 minutes, including start up and shut down times. The cardiothoracic surgeon is just coming to the phone. The patient can go to CT whenever you want."

C: "Nurse, please administer 80 mg of IV labetalol and 2 mg of IV morphine and accompany the patient to CT. May I talk to the cardiothoracic surgeon now? Please ask the helicopter transport service to remain on standby for us and ready to launch."

E: "Done. The cardiothoracic surgeon is on the line."

C: "Dr. Surgery, this is Dr. Emergency at west side suburban hospital. I have in my ER an otherwise healthy 40-year-old man who I believe has an aortic dissection. His history and presentation are fairly classic. He is a smoker and had some kind of open-heart surgery at age 29 to repair what sounds like a VSD or symptomatic ASD. Since we have been treating him with morphine and labetalol his symptoms have diminished and his blood pressures improved, currently at 162/88 in the right arm and 138/75 in the left. His chest x-ray shows a somewhat hazy and wider than normal mediastinum, which supports the diagnosis. His ECG does not have any specific findings. I have just finished examining him and he rolled out the door a minute ago heading for CT angiogram."

E: "Okay, we will be ready. Call me when the CT is done. If the patient has an aortic or other cardiothoracic problem confirmed by CT, I will gladly accept him here as a transfer."

C: "Sounds good, I will be in touch."

E: "Dr. Emergency to CT scanner #1 **stat**!"

C: "I request that a second nurse accompany me. We will take with us the 'crash cart' and 'airway bag/cart'—including all resuscitation medications, and all medications needed for RSI and sedation. We will take multiple ET tubes, sizes including 7-0, 7-5, 8-0 and will make haste to the CT scanner."

E: "You arrive in the CT scanner which is 2 floors up and 3 hallways away, to find your patient semiconscious, diaphoretic with thready pulses and a BP of 80/40 and HR 100."

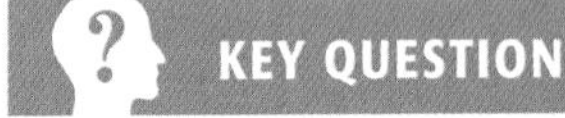

Intubating this decompensating patient is a critical action.

C: "I would like to immediately intubate the patient. Nurse, please draw up 20 mg etomidate and 125 mg succinylcholine. Tell me when you are ready with the drugs. I will prepare and test my equipment, including bag valve mask, suction, oxygen, several ET tubes sizes 7-0, 7-5, and 8-0, stylet, and laryngoscope blades—and begin pre-oxygenating and assisting the patient's ventilation efforts using the BVM and oxygen at 15 LPM. I will place a nasal airway if needed."

E: "The medications are ready."

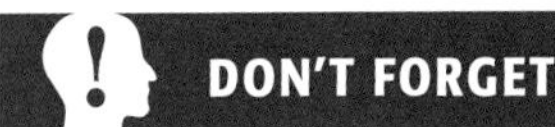

You will need to be able to describe emergent procedures such as chest tube, intubation, pericardiocentesis, etc. This is a good outline for how one describes an emergent intubation—memorize this.

C: "Please administer 20 mg etomidate immediately and in that order. 20 seconds after the etomidate is in, administer 125 mg succinylcholine. Nurse #2, please provide cricoid cartilage pressure."

E: "Done."

C: "I will now endotracheally intubate the patient with a 7-5 French tube. After placing the tube I will confirm the presence of bilateral breath sounds and use the colorimetric end-tidal CO_2 device to further confirm proper placement."

E: "Done. What now?"

C: "What are the patient's vital signs after intubation?"

E: "BP 115/68 (left), HR 84, oxygen saturation 100%."

C: "Was the scan completed?"

E: "Yes, the patient became acutely worse when transferring from the scanner table back to the ER cart."

C: "Can the radiologist give me a stat read on the CT?"

E: "It reveals an acute aortic dissection involving the proximal aorta extending from the aortic root to the take off of the left subclavian artery." The nurse asks you: "What is the preferred approach to further management of this type of acute dissection?"

C: "This is a Stanford A (or DeBakey Type I) acute thoracic aorta dissection which is best managed by control of HTN and acute surgical repair."

C: "I would like the helicopter transport service to lift off and head in our direction. I need to talk to the cardiothoracic surgeon again to update him. I would also like to talk to any family the patient might have waiting for him. I will need the unit coordinator to get the necessary COBRA/EMTALA transfer paperwork started and I will complete these forms together with the nurse."

E: "Done. The patient is being transferred and the case is now over."

CASE ASSESSMENT

The candidate managed the case well and achieved all critical actions. Note that the patient "coded" in the computed tomography (CT) scanner, a nightmare for any emergency physician. Intubating the patient prior to CT is not a critical action in this case because the patient appeared quite stable and was clearly improving after treatment in the emergency department (ED). In the "real world" if CT was truly that far from the ED an emergency physician would be expected to take this into account prior to sending a potentially unstable patient to the scanner. However, in a single coverage situation and under the described circumstances, making the judgment call to send the nurse with the patient while mentally preparing to act fast in case things went badly, as they did, is sufficient. The candidate responded quickly and appropriately to this challenge.

The candidate did a superb job of recognizing the severity of the patient's condition, implementing appropriate measures, both therapeutically and diagnostically, and did so without delay. Simultaneously she gathered information to plan her next steps and made an early presumptive diagnosis, a critical action in the case, and contacted the closest cardiothoracic surgeon while taking steps to ensure rapid transport if her presumptive diagnosis of aortic dissection proved correct. They met all standards of care including critical actions of pain control and blood pressure management using an appropriate agent, ie, labetalol. Had they chosen to use the traditional approach of a beta-blocker + nitroprusside it would have been important that they start the beta-blocker (ie, metoprolol) before the nitroprusside.

They performed a focused physical examination after initiating treatment on the basis of history and presentation, which is entirely appropriate in these cases. They interpreted data (labs, electrocardiogram [ECG], chest x-ray [CXR]) correctly and demonstrated a caring and compassionate approach when managing the patient, explaining her concerns to him, and later asking to speak with his family.

Critical Actions

1. Recognizing the possibility of aortic dissection and pursuing the diagnosis.
2. Avoiding a dangerous action, specifically not administering anticoagulant medications that could be fatal in this case.
3. Blood pressure control with either labetalol (as done) or using beta-blockers + nitroprusside (in that order).
4. Ensuring adequate pain control.
5. Early consultation with a cardiothoracic surgeon.
6. Proper and early arrangements to transfer the patient to a higher level of care.
7. Perform intubation when indicated.

Test Performance

1. *Data acquisition:* The candidate was thorough and appropriately focused on data acquisition as the case evolved. Score = **7**
2. *Problem solving:* The candidate rapidly assessed the situation for severity and moved quickly to respond to data and changes in condition in an appropriate manner. She frequently asked for updates on the patient's condition and response to treatment, a good habit on oral examinations. Score = **8**
3. *Patient management:* The candidate's approach to the problem displayed excellent ability to rapidly synthesize the clinical picture and consider important life threats. Score = **8**
4. *Resource utilization:* Resources were used appropriately and cost-effectively. However, a transesophageal echocardiogram (TEE) is not typically the first line of imaging to make the diagnosis of aortic dissection, especially in a patient with normal kidney function. Score = **6**
5. *Health care provided (outcome):* The candidate was appropriately aggressive in treating the patient's blood pressure with anti-hypertensives and analgesics. Score = **8**
6. *Interpersonal relations and communication skills:* The candidate had very good interactions with the staff, as she was directive without being demanding. She also was able to address the patient's concerns with compassion and respect. Score = **7**
7. *Comprehension of pathophysiology:* The candidate demonstrated a clear understanding of the classifications of aortic dissection and their associated treatments. Score = **8**
8. *Clinical competence (overall):* The candidate handled this complicated case very well, quickly arriving at the diagnosis, stabilizing the patient, and arranging timely transport. Score = **7**

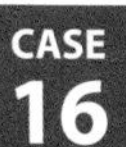

CASE 16 28 y/o Female With HIV, Back Pain, and Fever

Navneet Cheema, Fiona Gallahue, and Richard Sinert

INITIAL INFORMATION

Name: Marjorie Lucky

Mode of arrival: Brought by ambulance

Age: 28 years

Gender: Female

VS: T 39.7°C (103.5°F), BP: 140/80, HR: 110, RR:18, O_2 sat: 98%

CC: Back pain for 5 days, worse today

PLAY OF THE CASE

C: "What do I see as I walk into the patient's room?"

E: "The patient is a thin, diaphoretic female in moderate distress lying supine on the stretcher."

C: "Hello, Ms. Lucky, my name is Dr. Seethapic. What brought you to the hospital today?"

E: "I have really horrible back pain and it seems to be getting worse. Doc, please give me something for pain, I'm dying."

C: "Have you ever had back pain before?"

E: "Not really, a mild strain here and there but nothing like this type of pain. Doc, can you please give me something for my pain?"

C: "Just give me a minute, I'm worried about your pain and I'd like to figure out why you have your pain so I can treat it appropriately. Please answer a few more of my questions so I can give you the right medication. Can you describe the pain—is it in one spot or all over?"

E: "It's in the middle of my back, right about here." (The patient motions to approximately to the mid-thoracic level in the back at the level of the umbilicus.)

C: "Do you remember lifting anything heavy or any trauma to your back?"

E: "No."

C: "Does the pain move anywhere?"

E: "No, it's pretty much just there."

C: "Have you had any difficulty breathing or any shortness of breath?

E: "No."

C: "Have you had any abdominal pain or flank pain?"

E: "No."

C: "Do you have any numbness, tingling, or weakness in your arms or legs?"

E: "Well, I do have some numbness and weakness in my legs which started today and seems to be getting worse."

KEY QUESTION

Ask this open-ended question at the beginning of every case.

KEY QUESTION

Treating the patient's pain is often a critical action. While it is appropriate to conduct a short history and physical before administering opioids, you will get higher scores for interpersonal communication if you explain this and empathize with the patient.

C: "Have you have any episodes where you were incontinent of urine or stool?"

E: "Yes, this morning, I had urinary incontinence."

C: "Do you have any medical problems?"

E: "I'm HIV positive."

C: "Do you know your last CD4 count or viral load?"

E: "Actually, I haven't seen a doctor in a while, I've been living in a homeless shelter since I lost my job and it's been hard to schedule an appointment without a phone."

C: "We'll take good care of you here, don't worry."

E: "Thanks."

C: "How long ago were you diagnosed with HIV?"

E: "About 7 years ago."

C: "Are you on any medications?"

E: "I'm on methadone."

C: "Do you have any allergies?"

E: "No."

C: "Have you been using alcohol or any drugs?"

E: "I have a beer occasionally, I thought I kicked the heroin habit but I did use heroin a few weeks ago."

C: "Did you inject the heroin?"

E: "Yes."

C: "Any other drugs recently?"

E: "No."

C: "Have you ever had any surgeries?"

E: "No."

C: "Do you know when your last menstrual period was?"

E: "A week ago."

C: "Have you ever been to this hospital?"

E: "No, doc, the pain is really really bad, could you please give me something?"

C: "Nurse, I'd like Ms. Lucky to be started on oxygen 2 LPM by nasal cannula, put on a cardiac monitor and could you please place an 18-gauge IV, draw blood for CBC, PT/PTT, electrolytes, LDH, type and screen as well as two sets of blood cultures? I'd also like a UA, UCx, ECG, and a urine pregnancy test please. I'd like to send Ms. Lucky to radiology for a CXR, lumbar/thoracic spine x-ray and an MRI spinal survey. Could you also give Ms. Lucky 30 mg of IV ketorolac and let me know if she still is having significant pain."

E: "Those orders are being carried out. Doctor, radiology wants to know if you want the MRI or the x-rays first?"

C: "I'd like the MRI first, please. Thank you."

E: "OK."

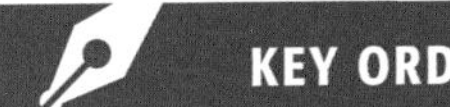

KEY ORDERS

Most of the patients you see during the exam will be unstable (or will become that way). Every unstable patient requires IV access (preferably two large-bore IVs), oxygen, and cardiac monitoring (and in most cases an ECG). As this patient likely has active infection, drawing blood cultures prior to antibiotic administration is also appropriate.

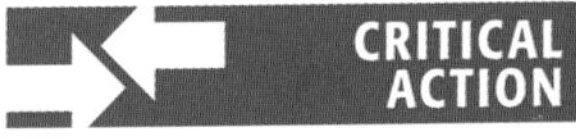

CRITICAL ACTION

There are two critical actions here. First, the examinee must treat this patient's pain, and secondly, they must order an MRI to rule out epidural abscess.

C: "How is your pain after that medicine?"

E: "It's a little better but it still really hurts, doc."

C: "Nurse, could we give Ms. Lucky 5 mg of morphine please."

E: "Yes, doctor."

C: "Ms. Lucky, I'd like to examine you now."

E: "OK."

C: "What do I see on HEENT exam?"

E: "What are you looking for?"

C: "I'm looking for any palatal lesions consistent with Kaposi sarcoma or oral lesions consistent with thrush, any pharyngeal erythema or exudate, any lymphadenopathy."

E: "The patient had lymphadenopathy along both the anterior and posterior cervical chains, she has white lesions on her tongue which can be scraped off easily, the rest of the exam is normal."

C: "What do I hear on chest exam?"

E: "Heart and lungs are both normal."

C: "How is the abdominal exam?"

E: "There is no rebound or guarding on exam, good bowel sounds."

C: "I'd like to do a rectal exam and check for rectal tone as well as guaiac the stool."

E: "The patient has poor rectal tone, brown stool which is guaiac negative."

C: "I'd like to examine the patient's back—are there any areas of step-off or point tenderness?"

E: "The patient has no step-off but she is point tender where she had indicated pain before in the midline."

C: "I'd like to do a full neurologic exam checking cranial nerves, reflexes, motor strength, sensation, gait, and cerebellar function."

E: "The patient's cranial nerves are intact; she is hyporeflexive in both lower extremities with diminished pain sensation to pinprick throughout both lower extremities. Her motor function is 5/5 in both upper extremities but 2/5 in the lower. She refuses to have gait tested reporting she feels too weak to walk and she has normal rapid alternating movements."

C: "I'd like to do a dermatologic exam to check for any rashes, evidence of cellulitis, or track marks."

E: "The patient has no rashes or evidence of cellulitis. She does have recent track marks along her left arm."

C: "Ms. Lucky, I'm worried about your back pain and I think you may need surgery right away but I can't be certain until I get an MRI of your spine. Are you claustrophobic or likely to have any problem being in an enclosed machine for a short period of time?"

E: "I don't think so, doc."

C: "I'd like to make sure that the patient is taken to MRI right away to rule out a cord compression. I'd also like to give the patient the appropriate antibiotics to cover an epidural abscess based on the Sanford guide that I carry in the department."

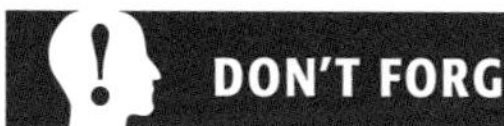

Remember—when the examiner says that an organ system is "normal" you are done. If they say "what are you looking for" that means that there is a specific finding in that organ system.

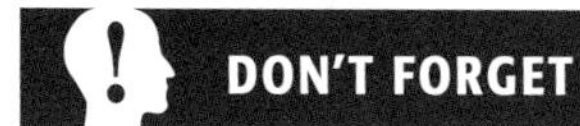

Remember to specifically ask about skin findings as they will often not be mentioned in the review of other organ systems.

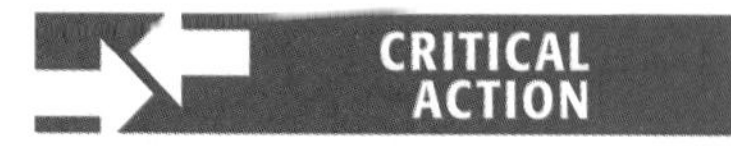

Giving antibiotics is a critical action in this case (and in any case in which infection is a serious concern).

E: "Those orders are being carried out. According to the guide, nafcillin 2 g IV and ciprofloxacin 400 mg IV are the appropriate empiric antibiotics."

C: "Thank you."

E: "Dr. Back is on the line for you."

C: "Dr Back, this is Dr. Seethapic calling from the emergency department, I'm concerned about a patient here. I believe she may have a cord compression from an epidural abscess. She's 28 years old, HIV positive with recent IV drug use, unknown CD4 count but probably low since she has evidence of thrush, a fever to 39.4°C (103°F) here, point tender at T10 with poor rectal tone, bilateral lower extremity weakness, loss of pain sensation, and hyporeflexia to my exam which started this morning. I've given her IV nafcillin and ciprofloxacin and she's in MRI to confirm right now but I'm very worried about her. I think she needs immediate decompression."

E: "I understand your concerns, I'm coming in to the hospital to perform surgery on another patient, do you think she can wait a few hours to be seen?"

C: "Dr. Back, I'm very concerned about the rapid progression of her symptoms, I think she will deteriorate further if she doesn't have an emergency decompressive laminectomy soon and I would really appreciate you seeing the patient as soon as you get to the hospital."

E: "If you feel that strongly about it, I'll see her as soon as I get there, about 10 minutes."

C: "Thank you."

E: "Doctor, the patient is back from MRI, her x-rays and labs are back."

UCG negative

WBC 7.0, neutrophils 90%

Hgb/Hct 9/27

Plt 110

Na 140

K 4

Cl 106

CO_2 19

BUN 16

Cr 1.0

Glu 110

LDH 550

PT/PTT 12/36

INR 1.0

CXR: Normal

Lumbar XR: Narrowed disk space at T10 with erosion of adjacent vertebrae

MRI: Intense enhancement at the T10 level with compression of the spinal cord

E: "Dr. Back is here, he's seen the patient and the MRI and he'd like to take the patient to the OR now for decompression. That concludes this case."

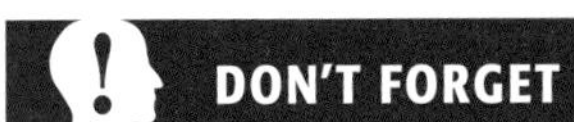

When you do not know the appropriate medicine or does it is acceptable to say that you will look them up in the appropriate reference.

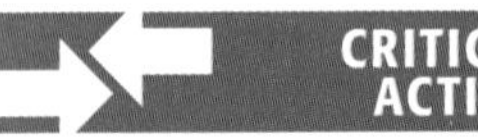

Getting the appropriate consultations is always a critical action. In this case, ensuring that the patient is seen in an emergent manner is also critical.

CASE ASSESSMENT

Overall, the candidate managed this case extremely well. Throughout the encounter, the candidate obtained an appropriate history and physical tailored for the back pain patient. The candidate did not let herself get thrown off by the patient's repeated requests for pain medication. She was able to incorporate managing the patient's pain with her focused history and physical. Notice that the candidate did not know the appropriate antibiotics for empiric coverage of an epidural abscess but was able to look them up during the examination.

The candidate did a good job of managing an HIV patient with a fever, sending the appropriate labs, and then tailoring down to the most likely diagnosis. Once the candidate realized that this patient had an emergent problem, she got the appropriate antibiotics started and the appropriate consultant on the line to see the patient. Notice that the candidate had to impress the emergent nature of the complaint on to the consultant. It is common in the oral boards to have to push the consultant to come when they are needed, so be prepared to know if the patient needs to be seen immediately or can wait a few hours to be seen.

Critical Actions

1. Adequate pain control.
2. Administer intravenous (IV) antibiotics.
3. Obtain emergent magnetic resonance imaging (MRI) to make the diagnosis.
4. Obtain emergent consultation for decompression.

Test Performance

1. *Data acquisition:* The candidate was able to quickly narrow down an extensive differential through an effective history and physical. Score = **6**
2. *Problem solving:* The candidate was able to rapidly assimilate data from the patient encounter, interpret test results, and synthesize information to direct further management. Score = **7**
3. *Patient management:* The candidate did an excellent job getting to the diagnosis and then quickly treating the infection and consulting for definitive management even prior to verification by imaging. Score = **7**
4. *Resource utilization:* The candidate ordered extensive testing, which is understandable for an ill-appearing immunocompromised patient. However, there is redundancy in obtaining an x-ray (XR) and magnetic resonance (MR) of the thoracic spine. Canceling the XR once the MR was done in a timely fashion, could have improved this score. Score = **6**
5. *Health care provided (outcome):* The candidate provided great care for this patient, arriving at the diagnosis efficiently and initiating early antibiotics. Score = **7**
6. *Interpersonal relations and communication skills:* The candidate eventually treated the patient's pain and was able to reassure the patient regarding her untreated human immunodeficiency virus (HIV). However, the candidate could have improved this score if it was clearer to the patient the reason pain control was being delayed. Score = **6**

7. *Comprehension of pathophysiology:* The candidate recognized the multiple risk factors this patient had for an epidural abscess and was able to make this a priority diagnosis that needed prompt evaluation. Score = **7**
8. *Clinical competence (overall):* The candidate was very effective in their management of this case, but could have improved their resource utilization and communication skills. Score = **6**

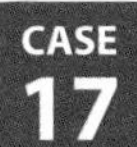

CASE 17 85 y/o Male With Abdominal Pain

Navneet Cheema, Thomas J. Regan, and Aleksandr Gorenbeyn

INITIAL INFORMATION

Name: Mr. Dyehard

Age: 85 years

Mode of arrival: Brought in by ambulance

Gender: Male

CC: Abdominal pain

VS: BP 118/90, HR 132, RR 26, T 37.7°C (99.9°F)

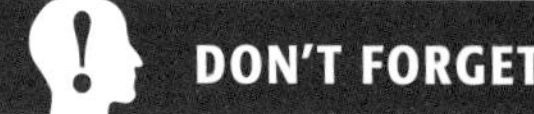

DON'T FORGET

When a vital sign is missing from the initial information—it is almost always abnormal—ask for it.

PLAY OF CASE

C: "What do I see as I walk into the patient's room?"

E: "The patient is a well-dressed older male lying on the hospital cart, who appears anxious, uncomfortable, and pale."

KEY QUESTION

Ask this open-ended question at the beginning of every case.

C: "Nurse, please undress the patient, put the patient on a cardiac monitor, show me a rhythm strip, begin oxygen via NC and titrate to keep sat above 97%, place a 16-gauge IV and begin NS and give a 500-cc bolus and draw blood for lab tests. Please obtain a stat 12-lead ECG and show it to me when ready. What is the saturation on room air?"

E: "Those orders are being done. The rhythm strip shows NSR in the 90s. His saturation is 97%."

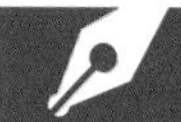

KEY ORDERS

Most of the patients you see during the exam will be unstable (or will become that way). Every unstable patient requires IV access (preferably two large-bore IVs), oxygen, and cardiac monitoring (and in most cases an ECG). In this case, as the patient has chest pain, sending cardiac labs and getting a stat portable chest XR is also appropriate at this time.

C: "Hello Mr. Dyehard, I am Dr. Apple. What brings you in today?"

E: "Doc, I have a really bad stomach pain. I woke up from a nap with it an hour ago. I thought a bowel movement would help, but it didn't."

C: "Have you ever had this pain before?"

E: "No, never."

C: "Are you nauseated or vomiting? Is your back hurting too?"

E: "I have nausea, but no vomiting. My back hurts a little bit."

C: "Do you also have chest pain or shortness of breath? Any light-headedness?"

E: "No, none of that. Only my stomach is hurting. It hurts quite a lot, doctor, right here in the middle. What is wrong with me?"

C: "That's what I am trying to figure out, sir. I need to ask you a few more questions. Is that OK?"

KEY ORDERS

When you order a test, always ask to be told the results when they come back. This places the responsibility for remembering to check the lab values on the examiner and relieves you of them—a good strategy.

E: "Patient: OK, go ahead. Nurse: Your ECG is done (Fig. C17-1)."

C: "Do you have any medical problems?"

E: "I have high blood pressure, and I had a heart attack a few months ago. They put two stents in my heart back then."

C: "Have you ever had any surgery on your abdomen?"

E: "No, I haven't."

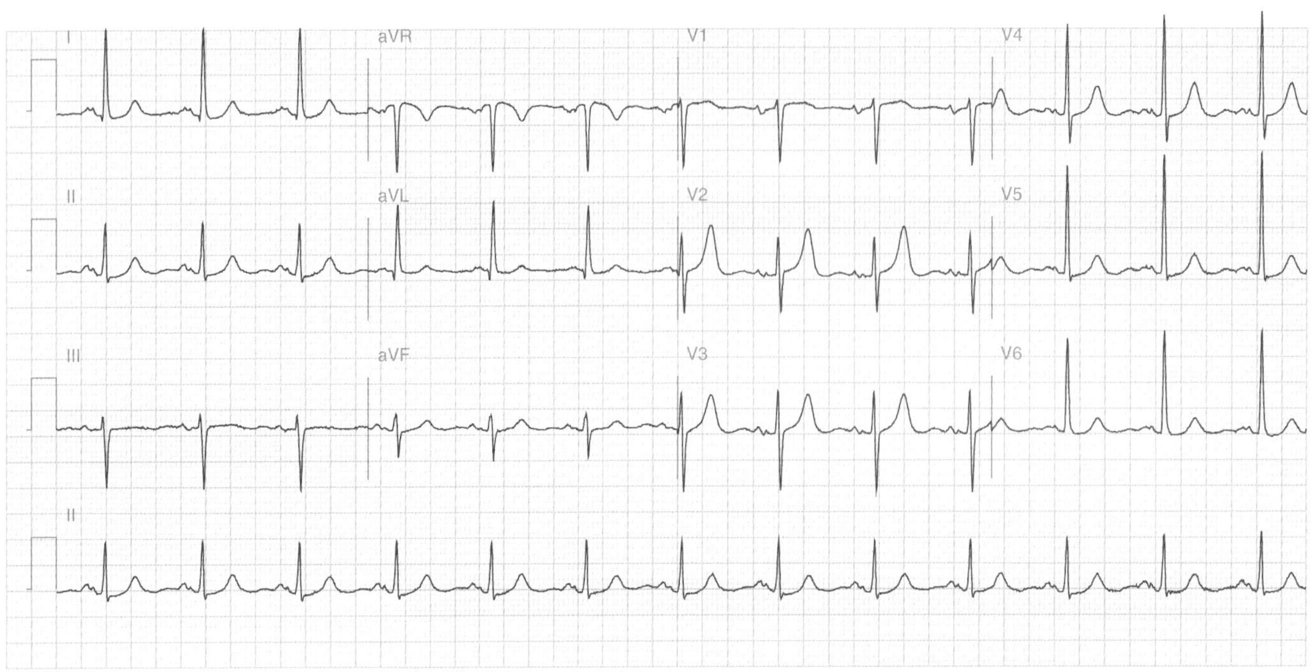

Figure C17-1. ECG with NSR and LVH, but no acute ST-T changes. (*Reprinted with permission from Fauci AS, Braunwald E, Kasper DL, et al.* Harrison's Principles of Internal Medicine. *17th ed. New York, NY: McGraw-Hill; 2008.*)

C: "Are you on any medications? Do you have any allergies?"

E: "I take some heart medications and an aspirin every morning. I have no allergies."

C: "Do you smoke or use alcohol or drugs?"

E: "No, I do not."

C: "I'd like to examine the patient. How is the patient's skin? Is the patient still pale? Is he cyanotic? Are the mucous membranes moist?"

E: "The patient remains pale, not cyanotic and mucous membranes are dry."

C: "Nurse, please perform a bedside hemoglobin test and send blood to the lab for CBC, electrolytes, BUN/Cr, glucose, coags, lactic acid, liver function tests, lipase, and a type and screen. I'd also like a urine analysis."

E: "The orders are being done."

C: "Is there any icterus or conjunctival pallor?"

E: "HEENT is normal."

C: "Are the patient's lungs clear, are there any abnormal heart sounds?"

E: "Normal."

C: "I'd like to do a vascular exam of all extremities."

E: "Pulses are present throughout and symmetric."

C: "I would like to examine the patient's abdomen."

E: "What are you looking for?"

C: "I am looking at the visual appearance for distention, listening for bowel sounds, and palpating for tenderness, guarding, rigidity or rebound, distention, or masses."

E: "The abdomen is flat and soft with hypoactive BS. It is not distended. There are no masses, and though there is diffuse tenderness it is not localized to any quadrant. There is no guarding or rebound."

C: "Rectal exam?"

E: "What are you looking for?"

C: "I'm looking for rectal tone, masses, presence of stool, and results of the stool guaiac."

E: "Rectal tone is normal. There is brown stool that is heme positive."

C: "Gross neurological exam?"

E: "There is no focal weakness or sensory disturbance found."

C: "Nurse, I'd like you to repeat the patient's vitals."

E: "Repeat vitals show a BP 120/90, HR 110, RR 24, sat 98%."

C: "Mr. Dyehard, how is your pain. Has it gotten any better?"

E: "No, it hasn't. What's wrong with me, doctor? Is there anything you can give me for the pain?"

C: "I'm not certain of your diagnosis but I think that you might have a problem concerning one of your blood vessels supplying your intestines. This problem is called mesenteric ischemia and it's like having a heart attack of your intestines. It's when an artery providing blood to your intestines starts to close off. Another problem could possibly be an aortic aneurysm. This concerns your aorta, which is a big artery that runs down the middle of your abdominal cavity. It may be leaking, which would also be a serious problem. It is also possible that you have appendicitis or an infection of your colon called diverticulitis, though that seems less likely. We will need to do some more tests to figure it out. In the meantime, I can give you something for the pain and nausea to make you feel comfortable."

E: "OK, doc, do what it takes."

C: "Nurse, please give Mr. Dyehard 4 mg of morphine and 4 mg of ondansetron IV, insert a second 18-gauge IV and **repeat a 500-cc saline bolus.** I would also like a Foley placed. Also, please order a flat and upright abdominal x-rays. When the x-rays are back, I would like the surgeon on call paged."

E: "This is being done, doctor."

C: "Also, I'd like you to repeat his vitals after his medications and repeat fluid bolus."

E: "His repeat vitals are BP 130/85, HR 88, RR 22, sat 97%. His x-rays are also back. The abdominal x-rays have a mild ileus pattern with calcifications of the abdominal aorta but there is no evidence of aneurysmal dilation."

C: "Nurse, please give a third 500-cc bolus of NS. How is the patient feeling now?"

E: "The patient says he feels a bit better. Dr. Knife is on the phone."

C: "Dr. Knife, I have an 85-year-old male here with abdominal pain for little over an hour, whose pain is out of proportion to his physical exam findings. His abdominal x-rays demonstrate a mild ileus and though there are calcifications of the abdominal aorta, there is no dilation present. I suspect that he is having mesenteric ischemia. I would like you to come in to evaluate him."

E: "Are you sure? I am at home now. Why don't you obtain a CT first and then call me back?"

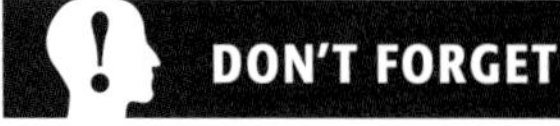

Remember—when the examiner says that an organ system is "normal" there are no pertinent findings, but when they say "what are you looking for" there is usually a finding there that is relevant.

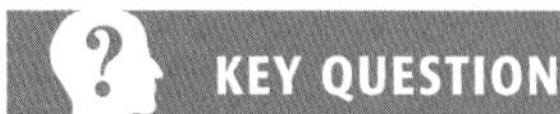

Remember to reassess your patient frequently.

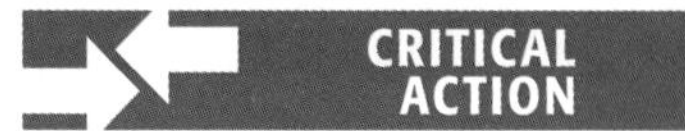

There are two critical actions taking place here. First, the examiner needs to consider and act upon both mesenteric ischemia and AAA. Secondly, they must act to rule out both diagnoses.

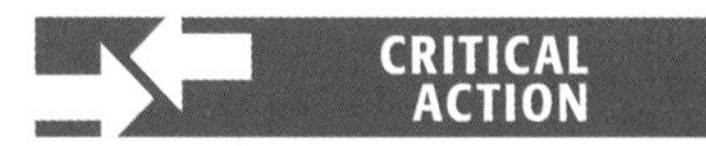

Giving ongoing fluid resuscitation is always a critical action when the patient is hypotensive (or borderline hypotensive).

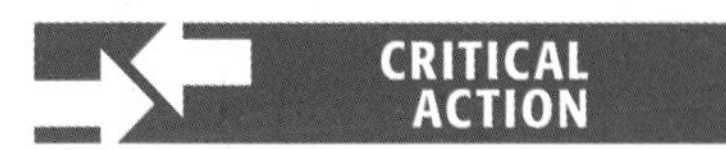

Getting an early surgical consultation is a critical action in this case.

C: "Dr. Knife, I think this patient needs your attention now."

E: "Well, do you have any labs back yet?"

C: "Not yet."

E: "Then call me when they are back. I'll talk to you later." (The surgeon hangs up.)

C: "Nurse, please order an abdominal CT. Is bedside ultrasound available?"

E: "Yes. What are you looking for?"

C: "Is an AAA present? Is there free fluid?"

E: "There is no free fluid and no evidence of an AAA."

E: "Labs and urine analysis are back, doctor."

UA is normal.

WBC 18,000, H/H 15/45.

Na 150, K 4.9, Cl 122, CO_2 19, glu 131, Ca 8.9.

Lactic acid 2.5.

Everything else ordered is normal.

C: "This patient has an acidosis and an elevated lactate. Nurse, please obtain ABG on room air."

E: "This is being done. Radiology reports that the CT scanner is down for repair."

C: "This patient needs an angiogram then. Please page the radiologist for me."

The examinee is completing the critical action from above in this section by getting an abdominal US and ordering tests for mesenteric ischemia.

E: "Doctor, the ABG results are back."

ABG (room air) 7.24/32/80/14.

E: "Dr. Apple, the patient is looking worse."

C: "Please repeat his vitals."

E: "His vitals are now: BP 95/50, P 120, RR 32, T 37.7°C (100°F), 94% on 2-L NC."

C: "Put this patient on a 100% oxygen non-rebreather mask, and infuse a liter of normal saline as fast as possible. What is his appearance now, can he respond to me?"

Intubating the patient when they become unresponsive is a critical action.

E: "He is tachypneic, diaphoretic, moaning, and appears confused."

C: "I am going to intubate him now. Please draw 20 mg of etomidate and 100 of succinylcholine and give it in quick succession when ready. I will use a Miller 3 blade and 8.0 ET tube. Call respiratory therapist for a ventilator."

E: "Patient is intubated successfully."

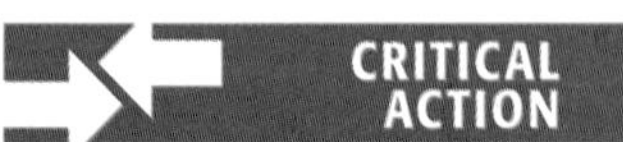

Giving antibiotics to this decompensating patient with an acute abdominal process is a critical action.

C: "I need a post intubation CXR. Please also insert a nasogastric tube and administer 1 g of ceftriaxone and 500 mg of metronidazole IV. What are the vitals now?"

E: "Vitals are 110/55, HR 110, RR 16 on ventilator, 100%. The CXR reveals clear lung fields with an endotracheal tube in good position. The radiologist, Dr. Vision, is on the phone."

C: "Dr. Vision, I have a critically ill patient with possible mesenteric ischemia. I need a stat angiogram."

E: "OK, bring him over right away."

C: "I'd like this patient to be accompanied by a nurse over to the radiology suite."

E: "The angiogram results are back, doctor."

Angiogram results: SMA occlusion, 6 cm from the origin, proximal to ileocolic artery take off.

C: "Nurse, please call Dr. Knife back."

E: "He is on the line."

C: "Dr. Knife, the patient I talked about earlier has an SMA occlusion on the angiogram. He decompensated briefly but has responded to intubation with mechanical ventilation and fluid resuscitation. He needs to be admitted to the ICU for stabilization and then will likely need to go to the OR for resection of necrotic bowel."

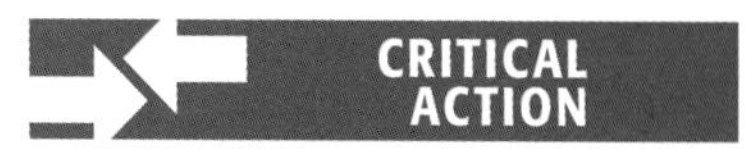

Admitting the patient to the appropriate level of care is always a critical action.

E: "OK, I will be right in. Please tell the ICU team the patient is being admitted."

C: "I'll call them right now. Nurse, please call the ICU team."

E: "This concludes this case."

CASE ASSESSMENT

This candidate managed this difficult case very well. He played the role of a physician smoothly, taking an appropriate history from the patient. He recognized immediately that the patient was sick and instituted proper monitoring. He formulated an appropriate differential for the presentation and communicated it well to the patient. He managed the patient's pain and symptoms and contacted the appropriate consultant.

Having encountered difficulties with consultant's availability, he moved on to additional available radiographic testing. Of note: bedside ultrasound (US) performed by the emergency medicine (EM) physician is helpful to rule out abdominal aortic aneurysm (AAA) and does not delay this patient's care.

Proper monitoring throughout the case was helpful in treating patient's relative hypovolemia early on and the candidate promptly intervened with intubation, mechanical ventilation, and continued fluid resuscitation when deterioration with hypotension and mental status changes occurred. He appreciated the patient's metabolic acidosis early and suspected mesenteric ischemia based on the history, physical examination, and preliminary laboratory findings, including the acidosis and elevated lactate level. The standard of care in treating mesenteric ischemia is considering the condition early on, obtaining further diagnostic testing in a timely manner, resuscitation, correction of underlying precipitants when appropriate, administration of antibiotics, and consideration of potential surgical intervention. The candidate met all these objectives in a timely fashion.

Critical Actions

1. Considering an abdominal crisis, including mesenteric ischemia and ruling out a leaking abdominal aortic aneurysm (AAA).
2. Performing a diagnostic procedure to confirm the diagnosis of mesenteric ischemia.
3. Initiate fluid resuscitation.

4. Intubation and mechanical ventilation when the patient deteriorates.
5. Administer antibiotics.
6. Admission to the intensive care unit (ICU).
7. Early surgical consultation.

Test Performance

1. *Data acquisition:* The candidate had an organized and logical approach to the history and physical. Score = **7**
2. *Problem solving:* The candidate was able to use available information to quickly narrow down the differential and evaluate for life threats. Score = **7**
3. *Patient management:* Great clinical judgment was evident with appropriate treatment decisions based upon available information and resources. Score = **7**
4. *Resource utilization:* The candidate had good use of resources that were available. He was cost-effective and did not compromise patient care. Score = **7**
5. *Health care provided (outcome):* The candidate was able to quickly recognize changes in the patient's condition and intervene appropriately. Score = **7**
6. *Interpersonal relations and communication skills:* Effective information exchange with the patient and nurse. The candidate provided excellent explanations of the differential to the patient. Score = **8**
7. *Comprehension of pathophysiology:* The candidate did an outstanding job of describing the underlying pathophysiology for mesenteric ischemia to the patient. Score = **8**
8. *Clinical competence (overall):* The candidate excelled in this case, being able to effectively obtain the history, arrive at the correct diagnosis, and keeping the patient updated during the process. Score = **7**

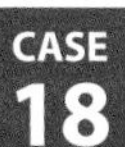

45 y/o Female With Shortness of Breath

Navneet Cheema and Mark P. Bogner

INITIAL INFORMATION

Name: Jane Smith

Mode of arrival: Husband/private car

Age: 45 years

Gender: Female

VS: T 38.0°C (100.4°F), BP 108/64, HR 98, RR 24, O_2 sat: 95% on RA

CC: Difficulty breathing

Setting: It is 10:00 AM Monday morning and you are working a single coverage shift in a busy rural hospital emergency department (ED) with an annual volume of 18,000 ED visits. You have excellent nursing and ancillary staff to assist you. The hospital resources and medical staff are superb for this environment. The nearest tertiary care center is 18 minutes away by helicopter (each way), and is a 60-minute trip by ground ambulance.

PLAY OF THE CASE

C: "What do I see as I walk into the patient's room?"

E: "The patient appears her stated age, well groomed, and dressed in professional attire. She appears reasonably comfortable but somewhat anxious. The patient is accompanied by her husband."

C: "Hello Mrs. Smith, I am Dr. Emergency. Nurse, please place the patient on a cardiac monitor and show me a rhythm strip when possible. Let's start her on oxygen via NC at 4 L, and place an 18-gauge IV with NS at 80 cc/h and draw blood for labs. For now, just have the lab hold the blood until I determine what tests we need."

E: "Your orders are being done. The patient's rhythm strip shows a sinus rate of 92 bpm."

C: "So Mrs. Smith, the triage nurse tells me you are feeling short of breath. Can you tell me some more about how you are feeling?"

E: "I started feeling ill late last night. It seems like I just can't get a full breath. I have never felt this way before, it is quite uncomfortable."

C: "Have you noticed anything that seems to make it worse or better, such as lying down flat, exerting yourself, coughing, or anything else?"

E: "When I walked up the stairs this morning it seemed a bit worse."

C: "Have you had a fever, cough, or any cold symptoms like sore throat or runny nose?"

E: "No, but I have felt warm."

C: "Nurse, could you please order a stat bedside ECG and CXR?"

E: "Your orders are being done."

C: "Have you noticed any swelling or pain in your legs?"

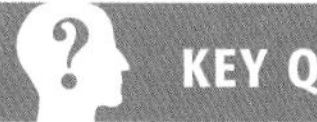

KEY QUESTION

Ask this open-ended question at the beginning of every case.

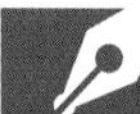

KEY ORDERS

Most of the patients you see during the exam will be unstable (or will become that way). Every unstable patient requires IV access (preferably two large-bore IVs), oxygen, and cardiac monitoring (and in most cases an ECG).

KEY ORDERS

When you order a test, always ask to be told the results when they come back. This places the responsibility for remembering to check the lab values on the examiner and relieves you of them—a good strategy.

E: "No."

C: "Have you fainted or felt like you might faint?"

E: "No."

C: "Any chest pain with a deep breath, cough, or otherwise?"

E: "Yes, it hurts right here (points to right lateral chest, mid-axillary line, at the level of ribs 6-12) when I cough or take a deep breath."

C: "Does it hurt there now?"

E: "No."

C: "Do you feel any better on the oxygen?"

E: "Perhaps a little bit better."

C: "Have you felt nauseated or sweaty?"

E: "No."

C: "Any abdominal pain or urinary changes?"

E: "No."

C: "Do you have any medical problems?"

E: "No, I just had a complete physical last month. Dr. Primary said everything was fine."

C: "Have you ever had surgery?"

E: "My appendix was removed when I was 12 and I had two C-sections many years ago."

C: "Have you ever had any form of cancer?"

E: "No."

C: "Do you smoke?"

E: "Yes, a little more than half pack a day."

C: "Are you on any medications?"

E: "My doctor recently put me on estrogen. He said it was for my bones and menopause."

C: "Anything else?"

E: "Other than occasional acetaminophen for aches and pain, no, nothing else."

C: "Any special supplements, vitamins, or herbal medications?"

E: "No."

C: "Are you allergic to any medications?"

E: "No."

C: "Have you ever used IV drugs or any other recreational drugs?"

E: "No."

C: "Have you taken any long trips in the past 6 weeks where you were sitting for more than 4 hours?"

E: "My husband and I returned from a trip to Europe last week."

C: "Is there anything else you think I should know?"

E: "No."

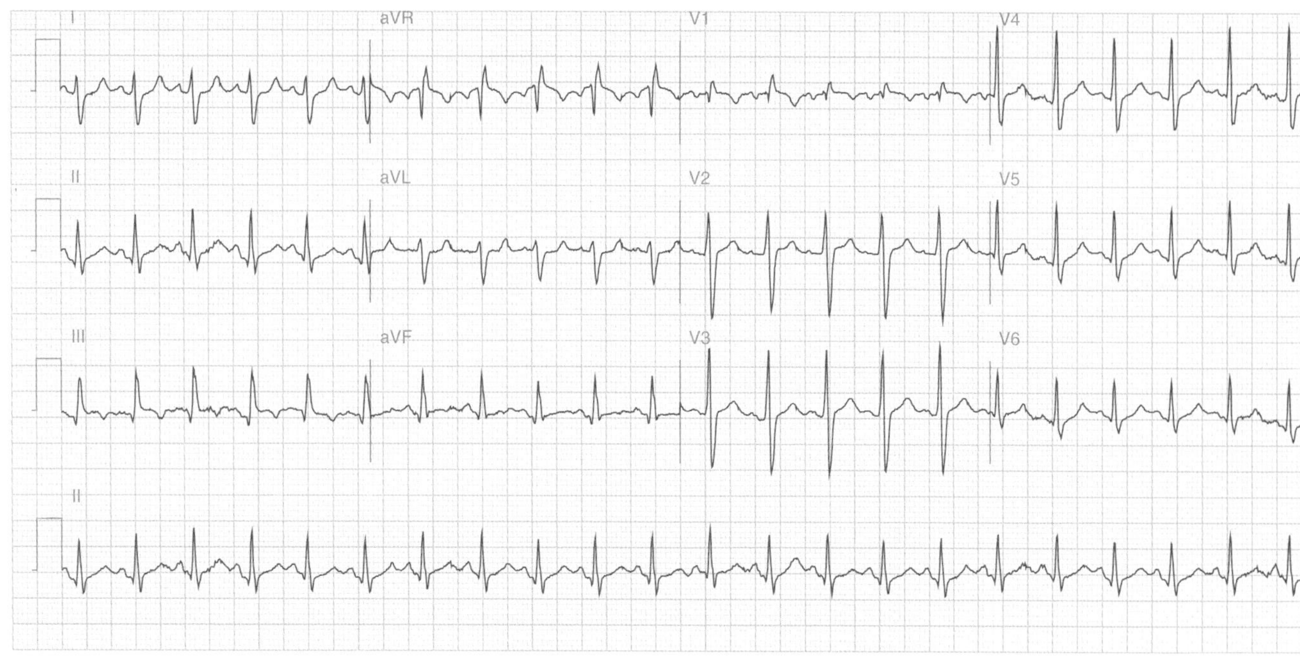

Figure C18-1. An ECG showing an S1Q3T3 pattern. (*Reprinted with permission from Fauci AS, Braunwald E, Kaspter DL, et al.* Harrison's Principles of Internal Medicine. *17th ed. New York, NY: McGraw-Hill; 2008.*)

E: "Your ECG is available (Fig. C18-1)."

C: "Thank you. While I look at that I would like the nurse to obtain a repeat complete set of vital signs and report them to me."

C: "Nurse, I would now like to order the following lab tests: CBC with differential, electrolytes, BUN, Cr, serum glucose, UA, cardiac enzymes including troponin, INR, PTT, BNP and a D-Dimer."

E: "Repeat vitals = T 38.1°C (100.58°F), BP 112/68, HR 102, RR 24, O_2 sat: 98% on O_2 at 4-L NC. The nurse will promptly take care of your orders."

C: "Mrs. Smith, my greatest concern from what you have told me so far is that you may have something called a pulmonary embolism, which is a blood clot in your lungs. These things can create big problems, or can be very minor. There are many other possible explanations for your symptoms and we will need to check into all of this further. More testing will be necessary and I want to warn both you and Mr. Smith that you may be here for several hours until we get to the bottom of this, and you may have to stay in the hospital overnight. My staff and I will try to keep you comfortable and answer your questions. We will keep you posted on things as best we can. Next I need to examine you, and then we will get on with the tests. When I have some results and hopefully some answers I will talk to you again. In the meantime, you can ask your nurse if you need anything. Would you like something for pain?"

E: "No doctor, I am comfortable just sitting here right now. My husband and I read about blood clots on the Internet when we searched 'trouble breathing' and I was actually quite worried I might have one when I decided to come in to the ER. I am glad you are checking to be sure either way."

C: "I would now like to proceed with my physical examination."

E: "Go ahead."

C: "Does the patient appear in distress, pale, or diaphoretic?"

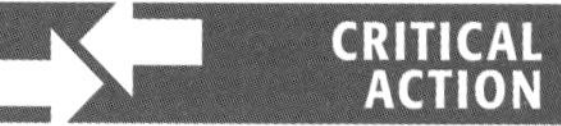

Considering PE in this febrile patient with shortness of breath and multiple risk factors is a critical action in this case.

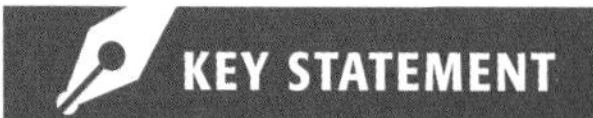

Remember to talk to your patient, explain test results, and describe the plan to them. Also, while treating pain is not always a critical action, it often is, so treat their pain.

E: "She does not appear pale or diaphoretic. Again, she seems mildly anxious but otherwise in no apparent distress."

C: "Are there any significant findings on the patient's HEENT examination?"

E: "No."

C: "How about her neck?"

E: "What are you looking for?"

C: "Tracheal deviation, JVD, subcutaneous emphysema, swelling or a hematoma."

E: "Neck examination is normal."

C: "When I auscultate her chest, do I hear wheezing, rales, rhonchi, diminished or asymmetrical breath sounds? Is there a pleuritic rub? Also, is there any chest tenderness or deformity?"

E: "Chest examination is normal except for a few scattered crackles heard intermittently in the right posterolateral lung base."

C: "On the cardiac examination, is her PMI displaced, are S_1 and S_2 clear, are there any murmurs, rubs, or gallops?"

E: "Cardiac examination is normal."

C: "When I examine her abdomen, do I palpate any masses, pulsatile or otherwise, tenderness, guarding, rebound? Are bowel sounds normal?"

E: "Abdominal examination is normal."

C: "In the extremities, are there any pulse deficits or asymmetries, deformities, swelling, or edema? Does she have a Homan sign or calf squeeze tenderness? When I measure her calves, is there a difference in circumference left to right of >1 cm? Are there any obvious venous cords or varicose veins?"

E: "Her right calf measures 1.8 cm greater than her left and she has slight calf squeeze tenderness on the right. Her extremity examination is otherwise normal."

C: "Any occult or gross blood in the stool on rectal examination?"

E: "No."

C: "Are there any neurologic deficits such as a difference in power between right and left arms, legs? Any cranial nerve deficits? Are there any gross sensory deficits, particularly unilateral loss or altered sensation? Her mental status can be stated as grossly normal from the history session."

E: "No deficits."

C: "I have completed my physical examination for now."

E: "The portable CXR is available for review (Fig. C18-2)."

C: "The CXR reveals a RLL infiltrate laterally versus atelectasis versus effusion. This may represent pneumonia, but I remain concerned about the possibility of a pulmonary embolus. I would like to order a PE protocol spiral CT angiogram of the chest with lower extremity run offs. Please administer dalteparin 200 IU/kg SQ."

E: The radiology department reports that the CT scanner is down."

C: "Is a V/Q scan available?"

E: "Yes. Would you like the patient to go now?"

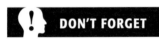

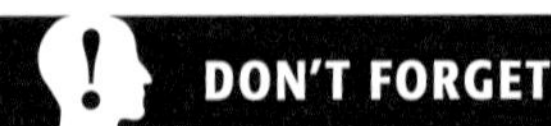

Remember—when the examiner says that an organ system is "normal" there are no pertinent findings, but when they say "what are you looking for" there is usually a finding there that is relevant.

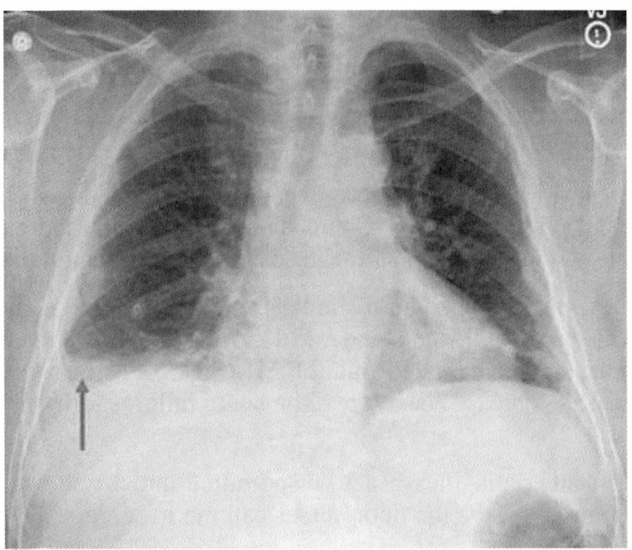

Figure C18-2. An AP CXR showing a small right-sided pleural effusion (arrow). (*Reprinted with permission from Fauci AS, Braunwald E, Kaspter DL, et al.* Harrison's Principles of Internal Medicine. *17th ed. New York, NY: McGraw-Hill; 2008.*)

C: "If the VS remain stable, the patient may go to the radiology department accompanied by an RN. Are any lab results available for me to review?"

E: "The following laboratory values are available:

CBC: WBC 12.8, 76 PMN, 12 bands, 12 lymph, H/H 13/39, Plt 378.

PT 13 (INR 1.0), PTT 29

BMP: Na 140, K 4.6, Cl 104, CO_2 23, BUN 14, Cr 1.1, Glu 111, Ca 9.9

CPK 121, 3.9 MB, troponin 0.18

D-Dimer 8.4

E: "The patient is just returning from her V/Q scan."

C: "May I review the V/Q scan or speak to the radiologist for a report."

E: "The radiologist sent a written 'preliminary report' with the patient. It states: the V/Q scan demonstrates large ventilation-perfusion mismatch involving the right lower lobe consistent with significant PE."

C: "Has the patient's condition changed?"

E: "No."

C: "I would like to speak to her physician please, to arrange admission."

E: "Hello Dr. Emergency, this is Dr. Primary."

C: "Dr. Primary, I have one of your patients here in the ED. Mrs. Smith came in with shortness of breath, pleuritic chest pain, right calf pain and has a positive D-Dimer and a V/Q scan demonstrating a right lower lobe PE. We have initiated anticoagulation with LMWH and she is currently comfortable. Mrs. Smith is a smoker, recently placed on estrogen and she just returned from a trip to Europe last week. Her slightly elevated troponin should be followed and she should be ruled out for MI, but as you know slight troponin elevations are

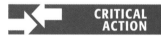

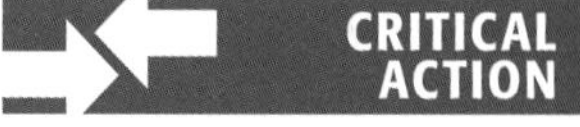

There are two critical actions here. First, the examinee has to order the appropriate test to diagnose PE, and second, they have to anti-coagulate the patient prior to the scan.

not uncommon with PE. Her ECG does show an S1Q3T3 pattern but no other acute ischemic changes. CXR shows a right pleural based density c/w the location of her PE. Given her age of 45, occult cancer will still need to be ruled out later. For now she needs admission for further anticoagulation, observation, and to be ruled out for MI."

E: "Dr. Emergency, I have a really busy schedule in clinic today. Would you consider writing her prescriptions for Coumadin and dalteparin and having her see me in clinic on Wednesday? I can arrange an outpatient stress test that same day."

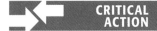

DON'T FORGET

On exam day, consultants will often "push back." You will be expected to advocate for your patient and demand the level of care you feel is appropriate.

C: "Well Dr. Primary, if she had a simple DVT that would be entirely appropriate, but with proven PE the standard of care is still inpatient management. And again, she should be ruled out for MI. She could throw a bigger clot and decompensate quickly, develop right heart failure, arrhythmia, or other complications."

E: "I think you are right. Please get her admitted and I will see her upstairs over my lunch break. Have the floor nurses call me for orders."

C: "Will do."

E: "Dr. Emergency, Mrs. Smith has become unresponsive! Please come see her!"

C: "What do I see when I look at the patient now. May I have a current set of vitals please? I would also like a repeat ECG."

E: "The patient is unconscious with rapid, shallow breaths. She is pale and diaphoretic. Her BP is 60/40, HR 140, RR 36, oxygen saturation is 84%. She moans in response to sternal rub."

Intubating the patient when they become unresponsive is a critical action.

C: "Nurse, please have someone call respiratory therapy and have them bring us a ventilator. Please also have someone get the airway equipment and crash carts. Also ask the unit secretary get in touch with the closest helicopter transport service and see if they are available and can standby. Please have the unit secretary get the tertiary care center ICU attending on the phone for me after checking on the helicopter. I would like to immediately intubate the patient. Nurse, please draw up 20 mg etomidate and 125 mg succinylcholine. Tell me when you are ready with the drugs. I will prepare and test my equipment, including bag valve mask, suction, oxygen, several ET tubes sizes 6-5, 7-0, and 7-5, stylet, and laryngoscope blades—and begin pre-oxygenating and assisting the patient's ventilation efforts using the BVM and oxygen at 15 LPM. I will place a nasal airway if needed."

E: "The medications are ready."

C: "Please administer 20 mg etomidate and then the 125 mg of succinylcholine in that order. Nurse 2, please provide cricoid pressure."

E: "Done."

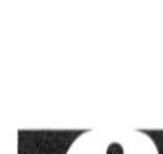
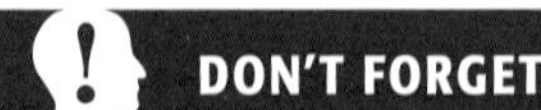

You will need to be able to describe emergent procedures such as chest tube, intubation, pericardiocentesis, etc. This is a good outline for how one describes an emergent intubation—memorize this. This examinee does not order a post-intubation CXR—which should always be done.

C: "I will now endotracheally intubate the patient with a 7-0 French tube. After placing the tube I will confirm the presence of bilateral breath sounds and use the colorimetric end-tidal CO_2 device to further confirm proper placement. Once intubation is completed and tube placement confirmed, I request that the nurse administer 5 mg midazolam IV."

E: "Done. What now?"

C: "What are the patient's vital signs after intubation?"

E: "BP 100/68, HR 110, oxygen saturation 100%."

C: "Has her ECG changed?"

E: "No."

C: "Is the helicopter service available?"

E: "Yes, but they won't launch in our direction until you have an accepting physician."

C: "Can I speak to the ICU attending at the tertiary care center?"

E: "She is on the phone."

C: "Dr. ICU, this is Dr. Emergency at nearby rural ED, I was just preparing to admit a 45-year-old woman to our hospital for further treatment of her PE when she decompensated and required intubation. The patient, Mrs. Smith, has a definite right lower lobe PE and may have thrown another clot. She is generally healthy, a smoker, on estrogen replacement therapy, and returned from a trip to Europe last week. She has no other known health issues or medications. She has had no recent surgeries and no known cancers. I would like to transfer her to your hospital via helicopter for further care given the sudden deterioration in her condition and my concern that she has a massive PE."

E: "I will be happy to accept the patient. We have a bed ready in the ICU."

C: "Great, thank you. Provided that it will not delay transport, while the helicopter is on its way here I would like to get a quick CT scan of her brain to rule out neoplasm and then start administering alteplase. I suspect she had a small PE when she presented here this morning but has now developed a massive PE given the sudden change in her condition."

E: "Sounds like a good idea."

C: "Nurse, please notify the helicopter service that Dr. ICU has accepted the patient and get them headed in our direction. Please arrange a stat head CT and have pharmacy prepare alteplase for weight-based bolus and infusion. Please have the unit secretary get the necessary COBRA/EMTALA transfer paperwork together and I will complete these forms along with the nurse. I would also like to talk to the patient's husband and any other family the patient might have waiting for her in a private consultation room."

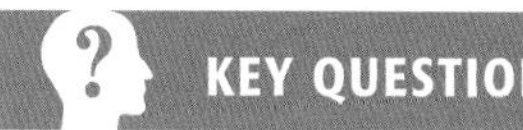

Remember to reassess your patient frequently.

E: "That is all done."

C: "Has the patient's condition changed? May I have a current set of vital signs?"

E: "No change in general condition. BP 108/72, HR 110, O_2 sat 100%."

C: "May I please speak to Dr. Primary again?"

E: "Dr. Primary is on the line."

C: "Dr. Primary, Mrs. Smith's condition has changed. Just after we spoke she became unresponsive and hypotensive and I had to intubate her. She has stabilized somewhat but I think she might now have a massive PE. I believe she will be best served at a tertiary care center. I have already made the necessary arrangements. I would have spoken to you first but her condition mandated rapid intervention and planning."

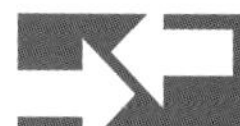

CRITICAL ACTION

Admitting the patient to the appropriate level of care is always a critical action.

E: "No problem. Thanks for the call and for arranging the transfer. Tell her husband I will check in with him later. The case is now over."

CASE ASSESSMENT

The candidate managed the case well and achieved all critical actions. He did an excellent job of eliciting key elements of history that are important in assessing the pretest probability of PE. Atypical presentations are more common than the "classic" story of dyspnea, tachypnea, pleuritic chest pain, and hemoptysis. Pulmonary embolism (PE) commonly presents as simple dyspnea with no other symptoms. It may also present as syncope with no warning. Because PE is not uncommon and has a high mortality rate, it must be considered in virtually all patients with any signs or symptoms of dyspnea, other respiratory complaints, new onset wheezing, weakness, syncope, chest pain, fever, acute right heart failure, and others. In any such case where a clear alternative diagnosis cannot be definitively assigned, PE must be considered. Suspicion is the first step in diagnosing PE and sets the physician on the right path of obtaining appropriate history, examination, and confirmatory studies. The candidate clearly kept PE on his differential diagnosis and elicited the history necessary to guide his actions through the rest of the case.

It is always wise to ask any patient "is there anything else you think I should know?" when you believe you are done with history taking. Not only will real patients frequently surprise you with critical information in response to this open-ended question, but the examiner might also; ie, if he or she feels you are on the right track but missed some little thing out of "nervousness" or due to the artificial nature of an oral exam, this is a chance for the examiner to "help" you. Give them this opportunity!

Remember that many patients do not consider dietary supplements, vitamins, or herbs as "medications." In this case it was not so important; however, in any toxicology case this history is critical and it is a good habit to ask. Many herbal remedies, teas, and supplements if used in excess can result in toxicity or may interact adversely with prescription medications, particularly anticoagulants—which this patient ultimately needed.

D-Dimer studies have become part of the standard of care in diagnosing deep vein thrombosis (DVT) and pulmonary embolism (PE). However, in this case the D-Dimer was unnecessary. The patient's presentation, recent travel, tachypnea, dyspnea, calf swelling, and pain result in a Wells Criteria Score of >6. In such cases, the pretest probability of PE is so high that a normal D-Dimer cannot be used to rule out PE and adds nothing to the workup. Anticoagulation followed immediately by V/Q or computed tomography (CT) angiography is mandatory in this case. Ordering the D-Dimer was the candidate's only significant error and would not hurt his score all that much if he were to comment while ordering that it probably wouldn't influence further testing all that much based on a high Wells Criteria Score.

The candidate did a good job of directing care without being overly authoritative. He communicated well with nurses, the primary physician, and the intensivist involved later. He made an effort to address the patient's concerns, comfort, and to communicate with her family. Please, thank you, and good manners count on exam day! "May I have" or "please obtain" are much better ways to ask than simply "get" or "get me."

Communicating detailed findings to a referring or primary physician and family members is an effective oral exam technique. This candidate applied this strategy masterfully to display his general understanding of the case, his interpretation of studies and figures, and his synthesis of the overall picture. He also used this approach to clarify his medical decision-making and demonstrate his solid understanding of current literature and standards of care in managing PE. It is worthwhile to study and remember this strategy as it will certainly be useful on exam day regardless of the cases you are presented with.

There is insufficient research data to prove that thrombolytics reduce mortality in PE. Thrombolytics have no role in treating "stable" patients with PE.

However, given the high mortality rate in patients with massive PE, and barring any absolute contraindications to thrombolysis, these agents may be life-saving in such cases and administering them in consultation with the intensivist was an elegant touch. The candidate initially requested PE protocol CT angiogram with lower extremity "venous run-offs" rather than V/Q. This is rapidly becoming the standard of care in appropriately equipped hospitals.

The candidate responded quickly and appropriately to the challenge when the patient's condition suddenly changed. Throughout the case, he did a superb job of recognizing the potential severity of the patient's condition, implementing appropriate measures, both therapeutically and diagnostically, and did so without delay. He definitely exceeded the standard of care and would score well on the case.

Critical Actions

1. Elicit appropriate historical information and suspect PE.
2. Initiate early anticoagulation before V/Q, using either unfractionated or low-molecular-weight heparin (LMWH).
3. Obtain V/Q or CT angiogram to prove PE in this highly suspicious patient.
4. Intubate and appropriately resuscitate the patient when she decompensates in ED.
5. Proper and early arrangements to transfer the patient to a tertiary care facility after she decompensates (ie, demonstrating evidence of massive PE).

Test Performance

1. *Data acquisition:* The candidate was very thorough with his history and physical, including asking about supplements, vitamins, and herbal products. Score = **8**
2. *Problem solving:* The candidate rapidly assessed the situation for severity and moved quickly to respond to data and changes in condition in an appropriate manner. He frequently asked for updates on the patient's condition and response to treatment, a good habit on oral exams. Score = **8**
3. *Patient management:* The candidate was thorough in his workup and treatment of this patient. Appropriately escalated treatment from LMWH to thrombolytics when the clinical condition changed. Score = **8**
4. *Resource utilization:* Resources were used appropriately and cost-effectively with the exception of the unnecessary D-Dimer. Score = **7**
5. *Health care provided (outcome):* The candidate was able to successfully advocate for the patient when he had push back from his consultant and expertly cared for the patient when the clinical condition deteriorated. Score = **8**
6. *Interpersonal relations and communication skills:* Very good interactions. Directive without being demanding. Also did a great job of setting expectations early on for the patient regarding workup and disposition. Score = **8**
7. *Comprehension of pathophysiology:* This candidate demonstrated great knowledge regarding the pathophysiology of PEs as he discussed the case with both the patient and consultants. Score = **7**
8. *Clinical competence (overall):* This case was excellent overall with the candidate excelling in data acquisition, health care provided, and communication skills. Score = **8**

CASE 19 2 y/o Fussy Male With Abdominal Pain

Navneet Cheema and Kip Adrian

INITIAL INFORMATION

Name: Jimmy Smith

Mode of arrival: Family

Age: 2 years

Gender: Male

VS: BP 80/40, P 175, RR 45, O_2 sat: 98% on RA

CC: Vomiting and fever

KEY QUESTION

Ask this open-ended question at the beginning of every case.

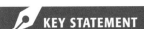

PLAY OF THE CASE

C: "What do I see as I walk into the patient's room?"

E: "The patient is lying in his mother's arms awake, but tired appearing, not moving or squirming."

C: "As I'm watching Jimmy how does his volume status appear? Specifically, are his mucous membranes moist, is his tongue/oropharynx moist, and what is his color like?"

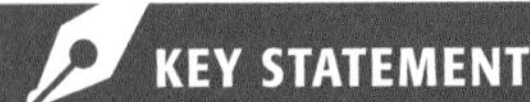

KEY STATEMENT

Remember to talk to your patient (or family in pediatric cases), explain test results, and describe the plan to them.

E: "The child appears pale, with dry mucous membranes and oropharynx."

C: "Ms. Smith, my name is Dr. Cramp and I'm the ER doctor today. Before we talk a little more, I'm concerned because Jimmy looks very dehydrated from all of his vomiting. I would like to start an IV and give Jimmy some fluids through it. At the same time I would like to collect a small amount of blood for some lab work. How does this sound to you?"

E: "Yes, that sounds fine."

C: "Nurse, please check the child's temperature and weight, and place the child on a cardiac and oxygen monitor."

KEY QUESTION

When a piece of information is missing, it is usually important. Make sure you have all five vital signs before you allow the case to go forward.

E: "The nurse checks the temperature which is 38°C (100.4°F). The child weighs 15 kg. The child is on the monitor which shows a sinus tachycardia with a heart rate in the 170s."

C: "Nurse, also please start a 20-gauge IV, giving a 300-cc NS bolus, and draw blood for labs. Please give 250 mg of Tylenol per rectum, and notify me when the bolus is finished."

C: "Hello Jimmy, my name is Dr. Cramp and I'm here to help you feel better. Ms. Smith what caused you to bring Jimmy to the ER today?"

CRITICAL ACTION

Recognizing that this patient is dehydrated and giving appropriate fluid resuscitation is a critical action in this case.

E: "Well, Jimmy has been vomiting for the past 3 days, and today I noticed he had a little fever."

C: "Have you noticed if there was any blood or green fluid in the vomit?"

E: "There was some green fluid in his vomit starting today."

C: "Has Jimmy reported any pain to you in the past several days."

E: "Yes, he has told me since even before the vomiting started that his tummy was hurting him."

C: "Jimmy, does your tummy hurt right now?"

E: (Jimmy quietly shakes his head to indicate no.)

C: "Nurse, please send the drawn blood for CBC, CMP, lipase, and coags."

E: "The nurse is carrying out these orders."

C: "Ms. Smith, has Jimmy had any colds recently?"

E: "Yes, he had a runny nose and a cough about a week ago."

C: "Has he been having normal bowel movements in the past several days?"

E: "Well, they have been slightly dark over the past several days, but on the whole they are fairly normal. As mom talks Jimmy throws up again."

C: "How much and does the emesis have any blood or bile in it?"

E: "Jimmy has thrown up approximately 200 cc of bilious fluid."

C: "Does Jimmy cry when he says he has pain, Ms. Smith?"

E: "Yes, he looks like he's in terrible pain."

C: "How long does the pain and crying seem to last?"

E: "The crying will last anywhere from a couple of minutes to maybe ten. He's been getting the episodes every 30-60 minutes. Although, today it seems to be getting more frequent."

C: "Ms. Smith, does Jimmy have any previous medical problems?"

E: "No."

C: "Is Jimmy allergic to any medications?"

E: "No."

C: "Jimmy, I'm going to take a look at your belly again. Ms. Smith, please keep holding Jimmy so that he's comfortable. Does the abdomen appear distended?"

E: "The abdomen does appear to be mildly distended."

C: "Are there bowel sounds in all four quadrants."

E: "There are diffusely diminished bowel sounds."

C: "Ms. Smith, please put Jimmy on the bed for me to finish examining him. As I palpate the abdomen is it soft? Is there any area of significant tenderness? Is there any guarding on the child's part? Is there any organomegaly? Are there any masses?"

E: "The abdomen is soft. There is diffuse mild tenderness with some voluntary guarding. There is no organomegaly nor any masses detected."

C: "As I continue my examination, are the TMs clear, the oropharynx clear, any cervical lymphadenopathy? Are the lungs clear, and is the heart regular sounding? Are there any murmurs noted?"

E: "The TMs and oropharynx are clear. There is no significant lymphadenopathy. The heart and lung exams are normal except for persisting tachycardia."

C: "Ms. Smith, I need to perform a rectal examination on Jimmy to see if the increased darkness of his stools is from some blood mixed in with them. It involves putting a finger in his bottom for a brief moment. It is uncomfortable, but will not hurt him."

E: "I understand."

C: "As I do a rectal examination are there any masses? Is the stool brown or red? Is the stool guaiac positive?"

E: "There are no masses on examination. The stool is dark, loose, and is guaiac positive. Of note the patient only whimpered with the examination."

C: "Are the testicles in normal position, tender?"

E: "No testicular abnormalities."

C: "Ms. Smith, based on Jimmy's symptoms over the past several days along with my physical examination findings I am concerned there may be a something causing a small blockage in Jimmy's bowels. I would like to do some x-rays on Jimmy and have one of our surgeons come and further evaluate him."

E: "That sounds like a good idea."

C: "Nurse, please order an obstructive series to be done stat here in the department. Also, please recheck the patient's vital signs. Ms. Secretary, please have the pediatric surgeon on call paged."

E: "Radiology has been notified, the surgeon is on page, and the repeat vitals are BP 85/50, P 160, RR 30. As the nurse is finishing the vitals the patient begins to scream. He has rolled into a ball in his mother's lap and will not let you touch his stomach."

C: "Nurse, please administer 2 mg of morphine to the patient."

E: "The nurse administers the morphine. Jimmy stops crying but still remains rolled in a ball in his mother's lap. The nurse also informs you the first bolus is through."

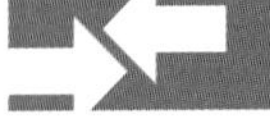
CRITICAL ACTION

There are two critical actions here. First, the examinee has to recognize the possibility of an intussusception and order an obstructive series. Secondly, they must get surgery involved early.

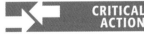

C: "Please start another 300-cc bolus of NS to again run over 30 minutes, and again notify me when this is through."

E: "The second bolus is started. Also, the obstructive series films return (Fig. C19-1)."

E: "The lab results have also returned:

CBC: WBC 17.2 with N 82, B 2, L 18; Hgb 15.5/Hct 46.5, plt 350

BMP: Na 142, K 3.7, Cl 110, CO_2 14, BUN 25, Cr 0.8, glu 110

Coags: PTT 35, PT 10.2, INR 1.0

CXR: Results are back (Fig. C19-1)"

CRITICAL ACTION

Treating the patient's pain is a critical action in this case.

E: "The surgeon, Dr. Steel, is on the phone."

C: "Hello, Dr. Steel, this is Dr. Cramp at ABEM General. I have a consult for you."

E: "Hello, what is the case."

C: "There is a 2-year-old child here who presents with symptoms and signs consistent with bowel obstruction, most likely from an intussusception. He has 3 days of vomiting that has become bilious, with associated severe colicky abdominal pain. He has a low-grade temperature, appears very dehydrated, and has a distended abdomen with mild, diffuse tenderness. His rectal examination showed dark brown stool with occult blood."

KEY ORDERS

Asking the nurse to inform you when fluid boluses are finished is a great way to ensure a quick recheck on vitals later in the case. The same should be done with laboratory or imaging studies.

E: "Yes, it sounds suspicious. Have you done any testing?"

C: "Yes, an obstructive series shows signs of obstruction consistent with intussusception. His lab work shows him to be dehydrated with a mild anion gap acidosis, and a mildly elevated WBC with a left shift."

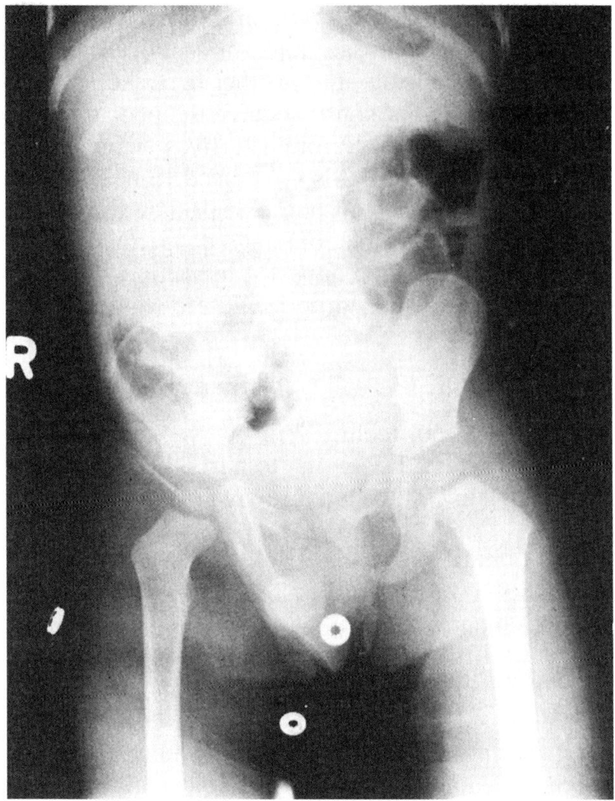

Figure C19-1. Abdominal x-ray. (*Reproduced with permission from Tintinalli JE, Kelen GD, Stapczynski JS, et al.* Emergency Medicine: A Comprehensive Study Guide. *6th ed. New York, NY: McGraw-Hill; 2004.*)

E: "Again, I agree this sounds like intussusception. Call radiology and have them do an air enema. Call me when it's done with the results."

C: "Dr. Steel, I agree an air enema is a good idea to diagnosis a possible intussusception, especially as it is usually therapeutic as well as diagnostic. However, the child's symptoms have been going on for several days and although there are no peritoneal findings or free air on the x-rays there is evidence of significant obstruction. The protracted course and small bowel obstruction are relative contraindications to the enema, and I think you should evaluate the child before any more diagnostic studies are done. In the meantime I'm going to place an NG tube and continue to fluid resuscitate the child."

E: "That sounds fair. I will be there shortly."

C: "Thank you very much Dr. Steel. Nurse, what are the patient's vital signs?"

E: "Vitals are T 37.1°C (98.9°F), P 150, RR 30, BP 95/60, O_2 sat 98% on RA, with almost all of the second bolus given."

C: "Very good. Please give a third bolus of 300 cc NS and notify me when it is through."

E: "Yes, Dr. Cramp."

C: "Ms. Smith, the x-rays confirmed that Jimmy does have a bowel obstruction. Further it shows that the blockage is likely caused by something called an intussusception. This is the most common cause of bowel obstruction in

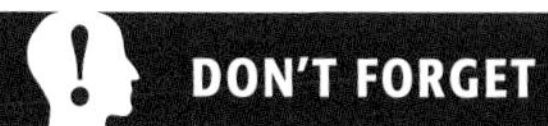

DON'T FORGET

On exam day, consultants will often "push back." You will be expected to advocate for your patient and demand the level of care you feel is appropriate.

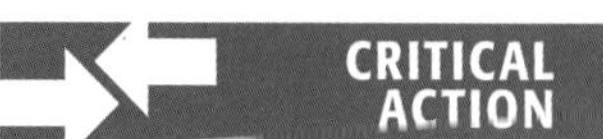

CRITICAL ACTION

Recognizing that this patient is dehydrated and giving appropriate and on-going fluid resuscitation is a critical action in this case.

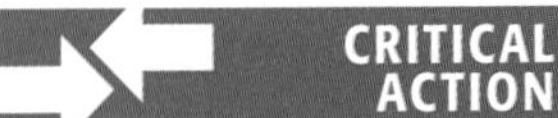

CRITICAL ACTION

Treating the patient's symptoms with an NG tube is also a critical action in this case.

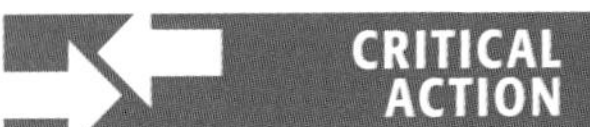

CRITICAL ACTION

Admitting the patient to the appropriate level of care is always a critical action.

child Jimmy's age. It happens when a portion of the bowel actually gets pulled ahead and essentially stuffed into an adjacent section of bowel. It's kind of like stuffing the edge of one straw into another one, and it causes a blockage. The next step in evaluating your son is to have the pediatric surgeon examine him. He will be here very shortly. Before he arrives we need to continue rehydrating him and treating his pain. Also, we need to help him stop vomiting. In order to do that it is necessary to put a small tube through his nose down into his stomach. It is uncomfortable, but not a dangerous procedure. Once the tube is in place we will be able to connect it to suction and take out all of the air and fluids that have been backed up because of the blockage. Is this OK, Ms. Smith?"

E: "Yes, I guess it sounds OK if it will help him feel better."

C: "Jimmy, I know you're not feeling well but the nurse is going to come in and put a tube into your nose. It is going to hurt a little bit and feel strange in your throat, but it will help you to stop throwing up."

E: "Jimmy nods slightly."

C: "Nurse, please place a 9 French NG tube into the patient; please call me to help evaluate its placement."

E: "The nurse goes to place the NG tube and the surgeon has evaluated the patient."

E: "Hello Dr. Cramp. I'm Dr. Steel. I evaluated Jimmy and his tests and agree it does seem he has an intussusception. I have explained to his mother that we will attempt the air enema and that if it does not work or there is any suggestion that there is a complication from the procedure Jimmy will need to promptly be taken to the OR."

C: "That sounds reasonable. I will contact the radiology department and arrange for a room on the pediatric surgical floor to observe him after the procedure."

E: "That sounds fine."

C: "Ms. Secretary, please order an air enema for suspected intussusception for Jimmy as well as a bed on the general pediatric floor for after the procedure. Also, nurse, what are Jimmy's repeat vital signs."

E: "T 37°C (98.6°F), P 135, RR 30, BP 105/60, O_2 sat 98%. The NG tube is placed, do you want to confirm placement?"

C: "Yes. As I listen over the stomach do I hear air as it is inflated into the NG tube?"

E: "Yes."

C: "Very good. Please connect the NG tube to suction at a low intermittent setting. Please keep Jimmy on a monitor and accompany him for his procedure."

E: "I will Dr. Cramp. The case is over."

CASE ASSESSMENT

Overall, the candidate did an excellent job of diagnosing a sometimes elusive entity, and managing a severely dehydrated child well. Abdominal pain in children is a diagnostic challenge even to the most seasoned clinician. The challenge is compounded in children who are unable or unwilling to talk. The candidate did a satisfactory job at immediately recognizing the child was significantly dehydrated from solely the vital signs and a brief look at the child. During oral boards, interventions should take place as soon as one entertains their need. Therefore, immediate IV, labs, and fluid were appropriately ordered in this case. Also, the candidate did well to ask for the missing set of vital signs. If vital signs are missing they are usually significant. Frequent reassessment of the vital signs is key, especially as resuscitative measures are in progress. The candidate kept asking the nurse to inform him when the fluid boluses were finished as a way to ensure that he was reminded to recheck the vitals later in the case. The same can be done with laboratory or imaging studies.

A critical action in this case was adequate fluid resuscitation, which was successfully done with repeated 20 cc/kg boluses of normal saline using updated vital signs as a guide as to how many were needed.

In addition to fluid resuscitating the child, the candidate was able to conduct a directed history and physical examination that led them to diagnose intussusception. It can be a challenge in such an artificial environment, but one has to make a concerted effort to make things happen in parallel. For example, the candidate was able to quickly address the volume status while at the same time asking questions and conducting the physical examination. Thinking in parallel is how a clinician works in the real world, but the skill must be learned for oral board cases as it is the key to keeping the case moving.

Also, key to this case was early notification of the surgeon. Any time a specialist is needed, prompt notification of that person should be the rule. In this case one may have argued that the surgeon could have been contacted based solely on the history and physical examination. Waiting a short time for the obstructive series was acceptable, but any further delays would not be justifiable. Additionally, the candidate did an outstanding job of discussing the case with the surgeon and the need for that person to come in to evaluate the patient sooner rather than later. This situation occurs fairly often at ABEM General as it is a good way to test the candidate's knowledge of the clinical course and potential morbidity of the disease process, but also his communication skills.

One must remember to talk with the patients and their family members. This applies to children as well as adults. The candidate in this case did a solid job of addressing both the child and mother at an appropriate level. In particular, the candidate made sure to explain each procedure to mother and child. They also made sure to explain intussusception in layman's terms so that the mother felt informed and able to make competent decisions regarding her child's care. Candidates must not forget to talk with the "patient" and "family" as failure to do so can significantly reduce scores in the communication category and possibly cause them to miss a critical action.

Critical Actions

1. Prompt and adequate fluid resuscitation.
2. Ordering an obstructive series and recognizing the small bowel obstruction.
3. Early surgical consult with recognition that the surgeon needs to see the patient before the air enema is performed (given risk factors for perforation present in this case).
4. Treatment of symptoms with pain medication and nasogastric (NG) tube.
5. Admission to the hospital for observation after the procedures.

Test Performance

1. *Data acquisition:* The candidate did an excellent job throughout the history and physical, being able to move through the case confidently and comprehensively. Score = **7**
2. *Problem solving:* The candidate quickly recognized the missing vital sign and obtained this important information. He was able to synthesize data as it was revealed to him to arrive at the diagnosis. Score = **8**
3. *Patient management:* Interventions were made in the correct order with due consideration to pain control and safety of the patient. Score = **8**
4. *Resource utilization:* The candidate had appropriate test ordering behavior and resource utilization. Score = **7**
5. *Health care provided (outcome):* The patient received timely care including adequate fluid administration, prompt imaging, and surgical consultation. Score = **7**
6. *Interpersonal relations and communication skills:* The candidate engaged in effective communication in an efficient manner. Score = **8**
7. *Comprehension of pathophysiology:* The candidate demonstrated a thorough understanding of the underlying pathophysiology of intussusception as evidenced by his conversations with the family and consultants. Score = **7**
8. *Clinical competence (overall):* The candidate performed very well on this case moving through it easily, administering appropriate care, and communicating effectively with the patient and family. Score = **7**

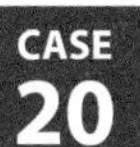

CASE 20 24 y/o Female Who Has a Fall

Navneet Cheema, Charles Maddow, and James I. Syrett

INITIAL INFORMATION

Time: 16:30

Name: Miss Red

Age: 24 years

Mode of arrival: Basic life support ambulance

Gender: Female

VS: P 100, BP 138/79, RR 18, O_2 sat: 96%

CC: Lower leg weakness and pain after falling

KEY QUESTION

Ask this open-ended question at the beginning of every case.

PLAY OF THE CASE

E: "Welcome to ABEM General. Do you have any questions?"

C: "No, thank you."

E: "The triage nurse asks you to see a patient that has just arrived in the emergency department. Here is her triage sheet."

C: "What do I see as I walk into the patient's room?"

KEY ORDERS

Remember to use your EMTs and family members to get additional history if needed.

E: "You see a young female on an EMS backboard, wearing a C-collar. She is crying. There are no unusual smells. An EMT is still with the patient."

C: "I would ask the EMT to stay, I may need to speak to him in a minute."

E: "The EMT will remain in the room."

C: "Ms. Red, My name is Dr. Jones, what happened to you today?"

KEY ORDERS

Most of the patients you see during the exam will be unstable (or will become that way). Every unstable patient requires IV access (preferably two large-bore IVs), oxygen, and cardiac monitoring (and in most cases an ECG).

E: "I fell off the roof of my house. I have a lot of pain in my back and I can't feel my legs."

C: "How far do you think you fell?"

E: "About 15 ft."

C: "Did you lose consciousness?"

E: "I don't know. I don't think so."

C: "OK Ms. Red, I am going to ask our nurses to do a couple of things and I want to speak to the EMT. Nurse, can you put the patient on a cardiac monitor, run a rhythm strip, and give it to me. Put her on 100% NRB oxygen, start two large-bore IV lines, and draw off blood for labs. Also can we remove her cloths and then cover her with blankets to keep her warm. Can I speak to the EMT?"

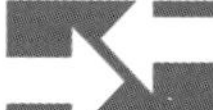

CRITICAL ACTION

In this case, establishing large-bore IV access is a critical action. Remember that this case is a trauma and should be treated by ATLS protocols, which includes IV access and fluids.

E: "I am the EMT."

C: "Can you tell me what happened?"

E: "She fell about 20 ft off a roof onto concrete."

C: "Did she lose consciousness?"

E: "No, someone saw her do it."

C: "Does she have any injuries?"

E: "Her only complaint was lower back pain."

C: "Thank you for the information. Ms. Red, I have some other questions for you. Do you have any allergies?"

E: "No. I have a lot of pain in my back."

C: "Are you on any medications?"

E: "No."

C: "Do you have any medical problems that we should know about?"

E: "No, I am really very fit. Why can't I move my legs the way I want to? I am really scared."

C: "We will figure that out in a minute. Could you be pregnant?"

E: "No, I don't think so."

C: "When was your last meal?"

E: "I had lunch at 1 o'clock."

C: "I would like to do an examination now. Does she have bilateral breath sounds?"

E: "Yes."

C: "Is her abdomen soft and non-tender?"

E: "Yes."

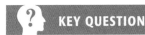

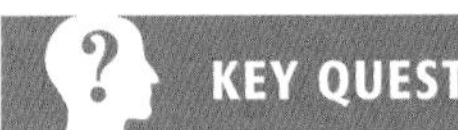

Since this is a trauma case, the examinee is taking the AMPLE history here—**A**llergies, **M**edications, **P**ast history, **L**ast meal, and **E**vents.

C: "Is the pelvis stable? Is there tenderness in her lower back when you stress the pelvis? Are there obvious long bone deformities, tenderness, instability?"

E: "The pelvis is stable; there are no obvious deformities or tenderness."

C: "I would like to do my secondary survey. Also at this time I want to get a chest and pelvis x-ray."

E: "The x-rays have been ordered. What do you want to do next?"

C: "I would like to examine the head for abrasions, tenderness."

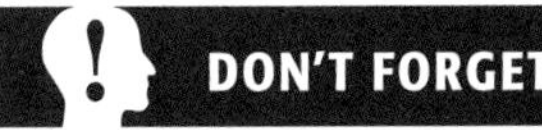

The examinee is failing to communicate appropriately with the patient here. They are not addressing her pain or answering her questions. Their score for communication will reflect this.

E: "There is an abrasion to the forehead, but nothing else."

C: "Any tenderness or bleeding from the TMs, nares, or mouth?"

E: "Normal."

C: "Her neck?"

E: "No midline pain or steps-offs."

C: "Chest examination with attention to breath sound symmetry and crackles. Any tenderness, swelling, abrasions, or bruises?"

E: "Multiple bruises on the posterior chest, no flail segments, and good air entry bilaterally."

C: "Are the bowel sounds present? Is there any abdominal tenderness?"

E: "The abdomen is soft and non-tender."

C: "Skin?"

E: "There is bruising and abrasions as I told you."

C: "I would like to logroll the patient to examine her back and rectum."

E: "You logroll the patient. What do you want to know about the back examination?"

C: "I would like to look for any bruising or abrasions, I would like to feel for any step-offs or any point tenderness in the midline. I would like to do a rectal examination to assess for sphincter tone, frank blood, and perianal sensation."

E: "There is bruising in the lumbar spine area. There is point tenderness over L4 and L5 with a possible step-off at that level. There is no sphincter tone and no rectal blood. There is saddle anesthesia."

C: "Completing the neurological examination?"

E: "What do you want to know?"

C: "The extremity examination looking at power, tone, reflexes, and sensation in the arms and legs."

E: "The arms are normal. There is decreased power in the L4/5 distribution and sensation is altered in those dermatomes as well."

C: "I would like to do a FAST scan of this patient."

E: "The x-rays that you ordered are back and a FAST scan is done. The radiology read of the XRs are normal. The FAST scan is negative."

C: "I would like to order steroids for this patient because of a presumed spinal cord injury. I would also like to give the patient 4 mg of morphine for pain and order a CT and an MRI of the lumbar spine area. I would also like to speak to the spine surgeon once the CT is done. I would also like to send my labs now, please send a CBC, electrolytes, coagulation studies and cross match the patient for 4 U of blood. I would also like a urine dip test and urine pregnancy test."

E: "Your CT is done. All of the labs have been sent. The UCG is negative for pregnancy. What dose of steroids do you want?"

C: "I would like to give her 30 mg/kg of methylprednisolone as a bolus and then start a drip at 5.4 mg/kg/h for the next 23 hours. I would also like to speak to Ms. Red. "Ms. Red, I think that when you fell you injured your lower spine. I have ordered additional special x-rays called a MRI that will allow us to look more closely at your spine. I am also going to speak to a neurosurgeon now."

E: "Here is your CT of the L-spine (Fig. C20-1). The MRI has been ordered and we have Dr. Spine on the phone for you."

C: "The L-spine CT shows a comminuted fracture of L4. Dr. Spine, this is Dr. Jones. I have a healthy 24-year-old female who fell approximately 15-20 ft on to concrete. She presented with severe lower back pain, leg weakness and numbness, no rectal tone, and saddle anesthesia. She has a normal chest and pelvis XR and we have started IV steroids and ordered an MRI."

E: "It sounds like she needs surgery. I will be in to see her immediately. This concludes the management portion of this case."

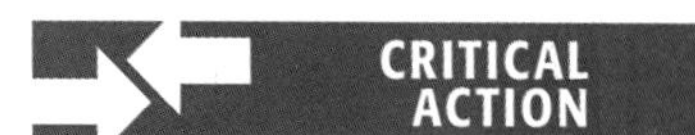

There are several critical actions taking place at this point. First, recognizing that there is a probably spinal cord injury and getting tests to asses it is a critical action. Second, the examinee is giving steroids for that injury. Third, they are calling a spinal surgeon for definitive management, and fourth, they are treating the patient's pain (albeit late in the case).

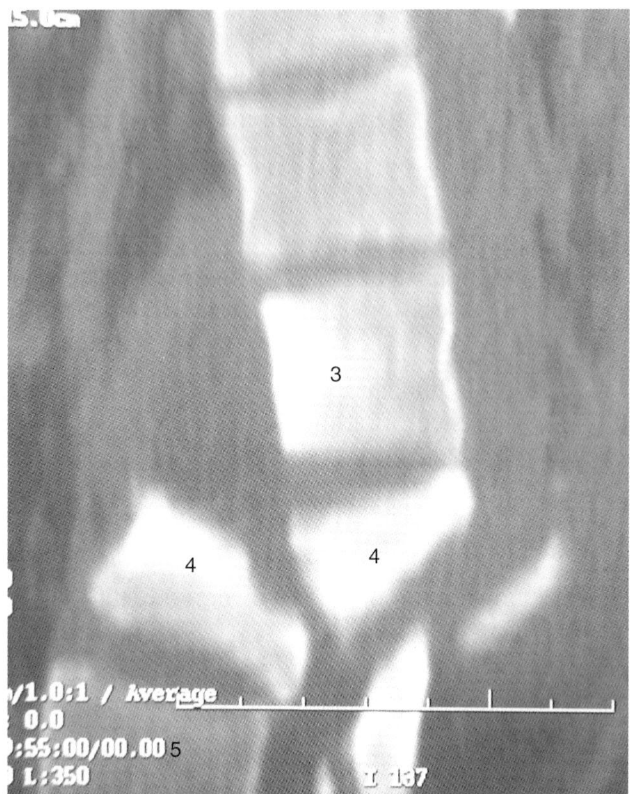

Figure C20-1. Sagittal reconstruction of an axial fine-slice CT scan through the lumbar spine demonstrating a severe fracture-dislocation through the body of L4. (*Reprinted with permission from Bruncardi FC, Andersen DK, Billiar TR et al.* Schwartz's Principles of Surgery. *8th ed. New York, NY: McGraw-Hill; 2005.*)

CASE ASSESSMENT

This patient presents with trauma and neurological deficit. This case is short and in the oral examination the patient may have additional injuries that would have to be managed, however, this case is presented here to illustrate the cauda equina syndrome and the use of steroids.

All trauma cases should be managed in the same way and the candidate should resist the temptation to jump to specific complaints in the case. Using the standardized approach to trauma will ensure that no important injuries are missed. In addition, life-threatening injuries should be dealt with as soon as they are detected. Other important aspects of the general trauma patient would be to secure early large-bore IV access, have the patient on a cardiac monitor, and provide high-flow oxygen.

As the case progresses a short history (AMPLE—**A**llergies, **M**edications, **P**ast medical history, **L**ast meal, and explanation of **E**vents) should be obtained either from the patient or other sources followed by a primary and then secondary survey. In the event the history cannot be taken either due to patient acuity or unresponsiveness then the case should be managed from the primary survey point.

Other aspects of a trauma case that may be forgotten include missing the need for IV antibiotics, tetanus booster or failing to do a pregnancy test. Another important aspect is to ensure that the C-spine is immobilized. Had this patient self-presented to the emergency department, the candidate would have to initially secure the C-spine with collar and immobilization.

In this case, there was a lack of communication with the patient and IV fluids were not started although IV access was obtained. Communication is an important aspect of the oral board exam since it is a section that can be easy to score in and easy to drop points. In this case the candidate did talk to the patient when a diagnosis was made.

Analgesia is essential in the board exam when a patient is complaining about pain. Often the examiner will attempt to prompt the candidate, and if the patient continues to complain, it means that the examiner is expecting the candidate to ask. In this case, analgesia was late in the management of the patient's pain.

Finally, while the topic of steroids remains controversial, it is generally safer (in the board exam) to give the steroids if indicated. If you are uncomfortable with that decision you can say to the examiner that you would consider steroids and could point out that this topic is controversial, however, it could be a critical action to initiate them.

Critical Actions

1. Secure large bore IV access.
2. Diagnose potential spine injury; suspect cauda equine syndrome.
3. Provide analgesia for pain.
4. Initiate steroids for spinal cord injury.
5. Consult a spine surgeon to further manage the case.

Test Performance

1. *Data acquisition:* The candidate performed a good basic trauma management and showed specific knowledge of spinal cord injury. A structured approach to assessment was demonstrated and all the pertinent points were found on examination. Score = **6**
2. *Problem solving:* The candidate was able to systematically evaluate for traumatic injuries, synthesizing new information as it was presented to confirm the suspected diagnosis. Score = **7**
3. *Resource utilization:* Tests were ordered in a timely and cost-effective manner. Tests were appropriate for the case. Score = **7**
4. *Patient management:* The candidate was late to provide analgesia; however, other aspects of the case were managed well. Score = **6**
5. *Health care provided (outcome):* The candidate appropriately initiated steroids for a presumed spinal cord injury. Score = **7**
6. *Interpersonal relations and communication skills:* The candidate showed fairly good skill in this area, although did not provide the patient with timely or complete information. It is important to involve the patient in the case to score highly in this area. Score = **5**
7. *Comprehension of pathophysiology:* The candidate demonstrated good understanding of the pathophysiology as evidenced by prompt initiation of steroids and discussion with the consultant. Score = **6**
8. *Clinical competence (overall):* This case overall was well managed, but could have improved with more attention to communication skills and addressing the patient's pain. Score = **6**

CASE 21 55 y/o Male With Sore Throat

Navneet Cheema, Reb Close, and Fred Abrahamian

INITIAL INFORMATION

Name: John Doe

Mode of arrival: Private auto

Age: 55 years

Gender: Male

VS: T 38.9°C (102.02°F), BP 150/95, HR 110, RR 24, O_2 sat: 96% on RA

CC: Sore throat

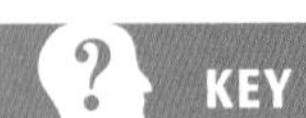

KEY QUESTION

Ask this open-ended question at the beginning of every case.

KEY ORDERS

Most of the patients you see during the exam will be unstable (or will become that way). Every unstable patient requires IV access (preferably two large-bore IVs), oxygen, and cardiac monitoring (and in most cases an ECG).

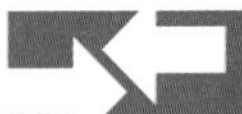

CRITICAL ACTION

Giving this patient oxygen is a critical action.

PLAY OF THE CASE

C: "What do I see as I walk into the patient's room?"

E: "The patient is a well-nourished male, sitting on the gurney, mouth breathing, and appears anxious."

C: "Nurse, please place the patient on oxygen by nasal cannula and titrate to keep the saturations >97%, place him on a cardiac monitor and show me a rhythm strip when available, start an 18-gauge IV in an antecubital vein with NS TKO, and draw and hold blood for lab tests."

E: "Here is your rhythm strip showing a sinus tachycardia at a rate of 114."

C: "Hello Mr. Doe, I'm Dr. Ellingson, can you please tell me what brings you into the emergency department today?"

E: "Dr. Ellingson, I have this terrible sore throat, never had anything like it before, hurts to talk, hurts to eat."

C: "When did the symptoms start?"

E: "I noticed it this morning when I woke up, got much worse throughout the day, doc I just can't stand it, it's even hard to breathe."

C: "Have you been sick lately with fevers, cough, or cold symptoms?"

E: "No doc, felt fine last night, now this is just killing me."

C: "Are you currently feeling any chest pain, nausea, or other symptoms?"

E: "Just hard to breathe doc, can't seem to get the air in."

C: "Do you have any medical problems?"

E: "None as far as I know."

C: "What medications are you currently taking?"

E: "None right now."

C: "Any allergies to medicines?"

E: "Sulfa."

C: "What happens when you take sulfa?"

E: "Bad rash."

C: "Mr. Doe, I need to examine you now."

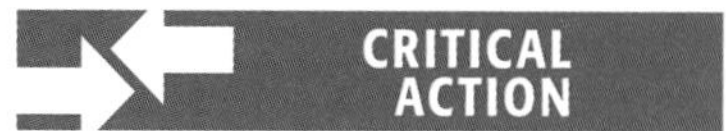

Getting a soft tissue lateral XR of the neck is a critical action in this case.

C: "HEENT examination?"

E: "What are you looking for?"

C: "Pupil size and reactivity, conjunctiva, external auditory canals for erythema, swelling, tympanic membranes for bulging, erythema, air-fluid level, oral cavity for dental abscess, tongue swelling/elevation, swollen or deviated uvula, enlarged tonsils, erythema, swelling, exudates over oropharynx, facial swelling, and erythema."

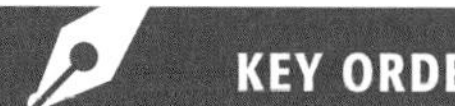

Always begin by treating any vital sign abnormality—this means fluids to people who are hypotensive, oxygen to people who are hypoxic, and antipyretics to people who are febrile.

E: "The pupils are equal and reactive to light, conjunctiva clear, normal ear examination. No facial cellulitis. Oropharynx is mildly erythematous without exudates or swelling. No evidence of uvulitis or peritonsillar abscess."

C: "Neck examination?"

E: "What are you looking for?"

C: "Swelling, induration, lymphadenopathy, trachea position, tenderness over the thyroid cartilage."

E: "Mildly tender anterior lymph nodes, the area over thyroid cartilage is also mildly tender but there is no swelling or induration, trachea midline."

C: "Lung examination?"

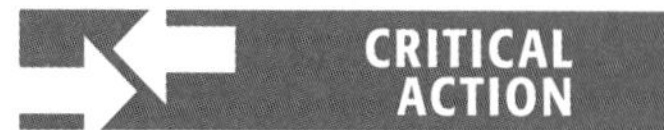

Giving pain medication is a critical action in this case—it could have been done before the physical examination.

E: "Tachypnea, scattered wheezes, symmetric lung sounds."

C: "Heart examination?"

E: "Normal except for the tachycardia"

C: "Abdominal examination?"

E: "Limited as the patient is unable to lie supine for the examination and complains of worsening pain and trouble breathing."

C: "Skin examination?"

E: "Warm, diaphoretic, no rashes."

C: "Extremity examination?"

E: "Normal."

C: "Nurse, please administer 500-cc bolus of NS and 1 g of acetaminophen PR, and have the blood sent for CBC and blood cultures. I need a cross-table soft-tissue lateral x-ray of the neck."

E: "The fluid bolus is started."

C: "What are the repeat vital signs after the fluid bolus?"

E: "BP 130/90, HR 100, RR 30, O_2 sat 100% on 4-L NC."

C: "How does the patient look?"

E: "He looks tired."

C: "Mr. Doe, how are you feeling?"

E: "Doc, can't you give me something for pain, this is killing me."

C: "Nurse, please administer fentanyl 50 μg IV and let me know the patient's response to the medication."

E: "Pain medication is given. Do you want to send the patient to x-ray now?"

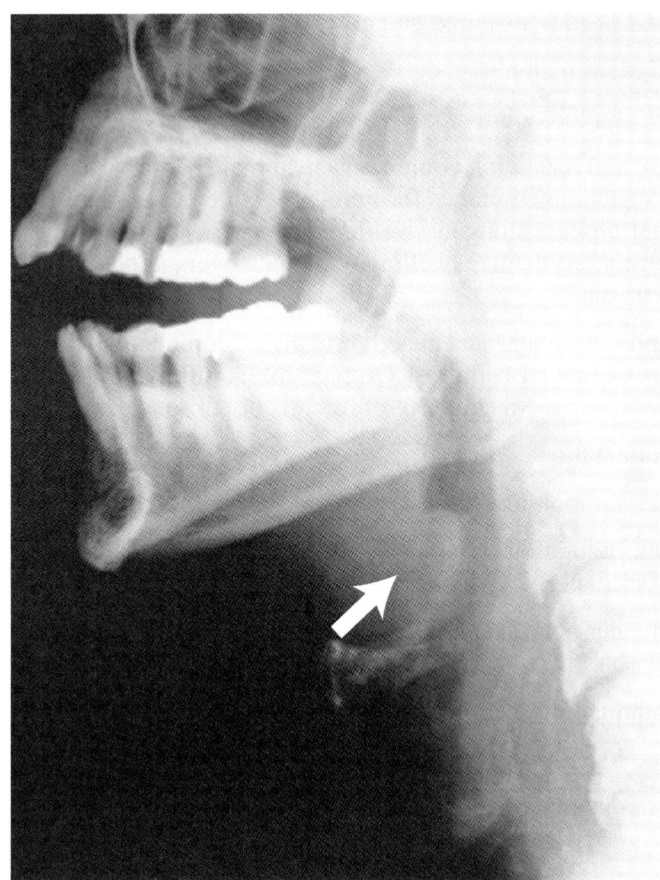

Figure C21-1. Lateral neck x-ray. *(Reproduced with permission from Tintinalli JE, Kelen GD, Stapczynski JS, et al.* Emergency Medicine: A Comprehensive Study Guide. *6th ed. New York, NY: McGraw-Hill; 2004.)*

Having equipment at the bedside for an emergent airway is a critical action in this case.

C: "No, I need the x-ray performed as a portable. I will stay in the room with the patient, and I need intubation and surgical airway trays to the bedside."

E: "The patient seems more comfortable with the medication, here is your x-ray (Fig. C21-1)."

C: "Nurse, please administer ceftriaxone 2 g IV and call the ENT specialist for me. Mr. Doe, you have an infection in the lower part of your throat. This infection can be very serious and needs to be treated with antibiotics. I am calling the specialist to admit you to the hospital."

E: "Is it that bad?"

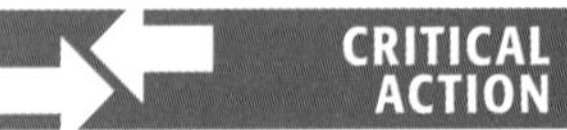

There are two critical actions taking place here—first, the examinee must place the patient on antibiotics, and second, they must call ENT for emergent management.

C: "It can be very serious which is why we need to keep you in the hospital."

E: "Whatever you say doc."

E: "Dr. Jones from ENT is on the phone."

C: "Hi Dr. Jones, this is Dr. Ellingson from the emergency department, I have a 55-year-old male in the ED with epiglottitis, I need you to evaluate this patient."

E: "How do you know he has epiglottitis?"

C: "He presents acutely toxic with a severe sore throat, minimal abnormalities on examination of the oropharynx, and a lateral soft-tissue x-ray of the neck shows a swollen epiglottis. I have administered antibiotics, fluids, and pain medication. I also sent blood for CBC and cultures."

E: "Great, I'll see him on the floor after I finish my clinic."

C: "This gentleman is too sick to go to the floor; he needs emergent evaluation and an ICU bed."

E: "Fine, I'll be over shortly."

E: "This case is now over."

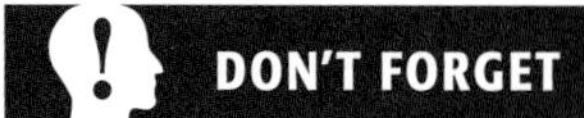

DON'T FORGET

On exam day, consultants will often "push back." You will be expected to advocate for your patient and demand the level of care you feel is appropriate.

CASE ASSESSMENT

Overall this case was managed very well. The candidate immediately interpreted the vital signs and started stabilizing measures with the IV, O_2, and monitor. The history and physical examination were adequate and the physician had enough information at that time to initiate therapy and call for intubation and surgical airway trays to be available at the bedside. The candidate needed some prompting from the examiner regarding pain management, as well as having the patient leave the department for x-ray without physician supervision. The candidate picked up on these clues and managed the patient appropriately.

Historical clues that were useful to the candidate were the sudden onset of severe symptoms with a relatively unimpressive oropharynx. The candidate did not inquire about stridor, voice change, drooling, neck stiffness, and swallowing difficulties and as a result the examiner did not offer this very important information. If there is a specific finding on history or physical examination that would help you "cinch" the diagnosis, ask for it specifically.

During the physical examination, when the examiner tells you that the examination is "normal" that means no need for additional questioning or investigation within that system. However, if the examiner asks "what are you looking for?" this is often a clue to ask for all of the possible findings that will help you focus on your differential diagnosis and management. Also, when part of the physical examination is made difficult, this is usually a significant finding. In this case, the abdominal examination was difficult as the patient preferred to be sitting upright. That finding should be decoded by the candidate as an indicator of the degree of respiratory distress.

Always remember to reassess the patient's overall status and repeat the vital signs, especially those that are abnormal. The candidate did well in reevaluating the patient and asking for repeat vital signs. However, he failed to see that the repeat temperature was not given to him. Always ask for complete set of vitals, if some are missing make sure to ask for them. Missing vital sign is often a clue to worsening condition or a diagnosis.

The candidate further expressed an understanding of the severity of the patient's problem when he specified that he would like the patient to remain in the emergency department and for him to be present at the bedside during the x-ray. Anticipating potential airway obstruction, it was appropriate to ask for intubation and surgical airway trays. This should be done as soon as the diagnosis of epiglottitis is considered. You will not be faulted for calling for it too early but may have a patient crash if it is not available.

Due to potential airway obstruction (especially in children) with direct visualization, it is best to perform this procedure in the operating room with personnel experienced in rapid airway management. In this patient there was no immediate need for airway management, so it was appropriate to start with soft-tissue lateral neck x-rays with the physician in attendance.

Once the diagnosis was made, antibiotics were ordered immediately. The administration of antibiotics is often a critical action and it is always best to initiate them early in the emergency department. For the purpose of oral boards, if you cannot remember the proper antibiotic(s) or dosage(s), it is acceptable to say, "I will look it up in a reference." It is possible the examiner may make this difficult so be resourceful (eg, look dosing up online, in a PDA, call the ID consultant, discuss with hospital pharmacist, use the Sanford guide).

The ENT consultation was handled very well by this candidate. When the specialist stated he would see the patient on the floor after clinic, the candidate was aware that this was not acceptable and requested immediate evaluation and intensive care unit (ICU) admission. It would also be reasonable to prepare the patient for the operating room if his clinical presentation was unstable or deteriorating.

Always remember to let the patient know of what is going on, what you are doing, and what the working diagnosis might be. If there are friends or family members present, talk to them as well. In this case, the candidate did not initially explain to the patient why he was giving him intravenous (IV) fluids, drawing blood, or getting an x-ray. Later on, the candidate explained to the patient what his diagnosis was and why he needed to be admitted. However, the candidate could have further asked the patient if he had any more questions, concerns, or needed any other help such as notifying family or friends that he was going to stay in the hospital.

Critical Actions

1. Oxygen therapy
2. Pain management
3. Intubation and surgical airway trays to the bedside
4. Cross-table soft-tissue lateral x-ray of the neck for diagnosis with the physician in attendance
5. Administration of appropriate antibiotic(s)
6. ENT consultation for ICU admission

Test Performance

1. *Data acquisition:* The data acquisition was appropriate, but the candidate failed to ask important historical information. The candidate did not inquire about stridor, voice change, drooling, neck stiffness, and swallowing difficulties which can all be clues to how sick the patient is and potential other diagnoses. Also other than looking at the reactivity of the pupils, the candidate did not perform a thorough neurological examination (specifically looking at the cranial nerves). Score = **5**
2. *Problem solving:* Problem solving was excellent and the candidate immediately used the information given to stabilize and manage the patient. Score = **7**

3. *Patient management:* The candidate demonstrated understanding of this potentially life-threatening condition and was able to treat the condition quickly and appropriately. Score = **7**
4. *Resource utilization:* The candidate was resourceful and efficient in the use of diagnostic methods without compromising patient care. Score = **7**
5. *Health care provided (outcome):* Patient care was appropriate and met the standard of care. It could have been improved by administering pain medications earlier without the examiners coaching. In addition, the candidate failed to reevaluate the elevated temperature. Score = **6**
6. *Interpersonal relations and communication skills:* The candidate's interactions with the patient, nurse, and consultant were appropriate. Initially, the candidate did not explain to the patient why he was giving him IV fluids, drawing blood, or getting an x-ray. After notifying the patient that he would be admitted, the candidate could have in addition asked the patient if he had any more questions, concerns, or needed any other assistance such as notifying family or friends that he was going to be admitted to the hospital. Score = **6**
7. *Comprehension of pathophysiology:* The candidate demonstrated a good understanding of the underlying disease process as evidenced by the discussion with ENT, ordering appropriate antibiotics, and having emergency airway equipment available. Score = **7**
8. *Clinical competence (overall):* The candidate excelled in problem solving, patient management, and comprehension of pathophysiology. The overall score could have been improved by more effective communication, addressing pain early, and a more targeted, thorough history. Score = **6**

CASE 22 33 y/o Female With Headache and Weakness

Navneet Cheema and Catherine Johnson

INITIAL INFORMATION

Name: Kelly Smith

Mode of arrival: Brought in by family

Age: 33 years

Gender: Female

VS: T 37.4°C (99.32°F), BP 155/95, HR 92, RR 20, O_2 sat: 99%

CC: Headache and weakness

PLAY OF THE CASE

> **KEY QUESTION**
>
> Ask this open-ended question at the beginning of every case.

C: "What do I see as I walk into the patient's room?"

E: "The patient is a young-appearing woman with a prominent abdomen who is lying on the stretcher with her eyes closed."

C: "Hello, I am Dr. Jones. What brings you in today?"

E: "Mmmm…my head hurts." (The patient sluggishly opens her eyes.)

C: "When did the headache start?"

> **KEY ORDERS**
>
> Most of the patients you see during the exam will be unstable (or will become that way). Every unstable patient requires IV access (preferably two large-bore IVs), oxygen, and cardiac monitoring (and in most cases an ECG). In this case, as the patient is pregnant, getting a UA, LFTs, and coags is also a good idea at this point.

E: (Her husband interrupts the conversation.) "She has just been lying in bed and feeling sick, she has been feeling dizzy when she stands up and her walking is unsteady."

C: "Mr. Smith, I am glad you are here to tell me about your wife's condition. I am Dr. Jones, is your wife pregnant?"

E: "She is 30-weeks pregnant, her first pregnancy."

C: "Does she have any medical problems?"

E: "No, she has been healthy."

C: "Has she been getting prenatal care?"

E: "Yes, she is seeing Dr. Sherman, she last saw him 2 weeks ago. She was concerned that her legs are getting more swollen."

C: "Has she had any seizures?"

E: "No, just this headache that started a few days ago and has just been getting worse for her."

C: "Is she on any medications or allergic to any medications?"

> **KEY ORDERS**
>
> When you are concerned about a patient, ask for vitals every 5-15 minutes. This places the responsibility for remembering to reevaluate the patient on the examiner—a good strategy.

E: "She only takes prenatal vitamins and she has no medication allergies."

C: "OK, I would like to examine her now. I am going to ask the nurse to put her on a cardiac monitor and show me a rhythm strip as soon as it is available. I would like her blood pressure to be checked every 10 minutes. Nurse, please start an 18-gauge IV with NS at TKO rate in the right antecubital fossa. Please draw her blood, and order a CBC with platelet count, electrolytes with BUN/Cr, Mg level, PT/PTT, and liver function tests. I would like to get a UA. Please check fetal heart tones as well."

E: "OK, the labs are sent. The FHTs are 145. The rhythm is NSR and her BP is 150/95."

C: "I just want to ask you a few simple questions to make sure that you are OK. Would you state your name, tell me where you are right now, and give me the date, please?"

E: "I'm Kelly Smith. I'm at the hospital." (She gives the correct date.)

C: "I would like to examine her head and neck. Is there any evidence of trauma, any hematomas, lacerations, abrasions, or contusions?"

E: "No, there is not."

C: "Does shc have any sinus tenderness or skin changes on the face?"

E: "No, she does not."

C: "Are the pupils equal and reactive to light and accommodation bilaterally? Are the cranial nerves intact and is there papilledema?"

E: "The examination is normal for those findings."

C: "Is the neck supple? Is there any C-spine tenderness?"

E: "Neck is supple, no C-spine tenderness."

C: "Are the breath sounds clear and symmetric? Are there any murmurs, rubs, or gallops on the cardiac examination?"

E: "Heart and lung examination is normal."

C: "Is the abdomen soft, is it tender to palpation, and are bowel sounds present on auscultation?"

E: "The abdomen is full and gravid, appropriate to gestational age. There is no focal tenderness and bowel sounds are normal."

C: "I would like to perform a pelvic examination. Is there any blood in the vaginal vault?"

E: "No."

C: "I would like to do a bimanual examination. Is the cervix open or closed? Is the uterus tender or boggy?"

E: "The cervix is open to fingertip and the uterus is nontender."

C: "I would like to perform a rectal examination. Is the rectal tone normal? Is there blood in the stool?"

E: "The rectal tone is normal; the stool is brown and guaiac negative."

C: "Is there any clubbing, cyanosis, or edema? Are the pulses and pressures equal and symmetric in all extremities?"

E: "There is no cyanosis; the patient has 3+ edema extending to the knees bilaterally. Pulses are palpable in all distal extremities and symmetric."

C: "Does the patient have any sensory or motor deficits? Are the cranial nerves intact? Are there any cerebellar signs when I test finger-nose or heel-shin maneuvers? Is the patient's gait steady?"

E: "The patient has no sensory or motor deficits. She has no cerebellar signs. Her gait is deferred as she feels very weak and it would be difficult to get out of bed."

C: "How are the patient's deep tendon reflexes?"

E: "She has hyperactive (4+) reflexes bilaterally."

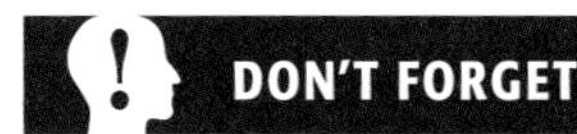

This examinee would have gotten high points for professionalism if they had explained and asked permission for the pelvic and rectal examinations before performing them.

C: "What is her BP now?"

E: "The BP is 160/95."

C: "I would like to give 4 g of magnesium over 10 minutes IV to this patient. I would also like to give 10 mg of hydralazine IV to the patient. Please recheck her blood pressure every 10 minutes and order an OB bed with fetal and maternal monitoring."

C: "Mr. Smith, your wife has a serious condition associated with her pregnancy. Her blood pressure is dangerously high. We will treat her aggressively and she will need to be admitted to the hospital. I will call Dr. Sherman to come and see her."

H: "Doc, is she going to be OK?"

C: "We will do everything we can for her and for the baby. I am glad you brought her in."

E: "Dr. Sherman is on the phone."

C: "Hello Dr. Sherman, it is Dr. Jones here. I have your patient Mrs. Smith here, a G1P0 who presents at 30 weeks with hypertension, edema, headache, and confusion but no history of seizure. We are treating her with IV magnesium and hydralazine. The fetal heart tones are normal, and there is no vaginal bleeding, abdominal pain, or tenderness at this time. I would like you to see her and admit her to the hospital."

E: "I will be right in. The case is now over."

CRITICAL ACTION

There are four critical actions taking place at this point in the case. First, the examinee must identify preeclampsia. Second, they must treat the blood pressure. Third, they must treat with magnesium and finally, they must admit to an OB bed with fetal and maternal monitoring.

CASE ASSESSMENT

The candidate handled the case fairly well. In this case, the candidate was told that the patient was pregnant. The examiner may not always provide this information. Remember to always inquire about pregnancy status on patients of child-bearing age, and screen for it. This patient could have easily been in status epilepticus and the candidate may have not been told the patient was pregnant. It is OK to ask, "Does this patient appear gravid?" If you aren't getting the answer, order a stat bedside UHCG.

The candidate realized that the patient was ill and was aggressive about getting the history from the husband. When patients are not good historians themselves, it is the candidate's obligation to seek out the history from available family, friends, or EMS personnel. In this case, the examiner introduced the husband to the candidate. The husband was able to give the history. Some historical elements were omitted from the history: Has there been vaginal bleeding or abdominal pain, chest pain or shortness of breath? Has her water broken? Has there been any trauma? (Remembering that pregnant women are more prone to domestic violence.) Does the patient have a history of headaches? Does the patient use or abuse drugs (specifically cocaine or amphetamines)? Obtaining this clinical information is important, and can be done quickly.

Many candidates make presumptive and assumptive diagnoses based on the vital signs and an incomplete history. In this case, there are many conditions that can cause this presentation. The candidate should be considering preeclampsia, infection, trauma, toxicology, or subarachnoid or intracranial hemorrhage in this patient. End-organ complications of systemic vasoconstriction can be screened for and should be considered in the diagnostic testing.

The candidate seemed to have taken note of the patient's blood pressure on presentation, but did not act on treating the patient's blood pressure until after he completed the physical examination and history taking. In this case, the patient did not decompensate because of a delay in treatment. The only feedback you get on the oral boards is how the patient is doing. The patient may have had a seizure if the examiner wanted you to treat the blood pressure more expeditiously or just to further test your ability to manage a patient with this complication.

The candidate performed all of the critical actions of this case and would have passed the case. To gain points, the candidate could have been more thorough in data acquisition, more prompt in treatment, and somewhat more professional to the patient and family. In this case, the examiner could have explained the pelvic and rectal examinations before beginning them.

Critical Actions

1. Identify preeclampsia.
2. Treat hypertension.
3. Give $MgSO_4$ for seizure prophylaxis.
4. Admit patient to monitored bed with OB physician.

Test Performance

1. *Data acquisition:* The candidate could have been more thorough in history taking. These "style points" would include: History of trauma, drug or alcohol abuse, directed questioning of headache characteristics, screen for third trimester vaginal bleeding or pain, and screen for risk factors of preeclampsia. Score = **6**
2. *Problem solving:* The candidate gathered information in an organized approach, ordered appropriate labs and diagnostics, and involved the proper consultants. Score = **7**
3. *Patient management:* The candidate made appropriate treatment decisions regarding the magnesium and antihypertensive administration. Score = **7**
4. *Resource utilization:* The candidate made good use of resources in a cost-effective manner. The candidate considered end-organ complications of the diagnosis and ordered tests that would be important for her care on admission. Some candidates would have ordered a head computed tomography (CT) scan on this patient, which would not be considered overutilization given the history and the neuro examination. Score = **7**
5. *Health care provided (outcome):* The candidate arrived at the diagnosis efficiently and treated the life-threatening condition appropriately. Score = **7**
6. *Interpersonal relations and communication skills:* The candidate was able to gather information from husband and relate to him effectively. The orders to nurses were clear and concise. The candidate could have been more thoughtful of telling patient of her condition, seeing if there were any questions, and preparing patient for rectal and pelvic examinations. Score = **6**
7. *Comprehension of pathophysiology:* The candidate demonstrated a thorough understanding of the disease process as evidenced by the workup and treatments provided in the case. Score = **7**
8. *Clinical competence (overall):* The candidate did an excellent job managing a life-threatening illness with effective resource utilization and appropriate diagnostic workup and treatment. Score = **7**

CASE 23 1½ y/o Male With SOB

John Dayton and Eileen Allen

INITIAL INFORMATION

Name: Paul Thomas

Mode of arrival: Brought in by parents on a snowy evening

Age: 18 months

Gender: Male

VS: T 38.2°C (100.76°F), BP 98/palp, HR 170, RR 60

CC: Noisy, rapid breathing

KEY QUESTION

Ask this open-ended question at the beginning of every case.

PLAY OF THE CASE

C: "What do I see as I walk into the patient's room?"

E: "The patient is a well-developed male toddler sitting on his mother's lap. He appears to be in moderate distress with audible grunting and rapid respirations."

KEY ORDERS

Most of the patients you see during the exam will be unstable or will become that way.

Every unstable adult patient requires IV access, oxygen, and cardiac monitoring. However, not every pediatric patient will require IV access.

C: "Nurse, place the patient on a cardiac monitor and check a pulse ox on RA. What rhythm do I see on the monitor?"

E: "You see sinus tachycardia at 165 on the monitor and the RA sat is 90%-92%."

C: "Nurse, please give the patient 100% O_2 by non-rebreather mask and place on continuous oximetry. Let me know what his pulse ox is once this takes place. I would also like the patient disrobed and placed in a hospital gown."

E: "Pulse ox is now 98% now that he is on 100% non-rebreather."

C: "Mr. and Mrs. Thomas, I'm Dr. Duffy. I'll be taking care of Paul in the Emergency Department. What has been going on with Paul?"

KEY ORDERS

Always ask about any missing vital signs? The missing ones are often abnormal.

E: "He has had a runny nose and some congestion for a few days. Yesterday he started coughing a little and that got worse today. Tonight, he seemed to have trouble getting his breath and he was making a grunting noise when he was breathing."

C: "I just want to listen to Paul to see if he needs anything right away to help with his breathing, and then we will talk more about this illness."

C: "What do I hear when I listen to the lungs?"

E: "What are you listening for?"

C: "I want to know if his breath sounds are equal, if they are diminished in any field and if he has any crackles, wheezes, or rales."

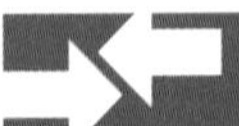

CRITICAL ACTION

There are two critical actions at this point. First, the examiner has to get a pulse ox measurement. Second, they must place this hypoxic child on supplemental oxygen.

E: "Breath sounds are decreased throughout bilaterally and distant inspiratory and expiratory wheezing is heard in all lung fields."

C: "Is there any nasal flaring, grunting, or retractions?"

E: "Yes. There is nasal flaring, both intercostal and subcostal retractions, and the patient has mild audible grunting on expiration."

C: "Is there anything remarkable when I listen to the heart?"

E: "Patient is tachycardic, but heart sounds are otherwise unremarkable."

C: "Nurse, please give the patient an albuterol nebulizer treatment. Let me know when it is finished."

C: "Mrs. Thomas, has Paul ever wheezed before or been diagnosed with asthma?"

E: "No."

C: "He is wheezing now. It is probably due to a viral infection he has. I am going to give him a breathing treatment. The medicine comes out as a mist and that may help his breathing. Has he been running fevers over the past few days?"

E: "He's felt warm since yesterday. I've been giving him Tylenol."

C: "Has he been around anyone who is sick?"

E: "Not at home but he is in daycare 3 days a week and I don't know if anyone has been sick there."

C: "Has he had any vomiting or diarrhea?"

E: "No."

C: "How has his appetite been?"

E: "He hasn't eaten anything since yesterday and today he only drank about half cup of juice."

C: "Is he still having wet diapers?"

E: "He had one wet diaper earlier today."

C: "Does Paul have any medical problems?"

E: "No."

C: "Has he ever been hospitalized or had surgery?"

E: "No."

C: "Does he take any medications on a regular basis?"

E: "No."

C: "In the past few days has he had any other medications other than Tylenol?"

E: "I gave him some Robitussin when he started coughing yesterday but it didn't seem to help."

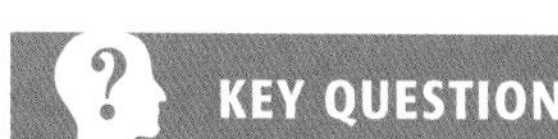

Remember to always go ask about medical history, medications, and allergies on all patients. Ask about immunizations for pediatric patients.

C: "Is he allergic to any medication?"

E: "Not that we know of."

C: "Are his immunizations up-to-date?"

E: "Yes."

C: "Now that he has had a breathing treatment, I want to re-evaluate Paul. Is he awake, alert, and interactive?"

E: "Yes."

C: "Are the mucous membranes moist? Does he have tears when he cries?"

E: "Mucous membranes are dry and he does not tear with crying."

C: "Tympanic membrane, oropharynx, eyes?"

E: "TMs are clear. Oropharynx is non-erythematous. There is no conjunctivitis."

C: "Is the neck supple?"

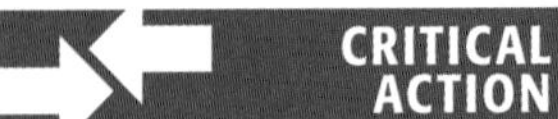

CRITICAL ACTION

Giving a fluid bolus is a critical action in this case. Any child breathing at this rate will have significant insensate losses.

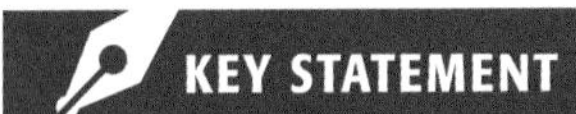

KEY STATEMENT

Remember to explain to patients and families what is going on, give test results, and answer any questions.

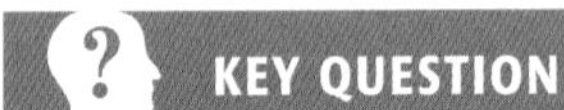

KEY QUESTION

Remember to reassess your patient's condition frequently—especially after any intervention has been completed.

E: "Yes."

C: "Has the heart or lung examination changed since I last listened? What is the capillary refill?"

E: "The heart exam is remarkable for a mild increase in heart rate, likely due to the albuterol. The lung examination hasn't changed. The cap refill is 1.5 seconds."

C: "Abdominal examination?"

E: "Unremarkable."

C: "Is there cyanosis or edema?"

E: "None present."

C: "Nurse, could you please recheck the patient's vitals and pulse ox. Now when I look at the patient what do I see?"

E: "What are you looking for?"

C: "What is his general appearance and mental status? Does he still look like he is in distress? Is he retracting? Is he grunting? Is he still wheezing?"

E: "He is awake, but appears tired while sitting on his mother's lap. He is still in moderate distress with intercostal and subcostal retractions. He is no longer grunting. He has persistent inspiratory and expiratory wheezing and decreased aeration throughout. Vitals are Temp 38.2, HR 180, RR 60, pulse ox back on 100% NRB is 97%."

C: "Nurse, I would like him to get a stat L-racemic epi neb treatment. I would also like an IV placed and the patient given a 20 cc/kg bolus of 0.9 NS. Finally, can you give 15 mg/kg of acetaminophen for his fever."

E: "The racemic epi neb is being started. IV is in."

C: "Mr. and Mrs. Thomas, Paul still has a lot of wheezes on examination and is still having to work hard to breath. I am going to give him another nebulizer treatment with a medication that addresses viral infections (like croup and bronchiolitis) that can also cause wheezing. Since this is Paul's first wheezing episode and he has a fever, I am also going to get a chest x-ray to be sure he doesn't have pneumonia. Do you have any questions?"

E: "No."

C: "Nurse, I'd like a portable upright chest x-ray."

E: "The x-ray is ordered."

C: "Is the epi neb finished?"

E: "The nebulized treatment and fluid bolus are done."

C: "Can I have a repeat set of vitals and pulse ox reading? When I look at the patient what do I see?"

E: "The patient is in less distress. He still has mild intercostal retractions. His fever has resolved, HR 145, RR 55, pulse ox on 100% NRB is 98%."

C: "When I listen to the lungs what do I hear?"

E: "Aeration is slightly improved. Patient still has inspiratory and expiratory wheezes."

C: "In 30 minutes I would like the patient to receive a repeat epi neb. Could you also send a nasal aspirate for RSV antigen testing? Has the patient urinated?"

E: "His mother is changing a wet diaper now. The chest x-ray is back. What do you see?"

C: "The x-ray shows streaky perihilar infiltrates and hyperinflation, concerning for a viral infection called bronchiolitis. Who is Paul's physician?"

E: "Dr. Childers."

C: "I am going to call Dr. Childers to let him know what's going on and I am going to admit Paul to the hospital. He is doing better since the last breathing treatment we gave him. He is not working as hard to breath, but his breathing is still a little fast, and he is still wheezing quite a bit. I want him watched overnight to make sure he doesn't worsen again. Hopefully, it will be a short stay. He will also get another breathing treatment in half an hour. Do you have any questions?"

E: "No."

C: "Nurse, could you please have Dr. Childers paged and arrange for the patient to be admitted to the pediatric floor?"

E: "Dr. Childers is on the phone."

C: "Hi, Dr. Childers. This is Dr. Duffy. I am seeing your patient, Paul Thomas, in the ED. He came in because of trouble breathing. He was in moderate distress when he arrived and had significant wheezing on examination. He also had a new oxygen requirement. He had no response to an albuterol neb, but did improve somewhat following an epi neb. A chest x-ray showed hyperinflation and perihilar infiltrates. I suspect he has bronchiolitis. A rapid RSV test is pending. He still has some decreased, but persistent, retractions and continued wheezing so I would like to admit him. I plan to give him one more epi neb before he goes to the floor. I will also try to wean him down on the supplemental oxygen."

E: "Thank you. This case is now over."

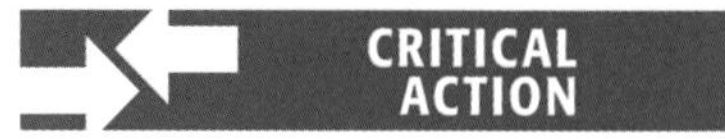

Admitting the patient to the appropriate level of care is always a critical action.

CASE ASSESSMENT

Overall the candidate managed the case very well. The candidate immediately recognized the patient was in respiratory distress and began a quick survey of the airway, breathing, and circulation (ABCs) to see if the patient needed emergent intervention. Although the pulse ox wasn't given initially, the candidate requested this information and supplemental oxygen appropriately given. This represented a critical action. The candidate then went on to address the patient's wheezing and respiratory status by initiating an albuterol neb treatment before obtaining a more thorough history and physical.

Given the time of year and the age of the patient, respiratory syncytial virus (RSV) bronchiolitis is the most likely diagnosis. In this case, an epinephrine neb treatment was required when the albuterol treatment was insufficient to manage symptoms. It would have been appropriate to tart with an epi neb in this scenario. The candidate also reassessed the patient following each treatment. Always reassess your patient after any intervention on exam day.

After completing a more detailed history and physical, the candidate recognized the patient was dehydrated and instituted appropriate treatment by starting an intravenous (IV) and administering normal saline (NS) bolus. Again, the patient was reassessed after this intervention.

Although the patient in this case improved following IV fluids and the epi neb, the candidate appropriately admitted the patient due to persistent signs of respiratory distress. Abnormal vitals, a new oxygen need, and persistent respiratory compromise are indications for admission and represent a critical action on exam day. The case closed as the candidate notified the patient's physician of the admission.

The case may have followed other paths. The patient may have decompensated and required rapid sequence intubation to stabilize. The patient may have dramatically improved following the first neb treatment. In that case, a period of observation would be warranted before making the decision to discharge the patient. The patient could then be discharged with a nebulizer with follow-up scheduled for the following day.

Critical Actions

1. Pulse ox check and supplemental oxygen
2. Nebulizer treatment with either epinephrine or albuterol
3. IV fluid bolus
4. Admission

Test Performance

1. *Data acquisition:* Dr. Duffy requested the missing vital sign, appropriately obtained a chest x-ray, and performed an efficient history and physical. Score = **8**
2. *Problem solving:* The examinee used vital signs and asked appropriate exam questions to form a differential diagnosis and treat the patient. Given the initial decrease in oxygen saturation, the placement was immediately placed on oxygen. Score = **8**
3. *Patient management:* The examinee immediately recognized the need for oxygen, and gave Tylenol for the fever. After two different neb treatments, the patient was doing better, but still needed further management. With this in mind, he was admitted to the appropriate physician. Score = **8**
4. *Resource utilization:* Dr. Duffy limited imaging and lab work to a chest x-ray and a respiratory antigen. The workup was logical, cost-sensitive, aided immediate diagnosis in the emergency department, and will be useful to the admitting physician. Score = **8**
5. *Health care provided (outcome):* After both nebulizer treatments, the patient's vital signs had improved. He received appropriate treatment and the candidate's interventions stabilized the patient. Score = **8**
6. *Interpersonal relations and communication skills:* Dr. Duffy communicated appropriately with the patient's parents to explain concerns, imaging results, and need for admission. The candidate also asked questions to make sure the parents were core comfortable with both the diagnosis and plan. Dr. Duffy also gave a succinct summary of his concerns and the treatment given when he spoke with Dr. Childers. Score = **8**
7. *Comprehension of pathophysiology:* The examinee conveyed understanding of the disease process by ordering appropriate studies and discussing results with the family. On exam day, demonstrate your comprehension of the case by your conversation with the patient, their family/friends, nursing staff, and consultants. Score = **8**
8. *Clinical competence (overall):* Overall, Dr. Duffy showed clinical competence by obtaining an appropriate history and physical, using early intervention to address concerns with breathing, developing a differential diagnosis, utilizing appropriate lab work and imaging, progressively stabilizing the patient, and making the appropriate disposition plan. Score = **8**

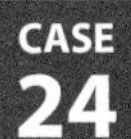

CASE 24 35 y/o Female Pedestrian Struck by an Auto

John Dayton, Jamie Collings, and Michael Gisondi

INITIAL INFORMATION

Name: Jennifer Small

Mode of arrival: EMS

Age: 35 years

Gender: Female

VS: T 36.2°C (97.2°F), BP 89/54, P 120, RR 16, O_2 sat: 95% on RA

CC: Pedestrian struck by a car

PLAY OF THE CASE

E: "You are at a Level 1 trauma center, with an ED team consisting of one recording nurse, two procedural nurses, a secretary, and an ED tech. Paramedics arrive with a 35-year-old female pedestrian who was struck by a motor vehicle going 45 mph. Initial vitals in the field were HR 125, BP 80/50, RR 20. The patient is alert and oriented, and complaining of pain in her right leg. One 16-gauge peripheral IV has already been placed by EMS."

KEY QUESTION

Ask this open-ended question at the beginning of every case.

C: "What do I see as I walk into the patient's room?"

E: "You see a young woman on a backboard wearing a cervical collar. She is softly moaning in pain. There is a cardboard splint applied to her right leg."

KEY ORDERS

Every trauma patient requires IV access (preferable two large-bore IVs), oxygen, and cardiac monitoring. In this case, as the patient is hypotensive, a fluid bolus should also be initiated.

C: "I'd like to initiate my primary survey, starting with the airway. I will ask the patient if she remembers the course of events. I will also have the secretary notify the trauma surgeon. 'What happened, Ms. Small?'"

E: "I was crossing the street, and this car turned and hit me on the right side and then ran over me. I couldn't walk afterward."

C: "Airway is intact. Now I will instruct the nurse and tech to disrobe the patient, while maintaining spinal immobilization, as I listen for breath sounds and palpate her chest. Meanwhile, I will request the nurse to place a second 16-gauge peripheral IV in an antecubital vein, draw blood for labs, and give a 1 L NS bolus. I will also ask that the patient be placed on both cardiac and oxygen monitors, obtain a rhythm strip, and to begin oxygen at 15 L via an NRB."

KEY ORDERS

Remember to reassess your unstable patients frequently and after every intervention.

E: "The patient has equal bilateral breath sounds and there is no crepitus or deformities of the chest wall. The IV is being placed and the patient is now fully disrobed. The patient asks, 'What's happening?'"

C: "'Ms. Small, please stay calm. Lots of team members are involved in your care and it's important to follow directions.' I will check carotid, femoral, and radial and dorsalis pedis pulses. Also, I would like the vital signs repeated and the results of the rhythm strip."

E: "The pulses are 1+ both centrally and peripherally in all extremities. The monitor shows sinus tachycardia. The second IV has been placed."

C: "What is the blood pressure and heart rate now?"

E: "After 1.5 L of NS the BP remains 88/50 with a pulse of 120."

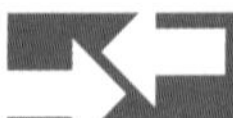

CRITICAL ACTION

Giving this hypotensive trauma patient blood products, after an initial fluid bolus, is a critical action in this case. The candidate could have waited to reassess BP and pulses after a full 2-L bolus. However, in a hypotensive trauma patient, hemorrhage is a major concern and you will not be penalized for giving blood products early.

KEY ORDERS

The candidate has now placed the responsibility of rechecking vitals on the examiner. This is a good strategy to use. The candidate forgot, however, to ask for the lab results when they are available. This candidate will forget to follow-up on the labs he orders, which will cause him to lose points on his "Resource Utilization" score.

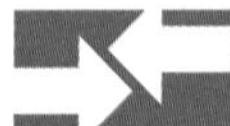

CRITICAL ACTION

Doing a FAST (or DPL) to assess the source of the hypotension is a critical action in this case. This candidate is, at this point, mixing the order of the primary and secondary surveys. They should have addressed the source of the hemorrhage (C for circulation) first before addressing the extremity injury. They should also finish their full primary survey before ordering radiology.

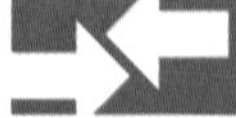

CRITICAL ACTION

Stabilizing this pelvic fracture in an unstable bleeding patient is a critical action in this case.

C: "I would like the nurse to continue to infuse the second liter of NS through the second IV and begin transfusing 2 U of PRBCs through the EMS IV."

E: "The nurse asks, 'What type of blood should I transfuse now?'"

C: "O negative uncrossmatched blood."

E: "The nurse asks what labs she should send."

C: "Type and cross for 6 U, CBC with differential, PT/PTT, basic chemistry panel, urine hCG, and UA. Please repeat vitals every 5 minutes and let me know of the results. I am concerned her hypotension is due to bleeding. Are there are any areas of obvious areas of hemorrhage, swelling, or deformity?"

E: "There are no obvious external sources of bleeding, though the right mid-lower leg is swollen, tender, and deformed."

C: "Is there a laceration in the area of deformity? Is the peripheral pulse intact distal to the area of lower leg injury? Can she wiggle her toes? Is she able to move all other extremities as well?"

E: "There is a small laceration in the area, but there are no bony fragments protruding from the wound. The pulse is present and she can wiggle her toes. She is neurovascularly intact."

C: "I will ask the nurse and a tech to dress the skin wound and apply a long-leg posterior plaster mold to the right leg and to check the neurovascular function post splinting."

E: "That is being done."

C: "To look for sources of internal bleeding, I would like to perform a FAST exam at the bedside. If that is not available, I will perform a DPL. Would the radiology tech perform the following x-rays: cervical spine, chest x-ray, pelvis x-ray, and a right tib/fib?"

E: "The FAST scan is available—which views would you like to look at?"

C: "The RUQ Morrison pouch, LUQ splenorenal recess, subxiphoid cardiac view, and suprapubic views. I am looking specifically for free fluid indicative of internal bleeding."

E: "The FAST scan is negative in all views."

C: "I would now like to palpate the pelvis to assess for any instability."

E: "The pelvis is tender and feels unstable and mobile."

C: "Does the ED have any pelvic binders?"

E: "No. By the way, the first unit of O-negative blood is now running."

C: "I would first place a Foley catheter in this female patient (unless there is a trauma near the urethra) and then place a sheet under the patient and tie the sheet tightly around the pelvis. I would like to repeat the vitals afterward."

E: "The sheet is in place. The repeat vitals are HR 110, BP 100/65, RR 20, SPo_2 98%."

C: "I would like to call the orthopedics service and request their assistance to treat our trauma patient, who may have an unstable pelvic fracture and right tib/fib."

E: "The orthopedist is on the phone and asks if the trauma surgeon has seen the patient yet."

C: "My reply is that the trauma surgeon has been paged and we are awaiting his return call. However, my assessment is that the patient needs consideration for external pelvis fixator along with ongoing evaluation for other sources of bleeding."

E: "The orthopedist says that he will come down. The trauma surgeon is now available for your consultation. What do you tell him?"

C: "We have a 35-year-old female who was a pedestrian struck by a motor vehicle, initially hypotensive to 80s systolic but responsive to fluids and blood products. Airway and breathing are intact. Lungs are clear and her FAST scan is negative. Chest and pelvis x-rays are about to be performed. There was obvious instability of the pelvis and I suspect substantial pelvic bleeding with possible retroperitoneal hematoma as well. She has an open right tib/fib fracture clinically—I've splinted the leg. There are no obvious femur fractures. After temporarily stabilizing the pelvis and the fluid/blood resuscitation I mentioned, the patient's SBP is now in the 100s."

E: "The trauma surgeon asks if the C-spine has been cleared. What is your response?"

C: "No I haven't yet cleared the C-spine because I felt that the pelvic and likely tib/fib fractures were distracting injuries. I have left the C-collar in place for now."

E: "The radiology technician is performing C-spine, chest, pelvis, and right tib/fib x-rays. Orthopedics is now here and is examining the patient's pelvis. The patient continues to be awake and alert and the vital signs are stabilizing. What is your next course of action?"

C: "Maintaining cervical spine precautions, I will logroll the patient with the help of the ED tech and nurses to examine her spine and perform a rectal examination."

E: "There is no tenderness in her spine, and the rectal examination shows normal tone without blood. Your CXR and pelvic XR are now available." (See Figs. C24-1 and C24-2.)

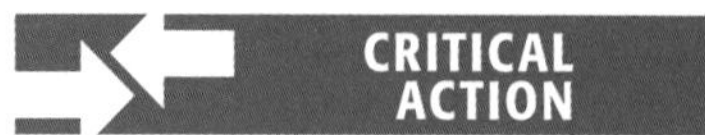

Consulting both trauma and orthopedics for this patient is a critical action.

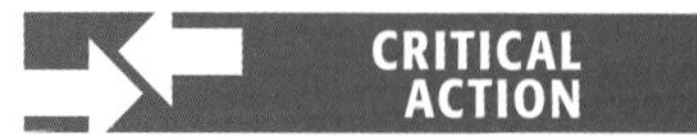

Recognizing that the patient has a distracting injury and cannot have her collar cleared yet is a critical action in this case.

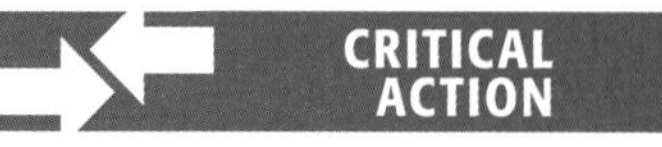

Managing the patient's pain is a critical action in this case. This candidate will lose points for having to be prompted by the nurse to give pain meds almost at the end of the case. Do not forget to manage pain.

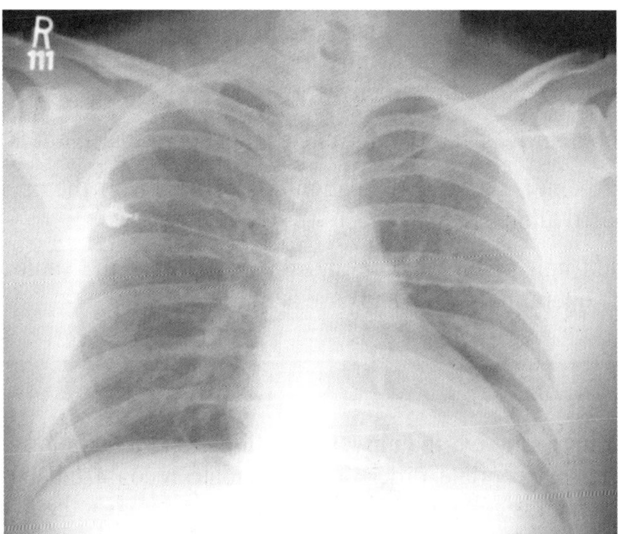

Figure C24-1. Normal CXR. (*Reproduced with permission from Schwartz DT.* Emergency Radiology: Case Studies. *New York, NY: McGraw-Hill; 2008.*)

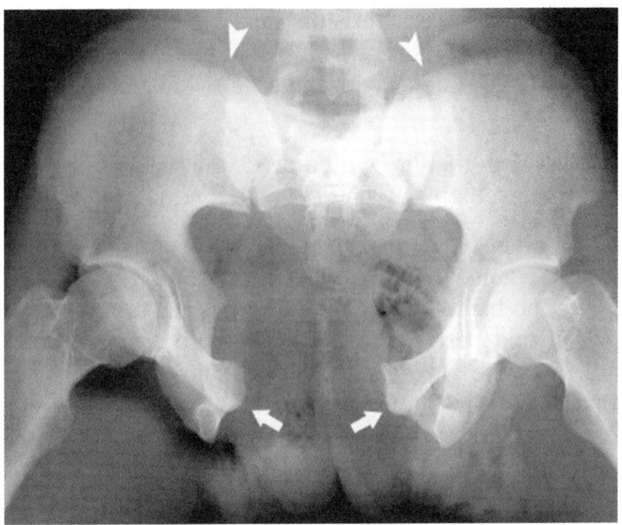

Figure C24-2. Pelvis x-ray with an open book fracture. (*Reproduced with permission from Schwartz DT.* Emergency Radiology: Case Studies. *New York, NY: McGraw-Hill; 2008.*)

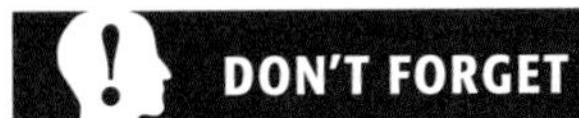

DON'T FORGET

The candidate has not followed up on their labs, and is in the process of disposition without having finished the secondary survey. This will lower their scores.

C: "I will show the pelvis x-ray to the orthopedist and discuss placement of an external pelvic fixator in the trauma bay versus immediate operative management. Is interventional radiology available for angiography?"

E: "The trauma and orthopedic surgeons decide to take the patient to the operating room for pelvis repair and exploratory laparotomy because angiography is unavailable. They contact the operating room to make arrangements for transfer. The nurse asks if she can give the patient morphine for pain."

C: "I will conduct an AMPLE history of the patient—Allergies, Medicines, PMH, Last meal, and Events prior to trauma—and give the patient 4 mg morphine sulfate IV if not allergic. I will make sure the patient gets a tetanus shot if they are not up-to-date."

E: "The patient has no allergies, takes no medicines, has no past medical history, and ate 6 hours prior."

C: "I will now return to the deformity to the right tib/fib. Is she neurovascular intact distally? Are the compartments soft?"

E: "There is no neurovascular compromise and the compartment is soft."

C: "I will ask the nurse to give the patient 2 g of Ancef for the open fracture as she has no stated allergies."

E: "The second unit of blood is in and the VS remain the same. The patient goes up to the operating room. The case is now over."

CASE ASSESSMENT

During the primary survey, the airway, breathing, and circulation (ABCs) were addressed in an appropriate order. The candidate recognized that despite the hypotension (which is certainly serious and life-threatening), the first step in any resuscitation is to address the airway and breathing. The pulmonary examination is important, as hemothoraces and pneumothoraces can be sources of hypotension in trauma patients. Circulation was managed appropriately as the third step. However, the candidate had difficulty working in a sequential manner after the primary survey, forgot to manage pain, and ask for lab and all imaging results.

Hypotension in trauma patients is almost always due to blood loss and most commonly involves the peritoneum, retroperitoneum, pelvis, chest, or femurs. Trauma associated with hypotension usually indicates stage III of hemorrhagic shock, or a blood loss of at least 1.5 L. This extensive loss of blood often requires the addition of blood products after an initial 2 L normal saline (NS) bolus. The candidate should have asked how much crystalloid had infused to establish that an adequate fluid challenge was given before giving blood products. However, he responded appropriately to the persistent hypotension. The candidate performed these actions expediently, not being sidetracked by the lower leg complaints. While the extremity deformity may appear dramatic, it does not represent a cause of life-threatening hemorrhage.

Before the advent of ultrasound and the focused assessment sonography for trauma (FAST), diagnostic peritoneal lavage (DPL) was considered the gold standard for determining the presence of intraperitoneal blood—the candidate offered to perform either procedure and described one in detail. If asked to describe a DPL for this case (or other cases with concern for pelvic fracture), the candidate should describe performing the DPL above the umbilicus, after placing an NG tube to decompress the stomach. Examination of the pelvis and prompt correction of the defect with seemingly simple equipment was done efficiently. The candidate called the orthopedic consultant afterward, recognizing that definitive management of a potentially serious pelvis fracture will require surgery. The transfer of information rapidly from one physician to another is of the utmost importance, and the candidate displayed sound professional interpersonal skills when discussing the case with his colleagues.

There is also room for improvement. The candidate ordered appropriate tests, but didn't follow up with the results before the end of the scenario. The candidate's response to the patient's question was condescending and he did not keep the patient updated and informed. Pain meds were given only after the nurse requested them, and the candidate should have recognized the need for pain control in the awake and stabilized trauma patient. The candidate should have completed the entire secondary survey soon after the primary survey and initial stabilization. The secondary survey was performed in a number of pieces, with the AMPLE portion coming late in the case. The x-rays were ordered and completed, with consultants present, before the candidate adequately completed the secondary survey. Lastly, the candidate did not ask if the patient was pregnant and didn't follow-up on the urine pregnancy test.

This is something the candidate did well. The candidate also did a good job with the tetanus and antibiotics for the open tibia fracture. He also prevented unnecessary trauma to the potentially injured urogenital tract by examining the introitus prior to placing a urinary catheter. While this may be more important in the male patient, given the longer urethral length, the candidate was right to address this issue in the female patient as well.

Critical Actions

1. Administration of blood products.
2. Establish cause of blood loss by physical examination and adjunct studies (FAST +/or DPL, plain films).
3. Stabilize pelvic fracture with sheet or pelvic binder.
4. Avoid C-spine clearance with distracting injury.
5. Pain management.
6. Consultation with trauma surgery and orthopedics.

Test Performance

1. *Data acquisition:* The candidate did not perform the primary and secondary surveys in an orderly fashion, but he did manage to get all the necessary information. He also did not follow-up on the results of the labs he ordered. Score = **5**
2. *Problem solving:* The candidate reacted appropriately to hypotension and knew the necessary interventions for both examination and x-rays findings. Score = **7**
3. *Patient management:* The patient made appropriate treatment decisions to address hypotension, and obtained appropriate consultations, though not always in an orderly fashion. He did not perform the secondary survey in an orderly fashion. Score = **6**
4. *Resource Utilization:* Even though he didn't ask for results, the lab and imaging requests were appropriate. Score = **5**
5. *Health care provided (outcome):* Although he could have been more efficient, the patient received appropriate treatment, the candidate's interventions stabilized the patient, and immediate concerns were addressed appropriately in the primary survey. Score = **6**
6. *Interpersonal relations and communication skills:* The candidate did not introduce himself, talked down to her, did not keep her updated about imaging findings or operative plans, did not discuss blood transfusion, and initially forgot to order pain medication. His interaction with consultants, however, was appropriate. Score = **5**
7. *Comprehension of pathophysiology:* The examinee conveyed their understanding of hypotension in a trauma setting, checked for complications and neurovascular integrity with the fracture, and used appropriate interventions. Appropriate lab studies and imaging were requested. The patient could have received better scores for this section and the "Interpersonal Relations" section by explaining his concerns and treatment plans to the patient. Score = **7**
8. *Clinical competence (overall):* Overall, the examinee showed clinical competence by appropriately completing the primary survey, utilizing appropriate lab work and imaging, explaining the FAST study and how he would apply a pelvic binder. Though his secondary survey was not concise, he completed all critical actions, obtained appropriate consultations, and made the appropriate disposition plan. Score = **7**

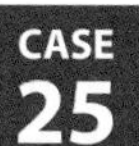

CASE 25 24 y/o Male With Gunshot Wound to Chest and Neck

John Dayton, Jamie Collings, and Michael Gisondi

INITIAL INFORMATION

Name: Charlie Oak

Mode of arrival: EMS

Age: 24 years

Gender: Male

VS: T: 36.2°C (97.2°F), BP 110/65, HR 126, RR 38, O_2 sat: 92% on RA

CC: Gunshot wound (GSW) to neck and chest

PLAY OF THE CASE

E: "You are at a Level I trauma center and the charge nurse approaches you: The paramedics are transporting a 24-year-old male shot in the chest and neck, alert, and oriented times three, HR 126, BP 110/65, RR 32, O_2 sat 93% room air, 98% on face mask. They will be here in 10 minutes, what would you like me to do doctor? You have two nurses, an ED technician, and an ED secretary."

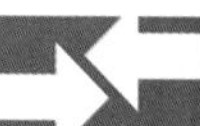

CRITICAL ACTION

There are two critical actions beginning at this point—early surgical consultation and preparation for a difficult airway.

C: "Please notify the trauma surgeon and have both a chest tube kit and a difficult airway cart ready. Please prepare for blood product infusion while I set up for intubation."

E: "Those preparations are underway as the paramedics arrive with the patient several minutes later."

C: "What do I see as I walk into the patient's room?"

E: "A young adult male, approximately 70 kg, eyes open, oxygen being delivered by face mask, moving all four extremities, tachypneic, blood-soaked gauze covering the right side of his neck, blood-soaked gauze covering the right side of his chest over a bloody T-shirt. You notice IV access in his left antecubital fossa with NS running wide open."

KEY QUESTION

Ask this open-ended question at the beginning of every case.

C: "Hello, I'm Dr. Joseph. Sir, what is your name?"

E: "As the paramedics transfer the patient to the ED trauma gurney, the patients states, 'Charlie…get this mask off me, I can't breathe!'"

C: "I will have the tech maintain in-line stabilization as I continue to assess the airway by examining his neck, looking for the location of any wounds, while assessing for pulses, crepitus, tracheal deviation, or hematoma. As I am doing this I will inform the nurses to start another 14-gauge antecubital IV, place the patient on the monitor and to provide a rhythm strip when available, place pulse oximeter, and obtain a blood pressure. What does my neck examination reveal?"

KEY ORDERS

Every trauma patient requires IV access (preferably two large-bore IVs), oxygen, and cardiac monitoring. This candidate does a very good job of starting these orders while assessing the patient airway.

E: "There are two neck wounds noted. One wound is 2 cm right of midline, 1 cm superior to the cricoid cartilage; no crepitus is noted. A non-pulsatile hematoma is appreciated deep to the medial wound, trachea is midline, bilateral strong carotid pulses are present. A second wound is noted 1 cm posterior and 1 cm superior to the angle of the right mandible without crepitance or apparent hematoma. The monitor shows a sinus tachycardia at a rate of 122, BP of 115/70, pulse oximetry of 98% on 100% face mask."

KEY ORDERS

Saying that you are in the process of addressing the airway while you complete the primary survey is an excellent way to buy time during the exam. Performing the rest of the primary survey is important for patient management, but technically speaking it should wait until "A" is finished. By doing this, you gain valuable information without losing the order of your primary survey.

C: "Although the airway currently appears intact, I am concerned about potential complications given the penetrating neck trauma and will prepare for intubation. While the nurse draws up the medications for intubation, I will perform the remainder of the primary survey. I will next listen for breath sounds and assess respirations."

E: "The patient is tachypneic at 32, with breath sounds present bilaterally."

C: "Is there any crepitus or signs of trauma?"

E: "Two right-sided chest wounds are noted. One wound is midclavicular, 2 cm superior to the nipple, without crepitance. The second wound is in the midaxillary line, 4 cm inferior to the apex of the axilla, also without crepitus."

C: "I will palpate for central and peripheral pulses."

E: "Strong femoral and radial pulses are present bilaterally."

C: "Because I'd like to evaluate his neurologic status before intubation, I will quickly assess pupils and ask the patient to move all his extremities."

E: "Pupils are 3 mm, reactive, equal. He speaks clearly and coherently, moving all fours on command."

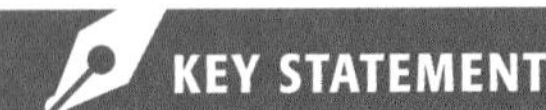

KEY STATEMENT

Remember to always inform the patient and get consent for any procedure you are planning to do.

C: "The patient has a GCS of 15. I will have the ED tech maintain in-line stabilization throughout the intubation, to be followed by a cervical collar after airway control. I will have the nurse run the second IV wide open with 1 L NS, draw up 20 mg of etomidate, and 150 mg of succinylcholine. I will ask the unit secretary to page the surgeon again and page the respiratory therapist for a ventilator. 'Charlie, you have some serious injuries that may require repair in the operating room. I need to give you medicine to put you to sleep, as well as place a breathing tube down your throat. Do you have any medical problems or take any medications? Are you allergic to any medications?'"

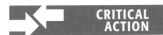

CRITICAL ACTION

Keeping C-spine immobilization in place throughout the case is a critical action.

E: "Charlie denies any medical problems, medications, or any allergies and states, 'just do what you have to, you are the doctor.'"

C: "After the induction and paralytic medications are given, I will orotracheally intubate the patient with an 8.0 ET tube and assess for breaths sounds and end-tidal CO_2 color change."

E: "Breath sounds present bilaterally, good color change on end-tidal CO_2, pulse oximeter reads 98%."

CRITICAL ACTION

Intubating this patient is a critical action.

C: "I will ventilate the patient with a bag valve mask on 100% oxygen at 14 times per minute while awaiting respiratory therapy with a ventilator. Have a post-intubation portable chest x-ray ordered stat. I will place a cervical collar on the patient and ask the nurse to take another full set of vitals."

E: "Temperature 36.4°C (97.6°F), HR 110, BP 115/70, RR 14, pulse ox is 98% on 100% oxygen."

C: "I'll ask the nurse to send blood for a complete blood count, basic chemistry profile, PT/PTT, and type and cross for 4 U. Also administer a tetanus and Ancef 2 g IV."

E: "The nurse informs you that the surgeon is on the phone."

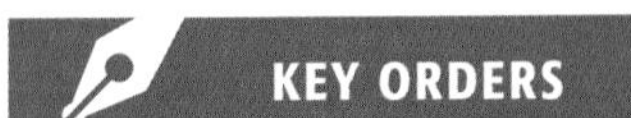

KEY ORDERS

Remember to reassess your unstable patients frequently—especially after any intervention.

C: "Dr. Chestnek, this is Dr. Joseph in the ER. I have an intubated 24-year-old male with apparent GSW injuries to the neck and chest who will need immediate surgical evaluation. He has a Zone II neck injury with hematoma that likely has penetrated the platysma. He also has a right-sided zone three injury. There are two right-sided chest wounds, but he has good aeration of the lungs bilaterally. Current vitals are T 36.6°C (97.9°F), HR 110, and BP 115/70, with

O_2 sat of 98% on an FIO_2 of 100%. I have two large-bore IVs running wide open and his pulse is responding to fluid resuscitation. A CXR is ordered. Prior to intubation the patient had no dysphonia, hemoptysis, crepitus, expanding hematoma, or facial droop. He has strong carotids appreciated bilaterally. If the patient remains stable, we will continue his evaluation with angiography, esophagoscopy, and bronchoscopy for the Zone II injury. The Zone III injury will also be addressed by the angiogram."

E: "Dr. Chestnek states, 'I am on my way.' As you get off the phone the nurse states the she does not feel a radial pulse and the sat dropped to 86%."

C: "I will reexamine the neck and reassess the airway, breathing, and circulation. What do I see and hear when I reexamine the neck and listen to the lung sounds?"

E: "No breath sound on the right side of the chest, and the medial neck hematoma appears larger."

C: "I will needle the chest for a tension pneumothorax. 14 gauge, 2nd intercostal space, midclavicular line. The nurse should begin infusing O-negative blood through the rapid infuser."

E: "A rush of air is heard with needle decompression, the oxygen saturation rises to 95% with continued ventilations."

C: "I will reassess pulses, what is the blood pressure?"

E: "Blood pressure reads 110/82, HR 110. Radial and femoral pulses are appreciated bilaterally."

C: "I will prepare to place a 36 French chest tube for a now open pneumothorax."

E: "The initial chest tube output is 150 cc of blood, there is no apparent air leak, the blood pressure is 126/82, the heart rate is 105, and the pulse oximeter reads 98%. Two antecubital large-bore IV continue to run wide open NS. The nurses are still setting up the rapid infuser and have yet to deliver any blood."

C: "Maintaining cervical stabilization I would like to turn the patient, palpate C, T, and L spine, perform a rectal, and look for any other injuries."

E: "No apparent injuries. No step-offs. Rectal negative."

C: "If there is no blood at the urethral meatus, I will instruct the nurses to insert a Foley catheter. I will place a right femoral central line in preparation for potential further hemodynamic decompensations."

E: "Foley is in. Right femoral central line is in. Dr. Chestnek arrives and states, 'The OR is ready but the patient looks stable and I would like to continue evaluation in the ED, wait for the angiogram, esophagoscopy, and laryngoscopy.'"

C: "Dr. Chestnek, I agree the patient needs those studies, but the Zone II injury, with an expanding hematoma, needs prompt surgical exploration. I am happy to call ENT and interventional radiology and get them to meet you in the OR to perform those studies."

E: "Dr. Chestnek agrees and the patient is taken to the operating room. This case is now over."

CASE ASSESSMENT

The candidate managed this case well. Throughout the encounter he followed advanced trauma life support (ATLS) protocol, moving through the case with critical and continuous attention to the airway, breathing, and circulation (ABCs).

KEY ORDERS

In the trauma setting, when the patient decompensates begin with "A" again and work your way down.

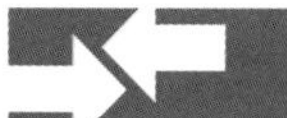

CRITICAL ACTION

Recognition and treatment of the tension pneumothorax is a critical action in this case. The candidate has also been giving the patient a 2-L fluid bolus for his tachycardia (remember that tachycardia is the first sign of shock) and is now switching to blood products. This fluid resuscitation is also a critical action.

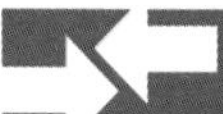

CRITICAL ACTION

Placement of a chest tube completes the treatment of the tension pneumothorax.

DON'T FORGET

On exam day, your consultants will often "push back" as a way to test your knowledge of the management of whatever disease process you are evaluating. Always insist on appropriate and prompt management of your patient.

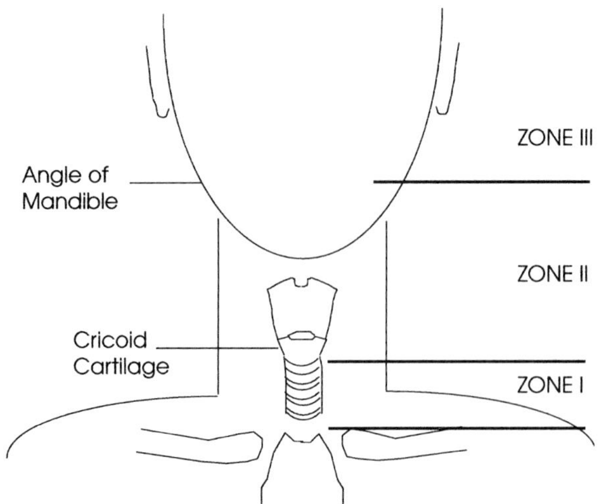

Figure C25-1. Zones of the neck. (*Reproduced with permission from Tintinalli JE, Kelen GD, Stapczynski JS, et al.* Emergency Medicine: A Comprehensive Study Guide. *6th ed. New York, NY: McGraw-Hill; 2004.*)

At the start of the case the candidate recognized the need for early surgical consultation. He efficiently identified penetrating injuries to the chest and neck, correctly anticipating airway compromise and potential shock. Zone II and Zone III injuries were properly identified. Anatomic zones are illustrated in Fig. C25-1 and Table C25-1.

The following signs must be appreciated and communicated clearly to surgical staff, as they are considered potential indications for immediate exploration without further diagnostic testing:

- Expanding hematoma
- Severe active bleeding
- Vascular bruit/thrill
- Lack of cooperation
- Subcutaneous air

Table C25-1. Penetrating Neck Injures: Imaging Considerations in Stable Patients

Zone	Imaging Guidelines
I	Angiogram of arch and great vessels Consider esophagram/esophagoscopy, bronchoscopy
II	Angiogram of carotid and vertebral arteries Combination of esophagram and esophagoscopy Consider bronchoscopy
III	Carotid angiogram Oropharynx examination

- Dysphonia/dysphagia
- Focal neurologic deficits/Horner syndrome
- Decreased carotid pulses
- Cerebral ischemia
- Airway obstruction
- Hemoptysis/hematemesis

Worsening vital signs in this case were properly addressed with a reevaluation of the ABCs. A tension pneumothorax had developed upon positive pressure ventilation and was correctly identified and managed with a chest tube. Important guidelines for chest tube output are as follows:

- Indications for thoracotomy.
- Initial chest tube drainage is >15-20 mL/kg of blood in children or 1000-1500 mL in adults.
- Persistent bleeding at a rate of 4 mL/kg/h in children or 200 mL/h for >3 hours in adults.
- Increasing hemothorax seen on chest x-ray.
- Persistent hypotension despite adequate blood replacement, if other hemorrhagic sources are excluded.
- Worsening vitals after initial response to resuscitation.

Although the vital signs improved with treatment of the tension pneumothorax, the candidate correctly obtained central venous access. Despite normalizing vital signs, the candidate identified the need for increased vascular access for definitive surgical intervention and exploration of a Zone II injury given the expanding hematoma.

Critical Actions

1. Early surgical consultation
2. Intubation/preparation for potential difficult airway
3. C-spine immobilization
4. Identification and management of early signs of shock
5. Recognition and management of a tension pneumothorax

Test Performance

1. *Data acquisition:* The candidate shows ability to obtain a directed history and examination in an efficient manner. Adhering to the Advanced Trauma Life Support (ATLS) guidelines, the candidate found appropriate time to get an AMPLE history without delaying resuscitative efforts. The patient could have elicited more information from the paramedics. Score = **7**
2. *Problem solving:* Problem solving is excellent as the candidate was able to make crucial decisions based on critical information. The candidate acted quickly and decisively to address the tension pneumothorax and performed appropriate resuscitative interventions. He efficiently stabilized the patient on arrival and after the tension pneumothorax and showed that he anticipated future problems by setting up a difficult airway cart before patient arrival and by placing the central line before transfer to the operating room (OR). Score = **8**
3. *Patient management:* The candidate makes appropriate treatment decisions based on patient information, ATLS protocols, and clinical judgment in an efficient manner. Patient care is excellent. Score = **8**

4. *Resource utilization:* Appropriate equipment was set up based on the emergency medical services (EMS) call, appropriate imaging was used to evaluate chest injuries and intubation. Appropriate trauma labs were ordered and blood products used. Labs and chest x-ray (CXR) may not have been available prior to transfer to the OR, but were also not requested or addressed with trauma surgeon. Score = **7**
5. *Health care provided (outcome):* The patient received efficient, appropriate treatment, and the candidate's interventions stabilized the patient. Score = **8**
6. *Interpersonal relations and communication skills:* The communication was appropriately tailored to the acuity of the case. Dialogue with the surgeon was non-confrontational, but acknowledged concerns over lengthy emergency department (ED) evaluations. Score = **8**
7. *Comprehension of pathophysiology:* The candidate demonstrated a highly detailed knowledge of penetrating neck injuries and surgical indications, tension pneumothoraces, and associated management, and anticipated the need for a more vascular access and placed a central line even after his patient had stabilized. Score = **8**
8. *Clinical competence (overall):* Overall, the examinee showed clinical competence by obtaining an appropriate history and physical despite the patient acuity, performing timely and appropriate interventions, working toward the appropriate disposition. Score = **8**

CASE 26 5 y/o Female With Abdominal Pain

John Dayton and Kip Adrian

INITIAL INFORMATION

Name: Nina Santiago

Mode of arrival: Brought in by mom

Age: 5 years

Gender: Female

VS: T 37.3°C (99.2°F), BP 110/50, HR 150, RR 45

CC: Abdominal pain

PLAY OF THE CASE

C: "What do I see as I walk into the patient's room?"

E: "A 5-year-old Hispanic female who appears lethargic, is lying on the bed and holding her abdomen."

C: "What is the oxygen saturation, and what is the patient's weight?"

E: "The child is breathing 45 times a minute at 99% on room air. She weighs 20 kg."

C: "Nurse, while I talk with the family please put the child on a monitor, 2 L of oxygen via NC, place a large-bore IV in the antecubital fossa and draw blood for lab work."

E: "The nurse does these things."

C: "Hello, my name is Dr. Doolittle and I am the ER doctor today. Nina, I noticed you are not feeling well, and that your tummy is hurting. While we talk, the nurse is going to put some stickers on your chest so we can make sure you're safe."

E: "The girl moans, but does not do much besides."

C: "Ms. Santiago, I want to ask you about what has been happening with Nina, but while we talk I'm going to have the nurse put Nina on a monitor, and start an IV and draw some blood."

E: "OK."

C: "Nurse, please start the IV, draw blood for chemistries and blood count. At the same time start a bolus of 20 cc/kg of NS. Ms. Santiago, how long has Nina's abdomen been hurting?"

E: "It started about 4 days ago, and has been slowly getting worse."

C: "Is it constant pain, or does it come and go?"

E: "It seems to be constant pain."

C: "Has Nina been throwing up, having diarrhea or difficulty urinating?"

E: "She has thrown up a few times over the past 2 days or so."

C: "Was there any green material in her vomit?"

KEY QUESTION

Ask this open-ended question at the beginning of every case.

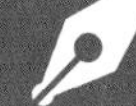

KEY ORDERS

Every patient with unstable vital signs requires IV access (preferably two large-bore IVs), oxygen, and cardiac monitoring.

KEY STATEMENT

Remember to introduce yourself to the patient and the family, explain procedures and lab results to them, and keep them updated regarding your treatment plan.

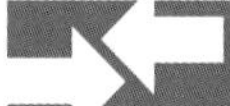

CRITICAL ACTION

Initiation of fluid resuscitation is a critical action in this case.

E: "No, it just seemed to be clear."

C: "Has Nina been able to eat or drink anything?"

E: "Not much over the past few days, but before that she was eating OK and constantly drinking."

C: "Was she drinking more than she usually does."

E: "Yes, she could not seem to get enough water."

C: "Is Nina urinating more or less than usual?"

E: "Actually, she is urinating much more than usual over the past week or so."

C: "Has Nina had any cold symptoms recently, like a runny nose, sore throat, or cough."

E: "No."

C: "Has Nina had any fevers that you have noticed?"

E: "No, she hasn't."

C: "Is it possible that Nina has eaten or drank something she wasn't supposed to recently?"

E: "Not to my knowledge."

C: "Nina, have you tried to eat or drink anything and you didn't know what it was?"

E: "She shakes her head somewhat vigorously."

C: "How long has Nina been so sleepy?"

E: "Really over the past day or so. She has just slept."

C: "Are you able to wake her up? And is she making sense when she talks when awake?"

E: "Yes, I seem to be able to wake her. She talks normally, but just falls right back asleep."

C: "Does Nina have any medical problems?"

E: "None that I know of."

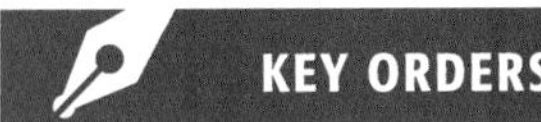

When you order a test, always ask to be told the results when they come back. This places the responsibility for remembering to check the lab values on the examiner.

C: "Are Nina's immunizations up-to-date, and does she have any allergies to medications?"

E: "Her shots are up-to-date, and she has no known drug allergies."

C: "Is the IV inserted and bolus running?"

E: "Yes, the IV is running and blood drawn."

C: "Thank you nurse, please let me know when the bolus is finished. Also, please send the blood for CBC with differential, BMP with magnesium and phosphate, beta-hydroxybutyrate, and acetone. Please check a fingerstick glucose level. Also, draw an ABG on the child, catheterize her for urine, hand dip it here in the ER, then send it for a formal urinalysis and urine culture. Let me know when any lab results are back."

E: "That is being done."

C: "When I examine the child, are her mucous membranes dry?"

E: "Yes, they appear dry."

C: "Is she breathing quite deeply and rapidly."

E: "Yes."

C: "Are the patient's TMs clear, nares clear, and is her oropharynx without signs of infection such as erythema or exudates?"

E: "Yes."

C: "Does the patient's breath smell fruity?"

D: "Yes, it does slightly."

C: "Are the patient's lungs clear to auscultation? Is her heart rhythm regular, with no murmurs, rubs, or gallops?"

E: "Yes."

C: "Nina, can you point to where your tummy hurts?"

E: "Nina, still sleepy, takes her hand and rubs it all around her abdominal area."

C: "Nina, I know it hurts all over, but can you show me one spot where it hurts the worst?"

E: "Nina takes her finger and again rubs it all over her abdominal area."

C: "Are her bowel sounds normal?"

E: "Yes, they are normal."

C: "When I palpate her abdomen is there apparent tenderness? If so, is there any one spot that seems to be more tender than the rest?"

E: "Nina moans slightly with the abdominal examination, but there is no point of maximal tenderness. The entire abdomen exhibits mild tenderness."

C: "Is there any guarding, rebound, or rigidity?"

E: "No."

C: "With the child fully undressed, is there any rash?"

E: "No."

C: "What is the child's skin turgor, and pulses?"

E: "The skin turgor is poor with significant tenting of her skin, and her pulses are thready and weak."

C: "What is the patient's capillary refill time?"

E: "About 3 seconds."

C: "Does the child wake up to the sound of my voice? Does she follow commands? Is her motor examination non-focal?"

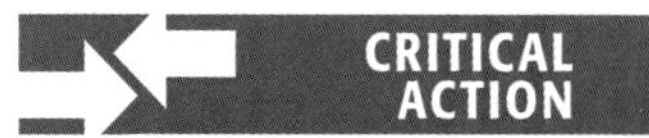

Recognizing DKA is a critical action in this case.

E: "Yes."

C: "Are the child's pupils reactive, extraocular movements intact, skin sensation intact, facial muscle activity intact, hearing intact, soft palate rise intact, tongue symmetric when it is stuck out, and ability to turn the head and shrug the shoulder symmetric and strong?"

E: "Yes, the child's cranial nerves are intact."

C: "Nurse, are the stat sugar and urine dip done yet?"

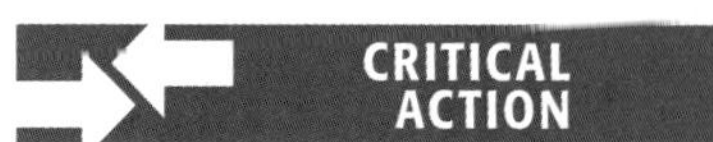

Initiation of insulin therapy is a critical action in this case.

E: "Yes, doctor, but the machine was unable to read a value. It just said 'critical high.' The urine dip shows large ketones and large glucose."

C: "Ms. Santiago, Nina's blood sugar is very high. It appears that Nina has developed diabetes. This happens when an organ called the pancreas stops

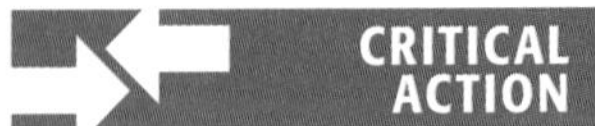

Admission to the appropriate level of care is always a critical action.

making insulin, which is necessary for the body to properly process sugars that it needs for energy. When the body doesn't have enough insulin, it runs out of sugars to use for energy and starts to feed on itself. When this occurs, patients develop changes like increased urination. That causes severe dehydration, which is why Nina has been so thirsty lately. We are going to watch Nina very closely in the hospital for the next several days while we replace the fluids she has lost. We also need to start giving her insulin through an IV so that Nina can begin to process sugars normally again and stop the body from breaking itself down. Do you have any questions?"

E: "No, that makes sense. Just help my daughter get better."

E: "The ABG comes back with the following information: pH 7.08, Pco_2 10, Po_2 110, HCO 6, base deficit 8."

C: "Ms. Santiago, how much does Nina usually weigh?"

E: "She weighed about 23 kg just 3 weeks ago."

E: "The nurse reports the first bolus is complete. The repeat vital signs are T 37.1°C (98.8°F), HR 125, RR 40, BP 110/65, O_2 sat 99% on RA."

C: "Thank you. Nurse, please change the fluid rate to 10 cc/kg/hr of NS and use this rate until Nina is hemodynamically stable. Please start a second IV for an insulin drip and start the drip at 0.1 unit/kg/h. Blood sugars should be rechecked every hour and a new BMP with magnesium and phosphate sent every 2 hours. Please let me know when the next bolus is finished, and please recheck vital signs at that time."

E: "The nurse goes to carry out the orders."

C: "I also need an ICU bed and to speak with the patient's primary doctor. Also, I would like to check a non-contrast head CT because of the patient's lethargy."

E: "This CT scan is ordered and Dr. Kinderdoc is on page."

E: "The labs have returned. The CBC shows WBC 20.5, Hct 18.0, Hgb 54.0, Plt 322. BMP: Na 118, K 5.0, Cl 91, CO_2 7, BUN 25, Cr 0.6, Glu 800. Beta-hydroxybutyrate present at 1:64, acetone present at 1:16. The UA shows large ketones, large glucose, large nitrites, and large leuk esterase with WBC 15-20/HPF, no squamous cells, and large bacteria."

E: "The nurse has returned and repeat vitals show T 98.6°F, HR 110, RR 30, BP 120/60, O_2 sat 99% on RA."

C: "When I re-examine the child, how are the cap refill, skin turgor, and pulse?"

E: "The skin turgor has improved, the pulse slower, and the cap refill is at 2 seconds."

C: Nurse, please change the rate of NS to 1.5 times the maintenance rate and add 20 mEq of potassium chloride to the NS (to replace the potassium deficit known to occur with DKA, even though Nina has an initially normal potassium level). When her serum glucose is below 300, we will change from NS to D5NS. Please accompany the monitored patient to the CT scanner when they are ready for her. Also, please give the patient 500 mg of ceftriaxone IV to treat her UTI."

E: "The nurse goes to do those things and the patient's primary doctor is on the phone."

C: "Hello Dr. Kinderdoc. Your patient, Nina Santiago, is here with us in the ED. She presented in DKA with an initial pH of 7.05, a serum glucose of 800, and an anion gap of 20. She was initially very dehydrated, with a fluid deficit of around 3 L, and is now on an insulin drip and receiving IV fluids to fix her fluid deficit without putting her at risk for developing cerebral edema. She is somewhat lethargic, but is responsive to voice, follows commands and had no focal findings on her initial examination. However, given concern for cerebral edema, I ordered a head CT, and she is there right now. Also, she has a UTI that may have contributed to this initial presentation of her diabetes by DKA, and I have started IV antibiotic treatment. I would like to admit her to the PICU and have an endocrinologist see her."

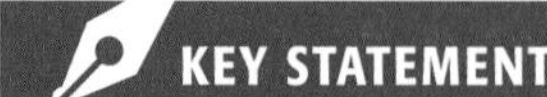

Remember to address the patient and the family, explain procedures and lab results to them, and update them on the plan as it changes.

E: "Well, that is quite a surprise as she is such a healthy little girl. I agree with your plan and will speak with an endocrinologist."

C: "Very good. I will notify you if there is anything abnormal on the CT scan."

E: "The primary doctor thanks you and hangs up. The child returns from her CT scan with a stat reading that says the study is normal, and that there is no radiographic evidence of swelling."

C: "Ms. Santiago, I just spoke with Dr. Kinderdoc and explained my concerns for Diabetic Ketoacidosis. The CT scan of the head is unremarkable, but the lab work confirms that this is an initial presentation of diabetes for Nina. Because she was very dehydrated and sleepy, we are going to watch her overnight in the Intensive Care Unit where Dr. Kinderdoc and an endocrinologist will follow her progress. Nurse, you may escort the patient upstairs on a monitor."

E: "Ms. Santiago thanks you and the case is over."

CASE ASSESSMENT

The candidate did an excellent job managing a common presentation of diabetic ketoacidosis (DKA). This diagnosis is often delayed in a patient with no prior history of diabetes. In this case, the candidate was careful to keep a broad differential diagnosis for abdominal pain, and remembered nonsurgical causes. By doing this, she was able to pick up on clues provided in the history including the polydipsia and polyuria. The candidate performed a directed physical examination that included attention to the patient's neurologic status, out of concern for cerebral edema which is the most common cause of death in pediatric patients with DKA.

The candidate was quick to initiate basic monitoring and fluid therapy to a child who was obviously in distress. The candidate must be able to gather a history, directed physical, and initiate fundamental therapies in a parallel and timely fashion. This candidate did all of these in an organized and efficient manner. With all patients, steps taken to direct initial stabilization are often "critical actions."

The candidate made sure to constantly reassess the patient after interventions were performed. She also did well to shift some of the management responsibility back to the examiner by using the "nurse" figure. By doing this, she was alerted when the initial fluid resuscitation was completed and then she began to correct fluid and electrolyte deficits with a balanced plan to hydrate the patient without increasing the risk of cerebral edema. Also, the candidate looked for underlying processes that may have precipitated the DKA episode. In this case it was a urinary tract infection (UTI) that was recognized and properly treated.

The candidate also did well with aspects of the case outside of just getting the diagnosis and treatment decisions correct. She continued to keep the family informed of the progression of the case and was very professional in her dealings with staff, family, and consulting doctors.

Critical Actions

1. Early recognition of dehydration and appropriate fluid therapy to resuscitate the patient.
2. Diagnosis of DKA.
3. Initiation of appropriate insulin therapy for DKA treatment.
4. Admission to the pediatric intensive care unit (PICU) for continuing treatment of severe acidosis, anion gap, and depressed neurological status.

Test Performance

1. *Data acquisition:* The data acquisition phase is superb as the candidate shows ability to obtain a comprehensive history and physical examination and order appropriate tests to assist in diagnosis. Score = **8**
2. *Problem solving:* Problem solving is excellent as the candidate is able to quickly assimilate data from the patient history and physical, interpret test results, and synthesize information to efficiently direct further management. Score = **8**
3. *Patient management:* The examinee recognizes when interventions needed to be made and adjusts fluid administration appropriately when she receives her first set of lab results. She obtains an appropriate consult and requests another (endocrinology), and admits the patient appropriately to the ICU. Score = **8**
4. *Resource utilization:* The candidate obtained the appropriate labs for a DKA workup. She proceeded in a manner that was logical, cost-sensitive, and showed patient concern. Score = **8**
5. *Health care provided (outcome):* The patient received efficient, appropriate treatment, and the candidate's interventions continued to evolve according to the patient's response to interventions. Score = **8**
6. *Interpersonal relations and communication skills:* The candidate demonstrates appropriate professionalism as all actions were performed in a manner that conveys respect, compassion, and integrity. The physician is solicitous of and responsive to the patient's needs and appropriate with ED staff and her consultant. Score = **8**
7. *Comprehension of pathophysiology:* This candidate demonstrated a detailed knowledge of the pathology of DKA, the appropriate treatment, looked for a potential infectious cause, and was wary of cerebral edema. Score = **8**
8. *Clinical competence (overall):* Overall, the examinee showed clinical competence by maintaining a broad differential diagnosis, asking questions to elicit DKA history, starting appropriate management and then changing that management as lab study results evolved. She explained why she was utilizing the treatments she chose in conversation with Nina's mother, nursing staff, and the admitting physician. Score = **8**

CASE 27 7 y/o Male With Asthma

John Dayton and Alan Kumar

INITIAL INFORMATION

Name: Louis Sobber

Mode of arrival: Brought by mother

Age: 7 years

Gender: Male

VS: T 37.2°C (98.96°F), BP 105/60, HR 125, RR 44, O_2 sat: 80% on RA, wt: 40 kg

PLAY OF THE CASE

C: "What do I see as I walk into the patient's room?"

E: "You see an obese young child sitting upright on the stretcher working very hard to breathe. You can hear audible wheezes."

C: "Have the nurse place the child on a cardiac monitor and pulse oximeter. Please place the child on 100% non-rebreather face mask."

KEY QUESTION

Ask this open-ended question at the beginning of every case.

C: "Have the child's oxygen saturations improved?"

E: "The child has been placed on a cardiac monitor, and the pulse-oximeter is reading 92%."

C: "I would like to talk to the mother."

C: "Hi Ms. Sobber, I am Dr. Breeze. What is going on with little Louis?"

KEY ORDERS

Every unstable patient requires IV access, oxygen, and cardiac monitoring.

E: "You have to help him doc! He has a history of asthma but this is the worst I've ever seen him."

C: "I will definitely help him. I would like to turn my attention to the patient and assess his ABCs and mental status. 'Hi, Louis. Are you having difficulty breathing?'"

E: "The child nods yes."

C: "What happened today?"

KEY QUESTION

When you ask about exam findings, and you are told that portion of the exam is unremarkable, no further questions involving that portion of the exam are needed.

However, if you are asked what you are looking for, this often signifies that there are abnormal exam findings that need to be discovered through further questions.

E: "The child is only able to talk in one-word sentences and turns to mom for help."

C: "Before I continue my interview with mom, I would like to quickly examine the child."

C: "I would like to get a general sense as to his breathing pattern and accessory muscle use."

E: "He is taking shallow breaths at 44-48 times a minute with audible wheezing and accessory muscle use. He appears to be working very hard."

C: "Are there any abnormalities in the oropharynx? Foreign bodies, exudative tonsillitis, swollen tongue/lips, etc.?"

E: "The oropharynx is normal."

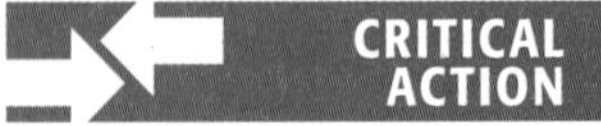

There are two critical actions here. First, the candidate has to begin continuous albuterol nebulizer treatments. Second, they should give a dose of steroids.

C: "Are the neck veins distended? Is the neck supple?"

E: "Normal neck examination."

C: "What do I hear on heart and lung examination?"

E: "What would you like to know?"

C: "Are the breath sounds symmetric? Is there good airway entry? Are there wheezes, crackles, or rubs? Are there murmurs or gallops? Can I hear heart sounds?"

E: "The breath sounds are distant, but symmetric. There is aeration and inspiratory and expiratory wheezes are noted on auscultation. Heart examination is notable for tachycardia with a normal rhythm."

C: "Please have the nurse start a continuous nebulized treatment of albuterol and Atrovent. Also, have her start a 22-gauge IV in the child's arm and draw off blood work for later tests. I would also like to obtain a stat portable CXR. Please give the child a 500-cc NS fluid bolus. Also administer Solu-Medrol 125 mg IV after I verify medication allergies."

C: "Ma'am, is Louis allergic to any medications?"

E: "No."

C: "In that case, please give the Solu-Medrol. I would like to continue my conversation with the mother while all these orders are being carried out. What has been going on today?"

E: "He's had a cold for the last couple days. He's had a cough and runny nose and seemed to be worse at night, so I have been using the inhaler. However, he got so much worse today."

C: "Has he had any fevers?"

E: "No, but he was hanging around his older sister and her friends today. They smoke, and I wonder if that made him worse."

C: "Possibly. Has he been coughing up any sputum?"

E: "No."

C: "What are his current medications? Has his inhaler use increased recently?"

E: "He only uses a rescue inhaler. Usually, he needs this a few times a week, but he has used it more frequently for the last few days."

C: "Has he ever had to take steroids for his asthma?"

E: "All the time. At least 2-3 times a year."

C: "Any inhaled steroids?"

E: "His doctor wanted him to take them but we can't afford those."

C: "Has he ever been admitted to the hospital for his asthma?"

E: "A couple times, but he has never been this bad."

C: "Was he ever admitted to the ICU? Did he ever needed a breathing tube put down his throat to help him breath?"

E: "Heavens, no!"

C: "Well, Ma'am, Louis looks pretty ill right now but we are going to do everything we can to make him better."

E: "Thank you so much, doctor."

C: "How is the patient doing now after the nebs and steroids?"

E: "Repeat vital signs are HR 140, BP 105/60, RR 40, O_2 sat 94%."

C: "How does he look? What are his breath sounds?"

E: "He is still using accessory muscles and taking rapid breaths. Lung sounds are slightly more audible on examination and he continues to have inspiratory and expiratory wheezing."

C: "Is he still alert and responding to questions?"

E: "He is still awake. He is responding with one word at a time."

C: "Have the nurse give 0.3 mg epinephrine SQ, 50 mg/kg of $MgSO_4$ over 20 minutes, and continue the albuterol neb."

E: "Epi is given and $MgSO_4$ is started."

C: "How is the child doing now?"

E: "The breathing seems to be slightly slower and not as labored."

C: "Do we have the CXR yet?"

E: "The CXR shows no infiltrates or pneumothorax."

C: "What are the vital signs now?"

E: "HR 140, BP 125/80, RR 36-40, O_2 sat 92%-94%."

C: "Place him in for a pediatric ICU bed and call his pediatrician."

C: "How does he appear now?"

E: "There continues to be incremental improvement."

E: "Dr. Kidd is on the phone."

C: "Hello, Dr. Kidd. This is Dr. Breeze at ABEM General Hospital. I have Louis Sobber, a 7-year-old patient of yours with a history of asthma, who presents today with a severe asthma exacerbation. His mom states he has been fighting a cold the last couple days and may have been exposed to cigarette smoke. He arrived in extremis with labored breathing and low O_2 sat. After oxygen and nebs, he improved slightly, so I gave epinephrine and $MgSO_4$. At this time, he seems to be doing slightly better, but he still needs to go to the ICU for intensive monitoring."

E: "Sounds good. Does he have a fever?"

C: "No fever, and his CXR was unremarkable."

E: "Did you give steroids?"

C: "Sorry, I forgot to mention that. Yes, I did."

E: "Sounds good. Send him upstairs."

E: "The case is now over."

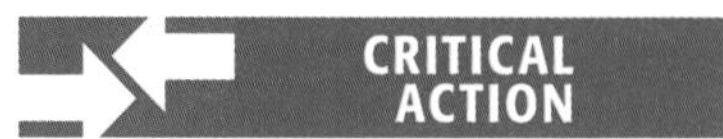

Treating with epinephrine is a critical action in this case.

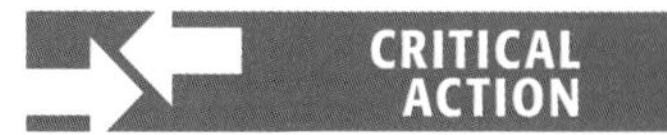

Admission to the appropriate level of care is a critical action in this case.

CASE ASSESSMENT

Overall, the candidate managed the case very well. He quickly recognized the severity of the patient's condition and began to manage his airway, breathing, and circulation (ABCs). When applying oxygen didn't provide sufficient relief, he used more aggressive therapy for dyspnea and proceeded to obtain more history. By doing this, he was able to form a differential diagnosis that he tested with questions, treatment, and a chest x-ray (CXR).

Based on additional history, the candidate focused on treating status asthmaticus, and his interventions were successful. Intubating the patient was an option, but the candidate was able to proceed without intubation. If intubation had been expected for this patient, the clinical picture would have worsened making the decision easy for the candidate.

The candidate managed this case well. As you are reviewing the case, do not worry if you would not have managed the case as efficiently. Remember the test requires each candidate to meet or exceed a national standard of care. Examinees do not need to provide perfect care.

Critical Actions

1. Administration of a continuous albuterol/Atrovent nebulizer
2. Steroid administration
3. Subcutaneous (SubQ) epinephrine
4. Admission to intensive care unit (ICU)

Test Performance

1. *Data acquisition:* The candidate obtained all of the information required to make the correct diagnosis. He did this in an orderly and organized fashion. Score = **8**
2. *Problem solving:* The candidate did a wonderful job of using vital signs and exam findings to create a differential diagnosis. He tested out that differential diagnosis through further questions and interventions, and each intervention further stabilizes the patient. Score = **8**
3. *Patient management:* The examinee recognized immediately that the patient needed oxygen. After recognizing and treating the asthma exacerbation, he obtained the appropriate consult for the appropriate disposition. Score = **8**
4. *Resource utilization:* The candidate used appropriate imaging and treatments and obtained information from the patient's mother. The workup was logical, cost-sensitive, and showed patient concern. Score = **8**
5. *Health care provided (outcome):* The patient received efficient, appropriate treatment, and the candidate's interventions stabilized the patient. Score = **8**
6. *Interpersonal relations and communication skills:* The candidate communicated appropriately with the patient's mother, the nursing staff, and the admitting physician. He gave a succinct history of the patient's disease, emergency department (ED) care, and answered questions appropriately. His only minor errors were forgetting to discuss the absence of a fever and initially omitting the use of steroids. Score = **7**
7. *Comprehension of pathophysiology:* The examinee conveyed his understanding of status asthmaticus by the choice of medication. He was able to check for other options on his differential diagnosis through history questions and a CXR. Score = **8**
8. *Clinical competence (overall):* This candidate demonstrated an efficient approach to dyspnea, was able to focus his differential toward asthma, used appropriate medication, and chose the appropriate disposition. Score = **8**

CASE 28 A 22 y/o Female With Abdominal Pain

John Dayton and Flora Waples

INITIAL INFORMATION

Name: Sally Smith

Mode of arrival: Brought in by friend

Age: 22 years

Gender: Female

VS: T 37.1°C (98.78°F), BP 90/50, HR 132, RR 20, O_2 sat: 95% on RA

CC: Abdominal pain

PLAY OF THE CASE

C: "What do I see when I walk in the room?"

E: "The patient is lying on the gurney moaning. She appears to be in moderate distress."

C: "Hello, I am Dr. Emergency. Before I start our examination, I would like to ask your nurse to do a few things. Nurse, can you please start two large-bore IVs in both the right and left antecubital fossa. Please bolus 1 L of 0.9 NS, place the patient on 2 L of oxygen via NC, and begin cardiac monitoring. After the bolus, please repeat her vital signs and let me know what they are. Thank you, nurse. Ms. Smith, what brings you in today?"

E: "Doctor, please help me. My belly hurts so much!"

C: "I'm here to help you, but I need to ask you a few questions before I will know the best way to treat your pain. Can you point to where your pain is the worst?"

E: "Patient points to her right lower quadrant."

C: "How long have you been having this pain?"

E: "I've been having mild pain for a few days, but it suddenly got worse an hour before I arrived."

C: "Have you been having fevers or chills?"

E: "No."

C: "Nausea and vomiting?"

E: "I have been nauseated for 2 days, and I started throwing up today."

C: "Diarrhea?"

E: "No, I have not gone to the bathroom for 2 or 3 days."

C: "Are you sexually active?"

E: "What does that have to do with anything? I am in pain doctor! Why can't you help me!"

C: "I am sorry, but this is an important question for female patients because there are very serious medical conditions that are caused by pregnancy and STDs. In order to help you, I need to know about these risk factors."

KEY QUESTION

Ask this open-ended question at the beginning of every case.

KEY ORDERS

Most of the patients you see during the exam will be unstable (or will become that way). This patient is hypotensive and tachycardic and requires IV access, oxygen, and cardiac monitoring. Notice how the examinee asked the examiner to reassess and report the patient's vital signs after the fluid bolus.

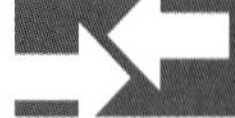

CRITICAL ACTION

Initiating early fluid resuscitation on this unstable patient is a critical action in this case. It is also critical to continue the resuscitation until the vitals normalize or the patient is admitted for more definitive care.

DON'T FORGET

Always begin by treating any vital sing abnormality. For this case, that means fluids to address the hypotension. Examples of other cases include starting oxygen for patients that are hypoxic and antipyretics for patients who are febrile.

KEY QUESTION

Remember never to give any medication without first asking about allergies.

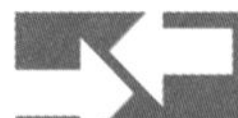

CRITICAL ACTION

Getting a stat pregnancy test is a critical action in this case.

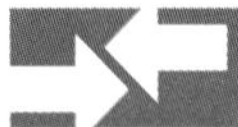

CRITICAL ACTION

Continuing fluid resuscitation is a critical action in this case.

DON'T FORGET

Remember that when the examiner states that an examination area is "normal" that means that you can move on. If they ask, "what are you looking for?" there is a good chance that there is a pertinent finding in that organ system.

E: "Okay, I understand. Yes, I am sexually active."

C: "Any new partners in the last 3 months? Do you use birth control?"

E: "I have had two new partners in the last 3 months. I usually use condoms, but not always."

C: "Have you had any vaginal discharge recently?"

E: "No."

C: "Do you have any history of ovarian cysts?"

E: "Yes."

C: "Have you ever had a cyst that required surgical treatment?"

E: "No"

C: "Okay. Just a couple more questions and then I'll get you some pain medication. Do you have any medical problems?"

E: "No."

C: "Have you ever had any surgeries or stayed overnight in the hospital for any reason?"

E: "No."

C: "Do you take any medications?"

E: "No."

C: "And any allergies to any medications?"

E: "No."

E: "Doctor, the initial bolus is complete, and your latest vital signs are HR 121, BP 98/54, RR 20, sating 98% on NC, T 37.1° C."

C: "Very good. Could you please start a second 1 L bolus of NS and give me another set of vitals when it is complete? After the fluids are hanging, I would like to get a stat urine pregnancy test. I would also like the patient to receive 1 mg of dilaudid IV. I would like to do a quick physical examination now."

C: "Can I get the results of the pregnancy test when it is available?"

E: "The pregnancy dip is negative."

C: "Thank you. HEENT examination?"

E: "Normal."

C: "Is the neck supple? Are there any signs of lymphadenopathy?"

E: "The neck examination is normal."

C: "I would like to examine the heart and lungs. Are the breath sounds clear and symmetric? Are there any murmurs, rubs, or gallops on the cardiac examination?"

E: "The lung examination is normal, the patient is tachycardic, and there are no murmurs, rubs, or gallops."

C: "Is the abdomen distended, tender to palpation? Are bowel sounds present on auscultation?"

E: "The abdomen is not distended, but bowel sounds are diminished. The abdomen is very tender in the right lower quadrant."

C: "Is there guarding or signs of peritonitis?"

E: "There is some guarding with rebound tenderness in the right lower quadrant."

C: "I would like to perform a pelvic examination."

E: "What are you looking for?"

C: "On bimanual examination is the cervix open or closed? Is there any CMT? Is there any discharge or bleeding? Is there any adnexal tenderness or fullness?"

E: "The cervix is closed and unremarkable. There is no CMT. There is fullness in the right adnexa and the patient is very tender to palpation of that area."

C: "I would like to perform a rectal examination. Is the rectal tone normal? Is there blood in the stool?"

E: "The rectal tone is normal. The stool is brown and guaiac negative."

C: "I would like to examine the extremities. Is the any clubbing, cyanosis, or edema? Are the pulses and pressures equal and symmetric in all extremities?"

E: "There is no cyanosis, clubbing, or edema. Pulses are slightly diminished, but symmetric, in all extremities."

C: "Is the patient neurologically intact? Gait OK?"

E: "The patient has no sensory or motor deficits. When she tries to stand she complains of dizziness and pain in her abdomen on trying to walk."

C: "We will defer gait testing since it is unsafe. Is there any rash or bruising on the skin examination?"

E: "Skin examination is normal."

C: "Is the second bolus of fluids finished? How is my patient's pain now?"

E: "The second liter of fluids is in and her new vitals are HR 113, BP 103/66, RR 18, satting 96% on NC, T 37.5°C. Her pain is now a 5/10."

C: "Based on the pelvic exam, I am not concerned about cervicitis or PID, but I am concerned about an ovarian cyst. Given her RLQ pain with rebound, I am also concerned about appendicitis. With this in mind, I would like to send the following labs: a CBC with diff, BMP, coags, UA, and a type and screen, and please let me know the results as soon as they come back. I would like the patient to be made NPO in case she needs surgical intervention. I would like to order a CT or the abdomen and pelvis. Please start a third liter bolus and re-vital the patient when it is finished."

E: "Those orders are being performed. The patient receives her third liter of fluid and rolls off to CT. By the time she gets back to the ER her labs are back."

CBC: WBC 17.4, Hgb 8.2, Hct 26.3, plt 354

BMP: Na 141, K 4.2, Cl 112, bicarb 25, BUN 31, Cr 1.1

Coags: nl

T & S: B+

UA: + leuks, otherwise normal

C: "What are her vital signs now? How is her pain?"

E: "After 3 L of fluid her HR is 115. Her BP is 96/62 and she is requiring 2 L of oxygen via NC to keep her sats in the 90's. Her pain is a 4/10. The CT has been read, and it shows a hemorrhagic ovarian cyst in her right adnexa."

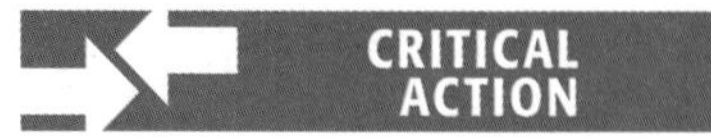

CRITICAL ACTION

Performing a pelvic examination is a critical action.

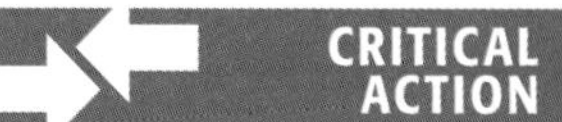

CRITICAL ACTION

Getting the appropriate imaging of the abdomen and pelvis is a critical action in this case. An US or a CT would both be accepted.

KEY ORDERS

Whenever you suspect that a patient may have a surgical emergency, always remember to make them NPO and request coags and run a T & S.

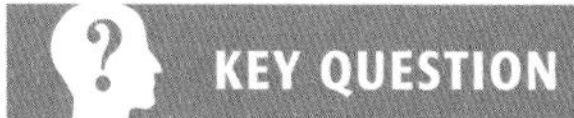

KEY QUESTION

Remember to reassess the vital signs of all unstable patients frequently.

CRITICAL ACTION

Admitting this patient to the OB service is a critical action.

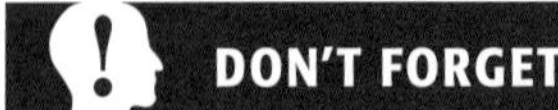

DON'T FORGET

The examiner may use the consultants or the nurse to question you about your management of the patient. This does not mean that you are wrong as there are often several ways to manage different pathology. Use this opportunity to explain your rationale and show your understanding of the disease process.

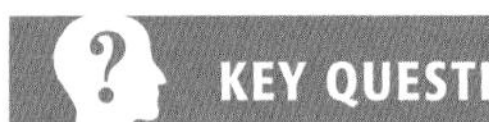

KEY QUESTION

Remember to talk to your patient. You get points for answering questions and keeping them updated about their condition.

C: "Is the appendix visualized on the scan?"

E: "Yes, it is normal. The OB on call is on the phone now."

C: "Hello, this is Dr. Emergency. I have a 22-year-old female down here with a hemorrhagic ovarian cyst and concern for active bleeding. On arrival, she was hypotensive with a blood pressure of 90s/50s, tachycardic to the 130s, and sats in the mid-90's. On physical examination, she had severe tenderness in the right lower quadrant with rebound and guarding. Her pelvic examination was positive for fullness and pain in the right adnexa. Given RLQ pain, I ordered a CT which showed the hemorrhagic cyst and a normal appendix. Despite 3 L of NS, her systolic BP is still below 100 and she continues to be tachycardic. I will order PRBCs, and I'm concerned she needs operative management. Can you come to the ED to evaluate her for surgery?"

E: "Thank you Dr. Emergency, I would be glad to take care of this patient. Why did you get a CT scan instead of an US?"

C: "While I know that US is the most recommended test for evaluation of the adnexa, I also needed to check for appendicitis. A CT allowed me to check for causes of both abdominal and pelvic pain simultaneously."

E: "Sounds good. I will come to the ED."

C: "Thank you. I would like to talk to the patient now. Ms. Smith, I have the results of your tests now. You have a hemorrhagic cyst and I am concerned that you will need to go to the OR. I have called the OB surgeons to come evaluate you. Do you have any questions for me?"

E: "No, thank you doctor. This case is now over."

CASE ASSESSMENT

While most hemorrhagic ovarian cysts resolve spontaneously, some continue to bleed and require surgical management. Because right lower quadrant (RLQ) pain can be caused by appendicitis, ectopic pregnancy, and ovarian cyst rupture, the decision about which imaging modality to obtain first is sometimes difficult.

The candidate chose to use computed tomography (CT) instead of ultrasound (US), and was able to defend that choice with a rational argument. Make sure that you find a way to explain your choices and rationale to the examiner. You can do this under the guise of talking to a consultant (as in this case), a nurse, or even the patient. You can also simply state your reasoning: "I am going to order a CT on this patient. Although US is the imaging modality of choice to evaluate the pelvic structures, a CT will also help me rule out abdominal pathology, like appendicitis."

The candidate handled the case extremely well. The candidate was aggressive with the fluid resuscitation and was always very professional and thoughtful of the patient and staff. The candidate used volume resuscitation, anticipated the need for a transfusion, and ordered laboratory tests that were needed to establish priorities in managing the patient.

The candidate performed all of the critical actions of this case and would have passed the case easily. The candidate picked also picked up "easy" points for professionalism and interpersonal skills by answering the patient's question, keeping her informed of her test results and the plan for care. The candidate was also sensitive to the patient's pain, which is often a critical action. Always go for these points on the exam and in real life.

Critical Actions

1. Appropriate and continuing volume resuscitation for this unstable patient
2. Getting a stat pregnancy test
3. Doing a thorough pelvic examination
4. Obtaining appropriate imaging of the pelvis
5. Recognizing this patient required surgery
6. Admitting the patient to OB for definitive management

Test Performance

1. *Data acquisition:* The candidate was concise and organized, and obtained all of the information required to make the correct diagnosis. Score = **8**
2. *Problem solving:* The examinee used vital signs, appropriate exam questions, lab work, and a CT to arrive at the diagnosis. He used aggressive fluid resuscitation to address hypotension, anticipated future need for transfusion by obtaining a Type and Screen. Lab studies could have been ordered earlier, and it would have been reasonable to order a Type and Cross after the patient continued to be hypotensive after a 2 L normal saline (NS) bolus. Score = **6**
3. *Patient management:* The examinee recognized when interventions needed to be made and obtained appropriate consults to create a safe disposition. An US could have been ordered and yielded a quicker diagnosis, but good rationale was used in explaining why a CT was ordered instead. Score = **7**
4. *Resource utilization:* The candidate ordered appropriate lab studies and imaging. The workup was logical, cost-sensitive, and showed patient concern. Score = 7
5. *Health care provided (outcome):* The patient received efficient, appropriate treatment, and the candidate's interventions stabilized the patient. All critical actions were met. Score = **8**
6. *Interpersonal relations and communication skills:* The candidate was respectful and effective in communications to staff, the patient, and the OB consultant. He did not ask permission or explain the pelvic and rectal examinations. Score = **7**
7. *Comprehension of pathophysiology:* The examinee conveyed their understanding of the differential diagnosis for RLQ/suprapubic pain, and used their conversation with the OB to further demonstrate their understanding of the associated diagnostic imaging. Score = **8**
8. *Clinical competence (overall):* Overall, the examinee showed clinical competence by obtaining an appropriate history and physical, developing a differential diagnosis, utilizing appropriate lab work and imaging, and arrived at the appropriate disposition. Score = **7**

CASE 29 A 68 y/o Male With Shortness of Breath

John Dayton and Joseph Peabody

INITIAL INFORMATION

Name: Ed Deema

Age: 68 years

Gender: Male

Mode of arrival: Ambulance

VS: BP 92/40, HR 100, RR 30, O_2 sat: 90% on RA

CC: Shortness of breath

PLAY OF THE CASE

KEY QUESTION

Ask this open-ended question at the beginning of every case.

C: "What do I see as I walk into the patient's room?"

E: "You see an overweight male in his 60s who is diaphoretic, breathing heavily, and leaning forward."

KEY ORDERS

Most of the patients you see during the exam will be unstable (or will become that way). Every unstable patient requires IV access (preferably two large-bore IVs), oxygen, and cardiac monitoring (and in most cases an ECG). In this case, as the patient is severely short of breath, getting a stat portable CXR is also appropriate at this time.

C: "Nurse, please place the patient on the monitor and show me a rhythm strip, let's start O_2 via NRB mask, place an 18-gauge IV and hang 0.9 NS at TKO rate (20 cc/h), and draw blood for labs. Nurse, please also obtain a temperature on the patient. Also order a stat bedside ECG and CXR."

E: "Your orders are being done. The nurse could only get a 22-gauge IV. Temp is 37°C. Rhythm strip shows NSR at 100."

C: "I would like to interview the patient. Hello Mr. Deema, I'm Dr. Koole, what brings you in to the ED today?"

E: "Doc....short.....of......breath................bad....."

C: "Nurse, call respiratory, let's start BiPAP mask ventilation at 10/5."

E: "BiPAP started."

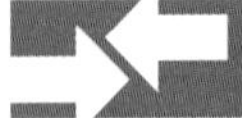

CRITICAL ACTION

Giving this patient appropriate ventilatory support is a critical action in this case.

C: "Is there any family here with the patient?"

E: "Yes, his wife just arrived at the bedside."

C: "Hello Mrs. Deema, I'm Dr. Koole, your husband had very hard time breathing, and we are assisting him with this mask until we can make him better. What has been going on with him?"

E: "He has been short of breath for the past 3 days, he couldn't even walk to the bathroom today. I have never seen him this bad. Help him, doctor."

KEY QUESTION

Remember to speak with family members, EMTs, or bystanders when the patient cannot give a history.

C: "What medical conditions does he suffer from? What medicines does he take?"

E: "He has high BP and congestive heart failure (CHF). He is on so many medicines that I don't remember them all, but I do remember furosemide and carvedilol."

C: "Is he on any inhalers?"

E: "No, only pills."

C: "Does he have any allergies to medications?"

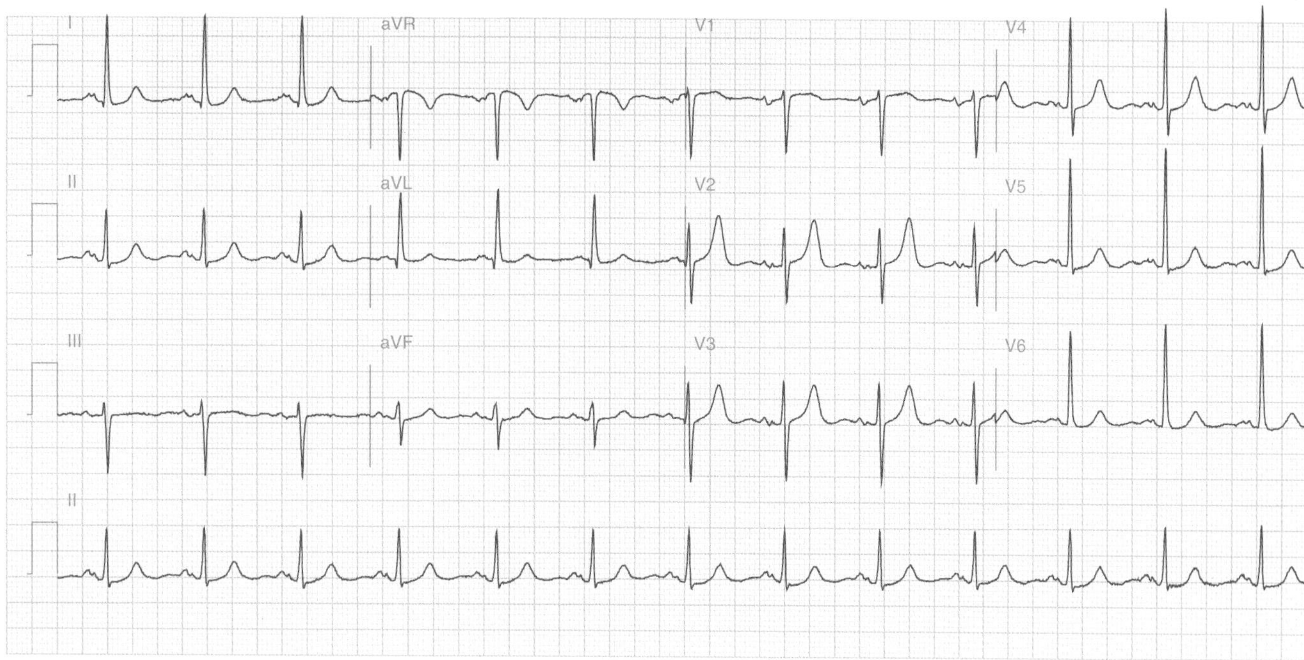

Figure C29-1. ECG (with sinus tachycardia and LVH). (*Reprinted with permission from Fauci AS, Braunwald E, Kasper DL, et al.* Harrison's Principles of Internal Medicine. *17th ed. New York, NY: McGraw-Hill; 2008.*)

E: "No, none. The ECG is available for your review. Please interpret the ECG" (see Fig. C29-1).

C: "The ECG reveals LVH and sinus tach."

E: "Thank you."

C: "I will examine the patient now. Can I get repeat vital signs? How is his breathing now?"

E: "Repeat VS are BP 90/40, HR 100, RR 20, O_2 sat 100%, breathing more comfortably on BiPAP although he is complaining of discomfort around his face due to the mask."

C: "Is there diaphoresis or cyanosis."

E: "Mild diaphoresis persists."

C: "Is there JVD or tracheal deviation?"

E: "JVP is elevated to the angle of the jaw, trachea midline."

C: "Are there any crackles/wheezes in the lung fields or unequal breath sounds?"

E: "Crackles throughout all lung fields."

C: "Are there any heart murmurs, rubs, or gallops? Are pulses equal?"

E: "II/VI systolic murmur at the left sternal border, good heart tones, pulses all symmetric."

C: "Is the abdomen distended or tender? Any pulsatile mass? Any blood in the stool?"

E: "No masses or tenderness, stool is guaiac negative."

C: "Is there any leg edema or tenderness?"

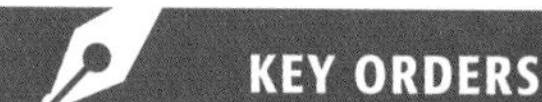

KEY ORDERS

Remember to reevaluate your unstable patients frequently.

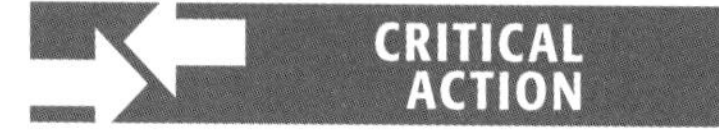

CRITICAL ACTION

Diagnosing CHF and pulmonary edema is a critical action in this case.

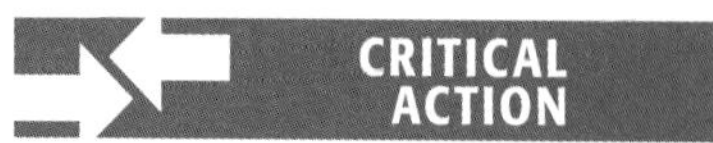

CRITICAL ACTION

There are several critical actions taking place at this point.

- First, the candidate is starting pressors on this patient in cardiogenic shock.
- Second, they are securing appropriate vascular access for this intervention (a central line).
- Finally, they are admitting the patient to the CCU.

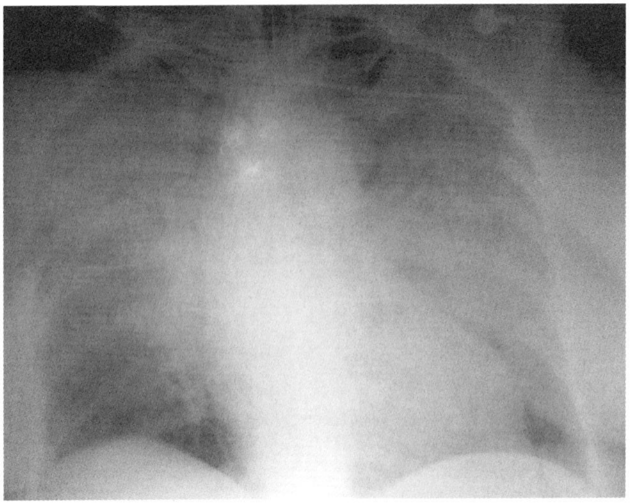

Figure C29-2. CXR. (*Reprinted with permission from Stone CK, Humphries RL.* Current Diagnosis and Treatment: Emergency Medicine. *6th ed. New York, NY: McGraw-Hill; 2008.*)

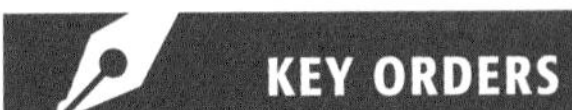

KEY ORDERS

When starting a vasoactive medication, it is a good idea to have the nurse titrate the medication to the desired change in vital signs. This relieves you of the responsibility of monitoring the effects of the medication.

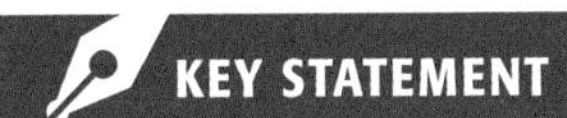

KEY STATEMENT

Remember to tell the patient the plan and the results of your tests.

E: "2+ edema in lower extremities bilaterally."

C: "Neurologic examination intact?"

E: "Grossly normal."

C: "Nurse, please give the patient 40 mg furosemide IVP and 325 mg chewable ASA PO. Send blood for CBC, BMP, PT, PTT, BNP, and troponin."

E: "Done."

C: "Is the CXR completed yet?"

E: "Yes, is has just been done" (see Fig. C29-2).

C: "The patient is in CHF and pulmonary edema. Can I get repeat vitals? Any urine output with the furosemide? How is his breathing?"

E: "BP now 80/38, HR 100, RR 20, minimal urine output (100 cc), breathing more comfortably with BiPAP, tolerating mask better."

C: "I'm glad he feels more comfortable, but I'm worried about his low pressure. Nurse, please start dopamine at 5 μg/kg/min and advance up to 15 μg/kg/min until SBP >100. Please also order an ICU/CCU bed for Mr. Deema and place a call to his cardiologist, Dr. Hart, for me. Also, I would like to place a right IJ central line to run the pressors."

E: "Done."

C: "Mr. Deema, you are in congestive heart failure with fluid in your lungs and your blood pressure is low. I am going to start a medication called dopamine through your IV to allow your heart to pump stronger. I would like to place a large IV into a vein in your neck to administer the medications safely. I will call Dr. Hart and you will need to be admitted to our ICU for close monitoring."

E: "Labs are back, troponin is negative at 0.04, Hgb 14.2, BUN 25, Cr. 1.4 (baseline for patient), BNP 6500."

E: "BP now 100/50 and HR 110 on dopamine 10 μg/kg/min, Dr. Hart is on the phone."

C: "Dr. Hart, this is Dr. Koole at ABEM General. I am taking care of your patient, Mr. Deema, who presented with 3 days of worsening shortness of breath. He presented in severe respiratory distress, his examination and CXR suggest acute pulmonary edema. His BP has been low and dropped to 80/38. I started dopamine and BiPAP. His breathing seems better and I am following his blood pressure. Troponin was negative, BNP is 6500, and renal function appears at baseline. I would like to admit him to the ICU."

E: "Very well. I will see him when he arrives in the ICU. The case is now over."

CASE ASSESSMENT

The candidate managed this complicated case very well. The overall approach of data acquisition and prompt intervention was outstanding. The candidate did an excellent job of quickly identifying a patient in respiratory distress and initiating oxygen and ventilatory assistance. As the patient couldn't speak, she immediately sought out the patient's wife to provide the key history, including meds and allergies. She asked specifically about medications related to shortness of breath, including inhalers. Diagnostic tests were appropriate and ordered in a timely manner. A complete physical examination was performed. When managing an acutely ill patient, it can be easy to forget this!

The medical management was excellent. BiPAP is an appropriate choice of ventilatory assistance for this patient who is awake and alert and has a condition that could be quickly improved. Intubation would have been appropriate if patient obtunded or suffered imminent respiratory arrest. The candidate gave furosemide despite the hypotensive state, but they also recognized the need for IV vasopressor/inotrope therapy and administered dopamine promptly. Dobutamine may be appropriate, but is more likely to lower the patient's blood pressure (BP). Nitrates and vasodilators were appropriately avoided due to the patient's low BP. The candidate also recognized the inadequate IV access for running vasopressors and placed an appropriate central catheter. Drugs were used in the appropriate dosage and route.

The candidate communicated well with the patient and his family and the cardiologist. They frequently reevaluated the patient which is key in a case such as this one. The disposition to cardiac care unit (CCU) was correct. Overall, the candidate showed excellent and efficient management.

Critical Actions

1. Diagnosis of congestive heart failure (CHF)/pulmonary edema
2. Providing immediate ventilatory assistance
3. Providing vasopressor treatment for hypotensive patient with CHF
4. Ensuring adequate IV access for vasopressors
5. Cardiology consult and CCU admission

Test Performance

1. *Data acquisition:* Excellent and efficient history taking and complete examination in this challenging situation. Although the patient was acutely ill, the candidate completed a full examination. Score = **8**
2. *Problem solving:* Again, excellent assimilation of data with very efficient analysis of the clinical picture. Score = **8**

3. *Patient management:* The candidate demonstrated excellent clinical judgment and provided prompt and appropriate treatment. The furosemide administration in this hypotensive patient could be questioned. Score = **6**
4. *Resource utilization:* The candidate checked appropriate labs, obtained a portable chest x-ray (CXR) given patient extremis, and obtained information from both hospital staff and the patient's wife. The workup was logical, cost-sensitive, and showed patient concern. Score = **8**
5. *Health care provided (outcome):* The patient received efficient, appropriate treatment, and the candidate's interventions stabilized the patient. Score = **8**
6. *Interpersonal relations and communication skills:* Excellent engagement and exchange of information with the patient, his wife, and the cardiologist. Candidate could have also spoken with emergency medical technicians (EMTs). Score = **7**
7. *Comprehension of pathophysiology:* The examinee conveyed their understanding of CHF and associated complications through their exam questions and by obtaining only germane lab work and imaging. She illustrated this knowledge by her communication with both the wife and the admitting cardiologist. She did, however, lose points for using furosemide in a hypotensive patient. Score = **6**
8. *Clinical competence (overall):* Overall, the examinee showed clinical competence by addressing immediate airway, breathing, and circulation (ABC) concerns, obtaining an appropriate history and physical, developing a differential diagnosis, utilizing appropriate interventions, and admitting the patient to the intensive care unit (ICU). Score = **7**

CASE 30 28 y/o Female in an MVA

John Dayton and Rohit Gupta

INITIAL INFORMATION

Name: Maya Patel

Age: 28 years

Gender: Female

VS: T 36.2°C (97.2°F), BP 90/60, HR 105, RR 28

CC: Motor vehicle accident

Setting: You are at a level 1 trauma center on a busy evening shift.

PLAY OF THE CASE

Prior to Arrival

E: "You respond to the following EMS call. This is ambulance 20. We are 5 minutes away with a 28-year-old pregnant woman who was the restrained driver of an SUV in a head-on MVA, SUV versus car. The driver of the car is dead on scene. The patient is complaining of difficulty breathing, headache, and abdominal cramping. VS: BP 90/60, HR 105, RR 28, O_2 sat 95% on RA. She says she is 30 weeks pregnant. The patient is boarded and collared. We have started an 18-gauge IV and are running NS."

C: "Are the breath sounds present and equal on examination? Is the patient alert and oriented?"

E: "Breath sounds are decreased on the R. Pt is speaking with us and is alert and oriented. Anything else? We're 5 minutes away."

C: "Place the patient on 100% oxygen by NRB. Also, while retaining in-line stabilization of the spine, please place the patient in the left lateral decubitus position by angling the backboard 30° up on the right. I want to order 2 U of O-negative blood from the blood bank. I need a chest tube tray setup in the trauma room with a 36 FR chest tube. I would like the secretary to notify the trauma surgeon and OB/GYN. I also want an ultrasound machine moved into the trauma room."

KEY QUESTION

Ask this open-ended question at the beginning of every case.

After the Arrival

E: "The patient arrives on a backboard, in a C-spine collar."

C: "As I begin my primary survey, can the nurses begin to obtain vital signs? As I walk into the room, what do I see?"

E: "You see a female patient who appears the stated age on a backboard with a cervical collar in place. She is breathing rapidly and moaning in pain."

C: "I will initiate my primary survey starting with the airway. Ms. Patel, I'm Dr. Jones, the emergency physician on duty this evening. Do you remember what happened?"

E: "I was driving down the street on my way home from work. Suddenly this car going the other way swerved out in front of me and hit me head on. I couldn't get out of my car and I waited until the ambulance arrived. Is the other driver okay?"

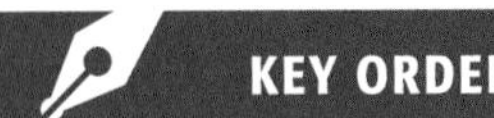

KEY ORDERS

Every trauma patient requires IV access (preferably two large-bore IVs), oxygen, and cardiac monitoring.

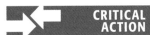

CRITICAL ACTION

Diagnosing and then treating the pneumothorax in this patient are two critical actions.

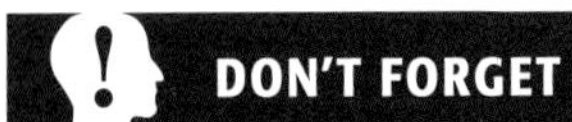

DON'T FORGET

In the course of the exam you may be asked to describe how you will do different invasive procedures like central lines, intubations, etc. This is an excellent description of how to place a chest tube.

C: "Ms. Patel, let's worry about the other driver later. We need to make sure that you and your baby are okay. We're going to do many things starting with getting all your clothes off. Airway is intact. I would like the patient to be completely disrobed. I want the nurse to draw blood for labs and place a second large bore peripheral IV in an antecubital vein, place the patient on the monitor, repeat the vitals, and provide a rhythm strip when available. Keep the patient on 100% oxygen by NRB mask. I want to examine the chest wall and listen for breath sounds."

E: What are you looking for?

C: Are breath sounds equal. Is there any sign of deformity, fracture, or crepitus?

E: "The patient has diminished breath sounds on the right side of her chest. Her chest wall is tender to palpation over the lower lateral ribs and you are able to palpate step-offs in the most tender area. There is no creptitus. The IV is being placed and the patient is now fully disrobed. The vitals are being recorded."

C: "The patient has broken ribs with a pneumothorax on the right. I will need to place a chest tube. Before placing the chest tube I would like to complete my ABCs. I will check carotid, femoral, radial, and dorsalis pedis pulses. Are the vital signs and a rhythm strip available?"

E: "The pulses are 1+ both centrally and peripherally in all extremities. The vitals are: BP 95/65, P 100, RR 26, oxygen at 100%. The monitor shows sinus tachycardia. The second IV has been placed. The thoracostomy tray is ready."

C: "I would like to ask the nurse to infuse a 1 L bolus of NS. Send the blood for a CBC with differential, PT/PTT, basic chemistry profile, and a type and cross for 4 U. Ms. Patel, you have broken ribs and a collapsed lung on the right and that is why you are having pain and difficulty breathing. I need to place a chest tube in order to re-expand your lung. Are you taking any medications and are you allergic to any medications? Do you have any medical problems?"

E: "Patient states that she is not allergic to any medications and that she is only taking prenatal vitamins. What is your technique for the tube thoracostomy?"

C: "I will place the tube in the third or fourth intercostal space in the anterior axillary line, going higher than normal because the patient is pregnant in the third trimester. After prepping the skin, I will anesthetize the skin and deeper tissues with lidocaine. I will make an incision overlying the rib one rib below my targeted interspace. Using forceps I will bluntly dissect the tissue until I reach my targeted interspace and pop through into the pleural space above the adjacent rib. I will insert my finger through the hole, ensure that there are no adhesions, and then place the 36 FR chest tube through the hole directing it superiorly and posteriorly. I will connect it to a pleurovac and secure it in place."

E: "The chest tube is in place. Your examination of the chest after placement indicates improved breath sounds on the right. Repeat VS: BP 100/65, HR 100, RR 20."

C: "I would like to order a stat portable CXR, lateral C-spine, and pelvis. Having secured the ABCs, I will check patient's GCS and check for disability and move to the secondary survey and in particular the abdominal examination. Is the patient able to move her extremities and does she have normal sensation?"

E: "GCS is 15 and the patient moves all extremities to command with normal sensation."

C: "Is there any evidence of head trauma? Are the pupils equal and reactive? Are the TMs intact?"

E: "Her right TM is perforated. Hemotympanum and clear fluid are seen on examination of her right external auditory canal. She states that you are hurting her during this exam. HEENT exam is otherwise unremarkable.

C: "I apologize for the discomfort. Your exam makes me concerned for basilar skull fracture. I would like to order a head CT, and instruct the tech to shield her abdomen during that study. Now, I would like to assess the abdomen and pelvis. Does the abdomen appear distended? Is it bruised? Is it tender to palpation? Are bowel sounds present? Are fetal heart tones audible? Is the pelvis stable on palpation?"

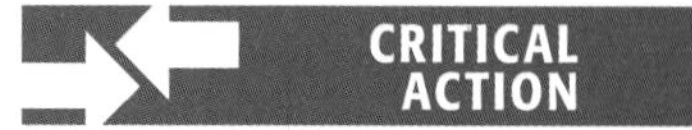

Recognizing signs of basilar skull fracture is a critical action in this case.

E: "The patient has a gravid abdomen. The uterus is palpable midway between the xiphoid and umbilicus. The abdomen is not tender to palpation. Bowel sounds are present. Fetal heart tones are not audible on examination. The patient states that she is having abdominal cramping. The pelvis is stable."

C: "Is there any evidence of vaginal bleeding or bruising on the perineum?"

E: "There is no vaginal bleeding and no bruising on the perineum."

C: "I would like to perform a FAST scan and ultrasound the fetus."

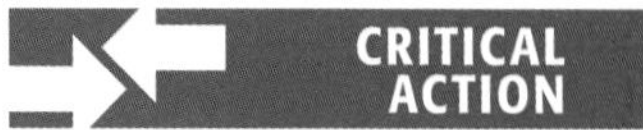

Doing a FAST examination and an US of the fetus is a critical action in this case.

E: "Which views will you include in your FAST?"

C: "The RUQ Morrison pouch, LUQ splenorenal recess, subxiphoid cardiac view, and suprapubic."

E: "The FAST scan is negative in all views. The radiology tech is ready to shoot the trauma series."

C: "I would like to examine the fetus by ultrasound before the x-rays. Is there fetal movement present and what is the fetal heart rate?"

E: "The US reveals an active fetus with a fetal heart rate of 120."

C: "The tech can shoot the trauma series and obtain the head CT. Then I will complete my secondary survey."

E: "The trauma series is performed."

C: "While maintaining cervical spine precautions, I want to logroll the patient with the help of the ED tech and nurses to examine her spine and perform a rectal examination."

E: "After rolling the patient, you discover no further trauma on the back. The rectal examination demonstrates normal tone and no gross blood."

C: "I want to examine the extremities. Are they deformed? Are pulses and sensation normal?"

E: "There is some bruising, but no deformity or sign of fracture. Pulses and sensation are normal."

C: "Are the x-rays and CT results available?"

E: "Your CXR shows a well-placed R-sided chest tube and fractures of the 7th and 8th right ribs. Your lateral C-spine and pelvis are normal. The head CT shows a basilar skull fracture involving her right-sided temporal bone. The trauma surgeon has arrived and would like to speak to you."

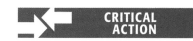

Consulting both trauma surgery and OB is a critical action in this case.

C: "We have a 28-year-old female who is 30 weeks pregnant and who was involved in a head-on MVA with a fatality in the field. The patient is mildly hypotensive and tachycardia, but her vital signs were normal for a third trimester pregnancy. Airway is intact. Breath sounds were decreased on the R and a

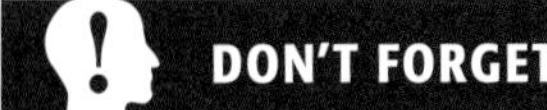

Remember that on exam day your consultants will often "push back" to test your knowledge of management of the patient's condition.

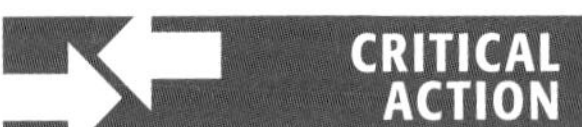

Making sure that OB sees this patient immediately is a critical action in this case.

32 FR chest tube was placed. CXR shows good position with re-expansion of the lung and right 7th and 8th rib fractures. She has a right-sided basilar skull fracture, associated hemotympanum, and possible CSF leak. Abdomen is not tender to palpation but the patient is having abdominal cramping. Her FAST is negative for internal bleeding and the US of the fetus shows movement and a normal FHR. Lateral C-spine and pelvis x-rays are normal. I would like to get the patient admitted to the ICU for close fetal monitoring and management of the PTX. The patient is alert and has no neurologic deficits, but I was about to call Neurosurgery because of the basilar skull fracture. Also, given the mechanism of injury, I would like to get an abdominal CT scan to rule out liver and spleen injuries."

E: "The trauma surgeon concurs and says she will speak with Neurosurgery. The OB/GYN is on the phone. After telling her the same story you told the trauma surgeon, the OB/GYN attending states that everything appears to be under control and that she will see the patient in the morning."

C: "Given the extremely high-risk mechanism and the patient's abdominal cramping during the third trimester of pregnancy, I feel strongly that you need to see her tonight. My US is limited and she needs a more definitive scan to rule out placental abruption. Also, she is going to need close cardiotocographic monitoring which is best interpreted by you."

E: "The OB/GYN agrees and will see the patient. The case is now over."

CASE ASSESSMENT

The candidate did an excellent job managing this difficult case. Serious trauma in pregnancy is not frequently encountered and many emergency physicians feel uncomfortable with managing it. The key to managing trauma during pregnancy is to strictly adhere to ATLS guidelines. You should also remember that what is good for the mother is good for the baby. First, assess and stabilize the mother according to ATLS guidelines. Save assessment of the pregnancy for the secondary survey. Involve the appropriate consultants early.

The candidate managed the trauma using strict ATLS protocols and incorporated assessment and evaluation of the pregnant fetus appropriately. The candidate was not distracted by the pregnancy and began by assessing the mother's ABCs. Having discovered a pneumothorax, the candidate managed it definitively before proceeding to the secondary survey. In a hemodynamically stable patient without tension pneumothorax, many physicians would advocate confirming the presence of a pneumothorax on chest x-ray (CXR) before placing a chest tube. Because a pneumothorax is a clinical diagnosis, it should be managed when discovered. The candidate rapidly assessed the ABCs before placing the chest tube. He also directed his team to obtain IV access and obtain blood work during his initial assessment.

The candidate took an appropriate, limited AMPLE history focusing on **A**llergies, **M**edications, **P**ast medical history, **L**ast meal, and **E**vents prior to the trauma. He also explained what he was doing to the candidate before performing any procedures. After completing his initial survey, the candidate called for radiographs and proceeded with the secondary survey. For the secondary survey, he began at the top moved down.

The candidate performed a limited emergency department (ED) ultrasound (US) to confirm that the fetus had a heartbeat and was moving. After completing the secondary survey, the candidate was asked to give report to his consultants who were on scene. His communication was rapid and thorough, detailing important features of the history, physical examination, management, and plan. Of importance, the candidate conveyed his desire to obtain a computed tomography (CT) scan of the head and of the abdomen. Limited CT scanning is generally considered safe in pregnancy, but should only be employed when the potential information is vital and cannot be obtained in other ways. The candidate provided rationale for the decision indicating the desire to check for basilar skull fracture and rule out solid organ injury in a patient with significant trauma. You should limit controversial treatments, as possible. As long as you provide clear evidence of understanding and a rational plan, you will be okay, but why take unnecessary risks?

Thought Battles sign and raccoon eyes are pathognomonic for basilar skull fracture, these findings are not usually seen until a few days after trauma. For this reason, ask about damage and rupture of the tympanic membrane and ask about cerebrospinal fluid (CSF) otorrhea or rhinorrhea if you suspect a basilar skull fracture.

Finally, in interacting with the OB/GYN surgeon, the candidate managed a difficult interaction capably. He was professional, but advocated strongly for the benefit of his patient. He conveyed that he understood the need and method to rule out placental abruption.

Some parts of the case could have been managed better. The candidate ordered many appropriate tests, but did not follow-up on all of the results. In many cases a smoothly flowing case will end before all of the results are back. However, if you order a test, always ask about the results. The candidate could have provided more information to the patient throughout the case. The candidate could also have provided better pain management.

Critical Actions

1. Clinical discovery of pneumothorax.
2. Tube thoracostomy.
3. Focused assessment with sonography for trauma (FAST) examination and US of fetus.
4. OB/GYN consultation with insistence that patient be seen urgently.
5. Identify signs of basilar skull fracture and consult Neurosurgery.

Test Performance

1. *Data acquisition:* The candidate followed advanced trauma life support (ATLS) guidelines and obtained appropriate imaging and lab studies, though he forgot to check the lab results. Score = **6**
2. *Problem solving:* The examinee used pre-arrival questions, asked appropriate examination questions and addressed abnormal findings in a systematic way. Score = **8**
3. *Patient management:* The chest tube was placed appropriately during the initial primary survey and appropriate consults were involved. However, the candidate could have done more patient education. Score = **7**
4. *Resource utilization:* Prior to arrival, the patient had a chest tube kit and an US ready to use. He also ordered appropriate lab work and explained his rationale for CT use. However, he did not use appropriate pain management. Score = **6**

5. *Health care provided (outcome):* The patient received efficient and appropriate treatment. The candidate's interventions stabilized the patient. Score = **8**
6. *Interpersonal relations and communication skills:* The candidate gave the consultants a concise summary of injuries, treatment, and further care needs. He was appropriate when the OB pushed back. However, the candidate could have talked more with the patient and addressed her pain.
7. *Comprehension of pathophysiology:* The candidate conveyed their understanding of pneumothoraces, basilar skull fractures, and trauma during pregnancy by his interventions, orders, and his conversations with consultants. Score = **8**
8. *Clinical competence (overall):* Overall, the examinee showed clinical competence by obtaining an appropriate history and physical, utilizing appropriate interventions, and working toward the appropriate disposition. However, the candidate made only minor errors with communication and forgetting to review lab studies in his stabilized patient. Score = **7**

CASE 31 2 y/o Female With Seizure

John Dayton and Janis Tupesis

INITIAL INFORMATION

Name: Jessica Smith

Mode of arrival: Brought in by parents

Age: 2 years, 5 months

Gender: Female

VS: BP 92/50, P 117, RR 32 T 37.9

CC: Seizure at home

PLAY OF THE CASE

C: "What do I see as I walk into the patient's room?"

E: "You see a female toddler lying in her mother's lap. She appears in no distress and appears sleepy but responds to her mother's gentle rubbing of her back."

C: "Nurse, could you please place the child into a small gown and place her on a monitor and pulse oximeter?"

E: "Her initial pulse oximetry reading is 98% and the pulse rate is 117."

C: "At the same time, could you please place the child on supplemental oxygen to keep her O_2 saturations above 95%, place an IV with 0.9 NS at a TKO rate and draw blood for lab tests and blood cultures."

E: "All of those tests are being done. The patient is now lying on the bed in a gown. She is sleeping and the monitor shows a normal sinus rhythm with a rate of 117."

C: "Hello Mrs. Smith. I'm Dr. Fitz, I am pleased to meet you. I am one of the emergency physicians and will be taking care of your little girl while she is in the ED. What brought you in today?"

E: "Well, I'm not really sure. Jessica was sitting on the couch playing with her doll when she started acting funny. She was playing and then she just stared off into space and her face started twitching. Then she fell back on the couch and started shaking all over. It was really scary."

C: "I'm sure it was, Mrs. Smith. I'd like to ask you some more questions to try to figure out a little more of what happened. What happened after Jessica fell back on the couch?"

E: "Well, she shook for a few minutes and was really stiff. She has some spit coming from her mouth and she wet her pants."

C: "How long did this whole episode last?"

E: "A couple of minutes. When it stopped Jessica started snoring and was really tired. I called her pediatrician Dr. Jones and she told me to come here right away."

KEY QUESTION

Ask this open-ended question at the beginning of every case.

KEY ORDERS

If you are not given all the vitals, the ones that are missing are usually important. Remember to ask for them.

KEY ORDERS

Every potentially unstable patient requires IV access, oxygen, and cardiac monitoring.

C: "I'm glad you did, Ma'am. Let me ask you some more questions. Has this ever happened to Jessica before?"

E: "No. This is the first time."

C: "Do you remember what Jessica was doing right before this episode happened?"

E: "She was just sitting on the couch playing."

C: "Has she been sick or had a fever lately?"

E: "She has been acting tired and sleeping a bit more than usual."

C: "Is Jessica on any medications?"

E: "No. She is really a healthy little girl."

C: "She has no other medical problems?"

E: "No, none."

C: "Has she had normal visits to her pediatrician?"

E: "Yes. Dr. Jones says that she is normal for her height and weight."

C: "Are there any prescription or over-the-counter medications that are in the house?"

E: "Yes, my husband takes a blood pressure pill, but the medications are in our medicine cabinet above the sink in the bedroom."

C: "Are there any over-the-counter medications that she can get to?"

E: "No. They are in the same medicine cabinet."

C: "Did you notice any open bottles of soap or cleaners or anything else when you were at home."

E: "No. All of our cleaners are locked up underneath the sink and in the garage."

C: "Does anybody else in the family have episodes like this?"

E: "I'm not sure. I think that her cousin has something called seizures. Is that what this is?"

C: "I'm not quite sure yet, Mrs. Smith. It sounds a like it, but we will have to do some further testing to let you know for sure."

E: "Oh my God! She is doing it again." At this time, you see patient having generalized seizure. She is having tonic-clonic activity with eyes deviated to the left. She is having copious secretions from her oropharynx.

C: "Nurse, could I please have some assistance. Mrs. Smith, I'm going to ask you to quickly step outside while we give Jessica some medications to make this seizure stop."

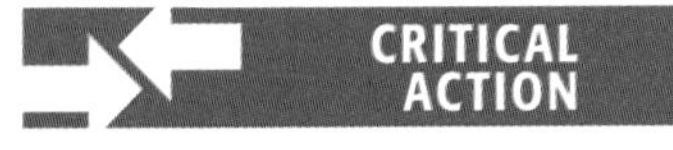

Treatment of the seizures with benzodiazepines is a critical action in this case.

E: "Please help her. This is terrible."

C: "Nurse, could we please put her on an NRB mask? Please suction her mouth and give her diazepam, 2 mg IV. Please do a bedside blood sugar determination as well."

E: "It is done doctor. The patient's blood glucose is 92." The patient stops seizing after the administration of the diazepam.

C: "Mrs. Smith, it seems like Jessica is having seizures. We are going to have to run some blood tests and do some radiographic tests. I am going to take you back into the room where I am going to do my physical examination."

C: "Nurse, can we please send off the blood for CBC with differential, electrolytes, BUN/Cr, coagulation labs, and blood cultures. Could we also order a stat head CT? Thank you."

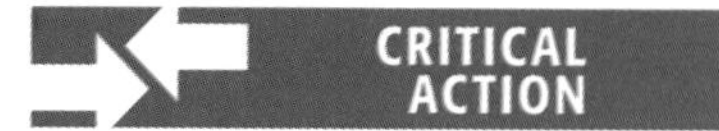

Getting a head CT to rule out a mass lesion or intracranial bleed is a critical action in this case.

C: "What do I see now when I look at the patient?"

E: "The patient is lying in the bed, attached to a monitor and a pulse oximeter. She is somnolent after the anxiolytics."

C: "What are the patient's vital signs now?"

E: "Pulse 122, RR 18, BP 90/60, oxygen saturation on NR facemask is 100%."

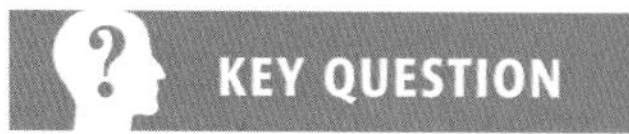

Remember to reassess any unstable patient frequently.

C: "Is there any evidence of head trauma, including bruising, scars, or hematomas?"

E: "There are none present."

C: "What do I see when I shine a penlight in the patient's eyes?"

E: "Her pupils are 5 mm and react briskly to 3 mm when light is shined into them."

C: "Is there an afferent or efferent pupillary defect?"

E: "No."

C: "Are the disk margins sharp when a funduscopic examination is done?"

E: "Yes."

C: "Are there any hemorrhages present?"

E: "No."

C: "What do I see when I look into the patient's ears?"

E: "What are you looking for?"

C: "Are there normal landmarks and are the tympanic membranes red and inflamed?"

E: "The external canals are normal, there are normal landmarks, and the tympanic membranes are not hyperemic."

C: "When I look in the patient's mouth, are her mucous membranes moist and does she have any injection of her posterior oropharynx."

E: "Her mucous membranes are moist and there is no injection in the posterior oropharynx. There are no exudates on her tonsils."

C: "When I examine her chest wall, is there any bruising and is it rising equally."

E: "There is no external evidence of trauma and there is equal expansion of both hemithoraces."

C: "Are breath sounds equal?"

E: "They are."

C: "Are there any crackles or wheezes?"

E: "There are none present."

C: "What do I hear when I listen to the patient's heart?"

E: "What are you looking for?"

C: "Is there a normal sinus rhythm? Are there any murmurs, rubs, or gallops?"

E: "Patient has sinus tachycardia. There are no murmurs, rubs, or gallops."

C: "Are there bowel sounds?"

E: "There are normoactive bowel sounds."

C: "Does the patient react to light or deep palpation?"

E: "She does not."

C: "Rectal examination?"

E: "There is a small amount of brown stool in the vault that is guaiac negative."

C: "When I look at her extremities, what is the temperature and what is the capillary refill like?"

E: "The extremities are warm and the capillary refill is under 3 seconds."

C: "Are there any rashes or other skin abnormalities?"

E: "There are no rashes, no petechiae, or other abnormalities."

C: "Is the patient moving her extremities?"

E: "She is sleeping."

C: "Before she seized, was she interacting appropriately?"

E: "She was lying in her mother's lap speaking with her."

C: "Can I please call over to CT to see if they are ready for the patient?"

E: "They are ready."

C: "I would like to ask the nurse to accompany the patient over to the CT scanner, while the patient remains on supplemental oxygen, continuous pulse oximetry, and cardiac monitor. I would also ask that she takes a pre-filled syringe with another 2 mg of diazepam. Please get a straight cath urine specimen before she leaves and send it for UA, culture, and toxicology screen. Thanks."

E: "The patient has gone to the CT scanner."

C: "Is the mother present?"

E: "She is."

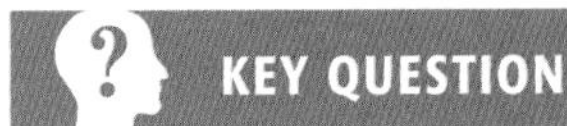

KEY QUESTION

Remember to follow-up on any labs you order. Write them all down as you will be penalized if you forget to follow-up on them.

C: "Mrs. Smith, Jessica has gone to the CT scanner so that we can get some pictures of her brain. She should be back in about 30 minutes. I'll ask you to have a seat in the waiting room and I will come get you when she gets back."

E: "OK."

C: "Are any of the lab tests back?"

E: "Yes. Her CBC shows a WBC count of 18.8, a Hgb of 12.2, and platelets of 234,000. Her electrolytes are: Na 138, K 4.2, Cl 112, CO_2 19, BUN 12, Cr 0.6, glu 82. Her UA is not back, but we have a urine dip. It shows a specific gravity of 1.025. There is no protein, leukocyte esterase, nitrites, or protein. A formal UA is pending and the urine has been sent for culture."

E: "Doctor, the patient has returned from the CT scanner with the nurse."

C: "What do I see when I look at the patient?"

E: "Patient is drowsy, but more interactive than when she went to the CT scanner. She awakens to name."

C: "Please place the patient back on the monitor and give supplemental oxygen."

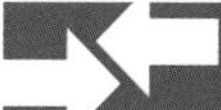

E: "It is done. At this time, a radiology tech arrives with the patient's CT scan and hand it to you."

C: "What do I see when I look at the CT scan of the brain?"

E: "What are you looking for?"

C: "Are there any bony abnormalities?"

E: "There are none. The sinuses are undeveloped. There are no fractures of the upper facial bones and the calvaria."

C: "Are there any fluid collections indicative of blood or infection?"

E: "No. There are no hyper or hypodense lesions."

C: "Is the grey/white matter well differentiated?"

E: "Yes."

C: "Are the ventricles normal in morphology and appearance?"

E: "Yes they are."

C: "It sounds like an unremarkable CT scan."

C: "Nurse, please place some EMLA cream on the patient's back on the lower lumbar area in preparation for a LP. Have the staff obtain a monitored bed on the pediatric step down/neurology floor in preparation for the patient's admission."

C: "I would like to speak to the mother, please."

E: "She has returned from the waiting room."

C: "Mrs. Smith, I have the preliminary results of Jessica's head scan and find it to be unremarkable. However, although there are no abnormalities such as a mass or blood in the brain, we still do not have a complete answer for what is going on. In such cases, we need to do a procedure called a LP. It entails numbing up the back and taking some fluid from the sac below the spinal cord. It gives us an idea of whether or not there might be an infection that is causing these seizures."

E: "Is it safe?"

C: "Yes it is very safe. Of course, as with any procedure there are some risks, such as bleeding and infection, but since we do it in a very sterile fashion these risks are very low."

E: "OK, when will you be doing this?"

C: "I will be starting as soon as we finish this conversation. As before, I will have you sit down in the waiting room and I will get you as soon as I am finished. Do you have any questions?"

E: "No."

C: "I would like to prepare the patient for a LP. I would have the nurse help me position the patient in the left lateral decubitus position with her knees drawn into the patient's chest while remaining on the cardiac monitor, pulse oximeter, and supplemental oxygen."

C: "Could I please review the patient's vital signs before we begin?"

E: "P 107, RR 18, BP 92/60, Sao_2 100% on 2 L per NC."

C: "Can I also get a temperature?"

E: "38.5."

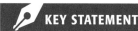

CRITICAL ACTION

There are two critical actions taking place here:

- Performing a LP
- Admitting the patient to a monitored bed.

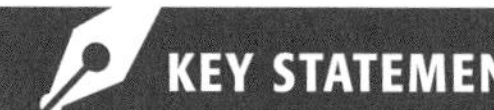

KEY STATEMENT

Remember to keep the patient and/or the patient's family apprised of lab results and updated on the plan. Also remember to get consent for any invasive procedures.

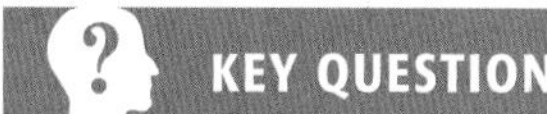

KEY QUESTION

Remember to reassess vital signs frequently on any unstable patient.

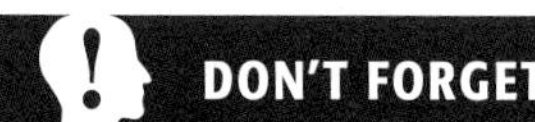

DON'T FORGET

You will need to be able to describe emergent procedures such as chest tube, intubation, pericardiocentesis, etc. This is a good description of a lumbar puncture.

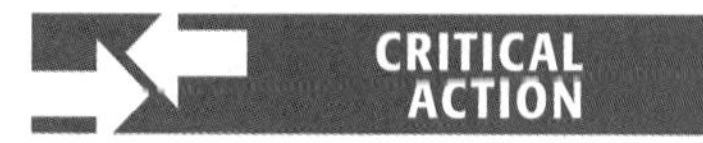

CRITICAL ACTION

Consulting neurology for this patient with new onset seizures is a critical action in this case.

C: "Please give a Tylenol suppository and administer vancomycin and ceftriaxone. We will not proceed with the LP: I would like to prep and drape the patient's back in a sterile fashion. I would like to anesthetize the L3/L4 and L4/L5 interspaces with 1 cc 1% lidocaine. I would then like to insert a 3.5 inch 22-guage spinal needle into the L3/L4 spinous interspace."

E: "It is done without difficulty. You obtain 5 cc of mildly cloudy fluid and note an opening pressure of 30."

C: "I would like to send the spinal fluid for the following: Tube #1 for cell count, tube #2 for Gram stain and culture, tube #3 for protein and glucose, and tube #4 for cell count and titers for viral titers. Can you let me know when those results are available?"

C: "I would also ask the secretary to get the patient's pediatrician, Dr. Jones on the phone for me."

E: "Dr. Jones is on the phone."

C: "Hi Dr. Jones. This is Dr. Fitz in the ER. I have one of your patients, Jessica Smith in the ED right now. As you know, she is an otherwise healthy little girl who came in today with a new seizure. She also had one while in the department which resolved with IV diazepam. There does not appear to be any head trauma or mass lesion on head CT. Her labs have been unremarkable, but she spiked a fever before I performed a LP. She is receiving antibiotics and I would like to admit her to the hospital for new seizure with concern for meningitis. Can I admit her to your service with Neurology consult? Do you have anything that you might like to add?"

E: "No, that sounds good. What was her neck exam like?"

C: "She is post-ictal and it is difficult for me to assess."

E: "Please admit her to my service and have Dr. Brain on consult as the pediatric neurologist."

C: "I would like to check the results of the LP."

E: "In tube #1, there are a 150 WBC (most are PMNLs) and 2 RBCs. In tube #2, the protein is elevated to 75 mg/dL and the glucose is 42 mg/dL. In tube #3, there are 151 WBCs and no RBCs. Other tests are still pending."

C: "I am concerned about bacterial meningitis and I would like to verify that antibiotics are going in. Can I please get Dr. Brain on the telephone?"

E: "Dr. Brain is on the telephone."

C: "Hi Dr. Brain. This is Dr. Fitz in the pediatric emergency department. I have one of Dr. Jones' patients in the ER and he wanted me to consult you. Her name is Jessica Smith, and she is a 2-year-old girl who presented with new onset seizure and her LP is concerning for meningitis."

E: "Thank you. I will see her on the floor tomorrow morning. Thank you for the consult."

C: "Is there anything else that we can do for you tonight?"

E: "No, thanks. If possible, could you please order an EEG for tomorrow morning?"

C: "No problem."

E: "At this time, the nurse lets you know that the patient's room is ready upstairs. The patient is admitted to the hospital. End of case."

CASE ASSESSMENT

Overall, the candidate managed the case reasonably well. He addressed the child's seizure appropriately. He also obtained a thorough history and physical examination that included questions about possible etiologies of seizure including trauma, ingestion, and infection.

However, he did not address the neck and check for meningismus. Also, though the patient was initially afebrile, she spiked a fever during the case, and the candidate did not discover this as quickly as he could have. It is important to remember that many cases evolve. By sticking to advanced trauma life support (ATLS) protocol and remembering to reassess the patient with any change in status, you will be able to manage and stabilize the patient.

In this case, the candidate could have done better by making sure the temperature was included when he asked for repeat vital signs, particularly after a repeat seizure. The patient had a low-grade temperature at triage and was presenting with a pathology that can be caused by infection. If the candidate had remembered to ask for repeat temperatures, he would have discovered the fever earlier and this would have led to earlier antibiotic use.

Critical Actions

1. Identify seizure history.
2. Treat active seizure with benzodiazepines.
3. Perform computed tomography (CT) to check for bleeding or structural lesions.
4. Perform lumbar puncture (LP) to R/O bacterial meningitis.
5. Recognize and treat bacterial meningitis.
6. Admit to hospital with Neurology consult.

Test Performance

1. *Data acquisition:* The candidate obtained all of the information required to make the correct diagnosis, but he should have made sure temperature was included when he asked for repeat vitals. Score = **6**
2. *Problem solving:* The candidate obtained a relatively thorough examination history, but should have asked about the neck examination during his secondary survey. To his credit, he proceeded in an appropriate stepwise fashion to CT and LP to find the source for the new seizure, and obtained appropriate lab work. Score = **6**
3. *Patient management:* The examinee treated the seizure appropriately and moved toward an appropriate disposition. Ideally, the antibiotic could have been started earlier. Score = **6**
4. *Resource utilization:* The candidate ordered symptom-specific studies and imaging. Score = **8**
5. *Health care provided (outcome):* The patient received appropriate treatment, and the candidate's interventions stabilized the patient. Points would be removed for an unnecessarily delayed diagnosis. Score = **6**
6. *Interpersonal relations and communication skills:* The candidate communicated appropriately with the patient's mother and with his consultants. These are easy points, so remember to keep patients aware of the plan and speak concisely and politely with consultants. Score = **8**

7. *Comprehension of pathophysiology:* The candidate showed comprehension of new seizure pathology by asking about ingestions, checking head CT for lesions, and asking about infectious pathology on exam. As noted above, he should have checked for meningismus on exam. Score = **6**
8. *Clinical competence (overall):* Despite a minor delay, the candidate arrived at the appropriate diagnosis and completed all critical actions. Score = **7**

CASE 32 8 mo/o Female With SIDS/PALS

John Dayton and Janis Tupesis

INITIAL INFORMATION

Name: Anna Lourdes

Mode of arrival: Ambulance

Age: 8 months

Gender: Female

VS: N/A

CC: Patient found unresponsive in crib

Background: It is 6:15 AM on a Thursday morning. You answer the EMS radio and find a frantic paramedic on the other line stating that they have been called to a private residence where they have found an unresponsive infant. They are only a block away and are asking to "scoop and run." They have not obtained vital signs, but are preparing to begin resuscitation. They are requesting to come to your level 1 pediatric trauma center.

PLAY OF THE CASE

C: "Do we know how old the child is?"

E: "The paramedics said that they thought that the patient was approximately 8 months old, but weren't sure."

C: "I would like to get the resuscitation room ready and alert the appropriate pediatric intensive care team. I would like to clear a resuscitation bay, get a Broselow tape on the bed, and make sure that I have all of my resuscitation equipment ready."

E: "What equipment would you like to prepare?"

C: "I would like to have a selection of pediatric endotracheal tubes with appropriate stylets, a blunt (Yankauer) suction catheter attached to wall suction, and an end-tidal carbon dioxide detector. I would like to get both size 2 and 3 Miller and Macintosh blades ready and would like to make sure that the laryngoscope light bulb is working. Prepare to place the infant on cardiac, oxygen, and BP monitoring on arrival."

E: "All of the equipment is functioning properly and it is all set up."

E: "At this time the ambulance arrives at the door of the resuscitation suite."

C: "What do I see?"

E: "You see the paramedics bagging an approximately 8 month-old female infant. She is unresponsive and cyanotic."

C: "Does the patient have vital signs?"

E: "BP unobtainable, pulse of 36, RR of 10 and shallow and the pulse ox is not registering."

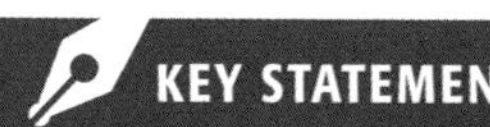

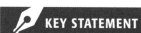

Know your resuscitation equipment and memorize the ET tube size for all age groups. This is not material you should be looking up in a code situation.

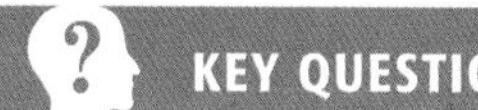

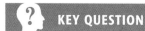

Ask this open-ended question at the beginning of every case.

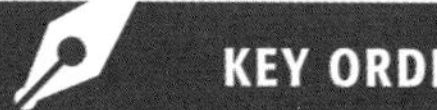

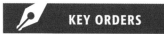

Every critical patient requires IV access (preferable two large-bore IVs, oxygen, and cardiac monitoring. In this case, the patient is hypotensive and a fluid bolus should also be initiated.

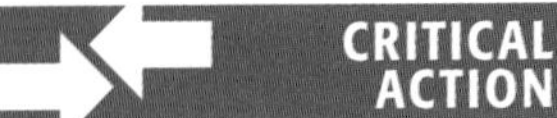

CRITICAL ACTION

Recognition of a shock state and treatment according to PALS criteria is a critical set of actions in this case.

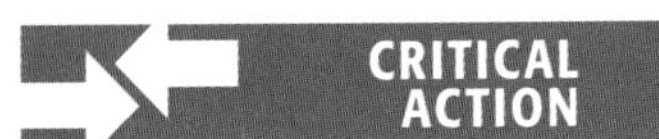

CRITICAL ACTION

Intubating this unresponsive patient is a critical action in this case.

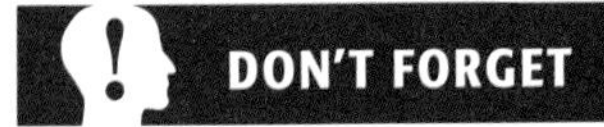

DON'T FORGET

For a pressure-cycled ventilator one might say: "SIMV at a rate of 20 with pressure control of 20, pressure support of 10 and a PEEP of 5."

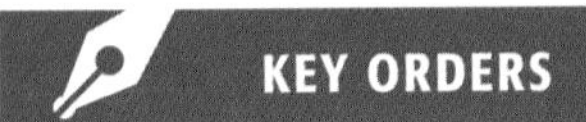

KEY ORDERS

Remember to reassess your unstable patients frequently—especially after interventions.

C: "I would like to transfer the patient to the bed and begin preparation for emergent endotracheal intubation. During this time I would like the nurse to put the patient on bag valve mask at 100% O_2, establish an IV, place the patient on a cardiac monitor, and place the child in a cervical collar."

E: "All of the above orders have been done. The patient is on the gurney next to the Broselow tape, has a 22-gauge established in the left antecubital fossa and is on a cardiac monitor."

C: "What does the Broselow tape say for the patient's weight?"

E: "It estimates the patient's weight at 8 kg."

C: "Is there any response to bagging?"

E: "The pulse is now 46 but the color hasn't changed."

C: "Please give epinephrine 0.01 mg/mg (0.08 mg) IV. Is there any response in the heart rate?"

E: "The heart rate is now 80."

C: "We will need to intubate this patient. We have already pre-oxygenated and prepared the appropriate equipment. Please position the patient by placing them in "sniffing position" with a rolled towel under the shoulders. Draw up the following medications:

- Lidocaine, 1.5 mg/kg (12 mg)
- Etomidate 0.3mg/kg (2.4 mg)
- Midazolam (Versed) 0.2 mg/kg (1.6 mg)
- Succinylcholine 2 mg/kg (16 mg)

E: "All of the medications are drawn up."

C: "First, I would like to pre-treat with lidocaine. I will sedate with Versed followed by the etomidate. During this time I would ask that one of the techs assist with in-line C-spine immobilization and apply cricoid pressure. I will continue to assist ventilations. Finally, please give the paralytic succinylcholine. While the tech continues to apply cricoid pressure I will attempt to intubate the patient."

E: "The patient has stopped breathing at this time."

C: "Using a Miller 1 blade, I will pass an uncuffed 3.5 ET tube through the vocal cords."

E: "It is done without difficulty."

C: "Nurse, please secure the airway with the ET tube at 13 cm at the patient's lips and apply the end-tidal CO_2 monitor. Do I see color change?"

E: "You see that the end-tidal CO_2 detector turns from purple to yellow."

C: "Listening over the stomach and over both of the lung fields?"

E: "You do not hear anything over the stomach and hear breath sounds bilaterally."

C: "Is there symmetric chest rise?"

E: "There is."

C: "Nurse, let's give the patient more sedation. Please administer diazepam, 1 mg, IVP."

E: "It is done."

C: "I would like to place the patient on mechanical ventilation with the following settings: SIMV Mode at a rate of 20 breaths/min, FIO_2 100%, TV of 75 cc, and PEEP of 5."

C: "Please give the patient a 20 cc/kg bolus of 0.9 NS and place a NG tube. Repeat the VS after the bolus is in. Also, please draw the following labs: CBC, BMP, LFTs, coagulation studies, and an arterial blood gas (ABG). Please obtain the following imaging: Stat portable CXR to confirm ET tube placement. Schedule a portable C-spine and pelvis and if the patient remains stable she is to go to the radiology department accompanied by an RN for a non-contrast CT scan of the head."

E: "The portable x-rays are being done and the CT is ordered. The current vital signs are pulse of 106, BP 73/42, respirations as per the ventilator settings, sat 98%."

C: "I would like to ask the paramedics that brought the patient in to wait so we can ask some questions, but at this time I would like to go ahead and continue with my secondary survey."

C: "Are there any external signs of trauma about the child's head? Swellings, lacerations, or hematoma?"

E: "No."

C: "Are the pupils reactive to light?"

E: "The pupils are 5 mm. They are reactive sluggishly when a pen light is shined into them."

C: "Are there any atypical eye movements or nystagmus?"

E: "None present."

C: "Looking in the ears—assess for blood or other fluid in the canal. I would also like to assess the landmarks in the inner ear."

E: "There is no blood in the ears and the landmarks are normal."

C: "Oropharynx?"

E: "There is a 3.5 ET tube, secured at the lip at 13 cm. There is fogging in the tube when the ventilator triggers."

C: "I would like to carefully take off the C-collar and assess the posterior cervical spine."

E: "What are you looking for?"

C: "I want to make sure that there is no step-off and no large soft tissue swelling."

E: "There is not."

C: "Is the trachea midline?"

E: "It is."

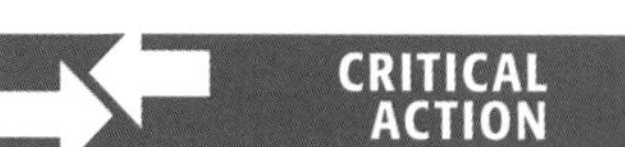

Throughout this section, the candidate is performing another critical set of actions, which is assessing this child for possible trauma.

C: "Is there any evidence of external trauma on the anterior chest wall?"

E: "There is not."

C: "Is there any evidence of subcutaneous emphysema?"

E: "There is not."

C: "Listening to the patient's heart sounds, are they regular with any murmurs, rubs, or gallops?"

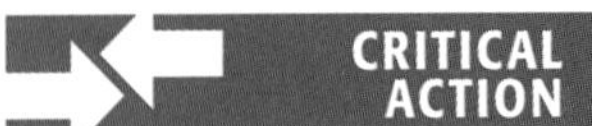

CRITICAL ACTION

Appropriate fluid resuscitation is almost always a critical action when it is required.

E: "Patient has a sinus tachycardia and no abnormal heart sounds."

C: "Looking at the patient, is there symmetric chest rise?"

E: "There is."

C: "Are there bilateral breath sounds? Any rales, rhonchi, or wheezing."

E: "The patient has bilateral breath sounds on auscultation. The breath sounds are diminished bilaterally with course crackles bilaterally. There are no rhonchi or wheezing."

C: "Signs of bruising or other evidence of external trauma to the abdomen?"

E: "There is not."

C: "Are the bowel sounds present."

E: "The bowel sounds are diminished."

C: "Palpating the abdomen, is it distended and are there any palpable masses?"

E: "The abdomen is mildly distended and there are no palpable masses."

C: "Is there any blood or bruising in the vaginal introital area or perineum?"

E: "No blood or other evidence of trauma."

C: "On rectal examination, is the rectal tone normal? Guaiac of stool for occult blood?"

E: "On rectal examination, the patient has mildly decreased tone and the stool is heme negative."

C: "With assistance, we will logroll the patient and evaluate the thoracic and lumbar spine for deformities, step-offs, and atypical swelling."

E: "The examination is normal."

C: "Are there signs of trauma to the extremities, deformities, or tenderness?"

E: "There are not."

C: "I would like to assess the patient's reflexes."

E: "They are diminished as the patient remains to be sedated."

C: "Does the patient respond to painful stimuli?"

E: "Yes, she responds to painful stimuli with a grimace and moving her arms and legs."

C: "Is the capillary refill normal? Skin color and temperature?"

E: "The capillary refill is under 2 seconds. The extremities are cool, dry, and normal color is returning as the fluid bolus is completed."

C: "Do we have the results of the blood gas?"

E: "Yes. pH 7.27, Po_2 166, Pco_2 43, HCO_2 21."

C: "I would ask the nurse to repeat a blood gas now that the patient has been on the ventilator."

E: "The nurse draws the ABG and sends it off to the respiratory lab."

C: "What are the patient's vital signs now?"

E: "T 36.8°C, BP 88/67, RR per vent setting, HR 116, Sao_2 99%."

C: "I would also like to put in a Foley catheter and give the patient a second 20/kg bolus of 0.9 NS."

E: "It is done."

C: "At this point, I would like to go talk to the paramedics and the family and obtain any further history."

E: "They are waiting for you in the EMS room."

C: "Hi guys. My name is Dr. Palmer. I am the physician taking care of Anna Lourdes. Are you the rig that brought the patient in?"

E: "We are."

C: "Can you guys tell me a little bit about what happened?"

E: "We really didn't get a long history. Basically, mom stated that she had just put the baby to bed about 45 minutes ago. She was washing the dishes when she said that she could not hear the little girl breathing on the baby monitor. She went in to check on the child and found her unresponsive."

C: "Is mom here?"

E: "No, she is on the way in."

C: "What did you guys see when you got there?"

E: "Nothing really. Mom had the child in her arms on the couch. The child was pale, cool, and mildly cyanotic. She was breathing on her own—but the respirations were shallow. We grabbed her, put her on some oxygen and brought her here. They live right around the corner."

C: "Do we know if the child has any medical problems?"

E: "I don't know. Mom said that she has no medical problems or allergies."

C: "Thanks guys, please let me know if you see mom come in."

C: "I would like to go back into the patient's room. What do I see when I walk into the room?"

E: "The radiology tech is finishing up the neck, chest, and pelvis films. The patient is on the ventilator without any untoward movements."

C: "I would like to see the x-ray films as soon as they are available."

E: "She states that they will be ready soon."

C: "What are the patient's vital signs?"

E: "The patient remains on the vent. T 37.1°C, BP 94/62, RR per vent setting, HR 100, Sao_2 100%."

C: "I would like to check to see if we have any of the labs back."

E: "The nurse says that the only lab that is back is the second ABG that was sent after the patient was put on the ventilator. They are: pH 7.37, Po_2 179, Pco_2 35, sat 99%."

E: "The nurse also states that transportation is here to take the patient to the CT scanner."

C: "I would like to examine the C-spine films and the CXR before the patient goes to the CT scanner to make sure that we do not to do any other imaging while the patient is in the scanner. I would, however, ask her to prepare the patient for transport by putting the patient on portable oxygen with the vent and respiratory therapy, a portable cardiac monitor, and some more midazolam for sedation."

E: "It is done and the x-rays are ready for review."

C: "I would like to first look at the CXR."

E: "What are you looking for?"

C: "First, I would like to systematically look from the outside in. Is it a good film? Can we see down to the thoracic ribs? Are there any bony abnormalities?"

E: "It is a good quality film and you can count 8-9 ribs. There are no bony abnormalities."

C: "Continuing in, at what position is the ET tube?"

E: "It is approximately 1.0 cm above the carina."

C: "When I look at the heart, are the heart borders regular?"

E: "They are."

C: "I would like to look at the lung fields and assess for the following: Any sign of pneumonia? Are both lungs equally inflated? Is there a pneumothorax?"

E: "Both lungs are inflated. There does not appear to be a pneumothorax as you can see vascular markings all the way lateral to the chest wall on both sides. There are no consolidations."

C: "Very well. I am satisfied that the ET tube is in the correct position above the carina."

C: "I would like to examine the patient's C-spine films. I am looking for symmetry of the vertebral bodies, normal anterior, and posterior laminar lines."

E: "The C-spines films show C1-C7 laterally. There are no obvious fractures. The posterior spinolaminar line is normal. There appear to be no abnormalities."

C: "I would like to leave the patient's C-collar on until further notice. I would also quickly like to look at the patient's pelvis films before she goes on to the CT scanner. I would like to make sure that there are no obvious fractures and that the joint spaces are appropriate for the stated age."

E: "There appear to be no fractures and the joint spaces are appropriate."

C: "OK, please let the CT tech know that the patient can go to the CT scanner with the nurse, the respiratory therapist and the portable cardiac monitor."

E: "The patient is wheeled off to the CT scanner."

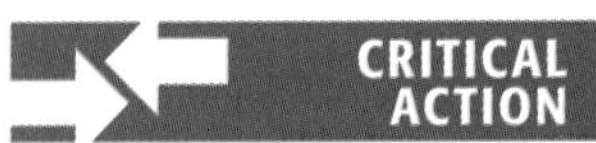

Admitting the patient to the appropriate level of care is always a critical action.

C: "At this point and time, I would like to ask the coordinator to request a PICU bed and start making arrangements for the patient's admission. I would also ask her to find out who is on call for the PICU and have them paged to my phone."

C: "Hi Dr. Child, this is Dr. Palmer, the attending in the ED. I am calling to tell you about a child that presented to the ED about 30 minutes ago that is going to need admission to the PICU."

E: "What happened?"

C: "The patient is an 8-month-old infant who was found unresponsive in her crib about 45 minutes after she was put to bed. The mother states that she did not hear the patient breathing on the apnea monitor and found her unresponsive. She stimulated the infant to breath and called 911. They were there within minutes and here a few minutes later. She was immediately intubated due to poor respiratory effort. She has baseline labs pending. She is on her way to get a head CT, but her C-spine, CXR, and pelvis x-ray and PE are negative."

E: "Are there any other injuries."

C: "No obvious ones. There appeared to be no trauma to the patient."

E: "Why did you image her spine?"

C: "Because of the possibility of unwitnessed injury."

E: "Are you suspicious of abuse?"

C: "There is no external evidence of trauma. There are also no bruises on the child's torso, back, and extremities. However, we have been unable to talk to the mother directly. We will as soon as she arrives here. At this time, it appears that the leading diagnosis is ALTE vs. SIDS. However, we will let you know if anything else comes back abnormal."

E: "OK, we'll be down to see her in a moment. Does she have any labs back?"

C: "Other than her ABGs, there is nothing back. Both of them are on the hospitals computer system if you would like to look at them."

E: "OK, we are on our way."

C: "Can I please check if any of the labs are back?"

E: "They are. The results of the CBC are as follows: WBC 11,900, Hgb/Hct 13.6/39, Plt 310,000. The results of the complete metabolic panel are as follows: Na 139, K 4.2, chloride 105, bicarb 22, BUN 12, Cr 0.6, glu 135, Ca 10.1. The results of the liver function tests are as follows: AST 17, ALT 31, alkaline phosphatase 82, GGT 29, total bilirubin 0.8, albumin 3.7. The results of the UA are not back at this time."

C: "It looks as though most of the laboratory results are normal. There are no signs of infection on lab assessment and imaging. There are no gross abnormalities with the patient's metabolic labs and her liver labs, so I am less worried about congenital metabolic derangements. I am continuing with my diagnosis being that of ALTE/SIDS."

E: "At this point, the patient returns from the CT scanner with the nurse."

C: "Any problems?"

E: "No, none at all. The patient has been adequately sedated and is tolerating the vent well."

C: "I would like to look at the CT results."

E: "The head CT is read as normal."

C: "I am less worried that there has been trauma to the child. **Are the parents here?**"

E: "Yes, they are."

C: "Hello, my name is Dr. Palmer. I am the supervising emergency doctor taking care of Anna. I want you to know that she is doing much better and that we are taking good care of her."

E: "Thank God. What happened?"

C: "We think that Anna had a period of what we call apnea. It means that Anna stopped breathing while she was sleeping. We are unsure exactly why it happened. When Anna came into the department she was barely breathing, so we had to put her on a breathing machine. She will probably be on this for a few days until her breathing improves. Otherwise, all of the rest of the test seem to be normal. She will be admitted to the PICU. Do you have any questions?"

E: "No, thank you. The PICU takes the patient. This is the end of the case."

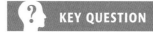

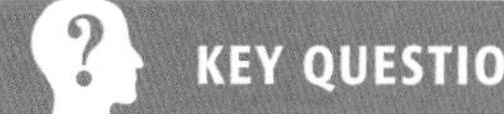

Remember that you will be penalized if you do not follow-up on the results of all your labs. Either write them down so that you remember them, or ask the examiner to notify you when they are back.

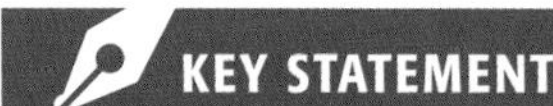

Remember to keep the patient and/or family updated on test results and the plan for the patient's disposition.

CASE ASSESSMENT

Overall, the candidate managed this case efficiently. Throughout the case, the actions were decisive and well thought out. In cases that include information from a pre-hospital care provider, it is important to start preparing for the patient before they arrive. As soon as the candidate was aware that he was going to get a critically ill patient, he began mobilizing his resources. He also started preparing for the resuscitation by getting airway equipment ready, thinking about what kinds of medication he would use for rapid sequence intubation, and preparing a Broselow tape.

Upon arrival, the candidate realized that the patient's mental status and poor vital signs necessitated early airway management and emergency intubation was performed. Because the candidate realized that there was a possibility of head trauma, he gave neuroprotective lidocaine.

One of the most important things to do in cases like this is to look for possible trauma. Early C-spine immobilization was achieved and appropriate imaging studies were done to evaluate for possible head and neck injuries. He also performed a Hx/PE screen for trauma. If labs are not back, that might give you a clue that there might be an additional injury. If the patient is already going to the computed tomography (CT) scanner for a CT of the head, one might consider doing a quick "trauma scan" of the abdomen and pelvis. Or, if the facility is equipped with an ultrasound machine, a focused assessment with sonography for trauma (FAST) examination might have been done as part of the secondary survey. Finally, the patient's disposition and consultation were performed in a timely manner.

Critical Actions

1. Recognize and treat the shock state.
2. Emergent intubation and resuscitation.
3. Consideration of trauma as a cause of patient's condition.
4. Admit patient to the pediatric intensive care unit (PICU).

Test Performance

1. *Data acquisition:* Data acquisition is excellent. The candidate has very little information but still considers all possible etiologies while resuscitating the patient. Score = **8**
2. *Problem solving:* Problem solving is excellent. The candidate was able to rapidly assimilate data from the patient encounter, interpret test results, and synthesize information quickly to direct further management. He could have considered further trauma workup, but this can be done as an inpatient. Score = **7**
3. *Patient management:* The examinee recognized the need for airway management, assessed for trauma, and admitted the patient to the PICU. Score = **8**
4. *Resource utilization:* Even before arrival to the ED, the candidate prepared for the resuscitation. Patient workup was focused and appropriate. However, he forgot to request the result of the lab studies he'd ordered. Score = **6**

5. *Health care provided (outcome):* The patient received efficient, appropriate treatment, and the candidate's interventions stabilized the patient. Score = **8**
6. *Interpersonal relations and communication skills:* The candidate did a good job of effectively communicating with the emergency medical services (EMS), the patient's mother, and the multiple professional colleagues in this scenario. Score = **8**
7. *Comprehension of pathophysiology:* The examinee conveyed his understanding of disease process through airway management, trauma assessment, ordering appropriate studies and imaging, and by his conversation with the consultant. Score = **8**
8. *Clinical competence (overall):* Overall, the examinee stabilized a critical patient, performed a focused evaluation, utilized appropriate lab work and imaging, and working toward the appropriate disposition. Score = **7**

CASE 33 38 y/o Male With Thermal Burns

John Dayton, Philip Shayne, and Daniel Wu

INITIAL INFORMATION

Name: Bob Smith

Mode of arrival: via EMS (basic ambulance unit)

Age: 38 years

Gender: Male

VS: T 37.5°C (99.5°F), BP 130/65, HR 110, RR 20

CC: Burned in a house fire

PLAY OF THE CASE

> **KEY QUESTION**
>
> Ask this open-ended question at the beginning of every case.

C: "What do I see as I walk into the patient's room?"

E: "The patient is a well-nourished, well-developed young man who appears uncomfortable. He smells of smoke and his clothes are burned and blackened."

C: "Nurse, please ask EMS to stay so that I can speak with them. Please place the patient on a cardiac monitor, start two large-bore IV catheters, draw blood for labs, and place the patient on mask oxygen at 15 L after getting a room air oxygen saturation level."

> **KEY ORDERS**
>
> Every unstable patient requires IV access (preferably two large-bore IVs), oxygen, and cardiac monitoring. Remember to use all possible resources to obtain medical history, and do not let EMS leave without asking them about the scene.

E: "Those orders are being done; the room air oxygen saturation is 95% and 99% on oxygen."

C: "Hello Mr. Smith, my name is Dr. Kandu. What happened to you today?"

E: "I just woke up this morning and my house was on fire. I couldn't get out of the house until the fire fighters rescued me."

C: "Did you get burned anywhere?"

E: "When I woke up the bed sheets were on fire and there was smoke everywhere. My chest and arms really hurt from being burned."

C: "Any difficulty breathing?"

E: "No."

C: "Are you coughing up any dark sputum?"

> **KEY QUESTION**
>
> Remember: If you are not given a full set of vitals at the beginning of the case, ask for what is missing.

E: "No."

C: "Does your mouth or throat hurt?"

E: "No."

C: "Do you have any difficulty swallowing?"

E: "No."

C: "Did you fall or jump out of a window to get away from the fire?"

E: "No, the firefighters had to come and get me out of the house."

C: "Do you have pain anywhere else?"

E: "No."

C: "Did you pass out?"

E: "No."

C: "Nurse, I would like to send basic labs including a CBC, basic metabolic profile, coags, type and screen, a troponin, an ABG with carboxyhemoglobin level, and a portable CXR. Please inform me as results come back."

E: "The labs have been sent."

C: "Do you have any medical problems?"

E: "High BP and migraine headaches."

C: "Do you take any medications?"

E: "HCTZ, Lisinopril, and pain medications when I need them."

C: "Do you have any allergies to medications?"

E: "No."

C: "When was your last tetanus shot?"

E: "I don't remember, but it was a long time ago."

C: "On a scale of 1-10 what is your pain now?"

E: "Eight."

C: "Nurse, please administer 4 mg of morphine sulfate IV and an IM tetanus booster. Please reassess the patient at 5 minute intervals and let me know if his pain scale has improved."

E: "The medications have been given and EMS is in the room."

C: "What was the report at the scene and what did you see?"

E: "The call was for a house fire and the patient was pulled out of the house by the firefighters. The house was totally burned down and the firefighters said the fire started from a cigarette in bed and the patient's clothes caught on fire."

C: "Did the patient receive any treatment in the field?"

E: "We just brought him here as fast as we could because we are a basic ambulance."

C: "Thanks."

C: "How is your pain now, on a scale of 1-10?"

E: "It is better; maybe a 5."

C: "Nurse, please give the patient another 4 mg of morphine IV."

C: "I would like to examine the patient. Has there been a change in his appearance or vital signs?"

E: "No."

C: "I would like to examine his HEENT."

E: "What are you looking for?"

C: "Are there any facial burns? Carbonaceous sputum? Singed facial hair? Lip or throat swelling?"

E: "The patient's eyebrows are singed. There are no obvious facial, nasal, or oral burns or throat swelling."

C: "Is there any cervical spine tenderness?"

E: "No."

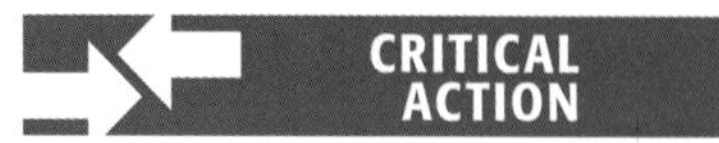

Giving pain medication is a critical action in this case. It often is, so do not ignore your patient's pain.

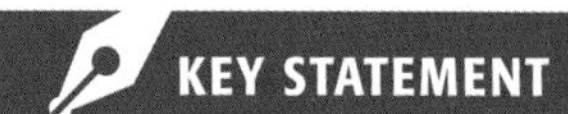

It is always a good strategy to have your examiner be responsible for reassessment of the patient after an intervention.

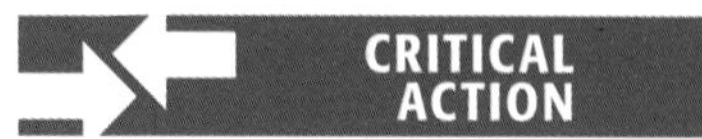

Assessing for smoke inhalation injury is a critical action in this case.

C: "Cardiac examination?"

E: "Slightly tachycardic but otherwise normal."

C: "Lungs?"

E: "What are you looking for?"

C: "Are breath sounds clear bilaterally? Wheezing? Rales?"

E: "The lungs are clear bilaterally with good air movement."

C: "Is there abdominal tenderness?"

E: "No."

C: "Neurologic exam?"

E: "GCS is 15. The patient is answering questions appropriately and there are no focal neurological findings."

C: "I would like to have the nurse fully undress the patient and examine the skin. Does the patient have skin burns?"

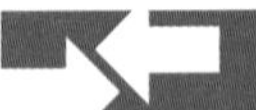

CRITICAL ACTION

Assessing the area of the burns is a critical action in this case. You should have the rule of 9s memorized.

E: "The patient has partial thickness burns with blisters over his entire anterior chest, the volar aspect of his right arm, and his entire left arm. The burns also extend to the upper portion of his abdomen where they appear whitish in color and are not painful to touch."

C: "Do the burns extend to his hands?"

E: "No."

C: "I would like to turn the patient over and examine his back."

CRITICAL ACTION

Giving adequate fluid resuscitation is a critical action in this case. You should have the Parkland formula memorized.

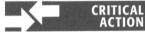

E: "There are no burns on the patient's back."

C: "Mr. Smith, how much do you weigh?"

E: "Around 175 lb."

C: "I will use the rule of 9s to determine the amount of body surface area affected by second- or third-degree burns. The patient is burned on the anterior chest which is 9%, upper portion of the anterior abdomen which is 4.5%, the volar surface of his right arm which is 4.5%, and his entire left arm which is 9%, giving him a total of 27%."

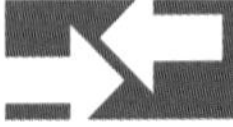

CRITICAL ACTION

Transferring this patient to a burn unit is a critical action in this case.

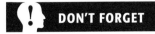

E: "The nurse asks how much fluid you would like him to receive."

C: "As he has had no fluids to this point in time, using the Parkland formula, I would like to give the patient 4 cc/kg of body weight multiplied by the percent of body surface area burned (4 cc × 80 kg × 27 = 8,640 cc). Our goal will be to give half of this in the next 8 hours and the other half during the following 16 hours. Although the Parkland formula provides a nice guideline, we will be focused on urine output as a measure of appropriate hydration."

DON'T FORGET

Remember: On exam day your consultants will often "push back" or ask you management questions as a way to test your knowledge of the management of whatever disease process you are evaluating. Be prepared for this.

E: "The IV fluids are started and several labs are back including a Hgb of 12.5, plt of 250,000, and a WBC 13. The coagulation profile is normal with an INR of 1.1 and the BMP reveals a Na 143, K 4.6, CO_2 19, Cl 105, BUN 17, Cr 1.2, Glu 156, Ca 8.9. The cardiac enzymes are pending. The ABG reveals a pH of 7.35, Po_2 455, Pco_2 31, HCO_3 19, sat 100%."

C: "Is the carboxyhemoglobin available?"

E.: "It is 27%."

C: "The patient's carboxyhemoglobin level is elevated due to smoke inhalation. Please continue the patient on 100% oxygen by NRB mask."

E: "That is done."

C: "Is there a burn unit available at this facility?"

E: "No."

C: "I would like to contact the nearest burn unit to transfer the patient. Please cover the patient, top and bottom with sterile, dry sheets for the time being. We may consider dressing the wounds with Silvadene if the burn unit personnel request this."

E: "The nurse is carrying out your instructions."

C: "Are the remainder of our lab studies available? Is the CXR available for review?"

E: "The cardiac enzymes are normal and the portable CXR is unremarkable."

E: "Dr. Burns is on the phone from Trauma General."

C: "Dr. Burns, This is Dr. Kandu. I have a 38-year-old man who was involved in a house fire today. He has second- and third-degree burns covering around 27% of his body surface area and his carboxyhemoglobin level is elevated."

E: "Does the patient need to go to the hyperbaric chamber?"

C: "I don't think he needs the chamber at this time. His level is not high enough, there was no loss of consciousness, and he has no neurological complaints."

E: "What have you done with his burn wounds?"

C: "We have placed him between sterile, dry sheets. Would you like us to go ahead and dress his wounds with Silvadene?"

E: "No, sterile dry coverings are best at this time and we really appreciate your thoughtfulness in waiting for our opinion on this matter. This will allow us to get a much better idea of the extent of tissue injury."

C: "Thanks."

E: "If the patient is stable you can send the patient to us for admission."

C: "Nurse, please recheck the patient's vital signs and prepare the patient for transfer to the burn center."

E: "The case is now over."

CASE ASSESSMENT

Overall, the candidate did a good job of managing the case. The candidate was able to correctly assess the extent of the burns and initiated appropriate fluid resuscitation. The candidate also recognized the risk for smoke inhalation in the setting of a fire in an enclosed space. The candidate also obtained a thorough history surrounding the events by interacting with emergency medical services (EMS). The candidate's also included thorough history and physical examination.

The physical examination was focused with special attention to the signs of potential inhalation injury and trauma to the neck and abdomen. The candidate gave analgesia early and often to the patient. A tetanus booster was also appropriately given. The candidate properly interpreted lab results and kept the patient on 100% oxygen when the carboxyhemoglobin level came back elevated. The disposition of the patient appropriately involves transfer to a burn unit due to due to the total body surface area (BSA) involved.

When a burn patient arrives, they should be placed on 100% oxygen and started on IV fluids. Our candidate used oxygen on arrival, but could have started the fluids earlier. However, the candidate performed all of the critical actions, did so in an efficient manner, and would have easily passed this case.

Critical Actions

1. Give pain medication.
2. Appropriately assess extent of burns.
3. Initiate appropriate fluid resuscitation.
4. Identify smoke inhalation.
5. Transfer patient to a burn unit.

Test Performance

1. *Data acquisition:* This phase was excellent. The candidate clearly understood what information was needed, given the chief complaint, and was able to obtain it in an efficient manner. Also, the candidate used outside resources such as EMS to acquire important information surrounding the events. Score = **8**
2. *Problem solving:* The candidate demonstrated excellent problem solving skills by investigating for inhalation injury, trauma, addressing the extent of burn, and addressing the patient's oxygen need. Score = **8**
3. *Patient management:* The patient care given in this case was great. The candidate could have improved the overall score by both addressing the patient's pain and starting IV fluids earlier. Score = **7**
4. *Resource utilization:* The candidate used appropriate lab work, imaging, and obtained information from the EMS crew. Her workup was logical, cost-sensitive, and showed patient concern. Score = **8**
5. *Health care provided (outcome):* The candidate clearly delivered the standard of care for this case and appropriately transferred the patient to a Burn Unit. Score = **8**
6. *Interpersonal relations and communication skills:* The candidate did a great job of communicating with the EMS team and the admitting physician. However, she could have done a better job of communicating with the patient about the extent of his injuries and need for transfer to a Burn Unit. Score = **6**
7. *Comprehension of pathophysiology:* The candidate demonstrated a very good understanding of burn management and associated trauma and inhalation injury. She included these in her screen and gave a concise history to the consultant. She also answered questions related to hyperbaric treatment appropriately. Score = **8**
8. *Clinical competence (overall):* Overall, the examinee showed clinical competence by obtaining an appropriate history and physical, utilized appropriate imaging and lab studies, provided appropriate interventions (sterile dressings, IV fluids, tetanus update, and pain management), and admitted the patient to the appropriate service. As noted above, she loses points only for not starting fluids earlier and not communicating with the patient about need for transfer. Score = **7**

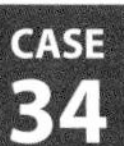

CASE 34 44 y/o Female With Fever and Bizarre Behavior

John Dayton, Fred Abrahamian, and Reb Close

INITIAL INFORMATION

Name: Jane Sturm

Mode of arrival: Brought in by her husband

Age: 44 years

Gender: Female

VS: T 39.0°C (102.2°F), BP 170/100, HR 135, RR 24, O_2 sat 99% on RA

CC: Bizarre behavior

KEY QUESTION

Ask this open-ended question at the beginning of every case.

PLAY OF THE CASE

C: "What do I see as I walk into the patient's room?"

E: "An anxious, thin female who is being comforted by her husband."

C: "Nurse, the vital signs are very abnormal. Please place the patient on a monitor, give me a rhythm strip, and start a large-bore IV. Set aside blood for lab work and blood culture, and give a 500-cc NS bolus. Please check blood glucose at the bedside. If there are no allergies, please give the patient acetaminophen, 1 g PO. Let me know what the repeat VS are in 10 minutes."

KEY ORDERS

Every unstable patient requires IV access (preferable two large-bore IVs), oxygen, and cardiac monitoring. In this case, as the patient is febrile, Tylenol is also indicated. As she is altered, a rapid bedside glucose is also appropriate.

E: "The orders are performed by the nurse. He reports that the blood glucose is 160 and hands you a rhythm strip that shows a sinus tachycardia."

C: "Mrs. Sturm, I'm Dr. Endoc. Can you tell me what brings you to the ED today?"

E: "I don't know, I don't know, I'm scared, my husband says something is wrong."

C: "OK, Mrs. Sturm, we are going to take good care of you, I'm going to talk to your husband about what has been happening."

KEY ORDERS

The candidate asked the examiner to keep them updated on vital sings in 10 minutes. This is an excellent strategy since it takes the responsibility for remembering to reassess off the candidate.

C: "Mr. Sturm, what has been going on with your wife?"

E: "She hasn't been right for about a week. She has been acting really weird, not doing the stuff she is supposed to be doing, not going to work. I don't know what is wrong. I've never seen her like this before."

C: "Mr. Sturm, have you noticed any recent complaints from your wife such as coughs, fevers, pain, or vomiting?"

E: "I did notice she was really shaky the other day and that she had been having some diarrhea the last 2 days with vomiting this morning. Also, last night, when I was talking to her about the house bills, she seemed to have no idea what I was saying."

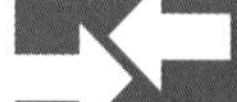

CRITICAL ACTION

Treating the patient's hyperthermia and beginning an immediate workup for altered mental status are both critical actions in this case.

C: "Are there any medications in the house?"

E: "I take BP medicines and something else that I can never remember."

C: "Could you please have someone bring all of the medicines to the ED?"

E: "Wow, sure, do you think this is a medicine problem? I don't think she takes any of my medicines."

C: "We just need to be sure we are evaluating all of the possibilities. Do you know if she has any medical problems?"

E: "Not that I know of, she doesn't even have a doctor as far as I am aware."

C: "Mrs. Sturm, have you been feeling sick lately?"

E: "I don't know."

C: "Mrs. Sturm, do you have any medical problems?"

E: "No."

C: "Mrs. Sturm, are you having any pain right now?"

E: "I feel weak."

C: "Are you on any medications?"

E: "No."

C: "Do you have any allergies to medicines?"

E: "No."

C: "Mr. Sturm, if any of her answers are different from what you know, please speak up."

E: "OK, so far I agree with what she has said. I know that she has no allergies to medicines."

C: "Any tobacco, alcohol, or drug use?"

E: "No."

C: "Do you know where we are now?"

E: "Maybe a hospital, but I'm not sure, I'm scared. I want to go home. Take me home."

C: "Mrs. Sturm, I'm going to examine you now."

C: "HEENT examination?"

E: "What are you looking for?"

C: "Any evidence of trauma, tenderness, swelling, hematomas?"

E: "No Battle sign, no raccoon's eyes; no external evidence of trauma."

C: "Eye examination, specifically pupil size and reactivity?"

E: "Normal."

C: "Is there icterus?"

E: "No."

C: "ENT examination?"

E: "Normal except for dry mucous membranes."

C: "Neck examination?"

E: "What are you looking for?"

C: "JVD, lymphadenopathy, suppleness, tenderness."

E: "No JVD or lymphadenopathy. Her neck is supple and non-tender over the spine."

C: "Heart examination? Any murmurs or gallops?"

E: "Normal except for tachycardia."

C: "Lung examination?"

E: "What do you want to know?"

C: "Are the breath sounds symmetric? Are there crackles or wheezing?"

E: "Tachypneic, but otherwise normal."

C: "Is there CVA tenderness present?"

E: "None present."

C: "Abdominal examination?"

E: "What do you want to know?"

C: "Are bowel sounds present? Is there tenderness, guarding, or masses?"

E: "Hyperactive bowel sounds are found. The abdomen is soft, non-tender, non-distended and there is no rebound or guarding. No masses are detected."

C: "Is there edema or cyanosis? Are the extremities intact? Is there tenderness?"

E: "The patient is diaphoretic. There is no cyanosis, clubbing, or edema."

C: "Is the patient oriented? What does the neuro examination show?"

E: "What would you like to know?"

C: "To the patient: 'I don't mean to insult you, but could you give me your full name and tell me the date today?'"

E: "Mrs. Jane Sturm. I'm not sure what day it is. I'm scared."

C: "Are there any focal findings related to motor strength, sensation, cerebellar examination, DTRs? Can she walk?"

E: "Sensation is grossly intact. Motor strength 4/5 throughout. A fine, resting tremor is noted. Reflexes are very brisk and symmetric. Patient is unable to perform cerebellar testing and gait is unsteady. Repeat vitals are T 39.9°C, BP 168/105, HR 130, RR 24, O_2 sat 99% on RA."

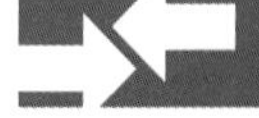

CRITICAL ACTION

There are several critical actions going on at this time:

- First, the candidate is initiating a full septic workup (including CT and LP), which is appropriate for a febrile and altered patient.
- Secondly, they are continuing to treat the patient's hyperthermia.

C: "Nurse, will you please administer Ibuprofen 600 mg orally for fever, give a repeat NS bolus of 500 cc and send blood for CBC, basic metabolic profile, liver function tests, a lipase, alcohol, aspirin, and acetaminophen levels. Check a bedside urine pregnancy test, send to the lab a UA, urine culture, and toxicology screen. Also get a stat ECG and portable CXR and arrange for a CT head scan. Please set up for a lumbar puncture (LP) as soon as the patient returns from radiology."

E: "Those orders are now done. The patient is not pregnant. The radiology department is calling for the patient. Is there anything else you would like to do before the patient goes to CT?"

DON'T FORGET

Do not let an unstable patient leave the ED for tests. Check an ECG and make sure vitals are stable before the patient leaves.

C: "Please administer ceftriaxone 2 g IV and then the patient can go for CT scanning accompanied by a nurse as long as the ECG shows no important changes and the potable CXR is unremarkable."

E: "The portable CXR has been done and is unremarkable. Here is your ECG" workup (see Fig. C34-1).

C: "If the vital signs have not deteriorated, the patient may go for CT scanning now."

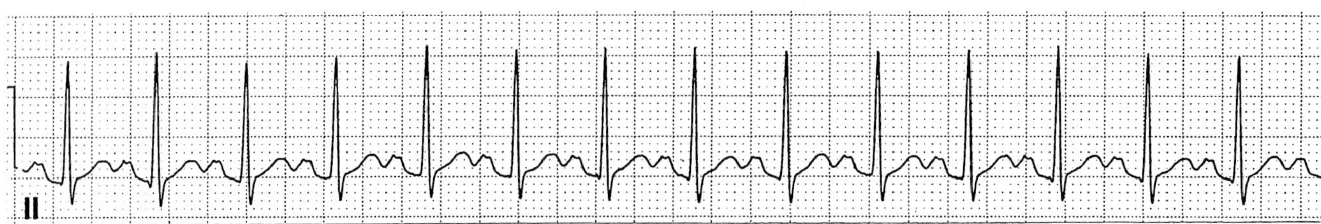

Figure C34-1. ECG with sinus tachycardia at 130, no acute ST- or T-wave abnormalities. (*Reprinted with permission from Stone CK, Humphries RL.* Current Diagnosis and Treatment: Emergency Medicine. *6th ed. New York, NY: McGraw-Hill; 2008.*)

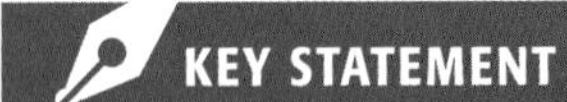

Remember to always inform the patient and get consent for any procedure you are planning to do.

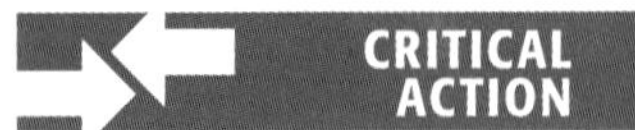

Continuing to treat the patient's persistent hyperthermia is a critical action in this case.

E: "The patient is back in the department and the radiologist called. The CT scan of the head is negative."

C: "Mr. Sturm, I'm concerned that your wife may have a serious brain infection. We need to perform a lumbar puncture to evaluate that possibility. We do this very frequently and there are rarely complications, but there is a small risk of infection at the puncture site. We use sterile equipment to decrease that risk. Do you have any questions about the procedure?"

E: "No."

C: "I will perform a LP using sterile technique. What is the opening pressure?"

E: "18."

C: "What does the fluid look like?"

E: "Clear and colorless."

C: "Please send the CSF for cell count and differential, glucose, protein, antigen panel, Gram stain, and culture."

E: "Your CSF is forwarded to the lab. The following laboratory studies are available: WBC 16,000, segs 89%, bands 5%, lymphs 5%. Hgb 16, Hct 48, plt 150,000. Na 140, K 4.5, Cl 102, HCO_3 20, BUN 25, Cr 1.3, glu 160, Ca 9.1. The LFTs are normal and the lipase is in the normal range. The UA is unremarkable."

C: "What are the repeat vital signs?"

E: "T 40°C, BP 158/102, HR 128, RR 22, O_2 sat 99% on RA."

C: "Let's start cooling measures with ice bags in the axilla and groin and a fan with water mist. Please repeat the temperature in 15 minutes and give me the result."

E: "The serum acetaminophen, aspirin, and alcohol levels are undetectable. The urine toxicology screen is negative. The CSF reveals RBC 0, WBC 0, glucose and protein normal, with a negative Gram stain."

E: "The nurse asks you a question: 'It doesn't seem that the patient has an obvious infection. What are your thoughts? What else could be going on?'"

C: "Her normal pulse oximetry and CXR indicate that pneumonia is unlikely, her urine is clear and her physical examination did not reveal focal findings of infection. Her CSF is also clear. I want to reexamine the patient."

E: "What else would you like to know?"

C: "Are there any rashes, specifically suggestive of cellulites or septicemia, like a petechial or purpuric rash? Is there thyroid enlargement or tenderness?"

E: "There is no evidence of cellulitis, petechiae, or purpura. There is an erythematous maculopapular rash over the bilateral shin areas. In addition, her thyroid is enlarged and tender."

C: "Nurse, please send a thyroid function panel. Is there any possibility of a stat TSH level?"

E: "Those tests have been sent and will be available in 2 hours."

C: "Mr. Sturm, it appears that your wife may have a thyroid problem that is causing her confusion and fever. We will begin treatment in the ED, and it will be continued in the ICU as this is a potentially life-threatening condition."

E: "OK, whatever you think is best."

C: "Nurse, please give Mrs. Sturm propranolol 80 mg PO and PTU 200 mg PO. I need to speak to the ICU attending on-call."

E: "That is Dr. James, and he is on the phone now."

C: "Hi Dr. James, this is Dr. Endoc in the ED. I have a 44-year-old female who presents with high fever, confusion, GI symptoms, and a negative sepsis workup in the ED, including normal CSF findings. She has an enlarged, tender thyroid gland. I believe she is likely to be in thyroid storm and I have started propranolol and PTU. She did receive one dose of ceftriaxone, 2 g IV, approximately one half hour prior to LP. Could you please come to the ED to see this patient and admit her to the ICU?"

E: "Certainly, I am on my way. Did you culture her urine and blood?"

C: "She has been fully cultured, including the CSF that I mentioned."

E: "The temperature has fallen to 37.6°C."

C: "You may discontinue the cooling fan and ice packs."

E: "This case is now over. Incidentally, the lab calls back 2 hours later—the TSH level is undetectable."

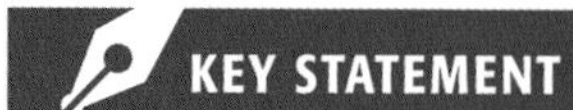

KEY STATEMENT

Remember to tell the patient and/or family about the plan and test results.

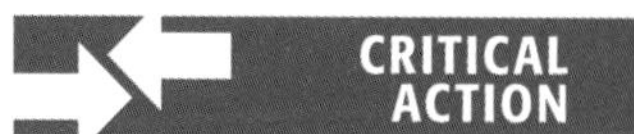

CRITICAL ACTION

There are two critical actions taking place here:

- First, the candidate has to discover and treat the thyroid storm.
- Secondly, they have to admit the patient to the ICU.

CASE ASSESSMENT

This was a tough case as the patient is very sick. There are many possible diagnoses and the final diagnosis is a rare condition. The candidate had a wide differential for fever and altered mental status (AMS) and was attempting to elicit as much historical information from both the patient and her husband as possible. In addition to questioning the patient and her husband, you can also ask for old charts, talk to paramedics or friends if available, and call other family members at home. Use any means possible to try and figure out what is going on.

Always pay attention to the vital signs. This patient's initial vital signs were abnormal (hypertensive, tachycardic, and febrile). Such patients need urgent intravenous (IV) access, oxygen, and placement on a monitor. The candidate initiated the basics and then did the best he could, under the circumstances, to obtain a history. When the VS are abnormal, delaying the basics for the history will be a disaster waiting to happen. For example, the patient could have been in atrial fibrillation associated with hyperthyroidism. If the candidate delays finding this out, you can bet that the examiner will have the patient "crash."

All patients with an AMS need an immediate bedside glucose. As a rule, during the oral board examination, any patient presenting with a depressed level of consciousness will require a bedside glucose check and naloxone (Narcan) administration. In this case, although the patient had AMS, her consciousness was not depressed and she had a normal pupil examination, so she was not given naloxone. However, because some synthetic opioids do not cause pupillary constriction, you will never be faulted for immediately giving it to an altered patient.

During the initial physical examination, the candidate did not perform a thyroid examination. When other causes of high fever and confusion had been ruled out, he returned to the bedside to assess the thyroid gland he'd initially overlooked. **It is important to appreciate that information not requested may not be given.** When the neck examination was elicited, the examiner asked, "What are you looking for?" This should have alerted the candidate that there was likely an abnormal finding that needed to be discovered. In this situation, you should continue asking questions about that portion of the exam until either you discover the abnormal finding or are told that there are no abnormal findings.

Additionally, regarding the physical examination, there may be an examiner prompt in those areas where one might reasonably look for a finding based on the chief complaint or additional history. For example, in this case, the patient had gastrointestinal (GI) complaints, so a detailed abdominal examination must be done. Also, the candidate could have performed a more thorough neurologic evaluation with regard to cranial findings. Any patient with AMS requires a full neurologic examination. You should ask about orientation, cranial nerves, muscle strength, deep tendon reflexes (DTRs), sensation including temperature, proprioception, gait, ataxia, speech, pronator drift, and Romberg test.

The candidate had a broad definition for infection and AMS and requesting appropriate labs and imaging. Even though most tests were negative, they could have helped the candidate find a source of infection or AMS: liver function tests (LFTs) (hepatitis), lipase (pancreatitis), urine analysis (UA), urinary tract infection (UTI), and tox screen results. Although not a critical action, the candidate obtained blood and urine cultures. Evaluation of fever and AMS includes a lumbar puncture (LP) for meningitis/encephalitis. A head computed tomography (CT) is also indicated for AMS and concern for infection. If meningitis is even a remote possibility, you must obtain blood cultures, initiate early empiric antibiotic therapy (and consider IV steroids). In this case, even though the cause of the patient's problem is thyroid storm, the early administration of antibiotics to treat a possible bacterial meningitis is a critical action. The addition of IV steroids and antiviral agents (to cover herpes encephalitis) would have been bonus points in scoring the "Health Care Provided" portion of the exam. Antibiotics must not be withheld until a CT of the head or LP has been performed.

The candidate may be asked to elaborate on planned procedures and asked to describe the procedure in detail. If not asked specifically for this information, it is acceptable to state, "I would perform a LP." The examiner will ask for any further information, if necessary. In addition, it is always a good habit to obtain informed consent from the patient for procedures. In this case, since the patient had AMS and was not in a capacity to sign consent, it was appropriate to explain the procedure to the husband and obtain consent from him.

It is very important to frequently reassess the patient's overall status and repeat the vital signs, especially those that were abnormal at any time during the case. A complete set of vitals should be requested periodically and after every intervention. A classic ABEM dodge is to omit abnormal vital signs. In this case, the candidate had to ask for the temperature. A missing vital sign is often a clue to a worsening condition or a diagnosis. It is important to reassess the patient's overall condition, including VS, prior to sending the patient out of the department for imaging, transfer or admission.

Ultimately, the initial history of confusion and fever, coupled with the lack of a positive sepsis workup and findings of both a pretibial rash and an enlarged, tender thyroid warrant the diagnosis of thyroid storm. The thyroid-stimulating hormone (TSH) screen is an appropriate study, but likely won't be immediately available at ABEM General. Cases like this will likely require a diagnosis on clinical grounds alone and treatment will initially be empiric. The candidate did this very well, starting propranolol and PTU. It is acceptable to look up dosing if necessary. Be resourceful if the examiner makes your first choice of reference unavailable. Remember that PTU is given before iodine.

This patient needed intensive care unit (ICU) admission and the ICU attending was appropriately consulted. Extra points would be given if the candidate discussed the case with an endocrinologist in addition to the ICU physician.

Always remember to let the patient know what is going on, what you are doing, and what the working diagnosis might be. If there are friends or other family members present, talk to them as well. In this case, the candidate did not initially explain to the patient or husband why she needed IV fluids, blood draws, and radiographic studies. However, later on, the candidate explained to the husband what her likely diagnosis was and why she needed to be admitted to the hospital.

Critical Actions

1. Use of antipyretics and cooling measures
2. Full sepsis workup, including LP for possible meningitis
3. Diagnosis and initiation of appropriate treatment for thyroid storm
4. ICU admission

Test Performance

1. *Data acquisition:* The data acquisition was appropriate, but should have included more thorough evaluation of the thyroid and a cranial nerve examination. To the candidate's credit, he returned to the physical examination when the infectious workup was negative. This second and more thorough, evaluation included questions related to rashes and the thyroid. Score = **7**
2. *Problem solving:* Problem solving was good and the candidate used the information given to stabilize and manage the patient. He performed an appropriate septic workup and circled back to the exam when that workup did not reveal the source of the AMS and fever. Score = **7**
3. *Patient management:* Patient care was appropriate. This patient's initial vital signs were abnormal (hypertensive, tachycardic, and febrile) and appropriately addressed. An appropriate septic workup was performed. The candidate sought repeat vital signs and responded appropriately by adding cool mist after oral antipyretics did not address the fever. The patient loses points for not using steroids empirically for meningitis and not covering for herpes encephalitis. Treating thyroid storm without a TSH level was appropriate. Score = **7**

4. *Resource utilization:* Although the workup was extensive, the candidate ordered tests that helped him rule out causes of fever and AMS and was logical in his approach. Score = **8**
5. *Health care provided (outcome):* The patient received appropriate treatment, and the candidate's interventions stabilized the patient. Score = **8**
6. *Interpersonal relations and communication skills:* The candidate's interactions with the patient, husband, nurse, and consultant were appropriate. However, the candidate did not initially explain to the patient why she needed IV fluids or blood draws and radiographic studies. Later on, the candidate explained to the husband his concerns, diagnosis, and need for admission. Score = **7**
7. *Comprehension of pathophysiology:* The examinee conveyed their understanding of appropriate AMS and septic workups and thyroid storm by the labs, imaging, and treatments they used. This was also conveyed during their consultation. Score = **7**
8. *Clinical competence (overall):* overall, the examinee showed clinical competence by obtaining an appropriate history and physical, developing a differential diagnosis, utilizing appropriate lab work and imaging, utilizing appropriate interventions, and working toward the appropriate disposition. Score = **7**

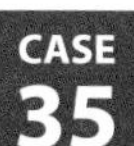

CASE 35 88 y/o Male With Fever and Change in Mental Status

John Dayton, Fiona Gallahue, and Richard Sinert

INITIAL INFORMATION

Name: Lawrence Best

Mode of arrival: Brought by ambulance

Age: 88 years

Gender: Male

VS: T 41.1°C (106°F), BP 80/40, HR 140, RR 8, O_2 sat: 94% on RA, wt: 70 kg

CC: Altered mental status

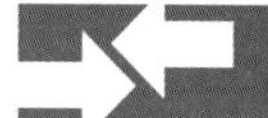

CRITICAL ACTION

In this case, obtaining an appropriate history is a critical action. If the patient is unable to speak with you, remember to talk with paramedics, family, friends, PMDs, and request charts.

PLAY OF THE CASE

C: "What do I see as I walk into the patient's room?"

E: "You see an elderly man lying supine on the stretcher not moving and not responding to you."

C: "I'd like to recheck the patient's responsiveness to voice first. I will perform a sternal rub if he is still unresponsive. I'd also like a blood glucose level."

E: "His blood glucose level is 120 mg/dL, he is unresponsive to both verbal and painful stimuli."

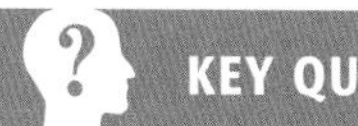

KEY QUESTION

Ask this open-ended question at the beginning of every case.

C: "I'll ask the paramedics to stay close so I can get more information from them in a minute. Is there anyone else with the patient who can help me obtain a history?"

C: "I'd like to check this patient to see if his airway is patent, check for stridor and any evidence of airway obstruction."

E: "His airway is patent, he has no stridor, he is moving air comfortably."

KEY ORDERS

Most of the patients you see during the exam are unstable (or will become that way). Every unstable patient requires IV access (preferably two large-bore IVs), oxygen, and cardiac monitoring (and in most cases an ECG). This part of the exam could have been handled better. The candidate should have asked for the "IV, O_2, monitor" part to be done while he assessed the airway.

C: "I'd like to start him on 100% NRB face mask, place him on a cardiac monitor, recheck a pulse ox on him, and listen to breath sounds. Do I hear and rales, rhonchi, wheezes? After oxygen is added, what is his new respiratory rate."

E: "He's on 100% NRB with a pulse ox of 96%, he has breath sounds with no rales, rhonchi, wheezes, and his respiratory rate is still 8."

C: "I'd like to start bag valve mask ventilating this patient, insert an oral pharyngeal airway (OPA), and see if he has a gag reflex."

E: "He is being bag valve mask ventilated, and an OPA is inserted with no gag reflex."

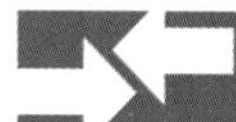

CRITICAL ACTION

Intubating this patient is a critical action. As he has no gag reflex (but is breathing appropriately), this is not an emergent intubation and taking a history first is appropriate.

C: "I'd like to get him set up for RSI intubation. Could the paramedics give me any medical history?"

E: "Certainly, they're here at the bedside."

C: "I'm going to need more information from you in a minute, but can you tell me if this man has any allergies to any medications?"

E: "No, he lives in an apartment above his daughter who reported that he had no allergies."

C: "Where is the daughter now?"

E: "She's still at home."

C: "OK. Do we have her number?"

E: "We wrote it down on our ambulance call report."

C: "Does he have any medical history?"

E: "BPH and HTN."

KEY ORDERS

Here the candidate is being very creative to get more information. Remember that you will not get information unless you ask for it! Ask for family members, and if they are not at the hospital ask if they can be contacted.

C: "What medications does he take for those?"

E: "He takes Ditropan, HCTZ, vitamin E, and Haldol every evening."

C: "What happened to him today?"

E: "His daughter said he seemed fine last night, but when she went to check on him in the morning he was still in bed. He felt very hot, and wouldn't respond to her, so she called 911."

C: "Was there any evidence of trauma or a fall?"

E: "No."

C: "Thank you for the help. Would you please continue to wait for me in the waiting room so I can get more history?"

E: "The paramedics are waiting in the waiting room."

C: "I'd like to perform RSI with lidocaine 100 mg pretreatment, a defasciculating dose of vecuronium of 0.01 mg/kg, etomidate 0.3 mg/kg, and then succinylcholine 1 mg/kg IV. I'd like to orotracheally intubate this patient. While we're getting the 18-gauge IV placed to give medications, I'd like to have the nurse draw blood for labs and blood cultures."

E: "The blood is drawn and the patient is now intubated."

C: "I'd like to recheck O_2 saturation, give 2 mg IV Ativan for sedation and muscle relaxation. I'd also like to given dantrolene since the patient is on a dopamine antagonist and could have neuroleptic malignant syndrome (NMS). Please check bilateral breath sounds, and check a post-intubation CXR as well as an ABG. I'd also like to have an NG tube and Foley placed."

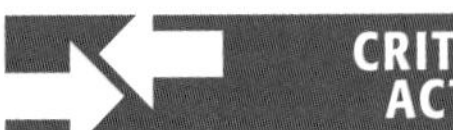

CRITICAL ACTION

Recognizing and treating the right main stem intubation is a critical action. If the candidate had not treated it promptly, the examiner would likely have crashed the patient.

E: "The saturation is 90% on 100% O_2, the breath sounds are greater on the right than the left, and the CXR is ordered. The ABG is pending."

C: "I'd like to deflate the cuff on the ET tube and move it back a few centimeters. Then I'd like to re-inflate the cuff and re-listen for breath sounds and check a pulse ox."

E: "He has good breath sounds bilaterally and 100% pulse oximetry reading now."

C: "I'd like to check circulation on this patient. Do I have a rhythm strip on this patient?"

E: "Rhythm strip shows sinus tachycardia at 140 with normal axis, QRS, ST segments, and T waves."

C: "I'd like to check this patient's capillary refill, mucous membranes, and skin color and temperature."

E: "His capillary refill is sluggish at >3 seconds, his mucous membranes are dry, and his skin is warm, reddish, and dry."

C: "I'd like to give this patient 1 L of NS bolus and listen to his chest halfway through to make sure he is not developing evidence of pulmonary edema while

I am bolusing him. Please let me know when his bolus is finished and what his repeat vital signs are at that time. I'd also like to have at least two fans in the room with the patient to make sure that he is sprayed with atomized water. Please place ice packs around his body to bring down the temperature. Please discontinue the fans, atomized water, and ice packs when the patient's temperature reaches 39°C (102.2°F)."

Treating the patient's hyperthermia is a critical action.

E: "That is being done."

C: "I'd like a 12-lead ECG on this patient."

E: "It looks the same as the rhythm strip. The patient's ABG and post-intubation CXR are back."

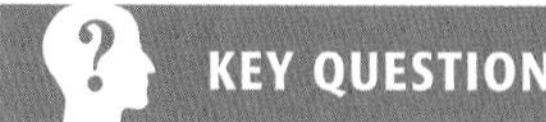

Remember to ask for vital signs after every intervention to assess whether or not it worked.

ABG 7.2/180/60, BE –6, bicarb 12, O_2 sat 100%

CXR: ETT in good position, NGT seen in stomach, no infiltrates, no effusions

C: "I'd like to send the patient's blood for CBC, electrolytes, two sets of blood cultures, BUN/Cr, LFTs, CPK, troponin, EtOH level, TSH, T4, PT/PTT, and type and screen."

E: "That's being done."

KEY ORDERS

Remember that you can request for orders to stop when a goal is reached. In this case, the candidate tells the nurse to stop the active cooling at a certain temperature. Do not allow treatments to be carried on indefinitely.

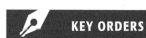

C: "I'd like to recheck his neurologic status. Is he still unresponsive to verbal and painful stimuli?"

E: "He is."

C: "I'd like to check his pupils for anisocoria and reactivity to light."

E: "There is no evidence of anisocoria and his pupils are 3 mm bilaterally and reactive to light."

C: "I'd like to make sure the patient is fully undressed and I'd like to look for any evidence of trauma, bleeding, medic alert tags, or deformity and roll him so I can visualize his back for the same."

E: "He's fully undressed with no bleeding, deformity, medic alert tags, or evidence of trauma."

C: "I'd like to check a rectal examination and a guaiac test."

E: "Rectal examination is normal except for an enlarged prostate; his guaiac is negative with brown stool."

C: "I'd like to have a rectal probe placed to monitor his temperature. I'd like to monitor urine output from the Foley. Has the patient made urine since placement of the Foley?"

E: "Patient has 30 cc of dark urine output."

C: "Please send it for UA, tox screen, and urine culture."

E: "Doctor, the patient's bolus is finished. His repeat vital signs are T 40.2°C (104.5°F), BP 90/60, HR 125, and ventilated at a rate of 12 on the ventilator, his pulse ox is 100%."

C: "I'd like Mr. Best to get a non-contrast head CT and one more liter of NS bolus."

E: "He's going to CT right now with the bolus started."

Do not send an unstable patient to the scanner unescorted!

C: "Could we please make sure another doctor accompanies Mr. Best to CT?"

E: "That's being taken care of."

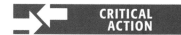

C: "I'd like to get the paramedics back to get more history."

E: "They got called back to the station."

C: "I'd also like to call the daughter."

E: "She's on the line."

C: "Hello, this is Dr. C. Are you Lawrence Best's daughter?"

E: "Yes, my name is Angela Carter."

C: "Ms. Carter, can you tell me more about what happened to your father?"

E: "I'll try."

C: "What did you notice about your father today when you called 911?"

E: "He wasn't moving or speaking this morning and last night he was totally fine! I was really worried about him, especially because of this heat wave and him not having air conditioning in his apartment."

C: "Ms. Carter, did your father complain of feeling ill yesterday? Did he talk about a having a cough or abdominal pain?"

E: "No, he seemed to be doing just fine."

C: "Does your father use drugs or alcohol?"

E: "No."

C: "Did he have any recent falls that you know of or did he complain of a headache?"

E: "No."

C: "Does your father have a regular doctor at this hospital?"

E: "Yes, Dr. Smith is his doctor."

C: "Does he have any other medical problems besides HTN and BPH?"

E: "No."

C: "Does he take any other medications besides HCTZ, Ditropan, Haldol, and vitamin E?"

E: "No."

C: "Does he have any allergies to medications?"

E: "No."

C: "Thank you so much for your help. Your father is going to have to stay in the hospital for a while until we stabilize him."

E: "Doctor, your patient is back from the CT scanner. His CT scan is ready and his labs are available. His repeat VS are T 39°C (102.2°F), HR 110, BP 110/80, pulse ox: 100%."

- CBC: WBC 9, Hgb/Hct 13/39, Plt 200
- Electrolytes*:* Na 140, Cl 108, K 4, CO_2 20, BUN 26, Cr 1.4, Glu 110
- LFT: ALT 200, AST 250
- CPK: 50
- Troponin <0.1
- CK-MB 2
- UA: SG 1.010, no blood, no leukocytes, no nitrites, no bili

- Urine tox negative for cocaine, opioids, methadone, barbiturates, or benzodiazepines
- CT head: normal, no blood, mass shift, or infarcts seen. Normal age-related atrophy

C: "I'd like to use antibiotics to cover the patient for possible meningitis. I'm going to give him ceftriaxone, vancomycin, ampicillin. I will add dexamethasone to cover possible bacterial meningitis. I'd also like to perform a LP on this patient after getting consent from the patient's daughter."

E: "Those orders are being carried out. The LP is done."

C: "I'd like to send CSF for Gram stain, culture, cell count, protein, and glucose. I'd like to finish the rest of my secondary survey. Can I quickly resurvey the HEENT examination? Earlier, he had dry mucous membranes. How does the patient appear now?"

E: "His mucous membranes are less dry now."

C: "I'd like to check CV and chest exams."

E: "He's tachycardic with no murmurs, rubs, or gallops. Chest examination sounds clear with no rhonchi, rales, or wheezing."

C: "Abdominal examination?"

E: "Normal."

C: "His extremities had poor capillary refill, how do they look now?"

E: "His capillary refill is improved to <3 seconds."

C: "His neuro examination was remarkable for no response to verbal or noxious stimuli. How is he now?"

E: "He's responding to pain now by withdrawing to painful stimuli."

C: "I'd like to recheck his vital signs."

E: "T 39°C (102.2°F), HR 100, BP 120/70, RR at 12 via ventilator. We're holding the atomized water, fans, and ice packs."

C: "Thank you. I'd like to start a NS drip of 100 cc/h for Mr. Best. I'd also like to call Dr. Smith."

E: "He's on the line."

C: "Dr. Smith, this is Dr. C. I have your patient, Lawrence Best here in the ED. He came in from home with a temperature of 41.1°C (106°F), hypotensive, tachycardic, and unresponsive. According to his daughter, he was fine when she last saw him the night. His apartment has no air conditioning and the temperature in his apartment is quite hot. He's on Ditropan and HCTZ, which would also predispose him to hyperthermia. He may have neuroleptic malignant syndrome since he's on Haldol QHS. On examination, he was unresponsive with no gag reflex. I intubated him in the ED, got a CT scan of his head which shows no acute abnormality, performed a LP with the results pending, covered him with antibiotics for possible meningitis, gave him 2 L of NS and cooled him using water and fans. He's showing some improvement now, but he needs to be admitted to the ICU for further monitoring and management."

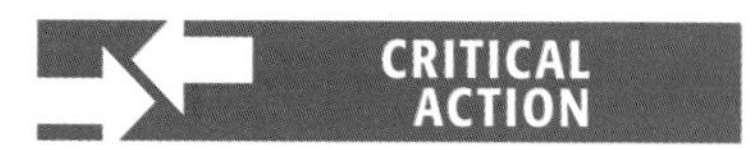

Admitting the patient to the appropriate level is a critical action.

E: "I agree, I'll follow the cultures and the patient. Please admit the patient to my service. That concludes this case."

CASE ASSESSMENT

This was a challenging case with multiple problems to manage. The candidate did a good job of addressing all of the emergent issues and prioritizing the airway, breathing, and circulation (ABCs). As this patient was unable to give a history, the candidate did a great job of speaking with the paramedics and the patient's daughter. Remember to use several resources to obtain patient history: family members, medical records, private doctors, and bystanders, etc.

The candidate did an excellent job of moving rapidly through the ABCs and addressing each issue that came up in the patient's scenario. The cause of altered mental status (AMS) was unclear, so the candidate focused on the patients presenting symptoms and medical history, kept the differential wide, treated the most likely causes, sent labs to help rule in/out certain problems, and used the historians to try to help narrow the differential. The patient could be altered for any number of reasons: sepsis, myocardial infarction (MI), rhabdomyolysis, neuroleptic malignant syndrome (NMS), heat stroke, drug intoxication, or meningitis. The diagnosis is still unclear at the end of the scenario, just as it often is in the emergency department (ED).

In order to manage this patient appropriately, the candidate focused on the ABCs of the case. While managing the ABCs, the candidate needed to intubate this patient and intubated the right main stem bronchus. She recognized the error right away and corrected it immediately.

This scenario also required the candidate to keep rechecking vital signs and neuro status to monitor the patient's progress. This is very helpful in the unstable patients in order to make sure their management is appropriate. As an examinee, you can never recheck vital signs too often.

Critical Actions

1. Address and treat potential causes of AMS.
2. Intubate the patient.
3. Recognize a right main stem intubation and correct it.
4. Use rapid cooling of the patient.
5. Speak with historians.
6. Admit the patient to the ICU.

Test Performance

1. *Data acquisition:* Data acquisition is excellent. The differential diagnosis for this patient is very broad, requiring the candidate to narrow it with her history and physical examination. She ordered a number of tests, but given the wide differential, this was appropriate. Score = **8**
2. *Problem solving:* Problem solving is excellent. The candidate was able to rapidly assimilate data from the patient encounter, interpret test results, and synthesize information quickly to direct further management. She was also able to remember that there was another historian when her original historians disappeared. Score = **8**
3. *Patient management:* The examinee recognized when interventions needed to be made and intubated and cooled the patient appropriately. She also obtained the appropriate consultation to admit the patient to the ICU. Score = **8**

4. *Resource utilization:* Although the patient ordered several lab and imaging studies, they were all appropriate and based on her differential diagnosis for AMS with fever. She remembered to ask for the results and directed care based on her findings. She was also resourceful in obtaining history from paramedics and the patient's daughter. Score = **8**
5. *Health care provided (outcome):* The candidate did an excellent job of working with little information. She made the appropriate treatment decisions based on patient information, scientific evidence, and clinical judgement. She did an excellent job of rechecking vital signs and adjusting therapy appropriately. Score = **8**
6. *Interpersonal relations and communication skills:* The candidate did a good job of effectively communicating with the daughter and her professional colleagues in this scenario. She could have provided more information to the daughter and her consultation could have been a bit more concise. Score = **7**
7. *Comprehension of pathophysiology:* The examinee developed, and tested, a broad differential for AMS and fever in an elderly patient. She made appropriate interventions and used test results to guide appropriate therapy. Score = **8**
8. *Clinical competence (overall):* Overall, the examinee showed clinical competence by her interventions, work-up, treatment, consultation, and admission to the ICU. Score = **8**

CASE 36 80 y/o Female With Weakness

Rohit Gupta and John Dayton

INITIAL INFORMATION

Name: Mary Jones

Mode of arrival: Brought in by family

Age: 80 years

Gender: Female

VS: BP 158/82, HR 77, RR 16, T 36.5°C (97.7°F), sat: 96% on RA

CC: Weakness

KEY QUESTION

Ask this open-ended question at the beginning of every case.

PLAY OF THE CASE

C: "What do I see as I walk into the patient's room?"

E: "The patient is a well-appearing, small, thin female. She is lying on the stretcher fully dressed."

C: "Hello, Mrs. Jones. I am Dr. Acsdrome. I'm going to take care of you today. What brings you in to see us?"

E: "I'm not feeling well. I've been tired all weekend, and I don't have any energy."

C: "How long have you been feeling weak?"

E: "All weekend, doc. When I woke up on Saturday, I felt like I hadn't slept. I just haven't felt right."

C: "What exactly do you mean by feeling tired? Is it that you have no energy?"

E: "That's right, doc. I have no energy. I feel like I don't have the strength to stand."

C: "Are you having any pain in your chest or abdomen?"

E: "No."

C: "What makes the weakness better or worse?"

E: "I feel more tired if I walk. The only thing I want to do is rest."

C: "Anything else you notice when you walk?"

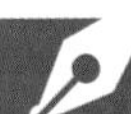

KEY ORDERS

Most of the patients you see during the exam are unstable (or will become that way). Every unstable patient requires IV access, oxygen, and cardiac monitoring (and in most cases an ECG). In this case, as the patient is stable at the moment, getting a brief history before initiating these orders was appropriate.

E: "I feel a little sick to my stomach when I walk, but it goes away when I rest."

C: "Are you short of breath?"

E: "Only after I walk a bit."

C: "Nurse, please place the patient on a cardiac monitor and give me a rhythm strip, start a NS IV at a KVO rate, check a pulse ox on RA, and then place the patient on 2-L O_2 NC. Send labs for CBC with diff, BMP, liver function tests, lipase, D-dimer, and cardiac labs including troponin and BNP. Also, please check a UA and a fingerstick glucose. I would like the tech to get an ECG. I would like to order a CXR."

E: "That is being done. The rhythm strip shows a normal sinus rhythm at 82 bpm. Pulse ox is 94% on RA which improved to 98% on O_2. The glucose is 100."

C: "Mrs. Jones, have you had any fevers or chills?"

E: "No, no chills. If anything, I feel like I've been sweating."

C: "Do you have a runny nose, sore throat, or cough?"

E: "I thought I might have been coming down with something last week, but then I felt better and didn't really get sick."

C: "Are you eating okay? Any nausea or vomiting?"

E: "I don't have much of an appetite. The thought of food makes me sick."

C: "Have you vomited?"

E: "No."

C: "Any diarrhea or constipation?"

E: "No."

C: "Any abdominal pain?"

E: "No pain, doctor."

C: "Any burning or pain when you urinate? Any back pain?"

E: "I haven't been peeing that much, but no pain or burning."

C: "Any numbness or weakness in your arms or legs?"

E: "No, I'm moving fine."

C: "Any dizziness or light-headedness? Do you feel like the world is spinning?"

E: "No."

C: "So you've been feeling weak since Saturday. Walking makes the weakness worse. You feel a little nauseated. Nothing else seems to be bothering you. Is that correct?"

E: "That's right doctor."

C: "What medical problems do you have?"

E: "I have high blood pressure, diabetes, and heart problems. I had bypass surgery 5 years ago."

C: "Are you taking any medications?"

E: "ASA, metoprolol, Lisinopril, glyburide, metformin, and eye drops for my glaucoma."

C: "Are you allergic to anything?"

E: "No."

C: "I would like to perform a physical examination. Is the patient's oral mucosa moist, is there mucous in her nose, is there erythema on oropharyngeal exam?"

E: "The oral mucosa is dry. No mucous in the nose. No pharyngeal erythema."

C: "Neck examination?"

E: "What are you looking for?"

C: "Is the neck supple? Are there bruits, masses, or a goiter? Is there JVD or lymphadenopathy?"

E: "Normal neck examination except for minimal JVD."

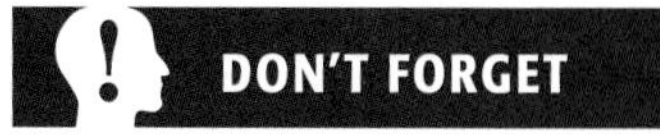

During the ABEM exam, expect each encounter to involve a patient with pathology. Workups will reveal disease. If the pathology is not clear from the history and physical examination, broaden your differential and order more tests. There are no negative workups on exam day!

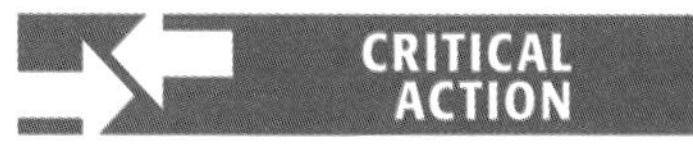

An elderly person with weakness can have just about anything. Casting a wide net, including cardiac and infectious etiologies is a critical action in this case.

C: "I would like to examine the patient's heart and lungs. Are there crackles or wheezes? Any murmurs, rubs, or gallops?"

E: "On the lung examination, there are fine bibasilar crackles. The heart examination is normal."

C: "Is the abdomen soft? Any tenderness, rigidity, guarding? Any flank pain? Are bowel sounds present?"

E: "The abdomen is mildly tender to palpation in the epigastrium. No flank or back tenderness. No RUQ tenderness. BS are present."

C: "Extremity examination? Pulses, cyanosis, edema, or rash?"

E: "Normal."

C: "Neurologic examination? Is the patient's gait normal? Is the cranial nerve examination normal? Are the sensory and motor examinations normal? Cerebellar function examination?"

E: "The sensory, cranial nerve, and cerebellar function examinations are normal. When the patient stands to walk, she gets noticeably short of breath and has to sit down. She is unable to cooperate with your examination saying that she is too tired."

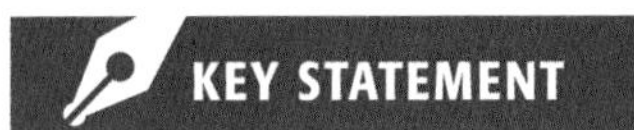

Remember to communicate with your patient. Tell them about your concerns, the plan, test results, etc.

C: "Mrs. Jones, I'm not quite sure what is wrong. There are several things that I want to check. I want to make sure you do not have an infection. I want to make sure your kidney function is normal and that you don't have low blood counts. Your blood sugar is OK, but we will look for other blood chemistry problems. Finally, I want make sure that you are not having a problem with your heart."

E: "Your ECG is performed (see Fig. C36-1)."

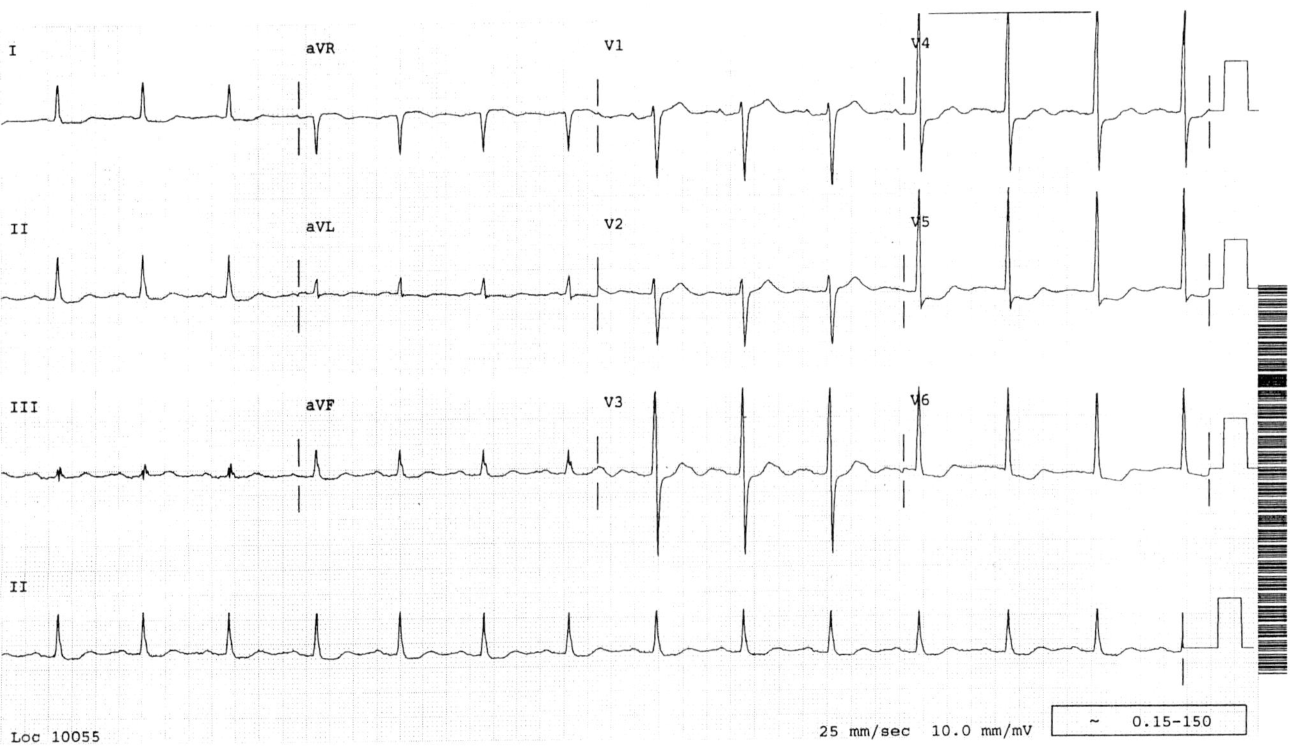

Figure C36-1. ECG. *(Reproduced with permission from Fuster V, O'Rourke RA, Walsh R, Poole-Wilson P.* Hurst's The Heart. *12th ed. New York, NY: McGraw-Hill; 2008.)*

C: "The ECG demonstrates LVH with strain. I cannot rule out ischemia. Is an old ECG available for comparison?"

E: "No old ECG is available."

C: "Mrs. Jones, where do you get your regular medical care?"

E: "I see Dr. Penn. He's my heart doctor."

C: "I would like the secretary to speak to Dr. Penn on the phone and have his office fax a copy of her most recent ECG."

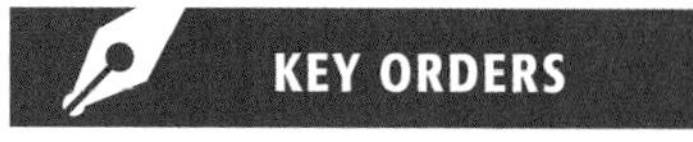

KEY ORDERS

This is a good strategy—you can usually get information if you continue to dig for it.

E: "That is being done. The following results are back."

Blood sugar: 257

UA:		CBC:		Chem 7:	
SG:	1.015	WBC	12.5	Na	142
Gluc:	negative	Hgb	11.7	K	4.3
Prot:	trace	Hct	35.1	Cl	105
Bili:	negative	Plt	457	HCO_3	24
Heme:	negative			BUN	27
Nit:	negative			Cr	1.8
LE:	negative			Gluc	263

C: "There is no evidence of a urinary tract infection (UTI). The WBC count is slightly elevated. Is a differential available?"

E: "The differential is pending. Here is your CXR (see Fig. C36-2)."

C: "The CXR is consistent with mild interstitial edema. No obvious infiltrate or consolidation."

E: "The following labs are back."

BNP: 475   Total CK: 400   Troponin T 4.1

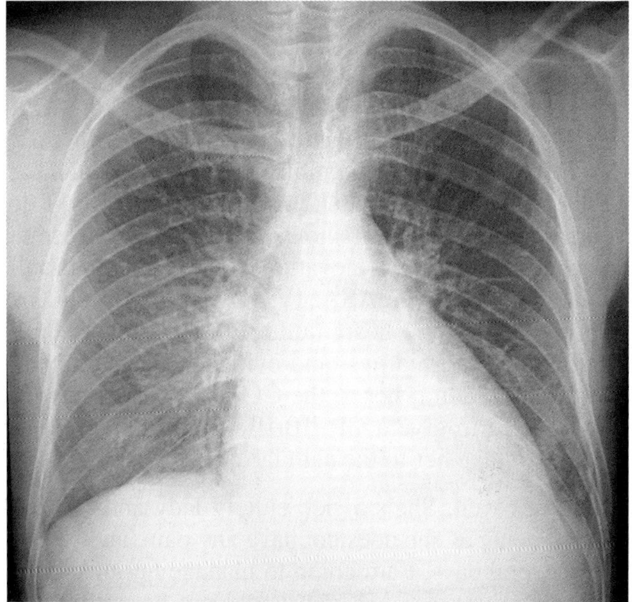

Figure C36-2. CXR showing mild interstitial edema. (*Reproduced with permission from Schwartz* DT. Emergency Radiology: Case Studies. *New York, NY: McGraw-Hill; 2008.*)

C: "The patient is having a non–ST-elevation MI (NSTEMI). Mrs. Jones, your blood work shows that you are having a heart attack. Patients with diabetes can have heart attacks without chest pain. I think it is what is making you feel so weak and SOB. The heart attack has weakened your heart muscle and is causing fluid to back up into your lungs. Did you take your medications, especially your ASA, today?"

E: "No, I didn't take any of medications today."

C: "We are going to have to give you several medications to begin treating your condition. I will also speak to your cardiologist to get you admitted to the CCU. Nurse, please have the patient chew on 325 mg of ASA. Recheck vital signs and repeat an ECG. Has an old ECG arrived?"

E: "No old ECG is available. The ASA is given and repeat vital signs are BP 145/88, HR 82, RR 20, O_2 sat: 98% on 4 L via NC. Repeat ECG is unchanged."

C: "I would like the patient's cardiologist paged."

E: "The cardiologist is paged."

Diagnosing the NSTEMI is a critical action in this case.

C: "Administer Lasix 40 mg IV. Begin a nitroglycerin drip at 50 µg/min, titrate upward by 10 µg/min as long as the patient's BP remains >100/60 mm Hg."

E: "It is being done."

C: "Mrs. Jones, I have given you a medication to make you urinate. It should help get some of the fluid off your lungs. I'm also starting a second medication to lower your BP and dilate your blood vessels, reducing the workload for your heart. In order to give you blood thinning medications, I need to perform a rectal examination to make sure you are not bleeding. Have you ever had bleeding in your brain or recent surgery."

Treating this NSTEMI with ASA and nitro titrated to comfort and control of blood pressure is a critical action in this case.

E: "No I've never had bleeding in my brain or any surgery."

E: "Patient complies for a rectal examination which reveals guaiac negative, brown stool."

C: "Please administer Lovenox 1 mg/kg SC."

E: "That is done. Mrs. Jones' cardiologist, Dr. Heart, is on the phone."

C: "Hello Dr. Heart, I am Dr. C. I have an 80-year-old female with dyspnea on exertion and weakness for several days. She is not having, and has not had, any chest pain. As you know, she has extensive CAD, s/p cath and CABG, HTN, and DM. Her physical examination reveals pulmonary basilar crackles and O_2 sat of 94% on RA. Her ECG shows LVH with strain. I do not have an old ECG for comparison. Her CXR shows mild interstitial edema. Her troponin is 4.1. She is having a non–ST-elevation MI with resultant mild congestive heart failure (CHF). I have given ASA, IV nitroglycerin, and Lovenox. I have withheld metoprolol, given the heart failure, though she is on metoprolol at home. Given her age, comorbidities, and evidence of significant cardiac dysfunction, I would like to admit her to the CCU. Also, she may need a cardiac catheterization. I waited to give a GP IIB/IIIA inhibitor or clopidogrel until I knew if you wanted to take her to the cath lab."

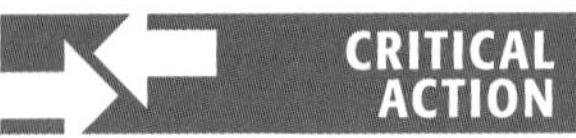

Admitting the patient to an appropriate level of care is a critical action.

E: "I know Mrs. Jones well. She's a sick elderly lady and she has had a lot of problems recently. Seeing as she does not have any pain, and her symptoms have been ongoing for several days, I am going to manage her medically. I know that she has extensive three-vessel CAD and would not be willing to have another bypass. Go ahead and give her the clopidogrel. I'll be in to see her immediately."

E: "This case is now over."

CASE ASSESSMENT

The candidate managed this case extremely well. In general, most ABEM cases are straightforward. Patients present with typical histories, classic physical examinations, and expected labs. Most cases are not as straightforward in the real world. The goal of this case is to demonstrate what to do when the diagnosis is not clear. The initial decision that must be made based on vital signs, age, and chief complaint, is whether the patient is sick. If the patient seems sick, stabilize the patient immediately. Assess the airway, breathing, and circulation (ABCs), start an IV (or two), and place the patient on the monitor. If the patient seems stable, then begin your evaluation as you normally would in the emergency department (ED), with a thorough history and physical examination.

In this case, the candidate appropriately assessed that the patient was stable. He proceeded to take a very thorough history and perform a complete physical examination. The patient provided a nonspecific chief complaint that was not clarified despite the excellent history and physical examination. The candidate noted the potential problems highlighted by the history (weakness, dyspnea on exertion, subacute course, extensive cardiac history, and crackles on examination) and generated an appropriate differential. He then ordered appropriate tests to evaluate each item on his differential.

During the ABEM exam, expect each encounter to involve a patient with pathology. Workups will reveal disease. If the pathology is not clear from the history and physical examination, re-examine the patient, broaden your differential, and order more tests. You are graded on efficient resource utilization, but do not miss making the diagnosis because you are trying to avoid ordering a few additional tests.

Throughout the encounter, the candidate played the role of the physician well, issuing commands, addressing the patient, and moving through the case. In particular, the candidate did a very nice job of telling the patient what he was thinking and giving her updates as information became available.

Having diagnosed a non–ST-elevation myocardial infarction (NSTEMI) with congestive heart failure (CHF), the candidate capably managed the MI. He instituted oxygen, acetylsalicylic acid (ASA), and IV nitroglycerin. IV nitro in the setting of ischemia and CHF is absolutely indicated. The patient started a relatively high dose with parameters, which is also appropriate. He withheld an IV beta-blocker because the patient had evidence of CHF. Some may argue that with mild CHF and definite ischemia, a beta-blocker may be indicated. We would advise that you avoid actions that can be debated or that could be potentially harmful.

The candidate appropriately risk-stratified the patient, determined that she was high risk, and admitted her to the cardiac care unit (CCU). In discussing the case with the cardiologist he suggested the need for coronary catheterization and offered to start a GP IIB/IIIA inhibitor. When the cardiologist opted for medical management, the candidate deferred. Finally, the patient knew the indications for clopidogrel.

Critical Actions

1. Diagnosis of NSTEMI
2. Nitroglycerin and ASA for management of ischemia and CHF
3. Admission to CCU
4. Broad differential for weakness with evaluation of multiple potential etiologies

Test Performance

1. *Data acquisition:* This phase is superb as the candidate shows ability to obtain a more than adequate history and physical examination in an efficient manner and orders appropriate tests to assist in diagnosis. Score = **8**
2. *Problem solving:* Problem solving is excellent as the candidate is able to quickly assimilate data from the patient encounter and interprets test results to efficiently direct further management. Score = **8**
3. *Patient management:* The candidate makes appropriate treatment decisions based on patient information, scientific evidence, and clinical judgment. Score = **8**
4. *Resource utilization:* The candidate demonstrates a sound, systems-based practice with an efficient use of tests that does not compromise patient care. He may be criticized for ordering too many tests, but given the vague history, it is appropriate to evaluate for several etiologies of his broad differential diagnosis. Score = **7**
5. *Health care provided (outcome):* The patient received appropriate treatment, consultation and disposition to the CCU. Score = **8**
6. *Interpersonal relations and communication skills:* The candidate engages in effective information exchange with both the patient and professional associates. Score = **8**
7. *Comprehension of pathophysiology:* The examinee conveyed their understanding of an atypical presentation of acute coronary syndrome (ACS) in an elderly patient with cardiac risk factors. This was shown in both the workup and in the conversation with the cardiologist. Score = **8**
8. *Clinical competence (overall):* Overall, the examinee obtained a thorough history and physical, created and tested an appropriate differential diagnosis, made the diagnosis and the appropriate disposition. Score = **8**

CASE 37 38 y/o Male With Sore Throat and Fever

John Dayton and Fiona Gallahue

INITIAL INFORMATION

Name: William Brown

Mode of arrival: Walk in

Age: 38 years

Gender: Male

VS: T 39.1°C (102.5°F), BP 130/80, HR 120, RR 18, O_2 sat: 98% on RA

CC: Sore throat

PLAY OF THE CASE

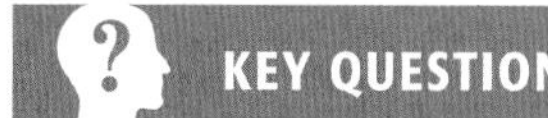

Ask this open-ended question at the beginning of every case.

C: "What do I see as I walk into the patient's room?"

E: "You see a well-developed, athletic-looking man in moderate distress."

C: "Hello Mr. Brown, I'm Dr. E. What can we do for you today?"

E: "I'm having a terrible sore throat. I can't swallow, and I think I have a fever."

C: "When did these symptoms start?"

E: "Yesterday, but I woke up today feeling like I couldn't breathe when I was lying down. It really scared me."

C: "Tell me about that."

E: "Yesterday, it hurt to swallow. Today, when I try to swallow, not only do I have pain, but I also feel like there is swelling in my throat. It's embarrassing to say, but I feel like I've been drooling."

C: "Have you had any other problems like a cough or body aches?"

E: "No, no cough or body aches."

C: "Is anybody sick at your home or work?"

E: "No, nobody that I can think of."

C: "Do you have any medical problems?"

E: "No."

C: "Do you take any medications, including over-the-counter and herbal medications?"

E: "No."

C: "Do you have any allergies to medications?"

E: "No."

C: "Do you have a regular doctor?"

E: "No, I don't go to doctors often."

DON'T FORGET

Remember that when an examiner states that part of the examination is "normal," it means that there are no findings.

When they say "What are you looking for?" it means that there is likely an important finding during that part of the exam.

KEY ORDERS

Most of the patients you see during the exam are unstable (or will become that way). Every unstable patient requires IV access (preferably two large-bore IVs), oxygen, and cardiac monitoring (and in most cases an ECG).

As this patient was stable, it was appropriate for the candidate to delay these orders until they noticed a potential life-threat on the physical examination.

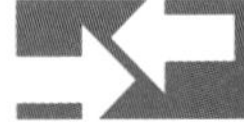

CRITICAL ACTION

Recognizing the potential life- and airway threat is a critical action in this case.

KEY ORDERS

Remember that if you are unsure of a dose of any drug, you can say that you will look it up. The only drugs for which this is not acceptable are code drugs.

C: "OK, I'd like to examine Mr. Brown. What do I see when I do my HEENT examination?"

E: "What are you looking for?"

C: "I'm looking for pharyngeal erythema or exudate, peritonsilar abscess, caries, uvular deviation, deformity of the neck, or cervical lymphadenopathy."

E: "Examination is difficult because Mr. Brown is unable to fully open his mouth. When he opens as far as he is able, you note diffuse pharyngeal erythema but do not see exudate, uvular deviation, or cervical lymphadenopathy. However, you do note that his posterior oropharynx has an abrasion and irritation."

C: "I would like to ask him about the abrasions. 'Mr. Brown, the back of your throat looks like it's scratched. Can you tell me about that?'"

E: "I like to eat chicken wings. When I was eating one 2 nights ago, one of the bones broke and it might have scraped me."

C: "Did you swallow it?"

E: "I don't think so."

C: "Have the nurse start a large-bore IV in the antecubital fossa, draw and hold blood work for possible tests, place the patient on 2 L O_2 by NC, place him on a cardiac monitor, and get me a 12-lead ECG. Please start with a 1 L bolus of NS and order a portable CXR and soft tissue x-ray of his neck."

E: "Those orders are being carried out."

C: "I'd like to visualize the neck carefully. Are there deformities on visual examination of the neck?"

E: "His anterior neck feels diffusely tender, and you note bilateral cervical lymphadenopathy, but you do not palpate any other abnormality. You note that he seems to prefer keeping his neck in a hyperextended position."

C: "I'd like to finish the rest of my examination, but make sure that the patient is sitting at all times. I'd like to listen to the heart and lungs, how do they sound?"

E: "Normal."

C: "I'd like to do an abdominal examination now, how does his abdomen feel?"

E: "Normal."

C: "I'd like to check the patient's extremities and skin especially looking for any rashes, cyanosis, or injury."

E: "His extremities and skin are normal."

C: "I'd like to give the patient antibiotics to an oral infection. I think clindamycin would cover it, but I'd like to double check that in my Sanford guide."

E: "Clindamycin IV, 600 mg, is recommended."

C: "OK, I'd like to give the patient 600 mg of clindamycin IV, and call the ENT surgeon on call. I'd like to send the labs for CBC, electrolytes, PT/PTT, type and screen, and two sets of blood cultures. Please make sure there is a difficult airway kit at the bedside. Thank you."

E: "Those labs are being sent. The soft tissue neck is ready for you. The CXR is normal with no sign of PNA, PTX, or foreign body" (see Fig. C37-1).

C: "This lateral neck x-ray shows increased thickness of the prevertebral space. Instead of just the 5 mm expected, the width is more than half the wide of the C4 vertebrae."

E: "Dr. Otolar is on the phone for you."

C: "Hello, Dr. Otolar, this is Dr. E. I have a patient here with retropharyngeal abscess. He was eating chicken wings 2 days ago and believes a bone may have scraped the back of his throat. He is having difficulty tolerating secretions, has a high fever of 38.8°C (102°F), and he's unable to breathe well lying down. I'm very concerned about the rapid progression of his disease and I think he may need operative management. I've already started him on IV clindamycin."

E: "Thank you, Dr. E. I'm in the OR right now. It sounds like he does need surgery but I'm concerned about possible mediastinal abscess. Do you think you could order a chest CT for the patient so we can make sure the infection hasn't tracked further?"

C: "Actually, Dr. Otolar, the patient cannot lie flat comfortably, and given the extent of the swelling, I don't think it's safe to have him lie flat for a chest CT. I have a surgical airway kit by the bedside in case he begins to have trouble breathing. When do you expect you'll be out of the OR?"

E: "Well, this case is pretty complicated, I think it'll take a few hours. My partner, Dr. Smith is in the hospital doing rounds currently. Could you page him and see if he can see your patient now since it seems to be fairly urgent?"

C: "OK."

E: "Dr. Smith is on the line."

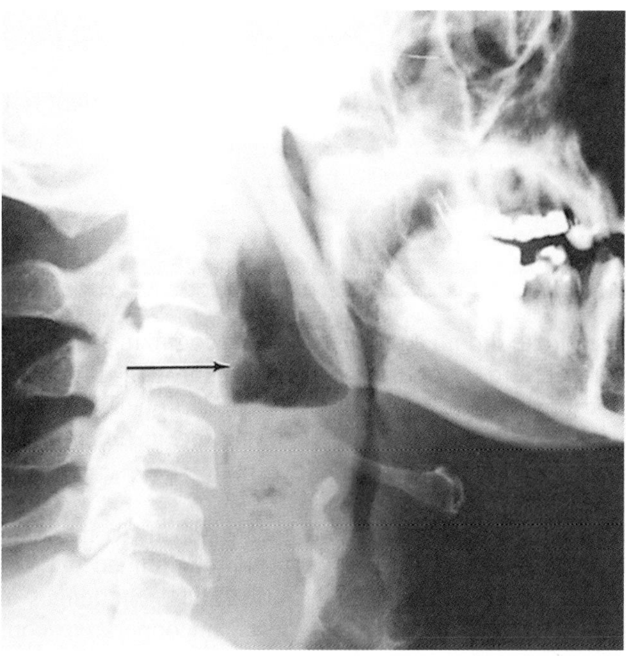

Figure C37-1 Soft tissue lateral x-ray. Retropharyngeal abscess in an adult. The airway is displaced anteriorly by a mass that contains an air-fluid level. *(Stone KS, Roger LH.* Diagnosis & Treatment: Emergency Medicine. *8th ed. New York: McGraw-Hill; 2017. Figure 32-6B.)*

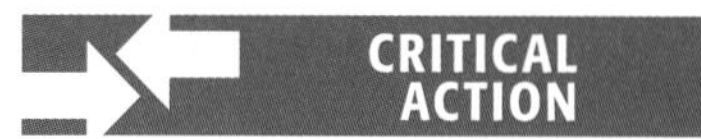

Giving antibiotics is a critical action in this case.

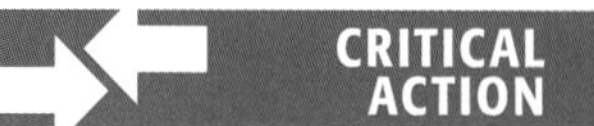

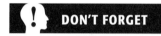

Calling an emergent ENT consult is a critical action in this case. Another critical action is recognizing the potential for airway concerns and obtaining a surgical airway kit.

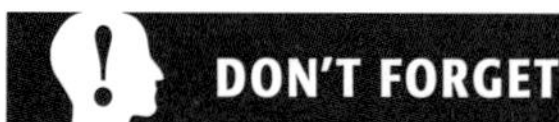

On exam day, your consultants will often "push back" as a way to test your knowledge of the best way to manage your current case. Always insist on appropriate and prompt management of your patient.

A patient with a potential airway threat should never go to the CT scanner.

If the candidate had let the patient go for CT, he would have lost his airway and would have required a surgical airway.

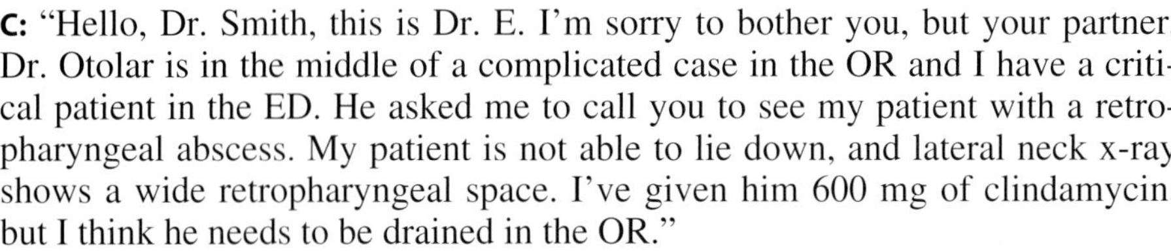

C: "Hello, Dr. Smith, this is Dr. E. I'm sorry to bother you, but your partner, Dr. Otolar is in the middle of a complicated case in the OR and I have a critical patient in the ED. He asked me to call you to see my patient with a retropharyngeal abscess. My patient is not able to lie down, and lateral neck x-ray shows a wide retropharyngeal space. I've given him 600 mg of clindamycin, but I think he needs to be drained in the OR."

E: "I'd be happy to come down. I'll be downstairs in just a few minutes."

C: "I'd like to talk to my patient and let him know what is happening. Mr. Brown, it looks like you have a very serious throat infection that can be life-threatening. I've called an ear, nose, and throat surgeon to come see you, and I believe you will need surgery to treat this infection."

E: "I know it's bad, doc. I wouldn't have come if it weren't, but I don't have insurance, and I'm really worried about how I'm supposed to pay for all of this. Surgery is really expensive and I don't think I can afford the bills."

C: "Why don't I call a social worker so they can help figure out if you qualify for financial assistance and see if there's anything they can do to help? I understand how upsetting this must be, but your health is really at stake, and this infection could kill you."

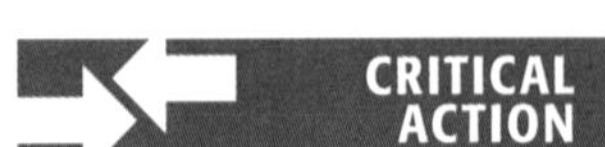

CRITICAL ACTION

Assuaging the patient's fears and getting them to consent to the operation is a critical action in this case.

E: "Yeah, the social worker sounds like a good thing. That would be great if I could get financial assistance. I don't want to jeopardize my life. Thanks."

C: "My pleasure. I'd like to ask the clerk to page social work for Mr. Brown."

E: "Ms. Andrews is on the line from social work."

C: "Hello Ms. Andrews. I have a patient with no insurance who has a serious infection and needs surgery and a hospital admission. He's very concerned about the costs involved and I was wondering if you could come to see him."

E: "I'd be happy to."

C: "Thank you so much."

E: "Dr. Smith is at the bedside, and he'd like to take the patient to the OR."

C: "Good."

E: "That concludes this case."

CASE ASSESSMENT

Overall, the candidate did an excellent job of recognizing a life-threatening illness. The candidate did a good job of moving through the encounter quickly and getting the appropriate treatment instituted properly. The difficulties of this case involve medical management, obtaining an emergent consultation, and addressing the patient's financial concerns.

Certain cases during the oral board exam are set up to make sure that candidates know how to handle themselves when challenged by social situations they are likely to encounter in the real world. These challenges might include violent patients, inability to get certain tests, uncooperative consultants, and uncooperative patients. Be sure to expect these challenges so that you are prepared to handle them. This candidate did a great job negotiating these challenges, empathizing with the patient, contacting another ENT consultant, and contacting social work for assistance.

Notice that the candidate prepared for a crash intubation in case the patient deteriorated. This is always a wise move, since it's impossible to know when the stable appearing patient will suddenly decompensate and require resuscitation. Had the patient allowed the patient to go to computed tomography (CT) or had delay in diagnosis, the patient would have become hypoxic and required surgical airway management.

Another issue that came up in this scenario, and may occur during the oral boards, is an inappropriate tests that the consultant wanted performed. The candidate did a good job in communicating her concerns to the consultant and explaining why she would not be able to comply with their request for a CT. During the oral boards, a test may be requested by a consultant that might place the patient at risk. Be sure to communicate your concerns and discuss why the test could be dangerous to the patient.

In this encounter, the labs were not important in making the diagnosis and waiting for them could have cost this patient valuable time getting to the operating room (OR). However, make sure you ask for the results for any test that you order. Also, the patient did not manage this patient's pain or fever. She also forgot to follow-up to make sure that the normal saline (NS) bolus was decreasing the patient's heart rate.

Critical Actions

1. Recognize the life-threatening potential of the disease and do not let the patient lie flat.
2. Obtain emergent ENT consultation.
3. Order IV antibiotics.
4. Address patient fears and consent for the OR.

Test Performance

1. *Data acquisition:* She got a very good history and physical examination on the patient and ordered the appropriate tests to assist in diagnosis. In addition to using appropriate imaging, she did not allow the patient to have an unsafe CT. Score = **8**
2. *Problem solving:* The candidate was able to rapidly assimilate data from the patient encounter, interpret the x-ray result, and synthesize information quickly to direct further management. However, she did not address the fever or follow-up on the pulse after the fluid bolus. Score = **7**
3. *Patient management:* The candidate did an excellent job of making appropriate treatment decisions, based on patient history, x-ray findings, and clinical judgment. Although she was not able to get the first ENT to come see the patient, she arranged for the other ENT to do so. However, she never addressed the patient's fever or pain, and pain management is often a critical action. Score = **6**
4. *Resource utilization:* The physician demonstrates very good use of resources with an efficient, cost-effective workup, and by speaking with two ENTs and a social worker. Score = **8**
5. *Health care provided (outcome):* The patient received efficient, appropriate treatment, and the candidate kept the patient stable by having him sit up until ENT evaluation. Score = **8**
6. *Interpersonal relations and communication skills:* The candidate did a good job of effectively communicating with the patient and the professional colleagues in this scenario. She also did a good job of alleviating the fears of the patient and getting social work involved. Score = **8**

7. *Comprehension of pathophysiology:* The examinee conveyed their understanding of oropharyngeal infections by asking appropriate history and physical questions, discussing imaging results, and consulting the ENTs. Score = **8**
8. *Clinical competence (overall):* Overall, the examinee showed clinical competence by obtaining an appropriate history and physical, developing a differential diagnosis, utilizing appropriate imaging, antibiotics, and consultations. She could have addressed pain and fever more effectively. Score = **7**

CASE 38 55 y/o Female With Hematemesis

John Dayton and Philip Shayne

INITIAL INFORMATION

Name: Joan Smith

Mode of arrival: EMS

Age: 55 years

Gender: Female

VS: BP 90/50, HR 70, RR 22, T 37.2°C (98.96°F)

CC: Hematemesis at home

PLAY OF THE CASE

C: "What do I see as I walk into the patient's room?"

E: "The patient is a well-nourished female who appears anxious, pale, and weak."

C: "Please request that EMS stay so I can speak to them. Nurse, please place the patient on a cardiac monitor and show me a rhythm strip. Please cycle the blood pressure every 5 minutes and let me know if it falls. Give the patient oxygen via NC at 5 L/min and place the patient on continuous pulse oximetry monitoring and let me know if it falls below 97%. Place two large-bore IVs (18-gauge or larger), draw blood for lab work including tubes for coagulation studies and type and cross, and give a 1 L NS bolus stat. Please obtain a 12-lead ECG and show it to me when ready."

E: "Those orders are being done. The rhythm strip shows a NSR at about 70."

C: "Hello Ms. Smith, my name is Dr. Trueblood and I will be caring for you today. What's going on?"

E: "I threw up a large amount of blood this morning. I don't feel well. I feel really weak."

C: "Has this ever happened to you before?"

E: "No, I am very healthy. I never had a problem with bleeding."

C: "How many times did you vomit?"

E: "Three, I think, one right after another."

C: "What did it look like?"

E: "It was just pure blood."

C: "Can you give me an idea of how much blood?"

E: "It looked like a lot."

C: "How where you feeling before that?"

E: "I had a bit of a stomach ache, but not bad. It was breakfast time, but I wasn't hungry. My stomach was fine yesterday."

KEY QUESTION

Ask this open-ended question at the beginning of every case.

KEY ORDERS

Most of the patients you see during the exam are unstable (or will become that way). Every unstable patient requires IV access (preferably two large-bore IVs), oxygen, and cardiac monitoring (and in most cases an ECG). In this case, as the patient is hypotensive and should receive a fluid bolus.

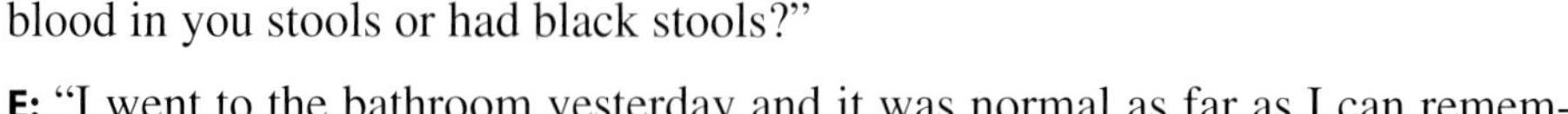

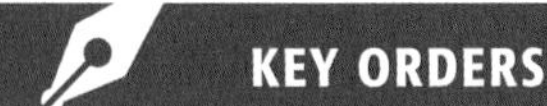

KEY ORDERS

Remember to ask the examiner to keep you apprised of changes in your patient's vital signs.

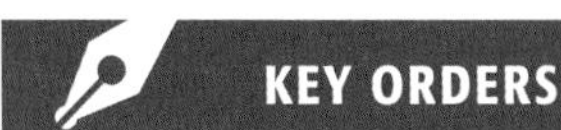

KEY ORDERS

Remember to get as much history from EMS and family members as possible.

C: "When was your last bowel movement? Was it normal? Have you ever had blood in you stools or had black stools?"

E: "I went to the bathroom yesterday and it was normal as far as I can remember. I have never had bloody or black stools."

C: "Do you have any pain now?"

E: "Yes, my stomach hurts, near the top. It is a dull, burning pain. I also feel like I might vomit, but I haven't."

C: "What medical problems do you have?"

E: "I have high blood pressure, but my doctor says it is well controlled with the medication."

C: "Ever had surgery?"

E: "No."

C: "What medication are you on?"

E: "I take atenolol and aspirin."

C: "Any other over-the-counter medications?"

E: "I have been taking Motrin for the last 5 days for a twisted ankle."

C: "How much Motrin have you taken?"

E: "Oh, my ankle was pretty bad so I was taking 2-4 tablets every few hours. But only for the last five days."

C: "Do you have any allergies?"

E: "No."

C: "For EMS: what did you guys find?"

E: "Doc, it was a mess…I would guess a liter of blood on her bed. She looked pale. Her initial BP was 90/40, but her pulse was only about 70. We gave her a 500 cc NS bolus and her pressure came up to 100/50. Blood glucose was 105. Cardiac monitor showed sinus rhythm. She was transported without incident."

C: "Thanks, guys. Nurse, how are the vitals?"

E: "Her BP is still 90/50, and her pulse is 75. Pulse ox steady at 99%. Your ECG is ready." (see Fig. C38-1)

C: "Please perform an immediate bedside hemoglobin check and obtain the following studies: CBC with differential, platelet count, BMP, LFTs, and a coagulation profile. I would also like a portable, upright CXR."

E: "The bedside hemoglobin is 7 g."

C: "Please have the patient typed and cross matched for 4 U of PRBC and repeat the 1 L NS bolus IV."

C: "Ms. Smith, I have a couple more questions. Do you drink alcohol?"

E: "I occasionally have a glass of wine at dinner."

C: "Do you smoke?"

E: "No."

C: "Do you use any street drugs?"

E: "No."

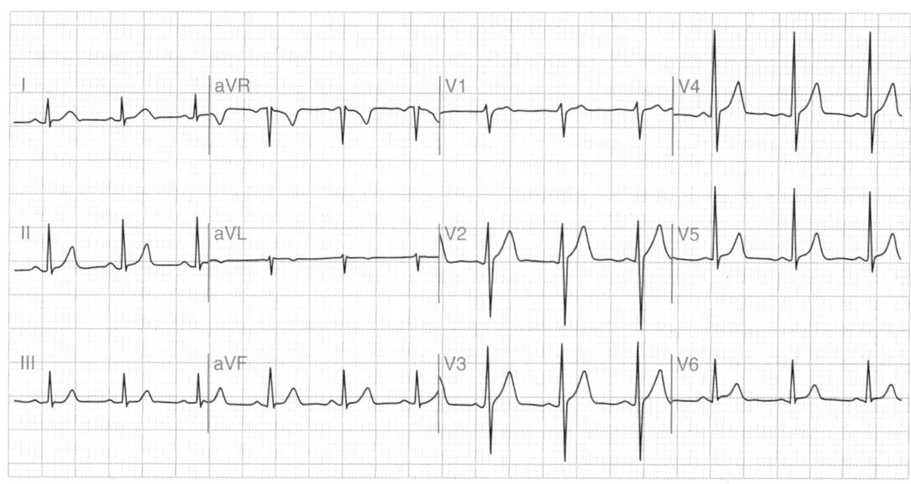

Figure C38-1. Normal ECG from a healthy subject. Sinus rhythm is present with a HR of 75 beats/min. PR interval is 0.16 second; QRS interval (duration) is 0.08 second; QT interval is 0.36 second; QTc is 0.40 second; the mean QRS axis is about +70°. The precordial leads show normal R-wave progression with the transition zone (R wave = S wave) in lead V3. *(Reprinted with permission from Fauci AS, Braunwald E, Kasper DL, et al.* Harrison's Principles of Internal Medicine. *17th ed. New York, NY: McGraw-Hill; 2008.)*

C: "Have you had any of the following problems today: headache, dizziness, weakness, shortness of breath, chest pain, cough, diarrhea, vaginal bleeding, or other bleeding?"

E: "I do feel weak and dizzy, but otherwise no."

C: "Have you fainted?"

E: "No."

C: "I will examine the patient. Has there been any change in her appearance?"

E: "No."

C: "Does she have any jaundice, icterus, pale conjunctiva, or signs of bleeding from the nose or mouth?"

E: "Her conjunctiva appear pale."

C: "Does she have JVD?"

E: "No."

C: "On chest examination, are there good, symmetric breath sounds? Are there murmurs or gallops?"

E: "Pulmonary and cardiovascular examinations are normal."

C: "Is the abdomen distended? Are there any surgical scars, areas of tenderness, or masses?"

E: "The abdomen is non-distended with no surgical scars. There are hyperactive bowel sounds. The abdomen is soft with tenderness in the midepigastric region. No masses are appreciated."

C: "Is there guarding or rebound tenderness?"

E: "None present."

C: "Please describe the genitalia."

E: "The external genitalia are grossly normal."

C: "I would like to explain to the patient that I'm going to do a pelvic and rectal examination, and asked the nurse to prepare for this examination."

E: "Explained and ready."

C: "Is there active bleeding observed on speculum examination? Is there tenderness or any fulness found on bimanual examination?"

E: "Speculum and bimanual examination are performed and unremarkable."

C: "Is there rectal tenderness or any mass? Is there gross or occult blood present? Any sign of anal fissure or hemorrhoid?"

E: "There is good sphincter tone and a large amount of soft stool in the rectal vault, which is reddish-black. It is strongly guaiac positive."

C: "Are the extremities pale or cool? What is the capillary refill? Are there strong distal pulses?"

E: "Her extremities are pale and cool and she has a delayed capillary refill. Her peripheral pulses are symmetric."

C: "I note that the patient is awake, alert, and appropriate. Does she know the date today? Is the strength symmetric with intact sensation?"

E: "Yes, she is fully oriented and moving all four extremities appropriately with intact strength."

C: "How has she responded to fluids? What are her vitals now?"

E: "BP remains 90/50. Her pulse is 75."

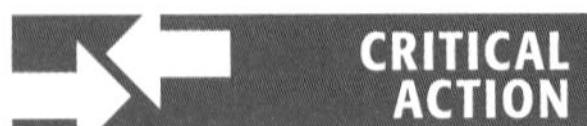

There are three critical actions ongoing at this point:

- the candidate has diagnosed hemorrhagic shock,
- treating aggressively with fluids, and
- initiating resuscitation blood products.

C: "Please bolus another L of NS and I want to transfuse 2 U of pRBCs stat. If the blood has not been cross-matched, please use 2 U of Type O-Negative blood. Please also start Protonix with 80 mg IV and a drip at 8 mg/h. Finally, please also insert an NG tube, connect it to suction, and let me know what is returned."

E: "Two units of uncross-matched blood are transfusing. NG tube returned 500 cc of red blood, and then stopped. I have lavaged the NG tube with saline and got a small amount of blood which cleared. The bolus of saline is in and the patient appears the same."

C: "Can you give me repeat vital signs? Also, please review her chest, abdominal, and extremity examination."

E: "Her BP is now 100/55 after the first unit of pRBCs. Her extremities remain cool with delayed capillary refill. Her chest and abdominal examination remain the same. Chest x-ray is normal, with an NG tube in the stomach and no free air under the diaphragm. Also, we just received 2 U of cross-matched blood. We have some lab values back."

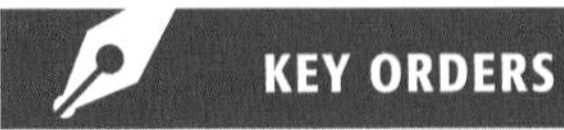

Remember to reassess vitals frequently in your unstable patients—especially after each intervention.

C: "Please infuse both units of cross-matched blood as rapidly as you can. Are my labs back?"

E: "CBC shows a WBC count of 12,000 which is 85% neutrophils and no bands. The laboratory Hgb is 7.0 g and confirms the bedside value; the Hct is 21%. Her PT is 21 with an INR elevation of 2.4 with a PTT of 50. Her BMP reveals the following: Na 147, K 4.6, Cl 110, CO_2 18, BUN 38, Cr 1.4, glu 121, Ca 9.1. The liver function tests are normal."

C: "She is very anemic, and has developed a coagulopathy. Please order 10 U fresh frozen plasma (FFP) to be transfused. Also transfuse two more units of typed and cross-matched blood when available. What are her vital signs now?"

E: "Her BP is now 110/60 and pulse is 65. She appears more comfortable and a less pale. There has been no further output from the NG tube."

C: "Please call the gastroenterologist on call. Also please arrange to make an ICU bed available."

E: "Dr. Liverblue is on the phone."

C: "Hello Dr. Liverblue. This is Dr. Trueblood. Are you on call today for the ED?"

E: "Yes I am."

C: "I have an ill 55-year-old female with an upper GI bleed who presented in shock. I would appreciate your admitting her to the ICU and I believe that she would benefit from immediate endoscopy. Prior to today, she had no medical problems except for hypertension. She has been taking a lot of Motrin for the last 5 days for an ankle sprain. She threw up a large volume of blood this morning at home and EMS reports that she was hypotensive when they arrived. On arrival to the ED she was hypotensive with a BP of 90/50 and HR of 75, with a blunted pulse response likely due to her beta-blocker. She has epigastric tenderness, melena, and we got 500 cc of blood via gastric lavage which subsequently cleared. She has been fluid resuscitated with 2 L of saline, we've started transfusion with pRBCs, and we've ordered FFP. Her pressure is now up to 110/60, she feels better and appears improved. There's been no further blood from the NG tube. Her initial bedside and lab confirmed a Hgb of 7 with Hct of 21. Her INR is 2.4 and I believe this is due to the rapid GI bleed she has experienced today."

E: "Dr Liverblue accepts the patient, and the room is available. Is there anything else?"

C: "No, she may go up."

E: "This case is now over."

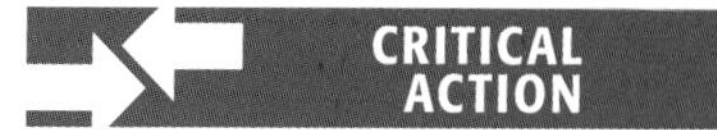

There are two critical actions ongoing at this point:

- The candidate is calling a GI consult, and
- She is admitting this patient to the ICU.

CASE ASSESSMENT

The candidate managed the patient's care very well. She correctly diagnosed a massive upper gastrointestinal (GI) bleed due to nonsteroidal anti-inflammatory drugs (NSAIDs). The patient presented as hemorrhagic shock with a falsely normal pulse rate due to beta-blocker therapy. The candidate properly fluid-resuscitated the patient using two large bore IVs with immediate 2 L bolus of normal saline (NS), and then used blood products when the patient's blood pressure (BP) did not improve. She correctly diagnosed a coagulopathy and ordered fresh frozen plasma (FFP). Proton pump inhibitor (PPI) therapy has been shown to be helpful for upper GI bleeding from ulcers. Though it was not a critical action, it was indicated in this case. The patient did not have liver disease, so somatostatin was not indicated. Though the patient improved, she is still in critical condition and requires intensive care unit (ICU) admission.

The candidate gets high marks for diagnosing shock, aggressive care, orderly and thorough evaluation, frequent reevaluation of vital signs, and appropriate responses to continued abnormal VS findings. The candidate properly interpreted the lab findings and demonstrated a good fund of medical knowledge and ability to synthesize clinical data. The candidate also did a very good job utilizing appropriate healthcare resources.

However, the candidate did not do as well with communication. There was no attempt to explain to the patient what was going on, diagnosis, prognosis, or the disposition. The candidate would be expected to continue the role model playing and deliver this information as they would in a real clinical setting. Also, nothing was done to assess and treat the patient's pain. There might be legitimate concerns about using pain medication that can either exacerbate hypotension or cause further damage. However, if it is really necessary to withhold pain medication, this should be explained to the patient. A small dose of a parenteral opioid pain medication, like morphine, may be given once the clinical condition is more stable.

Overall, the candidate managed this case well. Pay special attention to how the candidate reassessed the patient's response to each intervention, and then acted accordingly.

Critical Actions

1. *Data acquisition:* This phase was excellent as the candidate shows the ability to obtain a thorough history and physical examination, as well as order correct tests for the diagnosis. Score = **8**
2. *Problem solving:* Problem solving was also excellent as the candidate simulated clinical data, interpreted lab findings, and made the proper resuscitative interventions. She asks appropriate questions about abdominal history and both prescription and over-the-counter (OTC) meds to discover the source of the patient's upper GI bleed. Score = **8**
3. *Patient management:* Patient care was excellent. The candidate performed all the critical actions, made appropriate decisions, and provided care in an efficient manner. However, she could have been more attentive to patient comfort. Score = **6**
4. *Resource utilization:* The candidate used appropriate interventions, lab studies, imaging, and blood products. She also obtained information from paramedics and made the appropriate consultation. Score = **8**
5. *Health care provided (outcome):* The patient received efficient and appropriate treatment, and the candidate's interventions stabilized the patient. Score = **8**
6. *Interpersonal relations and communication skills:* Interpersonal and communication skills were not adequate. The candidate started off in an appropriate interactive manner, but got absorbed in the resuscitation and stopped communicating concerns and offering explanations to the patient. This is a common mistake in this artificial setting and must be avoided! Score = **4**
7. *Comprehension of pathophysiology:* The examinee conveyed their understanding of both the etiology and treatment of gastrointestinal bleeds by her lab requests, interventions, and discussion with the consultant. Score = **8**
8. *Clinical competence (overall):* Overall, the examinee showed clinical competence by stabilizing and admitting this patient. Score = **7**

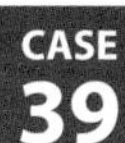

CASE 39 28 y/o Male With Sickle Cell Disease and Chest Pain

John Dayton, Philip Shayne, and Daniel Wu

INITIAL INFORMATION

Name: John Chespane

Mode of arrival: Ambulatory

Age: 28 years

Gender: Male

VS: BP 110/65, HR 115, RR 24, T 38.8°C (101.84°F)

PLAY OF THE CASE

C: "What do I see as I walk into the patient's room?"

E: "The patient is a young man lying on the stretcher. He appears uncomfortable and short of breath. You note nasal flaring and accessory muscle use."

C: "Nurse, please place the patient on a cardiac monitor, obtain IV access with an 18-gauge needle, draw blood for labs (including a type and screen) and place the patient on 3 L oxygen via NC, after getting a room air oxygen saturation level."

E: "Those orders are being completed; the room air oxygen saturation is 88% and 94% on oxygen."

C: "Hello Mr. Chespane, my name is Dr. Kindly. What happened to you today?"

E: "My chest hurts and I feel short of breath."

C: "How long have you had these symptoms?"

E: "The pain started last night and it is getting worse."

C: "Have you had this pain before?"

E: "Yes, this is my typical sickle cell type pain. Usually I feel it in my arms and legs, but my chest is really sore today."

C: "On a scale from 0 to 10, how high is your pain?"

E: "10."

C: "What medications do you usually take for pain?"

E: "I take hydrocodone and Tylenol at home but I ran out of medicine last night. When I come to the hospital they usually give me something in the IV."

C: "Do you have any allergies to medications?"

E: "Penicillin."

C: "Do you have any other medical problems?"

E: "No."

C: "Do you take any other medications besides the pain medicine?"

E: "Folic acid."

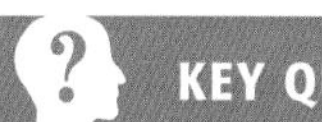

KEY QUESTION

Ask this open-ended question at the beginning of every case.

KEY ORDERS

Most of the patients you see during the exam are unstable (or will become that way). Every unstable patient requires IV access, oxygen, and cardiac monitoring (and in most cases an ECG).

DON'T FORGET

When any part of the vital signs is absent, it is usually abnormal. Be sure to make sure that you have a complete set of vital signs, including temperature and oxygen saturation on RA.

 **KEY QUESTION**

Always remember to get an AMPLE history on all patients:

- **A**llergies,
- **M**edications,
- **P**ast medical/surgical history,
- **L**ast meal (if surgery or intubation is a possibility), and
- **E**vents surrounding ED admission.

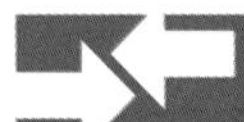 **CRITICAL ACTION**

Treating this patient's pain is a critical action in this case. It often is, so do not forget to treat pain when it is present.

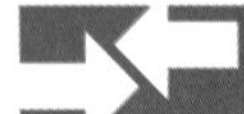 **CRITICAL ACTION**

Treating the fever with acetaminophen and the hypoxia with oxygen are critical actions in this case.

 **DON'T FORGET**

When the examiner states that the examination for a certain organ system is "normal," you can safely move on.

However, if they ask "what are you looking for," there is likely a significant finding and you should dig deeper.

C: "Nurse, please administer 10 mg of IV morphine sulfate with 10 mg of IV Compazine and 1 g of oral acetaminophen. Please start a 1 L bolus of 0.9 NS, then run the fluids at 150 cc/h, and send labs including a CBC with reticulocyte count, chemistry, type and screen, ABG, blood cultures, UA, and CXR. Please let me know when the tests results come back."

E: "Your orders are being done."

C: "Mr. Chespane, I am going to give you some pain medication, I want you to let us know if this helps with your pain. In the meantime I would like to ask you some more questions."

C: "Do you know what type of sickle cell disease you have?"

E: "SS disease."

C: "Are you immunizations up-to-date?"

E: "Yes."

C: "Have you been feeling sick lately?"

E: "I just got over a sore throat last week. For the last few days, I've had a fever, cough and runny nose."

C: "How high have the fevers been? Any chills?"

E: "Not sure, but I've felt warm. Yes, I've felt both hot and cold."

C: "Any pain when you urinate or back pain?"

E: "No."

C: "When you cough, do you cough up sputum?"

E: "Yes."

C: "What color is it?"

E: "It was white last week, but now it's dark and green."

C: "How is your pain now?"

E: "It is better."

C: "I would like to examine the patient, has there been a change in his appearance or vital signs?"

E: "No."

C: "I would like to examine his HEENT, specifically looking for signs of infection in his ears and throat."

E: "The HEENT examination is negative, both throat and ears are clear. Nasal flaring has resolved."

C: "Is the neck supple and is there lymphadenopathy?"

E: "Normal neck exam."

C: "Cardiac examination?"

E: "Slightly tachycardic but otherwise normal."

C: "Lungs?"

E: "What are you looking for?"

C: "Are the breath sounds clear bilaterally? Wheezing? Rales? Does the patient still have accessory muscle use for breathing?"

E: "The lung sounds are coarse bilaterally and appeared slightly decreased, there are no wheezing or rales. He no longer has accessory muscle use."

C: "Abdominal examination?"

E: "Soft, non-tender, non-distended, and there is no palpable liver or spleen."

C: "Extremity examination specifically looking for signs of infection, swelling, or erythema?"

E: "The extremities are normal. There is no erythema or swelling"

C: "GU examination, specifically looking for priapism."

E: "Negative."

C: "Neuro, specifically to assess mental status."

E: "GCS: 15, patient is answering questions appropriately and strength and sensation are intact, the examination is normal."

C: "On a scale of 1-10 what is your pain now?"

E: "Eight, the pain medication helped but it is starting to come back again."

C: "Nurse, please administer 10 more mg of morphine sulfate IV and please reassess the patient to let me know if his pain scale has improved."

E: "The patient's results are back. The Hgb is 5.5 with an elevated reticulocyte count and the WBC count is 18.5. The patient's ABG results are Ph 7.33, Po_2 80, Pco_2 30, HCO_3 18. The UA is negative for leukocytes and blood and positive for ketones; the BMP is normal."

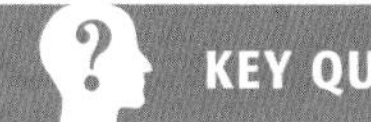

KEY QUESTION

Remember to be resourceful. If you keep coming up with ways to look for a piece of data, you will probably get it. Ask for old records, contact the primary physician, or ask for family members.

C: "What is his typical Hgb?"

E: "The patient is not sure."

C: "Do we have old lab values available?"

E: "A review of the electronic lab record at the hospital reveals that his Hgb 2 months ago was 8.5."

E: "Here is the CXR (see Fig. C39-1)."

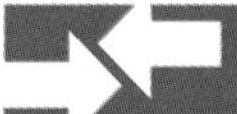

CRITICAL ACTION

Diagnosing acute chest syndrome in this sickle cell patient is a critical action in this case.

C: "There appears to be a new infiltrate. The patient is hypoxic with a respiratory acidosis, which makes me concerned for acute chest syndrome. I would like to start antibiotic therapy after obtaining sputum cultures."

E: "Which antibiotic would you like to start?"

C: "Since the patient has a penicillin allergy, I'd like to use a fluoroquinolone. Please start the patient on 400 mg of moxifloxacin to cover both community-acquired and atypical pneumonias. I would also like to start blood transfusion. Can you start transfusing 2 U of pRBCs?"

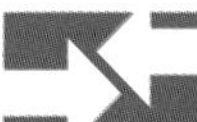

CRITICAL ACTION

Treating acute chest syndrome with appropriate antibiotics and transfusion is a critical action in this case.

C: "I would like to call the ICU physician on call and please recheck the vital signs."

E: "The patient's HR is 95, BP 135/85, RR 20, O_2 sat on 3 L is 96%. Dr. Iceeyu is on the phone."

C: "Please increase the oxygen to 4 L. Dr. Iceeyu, this is Dr. Kindly in the ER. I have a patient whom I would like to admit to the ICU. The patient is a 28-year-old man with known SS hemoglobinopathy (sickle cell) disease who presented with a chest pain, fevers, and SOB. Here he is febrile to 38.8, tachypneic, and hypoxic by oxygen saturation and by ABG. The CXR shows bilateral interstitial markings, so I am worried about acute chest syndrome versus pneumonia. I have already started the patient on antibiotics. I'd like to admit

KEY QUESTION

Remember to reassess vital signs frequently during the case.

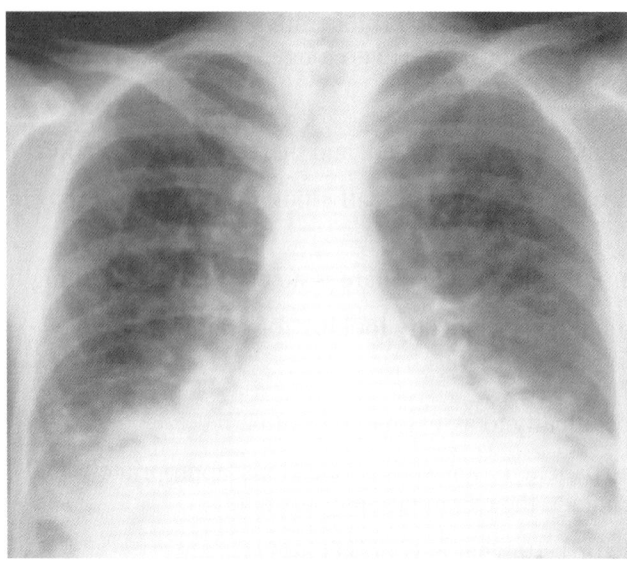

Figure C39-1. CXR with an infiltrate on it. *(Reprinted with permission from Fauci AS, Braunwald E, Kasper DL,* et al. Harrison's Principles of Internal Medicine. *17th ed. New York, NY: McGraw-Hill; 2008.)*

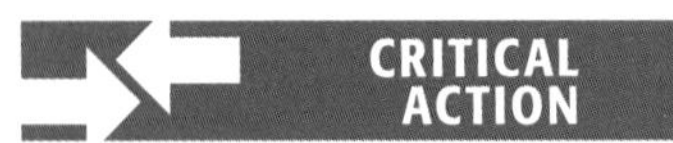

Admitting the patient to the appropriate level of care is always a critical action.

him to the ICU. I've started him on 2 U pRBC, but I also would consider an exchange transfusion because of his falling hemoglobin. He is at 5.5 and it was 7.9 just 2 months ago."

E: "Dr. Iceeyu has accepted the patient. Is there anything else you would like to do?"

C: "No."

E: "The case is now over."

CASE ASSESSMENT

Overall the candidate did an excellent job managing this case. The candidate quickly identified infection as a possible source of acute pain crisis and made the diagnosis of acute chest syndrome in a timely manner. The history was direct and appropriate and once a problem was identified, the necessary workup and therapy was quickly initiated.

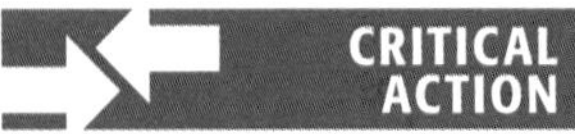

Considering and/or discussing exchange transfusion is a critical action in this case.

The candidate displayed a direct approach to the problem, yet was thorough, and even elicited the allergy history before antibiotics were given. The physical examination was focused with special attention to the signs of possible infection and sickle crisis. Given the hypoxia and chest x-ray (CXR) findings, the candidate promptly provided broad antimicrobial coverage for both common and atypical bacteria. The candidate also properly interpreted lab results and requested an old hemoglobin level. He determined that the falling hemoglobin, which may be due to acute chest syndrome, could require an exchange transfusion. The candidate communicated easily with the patient and nursing staff, but could have improved his score by continuing to reassess the patient, requesting permission to do genital examination, and discussing risks and benefits of transfusion. The patient did not have a second set of vital signs taken until the case was almost completed, despite numerous interventions such as IV fluids, pain medications, and supplemental oxygen.

The candidate would have easily passed this case as he clearly delivered the standard of care.

Critical Actions

1. Give pain medication.
2. Identify and treat fever and hypoxia.
3. Identify allergies and give appropriate antibiotics.
4. Diagnose acute chest syndrome.
5. Consider exchange transfusion therapy and implement or discuss with consultant.
6. Admit to the intensive care unit (ICU).

Test Performance

1. *Data Acquisition:* The candidate clearly understood what information needed to be obtained, given the chief complaint and patient history. He took a focused approach to the physical examination, investigating possible causes of the patient's fever and sickle crisis. Score = **8**
2. *Problem Solving:* The candidate demonstrated excellent problem solving skills by investigating both the patient's history of pain crises and realizing that the current crisis was due to a different etiology. He also reacted appropriately to lab findings. Score = **8**
3. *Patient Management:* The candidate clearly delivered the standard of care for this case and reacted appropriately to history and physical information and lab results. The candidate could have improved the score by following up on his interventions more frequently and reassessing the patient's pain, as mentioned above. Score = **6**
4. *Resource Utilization:* The candidate used appropriate lab work, imaging, and obtained information from both the patient and hospital records. The workup was logical and cost-sensitive. Score = **8**
5. *Health Care Provided (Outcome):* The candidate stabilized the patient, treated pain, diagnosed acute chest syndrome, and started appropriate antibiotics and transfusion. The patient was admitted to the proper service. Score = **8**
6. *Interpersonal Relations and Communication Skills:* The interpersonal skills demonstrated by the candidate in this case were very good. He interacted well with both the patient and the nursing staff. He could have been better about asking for updates with pain and explaining risks and benefits of transfusion. Score = **6**
7. *Comprehension of Pathophysiology:* The examinee conveyed their understanding of sickle crisis and infection by ordering appropriate studies and discussing both results and further admission needs with the consultant. Score = **8**
8. *Clinical Competence (Overall):* Overall, the examinee showed excellent clinical competence. He would have lost points for not repeating vitals and pain assessments, and also for not discussing risks and benefits of transfusion with the patient. Score = **7**

CASE 40 68 y/o Female With Palpitations

John Dayton and Mark P. Bogner

KEY QUESTION

Ask this open-ended question at the beginning of every case.

KEY ORDERS

Most of the patients you see during the exam are unstable (or will become that way). Every unstable patient requires IV access, oxygen, and cardiac monitoring (and in most cases an ECG).

DON'T FORGET

Remember to ask for the results of labs/studies as soon as they are available. You will be penalized for not following up on your orders, so use the note paper to write down all your lab and imaging requests and cross them off when you receive results.

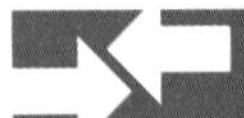

CRITICAL ACTION

Placing pacer pads as soon as the ECG is seen as a critical action in this case.

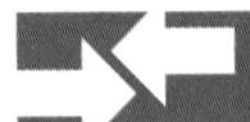

CRITICAL ACTION

Consulting cardiology early is a critical action in this case.

INITIAL INFORMATION

Name: Jane Smith

Mode of arrival: EMS (paramedics)

Age: 68 years

Gender: Female

VS: T 37.1°C (98.78°F), BP 108/64, HR 48, RR 18, O_2 sat: 97% on RA

CC: Irregular heart beat

Setting: It is 5 AM on Monday morning and you are nearing the end of a single coverage overnight shift in a busy suburban "comprehensive" general hospital emergency department (ED). You have excellent nursing and ancillary staff to assist you. The hospital's resources are state of the art and the medical staff is superb.

PLAY OF THE CASE

C: "What do I see as I walk into the patient's room?"

E: "The patient appears her stated age, is well-kempt and is wearing pajamas. She appears anxious and in some distress. The patient is accompanied by her husband who drove in separately after calling 911."

C: "Hello Ms. Smith, I am Dr. Emergency. Nurse, please place the patient on a cardiac monitor and show me a rhythm strip. Let's start her on oxygen at 3L via NC, place an 18-gauge IV with NS at 100 cc/h and draw blood for labs. We will need cardiac enzymes, including troponin, a CBC, lytes, BUN, Cr, glu, UA, and a BNP. Please have the unit coordinator order a stat ECG and please hand it to me when it is done. Also, please get us a stat bedside CXR."

E: "Your orders are being done."

C: "May I look at the rhythm strip?"

E: "The patient's rhythm strip shows an irregular rhythm with an average rate of 62 bpm. The 12-lead ECG is available for your review (Fig. C40-1)."

C: "Nurse, please assist me in placing transcutaneous pacer pads on the patient's chest and back and hook them up to the pacer/defibrillator. Turn the device on and set it in 'monitor' mode for now. Also, please administer atropine, 0.5 mg IV and then ask the unit coordinator to get the cardiologist on-call on the telephone. Also please get the patient's primary doctor on the phone if possible."

E: "Okay."

C: "Has the patient's heart rate or rhythm changed?"

E: "No."

C: "Nurse, please administer another dose of atropine, 0.5 mg IV. If the patient's HR does not increase to 55 or higher within 5 minutes, please repeat the atropine in 0.5 mg increments up to a total dose of 2 mg."

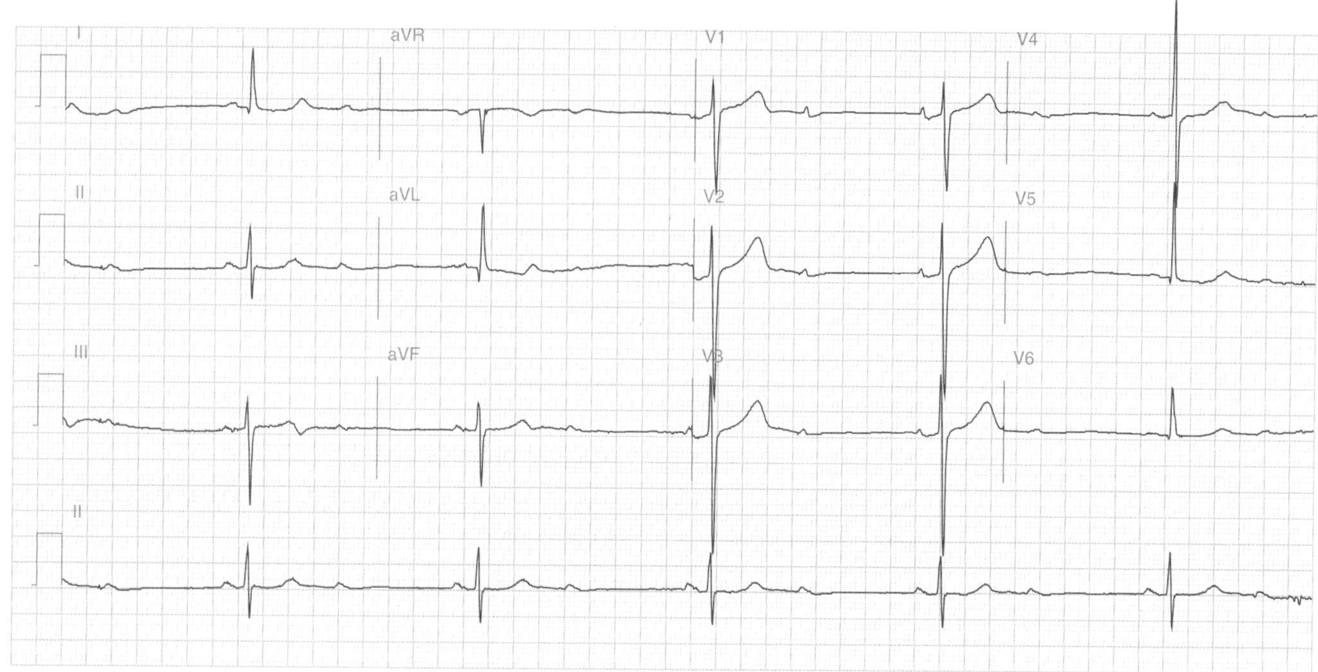

Figure C40-1. ECG showing an idiojunctional rhythm. *(Reprinted with permission from Fauci AS, Braunwald E, Kasper DL, et al.* Harrison's Principles of Internal Medicine. *17th ed. New York, NY: McGraw-Hill; 2008.)*

C: "Ms. Smith, the triage nurse tells me you are experiencing an irregular heartbeat. Can you please tell me some more about how you are feeling?"

E: "It is okay to call me Mrs. Smith, doctor. I woke up in the middle of night feeling strange. I got up to use the bathroom and felt very weak. I almost fainted. I barely made it back to our bed and woke up my husband. He called 911 and here we are. I have never felt this way before. My heart seems to be beating slowly and it feels odd. I really don't feel well in general."

C: "Are you having any pain, particularly in your chest?"

E: "No."

C: "Do you feel short of breath or nauseated?"

E: "Yes, I had a hard time breathing when I tried to get up at home. I felt nauseated and broke out in a cold sweat. I feel a little better now."

C: "Did they give you aspirin in the ambulance?"

E: "Yes, they had me chew four baby aspirin."

C: "Have you been on oxygen since the paramedics picked you up at your home?"

E: "Yes."

C: "Is it helping."

E: "I think so, yes."

C: "Did you feel okay when you went to bed last night?"

E: "Yes. We just returned from visiting our daughter and new grandson over the Holidays. I have felt wonderful these past few days. I haven't even had my usual winter cold."

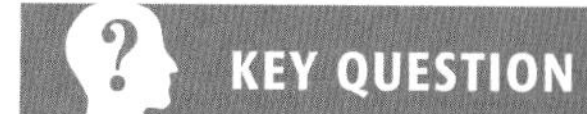

Remember to reassess vital signs frequently during the case.

C: "Have you noticed any fever or cough?"

E: "No."

C: "Do you feel weak anywhere in particular, such as on one side of your body more than the other?"

E: "No, I just feel wiped out in general."

C: "Any swelling in your feet or legs."

E: "Yes, a little, but I have had that for a few years. My doctor is treating me for it."

C: "Is the swelling worse?"

E: "Not noticeably."

C: "Have you noticed any black or bloody stools?"

E: "Yes, my stools have seemed very dark in color, almost black these past few days. I figured it was the Holiday diet."

C: "Have you had any pains in your legs or calves?"

E: "No."

C: "Have you been on any long trips lately, such as long plane, car, or train ride where you were sitting for an extended period?"

E: "Not really. Our daughter's home is a 2-hour drive away. We always stop at a rest area so my husband can use the restroom and we can walk around a bit to stretch our legs."

C: "Have you noticed any other new symptoms or concerns recently?"

E: "No, like I said, I have been feeling great up until about an hour ago."

C: "I know this seems a silly question, but have you used any alcohol or recreational drugs recently?"

E: "No doctor, I never drink and have never taken drugs of any kind except those prescribed by my doctor."

C: "Do you smoke or did you in the past?"

E: "No, never."

C: "Have you ever had a blood clot in your legs, arms, or lungs?"

E: "No."

C: "Have you ever had any form of cancer?"

E: "No."

C: "Have you ever had surgery?"

E: "I had two C-sections many years ago. My appendix was removed when I was 20 and my gallbladder when I was about 40. I haven't had surgery since the gallbladder problem."

C: "Have you been hospitalized in the past 5 years for any reason?"

E: "No."

C: "Do you have any heart problems?"

E: "Only very mild heart failure that my doctor is treating and tells me is stable."

C: "Has your doctor ever said you had a 'heart attack,' even a so-called 'silent heart attack?'"

E: "No."

C: "Have you ever had an ECG before now?"

E: "Yes, my doctor did an ECG and a stress test about 2 years ago when I first noticed the swelling in my feet. He said everything was fine but I needed to go on medication for what he called very mild heart failure."

C: "Is your doctor treating you for any other medical conditions?"

E: "Yes, I take Glucotrol for mild diabetes and have to watch my diet. I also take atenolol for my blood pressure, lovastatin for high cholesterol, Lotensin for my mild heart failure, and a baby aspirin every day for 'good measure,' as my doctor puts it."

C: "Do you take any other medications, including dietary supplements, vitamins, herbal medicines or teas or other holistic therapies?"

E: "No."

C: "Are you allergic to any medications?"

E: "No."

C: "Is there anything else you think I should know?"

E: "No."

C: "I would like to examine the patient now."

E: "Go ahead."

C: "Does the patient appear in distress, pale, diaphoretic, or 'shocky'?"

E: "She appears anxious and somewhat pale, but otherwise is in no apparent distress."

C: "Are there any significant findings on the patient's HEENT examination?"

E: "No."

C: "How about her neck?"

E: "What are you looking for?"

C: "Tracheal deviation, bruits, JVD, subcutaneous emphysema, swelling, or hematoma."

E: "Neck examination shows mild JVD, but is otherwise normal."

C: "When I auscultate her chest, do I hear wheezing, rales, rhonchi, diminished or asymmetrical breath sounds? Is there a pleuritic rub? Also, is there any chest tenderness or deformity?"

E: "Chest examination is normal."

C: "On the cardiac examination, is her PMI displaced, are S1 and S2 clear, and are there any murmurs, rubs, or gallops."

E: "Cardiac examination is normal."

C: "When I examine her abdomen, do I palpate any masses, pulsatile or otherwise? Do I notice tenderness, guarding, or rebound? Are bowel sounds normal?"

E: "Abdominal examination is normal."

C: "In the extremities, are there any pulse deficits or asymmetries, deformities, swelling, or edema? Does she have a Homan sign or calf squeeze tenderness? Is capillary refill delayed?"

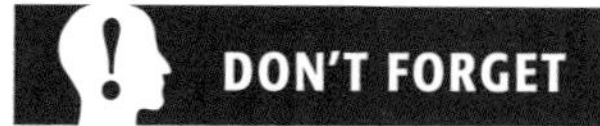

Remember that when the examiner states that the examination for a certain organ system is "normal," you can safely move on. However, if they ask "what are you looking for," there is likely a significant finding and you should dig deeper.

E: "She has minimal non-pitting edema to the ankle level bilaterally. Capillary refill is 3 seconds in her fingers. Her extremity examination is otherwise normal."

C: "Any occult or gross blood in the stool on rectal examination?"

E: "Her stool is formed, black, and positive for occult blood."

C: "Are there any neurologic deficits such as a difference in power between right and left arms and legs? Any cranial nerve deficits? Are there any gross sensory deficits, particularly unilateral loss or altered sensation? Is her mental status is grossly normal?

E: "There are no focal deficits."

C: "As I examine her skin, are there any significant rashes, bruising, petechiae, purpura, changes indicating chronic peripheral vascular disease, pallor, or jaundice?"

E: "There are no significant skin changes except as noted previously. She appears pale."

C: "I have completed my physical examination for now. Are the CXR and lab results available for me to review?"

E: "The portable CXR is available for your review (Fig. C40-2)."

C: "Thank you. I would like the nurse to obtain a repeat set of vital signs and report them to me. Also, have the patient's general condition or apparent distress level changed?"

E: "Repeat vitals = BP 98/60, HR 46, RR 16, O_2 sat: 99% on O_2 at 3 LPM via NC. Her appearance and distress level are unchanged. The nurse reports that she has now received a total of 2 mg of atropine over a 20-minute period without change in her rhythm. The following laboratory information is available:

- CBC: WBC 10,000, PMNs 65, bands 8; H/H 8.6/26; plt 195,000,
- PT 13 (INR 1.3), PTT 34,
- BMP: Na 142, K 4.5, Cl 106, CO_2 19, BUN 23, Cr 1.4, glu 134, Ca 9.7,
- CPK 121, MB 3.4, troponin 0.4,
- BNP 150, and
- UA unremarkable"

C: "Thank you. Mr. Smith, you might want to hear this too. Mrs. Smith, after examining you and reviewing your test results, my primary concern is that your heart is indeed beating too slowly and this has resulted in a drop in your blood pressure that is making you feel very weak, particularly when you stand up. Your blood count is low, which means you have anemia. This could be part of what is causing your symptoms. You are losing blood in your stool, which is why it is black, and this will have to be evaluated further by a gastroenterologist. Your kidney function is a bit below normal. At this point, there is no definite evidence that you are having a heart attack, but all these other problems are making your heart work harder than it should and some parts of your heart muscle may not be getting all the oxygen they need. This may have caused your heart's natural pacemaker to stop working properly. The atenolol you are taking may also be a factor. We will need to admit you to the cardiac ICU. The cardiologist will talk to you more about this, but it appears you will need a pacemaker. We need to correct these underlying problems and also make sure that your symptoms are not early signs of a heart attack. I am very sorry to have to tell you all this unpleasant news. The good news is that, so far, nothing really bad has happened. In most cases, all of these problems can be

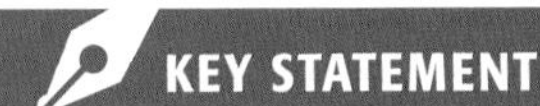

Remember to keep the patient and family aware of your concerns, test results, and the disposition plan. Answer any questions that they have and be respectful.

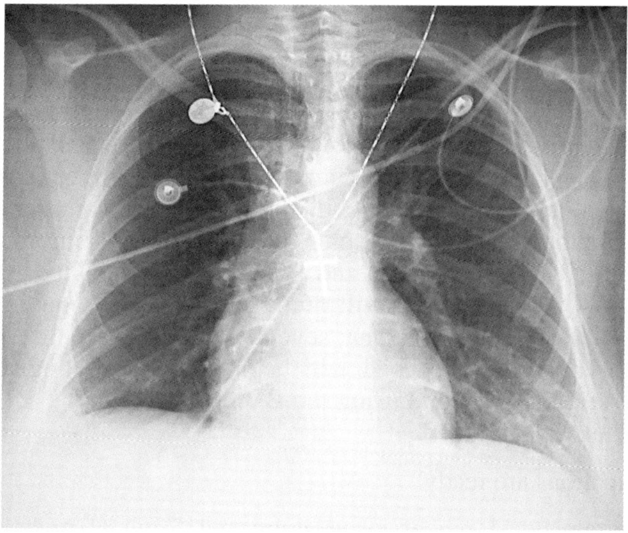

Figure C40-2. Normal CXR. *(Reprinted with permission from Schwartz DT.* Emergency Radiology: Case Studies. *New York, NY: McGraw-Hill; 2008.)*

effectively treated. It is very important that you let us know right away if you are having any pain in your chest or are feeling worse in any way. My staff and I will try to keep you comfortable and answer your questions. We will keep you and your family posted on developments as best we can."

E: "The patient's doctor is on the phone for you."

C: "Hello Dr. Primary, this is Dr. Emergency. I have your patient Mrs. Smith in the ED. She presented shortly after the onset of palpitations and weakness that began last night when she got up to use the bathroom. She is mildly hypotensive, but there are not mental status changes and she is stable. Her heart rate is in the mid-40s and her ECG shows an idiojunctional rhythm alternating every two beats with a captured atrial beat. She has a modestly elevated troponin of 0.4, there are no acute T-wave or ST-segment changes suggesting acute MI, but ischemia is still a concern. She does not appear to be in significant heart failure. She is anemic with a hemoglobin of 8.6, and she has mild renal insufficiency with a creatinine of 1.4. Her stool is black and positive for occult blood. I believe the patient needs a pacemaker and should be admitted to cardiology in the CCU, unless you wish to coordinate her care on your service. She has had a total of 2 mg of atropine with no response."

E: "No, cardiology and the CCU sound appropriate. I will follow-up on the other medical issues and arrange a GI consult. Thanks for seeing her."

C: "Certainly."

E: "The cardiologist called back while you were on the line with Dr. Primary. The nurse told her what you were telling Dr. Primary. She says she will be right down and to go ahead and arrange a CCU bed on her service."

E: "Dr. Emergency, Mrs. Smith has become unresponsive!"

C: "What do I see when I look at the patient now? May I have a current set of vitals please? I would also like a repeat ECG."

E: "The patient is unconscious with rapid, shallow breaths. She is pale and diaphoretic. Her BP is now 60/40, HR 32, RR 36, O_2 sat 82%."

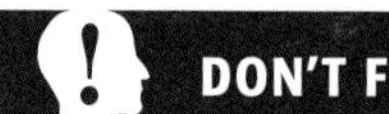

DON'T FORGET

Communicating detailed findings to a referring or primary physician and family members is an effective oral exam technique for displaying your understanding of a case.

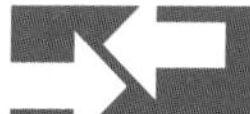

CRITICAL ACTION

Admission to the CCU is a critical action in this case.

DON'T FORGET

When a patient decompensates early in the case, it is most commonly due to a misstep in management. Make sure that you are not missing anything simple.

When a patient decompensates later in the case, it is usually and planned "crash."

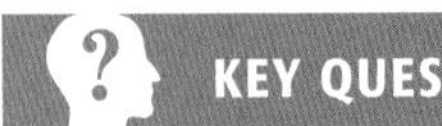

KEY QUESTION

Always reassess vital signs, especially when there is a change in the patient's condition or after you make a significant intervention.

C: "Does she respond to verbal stimuli? To sternal rub?"

E: "She does not respond to either stimulus."

C: "Nurse, please have someone call respiratory therapy and have them bring us a ventilator. Please set the pacer/defibrillator to transcutaneous pacing mode at a rate of 70 bpm and turn up the gain as needed until we get capture. Please also have someone get the airway equipment and crash carts. I would like to immediately intubate the patient. Nurse, please draw up 5 mg midazolam, 50 μg of fentanyl, 10 mg vecuronium, and 125 mg succinylcholine. Tell me when you are ready with the drugs. I will prepare and test my equipment, including bag valve mask, suction, oxygen, several ET tubes sized 6-5, 7-0, and 7-5, stylet, and laryngoscope blades. I will begin pre-oxygenating and assisting the patient's ventilation efforts using the BVM and oxygen at 15 LPM. I will place a nasal airway if needed."

CRITICAL ACTION

Appropriately resuscitating this patient is a critical action. In this case, that means supporting her heart with pacing.

E: "The medications are ready."

C: "Please administer 1 mg of vecuronium and 5 mg of midazolam immediately and in that order. 20 seconds after the midazolam is in, administer 125 mg succinylcholine. If possible, I would like a second nurse to provide cricoid cartilage pressure."

E: "Done."

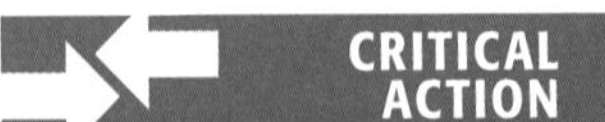

CRITICAL ACTION

Intubating the patient when she decompensates is a critical action in this case.

C: "I will now endotracheally intubate the patient with a 7-0 French tube. After placing the tube I will confirm the presence of bilateral breath sounds and use the colorimetric end-tidal CO_2 device to further confirm proper placement. Once intubation is completed and tube placement confirmed, I request that the nurse administer 9 mg vecuronium IV."

E: "Done. What now?"

C: "What are the patient's vital signs after intubation?"

E: "BP is now 105/68, HR successfully paced at 70, O_2 sat 100%."

C: "Has her ECG changed?"

E: "It shows a paced rhythm at 70 bpm."

C: "Is the cardiologist here?"

E: "Yes, and she wants to take the patient to the OR for immediate placement of an internal pacemaker. She is on the phone with the OR and with anesthesiology."

C: "May I please speak to Dr. Primary again? I would also like to update the patient's husband and any other family members on recent developments. If possible, I would like to speak to them all at once in a private consultation room."

E: "Dr. Primary is on the line."

C: "Dr. Primary, Mrs. Smith's condition has changed. Just after we spoke, she became unresponsive and hypotensive and I had to intubate her and initiate transcutaneous pacing. She has stabilized somewhat. The cardiologist is here and planning to take her to the OR for a transvenous pacer. I will update her family shortly."

E: "Thanks for the call. Please tell the cardiologist and Mrs. Smith's family that I will check in with them later when she is in the CCU. The case is now over."

CASE ASSESSMENT

The candidate managed the case well and achieved all critical actions. She recognized the potential for rapid deterioration in the patient. She placed transcutaneous pacer pads after the first electrocardiogram (ECG), and she initiated appropriate studies and interventions while proceeding with the interview and examination.

She also used atropine appropriately by making sure that the patient had no new ischemic changes on ECG or chest pain prior to use. On test day, atropine may not be effective and the patient will likely require transcutaneous pacing (TCP) for bradycardia. Like this patient, bradycardic patients who are stable do not need aggressive interventions such as TCP, pressors, and glucagon for potential beta-blocker toxicity. However, aggressive measures should be taken if the patient becomes unstable. While you must be careful about when you give atropine, aspirin is always appropriate.

For arrhythmia cases, particularly sudden and new-onset arrhythmias, you should focus your history, examination, and studies on discovering the underlying etiology or etiologies. Just like this case, many arrhythmias are multifactorial. The candidate did a good job of eliciting appropriate history, performing a focused and thorough examination, and ordering studies that demonstrated that she was considering a broad differential diagnosis for the etiology of the new bradyarrhythmia. Toxicology concerns, medication effects and interactions (including herbal medications), pulmonary embolism (PE), anemia, stroke, electrolyte imbalances, and endocrine etiologies must all be considered. It may not be important for you to identify the exact cause to pass a case, but it will be important to demonstrate that you are considering a wide differential diagnosis and that you act accordingly in your data acquisition and interventions. On exam day, keep in mind that all new arrhythmias are ischemic until proven otherwise. Also, the treatment for a dangerous bradyarrhythmia will involve an intervention like a pacemaker. Early placement of TCP pads will be a critical action in all bradyarrhythmia cases.

More aggressive measures should be implemented immediately if the patient presents in frank shock or deteriorates in the emergency department (ED). Understand that patients will deteriorate in oral exam cases for one of two reasons:

1. You are missing something or doing something wrong, or
2. You have proceeded properly in the early stages of the case and eventual deterioration is a planned "crash" to test your response.

Generally, the first scenario will occur early in a case if you are off target. If a patient deteriorates well into the case, this is likely a planned "crash." For both situations, you should go back to a primary survey and address any concerns. If you intervene and the patient does not improve, you are off target and must rapidly reconsider all data and assumptions to that point. If a patient suddenly deteriorates late in a case, but then responds rapidly to intervention (ie, intubation, resuscitation), then you are probably dealing with a planned "crash" and should keep moving forward. In this case the patient improved after pacing and intubation. Had she not improved, or only improved slightly, a fluid challenge and pressors would have been the next recommended interventions. The cases you face will be challenging, but not deliberately misleading.

The candidate directed the patient's care without being overly authoritative. She communicated well with nurses and the primary physician. She also made an effort to address the patient's concerns and to communicate with her family. Communicating detailed findings to a consulting physician and family members is an effective oral exam technique for displaying your understanding of the case.

Throughout the case, the candidate did a superb job of recognizing the potential severity of the patient's condition, implementing appropriate measures, both therapeutically and diagnostically, and did so without delay. She clearly exceeded the standard of care and would score well on the case.

Critical Actions

1. Obtain appropriate history, examination, and studies to seek potential underlying/reversible causes of bradycardia with weakness and hypotension—eg, medication adverse reaction(s), PE, myocardial infarction (MI), stroke, anemia, electrolyte abnormalities, diabetes ketoacidosis (DKA), etc—and make sure that ASA was given.
2. Apply transcutaneous pacer pads immediately after seeing rhythm strip.
3. Intubation and appropriate resuscitation if patient decompensates in ED.
4. Proper and early consultation with cardiology including plans for transvenous pacemaker and Cardiac/Coronary Care Unit (CCU) admission.

Test Performance

1. *Data acquisition:* Data acquisition was thorough and appropriately focused as the case evolved. Score = **8**
2. *Problem solving:* The candidate rapidly assessed the situation for severity and moved quickly to respond to data and changes in condition in an appropriate manner. She frequently asked for updates on the patient's condition and response to treatment, a good habit on oral exams. Score = **8**
3. *Patient management:* Excellent in all aspects. All critical actions met. See case assessment. Score = **8**
4. *Resource utilization:* Resources were used appropriately and cost-effectively. Score = **7**
5. *Health care provided (outcome):* The patient received appropriate treatment. The candidate met all critical actions, and rapidly stabilized the patient before admitting her to the appropriate service. Score = **8**
6. *Interpersonal relations and communication skills:* Appropriately directive, but not demanding. Good interactions with the patient's primary physician, nurses, and the patient's family. She did a good job addressing the patient's concerns. She should have requested permission before the rectal exam. Score = **7**
7. *Comprehension of pathophysiology:* The examinee conveyed her understanding of bradyarrythmias by her history and physical, workup and treatment. She displayed her understanding during her consultations and while speaking with the family. Score = **8**
8. *Clinical competence (overall):* The candidate did an excellent job as noted above. Score = **8**

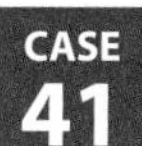

CASE 41 58 y/o Male With Shortness of Breath

John Dayton, Charles Maddow, and James I. Syrett

INITIAL INFORMATION

Time: 6:20 PM

Name: Mr. Yellow

Age: 58 years

Mode of arrival: Own vehicle

Gender: Male

VS: Pulse 92, BP 240/180, RR 26, sat: 90%

CC: Shortness of breath

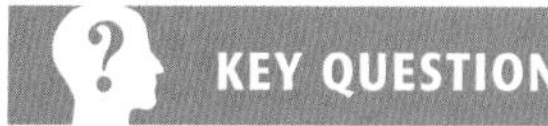

KEY QUESTION

Ask this open-ended question at the beginning of every case.

PLAY OF THE CASE

E: "The triage nurse asks you to see a patient that has just arrived in the ED. Here is his triage sheet."

C: "As I walk into the room what do I see, hear, and smell."

E: "You see an obese male sitting on the bed breathing fast. There are no abnormal sounds or smells."

C: "Sir, my name is Dr. Smith, I am going to ask our nurses to do some things and then I will speak to you."

E: "OK doctor, whatever you say."

C: "Nurse, can you place this patient on a NRB oxygen mask at 15 L. Also, place him on the cardiac monitor, run a rhythm strip, and give it to me. Start an IV and draw some blood for labs. Once the patient is on oxygen can you repeat his vital signs?"

E: "Your IV has been started, that patient is on the monitor and the rhythm strip shows sinus tachycardia, and the patient is on high flow oxygen. Repeat vital signs are pulse of 104, BP 252/190, RR 20, and sat 95%."

C: "Thank you. Mr. Yellow, my name is Dr. Smith. Why did you come up to hospital today?"

E: "Well, I have been short of breath for the last 4 hours, but it got really bad in the last hour."

C: "Have you ever had anything like this before?"

E: "Yes, a few years back, but I don't know what caused it."

C: "Sir, your blood pressure is very high. Do you have high blood pressure?"

E: "Yes, my doctor has been trying to treat me for it but I have not been able to afford the medicine, so I just do what I can."

C: "How long have you been off your medicines?"

E: "I ran out about 3 or 4 days ago."

C: "Do you remember what medicines you were prescribed?"

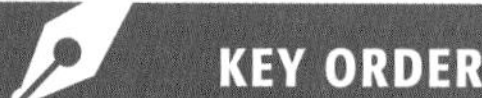

KEY ORDERS

Most of the patients you see during the exam are unstable (or will become that way). Every unstable patient requires IV access, oxygen, and cardiac monitoring (and in most cases an ECG).

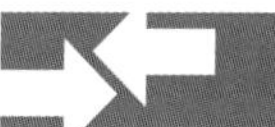

CRITICAL ACTION

Putting this hypoxic patient on the appropriate dose of oxygen is a critical action in this case.

DON'T FORGET

Always begin by treating any vital sign abnormality. Give fluids to people who are hypotensive, oxygen to people who are hypoxic, and antipyretics to people who are febrile. In this case, lower the blood pressure of people who are profoundly hypertensive.

E: "Yes, I was on HCTZ, Lasix, clonidine, atenolol, and Norvasc."

C: "And you stopped taking all these meds in the last few days?"

E: "Yes, do you think that is why I am short of breath?"

C: "It probably has something to do with it. Have you had any other symptoms, like headaches or chest pain?"

E: "Yes. I have had a headache for the last day and every now and then I have chest pain."

C: "Do you have pains in your chest now?"

E: "Yes, but that is not as bad as my breathing problem."

C: "OK Sir, I want to order some medications and tests now, and then I want to examine you. Do you have any allergies?"

E: "No."

C: "OK. Nurse, can you please give Mr. Yellow four baby aspirin tablets, and 0.4 mg of sublingual nitroglycerine. Also, can you get an ECG?"

E: "The nitro and aspirin are given, here is your ECG." (You are presented with an ECG showing sinus tachycardia and LVH with lateral ST depressions and highly peaked T waves.)

C: "Sir, have you ever had any problems with your kidneys?"

E: "Yes, I think they said that I have insufficiency."

C: "Have you been making urine?"

E: "Not really."

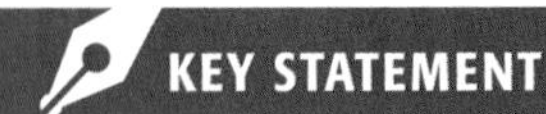

KEY STATEMENT

You need to know dosing for medications you would use in a code situation (ACLS, PALS, intubation meds). For all other medications, if you do not know the dose, it is OK to say that you will look them up.

C: "Sir, I am concerned that your blood pressure is causing a lot of your symptoms. Nurse, can you give Mr. Yellow 1 amp of calcium gluconate and some Kayexalate?"

E: "What dose do you want?"

C: "I am not sure, I would check the dose with the hospital pharmacy or the package insert."

E: "What is wrong doctor?"

C: "I am worried that your kidneys are not working very well and this is causing high levels of potassium in your blood. I am giving you some medications that help when you have too much potassium, but I still need to examine you."

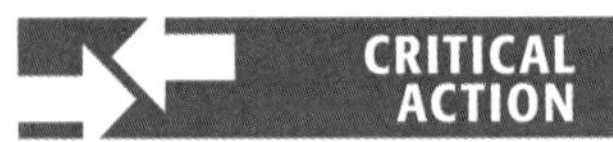

CRITICAL ACTION

Treatment of hyperkalemia with calcium is a critical action in this case.

E: "OK doctor. I still feel short of breath and my headache is worse since you gave me that stuff under my tongue."

C: "Yes, that is a side effect of the nitroglycerine. Sir, do you smoke or drink?"

E: "Yes, I drink a beer a night and smoke a pack of cigarettes every 3 days."

C: "Do any medical problems run in your family?"

E: "Yes, my dad died of a coronary when he was 52."

C: "OK, well, I would like to examine you now."

E: "OK doctor. The nurse wants to know what to do with the blood she just drew."

C: "Nurse, can you send the blood you drew for the following labs: CBC, BMP, coagulation studies, and a troponin."

E: "Your labs have been sent."

C: "When I examine the HEENT, what do I find?"

E: "What are you looking for?"

C: "I would like to examine the eyes and do a funduscopic examination. I would also like to palpate the neck for any masses and assess the JVP."

E: "The fundi show large soft and hard exudates. There are no masses in the neck. The JVP is slightly elevated."

C: "The chest examination?"

E: "Again, what do you want?"

C: "I would like to visualize the chest, percuss and then auscultate."

E: "The chest looks normal, there is bibasilar dullness and fine crackles on auscultation."

C: "I would like to give Mr. Yellow 40 mg of IV Lasix."

E: "The drug is given."

C: "The cardiovascular examination?"

E: "What do you want to know?"

C: "I would like to feel for heaves, then auscultate the heart and carotids."

E: "There is a left ventricular heave, the rate is tachycardic, and there are no murmurs."

C: "The GI examination?"

E: "Normal."

C: "Is there abdominal tenderness, organomegaly, or ascites?"

E: "None found."

C: "Is there swelling in the scrotum? Is the rest of the GU examination normal?"

E: "The patient is now making some urine. Otherwise normal."

C: "Can we send the urine for a urine dip?"

E: "The urine has been sent."

C: "The skin and neurologic examination?"

E: "The skin and neuro exams are normal."

C: "Thank you. I would like to order a repeat ECG, a CXR and also give Mr. Yellow something more for his high blood pressure."

E: "The ECG is done and shows some resolving of the peaked T waves. The CXR is done and here it is (Fig. C41-1). What do you want to give to the patient?"

C: "The CXR shows severe fluid overload. I would like to start this patient on a nitroglycerin drip. We can also give him 0.1mg of clonidine, in case he is withdrawing from it. I would also like to put this patient on BIPAP."

E: "What dose of nitroglycerin do you want to give?"

C: "I want to start an infusion, but I would look up the starting dose and titrate it to reduce his MAP by 20%. I would also like to put in an arterial line in this patient so I can closely follow his blood pressure. I would like to review the results of the labs I sent."

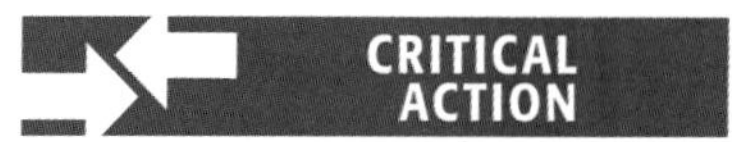

Initiating IV blood pressure control is a critical action in this case. The examinee could have done this earlier, as the diagnosis of hypertensive emergency is obvious from the initial vitals and presentation. However, they were not wrong to initiate SL nitro to buy time for a physical examination.

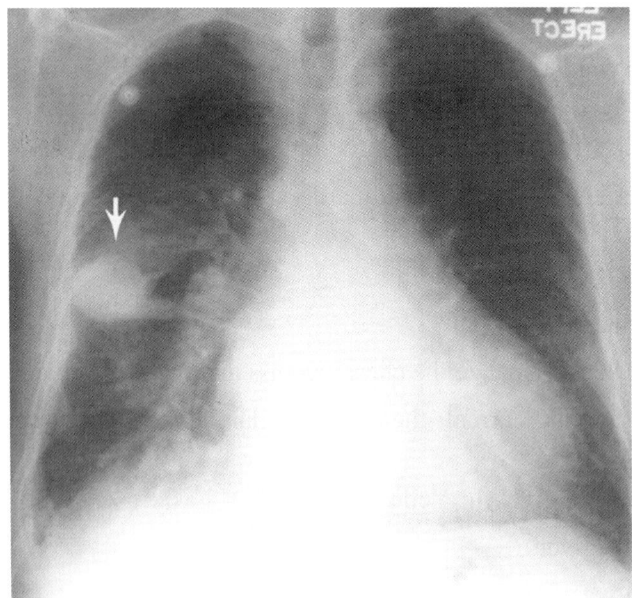

Figure C41-1. CXR. *(Reprinted with permission from Stone CK, Humphries RL.* Current Diagnosis and Treatment: Emergency Medicine. *6th ed. New York, NY: McGraw-Hill; 2008.)*

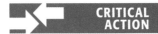

Getting this patient emergent dialysis for his renal failure is a critical action in this case.

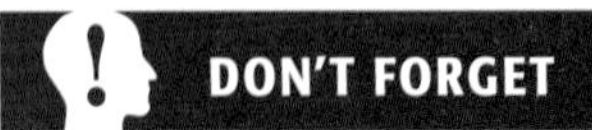

Remember that consultants will often "push back" as a tool to test your knowledge of patient management. Do not be afraid to insist on appropriate care.

E: "The patient is on BIPAP. The arterial line is working, the nitroglycerin is running. Your lab tests are now back. The CBC, coags, and troponin are unremarkable. His basic metabolic panel is remarkable for a potassium of 6.8 and a creatinine of 7.1."

C: "I would like to speak to the renal attending on call because I am concerned that the patient is in renal failure with CHF and hypertensive emergency."

E: "Dr. Kidney is now on the phone."

C: "Dr. Kidney, my name is Dr. Smith and I am covering the ED tonight. I have a 58-year-old male that has presented with hypertensive emergency, CHF, and acute chronic renal failure. I have given him calcium gluconate and Kayexalate for peaked T waves on his ECG and a potassium of 6.8. I have also given him Lasix and a nitroglycerine drip for the pulmonary edema and started BIPAP. I think he needs emergent dialysis and would like you to admit him to the ICU."

E: "OK, admit him to my service and I will see him in the morning."

C: "Sir, you need to see him tonight. He needs dialysis now due to his highly elevated potassium with ECG changes and fluid overload."

E: "OK, I will come in now to see him. This ends the management portion of this case."

CASE ASSESSMENT

This case had a rapid progression and incorporated several disruptors to its flow. The case presented as shortness of breath but developed into acute renal failure and hypertensive emergency. It is often the case that presenting complaints develop into other pathologies in the oral board exam.

This case started with abnormal vital signs on the triage sheet. Abnormal vital signs **must** be dealt with immediately. In this case the candidate initiated oxygen and monitoring and then proceeded with a quick history and physical examination. The candidate also initiated testing before starting the examination. This is appropriate in this circumstance. In this case, the candidate requested, and got, an electrocardiogram (ECG) immediately. They were then required to act on the ECG finding before lab results were available.

Examination of the patient revealed several medical issues. The candidate recognized that the patient could be withdrawing from clonidine and medicated appropriately. In addition, appropriate management was initiated for congestive heart failure (CHF), hyperkalemia, and hypertensive emergency.

Throughout this case, the examiner asked for specific drug doses. If you are unsure of dosing, it is appropriate to check either with the hospital pharmacy or the package insert. The package insert should always be available. While this approach may be less than optimal, giving the incorrect dose of the drug could be far more damaging.

This case developed quickly. This rapid development can sometimes throw an exam candidate. Often the first area that suffers is the required physician-patient interactions. In this case, the candidate neglected to inform the patient of developments. It is important to involve the patient as much as possible in order to maximize your score for "Interpersonal Relations and Communications Skills." These points are both easy to get and easy to lose.

Finally, this case ended with the difficult consultant. Often if a consultant refuses to come in to see the patient, the candidate must insist on them seeing the patient. Your response is a chance to show your interpersonal skills and understanding of the case.

Critical Actions

1. Initiation of oxygen
2. Recognition and management of hyperkalemia with calcium
3. Initiation of IV antihypertensive
4. Demanding emergent dialysis

Test Performance

1. *Data acquisition:* Data was acquired efficiently and in a timely manner. Diagnostic lab studies, imaging, and ECG were included. Score = **8**
2. *Problem solving:* All of the important medical conditions were treated in a timely manner, although the candidate was not familiar with some drug doses. Score = **6**
3. *Patient management:* The patient care was fine. The patient was efficiently assessed and managed and the appropriate diagnostic testing and medications were ordered and administered. Am antihypertensive agent could have been started earlier in the case. Score = **7**
4. *Resource utilization:* Tests were ordered in a cost-effective manner and in an appropriate time frame. Appropriate consults were made and emergency conditions efficiently dealt with. Score = **8**
5. *Health care provided (outcome):* The patient received appropriate treatment, and the candidate's interventions stabilized the patient. As per above, blood pressure (BP) control could have occurred earlier. Score = **7**

6. *Interpersonal relations and communication skills:* While the candidate handled the difficult consultant interaction well, he could have communicated better with the patient. Score = **5**
7. *Comprehension of pathophysiology:* The examinee conveyed their understanding of hypertensive urgency, hyperkalemia, and acute kidney injury (AKI) by asking appropriate questions, ordering appropriate studies and using necessary interventions. Their understanding was further shown by their conversation with consultants. Score = **7**.
8. *Clinical competence (overall):* The candidate showed clinical competence by obtaining an appropriate history and physical, developing a differential diagnosis, utilizing appropriate lab work and imaging, utilizing appropriate interventions, and working toward the appropriate disposition. Score = **7**

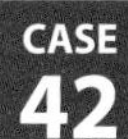

CASE 42 35 y/o Female With Depression and Suicide Attempt

John Dayton, Fred Abrahamian, and Reb Close

INITIAL INFORMATION

Name: Jane Smith

Mode of arrival: Brought in by husband

Time of arrival: 2:00 AM

Age: 37 years

Gender: Female

VS: T 38.8°C (101.84°F), BP 130/76, HR 120, RR 24, O_2 sat: 90% on RA

CC: Depression

PLAY OF THE CASE

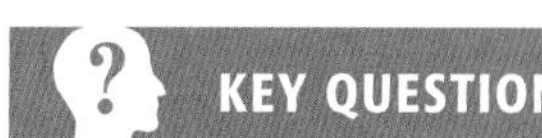

KEY QUESTION

Ask this open-ended question at the beginning of every case.

C: "What do I see as I walk into the patient's room?"

E: "A female who appears anxious and uncomfortable. Her husband is at the bedside."

C: "Before I begin with the history and physical, I would like to address the ABCs. I would like to ask the patient her name and what brings her to the ED today."

E: "She is able to tell you her name and states, 'I … just … can't … do it … anymore.' You note she seems short of breath, breathing rapidly and taking deep breaths."

C: "I would like to listen to her lungs."

E: "What would you like to know?"

C: "I would like to listen for rate and depth of breathing. I would also like to listen for rales, rhonchi, and wheezes."

E: "She is tachypneic, taking deep breaths, and you hear rales in the bases of her lungs."

C: "I would ask the nurse to please place the patient on 2 L of oxygen via NC, start a large bore IV, draw blood for labs, and start a bolus of NS at 500 cc/h. I would also like her to have 1 gram of Tylenol for her fever. How does the patient look and what are her vitals after these interventions?"

E: "Her temperature has come down to 38.3°C, BP is 125/85, HR is 105, and RR is 20 at 94% of 2 L NC. She seems less agitated, and she is breathing more comfortably."

C: "Since she is more stable, I would like to obtain a history from Mrs. Smith and her husband. 'Mrs. Smith, what do you mean you can't do it anymore?'"

E: "I just can't handle life. I'm worthless to my family and they would be better off without me."

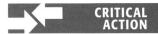

CRITICAL ACTION

Eliciting the patient's suicidal ideation is a critical action in this case.

C: "How long have you been feeling this way?"

E: "For years, but it's been worse over the last few months."

C: "Is there something that happened to make it worse?"

E: "Two of my siblings recently died and it just is too much to take right now."

C: "Are you having thoughts of hurting yourself?"

E: "Yes."

C: "Are you undergoing treatment for depression?"

E: "I was, but I stopped taking my antidepressants because they don't work."

C: "When did you stop taking them?"

E: "Two weeks ago."

C: "Did you take anything to commit suicide?"

E: "I took a handful of pills at home."

C: "What kind? How many?"

E: "I don't know."

C: "Can you tell me any more information?"

E: "I'm done talking about that."

C: "Nurse, please send the blood drawn earlier for a CBC, complete metabolic panel, coagulation studies, and send for serum levels of salicylates, acetaminophen, and alcohol. Please also check an ABG and TSH. Let's also obtain a urine sample for pregnancy and toxicology screen. I'd also like an ECG."

E: The ECG shows sinus tachycardia and the labs are running"

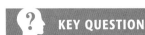

KEY QUESTION

Remember to use the resources around you. Ask family members and witnesses for any additional history.

C: "Mr. Smith, is there anything you would like to add?"

E: "We've been through this so many times. I got really scared tonight and wanted to bring her to the ER, but she locked herself in the bathroom. I was finally able to unlock the door and she agreed to come in. She threw up a few times on the way here. She's been acting dizzy and needed me to keep my arm around her so she wouldn't fall. She seems very agitated."

C: "Did you notice any open or empty bottles in the bathroom?"

E: "Yes, there was an empty bottle of baby aspirin on the counter."

C: "Thank you, that helps a lot. Before we can have you speak with Psychiatry, we need to make sure that you can safely be admitted to their service. Do you have any medical problems?"

E: "Chronic depression."

C: "What medicines are you taking?"

E: "I was taking Prozac until recently."

C: "Do you have allergies to medicines?"

E: "No."

C: "You had a fever when you got here. Have you had any recent infection, cough, sore throat, difficulty breathing, vomiting and diarrhea, or rash?"

E: "No"

C: "Do you have any chest pain, shortness of breath or other symptom?

E: "I feel dizzy, my ears are ringing, and I feel like I really need to keep taking deep breaths."

C: "I need to examine you now. What is the HEENT examination?"

E: "What do you want to know?"

C: "Are pupils constricted or dilated? Are they equal, round, react to light, with EOMs intact? Are there any abnormal findings on examination of the external ear, auditory canal and TMs? Any sign of infection?"

E: "Unremarkable HEENT exam."

C: "Is there scalp or facial soft tissue swelling, tenderness or sign of trauma?"

E: "Atraumatic."

C: "Is the neck supple or JVD present?"

E: "Supple without JVD."

C: "Are the lungs clear? Are there any murmurs, gallops, or rubs? Are the peripheral pulses full?"

E: "The patient sounds better than on initial exam, but still has tachypnea and basilar rales."

C: "Is the abdomen tender and are bowel sounds present? Any organomegaly or masses?"

E: "Here bowel sounds are active, but exam is otherwise unremarkable."

C: "Is there clubbing, cyanosis, edema, or joint soft tissue swelling or tenderness?"

E: "None found."

C: "Is there bruising, petechiae, or rashes? Is there any sign of infection? Any sign of IV drug use?

E: "There are no abnormal findings."

C: "Is there back or flank tenderness?"

E: "No."

C: "On neurologic examination, is the patient oriented × 3? Are the cranial nerves, motor, sensory, and cerebellar examinations intact? Are the deep tendon reflexes symmetrical?"

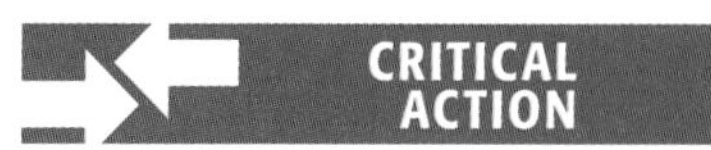

Sending toxicology and ingestion labs is a critical action in this case.

E: "She is becoming increasing agitated and has difficulty answering your questions. Given the information the husband gave earlier, you don't think it is safe to check her gait."

C: "Does she have a flat affect and depressed mood?"

E: "She did, but now she looks anxious and nauseated. She proceeds to vomit in the room."

C: "Nurse, please give the patient 4 mg of Zofran. What are her most recent vital signs?"

E: "Temp 37.9°C, BP is 115/80, HR is 105, and RR is 20 at 92% on 2 L NC."

C: "Nurse, please turn her oxygen up to 4 L NC, and please give 1 mg if Ativan. Have radiology shoot a portable upright chest X-ray in her room instead of having her leave the ED. Please give a bolus of 1 mEq/kg of sodium bicarb, and start her on a liter of D5W with 150 mEq of sodium bicarb. Are any of the labs back?"

E: "Some are. Here are your findings:

- ABG: Ph 7.46, PO_2 90, PCO_2 22, HCO_3 18.
- CBC: WBC 8.0, Hgb/Hct 13/39, plt 85,000
- CMP: Na 140, K 3.5, Cl 105, CO 17, BUN 45, Cr 2.5, glu 105, LFTs mildly elevated
- Coags: unremarkable

C: "What about the serum toxicology levels?"

E: "They are not finished yet."

C: "Do we have x-ray results?"

E: "The portable CXR shows fluid in the bases of her lungs. You notice that Mrs. Smith is trying to getting dressed and leave."

C: "Ms. Smith, is something wrong?"

E: "I'm sick of this. I'm leaving!"

C: "Mrs. Smith, we would like to help you with your depression. You have clearly expressed a desire to end your life, so I can't let you leave the ED."

Initiating an involuntary psychiatric hold is a critical action for this patient with active suicidal ideation.

E: "Screw you. I'm not staying!"

C: "Nurse, could you please get security to help, I'm putting Mrs. Smith on a psychiatric hold for danger to herself. Could you also give her another milligram of Ativan and 5 mg of Haldol?"

E: "Security is standing by."

C: "Mrs. Smith, we need to detain you in the ED for your own safety. These gentlemen are here to help you. Please understand we only want to keep you safe. Nurse, can you page Nephrology? I also need to speak with the psychiatry, please. How is she doing after those medications?"

E: "She is calmer. Nephrology is on the phone."

C: "Hello. I have a patient I'm concerned has salicylate toxicity and needs to be dialyzed. She is after an ingestion and her husband found an empty aspirin bottle in their bathroom. She presented tachypneic and febrile, she noted tinnitus and dizziness, she has fluid in the base of her lungs and her initial labs show a mixed respiratory alkalosis and metabolic acidosis with hypokalemia, and elevated creatinine. I've started her on oxygen and a bicarb bolus and drip, but I'm concerned she will need dialysis for definitive management."

E: "What is her salicylate level?"

C: "It is still pending."

E: "That sounds find. I'll come to the ED to assess her and start admission. Psychiatry is on the phone now."

C: "Hello Dr. Shrink. I have admitted a patient to nephrology for hemodialysis for salicylate toxicity. She has been placed on a psychiatric hold because of active suicidal ideation and an attempt prior to arrival. She is not yet medically cleared. Can you consult on her during this admission?"

E: "Yes. This case is over."

CASE ASSESSMENT

This is a difficult case about a suicidal patient. Although her depression is clear, there is some question about what she took and when she took it. It was important to try to elicit the history of the ingestion, but the history is often difficult to obtain in suicidal patients. The candidate was resourceful in talking with the husband to ask about any empty medication bottles. Because the patient was a poor historian, asking the spouse was the only way to get the needed information. This case is a good reminder to use all possible resources in obtaining a history. The candidate was aware of the ingestion and appropriately evaluated the patient for any evidence of toxicity. The candidate did a very thorough medical history and physical examination.

Without a history of ingestion, the candidate would have needed another source for the fever and had to do a more complete workup. The fluid on the chest x-ray (CXR) and hypoxia could have led to a possible misdiagnosis of pneumonia. Without a definitive source and altered mental status, the candidate may have needlessly pursued a lumbar puncture.

Although it may have been tempting to start collecting history, the patient did a great job of managing the airway, breathing, and circulation (ABCs) first. Once the patient was more stable, he proceeded with the history and physical and ordered the labs and electrocardiogram (ECG) to evaluate the possibility of a toxic ingestion. As this patient became agitated and tried to leave, the candidate appropriately initiated a psychiatric hold. The patient had clearly expressed her suicidal intent and could not be allowed to leave the emergency department (ED). Having security involved was necessary to keep the patient safe.

Even though the salicylate level was not available, the candidate correctly identified salicylate toxicity that would require hemodialysis. He had to be confident in this decision. Indications for hemodialysis for salicylate toxicity include the following:

- Altered mental status
- Fluid overload (particularly with concern for pulmonary and cerebral edema)
- Renal insufficiency
- Salicylate levels of >100 mg/dL
- Clinical worsening despite appropriate care

The candidate recognized these findings and called Nephrology for dialysis and the Psychiatrist for consultation. The candidate gave both consultants the appropriate information and showed his understanding of the case during the consultations.

Critical Actions

1. Elicit the history of suicidal ideation.
2. Check for ingestion.
3. Recognize salicylate toxicity.
4. Place the patient in psychiatric hold.
5. Admit for hemodialysis.

Test Performance

1. *Data acquisition:* The candidate obtained all of the information required to make the correct diagnosis. He requested additional information from the husband. He included concern for infection and toxidromic features during history and physical. Score = **8**
2. *Problem solving:* The examinee used vital signs, asked appropriate exam questions and used lab work to figure out that the patient had salicylate toxicity. He stabilized the patient, and both anticipated and prevented future problems. Score = **8**
3. *Patient management:* The examinee recognized when interventions needed to be made and obtained appropriate consultations to create a safe disposition. Score = **8**
4. *Resource utilization:* The candidate used appropriate lab work, imaging, and obtained information from both the patient and her husband. The workup was logical, cost-sensitive, and showed patient concern. Score = **8**
5. *Health care provided (outcome):* The patient received efficient, appropriate treatment, and the candidate's interventions stabilized the patient. Even though she had an evolving presentation, the candidate did a great job of making appropriate interventions and then following up to see if they had been effective. Score = **8**
6. *Interpersonal relations and communication skills:* Initially, the candidate communicated appropriately with the patient and her husband, though he could have done better to follow-up and explain the plan. His consultations with Nephrology and Renal were succinct, professional, and appropriate. Score = **6**
7. *Comprehension of pathophysiology:* The candidate conveyed understanding of toxic ingestions and indications for hemodialysis with salicylate toxicity. This was shown through orders, interventions, and consultations. Score = **8**
8. *Clinical competence (overall):* The candidate showed clinical competence by obtaining an appropriate history and physical, developing a differential diagnosis, utilizing appropriate lab work and imaging, using appropriate interventions, consulting with specialists, and working toward the appropriate disposition. As was mentioned before, he lost points only for not keeping the family more updated of the final disposition plan. Score = **7**

CASE 43 44 y/o Male With Weakness

John Dayton and Fiona Gallahue

INITIAL INFORMATION

Name: Ben Jones

Mode of arrival: Private car

Age: 44 years

Gender: Male

VS: BP 180/80, HR 110, RR 18, T 37°C (98.6°F), O_2 sat: 96% on RA

CC: Weakness and "not feeling right"

PLAY OF THE CASE

C: "What do I see when I walk into the room?"

E: "You see a middle-aged man sitting straight up on the stretcher in no apparent distress."

C: "Hello Mr. Jones, I'm Dr. Case. What seems to be the problem today?"

E: "Well, I just don't feel quite right. I've been gaining weight lately and just feeling poorly…and weak."

C: "Nurse, could we please put Mr. Jones on a cardiac monitor. Give him oxygen at 2 L via NC, and please place an IV drawing blood for labs? I'd like to get a 12-lead ECG and see it as soon as it's available, please."

E: "Those orders are being carried out."

C: "How long has this been going on?"

E: "A few weeks."

C: "Have you noticed any fevers, chills, nausea, or vomiting?"

E: "A little nausea sometimes, but no fevers, chills, or vomiting."

C: "Any abdominal pain, diarrhea, or bloating?"

E: "Sometimes I get some mild abdominal discomfort, but not exactly pain, and no diarrhea or bloating."

C: "Have you noticed any rashes or swelling in your extremities?"

E: "No rashes, but my legs have been getting a little swollen lately."

C: "What medical problems do you have?"

E: "HTN and DM."

C: "What medications do you use?"

E: "I take atenolol and insulin."

C: "Do you have any allergies to medications?"

E: "No."

C: "Do you have a regular doctor?"

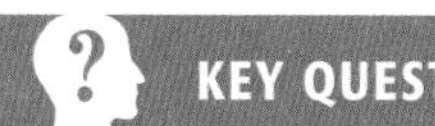

Ask this open-ended question at the beginning of every case.

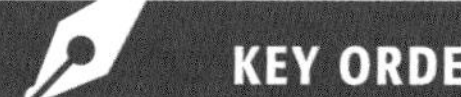

Most of the patients you see during the exam are unstable (or will become that way). Every unstable patient requires IV access, oxygen, and cardiac monitoring (and in most cases an ECG).

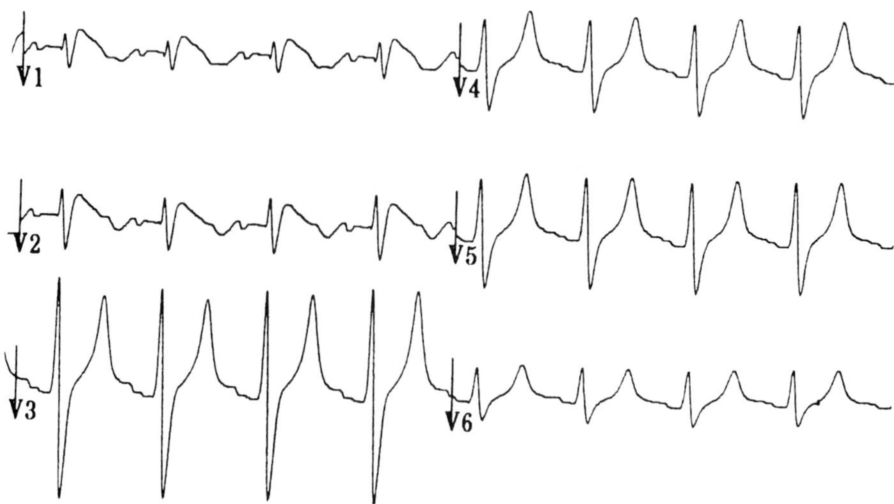

Figure C43-1. ECG showing severe hyperkalemia with widening of the QRS complex. *(Reproduced with permission from Fuster V, O'Rourke RA, Walsh R, Poole-Wilson P.* Hurst's the Heart. 12th ed. *New York, NY: McGraw-Hill; 2008.)*

E: "Yes, Dr. Brown."

C: "When was the last time you saw Dr. Brown?"

E: "About 3 months ago. He told me I needed to lose some weight, but otherwise everything was fine."

C: "Good. Do you have anyone with you today?"

E: "No, my wife is at work."

C: "OK."

E: "Doctor, that 12-lead ECG is ready for you (Fig. C43-1)."

C: "This ECG looks very worrisome to me for either a cardiac problem or hyperkalemia. I'd like to have blood sent for CBC, PT/PTT, electrolytes including Mg, P, and Ca, BUN, Cr, and troponin. I'd also like to give 10 cc of 10% calcium gluconate immediately, 44 mEq of sodium bicarbonate, nebulized albuterol, 10 U of regular insulin IV, 50 g of dextrose (2 amp of D50%) IV and 30 g of Kayexalate orally. I'd also like to make sure this patient receives 325 mg of ASA and chews it right away. He's on oxygen already, so let's make sure he stays on the oxygen. I'd also like to give the patient sublingual nitro of 0.4 mg to help with his blood pressure and possibly improve coronary artery blood flow if he's got an acute coronary syndrome. I'd like to order a portable CXR as well. Could we please repeat a 12-lead ECG as soon as all of those orders have been done please? Mr. Jones, are you sure you do not have any chest pain or shortness of breath right now?"

Recognizing and treating the patient's severe hyperkalemia immediately is a critical action in this case.

E: "I have very mild shortness of breath, but that's been going on for weeks and there's no change now. I don't have any chest pain."

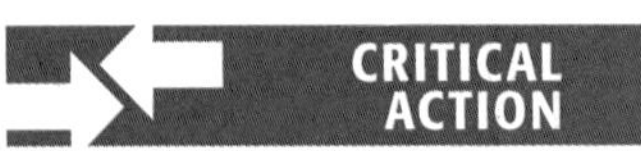

Getting a repeat ECG to assure success of the treatment is a critical action in this case.

C: "Have you had the feeling of having to urinate more often than you used to?"

E: "Yes, I've had to get up in the night a few times to go to the bathroom recently. I never used to have to do that."

C: "Besides urinating more frequently, do you have more urgency to urinate?"

E: "Yes, it's been a problem."

C: "Have you had a difficult time getting your urine to start or noticed a change in the stream of your urine?"

E: "Yes, it takes me a while to get started and the stream isn't very forceful."

C: "Do you have the feeling that after you urinated, you did not completely empty your bladder?"

E: "Yes."

C: "I'd like an HEENT examination especially looking for any JVD, or bruits in the carotids."

E: "The HEENT examination is normal."

C: "I'd like to do a cardiac examination looking especially for any murmurs, friction rubs, gallops, muffled heart sounds."

E: "Cardiac examination is normal with no murmurs, rubs, gallops, and a normal S_1/S_2."

C: "I'd like to do a lung examination listening for any rales, crackles, rhonchi, or wheezing."

E: "There are mild rales at bilateral lung bases, otherwise normal examination."

C: "I'd like to check an abdominal examination for hepatosplenomegaly, any evidence of tenderness, hepatojugular reflux, and bowel sounds."

E: "The abdominal examination is completely normal."

C: "I'd like to do a rectal examination, check the prostate, and guaiac the stool."

E: "Rectal examination reveals an enlarged prostate with no nodules, brown stool that is guaiac negative."

C: "I'd like to check the extremities for any clubbing, cyanosis, or edema and check for pulses in all four extremities. I'd also like to check the skin for any rashes or other abnormalities."

E: "There is +1 edema in both lower extremities, equal strong pulses in all extremities, and a normal skin examination."

C: "I'd like to check a neuro examination specifically looking for any focal areas of weakness. I'll also check cranial nerves, motor and sensory function, reflexes, gait, and cerebellar functions."

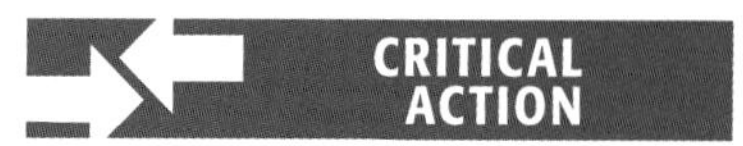

Continuing to treat the hyperkalemia is a critical action in this case.

E: "The neuro examination is symmetric, and though he is diffusely weak, there are no focal abnormalities. His cranial nerves are intact, sensation is equal, and he has symmetric, but depressed, DTR. No cerebellar findings."

C: "Do I have my repeat ECG?"

E: "It is available (Fig. C43-2). What are your concerns?"

C: "I'm concerned that this patient continues to have hyperkalemia, based on these peaked T waves, despite initial treatment. I'd like to repeat the doses of 10 cc of 10% calcium gluconate, nebulized albuterol, and give another 10 U of insulin with 2 amps of dextrose (50 g of dextrose) please and repeat another 12-lead ECG. Please place a Foley catheter, send a UA, and monitor urine output please."

E: "Those orders are being carried out."

C: "I'd like to place a call to Dr. Brown, please?"

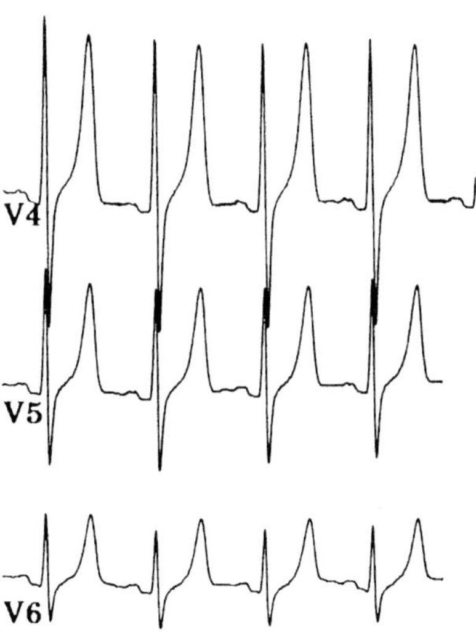

Figure C43-2. ECG showing severe hyperkalemia, with QRS narrower than the previous, but still with highly elevated T waves. (*Reproduced with permission from Fuster V, O'Rourke RA, Walsh R, Poole-Wilson P.* Hurst's the Heart. *12th ed. New York, NY: McGraw-Hill; 2008.)*

E: "Dr. Brown is on the line."

C: "Hello, Dr. Brown, this is Dr. Case. I have your patient Mr. Ben Jones here complaining of generalized weakness over the past few weeks without pain or focal weakness. On examination, he has bilateral rales and bilateral lower extremity edema. His initial ECG showed widened QRS complexes. I gave the patient aspirin, oxygen, nitroglycerine, calcium gluconate, bicarb, insulin, glucose, nebulized albuterol, and Kayexalate because I was concerned about possible hyperkalemia, although I'm concerned about the possibility of an acute coronary syndrome as well. I'm still waiting for his laboratory tests to come back. His repeat ECG after treatment continues to show peaked T waves with narrowing complexes, concerning for persistent hyperkalemia. I'd like to get additional medical history from you. I'd also like to contact a nephrologist in case he needs dialysis. I think he needs to be ruled out for acute coronary syndrome so I'd like to admit him to an ICU bed."

E: "Dr. Case. Thank you for your assessment. Mr. Jones has had evidence of chronic renal insufficiency for a few years, probably due to the fact that he's noncompliant with his antihypertensive medications. His baseline BUN/Cr are about 30/2.2 and they've been fairly stable there for the last year. He does have cardiac risk factors, so although he had a normal stress test 2 years ago, he could also have a cardiac cause for his weakness. I'd like to admit him to the ICU to monitor him. I'm a cardiologist and would be happy to follow him. Could you please call my partner, Dr. Nephron, a nephrologist, in case he needs dialysis? I'm rounding in the hospital and I'll be down in 10 minutes to see the patient. Thanks again."

C: "You're welcome."

E: "Doctor, your labs, CXR, and a third ECG are available (Fig. C43-3)."

- CXR: No infiltrates or effusions, mild vascular engorgement with cephalization, but a normal cardiac silhouette
- CBC: WBC 8.0, Hgb/Hct 13/39, plt 205,000

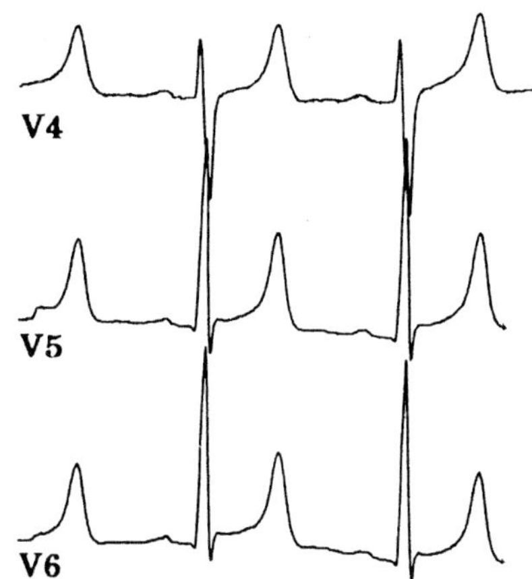

Figure C43-3. ECG showing hyperkalemia with narrow QRS complex with peaked T waves. (*Reproduced with permission from Fuster V, O'Rourke RA, Walsh R, Poole-Wilson P.* Hurst's the Heart. *12th ed. New York, NY: McGraw-Hill; 2008.)*

- Electrolytes: Na 140, K 8.2 non-hemolyzed, Cl 108, CO 14, BUN 88, Cr 7.5, glu 135, Ca 6.0, Mg 2.0, P 5.0
- Troponin <0.1
- UA: No leukocytes, nitrites, ketones, or bilirubin; trace blood and 2+ protein; no WBC or RBC

C: "I'd like to see if the Foley is putting out any urine?"

E: "The Foley has 300 cc of clear urine in the bag."

C: "OK, it looks like the ECG is improving. It looks like the source of hyperkalemia is renal failure. I'd like to give this patient 40 mg of Lasix for both fluid overload and hyperkalemia. I'd also like to re-check the potassium. Please recheck a blood pressure after those medications. I'd like to place a phone call to Dr. Nephron since I think Mr. Jones may need dialysis soon."

E: "Those orders are being carried out and Dr. Nephron is on the phone."

C: "Hello Dr. Nephron, this is Dr. Case. I just spoke to your partner, Dr. Brown about one of his patients, Ben Jones. He asked that I call you. Mr. Jones is a hypertensive, diabetic man who is noncompliant with his anti-hypertensive medications and with an enlarged prostate. He presents today with acute-on-chronic renal failure. His ECG initially had widened QRS complexes. I was concerned about hyperkalemia, so I treated him presumptively with nebulized albuterol, calcium gluconate, insulin, dextrose, sodium bicarb, and Kayexalate. His repeat ECG was better, but still showed significantly peaked T waves, so I repeated the albuterol, calcium, insulin, and dextrose and this led to improvement on his ECG. His labs came back with a BUN and Cr of 88 and 7.5 respectively with an initial potassium of 8.2 which we will repeat in a few minutes. Mr. Jones also has some evidence of mild fluid overload which I'm treating with nitroglycerine. Because he appears to be making urine, I've given him Lasix. However, I'm concerned he is going to need acute dialysis."

E: "OK, I'll be able to see him in 2 hours after I finish my clinic visits. Could you admit him to a general floor bed? His acute problem seems to have been taken care of and he sounds pretty stable to me."

Consulting nephrology and getting emergent dialysis are two critical actions in this case.

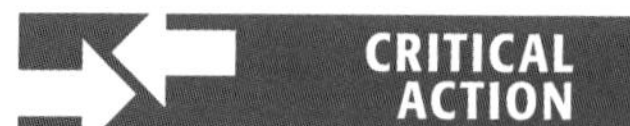

Admitting this patient into the ICU is a critical action in this case.

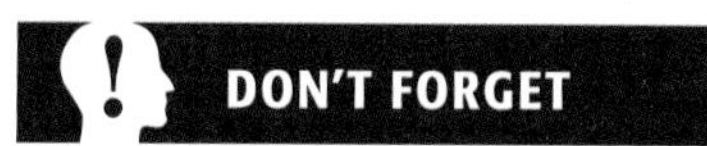

Remember—consultants will often "push back" as a tool to test your knowledge of patient management. Do not be afraid to insist on appropriate care. Use this opportunity to show your understanding of the case.

C: "Because of his life-threatening hyperkalemia, I believe an ICU bed would be more appropriate. I've discussed this with your partner and he agrees. I'd like to call the ICU consult now to get the patient admitted."

E: "OK, that's fine. Proceed."

E: "The ICU attending, Dr. Smith is on the line."

C: "Hello Dr. Smith, this is Dr. Case. I have a patient of Dr. Brown's by the name of Ben Jones who needs admission to an ICU bed. He's got acute-on-chronic renal failure, has a BUN/Cr of 88 and 7.5 mg/dL respectively along with hyperkalemia with a potassium of 8.2. I've treated him with calcium gluconate, bicarb, nebulized albuterol, insulin, glucose, and Kayexalate. His ECGs are improving, but his initial ECG was very worrisome with a wide QRS complex. After initial treatment, the QRS wave is narrowing, but the T waves are still peaked. He also has mild fluid overload which I'm treating with sublingual nitro and furosemide. Dr. Nephron said he'll be evaluating the patient shortly for dialysis and Dr. Brown will follow him as well. I'd like to have him admitted to the ICU for likely dialysis, monitoring of his cardiovascular status and hyperkalemia, and also to rule out a possible acute coronary syndrome as a contributing cause to his shortness of breath and weakness."

E: "I agree with that plan."

C: "Thank you."

E: "The repeat BP is 150/70 and there is an ICU bed ready. The patient is being wheeled up to the ICU. This concludes this case."

CASE ASSESSMENT

The candidate did an excellent job of managing this case, recognizing quickly that the patient had a potentially life-threatening issue, and addressing that issue well. She moved through the case well by asking for help from the nurse and her multiple colleagues. The candidate did an excellent job of rechecking the electrocardiograms (ECGs) to help direct management, as well as coordinating the multiple consultants who needed to be involved with this case. This was a complicated case requiring repeated checks on the patient and repeated doses of a multiple medications to successfully treat the hyperkalemia. The candidate included other causes in the differential including acute coronary syndrome (ACS) and treated the patient accordingly with aspirin, oxygen, and he checked cardiac enzymes and requested a cardiology consultation.

This patient had multiple reasons for renal failure including poorly controlled hypertension, use of s beta-blockers, diabetes, and an enlarged prostate. It is possible that his prostatic enlargement is the cause of his acute renal insufficiency.

This case demonstrates the need to continuously go back and re-address concerns with the patient. In this case, the ECG abnormality alerted the candidate to the likelihood of hyperkalemia. The candidate needed to recheck the ECG in order to be certain that her management was appropriate. This is a key component to patient care in the oral boards. Make sure you keep rechecking abnormal findings and vital signs after each intervention. This will be helpful in ensuring the patient is being managed correctly.

Critical Actions

1. Recognize the initial ECG as probable hyperkalemia.
2. Treat the hyperkalemia.

3. Recheck ECGs to ensure treatment appropriate.
4. Nephrology consultation.
5. Admit patient to the ICU (don't let a consultant talk you out of this, which was briefly attempted in this case).

Test Performance

1. *Data acquisition:* Data acquisition is excellent as the patient had some very serious ECG abnormalities which could have represented either hyperkalemia or ACS. She did a great job of getting information from the PMD and of rechecking the ECGs to help assess her management. Score = **8**
2. *Problem solving:* Problem solving is excellent. The candidate was able to rapidly assimilate data from the patient encounter, interpret test results, and synthesize information quickly to direct further management. Score = **8**
3. *Patient management:* The candidate did an excellent job. She made the appropriate treatment decisions based on patient information, scientific evidence, and clinical judgement. She rechecked abnormal ECGs and vital signs during the scenario to ensure that the patient was being given appropriate patient care. Score = **8**
4. *Resource utilization:* The candidate used ordered appropriate lab work and imaging, obtained information from the patient's PMD, the workup was cost-sensitive and showed patient concern. Score = **8**
5. *Health care provided (outcome):* The patient received efficient and appropriate treatment, evidence-based interventions, and was stabilized. Score = **8**
6. *Interpersonal relations and communication skills:* The candidate did a good job of effectively communicating with the patient and the multiple professional colleagues in this scenario. She was firm in requesting an appropriate urgent consult. However, she did not request permission or explain the rectal examination. Score = **7**
7. *Comprehension of pathophysiology:* The examinee conveyed their understanding of hyperkalemia, ACS and acute kidney injury (AKI) by ordering only appropriate studies and discussing the patient's presentation, workup and admission request with the consultant. Score = **8**
8. *Clinical competence (overall):* Overall, the examinee showed clinical competence by obtaining an appropriate history and physical, developing and tested a reasonable differential diagnosis, made appropriate interventions, and obtained the appropriate consults and disposition. Score = **8**

CASE 44 78 y/o Female With Paralysis

John Dayton, James I. Syrett, and Flora Waples

INITIAL INFORMATION

Time: 09:35 AM

Name: Mrs. Red

Age: 78 years

Mode of arrival: Basic life support ambulance

Gender: Female

VS: Pulse 100, BP 138/79, RR 18, sat 96%, T 37.6°C (99.68°F)

CC: Drooling, weakness

PLAY OF THE CASE

E: "The triage nurse asks you to see a patient that has just arrived in the ED. Here is her triage sheet."

C: "As I walk into the room what do I see, hear, and smell."

E: "You see an elderly looking female that is sitting on the bed, drooling out of the right side of her mouth and moaning. She is accompanied by her daughter. There are no unusual smells."

C: "Good morning, my name is Dr. Smith. I am going to ask my nurse to do some things and then I will speak to you. Nurse, can you put the patient on 4 L of oxygen by NC, start cardiac monitoring, run a rhythm strip, and give it to me when it is complete. Please start an 18-gauge IV and draw off blood for labs and also do a finger-stick blood glucose. I will tell you what labs I want in a moment."

E: "The IV has been started, the blood glucose is 153. Do you want any IV fluids started?"

C: "Just keep the IV at KVO for now. Ms. Red, why have you had to come to hospital today?"

E: "The patient attempts to talk but only moans."

C: "I would like to assess her airway. What does her breathing sound like?"

E: "She is drooling out of the right side of her mouth, her breathing sounds normal."

C: "Is she choking on her secretions?"

E: "No."

C: "Does she have a gag reflex?"

E: "Yes."

C: "OK, I am happy that she is protecting her airway."

C: "I would like to speak to the daughter now. Can you tell me what is going on today?"

KEY QUESTION

Ask this open-ended question at the beginning of every case.

KEY ORDERS

Most of the patients you see during the exam are unstable (or will become that way). Every unstable patient requires IV access, oxygen, and cardiac monitoring. In any patient with altered mental status, a fingerstick glucose and a dose of Narcan are also appropriate immediate interventions.

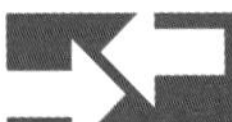

CRITICAL ACTION

Getting a rapid bedside glucose check is a critical action in this case.

DON'T FORGET

Always assess airway first before proceeding to any other aspect of the case.

E: "Yes doctor, we were out at breakfast and my mother dropped her coffee and slumped in her seat. She had not said anything since that happened."

C: "When did this happen?"

E: "It was about 9 AM—about 1/2 hour ago."

C: "Has anything like this happened to her before?"

E: "No, she is normally very well."

C: "Has she ever had a stroke before?"

E: "No."

C: "Does she have any other health problems?"

E: "Yes, she has high blood pressure and had a heart attack about 5 years ago."

C: "Is she on any medications?"

E: "Not really, she takes an aspirin every day and takes atenolol for her high blood pressure."

C: "Does she have any allergies?"

E: "No."

C: "Does she smoke or drink?"

E: "No."

C: "Thank you. I would like to examine the patient now. As I look at her, what do I see?"

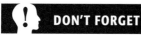

E: "She is an elderly looking female, drooling out of the right side of her mouth, and slumped over on the bed to her right side."

C: "When I examine her head, eyes, ears, nose, and throat what do I notice?"

E: "She has a right facial droop and lacks expression on the right. Her pupils are reactive, the rest of the examination is normal."

C: "Examining her chest?"

E: "Normal."

C: "Her cardiovascular examination?"

E: "What would you like to know?"

C: "What is her pulse rate and is it regular? Any extra heart sounds and does she have any carotid bruits?"

E: "Her pulse is regular and of good volume, her heart sounds are normal with no murmurs, and you hear a soft left carotid bruit."

C: "Her respiratory examination?"

E: "Normal."

C: "Her GI examination?"

E: "What do you want to know?"

C: "What does her abdomen look like, what do I feel when I palpate, and what do I hear when I listen? Is she guaiac positive?"

E: "Her abdomen looks normal, it is soft to palpation, her bowel sounds are active, and her guaiac is negative."

C: "Is dermatologic exam remarkable for any rash, bruising, or petechiae?"

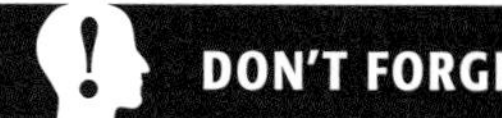

Remember that when the examiner states that the examination for a certain organ system is "normal," you can safely move on. However, if they ask "what are you looking for," there is likely a significant finding and you should dig deeper.

E: "Her skin examination is normal."

C: "Her neurologic examination?"

E: "What do you want to know?"

C: "Regarding her cranial nerves, are her eye movements, facial expression, facial sensation/power, and tongue deviation symmetric? Is her speech normal?"

CRITICAL ACTION

Getting a stat head CT, CBC, and coags in preparation for administering tPA is a critical action in this case.

E: "She has a right facial droop, her eye movements are intact and normal, and her tongue deviates to the left. She appears unable to follow commands or speak any words. Do you want any other information?"

C: "Are her motor strength, tone, and deep tendon reflexes in her arms and legs equal? What about her plantar reflexes?"

E: "Her right arm and leg have minimal power and tone, and her plantar reflex is up going on the affected side."

C: "Thank you, I would like to order an ECG, a stat head CT, a CBC, electrolytes, and coagulation studies. Please have the nurse notify me when we have these test results are available."

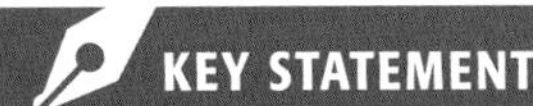

KEY STATEMENT

Remember to keep the patient and/or family aware of the test results. You will be expected to answer their questions, offer reassurance, get informed consent, and keep them updated regarding the patient's disposition plan.

C: "I would like to speak to the daughter. 'I think that your mother is having a stroke. We are going to get a CT scan to see if there is any bleeding in your mother's head. If there is not then we use a drug called tPA that will break up a clot that is probably casing her symptoms. I am going to speak to one of the neurology doctors to discuss if this would be an option in your mother. I do have some more questions though."

E: "Is she going to be OK?"

C: "Right now she is having a stroke and we have a time limit to give those medications I just mentioned. I will call the neurologists as well to come and see her and we will do everything that we can. Right now though, I need to get some more information to make sure that giving here these medications is safe."

E: "OK doctor, what else do you want to know?"

C: "Has your mother had any recent surgeries?"

E: "No."

C: "Has she had any recent trauma—such as a car accident or a fall?"

E: "No."

CRITICAL ACTION

Assessing the contraindications to tPA is a critical action in this case.

C: "Does she have any bleeding problems or does she take a drug called Coumadin."

E: "No."

C: "Has she ever had any bleeding in her head? Has she ever vomited blood or had a bloody bowel movement?"

E: "No."

E: "Your CT scan has been done and shows no bleeding. Your blood tests are also back and are all normal."

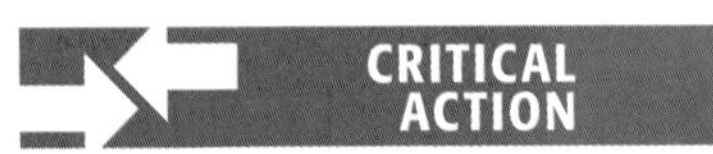

CRITICAL ACTION

Getting a neurology consult is a critical action.

C: "I would like to speak to the neurologist on call, please."

E: "Dr. Neurology is on the phone."

C: "Dr. Neurology, this is Dr. Smith in the ED. I have a 78-year-old female that has presented with a right-sided hemiparesis and aphasia. This was sudden onset at 9 AM this morning and was witnessed by a relative. Her blood glucose is normal, as is her ECG. Her CT shows no intracranial bleeding and she has no contraindications to thrombolysis. I think that this patient would benefit from tPA administration. Can you see her immediately, evaluate for tPA, and admit her to the ICU for frequent blood pressure and neurologic monitoring?"

E: "I am on my way now, but I can't make it in to the ED in time to give tPA before the window expires. You will have to make a decision to give tPA or not. Please arrange for an ICU bed and I will see the patient as fast as I can."

C: "I understand. Nurse, can we repeat a set of vital signs? How long has it been since the patient arrived in the ED?"

E: "The patient has been here for 45 minutes. Her current vital signs are pulse 104, BP 130/85, RR 18, sat 100% on 4-L NC, T 37.6°C."

C: "Has her neurologic examination changed during the time she has been here?"

E: "No."

C: "This patient has no evidence of intracranial hemorrhage on CT, has severe and unchanging symptoms, and no history of bleeding disorders with a normal CBC and coagulation studies. She has no recent surgery or trauma, no history of intracranial or GI bleeds, a normal blood glucose, and normal blood pressure. It has been 1 hour and 15 minutes since the onset of her symptoms. I think that she is an appropriate candidate for IV tPA. I would like to get informed consent from her daughter."

E: "The daughter is at the bedside."

C: "It appears that your mother is, in fact, having a stroke. There is a medication that we can give for strokes called tPA. It works by breaking up blood clots, and it has been shown to be effective in resolving symptoms of this kind of stroke. This medicine, however, has some serious side effects. Because it prevents the body from clotting, there is a risk that it can cause bleeding to occur. This bleeding can be severe, even life-threatening. Therefore, we require that you give your consent before we administer this medicine. Do you have any questions about this?"

E: "How often does that kind of bleeding happen?"

C: "About 10% of people who are given this medication will bleed at the site of the stroke, compared to about 3% of people who have this kind of stroke but do not get the medication. But, on the other hand, the chances of recovering from a stroke like this are 30% better if you get the tPA than if you do not."

E: "You have my consent to give the tPA."

C: "Nurse, can you administer tPA to this patient?"

E: "What is the dose doctor?"

C: "I will look up the appropriate dosing protocol on the NIH stroke website or using the package insert."

E: "The package insert indicates that the dose of tPA is 0.9 mg/kg infused over 60 minutes with 10% of the total dose administered as an initial IV bolus over 1 minute. This dose is given, and by the time that the ICU bed is available the patient is becoming more responsive. This case is over."

DON'T FORGET

Do not expect your consultants to help you manage the patient. While calling them is a critical action you will need to make all the clinical decisions on your own.

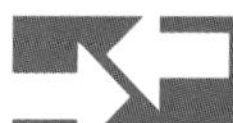

CRITICAL ACTION

Admitting the patient to the appropriate level of care is always a critical action.

DON'T FORGET

Administering thrombolysis to this patient is a critical action.

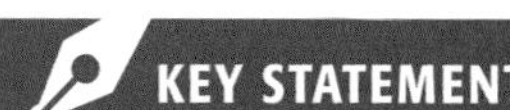

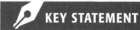

KEY STATEMENT

Remember that you can look up drugs and dosing if you do not know them.

CASE ASSESSMENT

This case illustrated the management of a patient who has presented with a presumed ischemic stroke and was managed very well. The patient presented soon after the initial symptoms and hypoglycemia was ruled out with a fingerstick blood glucose. It is essential to do this bedside test promptly in all patients presenting with neurological symptoms, and is almost always a critical action.

Once hypoglycemia has been excluded as a potential cause, the candidate quickly recognized the need for an immediate airway assessment, and this was done quickly and efficiently. The candidate also realized that because the patient was aphasic, it was essential to get history from other sources. Often these sources will be placed in the room with the patient and will be a relative, friend, or emergency medical service (EMS) provider. It is important not to let EMS providers leave before the candidate speaks to them. Often they will have helpful information.

Once it was clear that the symptoms were acute in onset, and within a 3-hour time window, the candidate progressed through a systematic focused examination. In general when the examiner asks what the candidate specifically wants to examine, it should be assumed that there is either something to be found that will be important later in the case. An example from this case was the gastrointestinal (GI) examination. Although there were no GI complaints, this part of the exam was important to discover that the rectal examination was remarkable for guaiac-negative stool.

The candidate also asked specific questions about possible contraindications to thrombolysis. All candidates taking the oral examination should be aware of these contraindications since they can easily be used in a critical actions requirement. In this particular case, the candidate consulted neurology early to request help in making the decision on thrombolysis. At ABEM General, your consultants will very rarely give you any practical advice for how to handle a patient. While calling them is a critical action, you will be expected to make clinical decisions on your own. The candidate did this very well, explaining their rational for giving tissue plasminogen activator (tPA) and using appropriate resources to find the dosing.

Another thing the candidate did well was keeping family members informed. Although it is easy to score well on the "Interpersonal Relations and Communication Skills" section, the stressful examination setting can make it hard to remember to have the necessary conversations with the patient and their family.

Critical Actions

1. Rapid blood glucose assessment
2. Stat computed tomography (CT) head, complete blood count (CBC), and coagulation studies
3. Stat neurology consultation
4. Initiation of thrombolysis
5. Assessment of contraindication to thrombolysis
6. Admission to the intensive care unit (ICU)

Test Performance

1. *Data acquisition:* The candidate did very well. Important and timely questions were asked and appropriate labs and imaging were requested. Score = **8**
2. *Problem solving:* The candidate used the patient exam and obtained medical history from the family to both form and test a differential diagnosis. The candidate could have also checked an electrocardiogram (ECG). Score = **7**
3. *Patient management:* The candidate did a great job of realizing that tPA could be used and making sure there were no contraindications. Score = **8**
4. *Resource utilization:* Tests were ordered in a cost-effective manner and in an appropriate time frame. The candidate also consulted the appropriate provider. Score = **8**
5. *Health care provided (outcome):* The patient was efficiently assessed and managed. The appropriate intervention (tPA) was used and the patient's symptoms began to resolve. Score = **7**
6. *Interpersonal relations and communication skills:* The candidate showed good skills in this area. The family was involved and informed. The candidate gave very thorough information about risks and benefits of tPA and obtained informed consent. Conversation with the neurologist was appropriate. Score = **8**
7. *Comprehension of pathophysiology:* The candidate showed understanding of ischemic stroke and for the indications for thrombolysis. Score = **8**
8. *Clinical competence (overall):* Overall, the examinee showed clinical competence by obtaining an appropriate history and physical, developing a differential diagnosis, utilizing appropriate lab work and CT, realizing that tPA was indicated, and working toward the appropriate disposition. Score = **8**

CASE 45 A 2 y/o Male Near Drowning

Navneet Cheema and Janis Tupesis

INITIAL INFORMATION

Name: William Jones

Mode of arrival: Ambulance

Age: 2 years 3 months

Gender: Male

VS: N/A

CC: Found in swimming pool

Setting: You are at the base station hospital for your local EMS system. Your charge nurse approaches you to let you know that ambulance 55 just radioed in a call that they are bringing in a small child who was found lifeless in a swimming pool. The paramedics are only 1-2 minutes out and are attempting to secure an airway and get an IV.

KEY ORDERS

Always have a Broselow tape ready for all pediatric trauma cases.

KEY ORDERS

Anytime you have to set up in anticipation of a trauma arrival you should get your airway equipment set up beforehand. This is a good example of how to describe your preparations.

PLAY OF THE CASE

C: "Do we have any vital signs?"

E: "The paramedics said that they just dragged the child out of the pool and are 'scooping and running.' They said that the child is unresponsive, but breathing shallowly on his own."

C: "Do we know how old the child is?"

E: "The paramedics said that they thought that the patient is approximately 2-3 years old, but aren't sure."

C: "I would go ahead and like to get the resuscitation room ready and alert the trauma team. I would like to clear a trauma bay, get a Broselow tape on the bed, and make sure that I have all of my resuscitation equipment ready."

KEY QUESTION

Ask this open-ended question at the beginning of every case.

KEY QUESTION

Always get vital signs first if possible. They are called "vital" for a reason.

E: "What equipment would you like to prepare?"

C: "I would like to get size 3.5, 4, and 4.5 ET tubes ready with stylets in place, a Yankauer suction catheter, and end-tidal carbon dioxide detector. I want an Ambu bag at the bedside attached to oxygen with an infant and pediatric-sized mask ready. I would like to get both size 2 and 3 Miller and Macintosh blades ready and would like to make sure that the bulb works in the laryngoscope. I would also like to have an appropriately sized oral airway ready as a backup."

E: "All of the equipment is functioning properly and it is all set up."

E: "At this time the ambulance arrives at the door of the trauma bay."

C: "What do I see?"

E: "You see the paramedics bagging an approximately 2-3-year-old male infant. He is unresponsive and cyanotic."

C: "Does the patient have vital signs?"

KEY ORDERS

Every trauma patient requires IV access (preferably two large-bore IVs, although that is not always possible in pediatric cases), oxygen, and cardiac monitoring. C-spine immobilization is also required—especially if the mechanism is unknown or the patient is unresponsive. In this case, as the patient is hypotensive a fluid bolus should also be initiated.

E: "The paramedics report a pulse of 60, RR of 26 and shallow, and the pulse oximetry is not registering."

C: "I would like to transfer the patient to the bed and begin preparations for emergent endotracheal intubation. While I am doing this I would like the nurse to assist the child's respirations with BVM ventilation with 15-L O_2 flow; make sure that an IV is established, put the patient on a cardiac monitor, and put the patient in a pediatric C-spine immobilization collar."

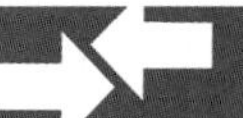

CRITICAL ACTION

Establishing an emergent airway in this child is a critical action.

E: "All of the above orders have been done. The patient is on the trauma gurney next to the Broselow tape, has assisted ventilations via BVM as requested and has an 20-gauge established in the left antecubital fossa; he is in a small pediatric hard C-spine collar and is on a cardiac monitor."

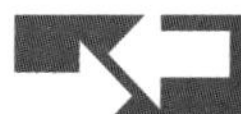

CRITICAL ACTION

Maintaining C-spine precautions in this child is a critical action.

C: "What does the Broselow tape say for the patient's weight?"

E: "It estimates the patient's weight at 30 kg."

C: "Nurse, please draw up the following medications: Lidocaine 1 mg/kg (30 mg), etomidate 0.3 mg/kg (10 mg), succinylcholine 1 mg/kg (30 mg), and midazolam 0.1 mg/kg (3 mg)."

E: "All of the medications are drawn up."

C: "I would like to go ahead and slowly push the lidocaine. I would then like to wait for approximately 1 minute and slowly push the etomidate. During this time I would ask that one of the techs assist with in-line C-spine immobilization and apply cricoid pressure. We will continue to assist ventilations for the patient and ask the nurse to slowly push the succinylcholine. I would ask that the tech continues to place cricoid pressure. I would then like to wait approximately 30 seconds and proceed with the intubation protocol."

DON'T FORGET

The candidate states that they are getting ready to intubate, and then uses the intervening time to get oxygen, labs, an IV, and a C-collar in place. This is a good strategy—as it allows you to follow the ABC correctly, but also allows you to initiate other important orders.

E: "The patient has stopped breathing at this time."

C: "I would like to assist with three tidal volume breaths with the BVM and proceed with the intubation. I would like to use the Macintosh 3 blade, pass a 4.5 ET uncuffed tube through the vocal cords."

E: "It is done without difficulty."

C: "I would like to ask the nurse to secure the airway with the ET tube at 15 cm at the patient's lips and at the same time apply the end-tidal CO_2 monitor. Do I see color change?"

E: "You see that the end-tidal CO_2 detector turns from purple to yellow."

DON'T FORGET

During the exam you may be asked to "talk through" several critical procedures. This is an excellent example of how to describe the sequence of events to follow for rapid sequence intubation. Memorize this.

C: "I would then like to listen over the stomach and over both of the lung fields."

E: "You do not hear anything over the stomach and hear breath sounds bilaterally."

C: "Is there symmetric chest rise?"

E: "There is."

C: "I would ask that the nurse go ahead and give the patient some more sedation. I would ask her to please give the diazepam, 3 mg IVP."

E: "It is done."

C: "I would like to place the patient on mechanical ventilation with the following settings: mode SIMV, FIO_2 100%, TV 200 cc, rate 20, PEEP 5."

KEY QUESTION

Remember to confirm tube placement, and get a CXR after every invasive procedure.

C: "OK. At this point I would like to do the following. I would like to ask the nurse to draw the following labs: CBC, Chem 7, LFTs, coags, ABG. I would ask for the following imaging to be done: STAT portable CXR to confirm ET

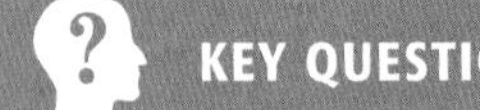

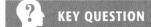

KEY QUESTION

Remember to reassess vital signs frequently—especially after any intervention.

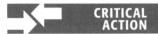

CRITICAL ACTION

After establishing the airway, having the correct ventilator settings is a critical action in this case.

tube placement. I would also ask that the following imaging be scheduled: x-rays of the C-spine, pelvis and a non-infused CT scan of the head. I would also ask that she give the patient a 20 cc/kg bolus of 0.9 NS and place a NG tube."

E: "That is being done."

C: "What are the patient's vitals?"

E: "HR 120, RR 20, satting 98% on the vent, BP 82/60, T 35°C."

C: "I would like to ask the paramedics that brought the patient in to wait so we can ask some questions, but at this time I would like to go ahead and continue with my secondary survey. Are there external signs of trauma about the child's head?"

E: "There is a small contusion above the right eye."

C: "Are there any other soft tissue swellings, hematomas, or lacerations?"

E: "There are none."

C: "Are the pupils reactive when a pen light is shined into them?"

E: "There is a normal pupillary response to light."

C: "Are there any atypical eye movements or nystagmus?"

E: "There are not."

C: "I would like to look into the child's ears and assess for blood or other fluid in the canal. I would also like to assess the landmarks in the inner ear."

E: "There is no blood in the ears and the landmarks are normal."

C: "Oropharynx?"

E: "There is a 4.5 ET tube, secured at the lip at 15 cm. There is fogging in the tube when the ventilator triggers."

C: "I would carefully like to take off the C-collar and assess the posterior cervical spine."

E: "What are you looking for?"

C: "I want to make sure that there is no stepoff and no soft tissue swelling"

E: "There is not."

C: "Is the trachea midline."

E: "It is."

C: "Is there any evidence of external trauma on the anterior chest wall?"

E: "There is not."

C: "Is there any evidence of subcutaneous emphysema?"

E: "There is not."

C: "I would like to listen to the patient's heart sounds assessing for type of rhythm, and the presence for any murmurs, rubs, gallops, or any other abnormal heart sounds."

E: "Patient has a sinus tachycardia without the presence of any abnormal heart sounds."

C: "Looking at the patient, is there symmetric chest rise?"

E: "There is."

C: "I would like to listen to the patient's chest assessing for the presence of bilateral breath sounds and the presence of rales, rhonchi, or wheezing."

E: "The patient has bilateral breath sounds on auscultation. The breath sounds are diminished bilaterally and there is presence of coarse rales bilaterally. There are no rhonchi and no wheezing."

C: "Is there any external trauma to the abdomen?"

E: "There is not."

C: "Auscultating the abdomen for the presence of bowel sounds?"

E: "The bowel sounds are diminished."

C: "Palpating the abdomen, is it distended and are there any palpable masses?"

E: "The abdomen is mildly distended and there are no palpable masses."

C: "Is there any blood at the patient's penile meatus or any other notable trauma to the genitourinary system?"

E: "There is no blood on the penile meatus and there does not appear to be any trauma."

C: "On rectal examination, I will assess the rectal tone and guaiac any stool for occult blood."

E: "On rectal examination, the patient has mildly decreased tone and there is no stool in the vault."

C: "I would like to get assistance and roll the patient and evaluate the thoracic and lumbar spine for deformities, step-offs, and atypical swelling."

E: "The examination is normal."

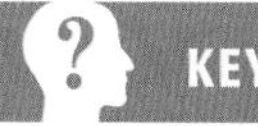

KEY QUESTION

Remember to ask for the results of any lab that you order. Make a list so that you can keep track of what you have back and what you do not.

C: "Is there any signs of trauma to the extremities?"

E: "There are not."

C: "The patient's reflexes."

E: "They are normal."

C: "Is the capillary refill normal?"

E: "The capillary refill is under 2 seconds, but the extremities are cool and clammy." (At this point and time, the radiology tech arrives in the trauma bay. He is there to take the C-spine x-rays, chest x-ray, and pelvis x-ray.)

C: "Do we have the results of the blood gas?"

E: "Yes. The pertinent values are as such: pH 7.21, Pao_2 166, Pco_2 53, CO_2 14."

C: "I would ask the nurse to repeat a blood gas now that the patient has been on the ventilator."

E: "The nurse draws the ABG and sends it off to the respiratory lab."

C: "What are the patient's vital signs now that the bolus has gone in?"

E: "T 35.8°C, BP 98/67, RR 20 (vent), HR 86, Sao_2 97% on vent/100% Fio_2."

C: "I would like to put a warming blanket, and/or a Bair hugger on the patient. I would also like to put in a Foley catheter and give the patient another 20-cc/kg bolus of 0.9 NS."

E: "It is done."

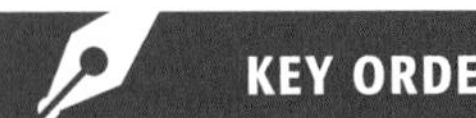

KEY ORDERS

Remember to use EMS, family members, or witnesses to get a history on unresponsive patients.

C: "At this point, I would like to go talk to the paramedics and the family and obtain any further history."

E: "They are waiting for you in the EMS room."

C: "Hi guys, my name is Dr. Commit. I am the physician taking care of William Jones. Are you the rig that brought the patient in?"

E: "We are."

C: "Can you guys tell me a little bit about what happened?"

E: "Basically, the kid was found in one of those small, portable plastic swimming pools in the backyard. The pool was right off of the back porch. Mom says that she took one of her plants inside and when she came back a few minutes later the kid was lying on his side in the pool."

C: "Is mom here?"

E: "No, she is on the way in with some family members."

C: "What did you guys see when you got there?"

E: "Well, mom had dragged the kid out of the pool and one of the neighbors was doing mouth to mouth. There was a hose next to the pool that they were using to fill it. Mom said that she thought the kid might have tripped over the hose and fallen into the pool. We took over, basically scooped the kid up and got here as soon as we could."

C: "Do we know how long the child could have been submerged?"

E: "I don't know, but I am guessing 5 minutes at the very most, by what the kid's mom told us."

KEY QUESTION

Remember to ask for the results of any lab that you order. Make a list so that you can keep track of what you have back and what you do not.

C: "Thanks guys, please let me know if you see mom come in. I would like to go back into the patient's room. What do I see when I walk into the room?"

E: "The radiology tech is finishing up doing the neck, chest, and pelvis films. The patient is on the ventilator without any untoward movements. He has a Bair hugger blanket on."

C: "I would like to ask the tech to let us know as soon as the films are available to review."

E: "She states that she will let you know."

C: "What are the patient's vital signs?"

E: "The patient remains on the vent. T 36.1°C, BP 100/62, RR 20 (vent), HR 90, Sao_2 100% on vent/100% Fio_2."

C: "I would like to check to see if we have any of the labs back."

E: "The nurse says that the only lab that is back is the second ABG that was sent after the patient was put on the ventilator. They are: pH 7.33, Pao_2 212, Pco_2 37, CO_2 17."

DON'T FORGET

Do not let an unstable patient go to the CT scanner alone, and do not let anyone out of the trauma bay before you have seen the chest and pelvis films.

E: "The nurse also states that transportation is here to take the patient to the CT scanner."

C: "I want to examine the C-spine films and the chest x-ray before the patient goes to the CT scanner, just to make sure that no additional imaging is needed while the patient is in the scanner. I would, however, ask her to get the patient ready to go—putting the patient on portable oxygen with the vent and respiratory therapy, a portable cardiac monitor, and some more midazolam for sedation."

E: "It is done. The radiology tech has the hard copies of the radiographs."

C: "I would like to first look at the chest x-ray."

E: "What are you looking for?"

C: "First, I would like to systematically look from the outside in. Is it a good film? Can we see down to the thoracic ribs? Are there any bony abnormalities?"

E: "It is a good quality film and you can count 8-9 ribs. There are no bony abnormalities."

C: "Continuing in, at what position is the ET tube?"

E: "It is approximately 1.5 cm above the carina."

C: "When I look at the heart, are the heart borders regular?"

E: "They are."

C: "I would like to look at the lung fields and assess for the following—are there any air space processes? Are both lungs equally inflated? Is there a pneumothorax?"

E: "Both lungs are inflated. There does not appear to be a pneumothorax as you can see vascular markings all the way lateral to the chest wall on both sides. There is a diffuse, four quadrant air space process involving both lungs. There is congestion with prominent vasculature in both lung fields. There are no consolidations."

C: "Very well. I am satisfied that the ET tube is in the correct position above the carina and that the patient most likely has an aspiration pneumonitis from his near-drowning episode."

C: "I would like to examine the patient's C-spine films (Fig. C45-1)."

C: "At this point, I would like to tell the nurse about the findings, assure myself that the patient has adequate spinal immobilization and let the CT tech know that we will have to scan the cervical scan as well as the brain. It appears that there is a subluxation at C2-C3."

E: "The nurse assures you that the patient is in a hard collar and that she has added on the non-infused scan of the patient's cervical spine."

C: "Very well, I would quickly like to look at the patient's pelvis films before they go on to the CT scanner. I would like to make sure that there are no obvious fractures and that the joint spaces are appropriate for the stated age."

E: "There appear to be no fractures and the joint spaces are appropriate."

C: "OK, please let the CT tech know that the patient can go to the CT scanner with the nurse, the respiratory therapist, and the portable cardiac monitor."

E: "The patient is wheeled off to the CT scanner."

C: "At this point, I would like to ask the coordinator to request a PICU bed and start making arrangements for the patient's admission. I would also ask them to find out who is on call for the PICU and have them page to my phone."

E: "Dr. Child, the pediatric intensivist, is on the phone for you."

C: "Hi Dr. Child, this is Dr. Commit, the attending in the ED. I am calling to tell you about an unfortunate child who presented to the ED about 30 minutes ago and who is going to need admission to the PICU."

E: "What happened?"

C: "The patient is a 2-3-year-old boy who suffered an unwitnessed fresh water submersion injury. The mother states that she left him unattended in

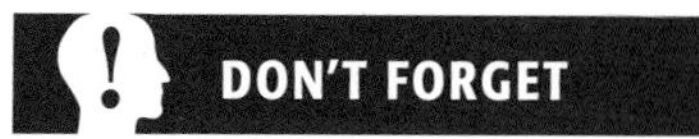

Be ready both to read x-rays, and to describe how you would read them.

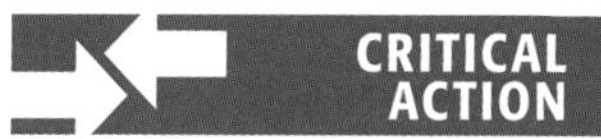

Finding the abnormality on x-ray, getting a CT of the C-spine, and continuing correct immobilization are critical actions in this case.

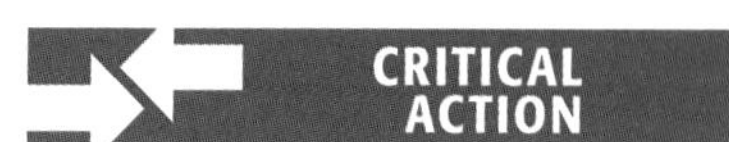

Admitting this patient to the PICU is a critical action.

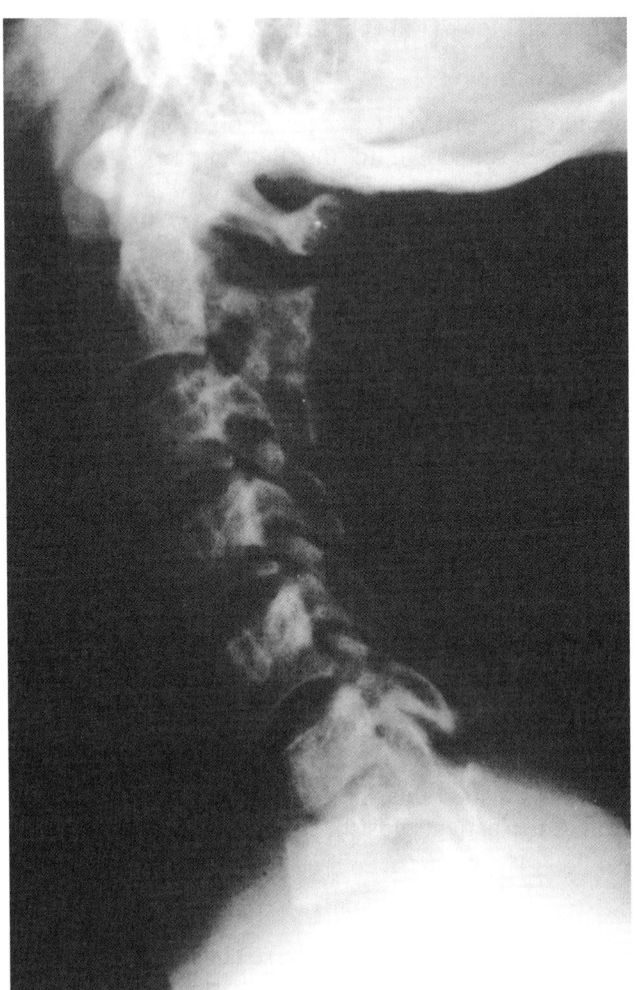

Figure C45-1. Lateral C-spine film showing a subluxation at C2-C3 (a large subluxation with at least half a vertebral body overhang. Pediatric would be nice, but not necessary if you have trouble finding it. Also, if you have trouble, we can have the subluxation be anywhere in the C-spine. *(Reproduced with permission from Shah BR, Lucchesi M.* Atlas of Pediatric Emergency Medicine. *New York, NY: McGraw-Hill; 2006.)*

the backyard and found him face down in the portable swimming pool behind their house. He was initially unresponsive in the field, but has spontaneous return of vital signs when he was picked up by the paramedics. He presented hypothermic, bradycardic, and hypoxic in respiratory distress. He was immediately intubated and his vital signs improved."

E: "Are there any other injuries?"

C: "No obvious ones. On secondary survey the patient had a little ecchymosis on his forehead and so is currently undergoing imaging of his cervical spine and his brain. There appears to be no other trauma to the patient."

E: "Why his cervical spine?"

C: "Because of the unwitnessed mechanism of injury and because on plain film there was a subluxation or a pseudosubluxation at C2-C3."

E: "Are you going to call neurosurgery?"

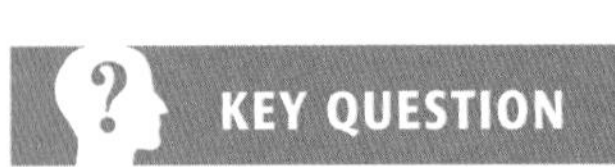

KEY QUESTION

Remember to ask for lab results. You can also ask that lab results be brought to you when they come back—which places the responsibility for remembering to check them on the examiner.

C: "We will as soon as we get the results of the CT scan back."

E: "OK, we'll be down to see him in a second. Does he have any labs back?"

C: "Other than his pre- and post-intubation blood gases, there is nothing back. Both of them are on the hospital's computer system if you would like to look at them."

E: "OK, we will be down in a second."

C: "Can I please check if any of the labs are back?"

E: "They are." (At this point the patient returns from the CT scanner with the nurse.)

WBC 17,000, Hgb 12.6 g/dL, Hct 37, plt 276,000

Na 139, K 4.2, chloride 99, bicarb 14, BUN 12, Cr 0.6, glu 135, Ca 10.1

AST 17, ALT 31, alkaline phosphatase 82, GGT 29, total bilirubin 0.8, albumin 3.7

UA is normal

E: "Dr. Commit, the patient is not doing that well. His sats are dropping even though we have not changed the vent settings. We finished the CT scans, but I thought I should get him here as soon as I could."

C: "What do I see when I look at the patient?"

E: "The patient is still on the vent. He is fighting the vent and the high pressure alarm on the vent is going off."

C: "What are the patient's vital signs?"

E: "The patient is overbreathing the vent at 28 bpm, his blood pressure has dropped to 64/40 and his heart rate is 92 and his oxygen saturations are 72% on 100% inspired oxygen."

C: "I would like to take the patient off the vent and attach him to an Ambu bag and give him two or three slow tidal breaths."

E: "You notice that the patient is much more difficult to bag than he was before he left."

C: "I would like to reestablish that the patient's ET tube is in the right place. I would like to reattach an end-tidal—CO_2 detector."

E: "It changes from purple to yellow."

C: "Is the patient's trachea midline?"

E: "It is."

C: "What do I hear when I listen to the patient's lungs? Are there equal breath sounds? Are there any rhonchi, wheezes, or rales?"

E: "The patient has equal breath sounds bilaterally. There is profound end expiratory wheezing with prolonged expiratory time. There are fine crackles throughout."

C: "At this point, the patient is probably having pneumonitis-induced bronchospasm. I would like to detach him from the Ambu bag and let the patient exhale until end expiration."

E: "It is done. The patient has one long end expiration lasting 15 seconds."

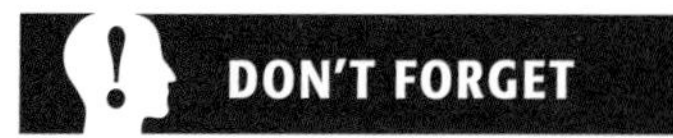

Often, when the patient "crashes" early in the case it means that you have missed something or are doing something wrong. Reevaluate. If the patient "crashes" when the case is almost over, it often means that the patient is supposed to crash so that you can show how you would manage that situation. Do not panic and remember your ABCs.

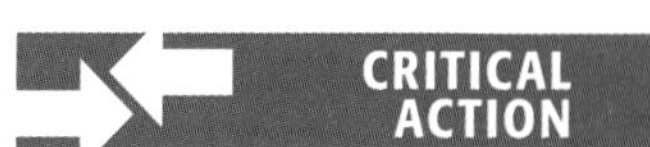

Managing the patient's bronchospasm, including checking tube placement, assessing for breath sounds, and changing the vent settings are critical actions in this case.

C: "I would like to switch the patient's ventilator settings at this time. I would like to decrease the child's RR to 14, prolong the end expiratory time to 3:1, and add in-line nebulized albuterol and atrovent."

E: "The patient appears much more comfortable and his sat come back up to 99%." (There is a telephone call from the radiologist at this time.)

E: "Hi, this is Dr. Radon. Are you the physician taking care of William Jones?"

C: "I am."

E: "Can you please tell me what happened?"

C: "He is a 2-year-old infant who was found unresponsive in a swimming pool behind his house. We don't know if he suffered any trauma, but presume that he had a near-drowning episode."

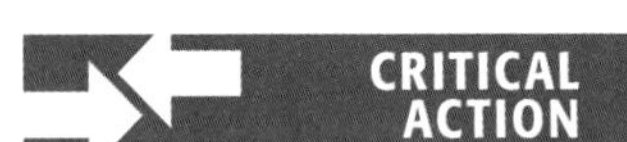

Calling neurosurgery for definitive management of a C-spine injury is a critical action in this case.

E: "Well, his head CT looks OK. It doesn't look like he has any intracranial pathology, but he has an abnormality on his C-spine CT. I can't tell for sure, but it looks as though there is a subluxation of C2 on C3. I know that the patient is intubated and sedated, but eventually he will either need flexion—extension views or a MRI of his cervical spine. Otherwise, there are no focal abnormalities or fractures."

C: "Thanks."

C: "At this point, I would like to page the neurosurgeon on call."

E: "I am from the neurosurgery service, I am Dr. Header."

C: "Hi, this is Dr. Commit in the ED. I just wanted to let you know about a little boy who will be going to the PICU that we will be consulting you on. He is a 2-year-old boy found unresponsive in a pool. We think that he might have tripped and sustained some head and neck trauma when he fell into the pool. He came to the ER, was emergently intubated, and just got back from radiology after head and neck CT were done. I just talked to Dr. Radon who says that while his head CT is normal, there is a subluxation at C2-C3."

E: "Is the patient in a collar?"

C: "Yes, of course. He is sedated, intubated, and will be going to the PICU shortly." (The PICU team arrives at the patient's bedside.)

E: "Hi, have there been any changes?"

C: "A little bit. He was having some post-aspiration bronchospasm in CT and desaturated, but we changed his vent setting to a lower respiratory rate and are giving him in-line nebs right now with improvement. We just talked to the radiologist who says that although he has a normal head CT, there is a subluxation on his cervical spine CT. We talked to Dr. Header of the neurosurgical service who will meet you when you go to the PICU."

E: "OK, can we take the patient upstairs?"

C: "Sure. Thanks for your help."

E: "This case is now over."

CASE ASSESSMENT

Overall, the candidate managed this case efficiently and effectively. Throughout the entire case, the actions were well thought out, organized, and decisive. In a case like this where information in provided from a pre-hospital care provider—it is important to start preparing for a patient before they arrive. As soon as there was information that the candidate was going to get a critically ill patient, he began mobilizing his resources including nursing and ancillary staff. He also started preparing for the resuscitation before the patient arrived by getting airway equipment ready, thinking about what kinds of medication he/she would use for rapid sequence intubation and preparing with a Broselow tape.

Upon arrival, the candidate realized that the patient's mental status and poor vital signs necessitated early airway management and emergent intubation was done. The candidate realized that there could be secondary trauma and gave appropriate premedications such as lidocaine and appropriate induction and paralytic agents.

One of the most important things to do in cases like this is to look for secondary trauma. The questions of "Why did this patient fall?" and "What happened when this patient fell in the pool?" needed to be answered. Early C-spine immobilization was achieved and appropriate imaging studies were done to evaluate head and neck injuries. One thing that might have been done a little better is that—without a witness or parent—the worse possible injury needs to be suspected. Although there was no bruising on the abdomen or abdominal distension, with an unresponsive patient it is difficult to evaluate intra-abdominal injury. If labs are not back that might give you a clue that there might be an abdominal injury and the patient is already going to the computed tomography (CT) scanner for a head and neck CT, one might consider doing a quick "trauma scan" of the abdomen and pelvis. Otherwise, if the facility is equipped with an ultrasound machine, a focused assessment with sonography for trauma (FAST) examination might have been done as part of the secondary survey.

Finally, the patient's disposition and consulting services were figured out in a timely manner. The candidate realized that the patient needed admission to the intensive care unit (ICU) and that the patient would need pediatric intensive care unit (PICU) and neurosurgical consultations.

Critical Actions

1. Airway management including intubation and setting-appropriate ventilator settings.
2. Cervical spine immobilization and continued work-up post initial abnormal plain films.
3. Appropriate management of desaturation upon return from the radiology department.
4. Consideration of potential traumatic injury to head, neck, chest, and abdomen in addition to addressing drowning aspects of the case.

Test Performance

1. *Data acquisition:* Excellent and efficient history taking and complete examination in this challenging situation. Score = 7
2. *Problem solving:* Again excellent assimilation of data with very efficient analysis of the clinical picture. Score = 7
3. *Patient management:* The candidate demonstrated an efficient yet thorough approach to the clinical picture. Score = 7
4. *Resource utilization:* Demonstrated very appropriate use of resources. Score = 7
5. *Health care provided (outcome):* The candidate demonstrated excellent clinical judgment and provided prompt and appropriate treatment. Score = 7

6. *Interpersonal relations and communication skills:* Great engagement and exchange of information with the paramedics, support staff, and the consultants. Never gets a chance to talk to the family—however, this is almost always done at ABEM General! Score = **7**
7. *Comprehension of pathophysiology:* Demonstrated comprehension of the underlying pathophysiology of drowning as evidenced by the interpretation of the chest x-ray (CXR) and quick recognition of post-aspiration bronchospasm. Score = **8**
8. *Clinical competence (overall):* This case was excellently managed with the candidate excelling in the data acquisition, patient management, and medical knowledge. Score = **7**

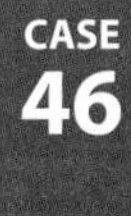

CASE 46 Situation Encounter: A 14 y/o Male With a Limp, a 45 y/o Male With Shoulder Pain, and a Woman With Abdominal Pain

Navneet Cheema, Catherine Johnson, and Flora Waples

INITIAL INFORMATION

Name: Jimmy Bender

Mode of arrival: Brought in by mother

Age: 14 years

Gender: Male

VS: T 37.4°C (99.32°F), BP 90/50, HR 82, RR 20, O_2 sat: 99%

CC: Limping

PLAY OF THE CASE (JIMMY BENDER)

C: "When I walk into the room, what do I see?"

E: "The patient is a young man who is moderately overweight sitting on the stretcher talking to his mom."

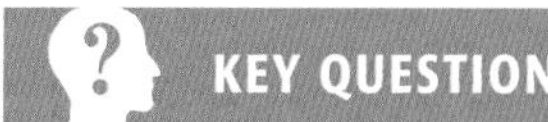

KEY QUESTION

Ask this open-ended question at the beginning of every case.

C: "Hello, I am Dr. Clemava. What brings you in today?"

E: "I've been having trouble with my hip, I've been limping for a couple days."

C: "Any falls or trauma?"

E: "No."

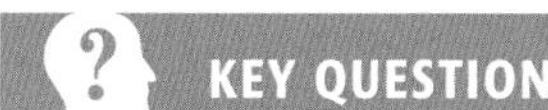

KEY QUESTION

Remember to introduce yourself by name—easy points for professionalism.

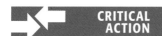

C: "Have you had any fever or rash?"

E: "No."

C: "Do you have any medical problems?"

E: "No, I'm healthy, I just see the doctor when I need my shots."

C: "Where does it hurt the most?"

E: "Here in my right hip, and I feel it in my knee, too."

C: "Well, how about if we have a look. Mom, do you have anything else to add?"

E: "No, doctor. I gave him some acetaminophen and called his pediatrician. They couldn't get him in today."

C: "I'm glad you brought him in. Does he take any other medications?"

E: "No, he's only ever had acetaminophen when he feels sick or has pain."

C: "OK, I am going to start by examining the head and neck. Is there any evidence of trauma? Is the neck supple?"

CRITICAL ACTION

Getting a hip x-ray with a frog-leg view is a critical action in this case.

E: "No evidence of trauma, neck is supple."

C: "Are the heart and lungs clear? Any murmurs?"

E: "Heart and lungs are clear."

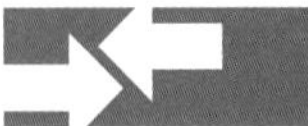

CRITICAL ACTION

Conducting a physical examination and ordering tests with slipped capital femoral epiphysis (SCFE) in mind are a set of critical actions in this case.

C: "Is there any rash or skin changes?"

E: "No."

C: "Are either of the hips tender or warm?"

E: "No."

C: "Can the patient flex and extend the hips painlessly?"

E: "Flexion is uncomfortable for the patient when examining the right hip."

C: "Do any of the other joints feel tender or warm?"

E: "No."

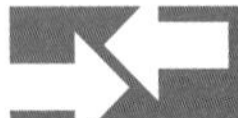

CRITICAL ACTION

Giving pain control is a critical action in this case. Analgesia is not always critical, but it can be, so always remember to treat your patient's pain.

C: "I would like to examine the patient's gait. Can the patient bear weight on the right leg?"

E: "The patient walks with a limp and favors the left leg. The nurse interrupts your examination to tell you that you are asked to see a patient in the next room."

C: "Well, I will have to step out. Nurse, can you please order a right hip and pelvis x-ray with frog view, a CBC, sedimentation rate, blood culture, and a urethral culture? The patient may have 400 mg of ibuprofen PO for pain."

E: "OK, these tests are ordered and the medication is given. There is another patient you need to see in room 2."

INITIAL INFORMATION

Name: Derek Thompson

Mode of arrival: EMS

Age: 45 years

Gender: Male

VS: T 37.1°C (98.78°F), P 114, BP 135/80, RR 18, O_2 sat: 98%

CC: Fall

PLAY OF THE CASE (DEREK THOMPSON)

KEY QUESTION

Ask this open-ended question at the beginning of every case.

C: "When I walk into the room, what do I see?"

E: "A man lying on the stretcher, backboarded in a C-collar. He is wincing."

C: "Mr. Thompson, I am Dr. Clemava. What happened?"

E: "Well, doc, I was sitting at the bar and I fell off the stool."

C: "What made you fall?"

E: "I was just rocking the stool and slipped on some beer on the floor."

KEY ORDERS

Remember to utilize your resources. Always ask to speak to EMS or family members to get a good history.

C: "Did you hit your head or blackout?"

E: "The back of my head hurts, but it's my arm that is really killing me. I think I was awake the whole time. A few ladies screamed and the bartender kind of freaked out."

C: "How much did you drink today?"

E: "Nothing, doc."

C: "Do you have any medical problems?"

E: "I have seizures and take phenytoin."

C: "Nurse, can you ask the paramedics to stand by please, I'll need to talk to them."

E: "OK, they are here."

C: "Thanks for staying. What happened?"

E: "The bartender said he started shaking and fell off the stool. He was waking up by the time we got there. He bumped the back of his head, so we immobilized him."

C: "Great job, thank you. Anything else I should know about?"

E: "No allergies, just takes phenytoin. Hadn't even taken a sip of his first beer yet."

C: "OK. I'll let you guys get going then. I would like to examine the patient now. I would like to look at the head. Is there any sign of trauma? Are the pupils equally reactive to light and accommodation? Are there any abrasions, contusions, or lacerations to the head or face? Are the tympanic membranes and oropharynx clear of blood or trauma?"

E: "He has a posterior scalp abrasion, about 2 cm circumferentially, otherwise the examination is normal."

C: "Is there any alcohol on the breath?"

E: "No."

C: "Is there any posterior C-spine tenderness? Mr. Thompson, do you have any numbness or tingling to your arms or legs? Any other part of your body hurt?"

E: "Oh, doc. It's my shoulder, just feels really bad."

C: "OK, I'll get you some pain medicine just as soon as I finish examining you. Are there any abrasions, lacerations, contusions on the chest wall?"

E: "No."

C: "Are the heart and lungs clear? No murmurs, gallops, or rub? No crackles or wheezing?"

E: "Heart and lungs are clear."

C: "Is there any abrasion, laceration, contusion to either shoulder? Are the shoulders symmetric? Is the range of motion normal?"

E: "The left shoulder is tender and appears full at the AC joint. The coracoid process appears prominent. The arm is held in adduction and internal rotation. Patient resists external rotation and abduction. The right shoulder is normal."

C: "Is there any deficit in sensation, strength, or pulse in the left arm?"

E: "No."

C: "Is the patient's abdomen soft? Is there any tenderness, rebound, or guarding in the abdomen?"

E: "No, the abdominal examination is benign."

C: "Are the pulses and pressures symmetric in the arms and legs? Is the pelvis stable? Are there any deformities, lacerations, abrasions, or contusions in the arms or legs?"

E: "All normal except as noted before in the left shoulder."

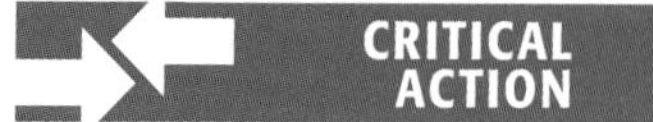

Getting a full history of the seizure is a critical action in this case, and it cannot be achieved by talking to the patient alone.

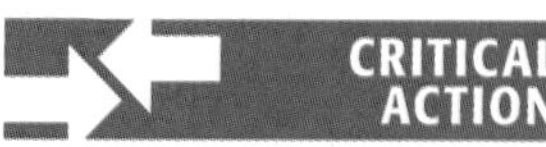

Maintaining C-spine precautions in this patient with blunt head trauma after a seizure is a critical action in this case. He has a distracting injury and the collar cannot be cleared clinically.

C: "Is the rectal examination normal? Is there any ecchymoses in the scrotum or perineum?"

E: "Rectal and perineal examinations are normal."

C: "Is the patient alert and oriented to time, person, and place? Are the cranial nerves intact? Are there any motor or sensory deficits?"

E: "The examination is normal."

E: "Doc, can we take this collar off my neck—it is killing me."

C: "I am sorry, but since it appears that you had a seizure and hit your head, we cannot be sure that you did not injure your neck. I would like to get x-rays of your neck, and a CT scan of your head, and if they are normal, we can take the collar off. I know that it is uncomfortable, but I am asking you to be patient."

E: "Okay doc, do what you have to do."

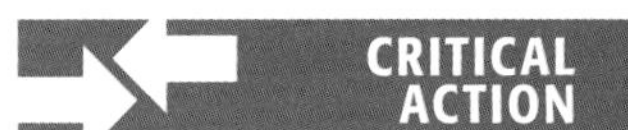

Giving pain control is a critical action in this case. Analgesia is not always critical, but it can be, so always remember to treat your patient's pain.

C: "Nurse, would you please give the patient 4 mg of morphine sulfate IV and order a head CT, non-infused, three view C-spine radiographic series and a left shoulder x-ray. Please send a phenytoin level as well. I would like to keep the patient on a cardiac monitor."

E: "Those orders will be carried out. In the meantime, your next patient is here, doctor."

INITIAL INFORMATION

Name: Lillian Elliott

Mode of arrival: Family

Finding and treating the patient's phenytoin level is a critical action in this case.

Age: 34 years

Gender: Female

VS: T 37.1°C (98.78°F), P 94, BP 130/70, RR 18, O_2 sat: 98%

CC: Abdominal pain

PLAY OF THE CASE (LILLIAN ELLIOTT)

C: "When I walk into the room, what do I see?"

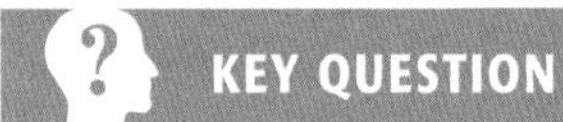

Ask this open-ended question at the beginning of every case.

E: "A woman lying on the stretcher, making a retching noise and holding an emesis basin."

C: "Hello, Mrs. Elliott, I am Dr. Clemava. How are you feeling, what can I do for you?"

E: "Oh doctor, I feel so sick."

C: "Where does it hurt?"

E: "The patient is pointing to her upper abdomen."

C: "When was your last period?"

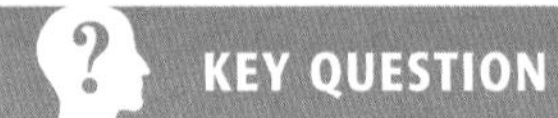

Remember to introduce yourself by name—easy points for professionalism.

E: "I'm on it now."

C: "Do you have any medical problems?"

E: "No."

C: "Have you had a fever?"

E: "No."

C: "Have you been vomiting?"

E: "No, I am just so nauseated."

C: "Are you having any problem with your urination—burning or blood in the urine?"

E: "No."

C: "Are you having any chest pain or shortness of breath?"

E: "No."

C: "When is the last time you ate?"

E: "I had some fried chicken for dinner, which was about 3 hours ago. Is there anything you can give me for the pain?"

C: "Yes, I'll get you some pain medicine just as soon as I finish examining you. Are you allergic to any medications or take any medications regularly?"

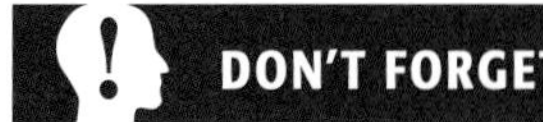

If the examiner asks more than once for pain medication—give it. They are reminding you for a reason. In fact, in some cases, points will be deducted if they have to ask more than once for analgesia.

E: "No."

C: "Have you had any surgeries?"

E: "No."

C: "OK, very good. I would like to examine you now, but first I will have the nurse start an 18-gauge IV in the left antecubital fossa and draw your blood. We will also need a urine sample. Nurse, can you please send a CBC, electrolytes, BUN/Cr, LFTs, lipase, and a stat urine pregnancy test. Set up for a pelvic examination."

E: "Doctor, can you give me something for the pain?"

C: "Yes, let me examine you first so that I can best treat you. Is there any evidence of trauma to the head or neck? Are the pupils equal and reactive? Are the conjunctivas pale or is there scleral icterus?"

E: "No evidence of trauma, the papillary examination is normal, there is no scleral icterus, and the conjunctivas look healthy."

C: "Is the neck supple?"

E: "Yes."

C: "Are there any skin changes, jaundice, or rash; is the turgor of the skin normal?"

E: "The skin examination is normal."

C: "When I do the lung and cardiac examination, are there any murmurs, rubs, or gallops? Is the rhythm normal? Are there any crackles, wheezes in the lungs; are the breath sounds equal?"

E: "The cardiac and lung examinations are normal."

C: "Is the abdomen soft, is there any tenderness, rebound, or guarding? How are the bowel sounds? Is there any tympany to percussion?"

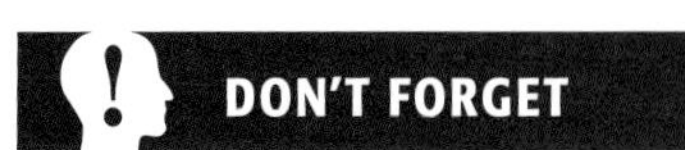

Before you do a personal examination (such as a pelvic) it is a good idea to address the patient, explain what you are about to do and get their permission.

E: "The abdomen is soft and obese, with tenderness in the RUQ. There is no rebound or guarding. The bowel sounds are normal, and there is no tympany."

C: "I would like to perform a pelvic examination. Is there any vaginal discharge, cervical motion tenderness, adnexal fullness, or abnormal uterine findings to palpation?"

E: "The pelvic examination is benign."

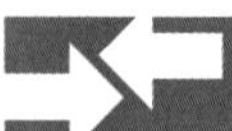

CRITICAL ACTION

Giving pain control is a critical action in this case. Analgesia is not always critical, but it can be, so always remember to treat your patient's pain.

KEY ORDERS

In the triple cases remember to reassess your patients and to follow-up on the labs/studies for each one. It is useful to go in order of presentation to keep organized, and make sure that you do not skip anyone.

DON'T FORGET

The examiner will often use questions from the nurse or family in order to "pimp" you on your knowledge of a subject.

C: "I would like to perform a rectal examination, is there any blood in the stool, any tenderness to digital examination?"

E: "There is no blood in the stool, and no tenderness on examination."

C: "I would like to check the patient's neurologic examination. Are the cranial nerves intact? Is her strength and sensation in the upper and lower extremities normal and symmetric?"

E: "The examination is normal."

C: "Nurse, I would like to order ondansetron 4 mg IV and ketorolac 30 mg IV if the patient is not pregnant. Mrs. Elliott, I have ordered you some pain medicines and I will be back to tell you what the laboratory tests show. I am hopeful you will be feeling better soon and we should have some more information about your abdominal pain when the laboratory tests come back."

E: "OK, doctor, thanks."

C: "Nurse, I would like to reexamine my patient Jimmy Bender. Have the labs and x-rays returned?"

E: "The right hip and pelvis x-ray with frog view are done, the CBC is normal, the sedimentation rate is 5, and the blood and urethral cultures have been sent. The patient feels better after the dose of ibuprofen he has received (Fig. C46-1)."

C: "This x-ray concerns me for the diagnosis of a slipped capital femoral epiphysis. I would like to get an orthopedic surgeon on the phone. I will talk to the family now."

E: "Doctor, how do the films look?"

C: "Well, I am concerned that your son has a problem with the hip joint. The joint surfaces seem to have slipped while he was growing and he will need to see a bone specialist."

E: "Oh my, will he be able to walk again? Will he be OK?"

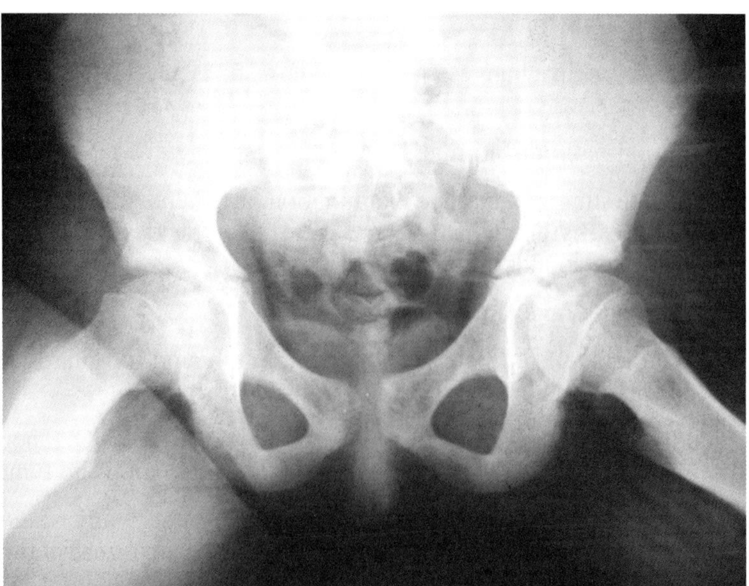

Figure C46-1. Hip x-ray showing SCFE. *(Reproduced with permission from Simon RR, Sherman SC, Koenigsknecht SJ.* Emergency Orthopedics: The Extremities. *5th ed. New York, NY: McGraw-Hill; 2007.)*

C: "He will need to have surgery to correct this problem as soon as possible. The good news is that we have caught this early. The sooner his hip is pinned into place the better his prognosis is. He will be in crutches for about 2 months, and after that he will likely be able to go back to his daily activities. I am calling an orthopedic surgeon now to get him the care he needs."

E: "Dr. Hipop is on the phone."

C: "Hello, it's Dr. Clemava. I am seeing Johnny Bender, a 14-year-old boy who presented with a painful right hip. He has a limp and his frog-leg views are consistent with SCFE. Could you please see him?"

E: "OK, I will be down to see the patient."

C: "Thank you."

E: "This part of the case is over now."

E: "The nurse tells you that Mr. Thompson has a phenytoin level of 5 mg/dL. The shoulder and C-spine x-rays are done. The radiologist reads the C-spine films as normal, but he has not read the shoulder films yet (Fig. C46-2)."

C: "Please give the patient 1 g of phenytoin IV, and keep him on the cardiac monitor, checking his blood pressure q15min during the infusion. His x-rays show an anteriorly dislocated shoulder. Please start a second IV and prepare for conscious sedation and shoulder reduction. Draw up 10 mg of etomidate, place the patient on a cardiac monitor and continuous pulse oximeter. We should have suction and bag valve mask equipment at the bedside prepared. While that is being set up, can I review Mrs. Elliot's labs please?"

Hgb 13.3, WBC 17.5, electrolytes are WNL, BUN 32, Cr 1.3, alkaline phosphatase 435, AST 65, ASP 72, lipase 65

C: "I will go into the room to reassess her. Mrs. Elliott, how are you feeling?"

E: "Oh, the medication has helped, but I still feel uncomfortable. How do my tests look?"

C: "Well, you are not pregnant, and your urine looks healthy. You have some signs of infection and some of your liver tests are concerning for an infection in your gallbladder—which is usually due to stones. I would like to order a

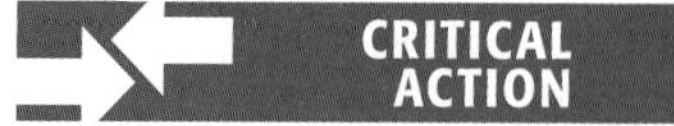

CRITICAL ACTION

Getting an orthopedic referral is a critical action in this case. In every case getting the patient the appropriate follow-up and/or admitting them to the appropriate level of care is critical. Do not forget to disposition patients appropriately.

KEY ORDERS

In the triple cases remember to reassess your patients and to follow-up on the labs/studies for each one. It is useful to go in order of presentation to keep organized, and make sure that you do not skip anyone.

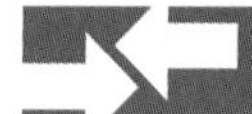

CRITICAL ACTION

Getting imaging of the RUQ is a critical action in this case.

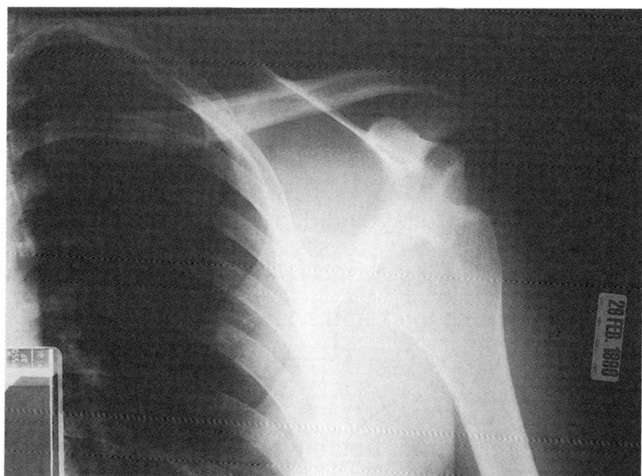

Figure C46-2. X-ray of shoulder showing an anterior dislocation. *(Reproduced with permission from Knoop KJ, Stack LB, Storrow AB.* Atlas of Emergency Medicine. *2nd ed. New York: McGraw-Hill; 2002.)*

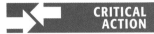

Getting a surgical consult is a critical action in this case.

Treating this patient with appropriate antibiotics is a critical action in this case.

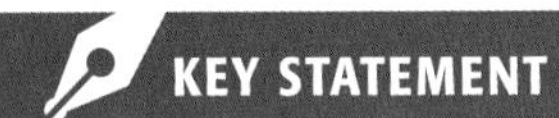

Remember to explain procedures to your patients, and to get consent before you perform them.

Reducing this dislocated shoulder is a critical action.

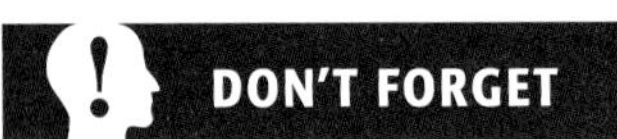

Be ready to explain procedures to the examiner. They will not always require it, and if so they will state, "The procedure was successful" or words to that effect. You should be able to "talk through" intubation, central line placement, chest tube placement, pericardiocentesis, paracentesis, thoracentesis, lumbar punctures, joint aspirations, and basic reductions.

RUQ ultrasound to confirm the likely presence of gall stones and talk to a surgeon about operating to remove the gall bladder."

E: "Oh, I have had an ultrasound before; they said I had some gallstones. They told me I should have my gallbladder taken out, but I just haven't had the chance to schedule it."

C: "Well, it looks like we'll have to make some time now."

E: "Dr. Cutter is on the phone now."

C: "Dr. Cutter, I am seeing Mrs. Elliott, a 34-year-old female with a history of symptomatic cholelithiasis. Today she has significant pain, RUQ abdominal tenderness on examination, an elevated WBC, elevated alkaline phosphatase and transaminase enzymes, and normal lipase. I am getting a RUQ US to assess for cholecystitis. I am also going to start her on cefoxitin 2 g IV unless there is another antibiotic you would prefer."

E: "OK, I will admit her; you can send her upstairs after the US and I will see her there."

C: "Nurse, can you please give Mrs. Elliott 2 g of cefoxitin IV and a bed on the general surgical floor? Are we ready for the shoulder reduction in room 2?"

E: "Yes, doctor. This part of the case is now over."

C: "Excellent. Mr. Thompson, It looks like your x-rays of your neck are clear. You did dislocate your shoulder and I will have to do a procedure to realign the shoulder joint. It is a painful procedure, so I will give you some medicine to knock you out briefly. When you wake up, the shoulder will be immobilized and we will repeat your x-rays to ensure we were successful. Do you have any questions?"

E: "No, doc, thanks. Whatever you think is best, I agree."

C: "OK, nurse, let's quickly check the patient's vital signs, ensure he is successfully being monitored and check his IV sites."

E: "Vitals are: 135/90, 89, 100%, and 16. Rhythm is normal sinus and he has a good wave form on the pulse oximeter."

C: "OK, let's use 10 mg of etomidate IV. I will ask the tech to provide countertraction while I attempt to reduce the dislocation using traction."

E: "It sounds like the joint is in and it looks better already."

C: "OK, let's place the shoulder immobilizer on and check a portable left shoulder x-ray. We will stay in the room with him until he regains consciousness."

E: "Is it all over, doc?"

C: "Looks like it, Mr. Thompson, you did great."

E: "It feels much better, thanks."

C: "In that case, I would like to examine your neck. Does it hurt when I press along the midline?"

E: "No."

C: "Do you have any numbness or tingling in your arms or legs?"

E: "No."

C: "OK, I will remove the C-collar."

E: "The portable x-ray has been shot. The results are normal. The patient asks, 'Can I go home now?'"

C: "Well, it looks like your repeat x-ray shows that our procedure was successful. I will need you to wear the immobilizer until you follow-up with your doctor. You must take your phenytoin, and avoid alcohol."

E: "I will, doc, thanks. The case is now over."

SITUATION ENCOUNTER ASSESSMENT (JIMMY BENDER)

The candidate handled the situation encounter very well. The candidate was organized and did not move on to the next patient unless they gave appropriate orders for the previous patient. This is a good thing to remember—when the examiner prompts you to move on (usually by saying "there is another patient, doctor"), order all the tests and medications you want for the patient you are seeing before you go. That way, when you are finished seeing the other patients the results will be ready for you to review. The evaluation was thorough, and the candidate did not give in to the common urge to rush (which happens often in the triple cases).

Slipped capital femoral epiphysis (SCFE) is a fairly uncommon childhood disorder, which classically presents with displacement of the femoral head posteriorly and inferiorly in relation to the femoral neck while still within the confines of the acetabulum as was seen in this x-ray. Definitive treatment is internal fixation with the goal to prevent complications such as avascular necrosis. In general, about 20% of patients will have bilateral involvement at the time of presentation and an additional 20%-40% will subsequently progress to bilateral involvement. Obese children are at increased risk. On physical examination, while external rotation is usually preserved, internal rotation is decreased and often painful.

The prognosis of a SCFE is determined in part by whether it is acute (<3 weeks) or chronic (>3 weeks) and stable (weight-bearing) or unstable (unable to bear weight). The rate of complications such as avascular necrosis goes up with increase in time from onset to surgery, so this process should be treated as an emergency. Most patients with SCFE who are treated with urgent in situ fixation do well. However, in those cases with severe slippage and resultant deformity, long-term sequelae such as leg-length discrepancy, avascular necrosis (AVN), or osteoarthritis may result. Following fixation of SCFE, the patient is given crutches with protected weight-bearing for 6-8 weeks and can return to full activity when they are pain free.

The candidate performed all of the critical actions of this case and would have passed easily. The candidate picked up all of the "easy" points for professionalism and interpersonal skills. She was always sensitive to the patient's pain, which can be a critical action. Always go for these points, both on the exam and in real life, for these are always of high yield.

Critical Actions (Jimmy Bender)

1. Elicit history and perform focused physical examination to raise level of suspicion for SCFE.
2. Order x-ray of hip and pelvis with frog view.
3. Administer analgesia.
4. Discuss case with orthopedic consultant.

Test Performance (Jimmy Bender)

1. *Data acquisition:* The candidate was concise and organized. Score = **7**
2. *Problem solving:* The candidate ordered labs and diagnostics appropriately. Score = **7**
3. *Patient management:* The candidate made appropriate treatment decisions very efficiently and timely. Score = **7**
4. *Resource utilization:* The candidate made good use of resources in a cost-effective manner. Score = **7**
5. *Health care provided (outcome):* The candidate made appropriate consultation and disposition decisions. Score = **7**
6. *Interpersonal relations and communication skills:* The candidate was very thoughtful of her patient's needs with regard to appropriate updating of medical conditions and discussions with the patient and consultants. Score = **7**
7. *Comprehension of pathophysiology:* Demonstrated good medical knowledge as evidenced by appropriate consultation and follow up. Score = **7**
8. *Clinical competence (overall):* This case was handled very well overall. Score = **7**

SITUATION ENCOUNTER ASSESSMENT (DEREK THOMPSON)

The candidate handled the situation encounter very well. She conducted reasonably thorough evaluations for each patient and did not rush through the process. The candidate did a good job uncovering the patient's seizure history and getting additional history from the emergency medical services (EMS) personnel, but should have asked about whether the patient had been taking his phenytoin regularly. The candidate ordered the necessary tests before moving on to the initial evaluation of the final patient—and this is a good thing to remember. That way, when you are finished seeing the other patients the results will be ready for you to review.

Shoulder dislocations are a very common problem in the emergency room (ER). While 95%-98% are anterior (as this one was) seizures can also produce posterior dislocations. Most reduction techniques involve trying to manipulate the humeral head back into its position in the glenoid through combinations of traction (to overcome the muscle spasm that almost inevitably ensues once the shoulder loses its usual anatomical integrity) and leverage (to manipulate the humeral head back into its anatomical position). While this candidate was not asked to describe the procedure, had the examiner asked, it could have been described as follows: "I will have an assistant hold counter-traction with a sheet around the patient's torso while I apply downward traction and abduct the arm until I feel the joint reduce into the appropriate position. I will then place the patient in a shoulder immobilizer and order post-reduction films of the joint."

The candidate performed all of the critical actions of this case and would have passed the case easily. The candidate picked up all of the "easy" points for professionalism and interpersonal skills by taking particular attention to the patient's need to be informed of treatment and procedures. They were sensitive to the patient's pain, and explained the need for cervical immobilization well.

Critical Actions (Derek Thompson)

1. Maintain C-spine precautions.
2. Get full story from EMS.

3. Identify and reduce shoulder dislocation using conscious sedation.
4. Administer analgesia.
5. Discover and remedy sub-therapeutic phenytoin level.

Test Performance (Derek Thompson)

1. *Data acquisition:* The candidate was concise and organized, but the history could have included a more detailed history regarding alcohol use and his phenytoin regimen, as well as inquiry as to other potential drug use/toxin exposure. Score = **6**
2. *Problem solving:* The candidate ordered labs and diagnostics appropriately and made an appropriate disposition decision. Score = **7**
3. *Patient management:* The candidate made appropriate treatment decisions very efficiently and timely. Score = **7**
4. *Resource utilization:* The candidate made good use of resources in a cost-effective manner. Score = **7**
5. *Health care provided (outcome):* The candidate was able to recognize the sub-therapeutic phenytoin level and evaluated for evidence of traumatic injury related to the seizure in an appropriate manner. Score = **7**
6. *Interpersonal relations and communication skills:* The candidate was very thoughtful of the patient's needs with regard to appropriate updating of medical conditions and answering questions. Score = **7**
7. *Comprehension of pathophysiology:* The candidate appropriately evaluated for nerve injury related to the shoulder dislocation. Score = **7**
8. *Clinical competence (overall):* This case was handled very well and could have been even better with more thorough data acquisition. Score = **7**

SITUATION ENCOUNTER ASSESSMENT (LILLIAN ELLIOT)

The candidate handled the situation encounter well. The candidate conducted a reasonably thorough evaluation of the patient and did not rush through the process. Many candidates will feel rushed during situation encounters (often called "triples") and miss key physical examination findings or historical findings.

Cholecystitis is in the spectrum of biliary tract disease which runs from asymptomatic gallstones to biliary colic, cholecystitis, choledocholithiasis, and ascending cholangitis. The inflammation in cholecystitis may be sterile or bacterial—and bacterial infection is thought to be a consequence, not a cause, of cholecystitis. When infection is present, common pathogens include *Escherichia coli, Klebsiella*, enterococci, and *Streptococcus*. Currently, practice is to "cool off" the infection and perform a cholecystectomy after several days or readmit the patient at a later date. Emergent cholecystectomy is performed in about 20% of cases of acute cholecystitis that has become complicated (ie, gangrene, perforation, ascending cholangitis, etc). Antibiotic therapy should be broad-spectrum—ampicillin/gentamicin/Flagyl is a good combination, and single-agent treatment with Zosyn or a third-generation cephalosporin is also appropriate.

The candidate performed all of the critical actions of this case and would have passed the case. They ordered appropriate tests, medication, and consults, and gave the patient the appropriate disposition. They could have improved, however, by having explained the procedure of pelvic and rectal examination to Mrs. Elliott, as well as taking a more careful history of her symptoms that would more strongly suggest the diagnosis of cholelithiasis. The candidate also did not treat the patient's pain until reminded twice by the examiner.

Critical Actions (Lillian Elliott)

1. Administer intravenous (IV) analgesics.
2. Elicit findings on history and physical examination to support diagnosis of acute cholecystitis.
3. Order appropriate diagnostic testing to support diagnosis of cholecystitis, eg, ultrasound (US) or computed tomography (CT).
4. Administer antibiotics to cover "gut" flora.
5. Obtain surgical consultation.

Test Performance (Lillian Elliot)

1. *Data acquisition:* The candidate was concise and organized, but did not obtain an adequate history about Mrs. Elliott's history of cholelithiasis. Score = **5**
2. *Problem solving:* The candidate gathered information in an organized approach, but had they gotten a better history they could have ordered the right upper quadrant (RUQ) US earlier. Score = **6**
3. *Patient management:* The candidate made appropriate treatment decisions very efficiently and timely. Score = **7**
4. *Resource utilization:* The candidate made good use of resources in a cost-effective manner. Score = **7**
5. *Health care provided (outcome):* The candidate eventually arrived at the correct diagnosis and administered appropriate care with antibiotics and surgical consultation. Score = **6**
6. *Interpersonal relations and communication skills:* The candidate was respectful and effective in communications to staff, patient, and consultant, but did not address and treat her patient's pain initially or explain invasive physical examinations. Score = **5**
7. *Comprehension of pathophysiology:* The candidate was able to demonstrate underlying knowledge of the disease process by ordering appropriate antibotics. Score = **6**
8. *Clinical competence (overall):* The candidate performed well overall, but could have greatly improved the score with more detailed history and more effective communication with the patient. Score = **6**

CASE 47 Situation Encounter: A 24 y/o Male With a Hand Laceration, a 62 y/o Female With SOB, and a 2 y/o Male With SOB

John Dayton, Catherine Johnson, and Flora Waples

INITIAL INFORMATION

Name: Joe Harris

Mode of arrival: Brought in by self

Age: 24 years

Gender: Male

VS: T 37.4°C (99.32°F), BP 120/80, HR 82, RR 20, O_2 sat: 99%

CC: "Cut on hand"

PLAY OF THE CASE (JOE HARRIS)

C: "What do I see when I walk in the room?"

E: "The patient is a young man who is sitting on the stretcher."

C: "Hello, I am Dr. Sanders. What brings you in today?"

E: "I got a cut on my hand and it's starting to swell up a bit."

C: "How did this happen?"

E: "I just scraped it when I almost fell. I was going down the steps, lost my footing, but I caught myself."

C: "Any other injuries?"

E: "No."

C: "Do you have any medical problems?"

E: "No."

C: "When did this happen?"

E: "Yesterday morning."

C: "Let me have a look. Have you taken anything for the pain?"

E: "No."

C: "Do you take any medications? Have you had a tetanus shot in the last 10 years?"

E: "No meds, I think my last shots were when I was in high school."

C: "Are you allergic to anything?"

E: "No."

C: "OK, well, let's see your hand? Show me where it hurts."

E: "The patient points to the dorsum of his right hand at the base of the second and third proximal metacarpal joints. There is an irregular abrasion at the joints with significant soft tissue swelling and erythema. The swelling extends about 5 cm circumferentially from the abrasions and down the index finger. It is warm to the touch."

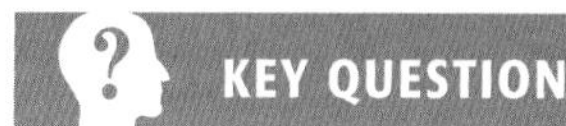

KEY QUESTION

Ask this open-ended question at the beginning of every case.

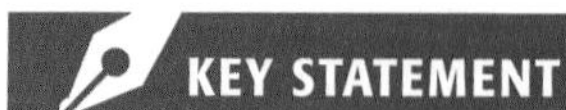

KEY STATEMENT

Remember to introduce yourself by name to all awake patients.

Giving appropriate antibiotics and a tetanus shot is a critical action.

Getting an x-ray to make sure that this is not an open fracture is a critical action in this case.

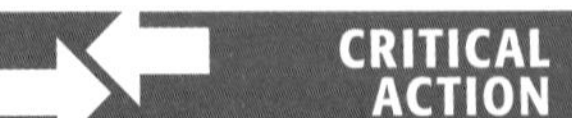

Getting a surgical consult and admitting for IV antibiotics is a critical action.

Placing the patient in a splint and irrigating/dressing the wound is a critical action in this case.

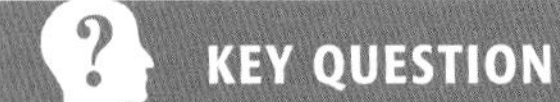

Ask this open-ended question at the beginning of every case.

C: "Can the patient extend or flex the finger?"

E: "No."

C: "Is there pain on passive range of motion of the finger?"

E: "Yes, any motion is exquisitely painful."

C: "Are the heart and lungs clear? Any murmurs?"

E: "Heart and lungs are clear."

C: "Is there any rash or skin changes?"

E: "No."

C: "Are any other joints tender or warm?"

E: "No."

C: "Does the patient have FROM in all other joints?"

E: "Yes."

C: "Mr. Harris, the infection on your hand is very serious. I will have to keep you in the hospital for antibiotics and consult with a hand specialist. You may even need surgery."

E: "Boy, I'm really going to get Henry for this!"

C: "What do you mean?"

E: "I got so angry at him yesterday that I punched him, and now look at my hand! Surgery? I'm pretty upset, doctor."

C: "Well, I am glad you came in, I will make the arrangements for you. Nurse, can you please give the patient 3 g of Unasyn IV, 4 mg of morphine sulfate IV, a tetanus shot, and keep the patient NPO. I will order an AP/lateral of the hand, a CBC, and two peripheral blood cultures. Let's call the hand surgeon on call and let him know he has a patient here. Please irrigate the wound with 500 cc of 0.9 NS under pressure with an 18-guage angiocath, then place a bulky dressing on the patient's hand and splint it in neutral position."

E: "Dr. Hand is on the phone."

C: "Hi Dr. Hand. I have a patient with a "fight bite" injury who presents about 12 hours after a fight. He has a significant cellulitis of the hand and has compromised flexion and extension of the primary metacarpal joint secondary to soft tissue swelling a pain. He may have infectious tenosynovitis. I would like to admit him for IV antibiotics and I would like for you to see him."

E: "Fine, put him on the surgical floor."

C: "Will do. Thank you. Nurse, please do not send him up until I have the lab results and x-rays back."

E: "Sounds good. We need you in room 2 right away, doctor!"

INITIAL INFORMATION

Name: Rose Williams

Mode of arrival: Brought by EMS

Age: 62 years

Gender: Female

VS: T 37.4°C (99.32°F), BP 90/50, HR 132, RR 28, O_2 sat: 88% on RA

CC: Shortness of breath

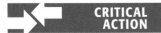

PLAY OF THE CASE (ROSE WILLIAMS)

C: "When I walk into the room, what do I see?"

E: "The patient is a 62-year-old woman named Mrs. Williams. The woman is sitting upright, leaning forward, and looks uncomfortable. There is audible wheezing. Her eyes and cheeks are very swollen; her skin is red and she is scratching herself. Her skin looks red everywhere."

C: "Ask the paramedics to stand by. Please place the patient on a 100% NRB mask, place two large-bore 18-gauge peripheral IVs, start a 500-cc bolus, and place the patient on a cardiac monitor. May I have another set of vitals?"

E: "Yes, doctor, her BP is 90/50, pulse 128, RR 24, and is coming up on the NRB mask O_2, now at 94%.

C: "I would like to assess her airway. Is there any stridor, pooling of secretions, or evidence of angioedema or upper airway obstruction?"

E: "No."

C: "Mrs. Williams, what happened?"

E: "The patient pants and grasps her throat, pointing to her husband."

C: "Mr. Williams, what happened?"

E: "Well doctor, we were at a luncheon and she mistakenly ate some fried shrimp."

C: "Has this ever happened before?"

E: "It's been a long time. She's usually very careful. It all happened so fast."

C: "Any medical problems? Heart disease?"

E: "She's pretty healthy: no other allergies, doesn't take any medications or have any medical problems. Her heart is fine."

C: "In addition to wheezes on examination, are there any crackles and are the breath sounds symmetric? Do I hear any murmurs or gallops?"

E: "There are symmetric breath sounds, wheezes throughout, and no crackles, murmurs, or gallops."

C: "Nurse, please give the patient epinephrine 1:1000, 0.3 mg IM, 50 mg Benadryl IV, 20 mg IV Pepcid, 125 mg of Solu-Medrol IV, and a liter of NS bolus."

E: "OK, doctor, anything else?"

C: "Please give her an albuterol nebulizer treatment. Repeat her blood pressure after the bolus and let's get an ECG. I would like to examine the patient. Is her breathing improving with the treatments?"

E: "Her respiratory rate is now 22 and her wheezing is less audible. She looks more comfortable. Repeat BP is 135/70 and pulse is 104 with a saturation of 96% on the NRB mask."

C: "Mrs. Williams, do you feel better?"

E: "Oh, yes, doctor, thank you."

C: "Do you have any medical problems?"

E: "No."

KEY ORDERS

Most of the patients you see during the exam are unstable (or will become that way). Every unstable patient requires IV access, oxygen, and cardiac monitoring (and in most cases an ECG).

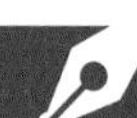

KEY ORDERS

Always repeat vitals after every intervention. This includes giving a fluid bolus or putting a patient on oxygen.

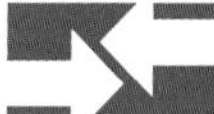

CRITICAL ACTION

Administering oxygen and monitoring the patient carefully is a critical action in this case.

DON'T FORGET

For any airway complaint, examine the airway before getting the history or the rest of the physical. Remember your ABCs.

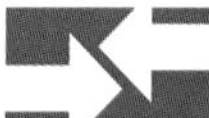

CRITICAL ACTION

Addressing whether the patient has any heart disease before giving epi is a critical action in this case.

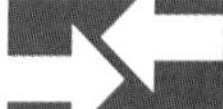

CRITICAL ACTION

Treating the anaphylaxis with appropriate meds and IV fluids is a critical action in this case

C: "I want to thank the paramedics for standing by and ask them what happened."

E: "We were called at a restaurant for an allergic reaction. She was really tight when we first got to her, so we gave her a few breathing treatments and a dose of Benadryl 50 mg on the way in."

C: "Great job, thank you. Anything else I should know about?"

E: "No allergies, no meds, no medical problems."

C: "OK, I'll let you guys get going then. I would like to complete my examination of the patient now. I would like to look at the head. Is there any sign of trauma? Are the pupils equally reactive to light and accommodation? Is there any swelling or lesions at the skin? Is there any trismus? Can I see the patient's posterior pharynx?"

E: "The examination of the head is normal. The patient has bilateral periorbital soft tissue swelling. Her cheeks are very flushed and red. There is no trismus and the patient's posterior pharynx is well visualized with normal abnormal findings."

C: "Does she have any swelling of her neck or JVD?"

E: "No."

C: "Is her lung examination clear? Does she still have any wheezing? Are the heart sounds regular? Are there any murmurs?"

E: "The patient has expiratory wheezing in all lung fields with good airway entry throughout. Her heart examination reveals a regular rate and rhythm, no murmurs or gallops."

C: "Is the abdomen soft, non-tender, non-distended without rebound or guarding?"

E: "Yes."

C: "How does her skin look? Does she have any petechia, urticarial lesions, vesicles or warmth on the skin? Is the skin intact?"

E: "The patient has diffuse, erythematous lesions on her upper chest, back, and neck that are raised, non-tender, and urticarial in nature. There are no vesicles or petechiae and the skin is intact."

C: "Does she have any swelling to her joints?"

E: "No."

C: "Is there any deficit in sensation, strength, or pulse in the extremities?"

E: "No."

C: "Is her cranial nerve examination normal? Is she alert and oriented × 3?"

E: "Her cranial nerve examination is normal and she is fully oriented."

C: "Is the rectal examination normal? Is the perineum normal to inspection, without any skin lesions?"

E: "Rectal and perineal examination are normal."

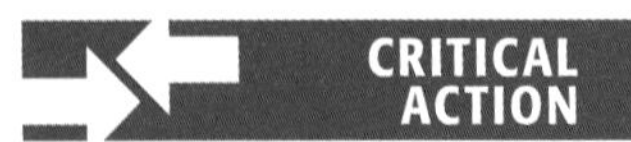

Admitting this patient for observation is a critical action in this case.

C: "Mrs. Williams. You are improving nicely after the treatments we have given you. It looks like you had a serious allergic reaction to the shrimp you ate. Although you are improving, because your attack was so severe, we will need to observe you in the hospital for at least a brief period to be sure that you do not relapse or have any further trouble. Would that be OK with you?

Nurse, would you please keep the patient on a continuous pulse oximeter and cardiac monitor, give her one albuterol per nebulizer now and, q20min × 3 treatments. I would like to request an observation admission. Please put a call into her doctor."

E: "This will be done. Your next patient is here, doctor."

INITIAL INFORMATION

Name: Jake Foster

Mode of arrival: Family

Age: 2 years

Gender: Male

VS: T 38.5°C (101.3°F), P 154, BP 90/70, RR 34, O_2 sat: 98%

CC: Cough

PLAY OF THE CASE (JAKE FOSTER)

C: "What do I see as I walk into the patient's room?"

E: "A 2-year-old child who is coughing intermittently. He is here with his two parents, Mr. and Mrs. Foster."

C: "Hello, Mr. and Mrs. Foster. I am Dr. Sanders. How is Jake doing today?"

E: "Oh doctor, he's been coughing and it's a really harsh cough that is keeping him up at night. I just don't like the way he is breathing."

C: "I would like to examine the patient's airway. Is it patent? Is there any stridor or drooling? Are the breath sounds clear? Are there any retractions?"

E: "The child's airway appears clear to visual inspection, he has a faint inspiratory auditory wheeze, his lungs are clear. There are no retractions present."

C: "Mr. and Mrs. Foster, when did these symptoms start?"

E: "This is the third day. He has had fevers only today, this is the highest temp now, he was about 38°C (100.4°F) at home this afternoon."

C: "How is he eating? Is he still playful?"

E: "He ate less today than usual, but he kept it down. He hasn't thrown up or had diarrhea. He was playful and acting like himself until a few hours ago. Now he looks a little tired."

C: "Does he have any medical problems? Are all of his vaccinations up-to-date? Was he a full-term baby?"

E: "No medical problems. He was born after his due date and we brought him home the next day. He's had all of his shots and the doctor says his growth is off the charts."

C: "Has he ever wheezed or had asthma?"

E: "No. Sometimes I feel like I hear a wheeze today, though."

C: "Have you given him anything at home?"

E: "No."

C: "Any other children at home that are sick or at day care?"

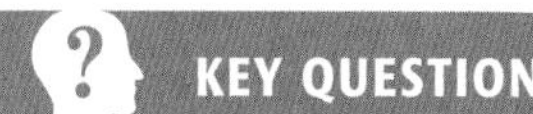

Ask this open-ended question at the beginning of every case.

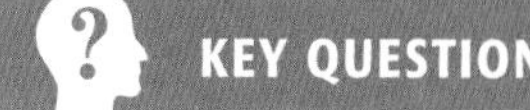

Remember to introduce yourself by name and get easy points for "Interpersonal Relations and Communication Skills."

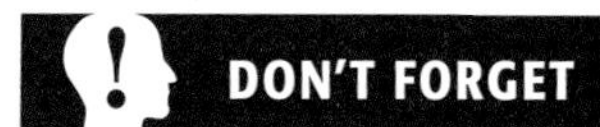

In any airway complaint, examine the airway before getting the history or the rest of the physical. Remember your ABCs.

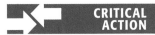

CRITICAL ACTION

Treating this case of croup with steroids and a racemic epi neb is a critical action in this case.

E: "No, he's our only child. At day care, there have been a lot of colds. He goes twice a week."

C: "Has he had any rash?"

E: "No."

C: "When is the last time he ate?"

E: "He had some juice about 2 hours ago, probably 6 oz?"

C: "Does he take any medications or have any allergies to medications?"

E: "No."

C: "Has he had any surgeries?"

E: "No."

C: "OK, I would like to finish my examination now, but first I will have the nurse keep him on the monitor, so we can watch his vital signs. Can we have respiratory come down to bring him a racemic epi neb? I would like to give him a shot of Decadron 0.6mg/kg IM, Tylenol suppository, 15 mg/kg PR, and get a portable CXR and neck x-ray."

E: "Will he get better?"

C: "Of course, we expect that the treatments will help. We will see how the tests look as well. I will do a thorough examination and then decide if he needs more treatment or if he can go home. Is there any evidence of trauma to the head or neck? Are the pupils equal and reactive? Are there any oral lesions? Any foreign bodies seen in the nose or mouth?"

E: "No evidence of trauma, the pupillary examination is normal, nose and mouth are clear."

C: "Is the neck supple? Any audible stridor?"

E: "The neck is supple, the patient has faint inspiratory stridor."

C: "Are there any skin changes, jaundice, or rash. Is skin turgor normal?"

E: "The skin examination is normal."

C: "When I do the lung and cardiac examination, do I hear any murmurs, rubs, or gallops? Is the rhythm normal? Are there any crackles or wheezes in the lungs? Are the breath sounds equal?"

E: "The cardiac and lung examinations are normal."

C: "Is the abdomen soft, is there any tenderness, rebound, or guarding? How are bowel sounds?"

E: "Abdominal exam is normal."

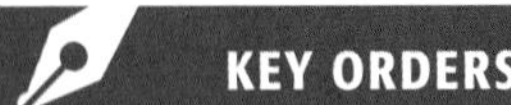

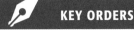

KEY ORDERS

In the triple cases remember to reassess your patients and to follow-up on the labs and imaging studies for each one. It is useful to go in order of presentation to keep organized, and make sure that you do not skip anyone.

C: "Is examination and inspection of the genitalia, testis, rectum, and perineum normal?"

E: "The examination is normal."

C: "I would like to check the patient's neurologic examination. Is the child interacting appropriately for his age? Is his gait normal for his age and is he sitting up in bed OK? Does he move all of his extremities?"

E: "The neurologic examination is normal. The respiratory therapist is here and the nurse has the medications."

C: "OK, Mr. and Mrs. Foster, we will proceed with the treatments. I will be back to reexamine him and review his x-rays."

C: "I would like to reexamine my first patient, Joe Harris. Have the labs and x-rays returned?"

E: "The x-rays are done, the CBC shows a WBC of 16,000, Hgb 14, plt 234, and the blood cultures have been sent. The radiologist read the x-ray as normal, except for soft-tissue swelling. The patient feels better and is sleeping. He has a bed. Shall I send him upstairs?"

C: "Yes, he may go up. How is Mrs. Williams doing in room 2?"

E: "She feels better. Her rash is going away and her wheezing has diminished. Her ECG is here and Dr. Wood, her family doctor, is on the phone. The ECG shows sinus tachycardia."

C: "Hello, Dr. Wood, I am seeing your patient Mrs. Williams, who came in with an anaphylactic reaction after ingesting shrimp. She has responded to treatment with epinephrine, Albuterol, Solu-Medrol, Pepcid, and Benadryl. I would like to admit her for a 24-hour observation period. We did an ECG because she was a bit tachycardic, and it is remarkable for sinus tachycardia only. There are no PVCs."

E: "OK, you can admit her to me to the observation unit."

C: "Thank you. How is little Jake Foster doing in room 3?"

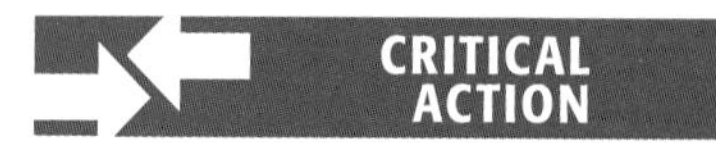

Reading the x-ray correctly is a critical action in this case.

E: "Well, he looks better. His temp is down to 37.2°C and he says he is hungry. His x-rays are done (Fig. C47-1)."

C: "Well, it appears that he likely has croup. His x-rays show a classic "steeple sign" in the trachea. Nothing on his CXR suggests a foreign body, infiltrate, or

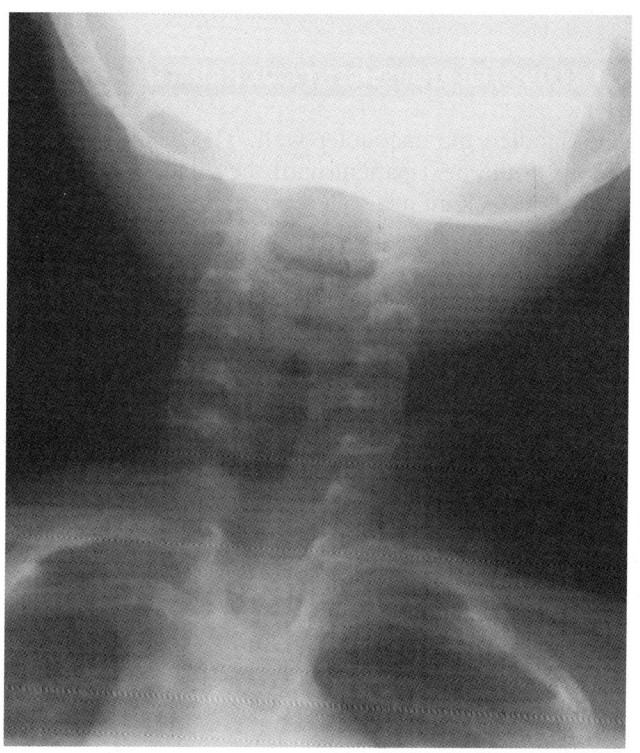

Figure C47-1. AP soft tissue neck revealing a "steeple" sign of the airway and a normal AP/lateral CXR. *(Reproduced with permission from Shah BR, Lucchesi M.* Atlas of Pediatric Emergency Medicine. *New York, NY: McGraw-Hill; 2006.)*

pneumothorax. I will reexamine him. Does he have stridor? How do the lung sounds now?"

E: "His stridor has resolved and his lungs are clear."

C: "Well, Mr. and Mrs. Foster, it looks like Jake has a viral infection called croup. The way he is coughing and the findings on the x-ray seem to fit. He has made a lot of improvement. How does he look to you?"

E: "He's back to himself. Thank you, doctor. Can we take him home?"

C: "How far away do you live from a hospital?"

E: "We live just a few blocks away."

C: "And when can he see his pediatrician?"

E: "I can make him an appointment for tomorrow. His doctor is really good about seeing us when we need to come in."

Checking the patient's social situation and ensuring adequate follow-up before discharging him to home is a critical action in this case.

C: "Well, sometimes children need to be hospitalized if they are not improving. Because he is improving, has been stable during an observation period, and you live close by, I will let you take him home. Keep a humidifier by his bed, and place him in the bathroom next to a steamy shower if his cough or breathing act up again. He will need to follow-up with his pediatrician tomorrow morning. If he gets worse or you have any concerns, bring him back ASAP. He may have fever on and off for another couple of days and you can treat that with Tylenol."

E: "OK, doctor, we can do everything you said."

C: "I would like to watch him for another 2 hours to be sure he is OK. We will reassess him before he goes."

E: "OK, thank you. The cases and situation encounters are now over."

SITUATION ENCOUNTER ASSESSMENT (JOE HARRIS)

The candidate handled the encounter well. The candidate was organized and did not move on to the next patient until they had started some orders on the patient they had just examined. They were reasonably thorough with each evaluation, and did especially detailed examinations.

The candidate performed all of the critical actions of this case and would have passed easily. The candidate could have done better by suspecting that this was a "fight bite" and pointedly asking Mr. Harris what happened. He was very lucky that the patient mentioned it spontaneously. This is a potentially disastrous injury that is likely to have a poor outcome if the infection is not suspected and the patient is discharged with a simple wound care plan. Thorough questioning is always a key.

The flexor tendons of the hand run in tight fibro-osseous tunnels. Infection can run along the tendon sheaths causing flexor tenosynovitis. This infection classically presents with

1. Fusiform swelling of the finger (often described as "sausage-like")
2. Flexed position of the finger
3. Severe pain with passive extension of the finger, and
4. Tenderness and swelling along the flexor tendon sheath.

Infection can be introduced directly into the tendon sheaths through a skin wound (most often) or via hematogenous spread, as occurs with gonococcal tenosynovitis. Note that the candidate inquired about the other joints to look for disseminated gonococcal disease. A history of recent trauma to the involved area is not uncommon. The complications of infectious tenosynovitis are a loss of active range of motion and, in severe cases, amputation.

The management of this infection differs from standard treatment of other soft-tissue infections and cellulitis, since the poor blood supply inside the tendon sheath reduces the efficacy of many antibiotics. Surgical incision and drainage in combination with IV antibiotics is the mainstay of treatment. *Staphylococcus aureus* and *Streptococcus* species are the most common etiologic agents, but infection is usually mixed. *Eikenella corrodens* occurs with human bites, so broad coverage antibiotics is a must.

Aside from missing the "fight bite," however, the candidate did a good job treating the patient, consulting the appropriate specialist, administering antibiotics, and providing appropriate wound care.

Critical Actions (Joe Harris)

1. Order x-ray of hand.
2. Administer an appropriate initial antibiotic and a tetanus shot.
3. Dress and splint the wound to prevent further movement of the hand and spread the infection with use.
4. Admit to surgery.

Test Performance (Joe Harris)

1. *Data acquisition:* The candidate was concise and organized except the candidate did not elicit from Mr. Harris the possibility of this being a "fight bite." Score = **5**
2. *Problem solving:* The candidate gathered information in an organized approach, ordered labs and diagnostics appropriately, and made appropriate consultation and disposition. Score = **7**
3. *Patient management:* The examinee recognized the need for IV antibiotics and appropriate wound dressing, obtained the appropriate consult, and arranged for admission for IV antibiotics ± surgery. Score = **8**
4. *Resource utilization:* The candidate made good use of resources in a cost-effective manner. Score = **8**
5. *Health care provided (outcome):* The patient received efficient, appropriate treatment, and the candidate's interventions stabilized the patient. Score = **8**
6. *Interpersonal relations and communication skills:* The candidate was respectful and effective in communications to staff, patient, and consultant. Score = **8**
7. *Comprehension of pathophysiology:* The candidate did not suspect a fight bite and could have missed this diagnosis without help from the examiner. However, the candidate did a good job screening for hematogenous spread of infection. Score = **6**

8. *Clinical competence (overall):* The candidate showed clinical competence by obtaining an appropriate history and physical, developing a differential diagnosis, utilizing appropriate lab work and imaging, utilizing appropriate interventions and consultation, and working toward the appropriate disposition. As noted above, points are lost for not anticipating and asking about a "fight bite." Score = **7**

SITUATION ENCOUNTER ASSESSMENT (ROSE WILLIAMS)

The candidate handled the situation encounter very well. The candidate was thorough with their evaluation, but could have avoided unnecessarily repeating treatment with Benadryl if they had spoken earlier with the paramedics. This is not a large error, however, since repeating the dose is not harmful to the patient. Always remember to get a brief history from emergency medical services (EMS) as soon as is practical, and detain them until all of your questions and concerns have been identified.

Anaphylaxis is a severe allergic reaction that is rapid in onset and may cause death. The full-blown reaction includes urticaria, hypotension (due to loss of smooth muscle tone and third-spacing), angioedema, and bronchospasm. Dyspnea is present when patients have bronchospasm or upper airway edema. Hypoxia and hypotension may cause weakness, dizziness, or syncope. Chest pain may occur due to demand ischemia secondary to hypotension and hypoxia. Upper airway compromise may occur when the tongue or oropharynx is swollen, so be sure to ask about stridor, hoarseness, or loss of speaking ability.

The candidate performed all of the critical actions of this case and would have passed the case easily. The candidate picked up all of the "easy" points for "Interpersonal Relations and Communication Skills" by keeping the patient informed of treatment and procedures. The ECG was probably not needed as tachycardia is expected in anaphylaxis. However, it is a cheap and rapid test, and the candidate would not lose points for it.

Critical Actions (Rose Williams)

1. Administer oxygen and monitor patient carefully.
2. Assess for the presence of heart disease before epinephrine administration.
3. Treat anaphylaxis with appropriate medications and IV fluids.
4. Admit patient for 24-hour observation period.

Test Performance (Rose Williams)

1. *Data acquisition:* The candidate was concise and organized. Mrs. Williams' history from the paramedics should have been requested earlier. Score = **6**
2. *Problem solving:* The candidate gathered information in an organized approach and ordered appropriate interventions. Score = **8**
3. *Patient management:* The examinee recognized when interventions needed to be made and obtained appropriate consults to create a safe disposition. Score = **8**
4. *Resource utilization:* The candidate made good use of resources in a cost-effective manner. A minor criticism could be made that an electrocardiogram (ECG) is not necessary if the tachycardia resolves after the anaphylaxis is treated and the epinephrine has worn off. Score = **7**

5. *Health care provided (outcome):* The patient received efficient, appropriate treatment, and the candidate's interventions stabilized the patient. Score = **8**
6. *Interpersonal relations and communication skills:* The candidate was respectful and effective in communications to staff, patient, and consultant. The candidate was very thoughtful of the patient's need to be updated regarding her condition. Score = **8**
7. *Comprehension of pathophysiology:* The examinee conveyed their understanding of anaphylaxis by their history and physical, interventions, and consultation with the admitting physician. Score = **7**
8. *Clinical competence (overall):* The candidate obtained an appropriate history and physical, ordered appropriate interventions, and obtained a safe disposition plan. Score = **7**

SITUATION ENCOUNTER ASSESSMENT (JAKE FOSTER)

The candidate handled the situation encounter very well. They did an especially detailed examination and never needed prompting by the examiner to ask for more detail. Many candidates will feel rushed during the "triple encounters" and may miss key history and examination findings.

Croup is a viral respiratory tract infection and the most common etiology for stridor in febrile children. It is a common pediatric illness, with the vast majority of children recovering with no sequelae. However, it can be life-threatening. Croup presents with a "seal-like" barking cough and a variable degree of respiratory distress. Morbidity is secondary to narrowing of the larynx and trachea below the level of the glottis, causing the hallmark inspiratory stridor. During inspiration, the supraglottic region can be suctioned closed because of negative intraluminal pressure generated. This same area is forced open during expiration. Stridor that occurs due to glottic disorders, such as croup, is often heard during both inspiration and expiration. The current cornerstones of treatment are glucocorticoids and nebulized epinephrine. Corticosteroids are beneficial because of their anti-inflammatory action, which causes decreased laryngeal mucosal inflammation. Antibiotics are not indicated.

The candidate performed all of the critical actions of this case and would have passed the case easily. The candidate picked up all of the "easy" points for professionalism and interpersonal skills by paying particular attention to the family's need to be informed of treatment and procedures. They also did a thorough evaluation of the patient's social situation and ability to ensure follow-up before sending him home. Always do a thorough evaluation before sending anyone home from ABEM General.

Critical Actions (Jake Foster)

1. Administer Decadron and racemic epi.
2. Order and correctly interpret x-rays of the neck and chest.
3. Make appropriate disposition based on patient's history, progress, and social situation.

Test Performance (Jake Foster)

1. *Data acquisition:* The candidate obtained all of the information required to make the correct diagnosis and this was done in an orderly fashion. Score = **8**

2. *Problem solving:* The examinee used vital signs, asked appropriate exam questions, obtained helpful imaging, and ordered appropriate interventions. Although croup is often diagnosed by history and physical, a history involving 3 days of symptoms made the x-rays a reasonable request. Score = **8**
3. *Patient management:* The examinee recognized the need for steroids and a racemic epi neb, monitored the patient for an appropriate observation period, and discharged the patient after making sure the parents were aware of return precautions and lived relatively close. Score = **8**
4. *Resource utilization:* The candidate used appropriate medication and intervention. Points are missed for not calling the Pediatrician to arrange follow-up. There will be some patients who can be discharged from ABEM General, but follow-up should be arranged. Score = **6**
5. *Health care provided (outcome):* The patient received efficient, appropriate treatment, and the candidate's interventions stabilized the patient. Score = **8**
6. *Interpersonal relations and communication skills:* The candidate was respectful and effective in communicating with the staff and the patient's parents. Score = **8**
7. *Comprehension of pathophysiology:* The candidate conveyed their understanding of croup by their history and physical, treatment provided, and observation period. Score = **8**
8. *Clinical competence (overall):* The candidate showed clinical competence by obtaining an appropriate history and physical, developing a differential diagnosis, utilizing appropriate imaging and treatment, and working toward a safe disposition. Score = **7**

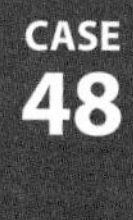

CASE 48

Situation Encounter: A 74 y/o Female With Mental Status Changes, a 45 y/o Male With a Headache and Syncope, and an 8 y/o Male With SOB

John Dayton and Alan Kumar

INITIAL INFORMATION

Name: Maude Redmond

Mode of arrival: Ambulance

Age: 74 years

Gender: Female

VS: T 39.2°C (102.56°F), BP 85/60, HR 115, RR 24, O_2 sat: 94% on RA, wt: 60 kg

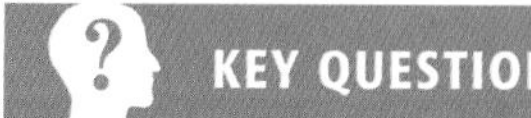

KEY QUESTION

Ask this open-ended question at the beginning of every case.

PLAY OF THE CASE (MAUDE REDMOND)

C: "What do I see as I walk into the patient's room?"

E: "You see an elderly frail female lying with her eyes closed on the stretcher."

C: "Are there any family members present?"

E: "No."

C: "Please ask the paramedics to remain so I may ask them questions in a moment."

C: "I would like to talk to the patient."

KEY ORDERS

Remember to use all available resources to get a history about patients with any altered mental status—including family, caregivers, and EMS.

C: "Hello, Ms. Redmond. I am Dr. Clearviz. Do you know where you are right now?"

E: "The patient opens her eyes and looks at you briefly before closing them again. There is no response."

C: "Ms. Redmond? Can you hear me? Are you in any pain?" Please shake the patient lightly."

E: "Again, the patient briefly opens her eyes, then closes them again."

KEY ORDERS

Most of the patients you see during the exam are unstable (or will become that way).

Every unstable patient requires IV access, oxygen, and cardiac monitoring (and in most cases an ECG).

C: "I would like to perform a brief examination. While I am doing this, I would like the nurse to place a large-bore IV, put the patient on a cardiac monitor, 4 L O_2 by NC, pulse oximeter, and draw blood work including two sets of blood cultures to be sent later. Given the fever, also place a Foley catheter and send off urine for analysis and culture and ask the secretary to order a portable chest x-ray."

E: "All of those things are being done."

C: "Give a 500 cc fluid bolus of NS and please tell me the repeat blood pressure after it is done. Also, give a Tylenol suppository to combat that temperature."

KEY ORDERS

Always begin by treating any vital sign abnormality: give fluids to people who are hypotensive, oxygen to people who are hypoxic, and antipyretics to people who are febrile.

C: "I will start by assessing the ABCs. What is her breathing pattern? Is her gag reflex intact?"

CRITICAL ACTION

Giving appropriate fluid resuscitation is a critical action in this case.

KEY ORDERS

Always assess the airway first in any patient who is unstable or altered. You can go back and do the rest of your examination after the patient is stable and the airway is secure.

KEY ORDERS

Remember to reassess any unstable patient frequently. It is also a good idea to instruct your "nurse" to bring you a new set of vitals after any intervention. This places the responsibility for remembering to reassess on the examiner.

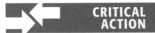

E: "She has a steady, deep breathing pattern without distress. Her gag reflex is intact."

C: "Are there any signs of trauma on the head, thorax, or extremities?"

E: "No."

C: "How are the pupils? TMs? Oropharynx?"

E: "Pupils are reactive, 4-3 mm bilaterally. The mucous membranes are dry. The rest of the HEENT examination is normal."

C: "I would like to assess the neck for JVD, stiffness, trachea, and bruits."

E: "Normal."

C: "Heart and lung examination?"

E: "Lungs are clear to auscultation and the heart sounds are normal S_1, S_2, without murmurs or rubs."

C: "Abdomen examination?"

E: "Soft, non-tender, non-distended, with decreased bowel sounds."

C: "Rectal examination?"

E: "Normal tone and guaiac negative."

C: "Extremity examination?"

E: "Normal tone, good distal pulses, no signs of pressure sores. Some chronic venous stasis changes to the lower legs."

C: "During this examination, has the patient spontaneously moved any extremities?"

E: "She is intermittently moving all four extremities."

C: "Is she at all verbal with any questioning?"

E: "She moaned slightly during the placement of the Foley, otherwise no."

C: "I would like to send blood for CBC, chem 7, blood and urine cultures, UA. Please order an ECG, and put the patient in for a head CT."

E: "All those things are being done. The nurse informs you that there is a 45 y/o male in examination room 2 complaining of a headache."

C: "Has the blood pressure come up with the fluid bolus?"

E: "After the 500-cc bolus, the pressure is now 90/60."

C: "Please give another 500-cc fluid bolus. I will go and examine the new patient."

INITIAL INFORMATION

Name: Todd Gaston

Mode of arrival: Car

Age: 45 years

Gender: Male

VS: T 37.2°C (98.96°F), BP 125/60, HR 105, RR 24, O_2 sat: 94% on RA, wt: 70 kg

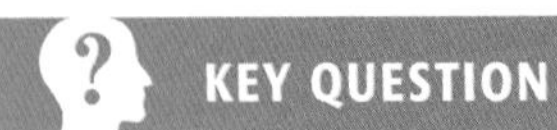

KEY QUESTION

Ask this open-ended question at the beginning of every case.

PLAY OF THE CASE (TODD GASTON)

C: "What do I see as I walk into the patient's room?"

E: "You see a well-developed male sitting in the stretcher in some discomfort."

C: "Hello sir. My name is Dr. Clearviz. What brings you to the ED today?"

E: "Doc, my head is killing me. I was working all afternoon and got this headache that slowly got worse and worse. I can barely stand it now."

C: "Do you have a history of headaches?"

E: "No, I never get them. This is horrible!"

C: "Is your neck stiff? Does the light bother your eyes?"

E: "My neck isn't stiff, but it's hard to keep my eyes open."

C: "Any nausea or vomiting? Any problems with talking, walking, or change in your vision?"

E: "No, but I stepped outside to get some fresh air and I passed out. Next thing I know, my next door neighbor is waking me up and brought me here."

C: "Did you have any palpitations or chest pain before passing out?"

E: "No. One minute I'm walking outside, and the next I'm on the ground."

C: "Does anything hurt from the fall?"

E: "No, Just my head, but I don't think that I bumped it as I have no sore spots."

C: "Anything else going on?"

E: "I am feeling fuzzy. You know, just not myself. Like I have to struggle to concentrate."

C: "Any other medical problems? Medications, allergies?"

E: "No, I'm usually healthy as a horse. No allergies either."

C: "Do you smoke or drink? Any other drug use?"

E: "No."

C: "I would like to perform an examination. Any external signs of trauma from the fall?"

E: "No."

C: "I would like to do an HEENT examination, paying special attention to the pupils and fundi."

E: "The examination is normal."

C: "Is there any JVD? Is there any midline tenderness found? If so, I will place the patient in a C-collar."

E: "There is no JVD or midline tenderness. The neck is supple."

C: "Are lung sound clear and symmetric? Any murmurs, rubs, gallops? Are the peripheral pulses full? Are there any neck bruits?"

E: "Lung sounds are normal and the cardiovascular examination is fine."

C: "Abdominal examination?"

E: "Normal."

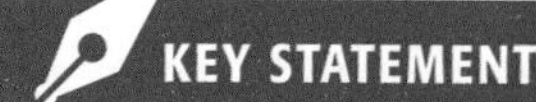

Remember to introduce yourself by name to the patient and family. Don't lose easy points for professionalism by forgetting to do simple things such as this.

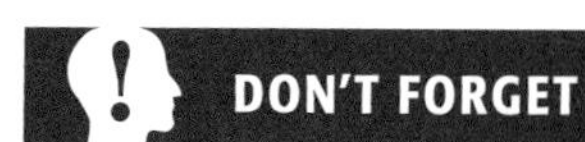

If the examiner states that an examination is "normal," that means there are no pertinent findings in that organ system and you can move on to the next.

If the examiner says "what are you looking for?" then there may be pertinent finding there and you should dig deeper.

Getting an ECG is a critical action in this case.

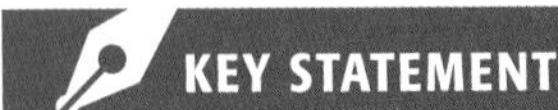

Remember to explain the plan to the patient and keep them updated about any test results.

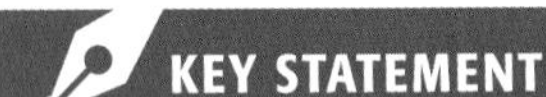

Remember to treat your patient's pain. Pain management is often a critical action, so don't miss it!

KEY QUESTION

Ask this open-ended question at the beginning of every case.

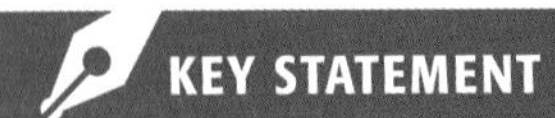

Remember to introduce yourself by name to the patient and family. Don't lose easy points for professionalism by forgetting to do simple things such as this.

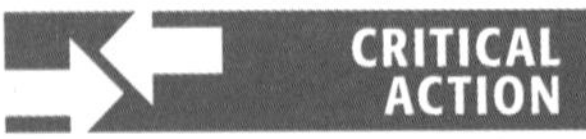

Giving this patient nebulizer treatments is a critical action in this case.

C: "Is there any clubbing, cyanosis, edema, joint tenderness, or deformity?"

E: "None found."

C: "Neurologic examination?"

E: "What would you like to know?"

C: "Cranial nerves, strength, sensation, reflexes, cerebellar signs, and gait."

E: "All normal."

C: "Mr. Gaston, what is the date today."

E. "He tells you the correct date."

C: "That is correct. Please have the nurse place an IV, draw extra blood samples, and send for a BMP, a CBC, and cardiac enzymes. Please order an ECG and a head CT."

C: "Mr. Gaston, I am not exactly sure why you have this headache but I want to make sure you are OK so we are going to do some tests including a head CT to make sure this is not an aneurysm. If that is negative, we might need to do a spinal tap to look for minute amounts of blood the CT scan can miss. This is all to make sure you're OK."

E: "Wow, that doesn't sound pleasant. But do what you have to do."

C: "Please give morphine, 4 mg IV for his headache and Zofran 4 mg IV to prevent nausea."

E: "All of the tests are ordered and the medications are administered. The nurse informs you that there is another patient in examination room 3."

INITIAL INFORMATION

Name: Rod Lever

Mode of arrival: Car

Age: 8 years

Gender: Male

VS: T 37.4°C (99.32°F), BP 105/60, HR 115, RR 34, O_2 sat: 90% on RA, wt: 30 kg

PLAY OF THE CASE (ROD LEVER)

C: "What do I see as I walk into the patient's room?"

E: "You see an 8 y/o boy with an increased respiratory rate sitting on the stretcher coloring in a book. Dad is at the bedside."

C: "Hi Sir. My name is Dr. Clearviz. What is going on?"

E: "Hi doc, Rod here has asthma and seems to be having an attack."

C: "How long has it been going on? Any fevers?"

E: "Well, he has had a cold for a couple days with a mild cough but nothing severe. His inhaler was working great, but we ran out this afternoon and weren't able to get a hold of his doctor to get a prescription refill. No fevers."

C: "Ask the nurse to give Rod an albuterol/Atrovent nebulizer treatment."

C: "Has he ever had attacks like this before? How does this one compare to others?"

E: "He seems to have one or two attacks every winter. Never anything serious. He has never been admitted to the hospital for them. But we didn't realize that we didn't have a proper supply today."

KEY ORDERS

Always remember to get your past medical and surgical history complete with medications and allergies.

C: "Has he been coughing anything up?"

E: "No, just a dry hacking cough."

C: "Any other medical problems?"

E: "He had pneumonia as a child a few years ago."

C: "Does he take any medications on a regular basis?"

E: "Just the inhaler when he needs it."

C: "Is he allergic to any medications?"

E: "Penicillin."

C: "Hi Rod. I'm Dr. Clearviz. I'm going to do a quick examination."

C: "Are there wheezes? Is the air entry good?"

E: "The lungs show average aeration with inspiratory and expiratory wheezing. No crackles."

C: "Are the mucous membranes moist? Are the tonsils enlarged? The ears OK?"

E: "The mucous membranes are moist. The tympanic membranes are normal. The oropharynx shows mildly enlarged tonsils without signs of erythema or exudate."

C: "Is there JVD? Is the trachea midline?"

E: "Normal findings."

C: "Are there murmurs, gallops, or rubs? Is there palpable pulsus paradoxus? Is capillary refill normal?"

E: "Tachycardia is noted. Otherwise cardiovascular examination is normal, though you note that the pulse strength varies with respirations."

C: "Any rash, petechiae, cyanosis, or edema?"

E: "None."

C: "Neurologic examination. How alert is he?"

E: "The patient is watching TV while the nurse starts the neb."

C: "Mr. Lever, I don't think Rod has pneumonia based on my examination. Let's see how he responds to the nebulizer, and I'll examine him again soon."

KEY ORDERS

In the triple cases, remember to reassess your patients and to follow-up on each of the labs and studies you order for each one.

It is useful to go in order of presentation to keep organized, and make sure that you do not skip anyone.

C: "What are Maude Redmond's vital signs? Have we gotten any of the tests back yet?"

E: "I was just going to tell you that Maude Redmond's BP is 70/40. The remainder of her VS after the second fluid bolus are: HR 110, RR 24, O_2 sat 94% on 4-L NC, and the BP of 70/40 that I mentioned."

C: "How is the temperature after the Tylenol?"

E: "The temperature has come down to 38.4°C."

E: "Here are the tests you ordered."

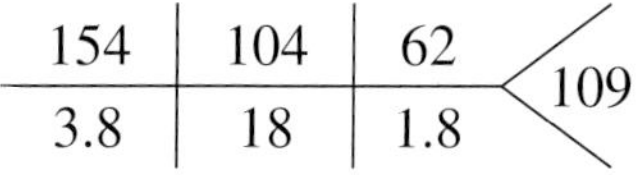

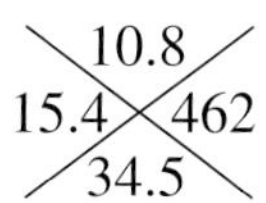

Segs: 89%
Bands: 4%
Lymphs: 4%

ECG: Sinus tachycardia with nonspecific changes unchanged from old ECG

Portable CXR: Clear lung fields, mild cardiomegaly

UA: Specific gravity is 1.03. No protein or bilirubin. Positive for blood, nitrates, and leukocyte esterase.

C: "What is her mental status at this time?"

E: "Unchanged from before."

C: "Lung examination?"

E: "Clear lungs."

C: "Change her oxygen supplement to a 100% NRB. Give another 500-cc fluid bolus. Is there any family present?"

E: "No."

C: "Are the paramedics still here?"

E: "They have remained as you requested."

C: "Hey guys, do you have any more medical information on her?"

E: "They inform you that they picked her up at an assisted living center. She is normally able to care for herself, but when she didn't come down for lunch, the nursing assistant went to her apartment and found her in bed confused and lethargic. She is on Aricept for mild Alzheimer disease, has a history of a hip replacement a couple years ago, and takes metoprolol for hypertension. She has an allergy to Cipro."

C: "Start the patient on Zosyn 3.375 g IV to treat urosepsis. I will place a central line in the right internal jugular to address the low pressures and need for IV antibiotics. Please send a urine culture."

E: "The central line has been placed."

C: "Check breath sounds to rule out a pneumothorax."

E: "Breath sounds are normal."

C: "Order a confirmation chest x-ray."

E: "Repeat chest x-ray shows the tip of the catheter at the entrance to the right atrium and no signs of pneumothorax. The pulmonary vasculature seems more congested than before."

C: "Start levophed at 5 μg/min and titrate up to a goal blood pressure of 90-100 systolic."

E: "The levophed drip is started and the blood pressure comes up to 95/60. The rest of the vital signs remain stable."

C: "Please place the patient in for an ICU bed and call her admitting doctor."

E: "Dr. Primo, the patient's primary care physician, is on the phone."

C: "Hi Dr. Primo, this is Dr. Clearviz at ABEM General and I have Ms. Redmond here. She is a 74-year-old female from an assisted living facility that was found to be lethargic and confused today and sent here for evaluation. She arrived here with a depressed mental status and a fever. Our evaluation included blood work and a sepsis workup based on the examination showing that she is suffering from urosepsis. She has received appropriate antibiotics, has a urine culture pending, and she is requiring pressors. I want to admit her

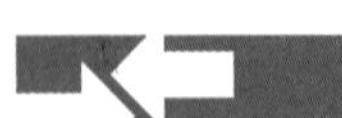

CRITICAL ACTION

Placing this septic patient on antibiotics is a critical action in this case.

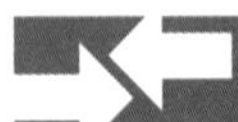

CRITICAL ACTION

Making the diagnosis of urosepsis is a critical action in this case.

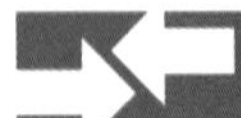

CRITICAL ACTION

Placing this septic patient on pressors after appropriate fluid resuscitation is a critical action in this case. For extra style points this candidate could have measured a CVP before starting dopamine.

KEY ORDERS

Having your "nurse" titrate meds to a specific goal is a good idea. This will help you adjust medication to the appropriate dose.

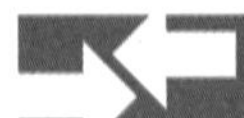

CRITICAL ACTION

Admitting this septic patient to the ICU is a critical action in this case.

to the ICU under your care. Given her altered mentation, I also ordered a head CT that is unremarkable."

E: "Thanks for your help. I'll take it from here. This case is now over."

E: "The patient in room 2 is getting anxious about his head CT results."

C: "Mr. Gaston, how is the headache after the pain medication?"

E: "Doc, it is still killing me!"

C: "Have the nurse give another 4 mg of morphine and set up for a lumber puncture."

E: "Is the spinal tap necessary, doc?"

C: "The final decision is yours, but this is one thing that I would like to rule out because it could be life-threatening if we miss it."

E: "OK."

C: "Do we have the blood work or the ECG?"

E: "All blood tests are normal. The ECG shows no abnormalities."

C: "Perform a lumbar puncture on this patient."

E: "The lumbar puncture is successful and results in clear fluid."

C: "Please send tubes 1 and 4 for cell count and differential. Tube 2 for glucose and protein and tube 3 for Gram stain and culture."

E: "Those tests are sent. His headache is getting better."

E: "The father of Rod Lever thinks they are ready to go home. He states his child looks much better."

C: "How does the child look when I walk back into the room?"

E: "His breathing is much more comfortable."

C: "Can I get a repeat set of vital signs? How is his lung examination?"

E: "His O_2 sat is now 98% on RA and other vital signs are normal."

E: "His lung examination shows scant expiratory wheezes intermittently, but he has marked improvement from before."

C: "Mr. Lever, Rod seems to be doing much better now. I want to write you a prescription for an albuterol inhaler with an Aerochamber to allow for better utilization of the metered dose inhaler. I also want to give Rod a short course of steroids to stop this attack in its tracks and make him better faster. You should follow-up with your physician shortly."

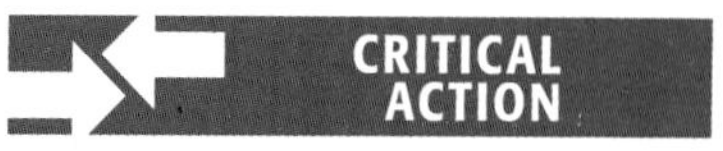

Assuring the patient's follow-up and giving him medication to go home on before sending him to home are two critical actions in this case.

C: "Please page Rod's pediatrician for me."

E: "Dr. Kidd is on the phone."

C: "Hi Dr. Kidd, this is Dr. Clearviz at ABEM General. Rod Lever came here tonight with a mild asthma attack after they ran out of his inhaler at home. After one neb, he looks and sounds much better. He currently has a minor cold but he is afebrile, has scant wheezing on lung examination without rhonchi, and now looks great. I was going to send them home with prescriptions for an albuterol MDI as well as a burst of steroids to help clear this up. I just wanted you to know so that they can confirm follow-up."

E: "Sounds good. Have them see me in 2 days in my office."

C: "Discharge Rod and his dad with clear asthma instructions and reasons to return."

C: "Are the LP results back on Mr. Gaston yet?"

E: "The LP results show no cells in either tubes 1 or 4, normal glucose and protein levels, and the Gram stain is negative."

C: "Mr. Gaston, how are you feeling?"

E: "Doc, I am still slightly fuzzy. The headache is better but still there. Have you figured out what is going on?"

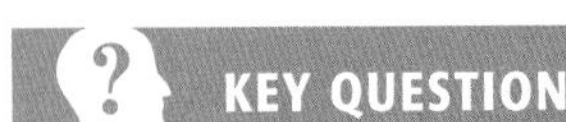

Remember to use all available resources to get a history on anyone with altered mental status—including patients with syncope.

C: "All the tests we have done so far are normal. Is there anybody here with you today?"

E: "Yeah, my neighbor who saw me pass out is in the waiting room."

C: "Please call him into the room so I can talk to him."

E: "Mr. Neighbor is now in the room."

C: "Mr. Neighbor, what did you see this afternoon?"

E: "Well, I was looking out my window and saw Todd come out of his garage, stumble, and then fall into the snow."

C: "How long was he out?"

E: "Maybe a couple minutes. I went out to see him, and he seemed pretty pale. He was cold too. I went into his garage and got his jacket. He had left a heater on and a generator running, so I turned them off and brought him here."

Getting a CO level and applying 100% oxygen by face mask are two critical actions in this case.

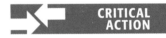

C: "Todd, what kind of work were you doing this afternoon?"

E: "I was doing some work out in the garage."

C: "Was the garage closed?"

E: "Yeah, doc. It's cold outside."

C: "Did you have the generator running the whole time?"

E: "No, but it was on and off while I was working."

C: "Have the nurse place the patient on a 100% O_2 NRB face mask and draw a CO level."

Arranging for hyperbaric therapy and admitting the patient to a monitored setting are two critical actions in this case.

C: "Mr. Gaston, working in an enclosed space and leaving a generator on can be very dangerous. I think the cause of your symptoms could be carbon monoxide poisoning from the exhaust from generator."

E: "Wow, I didn't think it could happen so quickly! I was only in there for an hour or so."

C: "Do we have hyperbaric capability at this facility?"

E: "Yes we do. And the CO level is 34%."

C: "Mr. Gaston, your carbon monoxide level is at dangerous levels. We are going to treat it aggressively with a dive chamber to force the carbon monoxide out of your blood. Given that you passed out today, we are going to need to watch you overnight as well."

E: "Thanks doc. I'll never do that again."

C: "Please inform respiratory that they need to accompany the patient to the hyperbaric chamber and perform a 90-minute dive to lower the CO levels in his blood. Put him in for a monitored bed overnight and place a call to his doctor."

E: "Dr. Ayre is on the phone."

C: "Hello Dr. Ayre. This is Dr. Clearviz at ABEM General. I am taking care of Todd Gaston here in the ED today. He came in after complaining of a headache and passing out. Initially, I was worried about subarachnoid hemorrhage, but the CT and LP were unremarkable. Further questioning revealed that he had been working in his garage this afternoon and using a generator to power a heater in an enclosed space. His CO level is 34% and he is currently in the dive chamber getting treated. One treatment should be enough to bring down levels sufficiently along with 100% O_2 overnight but given the syncope, I want to observe him on telemetry overnight."

E: "Did he have any ECG changes?"

C: "Luckily, no, and his labs were all normal, including cardiac enzymes. He was very lucky."

E: "OK. I'll see him within the hour. The case is now over."

CASE ASSESSMENT (MAUDE REDMOND)

Though this patient arrived to the emergency department and was not able to provide any information on her own, the candidate was still given clues to her diagnosis, given her age and vital signs. The candidate did a superb job of organizing the examination, tests, and treatments. The paramedics also gave helpful history that completed the clinical picture and provided for optimal care. Re-evaluation of the patient was also promptly done when she became hypotensive and after multiple interventions. As the patient became critically ill, the treatment course was logical and placing a central line for pressors was an appropriate intervention. Checking for complications of your procedures is also necessary and easily missed in the artificial environment of the oral boards.

Overall, the candidate did a wonderful job taking care of this patient. Even though the evaluation and treatment were done in phases between the management of other patients, the candidate did not skip a beat and appropriately managed this patient. The candidate was able to make it through the three cases successfully. You will notice that throughout the case, the examiner is responsible for guiding the candidate from room to room at appropriate points of the workup. A systematic approach to every patient will definitely help with patient management and help the examiner guide you more efficiently. Time becomes your main enemy in the multiple case encounters and the ability to organize the history, tests, and information exchange will benefit you greatly. If you notice throughout the encounters, the evaluation is always the same with the candidate addressing ABCs, obtaining history, and then performing an abbreviated head-to-toe physical examination. This systematic approach allows for fewer mistakes and provides for better organization, especially when managing multiple patients at once.

Critical Actions (Maude Redmond)

1. Fluid bolus for initial low blood pressure
2. Recognition of urosepsis
3. Antibiotic administration
4. Pressors for the hypotensive shock
5. Admission to the ICU

Test Performance (Maude Redmond)

1. *Data acquisition:* This phase is superb as the candidate shows ability to obtain a proper history from secondary sources and perform an examination on a patient who is unable to cooperate with the examination. Score = **8**
2. *Problem solving:* Problem solving is excellent, as the candidate is able to quickly assimilate data from the patient encounter, interprets test results and directs further management. Score = **8**
3. *Patient management:* The candidate directs appropriate interventions. Tylenol is given for the fever, fluids for the low blood pressure, and antibiotics for the urosepsis. More points could have been obtained by checking central venous pressure (CVP) after central line placement, but this was not required of the scenario. Score = **7**
4. *Resource utilization:* Even though an elderly patient with altered mental status (AMS) has a broad differential, the candidate was able to order only appropriate tests and imaging, spoke with paramedics, and appropriately consulted an admitting physician. Score = **8**
5. *Health care provided (outcome):* The patient received efficient, appropriate treatment, and the candidate's interventions stabilized the patient. Score = **8**
6. *Interpersonal relations and communication skills:* As the patient is unable to participate in the history taking, the candidate appropriately interviews the paramedics and has appropriate conversation with the admitting physician. Score = **8**
7. *Comprehension of pathophysiology:* The examinee conveyed their understanding of how to perform an efficient work-up for an elderly patient with fever and AMS. The candidate ordered appropriate studies and provided appropriate interventions. The candidate also used the conversation with the consultant to display her understanding of the case. Score = **8**
8. *Clinical competence (overall):* The candidate showed clinical competence by obtaining an appropriate history and physical, developing a differential diagnosis, utilizing appropriate lab work and imaging, utilizing appropriate interventions, speaking with paramedics, and working toward the appropriate disposition. Score = **7**

CASE ASSESSMENT (TODD GASTON)

In this case, the candidate started off on the wrong track in pursuing the headache and does not obtain an adequate history. This results is an unnecessary workup for a subarachnoid hemorrhage. When that entire workup comes up empty, the candidate does a wonderful job of starting over and pulling in new information and sources to figure out where he went off track. Finding a second source for history is often necessary in the oral board format. Whether it be from paramedics, family, friends, or a medical card in the patient's wallet, this information is often key in determining the underlying cause of disease. Once the candidate determines the environmental risk, a proper diagnosis is quickly made and proper therapy is initiated.

A systematic approach will help the examiner guide you more efficiently. Time becomes your main enemy in the multiple case encounters and the ability to organize the history, tests, and information exchange will benefit you greatly.

Critical Actions (Todd Gaston)

1. Get an electrocardiogram (ECG).
2. Get a CO level.
3. Apply 100% oxygen by face mask pending CO levels.
4. Arrange for hyperbaric therapy.
5. Admit patient to monitored setting.

Test Performance (Todd Gaston)

1. *Data acquisition:* This phase is limited, as the key history is not obtained until late in the patient's evaluation. Score = **5**
2. *Problem solving:* Problem solving is good. Even though initially incorrect, the candidate proceeds aggressively for a diagnosis and regroups well to get the proper diagnosis before the case finishes. Score = **6**
3. *Patient management:* Limited by a poor history, early tests and interventions do not help with the headache. However, once a better history is taken, the candidate makes appropriate interventions and stabilizes the patient. Score = **6**
4. *Resource utilization:* After the proper diagnosis is made, the candidate demonstrates appropriate utilization of 100% oxygen and the hyperbaric chamber. He also shows resourcefulness in speaking with the patient's neighbor. However, the computed tomography (CT) and lumbar puncture (LP) were unnecessarily performed. Score = **5**
5. *Health care provided (outcome):* The patient received delayed, but appropriate, treatment, and the candidate's interventions stabilized the patient. Score = **7**
6. *Interpersonal relations and communication skills:* Even though the candidate pursues the wrong diagnosis for much of the case, the patient is kept at ease with frequent updates and discussions of care. Score = **7**
7. *Comprehension of Pathophysiology:* The examinee conveyed their understanding of CO poisoning and management with appropriate interventions and by their conversation with consultant. Score = **7**
8. *Clinical Competence (Overall):* The examinee showed clinical competence once a more thorough history was obtained. He made appropriate interventions, and admitted the patient to the appropriate service. Score = **6**

CASE ASSESSMENT (ROD LEVER)

Usually, each "triple case" will have one simple patient encounter that isn't testing your breadth of knowledge but your ability to manage multiple patients simultaneously and efficiently. The approach used with this child was straightforward and the candidate did a splendid job of working up the patient. Treatment was administered appropriately and discharge (although rare at ABEM General) was the correct course of action after follow-up had been arranged with his pediatrician.

Critical Actions (Rod Lever)

1. Albuterol/Atrovent nebulizer treatment.
2. Discharge with an metered-dose inhaler (MDI) and steroids.
3. Arrange follow-up.

Test Performance (Rod Lever)

1. *Data acquisition:* This phase is performed well as the candidate shows ability to obtain a thorough history and physical examination in an efficient manner. Even though there is a history of medications running out, the candidate is still careful to check for infectious processes that could exacerbate the asthma. Score = **8**
2. *Problem solving:* Problem solving is excellent, as the candidate is able to quickly assimilate data from the patient encounter and efficiently direct further management. Score = **8**
3. *Patient management:* The examinee recognized asthma exacerbation related to lack of medication and provided appropriate treatment. This stabilized the patient. Score = **8**
4. *Resource utilization:* The candidate used an appropriate breathing treatment, obtained history from the parent, and arranged follow-up with the pediatrician. Score = **8**
5. *Health care provided (outcome):* The patient received efficient, appropriate treatment, and the candidate's interventions stabilized the patient. Score = **8**
6. *Interpersonal relations and communication skills:* The candidate was able to engage in effective information exchange with both the patient's father and professional associates. Score = **8**
7. *Comprehension of pathophysiology:* The examinee conveyed understanding of asthma exacerbation and common causes by making a rapid diagnosis, providing appropriate treatment, and in conversation with patient's pediatrician. Score = **8**
8. *Clinical competence (overall):* Overall, the candidate did a superb job and would not have lost any points on this encounter. Score = **8**

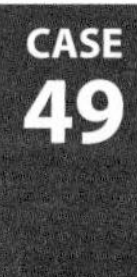

CASE 49 Situation Encounter: A 10 y/o Male Struck by a Car, a 22 y/o Male With Hemophilia and a Hand Laceration, and a 36 y/o Female With Acute Abdominal Pain

John Dayton, Phillip Shayne, and Daniel Wu

INITIAL INFORMATION

Name: Billy Jones

Mode of arrival: EMS

Age: 10 years

Gender: Male

VS: T 37.0°C (98.6°F), BP 110/65, HR 95, RR 16

CC: Struck by a car

PLAY OF THE CASE (BILLY JONES)

C: "What do I see as I walk into the patient's room?"

E: "The patient is a young boy lying on the stretcher, boarded with a cervical collar, and appearing scared. The boy's mother is by his side"

C: "Is EMS present?"

E: "Yes."

C: "Please ask them to stay until I can talk with them."

C: "Nurse, please place the patient on a cardiac monitor, obtain IV access, draw blood for labs including a type and screen, and place the patient on 2-L oxygen via NC after getting a room air oxygen saturation level."

E: "Those orders are being completed. The oxygen saturation is 100% on room air."

C: "Hello Mrs. Jones, hello Billy, my name is Dr. Cule. What happened today?"

E: "The mother responds: We were walking across the street and a car turned the corner and didn't see us and ran right into us. I tried to get Billy out of the way, but he got hit and knocked over."

C: "Where did Billy get hit?"

E: "The car struck the right side of his body."

C: "Was he able to get up and walk?"

E: "No."

C: "Did he lose consciousness?"

E: "Yes, it seemed like forever, maybe 2-3 minutes."

C: "I would like to ask EMS for any additional information."

E: "EMS: The boy was conscious and lying on the ground when we arrived. He was complaining of leg pain. Bystanders said he was hit on the side and then hit his head on the ground and passed out for about 2 minutes."

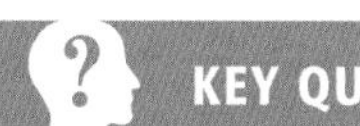

KEY QUESTION

Ask this open-ended question at the beginning of every case.

KEY ORDERS

Remember to use all available resources to get a history about patients with any altered mental status. Talk with family, caregivers, and EMS.

KEY ORDERS

Most of the patients you see during the exam are unstable (or will become that way). Every unstable patient requires IV access, oxygen, and cardiac monitoring.

C: "Thanks. Billy, are you hurting anywhere?"

E: "My leg hurts."

C: "Point to where it hurts."

E: "He points to the right thigh."

C: "Are you in pain anywhere else?"

E: "No."

C: "Mrs. Jones, does Billy have any medical problems?"

E: "No."

C: "Does he take any medications?"

E: "No."

C: "Any allergies to medications?"

E: "No."

C: "I would like to examine the patient. Has there been a change in his appearance or vital signs?"

E: "No."

C: "What is his Glasgow Coma Score?"

E: "15."

C: "Primary survey appears to be intact from my initial assessment. I would like to start with the HEENT examination focusing on lacerations, abrasions, and pupils."

E: "Normocephalic with a 3-cm abrasion over his right eyebrow. There is no active bleeding. The pupils are mid-range, equal, and reactive to light."

C: "Keeping in-line C-spine control, I would like to palpate the C-spine. Is the neck tender to palpation?"

E: "No."

C: "Please maintain the spinal immobilization. Is the chest tender?"

E: "No."

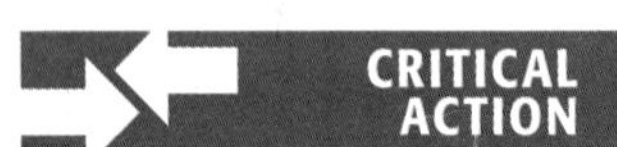

Doing a complete neurovascular examination on the injured extremity is a critical action in this case.

C: "Cardiac examination?"

E: "S_1, S_2, no murmurs, rubs, or gallops."

C: "Lungs?"

E: "Clear to auscultation bilaterally with good air movement."

C: "Abdominal examination?"

E: "Soft, non-tender, non-distended."

C: "Neuro and extremity examination, specifically focusing on his right leg where he says he is having pain?"

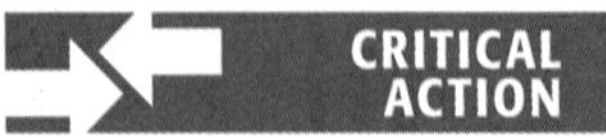

Taking C-spine precautions and getting appropriate imaging to rule out head and C-spine injury is a critical action in this case.

E: "The patient is answering questions appropriately and is alert and oriented. His strength and sensation are intact in the upper extremities and his left leg. He refuses to move his right leg and on visualization there is a hematoma over his upper thigh and it is extremely tender to palpation."

C: "Can he bend his knee or ankle?"

E: "He refuses to bend his knee because of the pain, but can bend his ankle and toes."

C: "I would like to do an extensive neurovascular examination distal to the injury including capillary refill, pulses, and sensation."

E: "There is no tenderness over his lower extremity, foot, or ankle. The DP and PT pulses are intact as well as sensation and capillary refill."

C: "I would like to roll the patient, supporting his right leg and palpate his T/L/S spine and perform a rectal examination."

E: "There is no spinal tenderness and the rectal examination is negative."

C: "We can remove the board, but maintain the cervical collar. I would like to send the labs and send the patient for a CT of his head and C-spine, and x-rays of his chest, pelvis, and right femur and knee."

E: "The patient is receiving the x-rays. Dr. Cule, there is another patient in room 2."

C: "Nurse, please inform me when any test results of Billy's return."

KEY ORDERS

Remember to ask for the nurse to give you test results as they come back. This will make the examiner give you results instead of you having to remember to ask for them.

INITIAL INFORMATION

Name: John Smith

Mode of arrival: Ambulatory

Age: 22 years

Gender: Male

VS: T 37.4°C (99.32°F), BP 135/85, HR 105, RR 18

CC: Hand laceration

PLAY OF THE CASE (JOHN SMITH)

C: "What do I see as I walk into the patient's room?"

E: "The patient is a young man sitting on the stretcher with a bandage on his left hand."

C: "Mr. Smith, my name is Dr. Cule. What can I help you with today?"

E: "I cut my hand."

C: "What happened?"

E: "I was making dinner and I cut my hand while preparing the food."

C: "Any other injuries?"

E: "No."

C: "When did this occur?"

E: "Around 3 hours ago."

C: "Have you lost a lot of blood?"

E: "The blood keeps soaking through the bandages I put on, I've had to change the dressing several times."

C: "Do you have any medical problems?"

E: "Hemophilia and asthma."

C: "What type of hemophilia?"

E: "Hemophilia A."

C: "Have you had bleeding problems in the past?"

KEY ORDERS

Ask this open-ended question at the beginning of every case.

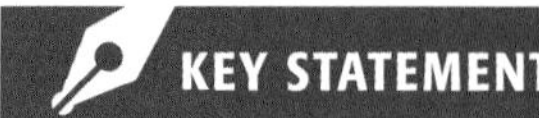

KEY STATEMENT

Remember to introduce yourself by name to the patient and family. Don't lose easy points for professionalism by forgetting to do simple things such as this.

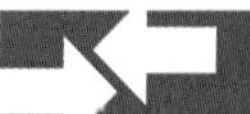

CRITICAL ACTION

Getting the appropriate history of hemophilia is a critical action in this case.

E: "Yes."

C: "Have you ever had to have a transfusion before?"

E: "No."

C: "Do you take any medications?"

E: "Albuterol."

C: "Do you have any allergies to medications?"

E: "No."

C: "Is you tetanus vaccination up-to-date?"

E: "I don't know."

C: "Nurse, please place a large-bore IV, place the patient on a monitor, and draw blood to be sent for labs."

CRITICAL ACTION

Doing a thorough neurovascular examination of the affected extremity is a critical action in this case.

C: "I would like to examine the patient, starting with the HEENT examination with focus on possible signs of active bleeding including epistaxis. And is there pallor?"

E: "No signs of active bleeding in the head and neck area, but there is pallor present."

C: "Cardiovascular examination?"

E: "S_1, S_2, regular rate and rhythm."

C: "Lung examination?"

CRITICAL ACTION

Giving this patient tetanus prophylaxis is a critical action in this case.

E: "Clear to auscultation bilaterally, good air movement."

C: "Abdominal examination?"

E: "Normal."

C: "Extremities?"

E: "There is a 4-cm laceration on the dorsal aspect on his mid-left hand, the other extremities are normal."

C: "Neurovascular examination distal to the injury? Is there active bleeding?"

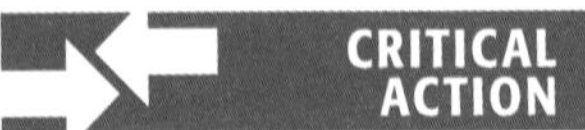

CRITICAL ACTION

Sending the appropriate labs including CBC, T & S, coags, and most importantly a factor VIII level is a critical action in this case.

E: "There is good capillary refill, full range of motion, and normal strength of his fingers. The radial pulse is strong and palpable. The wound is still oozing a moderate amount of blood, and the wound appears to be of moderate depth, but no bone is visualized."

C: "When I examine the wound does there appear to be any tendon damage?"

E: "No."

C: "I would like to ask the nurse to administer a tetanus booster and I would like to irrigate the wound, place a pressure dressing on the wound, and setup for laceration repair."

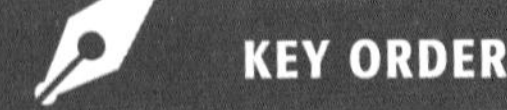

KEY ORDERS

Remember to ask for the nurse to give you test results as they come back. This will make the examiner give you results instead of you having to remember to ask for them.

E: "The pressure dressing has been applied. The nurse comes into the room to inform you that the results of Billy Jones' CT head and C-spine are negative and Billy is receiving his x-rays."

C: "Thank you. For John Smith, please place an IV and start 0.9 NS with a 1 L bolus of NS, then continue at 150 cc/h. Please send a type and screen, CBC, chemistry, coags, and a factor VIII level. Please inform me when the results are back."

E: "The labs have been sent. There is another patient who needs to be seen."

INITIAL INFORMATION

Name: Jane Doelful

Mode of arrival: EMS

Age: 36 years

Gender: Female

VS: T 37.7°C (99.32°F), BP 155/90, HR 110, RR 18

CC: Abdominal pain

KEY QUESTION

Ask this open-ended question at the beginning of every case.

PLAY OF THE CASE (JANE DOELFUL)

C: "What do I see as I walk into the patient's room?"

E: "The patient is a young woman lying on the stretcher in obvious discomfort."

C: "Nurse, please place a large-bore IV, place the patient on a monitor and 2 L of oxygen by NC, and draw blood to be sent for labs including a type and screen."

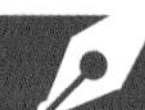

KEY ORDERS

Most of the patients you see during the exam are unstable (or will become that way). Every unstable patient requires IV access, oxygen, and cardiac monitoring.

C: "Ms. Doelful, my name is Dr. Cule. What can I help you with today?"

E: "My stomach is hurting."

C: "How long have you been having pain?"

E: "It started last night, but it got a lot worse this morning and is now unbearable."

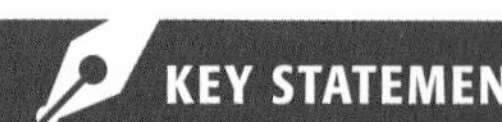

KEY STATEMENT

Remember to introduce yourself by name to the patient and family. Don't lose easy points for professionalism by forgetting to do simple things such as this.

C: "Where does it hurt, can you point to where the pain is?"

E: "It started around my belly button, but now it hurts everywhere."

C: "Are you vomiting?"

E: "Yes, and I am nauseated."

C: "Are you having any bowel movements?"

E: "Yesterday was the last time."

C: "Are you still eating?"

E: "I haven't eaten anything today."

C: "Are you having any fevers?"

E: "No."

C: "Do you have any medical problems?"

E: "Diabetes and ulcers."

C: "Do you take any medications?"

E: "Metformin, Lipitor, and Pepcid."

C: "Any allergies to medications?"

E: "No."

C: "Do you smoke tobacco, drink alcohol or take drugs?"

E: "I smoke just a few cigarettes a day and drink two beers a day. I don't do any drugs."

Getting an orthopedic surgery consult is a critical action in this case.

C: "On a scale of 1-10, with 10 representing the worst pain you have ever experienced, what number would you rate your pain now?"

E: "10."

E: "The nurse informs you that Billy Jones is back from the radiology department and that the radiologist wants you to know that the child's head CT, C-spine, chest, pelvis, and knee are fine but he does have a right femur fracture that is moderately angulated and displaced."

C: "Thank you, please recheck the distal pulses of Billy Jones and call the orthopedic surgeon on call."

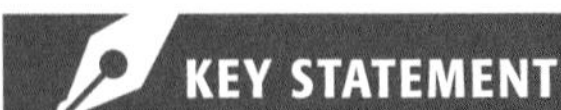

Note that the candidate explains their differential as they are giving their orders. This is a good strategy. The more the examiner knows about your thought process, the easier it will be for them to follow the strategy for the tests you are ordering.

C: "I would like to start my examination of Ms. Doelful, starting with the HEENT examination."

E: "What would you like to know?"

C: "Is there icterus, pallor, or evidence of recent bleeding? Are the pupils equal, round, and reactive to light? Are the membranes dry?"

E: "No evidence of bleeding or icterus, though the patient has pallor and is dry."

C: "Cardiovascular examination?"

E: "S_1, S_2, regular rate and rhythm."

C: "Lung examination?"

E: "Clear to auscultation bilaterally, good air movement."

C: "Abdominal examination?"

E: "What are you looking for?"

Identifying that this is a potential surgical abdomen is a critical action in this case.

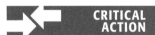

C: "Location of tenderness, distention, rebound, or guarding?"

E: "There is generalized tenderness throughout her entire abdomen. It is mildly distended and there is voluntary and involuntary guarding."

C: "Bowel sounds?"

E: "Markedly diminished."

C: "Rectal examination?"

E: "There is good tone, and guaiac of the stool is weakly positive."

Treating this patient's pain is a critical action in this case.

C: "Nurse, please administer 6 mg of morphine sulfate and 4 mg of Zofran. I am concerned that the patient may have an acute abdomen and cannot rule out appendicitis versus perforated viscus. Please perform a fingerstick glucose and a fingerstick hemoglobin and let me know the results ASAP. Also, send a CBC, BMP, lipase, PT/INR, LFTs, and type and cross the patient for 4 U of blood. I am going to send the patient for a CT scan of the abdomen with IV and oral contrast."

E: "The patient is being sent to the CT scanner."

E: "Dr. Bones from orthopedic surgery is on the line."

C: "Thank you, Dr. Bones. This is Dr. Cule from the ED. I have a 10-year-old boy, Billy Jones, who was involved in a low-speed pedestrian versus auto MVC. He has a moderately angulated and displaced femur fracture, but is neurovascularly intact."

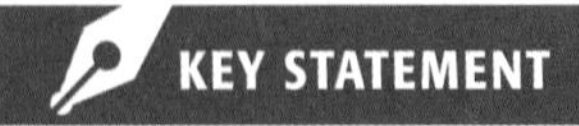

Remember to inform the family and patient about the plan and tell them about test results.

E: "Are there any other injuries?"

C: "Clinically, he has a minor concussion with a brief LOC but a normal examination and a normal CT head scan. Films of his neck, and x-rays of the chest and pelvis were all negative."

E: "Great, you can admit him to me? I will come examine him in the ER."

C: "Thanks. I would like to talk to Billy and his mother. Billy, all of your tests are back and it looks like you broke your leg. The good news is that it could have been much worse and you are very lucky."

E: "Mrs. Jones: What is going to happen now?"

C: "I have spoken with the bone specialist who is going to take care of Billy in the hospital. He said he will come down shortly to see him. Billy, are you still in pain?"

E: "Yes."

C: "We will make sure that you get pain medication to make your leg feel much better; do you have any other questions?"

E: "Mrs. Jones: No, Thank you."

C: "Nurse, please give the patient 2 mg of morphine via IV."

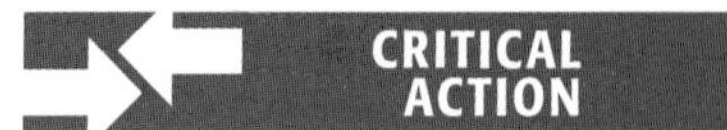

Treating this patient's pain is a critical action in this case.

E: "John Smith's laceration has been irrigated and a pressure dressing applied. Here are his labs: Hgb 10.3, WBC 9.0, unremarkable chemistry panel. Coagulation profile reveals a PT of 11.0, INR 1.5, and PTT 38.5. The factor VIII level is 18%."

C: "I will go see him now, is Ms. Doelful back from radiology yet?"

E: "Yes."

C: "Please repeat her vital signs and let me know if they change."

C: "I would like to examine Mr. Smith's laceration. When I look at the wound what do I see?"

E: "The wound appears clean but it is still oozing blood."

C: "Is there any arterial bleeding?"

E: "No."

C: "I would like to repair the wound now and then apply a pressure dressing. I would also like to administer Factor VIII. Do we have any?"

E: "No, the pharmacy says they don't have any and can't get any Factor VIII until tomorrow."

C: "In that case, please administer 5 U of FFP. I will repair the wound now with simple sutures after local lidocaine and sterile prep. Has the bleeding stopped?"

E: "Despite wound closure and a pressure dressing, the wound is still actively oozing blood."

C: "Mr. Smith, though we have closed your wound, you are still bleeding and your factor VIII level is low. I think it would be best to admit you so we can give you a transfusion and make sure the bleeding stops. Do you have a doctor who treats your hemophilia?"

E: "Yes, Dr. Blood"

C: "I would like to call Dr. Blood and please transfuse the patient when the FFP arrives."

E: "Dr. Blood is on the phone."

C: "Dr. Blood, this is Dr. Cule. I have a patient of yours in the ER. His name is John Smith. He cut his hand and is actively bleeding despite suture repair."

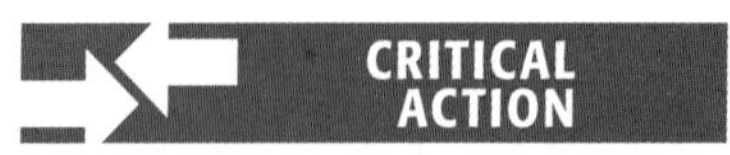

Admitting this patient for further care is a critical action in this case.

KEY ORDERS

Always begin by treating any vital sign abnormality. This means giving fluids to people who are hypotensive, giving oxygen to people who are hypoxic, and giving antipyretics to people who are febrile.

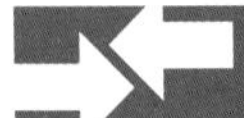

CRITICAL ACTION

Administering fluids is a critical action in this case.

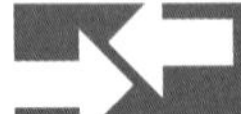

CRITICAL ACTION

Giving antibiotics and admitting the patient to surgery are both critical actions in this case.

E: "Does he need a factor VIII transfusion?"

C: "Well, his hemoglobin is a little low, but the bleeding is not brisk. I think he would benefit from a transfusion to help stop the bleeding. We do not have any Factor VIII available, so I am going to transfuse him with FFP. I'd like to admit him for transfusion and observation, to make sure the bleeding stops."

E: "That's fine. Admit him to me and I will see him on the floor."

C: "Thanks."

E: "I have repeated Ms. Doelful's vital signs. Her BP is 90/60, HR 115. In addition, her labs are back: her WBC is 15.1 with an Hgb of 11. The rest of her labs are normal."

C: "Is she febrile?"

E: "Her temperature is 38.7°C."

C: "Please administer a 1 L bolus of NS. In addition, please place her on 4L of oxygen via NC and administer 1 g of Tylenol."

E: "The radiologist is on the phone."

C: "This is Dr. Cule."

E: "Dr. Cule, this is Dr. Gamma from radiology. I am reading the CT for Mrs. Doelful. She has a perforated duodenal ulcer with a moderate amount of fluid in her abdominal cavity."

C: "Thanks."

C: "I would like reexamine the patient after the IV fluid bolus, what are her vital signs?"

E: "Her BP has increased to 110/75 with a HR of 95."

C: "She appears to be responding to the fluid resuscitation, please administer a dose of Zosyn and Flagyl and call the surgeon on call."

E: "Dr. Cutter is on the phone."

C: "Dr. Cutter, this is Dr. Cule. I have a young woman in the ER who has a perforated ulcer diagnosed by CT scan. She became hypotensive and tachycardic, but has responded to fluids."

E: "Has she received antibiotics yet?"

C: "Yes."

E: "Good, continue the fluids and send her up to the OR. I will call the OR team now."

E: "This ends the case."

CASE ASSESSMENT (BILLY JONES)

The candidate correctly identified the major injury (femur fracture) in this trauma case while appropriately investigating all other possible injuries. He follows his advanced trauma life support (ATLS) protocol appropriately and identified that the child sustained a minor concussion. The candidate maintained a good rapport with the patient and his mother and used other available resources, such as emergency medical services (EMS), to obtain a complete history of the events surrounding the injury. The candidate demonstrated a good knowledge of trauma assessment and evaluation and investigated other potential injuries to the patient. The candidate could have improved by addressing the patient's pain earlier. The candidate did not fully investigate and administer pain medications until the patient was dispositioned.

Critical Actions (Billy Jones)

1. Proper evaluation of possible head and cervical spine injuries.
2. Complete neurovascular examination of injured extremity.
3. Orthopedic surgery evaluation and disposition.
4. Administer pain medication as needed.

Test Performance (Billy Jones)

1. *Data acquisition:* The candidate clearly understood what information needed to be obtained and was also able to acquire it in an efficient manner. Score = **8**
2. *Problem solving:* The candidate demonstrated excellent problem solving skills by asking about the mechanism of injury and evaluating injuries in a complete and logical approach. Score = **8**
3. *Patient management:* The candidate followed ATLS protocols, and approached the management in a logical and thorough manner. While the candidate delivered the standard of care, he could have been more aggressive in administering pain medication and reassessing the comfort of the patient. Score = **6**
4. *Resource utilization:* The candidate used appropriate systems-based practice in the management of this case. The workup showed very good use of resources with respect to efficiency and cost-effectiveness. Score = **8**
5. *Health care provided (outcome):* The patient care given in this case was very good. All critical actions were taken and the patient was admitted to the appropriate service. Score = **8**
6. *Interpersonal relations and communication skills:* The interpersonal skills demonstrated by the candidate in this case were good. He interacted well with both the patient and the nursing staff and kept the patient and family informed about test results. He should have been more attentive to Billy's pain. Score = **7**
7. *Comprehension of pathophysiology:* The examinee conveyed their understanding of ATLS, femur fractures and concussion by ordering only appropriate studies and by their communication with the orthopedist. Score = **8**
8. *Clinical competence (overall):* Overall, the examinee showed clinical competence by obtaining an appropriate history and physical, identifying injuries, using appropriate lab work and imaging, and admitting the patient for orthopedic surgery. As noted earlier, the candidate could have done a better job addressing Billy's pain. Score = **7**

CASE ASSESSMENT (JOHN SMITH)

The candidate did a very good job of managing this portion of the case. Again the candidate was able to correctly identify the major injury (underlying bleeding disorder in the face of trauma). The candidate was able to obtain a focused and pertinent history and physical after quickly identifying the major problem. The candidate properly interpreted the lab results and the further risk of bleeding due to a low factor VIII level.

Factor VIII is the treatment of choice for acute or potential hemorrhage in a patient with hemophilia A, and treatment is titrated to the percent activity of factor VIII. The factor VIII activity level should be corrected to 100% of normal for potentially serious hemorrhage (central nervous system [CNS], trauma, gastrointestinal [GI] bleeding, severe epistaxis, etc) and to 30%-50% of normal for minor hemorrhage (hemarthrosis, oral mucosal, intramuscular bleeding). Minor hemorrhage requires one or three doses of factor VIII. Major hemorrhage requires multiple doses and continued factor VIII activity monitoring. Continuous infusions of factor VIII should be considered for major hemorrhage. If there is no factor VIII available, fresh frozen plasma (FFP) contains factor VIII and can be used as well until factor VIII is available. Cryoprecipitate, prothrombin complex concentrates, and DDAVP would also have been acceptable adjunct treatments.

The candidate manifested a strong knowledge of treatment modalities for hemophilia by administering FFP in the setting of an active bleed when factor VIII was not available. Although the laceration was not life-threatening, his hemoglobin (Hgb) was borderline low and hemostasis was not able to be achieved by a pressure dressing and repair, so the patient was appropriately admitted for blood product transfusion and observation.

Critical Actions

1. Identify history of hemophilia A.
2. Complete neurovascular examination of injured extremity.
3. Obtain tetanus history and administer booster.
4. Obtain appropriate labs (Hgb/Hct, coags, factor VIII level). Administer appropriate treatment in setting of active bleeding (factor VIII, FFP, cryoprecipitate, prothrombin complex concentrates, or DDAVP).
5. Admit patient for further treatment.

Test Performance

1. *Data acquisition:* The candidate clearly understood what information needed to be obtained and was also able to acquire the needed information in an efficient manner. Score = **8**
2. *Problem solving:* The candidate demonstrated excellent problem-solving skills by investigating labs for bleeding and hemophilia and used FFP when factor VIII was unavailable. Score = **8**
3. *Patient management:* The candidate recognized when interventions needed to be made and obtained appropriate consults to create a safe disposition. Mr. Smith was safe while the candidate attended to the other patients. Score = **8**
4. *Resource utilization:* The candidate used appropriate systems-based practice in the management of this case. The workup showed very good use of resources with respect to efficiency and cost-effectiveness. The candidate allowed labs to run for Mr. Smith while he treated other patients. Score = **8**
5. *Health care provided (outcome):* The patient received efficient, appropriate treatment, the candidate's interventions stabilized the patient, and he was appropriate admitted for further evaluation. Score = **8**
6. *Interpersonal relations and communication skills:* The interpersonal skills demonstrated by the candidate in this case were good. He asked about

hemophilia, discussed management concerns with the patient, and had a professional conversation with the consultant. Score = **8**

7. *Comprehension of pathophysiology:* The examinee conveyed their understanding of hemophilia by ordering only appropriate tests, using a compression dressing, and requesting factor replacement. Score = **8**
8. *Clinical competence (overall):* Overall, the examinee showed excellent clinical competence by obtaining an appropriate history and physical, developing a differential diagnosis, utilizing appropriate lab work and imaging, utilizing appropriate interventions, and working toward a safe and appropriate disposition. Score = **8**

CASE ASSESSMENT (JANE DOELFUL)

The candidate did a good job of managing this patient. He promptly identified this patient as the sickest of the three patients and was appropriately aggressive in his management. The candidate identified a potentially acute surgical abdomen from the history of ulcers, low blood pressure, and abdominal pain. He confirmed the diagnosis of a perforated peptic ulcer by computed tomography (CT) scan.

This diagnosis may have been confirmed with a bedside focused assessment with sonography for trauma (FAST) showing free fluid or an upright chest x-ray (CXR) showing free air, but the patient was stable enough for CT scanning. If the patient exhibits signs of instability that are not responsive to IV fluids, then the candidate should not allow that patient to go to the department of radiology as deterioration is certain, especially at ABEM General hospital. In this circumstance, portable plain abdominal films to include an upright CXR (or lateral decubitus of the abdomen) to detect free air should be done.

The candidate demonstrated the appropriate level of concern and was aggressive in reevaluating the patient. The candidate also instituted the appropriate therapy of fluid resuscitation in the setting of hypotension, and he anticipated the development of sepsis with hypoperfusion (shock) when the patient returned from radiology.

Critical Actions

1. Identify surgical abdomen.
2. Administer pain medications.
3. Initiate appropriate fluid resuscitation.
4. Administer antibiotics.
5. Admit to surgery.

Test Performance

1. *Data acquisition:* The candidate clearly understood what information needed to be obtained and was also able to acquire the needed information in an efficient manner. Score = **8**
2. *Problem solving:* The candidate diagnostic approach was systematic, organized, and appropriate. Score = **8**
3. *Patient management:* The candidate gave appropriate treatment, managed hypotension and addressed that with fluids and blood products, recognized bowel perforation, and called the appropriate consultant. Score = **8**

4. *Resource utilization:* The candidate used appropriate systems-based practice in the management of this case. The workup showed very good use of resources, but the candidate could have used an upright CXR to find the diagnosis more quickly. Score = **6**
5. *Health care provided (outcome):* The patient provided efficient and appropriate treatment and the candidate's interventions stabilized the patient. Score = **8**
6. *Interpersonal relations and communication skills:* The interpersonal skills demonstrated by the candidate in this case could have been improved. He did not request permission to do a rectal examination, tell the patient about her test results, or inform her that she was going to surgery. Score = **5**
7. *Comprehension of pathophysiology:* The examinee understood complications of peptic ulcer disease (PUD), anticipated imaging findings and risk for shock, and addressed these concerns. Score = **8**
8. *Clinical competence (overall):* Overall, the candidate did a great job, but could have done better communicating with the patient and used more rapid imaging studies. Score = **7**

CASE 50 Situation Encounter: A 2 y/o Febrile Child, an 85 y/o Male With Eye Pain, and a 48 y/o Male With CP

John Dayton, Reb Close, and Fred Abrahamian

INITIAL INFORMATION

Name: Jenny Yellow

Mode of arrival: Brought in by mom and dad

Age: 2 years

Gender: Female

VS: T 39.5°C (103.1°F) rectally, BP 90/50, HR 120, RR 27, O_2 sat: 99% on RA

CC: Fever

PLAY OF THE CASE (JENNY YELLOW)

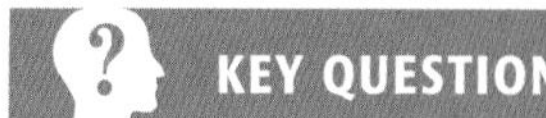

Ask this open-ended question at the beginning of every case.

C: "When I walk into the room, what do I see?"

E: "A 2-year-old female sitting quietly on dad's lap. She is in no apparent distress."

C: "Hi everyone, I am Dr. Emergency, what brings Jenny into the ED today?"

E: "She has a bad fever that has been going on for 2 days now."

C: "How high has the fever been?"

E: "Up to 40°C (104°F)."

C: "Does she have any other symptoms or complaints of any pain?"

E: "Like what?"

C: "Does she complain of ear pain, congestion, or runny nose?"

E: "No."

C: "Coughing?"

E: "A little bit."

C: "Vomiting or diarrhea?"

E: "She threw up part of her dinner last night and hasn't pooped in a few days."

C: "Any rashes or skin changes?"

E: "Not that we have noticed."

C: "Any change in her appetite or activities?"

E: "She hasn't wanted to eat much, when her fever is better she is more playful but she just watched TV all day yesterday."

C: "How many wet diapers today?"

E: "Three, last one just in the waiting room."

C: "Is anyone else at home sick?"

E: "Her little sister has a cold."

C: "Does she have any medical problems, any problems with her birth or previous hospitalizations?"

E: "She was hospitalized with pneumonia when she was 6 months old but has done really well ever since. She used a nebulizer for a few months, but not recently."

C: "Are her immunizations up-to-date?"

E: "Yes."

C: "Is she on any medicines right now?"

E: "I gave her Tylenol about 1 hour ago."

C: "Any allergies to medicines?"

E: "She gets a rash when she takes amoxicillin."

C: "I need to examine her. Can you hold her to keep her comfortable? HEENT examination?"

E: "Eye examination is normal, ear examination is limited as the canals are obstructed with cerumen, nose and throat examination are normal, and mucous membranes are moist."

C: "I need to irrigate and clean Jenny's ears to get a better look."

E: "This has been performed. There is mild erythema of the tympanic membranes bilaterally. Landmarks are well visualized."

C: "Neck examination?"

E: "Supple, without lymphadenopathy."

C: "Does the patient appear to be in any distress when I touch her chin to her chest?"

E: "No."

C: "Chest examination?"

E: "Lungs are clear to auscultation: no wheezing, crackles, or rales."

C: "Heart examination?"

E: "Tachycardic and regular with no murmurs, rubs, or gallops."

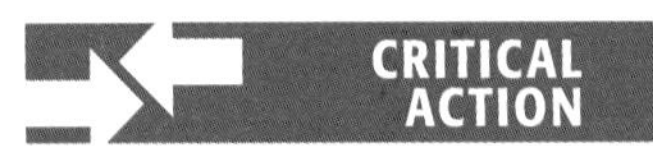

Treating the patient's fever is a critical action in this case.

C: "I need to fully undress Jenny and examine her on the hospital bed."

C: "Abdominal examination?"

E: "Soft, non-tender, no masses, no rebound, no guarding."

C: "GU examination?"

E: "Normal female anatomy. No erythema or rashes."

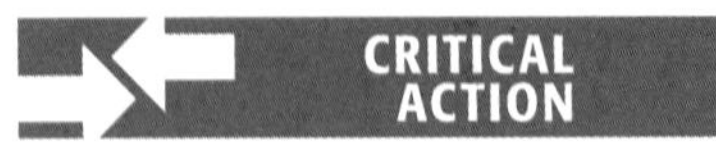

Getting labs (including blood and urine cultures) and a CXR is a critical action in this case.

C: "Skin examination?"

E: "Warm, dry, no rashes."

C: "How is Jenny interacting with me?"

E: "She cries through part of the examination, but she is easily consoled by her parents. She has age-appropriate behavior, no lethargy, moves all extremities."

C: "I'm not sure where Jenny's fever is coming from, let's check a few tests while we give her some medication to bring down the fever, and then we will discuss what we have found. Nurse, please draw a CBC and blood culture, catheter urine for UA and culture, PA and lateral chest x-ray. Please give Motrin 10 mg/kg orally once."

E: "Those orders are being carried out. Another nurse informs you that you need to see the gentleman in room 2."

INITIAL INFORMATION (JOE BLUE)

Name: Joe Blue

Mode of arrival: Brought in by EMS

Age: 85 years

Gender: Male

VS: T 37°C (98.6°F), BP 150/85, HR 100, RR 20, O_2 sat: 95% on RA

CC: Headache

PLAY OF THE CASE (JOE BLUE)

C: "What do I see as I walk into the patient's room?"

E: "You see an elderly appearing male, lying on his left side on the gurney, holding his head, and moaning in pain."

C: "Mr. Blue, I'm Dr. Emergency, what brings you into the ED today?"

E: "Oh doc, this is killing me. My head is going to explode!"

C: "When did this start Mr. Blue?"

E: "This morning when I went downstairs to work in my wood shop."

C: "Did this start suddenly or gradually?"

E: "Pretty fast and it makes me nauseated. I've thrown up my breakfast. I feel like throwing up again."

C: "Mr. Blue, have you ever had a headache like this before?"

E: "Never doc."

C: "Where is the headache located and what does it feel like?"

E: "Top of my head and behind my right eye. It feels like lots of pressure, like my eye is going to pop out."

C: "Do you feel any paralysis or numbness anywhere in your body?"

E: "No."

C: "Have you had headaches like this before?"

E: "No."

C: "Any fevers or chills?"

E: "No."

C: "Does your stomach hurt you?"

E: "No."

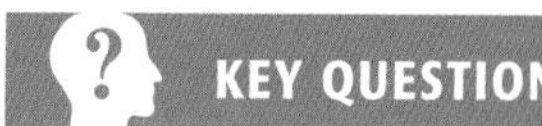

Ask this open-ended question at the beginning of every case.

KEY ORDERS

Most of the patients you see during the exam are unstable (or will become that way). Every unstable patient requires IV access, oxygen, and cardiac monitoring (and in most cases an ECG).

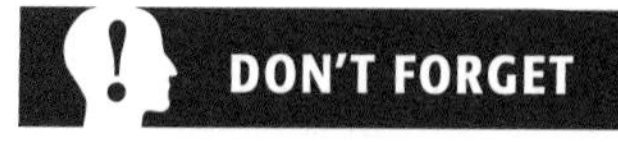

Never administer medication before asking if the patient has any allergies.

C: "Nurse, could you start an 18-gauge catheter in Mr Blue's antecubital fossa, draw and hold blood for labs, administer Reglan 10 mg IV and let me know his response to this."

E: "What type of fluid do you want me running?"

C: "Normal saline TKO until I finish evaluating him. Was his gait normal on arrival? Is he able to sit up now?"

E: "The nurse reports that he arrived ambulatory and the patient is able to sit up."

C: "Is the scalp tender?"

E: "No."

C: "Is there facial symmetry?"

E: "Yes."

C: "Is the neck supple?"

E: "Yes."

C: "Is the abdomen soft and non-tender?"

E: "Yes."

C: "Does the patient move all extremities equally?"

E: "Yes."

E: "The nurse reports that he is no longer vomiting after the Reglan."

C: "Nurse, I need a head CT scan for Mr. Blue."

E: "They can take him now. Do you want me to go with him?"

C: "Yes, take him on the monitor."

E: "As your patient is wheeling toward the CT scanner, another nurse tells you the patient in room 3 has to be seen now."

INITIAL INFORMATION

Name: John Red

Mode of arrival: Brought in by EMS

Age: 48 years

Gender: Male

VS: T 36.5°C (97.7°F), BP 110/50, HR 110, RR 28

CC: Chest pain

KEY QUESTION

Ask this open-ended question at the beginning of every case.

PLAY OF THE CASE (JOHN RED)

C: "When I walk into the room, what do I see? And may I please get room air oxygen saturation?"

E: "Thin male, appears stated age, anxious, diaphoretic, clutching chest with O_2 sat: 90% on RA."

C: "Please place Mr. Red on O_2 by NC, titrate the saturations to >95%, and inform me of his response to this."

E: "O_2 sat is 98% on 6 L via NC, breathing is less labored."

DON'T FORGET

Remember that missing vital signs are usually important. They are called "vital" for a reason!

C: "Mr. Red, I'm Dr. Emergency, what brings you in to the ED today?"

E: "Oh doc, I'm going to die, this hurts so bad."

C: "When did this start?"

E: "About 45 minutes ago."

C: "What were you doing when it started?"

E: "Walking to my car after work."

C: "Where in the chest is the pain?"

E: "Right here." (Patient points to anterior chest, left of sternum.)

C: "Does the pain radiate to any other place?"

E: "Feels tight in my neck."

C: "What kind of pain is it?"

E: "Sharp, piercing."

C: "Has it changed since it started?"

E: "No, it's just getting harder to breathe."

C: "Have you ever had pain like this before?"

E: "No."

C: "Do you have any medical problems?"

E: "High blood pressure, cholesterol, asthma."

C: "What medicines do you take?"

E: "Atenolol, Lipitor, and albuterol when I need it."

C: "Do you have any Allergies to medicines?"

E: "No."

C: "Do you smoke?"

E: "I was finally able to quit a year ago."

C: "Any drug use, specifically cocaine?"

E: "No."

C: "Do people in your family have heart or lung problems?"

E: "Dad died of a heart attack in his seventies, and mom is alive and healthy. Doc, can you give me anything for the pain?"

C: "I need to examine you and check a few tests in order to see what we are treating first. Nurse, could you please start an 18-gauge catheter in an antecubital vein, draw and hold blood for labs. We need the patient on a monitor and I need an ECG. Please show me the rhythm strip and ECG as soon as they are available."

E: "Here are your rhythm strip and ECG (Fig. C50-1)."

C: "HEENT examination?"

E: "PERRLA, EOMI, normal TMs bilaterally, and oropharynx clear."

C: "Neck examination?"

E: "Supple, no JVD, no lymphadenopathy."

C: "Chest examination?"

KEY ORDERS

Remember to reassess your patient after every intervention to make sure you are heading in the right direction.

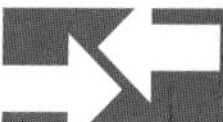
CRITICAL ACTION

Recognizing and treating this patient's hypoxia is a critical action in this case.

KEY ORDERS

Most of the patients you see during the exam are unstable (or will become that way). Every unstable patient requires IV access, oxygen, and cardiac monitoring (and in most cases an ECG).

KEY ORDERS

Remember to ask for test results to be brought to you when they are available.

DON'T FORGET

Treating the patient's pain is not a critical action in this case, but it often is. Remember to treat pain, or explain why you are not doing so.

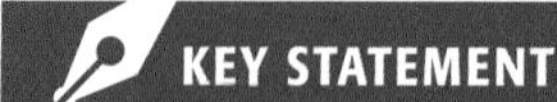
KEY STATEMENT

Remember to keep your patient informed about the diagnosis and plan.

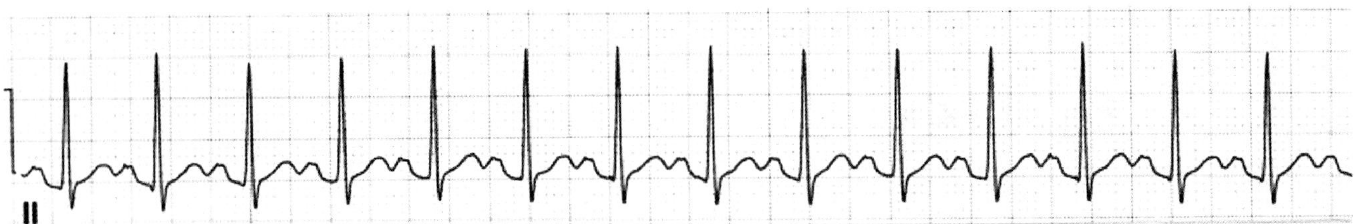

Figure C50-1. Rhythm strip and ECG showing sinus tachycardia at a rate of 125, no acute ST- or T-wave abnormalities. *(Reproduced with permission from Goldschlager N, Goldman MJ.* Principles of Clinical Electrocardiography. *13th ed. Originally published by Appleton & Lange. Copyright © 1989 by The McGraw-Hill Companies, Inc.)*

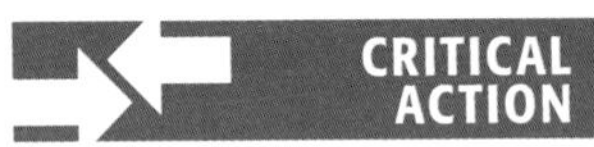

Diagnosis of a pneumothorax is a critical action in this case.

E: "Decreased breath sounds on the left. No crackles, wheezing, or rhonchi."

C: "Heart examination?"

E: "Tachycardic and regular rate at 120 with no murmurs, rubs, or gallops."

C: "Abdominal examination?"

E: "Normal."

C: "Extremity examination?"

E: "No cyanosis, clubbing, or edema."

C: "Skin examination?"

E: "Cool and diaphoretic."

C: "Nurse, I need a portable CXR please."

E: "Here is your x-ray doctor (Fig. C50-2)."

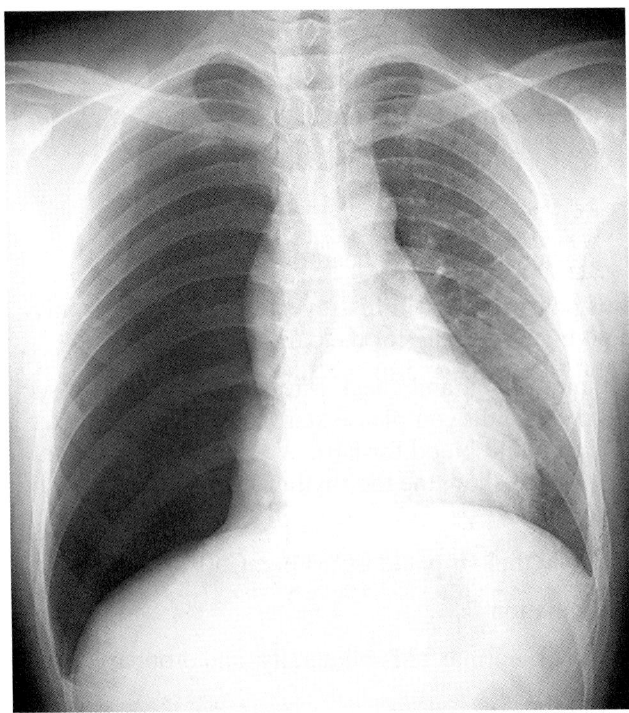

Figure C50-2. Portable CXR with a large pneumothorax on the R side. *(Reproduced with permission from Schwartz DT.* Emergency Radiology: Case Studies. *New York, NY: McGraw-Hill; 2008.)*

C: "Mr. Red, it looks like you have a collapsed lung. We need to re-expand that lung by putting a tube into your chest. I'm going to give you some medicines for the pain and then place the tube. You will need admission to the hospital while the lung re-expands."

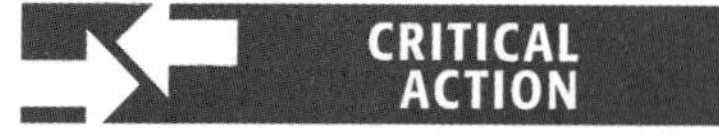

Placing a chest tube is a critical action in this case.

E: "Is this going to hurt?"

C: "I'm going to give you medicine for the pain in the IV, and then I'll numb the area of the chest where the tube will go in. Nurse, could you please administer 4 mg of morphine IV to Mr. Red and set up for chest tube placement?"

E: "That is being done."

E: "The nurse for Jenny Yellow informs you that the lab and x-ray results are back."

- WBC 17,000, Hgb 14, Hct 41, plt 250, segs 80%, bands 5%, lymphs 10%
- Urine with specific gravity 1.012, negative for glucose, protein, bilirubin
- RBC/HPF 0, WBC/HPF 0, bacteria 0
- CXR is negative

C: "When I walk into Jenny's room what do I see?"

E: "She is sitting on the bed, coloring with her dad, nontoxic, no apparent distress. Nurse informs you that the repeat temperature is 37.5°C."

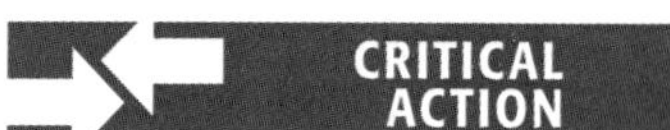

Treating this febrile patient with an elevated white count and a left shift is a critical action in this case.

C: "Mr. and Mrs. Yellow, the lab work shows that Jenny has an infection, but I'm still not sure where it is. Her chest x-ray looks good and I don't see pneumonia. Her urine does not appear infected and I didn't see the source of infection on my examination. We are waiting for the urine and blood cultures to be done to see if any bacteria grow. While we are waiting for those results we need to give her antibiotics. I'm going to give her the first dose here then I will talk with her pediatrician so she can be seen tomorrow for follow-up of the culture results and another dose of antibiotics if necessary."

E: "OK, we will see her doctor tomorrow."

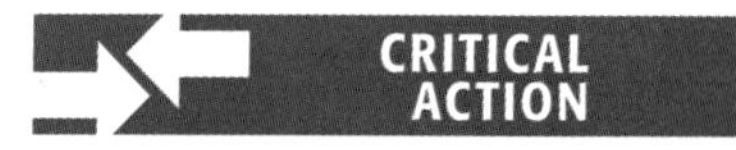

Getting appropriate follow-up for this patient is a critical action in this case.

C: "Nurse, please administer ceftriaxone 50 mg/kg IM. Observe Jenny for any reaction to the medicine as she does have an amoxicillin allergy. I need to speak with her pediatrician."

E: "Dr. Pediatrics is on the phone."

C: "Hi Dr. Pediatrics, this is Dr. Emergency in the ED. I have Jenny Yellow here with a temp of 39.5°C. Her repeat examination is normal, her chest x-ray and urine are also normal. Her WBC count is 17,000 with 80% segs and 5% bands. I've given her 50 mg/kg ceftriaxone and have sent urine and blood for culture. Can you see her tomorrow to follow-up on the cultures and re-dose the antibiotic, if necessary?"

E: "Sure, no problem. I know this family well. Thank you."

C: "Thank you."

E: "Jenny tolerated the antibiotic well, hasn't shown any sign of a reaction. Can she go home now?"

C: "Do her parents have any questions for me?"

E: "No, they said they will call the pediatrician's office for the appointment time."

C: "Then she can go."

CRITICAL ACTION

Measuring intraocular pressure is a critical action in this case.

E: "The case of Jenny Yellow is now over."

E: "The nurse for Mr. Blue informs you that he is back from CT, and that he is in a lot of pain."

C: "Mr. Blue, how are you feeling?"

E: "Awful doc, this headache is killing me."

C: "Do I have my head CT results?"

E: "The radiologist just called over and said the CT results are negative."

C: "What are his vital signs?"

E: "No change."

C: "I'm going to examine the patient in more detail now. HEENT examination?"

E: "What are you looking for?"

C: "Evidence of trauma, tenderness. Eye examination for pupil size, reactivity, funduscopic examination. I will look for any signs of trauma, infection, or tenderness."

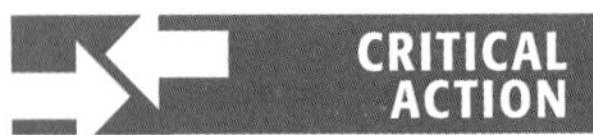

CRITICAL ACTION

Getting an emergent ophthalmologic consult is a critical action in this case.

E: "Normocephalic, atraumatic. No head tenderness. Here is a picture of his right eye (Fig. C50-3)."

E: "The pupil is 8 mm and not reactive to light and you are unable to evaluate the fundus on the right due to diffuse corneal haziness, but the funduscopic examination of left eye is normal. The left pupil is 4 mm and reactive. The remainder of the ENT examination is normal."

C: "What are his visual acuities?"

E: "20/20 corrected on the left, 20/100 corrected on the right."

C: "What are his intraocular pressures?"

E: "Pressure 15 left, 55 right."

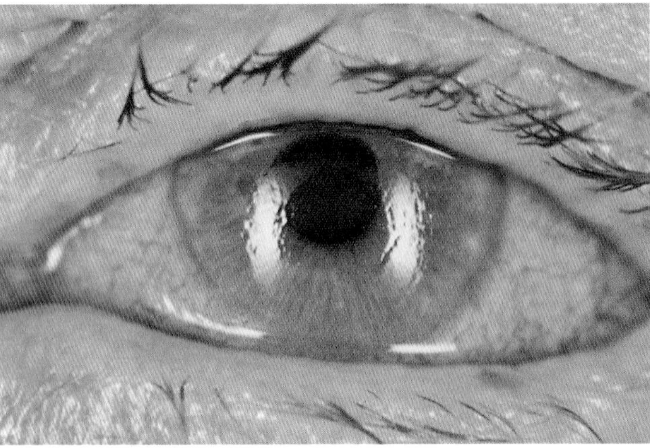

Figure C50-3. An image of acute closed-angle glaucoma showing conjunctival injection, mid-position pupil, hazy cornea. *(Reproduced with permission from Knoop KJ, Stack LB, Storrow AB.* Atlas of Emergency Medicine. *2nd ed. New York: McGraw-Hill; 2002.)*

C: "Mr. Blue, you have acute glaucoma of your eye, we need to start treatment in order to try to save your vision. Nurse, start an IV and give acetazolamide IV. I will also give ophthalmic pilocarpine and timolol drops. I need to speak to the ophthalmologist on-call. While I am waiting for the ophthalmologist to call back I will finish my examination."

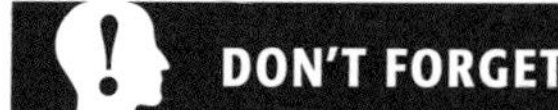

Remember that it is okay to look up medication doses if you do not know them off the top of your head.

C: "Is the neck still supple? JVD?"

E: "Normal."

C: "Are the lungs clear?"

E: "Normal."

C: "Heart examination?"

E: "Normal."

C: "Is the abdominal examination changed? Is he still soft and non-tender?"

E: "Normal."

C: "Extremity and skin examination?"

E: "Normal."

C: "Detailed neuro examination?"

E: "What would you like to know?"

C: "Is he alert and oriented × 4?"

E: "Yes."

C: "EOMI? Have the pupillary responses changed? Are the cranial nerves otherwise intact? Are the sensory, motor, and reflex examination normal? Is the gait steady without ataxia?"

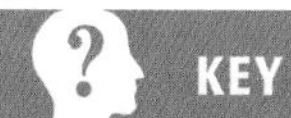

Remember to reassess the patient after every intervention to make sure you are on the right track.

E: "His neurologic examination is normal except for the right pupillary response."

E: "Dr. O is on the phone from ophthalmology."

C: "Hi Dr. O, this is Dr. Emergency from the ED. I have Mr. Blue here who has acute angle closure glaucoma. His pressure in the normal eye is 15 and the affected eye is 55. He also has marked decrease vision in the affected eye. I have given him acetazolamide IV, timolol one drop, and pilocarpine one drop. I need you to please see him in the ED."

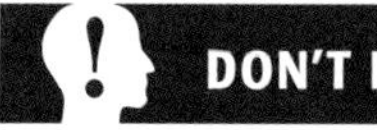

If the examiner does not ask for you to describe a procedure you do not have to.

E: "What time did his symptoms start?"

C: "This morning."

E: "I'm on my way."

C: "Thank you."

E: "The case of Mr. Blue is now over."

E: "The nurse for Mr. Red informs you that the chest tube tray is ready at the bedside. What size tube do you want doctor?"

C: "28 French, please. Hi Mr. Red, let's get this tube put in so you can breathe easier. After obtaining informed consent, I would place a chest tube on left side using standard technique. The tube would be connected to a Pleurovac and wall suction. What is the patient's response to the procedure?"

E: "His breathing is easier, but he is still feeling a lot of pain."

C: "How are his lung sounds?"

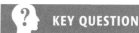

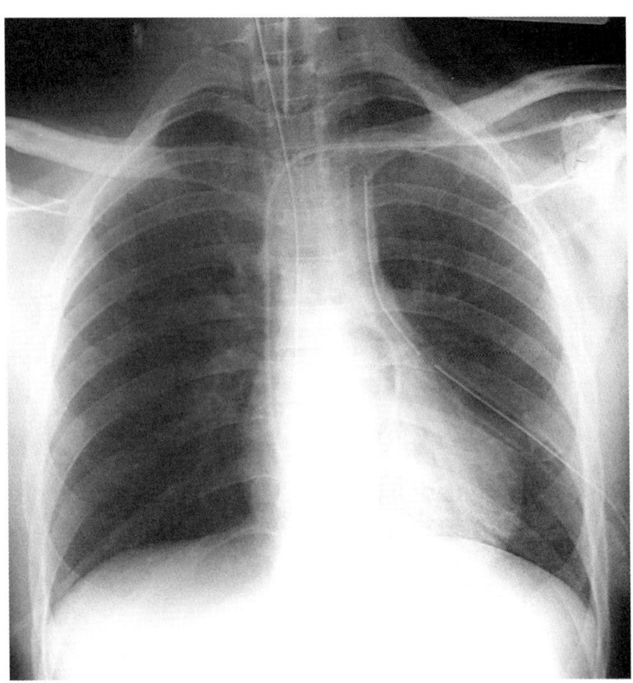

Figure C50-4. CXR showing chest tube in a good position with re-expansion of the lung. *(Reproduced with permission from Schwartz DT.* Emergency Radiology: Case Studies. *New York: McGraw-Hill; 2008.)*

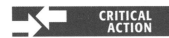

CRITICAL ACTION

Admitting this patient is a critical action.

E: "Symmetrical breath sounds bilaterally."

C: "I need a portable chest x-ray. Please administer another 4 mg of morphine. What is his response to this?"

E: "Much better. Your x-ray is back (Fig. C50-4)."

C: "I need to speak with Mr. Red's physician."

E: "Dr. Medicine is on the phone."

C: "Dr. Medicine, this is Dr. Emergency from the ED. I have Mr. Red here and he presented with a spontaneous pneumothorax on the left. I placed a chest tube with improvement in his breathing and lung sounds. He needs admission to the hospital."

E: "I'll see him on the floor."

E: "The case of Mr. Red is now over."

CASE ASSESSMENT (JENNY YELLOW)

The candidate did a thorough history and physical examination, looking for the source of fever. The tympanic membranes were red bilaterally without bulging and without a loss of landmarks. The candidate was correct in searching for another source of this fever. With the elevated white count, but no obvious source of infection on examination, negative urinalysis and chest x-ray, the candidate may have also chosen to perform a lumbar puncture. However, in this case, the index of suspicion for meningitis was not high since patient was 2 years old, did not appear toxic, had normal mental status, up-to-date vaccinations, and no evidence of meningitis on examination.

It is very important to always remember to reassess the patient's overall status and repeat the vital signs, especially those that were initially abnormal. Throughout the case, the candidate never asked for a complete set of repeated vital signs, but did ask for a repeat temperature, which could have led to many errors in management and misdiagnoses. A complete set of vitals should be asked for and any missing vital sign should be requested. A missing vital sign is often a clue to a worsening condition or diagnosis. Also, it is important to obtain a set of vitals before sending the patient out of the department for radiology, admission, discharge, etc.

The good rapport with the parents and pediatrician made this case conclude smoothly.

Critical Actions (Jenny Yellow)

1. Obtain blood and urine cultures.
2. Administer antipyretic.
3. Administer antibiotic.
4. Arrange follow-up.

Test Performance (Jenny Yellow)

1. *Data acquisition:* The candidate obtained all of the information required to make the appropriate disposition. This was done in an organized fashion. Score = **8**
2. *Problem solving:* The candidate used information to appropriately manage the patient. Though the patient had an elevated WBC, Jenny had no obvious source of infection on examination, and a negative urinalysis and chest x-ray. Performing a lumbar puncture (LP) would have been reasonable, but not required, as the child is so non-toxic and well-appearing. Score = **8**
3. *Patient management:* The examinee recognized when interventions needed to be made and obtained appropriate consults to create a safe disposition. Given no acute concerns, the patient was started on an appropriate antibiotic and follow up appointment with her pediatrician was arranged. However, rechecking vital signs could have aided diagnosis and disposition. Score = **6**
4. *Resource utilization:* The candidate used appropriate lab work, imaging, and obtained cultures to guide therapy. Score = **8**
5. *Health care provided (outcome):* While a firm diagnosis was not found, the candidate made sure that the fever was resolving and that the patient was stable. Jenny was discharged with cultures pending and follow up arranged. Score = **8**
6. *Interpersonal relations and communication skills:* The candidate's interactions with the patient, parents, nurse, and consultant were appropriate. Score = **8**
7. *Comprehension of pathophysiology:* The examinee conveyed understanding of both an infectious workup and appropriate management for fever of unknown origin. This was shown by the history and physical, workup, and conversation with the pediatrician. Score = **8**
8. *Clinical competence (overall):* Overall, the candidate showed clinical competence by obtaining an appropriate history and physical, developing a differential diagnosis, ordering appropriate studies and arranging for safe follow up. They could have done a better job of re-checking vitals after interventions, but they did a good job of reevaluating the patient. Score = **7**

CASE ASSESSMENT (JOE BLUE)

The candidate got distracted when the nurse informed him that computed tomography (CT) was ready for the patient. Had a complete physical examination been performed, the candidate would have made the diagnosis without the CT scan. In a patient with severe, sudden onset headache, a subarachnoid hemorrhage is high on the differential diagnosis and a CT scan of the head is clearly indicated. However, sudden headache associated with changing light environments (such as walking out of a building after work or a movie), is associated with acute angle glaucoma.

This case illustrates the importance of not losing focus. Immediate stabilizing measures for the airway, breathing, and circulation (ABCs) should be performed first, but remember that the majority of information obtained for these cases comes from the history and physical. A focused primary physical examination can be performed very quickly and then the complete secondary examination can be completed when appropriate. During the secondary survey, a full physical examination should always be performed.

The candidate also administered antiemetics prior to obtaining any history of allergy to medication. This is a major mistake and might lead the patient to having an anaphylactic reaction. Remember to always ask about allergies prior to giving any medications.

The candidate asked to look up the doses for acetazolamide, pilocarpine, and timolol. This is totally appropriate. If the examiner makes this task difficult be resourceful by checking a medication references or speaking with pharmacy.

Critical Actions (Joe Blue)

1. Measuring intraocular pressures
2. Diagnosis and treatment of acute angle-closure glaucoma
3. Ophthalmology consultation

Test Performance (Joe Blue)

1. *Data acquisition:* The data acquisition was acceptable. However, the candidate administered an antiemetic prior to obtaining any history of medication allergy. This is a major mistake and might lead the patient to having an anaphylactic reaction. Remember to always ask about allergies prior to giving any medications. Score = **6**
2. *Problem solving:* Problem solving was good and the candidate used the information given to manage the patient. However, the candidate became distracted when the nurse informed him that CT was ready for the patient. Had a complete physical examination been performed, the candidate would have made the diagnosis without the CT. Score = **6**
3. *Patient management:* As noted above, the examinee recognized pathology late because of the CT. However, when the acute angle closure was discovered, the candidate appropriately obtained intraocular pressure (IOP), visual acuity, started the correct meds and called the correct consultant. Score = **6**
4. *Resource utilization:* As noted above, the candidate did not need a CT scan, but did a good job of utilizing appropriate medication and

consultation. No lab studies were needed for this case and none were ordered. Score = **6**

5. *Health care provided (outcome):* The patient received appropriate treatment and the candidate's interventions stabilized the patient. Score = **8**
6. *Interpersonal relations and communication skills:* The candidate's interactions with the nurse and consultant were appropriate. Always remember to let the patient know what is going on, what you are doing, and what the working diagnosis might be. The candidate notified the patient of his diagnosis, but he never revisited the patient or notified him about the conversation with the ophthalmologist. It is a good idea to always make the patient and/or family members aware of final events or disposition. The candidate could have also asked the patient if he had any more questions, concerns, or needed any other help such as notifying other family members or friends. Score = **6**
7. *Comprehension of pathophysiology:* The examinee conveyed their understanding of causes of acute cephalgia by considering subarachnoid hemorrhage (SAH) and of acute angle glaucoma by recognizing examination findings and using the appropriate interventions. Using a more organized protocol would have helped him discover the diagnosis sooner. Always stick to the same evaluation protocol, even on a "triple case." Score = **6**
8. *Clinical competence (overall):* Overall, the examinee showed clinical competence by developing a differential diagnosis, eventually obtaining an appropriate history and physical, and appropriately treating the acute-angle glaucoma. Score = **6**

CASE ASSESSMENT (JOHN RED)

The candidate realized that the fifth vital sign (O2 sat) was not given and asked for this information immediately. Always make sure a complete set of vital signs is given. A missing vital sign is often a clue to a diagnosis or worsening condition. Appropriate oxygen administration was ordered and the candidate followed this up by asking the patient's response to the oxygen. Obtaining a new set of vitals and making sure the patient improves should be done after any intervention.

The history and physical examination suggested the diagnosis of pneumothorax and this was confirmed by x-ray. The procedure for chest tube placement was not described by the candidate. If the examiner wanted a detailed explanation of the procedure, they would have asked. Otherwise, it is appropriate to do as this candidate did and explain that the procedure would be performed using standard technique.

This patient needed urgent IV access, oxygen, and placement on a monitor. The candidate in this case took too much time obtaining a history without initiating these interventions. The patient could have been in an abnormal rhythm or having an ST-segment-elevation myocardial infarction. The candidate would not be faulted for obtaining an electrocardiogram (ECG) early in the case, but they may have a patient crash if this is not performed.

Always remember to let the patient know what is going on, what you are doing, and what the working diagnosis might be. If there are friends or family members present, talk to them as well. Like with the last patient, the candidate notified the patient of his diagnosis, but did not let them know about disposition plans or ask if they had any questions.

Critical Actions (John Red)

1. Recognize and treat hypoxia.
2. Obtain chest x-ray and recognize pneumothorax.
3. Chest tube placement.
4. Admission.

Test Performance (John Red)

1. *Data acquisition:* The data acquisition was appropriate. In this case, the candidate did not perform a neurological examination. Remember to always perform a full physical examination during your secondary survey. Score = **7**
2. *Problem solving:* The candidate requested missing vital signs and exam findings to discover pneumothorax (PTX) and confirm the diagnosis with chest x-ray (CXR). Score = **8**
3. *Patient management:* Given a chief complaint of chest pain, this patient needed urgent IV access, oxygen, and a monitor. The candidate took too much time obtaining a history without initiating these interventions. The patient could have been in an abnormal rhythm or having a STEMI during that time with the candidate unaware. Throughout the case, the candidate never asked for a complete set of repeat vital signs, which could have potentially led to errors in management. Always repeat vital signs. That being said, the PTX was managed appropriately. Score = **5**
4. *Resource utilization:* The candidate used appropriate lab work and CXR. The workup was logical, cost-sensitive, and showed patient concern. Score = **7**
5. *Health care provided (outcome):* Despite some errors, the patient received appropriate care for their PTX and was appropriately stabilized. Score = **7**
6. *Interpersonal relations and communication skills:* The candidate's interactions with the patient, nurse, and consultant were appropriate. The candidate notified the patient about his diagnosis, but could have been better about keeping him updated about disposition plans and asking if he had any questions. Score = **6**
7. *Comprehension of pathophysiology:* The examinee conveyed their understanding of pneumothorax through appropriate evaluation, interventions, conversation with the patient and consultation. Score = **8**
8. *Clinical competence (overall):* Overall, the examinee showed clinical competence by obtaining an appropriate history and physical, developing a differential diagnosis, utilizing appropriate lab work and imaging, utilizing appropriate interventions, and working toward the appropriate disposition. Score = **7**

Index

B

C

D

E

I

J

O

P

Q

R

S